AF540760

ENCYCLOPAEDIA OF BIOPHARMACEUTICAL

Vol. 4

PLANT PRODUCT PHARMACEUTICALS

By

Dr. S.K. Prasad
School of Studies of Zoology & Biotechnology
Vikram University
Ujjain (M.P.)
(India)

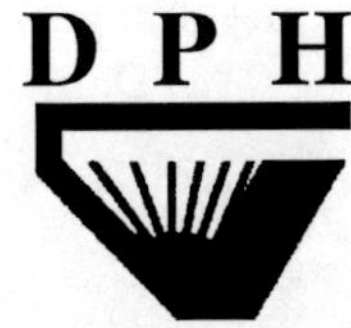

DISCOVERY PUBLISHING HOUSE PVT. LTD.
NEW DELHI-110 002

First Published: 2010

ISBN: 978-81-8356-594-3 (Set)

Encyclopaedia of Biopharmaceutical

Published by:

DISCOVERY PUBLISHING HOUSE PVT. LTD.
4383/4B, Ansari Road, Darya Ganj
New Delhi-110 002 (India)
Phone: +91-11-23279245, 23253475, 43596065
E-mail: discoverybooksindia@gmail.com
discoverypublishinghouse@gmail.com
orderdphbooks@gmail.com
web: www.discoverypublishinggroup.com

Printed at:
Infinity Imaging Systems
Delhi

PLANT PRODUCT PHARMACEUTICALS

Preface

The present title "Encyclopaedia of Biopharmaceutical" has been written for those in the pharmaceutical research and those responsible for the education and training in pharmaceutical science and technology of graduate and undergraduate students. Medicine is an ever changing science. As new research and clinical experience broaden our knowledge, changes in treatment and drug therapy are required. This branch of life science has progressed enormously in recent years and the significant advances in therapeutics and an understanding of the need to optimize during delivery in the body have brought about an increased awareness of the valuable role played by the dosage forms. This statement is as true as it was back in ninteenth century and perhaps more so, given the increasing emphasis being placed on discovery, development, and use of large molecular entities as therapeutic and diagnostic agents. Development of these abilities requires an integration of knowledge, skills, attitudes, and values that can be acquired only through structured learning process including independent study, hands on practice and the availability of advanced literature. This tittle has designed to meet such needs of learners in the health professions.

In the last two decades, the pharmaceutical industry has experimented and successfully adopted several integrated and multidisciplinary approaches in the research areas of dring compound screening, toxicological evaluation, and pharmaceutical product development. The book is written in a concise style that facilitates an in-depth level of understanding of the essential concepts. The objectives of the present title are three folds: (i) to serve as a useful tool to help guide scientists in research and development by out-lining the theory and successful practice of in vitro - in vivo correlation, (ii) to help formulators apply the tool in designing and developing prototypes that enable selection of clinical formulations, and (iii) to help formulate strategy(ies) for product life-cycle management.

To make the work more comprehensive and informative, the author has consulted many authoritative books, research journals, abstracts, monographs etc., so there can be no claim to originality except in the manner of treatment.

The author expresses his thanks to his friends and colleagues whose continue inspirations have initiated him to bring out this book.

The author expresses his gratitude to Mr. Wasan and staff of M/s Discovery Publishing House Pvt. Ltd. for their whole hearted co-operation in the publication of this book.

Author

CONTENTS

1

INTRODUCTION

Botanical or herbal products have been used extensively as drug treatments in the complementary and alternative medical (CAM) system in many regions of the world, but have not been subjected to the same rigorous evaluation by regulatory agencies as that for modern nonbotanical pharmaceutical agents. To facilitate further development of new drugs from botanical sources, the Center for Drug Evaluation and Research (CDER) of U.S. Food and Drug Administration (FDA) has published a draft Guidance for Industry: Botanical Drug Product in August, 2000. The Guidance has since been published in its final form in June of 2004. The new regulatory approaches in the Guidance take into consideration the unique features of the botanical drugs and the substantial past human experiences.

REGULATORY OBJECTIVES

To support approval as a nonbotanical drug, adequate and well-controlled clinical studies are required. Not only must the treatment be shown to be effective, with real patient benefits in morbidity and/or mortality to justify the safety risk of adverse reactions as observed, but the clinical data must also provide practical instructions for use, which can be reasonably followed by health care professionals. There is no reason why these requirements should be different for botanical drugs, because patient suffering and treatment benefits are independent of medical theory or practice. Regardless of medical systems and terminology used, courses of diseases/conditions should be established and treatment effects must be clinically meaningful. Incorporation of alternative medical practice into the clinical studies will be acceptable if the new set of instructions derived from such studies will be practical.

The objective of the new FDA regulatory approaches to new botanical drug development is not to create an additional category of products different from dietary supplements or nonbotanical drugs. Instead, the goal is to confer the botanical new drugs the same degree of confidence in quality and clinical usefulness, as that of nonbotanical drugs, and ultimately to bring the botanical drugs into the mainstream medical use.

DISTINCTIVE FEATURES OF PLANTS

From a regulatory perspective, botanical drugs have some unique features that demand special considerations. Clinically, there is a large quantity of anecdotal experience about the efficacy, which is not supported by modern scientific data, nor can it easily be dismissed. Likewise, extensive human usages also suggest that most of the botanical preparations are possibly safe, but confidence in such presumed safety can only be based on mostly poorly documented data. The pre-existing availability of most botanical products, although not marketed as drugs, also creates difficulties in their regulation. Concern about the quality of botanical products poses another regulatory challenge. Most botanical products are complex and variable mixtures of constituents too numerous to characterize individually. For many preparations, active ingredients have not been identified and it is thus difficult to quantify strength or potency of the botanical product. Because of the biological nature of botanical products, the assessment of their impurity and stability is often more problematic than that of nonbotanical pure drugs.

Beyond the natural mixtures in one part of a single plant, many botanical drugs are combinations of multiple botanical products. While the rationale of combining many plants is not easy to understand and contributions from ingredients remain to be elucidated, it is also not clear whether the ratio and composition have been optimized in many widely used formulations.

Plant Guideline

In the Guidance, the botanical drug products are defined as those that contain as ingredients vegetable materials, which may include plant materials, algae, macroscopic fungi, or combinations thereof, that are used as drugs. It may be available as (but not limited to) a solution (e.g., tea), powder, tablet, capsule, elixir, topical, or injectable. In the current version, fermentation products, highly purified (or chemically modified) botanical substances, allergenic extracts and vaccines that contain botanical ingredients are excluded. In essence, the Botanical Guidance provides that

1. Further purification of the botanical preparations is not required,
2. Identification of active ingredient(s) is not essential,
3. Chemistry, manufacturing and control (CMC) is extended to raw materials, not just regulations of drug substance and product, and
4. Nonclinical testing may be reduced or delayed for products with extensive history of human use.

It should be emphasized that, in the above new approaches, only different types of information are used in part of the safety assessment. This does not imply that overall standards for quality consistency and clinical efficacy/ safety are more or less stringent than that of nonbotanical drugs.

In general, requirements in CMC and nonclinical studies for initiating a clinical study of botanical drugs depend to a large extent on the marketing history, known safety concerns (if any), the degree of modification from past use, and the scale of proposed clinical trials. For a small early phase study, animal toxicity may not be needed if the preparation and usage are the same as in prior human experiences. On the other hand, for large scale, more definitive trials, greater assurance in product quality, consistency, and reproducibility is necessary, as well as the safe use in the clinical setting of the protocol.

As evidence of prior human use, documentation of marketing history (with volume of sales) and review of past and current references, compendia, and literatures should be provided. It is understandable that many of these publications are in variable format and quality, and often do not consist of modern scientific data. In this respect, the Agency will accept all types of documentation for consideration and determine the validity of support in individual cases.

As noted above, all botanical drugs contain many potentially active molecular entities and many preparations are combinations of multiple parts/plants. Because the current policy on fixed-dose combination products requires demonstration of contribution to overall efficacy and safety from each active ingredient, it could be impractical or impossible for botanicals to comply with this regulation in the development as a drug product. This issue was not addressed in the current version of Botanical Guidance. While the Agency is considering revision of the fixed-dose combination regulation to accommodate the difficulties encountered by the botanical drugs, the sponsor is encouraged to consult the CDER for assistance.

Plants Review Team in Center for Drug Evaluation and Research

To acquire and consolidate regulatory experiences on botanical drugs, a dedicated BRT has been established in CDER. The BRT will provide scientific expertise on botanical issues to other reviewing staff to ensure consistent interpretation and implementation of the Botanical Guidance and related policies. In addition, the BRT has the following functions:

1. Participates in all phases of reviews, meetings, and decision- making processes for all botanical drug applications and submissions as a collaborative scientific discipline, and serves as an expert resource for CDER on all botanical issues.
2. Collects information, maintains a database of botanical applications, and performs periodic analysis on the status of botanical new drug development.
3. Responds to external constituents who have general botanical drug development questions.
4. Responds as the expert resource for CDER to issues and meeting requests from the Office of the Commissioner and interfaces on common botanical issues and fosters communication with the FDA Center for Food Safety and Applied Nutrition and the National Center for Complementary and Alternative Medicine and the Office of Dietary Supplements at the National Institutes of Health (NIH).
5. Interfaces with external professional regulatory and scientific groups, makes presentations, and participates in workshops to promote and enhance botanical drug product development and knowledge.

The botanical reviews performed by the BRT cover the following area:

1. *Medicinal plant biology*: methods and problems in species identification; potential misuse of related but incorrect species.
2. *Pharmacology and toxicology of medicinal plants used in the proposed studies*: activities based on old, alternative theories and/or modern testing.
3. *History of prior human uses*: therapeutic effects in the CAM system; potential toxicities from past experience.

The BRT experts serve as members of the review teams, and provide scientific opinion on the botanical drug product in a role similar to that of other disciplines such as chemistry. Currently, the BRT is a team of experts consisting of a medical officer as team leader, a pharmacognosy reviewer, and a project manager.

Review Processes for Plant Applications

To implement the Botanical Guidance, a new set of review processes for botanical applications have been delineated in a new CDER MAPP. As described in the MAPP, the BRT will respond only to general inquiries on botanical-related issues and interpretation of the Botanical Guidance and related policies. For questions about individual botanical drug product with specific clinical indication, the sponsor should submit the application to the new drug review divisions in charge of the therapeutic area in the CDER's Office of New Drugs, and the applications will remain under the divisions' administration. For specific botanical drug applications, all regulatory decisions will be the responsibilities of the new drug division and all regulatory actions will be issued by the division directors. Communication between sponsors and all review team members, including BRT staff, will be conducted through the project manager of the new drug division. As a member of the review team, the BRT experts provide scientific opinion on the botanical drug product in a role similar to that of experts in other disciplines.

In principle, all botanical submissions will be managed in the same manner as nonbotanical drug products by all review disciplines. That is, primary and secondary reviews in CMC, pharmacology/

toxicology, biopharmaceutics, and clinical and statistical issues will be conducted by the respective primary reviewers and team leaders. To ensure consistency across different new drug review divisions, the supporting disciplines in CMC, pharmacology/toxicology, and biopharmaceutics have also designated one to three senior staff to serve as expert consultant(s) in botanical issues for the review divisions in each area. These review processes for botanical applications have been tested in CDER with approximately 100 submissions. Collaborations between BRT and the new drug divisions have been smooth and productive.

Plant Drug Applications in Center for Drug Evaluation and Research

As of April 30, 2004, there are a total of 203 botanical drug applications in CDER, including 167 investigational new drug (IND) applications and 36 pre-IND consultations. At least 75% of the total botanical applications were submitted after 1999, and about two per month were received by the Agency recently. Of these, 43% are commercial development programs and the remaining are academic research projects. These botanical submissions are distributed in all 14 therapeutic divisions, with most activities aggregated in the oncology, antiviral, and dermatology–dental drug areas. A great majority of botanical sponsors have taken advantage of the pre-IND consultation service provided by FDA. As a result, most IND applications were successful with initial submission and few (less than 20) were placed on clinical hold for safety concerns. However, despite the early success, many development programs and research projects have subsequently been suspended for various reasons. As of the above-mentioned cutoff date, nearly two-thirds (66%) of INDs still remain active (have not been placed on clinical hold, inactivated by FDA, or withdrawn by sponsor for lack of activities). To date, there have been no submissions of NDAs to FDA for marketing approval of botanical prescription drugs.

Challenges in the Review of Plant Drug Applications

Not surprisingly, quality of the botanical products is a frequent review issue in our regulatory experiences. Some sponsors had not presented accurate name/identification of the botanical plants and/or description of manufacturing processes. Because of the recent incidence of diethylstilbestrol containing PC-SPES, adulteration of botanicals with active chemical drugs has become a serious concern for both the study supporter (e.g., NIH) and the regulatory agency. For many botanical preparations, there are often uncertainties in the identity of the plant species and/or consistency of botanical raw materials. Complicated manufacturing processes add further possible variation to the drug substance and final products. While most contamination problems unique to botanicals are resolvable, purity/potency and stability are more difficult technical issues, without knowing the identity of active ingredients.

Both the industry and the regulatory agency have realized that, as complex mixtures, it is usually difficult to define or characterize botanical preparations and differentiate among similar products. The tough task for the reviewing staff is thus finding out how to apply the set of regulations designed for highly pure, small molecular entities to a less well-defined botanical system. Apparently, some allowance of imprecision will be needed for CMC of botanical drugs without sacrificing the therapeutic consistency of different batches. As provided in the Botanical Guidance, clinical studies have been permitted for many botanical preparations prior to a complete set of conventional animal toxicity testing. The decisions were not difficult for submissions with substantial and well-documented history of past human use. But some other applicants had not presented an adequate summary of the past human experiences and had failed even to document well-known toxicity of the herbal ingredients. Between these two extremes, how to adjust the requirements of animal toxicity data and substitute that with large quantity but poor quality of human experiences is another big challenge to the regulatory agency in the review of botanical applications. As noted above, all available information on the historical use of botanical preparations will be accepted for safety consideration. But for FDA clinical reviewers, such experiences are often poorly documented and difficult to interpret or correlate with the paradigm of conventional medicine. In the alternative medical system, almost all the diagnoses to be treated with herbal medicine are defined in imprecise and foreign terms. Typically, one herbal medicine is indicated for numerous seemingly unrelated conditions, most of which are symptomatic relief without clear mechanisms. For these reasons, integrating all the background information into the overall safety assessment for botanical applications has been difficult and required active participation of the BRT.

Prospects of Further Development

As noted above, there has been no botanical product approved as prescription new drug by the FDA. The slow pace of progress in botanical new drug development has been increasingly disappointing, possibly for the following reasons:

1. The industry is still struggling with technical difficulties in bringing a complex and ill-defined system to comply with regulatory requirements set for precision of pure chemical drugs.
2. Some of the diseases and conditions selected as indications for the botanical drugs are difficult to study. There are few exciting products to satisfy serious and unmet medical needs.
3. Many sponsors were inexperienced in new drug development and unrealistic about the resources required for the complicated processes.
4. There is no effective protection of intellectual property right and little incentive for further development of pre-existing preparations available on the market (albeit not yet as drugs).

Thus, while the Agency will in general use previous uncontrolled human experiences to expedite limited early stage testing to assess the therapeutic potential of herbal medicines, the overall progress has been slow. However, the technical difficulties in quality controls should be resolvable, and more clinical trials should be initiated. The sponsors of botanical applications should be prepared to go through a complicated scrutiny, the same as that for nonbotanical drugs, and plan ahead with an assessment of difficulties in clinical testing. Lastly, although market exclusivity may not be strictly enforceable for well-known botanical preparations, benefit of the first FDA-approved botanical drugs may still be significant but underestimated for the sponsor.

2

PLANT DRUGS

Nature, as a biochemist, is unparalleled. Mankind has harvested the benefits of her combinatorial talents for thousands of years as a source of novel medicinals. For more than half a century, however, natural products have been relegated to source materials for "*chemical libraries*" from which new "leads" are mined. In a grants announcement, the National Institutes of Health (NIH) stated: "Chemical libraries are a mainstay of drug discovery. Well-crafted libraries, consisting of collections of anywhere from a few compounds to millions of them, can help scientists sort quickly through a haystack of possibilities to find the shining needle that may be developed into a lifesaving drug". Once an "*active*" or "*new chemical entity*" (NCE), is found, it is isolated, "*optimized*," and then screened in receptor assays for further clinical development. To enhance the odds of finding clinically useful NCEs, the pharmaceutical industry has developed modern techniques, which include proteomics, bioinformatics, "high- throughput" screening techniques, combinatorial chemistry, and computer-aided design and prediction of drug toxicity and metabolism. These new approaches are based upon increasing knowledge of receptor sites in normal and disease states.

But "botanicals" do not fit easily into this development paradigm. As a drug class, botanicals have no rival for their structural complexicity or diversity of effects. Defined by their heterogeneity, botanicals have multiple actives, which in some cases are unknown and in others are too numerous to evaluate. Screening these products against individual receptor targets cannot begin to describe their rich activity profiles. Similar to biologic products, such as vaccines, the potential activity of botanicals as pharmaceutical products may be best illuminated in bioassays and, more importantly, in living systems.

Mainstream U.S. pharmaceutical development has thrived on regulatory policies that evolved over decades of experience with single NCEs. Therefore, the heterogeneous nature of botanicals engenders discomfort and uncertainty in those who are used to single-chemical entity drugs and the NCE regulatory structure. But the interest in botanicals and other heterogeneous products as pharmaceuticals has inspired a change in the U.S. perspective, resulting in a new regulatory paradigm that draws upon historical precedent and novel interpretations of regulatory policies. Only recently has the U.S. Food and Drug Administration (FDA) developed a regulatory definition of a "botanical," as any product that "contains ingredients of vegetable matter or its constituents as a finished product". For the purposes of US regulation, botanicals include drug products derived from one or more plants, algae, or macroscopic fungi, but does not include a highly purified or chemically modified substance derived from such a source. In the United States, botanicals can be regulated as foods, drugs, biologics, cosmetics, and medical devices. However, no botanical "*pharmaceuticals*," or more precisely, botanical "new" drugs are being marketed at this time. A "new" drug is defined by the Federal Food, Drug and Cosmetic

(FD&C) Act as any drug marketed after 1938 that is "...not generally recognized as safe (GRAS) and effective under the conditions prescribed, recommended or suggested in the labeling" or one that has become GRAS, but "which has not... been used to a material extent or for a material time". A "new" drug must be proven to be safe and effective for its intended use prior to marketing in the United States. To study a "new" drug, the product sponsor must file an "Investigational New Drug" (IND) application with the FDA, exempting the product from the requirements of safety and efficacy while it is being tested in an investigational setting. After sufficient evidence is obtained, the sponsor can submit the data to the FDA as part of a "*New Drug Application*" (NDA). If the information is deemed adequate, the FDA can approve the product for marketing.

Therefore, to be marketed as a pharmaceutical, a botanical must traverse the modern regulatory process resulting in an approved NDA. The fact that no botanical is currently "*NDA-approved*" has caused many to speculate whether a botanical could ever make it through the rigorous U.S. drug development process, and still others to ask "why" one would choose to pursue this avenue, given the panoply of regulatory options already available to botanicals in the United States.

Regulatory Options

When asked to describe a "botanical" product, food products come quickly to the mind. Fruits, vegetables, grains, herbs and spices, condiments, and teas are easily recognized as products from plant sources. Dietary supplements, defined by the Dietary Supplement Health and Education Act (DSHEA) of 1994, belong to the regulatory category of food products permitted to contain ingredients that are "... herbs or other botanicals, ... dietary substances or concentrates, metabolites, constituents, extracts, or combination of these ingredients ...." Products such as ginkgo, St. John's wort (SJW), and ginseng are examples of botanicals currently marketed in the United States as dietary supplements. Less commonly recognized as botanicals are the allergenic vaccines derived from grasses and pollens, which are regulated as biologics, and the dental alginates, poultices, and adhesives that are medical devices. Finally, botanicals are often ingredients of cosmetics, such as aloe-containing hand lotions and herbal shampoos.

Historical Perspective

To understand the current regulatory milieu of botanicals as drugs in the United States, one must revisit their historical use. Botanical medicine is an integral part of U.S. history. The democratic processes that governed this new nation extended to the practice of the healing arts. At the beginning of the 19th century, no single medical profession existed. Samuel Thomson, who had no formal education, received a patent for his system of "*botanic medicine*," which he described in the "New Guide to Health," published in 1822. His followers, known as "Thomsonians," practiced a form of naturopathy using plant-based medicines such as *Lobelia inflata* or "*Indian tobacco*"—a violent emetic to purge the system of obstructions—and red pepper, to induce perspiration. After Thomson's death in 1843, his disciples formed another botanic sect, known as the "*Eclectics*," deriving their name from their assimilation of the "best" from the various schools of medicine that were developing at the time.

By 1900, most drugs in the United States were derived from natural sources. Ingredients were pulverized and extracted with hot water and alcohol, and administered in the form of teas, suspensions, emulsions, and syrups. Fine powders were prepared for pills or ointments. Ingredients were combined in proprietary mixtures called "patent" medicines. Hawked by their inventors as "cure-all" medicinals, these secret formulas were not only concocted by uneducated consumers, but were also sold directly to the unsuspecting public. Preparations often contained dangerous and addictive substances, such as morphine, cocaine, and opium, which resulted in severe and sometimes fatal reactions. In 1906, the first comprehensive federal legislation in the United States was passed to address the quality and safety of food and drug products. This new law, known as the Pure Foods and Drugs Act, prevented the importation of "adulterated and spurious drugs and medicines," and required that all ingredients be identified on the drug label, thus ending the era of "secret" nostrums.

Passage of the 1906 act heralded the beginning of a new regulatory environment that would transform the U.S. drug industry. Many so-called drug "manufacturers" disappeared overnight, while others succeeded in complying with the new regulations. Those who did change would grow into a new industry, gaining further momentum with the passage of the comprehensive 1938 FD&C Act. Fueled by the 1937 tragedy in which a hundred or so individuals died following ingestion of a tainted formulation of an "*Elixir of Sulfanilamide*," the new act now required that drugs be demonstrated as safe in animals and humans prior to being marketed. This new Act also considerably expanded the federal government's jurisdiction over the food and drug industries and has become the cornerstone of modern food and drug regulation in the United States.

By this time, however, botanicals as a product class had the reputation of being mostly palliative. Many had a slow onset of action and were used to treat signs and symptoms, without improving the underlying disease process. A notable exception was quinine, an extract of the bark of the South American cinchona tree, traditionally used to ward off the symptoms of malaria. One natural product, however, would irrevocably change the U.S. drug industry. From its discovery as a product of fermentation, to its isolation, purification, and synthesis, penicillin set the stage for an entirely new industry based on single chemical entities. Penicillin belonged to a class of antibiotics that became known as the "miracle" drugs. Unlike the traditional botanicals, these drugs displayed a rapid onset of action and demonstrated remarkable therapeutic efficacy that would elevate the public's expectations for all future pharmaceuticals.

Following the passage of the FD&C Act, FDA was authorized to permit NDAs for "new" drugs, but the agency could not approve them affirmatively. One such NDA was for the botanical rauwolfia (Rauwolfia serpentina), first marketed in the United States in 1953. Used in India for centuries, root of rauwolfia was sold in the United States as a treatment for hypertension. More than a dozen NDAs were subsequently recorded for the drug, all of which were discontinued by 1982, as better antihypertensives came to market.

Passage of the Drug ("Kefauver-Harris") amendments in 1962 further tightened the federal government's control over the regulation of pharmaceuticals, increasing FDA's role in the testing of investigational drugs and providing the agency greater powers of enforcement. The legislation was precipitated by the thalidomide disaster that left hundreds of European infants malformed after their mothers took the drug as a sleeping aid during pregnancy. Drugs were now required to demonstrate proof of safety and efficacy for their labeled indications, prior to being marketed. Data collected from investigational studies would now be reviewed by FDA to determine whether the legal test of "*substantial evidence*" was met for approval. FDA was also required to review retrospectively all drugs that had entered the domestic market between 1938 and 1962. Those marketed under an NDA were reviewed by the Drug Efficacy Study Implementation or "DESI" program. Under DESI, more than 3400 drug products and 16,000 claims were reviewed. Thirty percent of the drugs lacked sufficient supporting evidence and were considered ineffective and removed from the U.S. market.

DESI also included 420 nonprescription ("over the counter" or "OTC") drugs, which had entered the US market through the "new" drug procedures during 1938 and 1962. OTC drugs not reviewed by the DESI program numbered in the hundreds of thousands and were considered to be "GRAS". The agency began its efficacy review of the OTC drugs in 1972. To conserve resources, FDA focused on active ingredients, which it grouped by therapeutic category. For each category, FDA promulgated regulations in the form of monographs, establishing conditions by which the ingredients were determined to be "generally recognized as effective" or "GRAE." Faced with the enormity of its task, FDA chose to limit its review to those ingredients that had U.S. marketing experience to support "material time" and "material extent". As a result of the agency's narrow interpretation of the statute, many botanical ingredients were ineligible for inclusion in the OTC review, because at that time they were only being marketed outside of the United States. However, products that had entered the U.S. market prior to 1938 were exempt from review, and included botanicals such as senna, cascara, and witch hazel, which continue to be marketed as OTC drugs today.

Complementary and Alternative Medicine

During the 1980s, U.S. interest in botanicals resurfaced under the guise of "complementary and alternative medicine" (CAM). By this time, botanicals had lost considerable credibility. Proponents of "Laetrile"—a concoction of cyanogenic glycosides extracted from peach pits—drew media attention when the FDA began seizing the product as an "unapproved" drug and as "ineffective cancer treatment". However, by 1991, in response to growing consumer interest, the U.S. Congress appropriated funds to the National Institutes of Health for the establishment of a federal research program for the scientific evaluation of CAM. Now identified as one of the "*biologically-based therapies*," botanical medicine became a research priority for the new NIH Office of Alternative Medicine (OAM).

This dramatic turnabout in the U.S. consumer attitude toward botanical medicine was not lost on foreign manufacturers. Many companies in Europe and Asia that had never stopped marketing botanicals were now eager to satisfy the growing U.S. demand. A rate-limiting step, however, was FDA's exclusion of foreign marketing experience as a threshhold criteria for inclusion in the OTC drug monograph process. Most botanicals had been discontinued from the US market in the earlier part of the century. Due to the 1962 amendments these same products would now have to undergo FDA approval as "new" drugs through the IND/NDA process—a process established based on single chemical entities. In July 1992, the European American Phytomedicine Coalition (EAPC), an alliance between the U.S. and European phytomedicine companies, submitted a petition to FDA requesting that foreign marketing histories be eligible for inclusion in the OTC review process. The agency took several years to respond to the petition, and when it did, its response was to request more information from the petitioners. This inaction led many in the industry to conclude that FDA either did not consider botanicals on equal footing with the single chemical entities, or would not seriously entertain their review under the IND/NDA process. According to Loren Israelsen, an attorney involved with the herb industry and EAPC cocounsel, "The issues raised by the EAPC are important policy considerations which deserve a thoughtful and affirmative response from FDA. We have tried to frame the problem and the solution squarely and FDA's silence is not only disappointing but gives support to the industry's belief that the Agency remains inflexible and unresponsive".

FDA's inaction may have been responsible in part for efforts leading to the passage of DSHEA in October 1994. The new law addressed "herbs and other botanicals" in the context of nutritional supplement ingredients. Over the next six years, botanical supplement sales doubled, peaking at over US $4 billion in 2000. Even so, the intent of Congress was clear from the language of DSHEA: unlike drugs, dietary supplements were not intended to diagnose, mitigate, treat, cure, or prevent disease, although similar to drugs they could make claims to "affect the structure or function of the body".

New Regulatory Paradigm

The legal limitations placed on dietary supplements with respect to disease claims did nothing to stem the increase in the consumer use of botanicals as an alternative means to prevent or treat disease conditions. A survey conducted in 1990 and repeated in 1997 found "*herbal medicine*" to be one of the leading alternative therapies responsible for a significant increase in CAM usage in the United States. In response to growing concerns over the safety and efficacy of botanicals, the OAM funded several grants that proposed to study botanicals for therapeutic indications. Although products could be purchased in local grocery and health-food stores, their evaluation as "new" drugs required that the trials be conducted under IND applications.

What criteria would the FDA use to determine whether the clinical trials could be allowed to proceed under an IND application? The test products were complex mixtures of botanical extracts with multiple or unknown actives. In the absence of a single known active, routine chemistry, pharmacology, and toxicology testing could not be easily conducted. The closest products resembling botanicals were biologics: vaccines and blood- derived products. Both product categories were defined by strict controls over the manufacturing process, rather than by chemical determination of the product in the final vial. Botanicals raised unique issues: not only were plant nomenclature and taxonomy not internationally harmonized, but also the common names for plants varied by country

FDA needed a new regulatory paradigm—one that would be consistent with current drug law, but could also address the unique characteristics and status of botanicals as a heterogeneous class of pharmaceuticals. Over the next six years, the FDA developed a "Draft Guidance for Industry on Botanical Drug Products," published on August 10, 2000, and finalized in June 2004. The FDA would also amend its regulations to allow foreign marketing experience as a basis for including foreign-marketed botanicals in the OTC drug monograph process.

Selecting a Route to Market

Although the new FDA guidance provides a broad outline for botanical drug development, it does not assume all botanicals to be drugs. Instead, manufacturers are presented with a "*decision-tree*" that describes the possible regulatory categories. How a product is regulated depends on several factors, which include product formulation and route of administration. Topically administered products can be sold as drugs, devices, or cosmetics, but not as foods or dietary supplements. Parenteral administration is reserved for drugs. Tablet or capsule formulations can be marketed as dietary supplements or drugs, but not as "conventional" foods.

Intrinsic safety can further define the regulatory possibilities. Foods, including dietary supplements, must be safe for the general public. Conventional foods are limited to ingredients that are "dietary," "GRAS," or approved food additives. In contrast, dietary supplements can contain both "dietary" ingredients and "new" dietary ingredients. "Dietary" ingredients must have been "present in the food supply in a form used for food, not chemically altered." Ingredients marketed in the United States after October 15, 1994, are considered to be "new dietary ingredients.""New" dietary ingredients must have "a 'history of use' or other evidence of safety ... that the new dietary ingredient would be reasonably expected to be safe under conditions of labeling." For products containing "*new dietary ingredients*," FDA must receive written notification at least 75 days prior to marketing, providing information to support the safety of the ingredients.

Unlike foods, including dietary supplements, the safety of a drug is based on a "benefit to risk ratio." "Benefit" is an assessment of the drug's efficacy, balanced against any negatives with respect to a particular indication in a target population. Thus, a drug that is deemed "safe" to treat leukemia may not be "safe" to treat osteoarthritis.

Intended Use

A defining principle of U.S. regulation is a product's "*intended use*." "Intended use" is determined by labeling claims. "Labeling" encompasses not only the required elements that make up the printed label on the bottle, but also any direct or implied claims made by the manufacturer or distributor in the product packaging, advertising, and promotional materials. "Intended use" defines the product category. For example, the FD&C Act defines drugs as "articles intended for use in the diagnosis, mitigation, treatment, cure or prevention of disease or to affect the structure or function of the body." Drug products may bear "disease," "sign," or "symptom-related" claims ("prevents migraine"; "lowers blood pressure"; and "relieves cough and fever").

Similar to drugs, dietary supplements can make claims to "affect the structure or function of the body." However, supplements are specifically prohibited from making "disease" claims. A dietary supplement bearing "structure or function" claims is also required to carry the following disclaimer on the product label: "The FDA has not evaluated this claim. This product is not intended to diagnose, mitigate, treat, cure or prevent disease".

Advantages of the Drug Route

If a botanical is shown to reverse an abnormal test result, modify another drug's adverse event, or act synergistically with another modality, it will usually be best developed as a "drug." This is especially true if the botanical provides a distinct benefit for a patient population, but would pose safety concerns if used by the general public. In contrast to prevention, risk-reduction, or health-maintenance trials, therapeutic studies are often able to demonstrate clinical benefit with smaller numbers of subjects and with more tangible measures of outcome.

But sponsors, enticed by the low cost of market entry for dietary supplements, often dismiss the potential advantages of pharmaceutical development. Because the regulatory schema for a drug is significantly more complicated than that for foods, US law provides many protections for those who choose the pathway of drug development, not the least of which is the confidentiality of the process. From the filing of the IND through the NDA approval, exchanges between sponsors and FDA are kept confidential by the agency. This is in stark contrast to the very public process of food applications, petitions, and notifications.

Patents, trademarks, and copyrights provide additional proprietary protection, which may have a more profound impact on pharmaceuticals than on products sold in most other categories. Although food and cosmetic ingredients may be afforded some protection through composition and process patents, an underlying premise behind marketing of food products is their similarity to prior foods and ingredients with known histories of safe use. The further a "*new dietary ingredient*" strays from a traditional food ingredient, the more documentation will be necessary to ensure "safety," thus undermining the ease and minimal cost at which most food products are allowed to come to the market. In contrast, pharmaceuticals exploit differences, capitalizing on the nuances between molecular analogs and minor alterations in formulation, dosing, and usage. "New" drugs do not have "GRAS/E" status. Generic equivalents of "new" drugs usually enter the marketplace only after an innovator's patent protection have expired. Under the "Price Competition and Patent Term Restoration" Act (also known as the "Hatch-Waxman" Act), not only can the term of a drug's patent be extended or "restored" to account for market-time lost while the product is under regulatory review, but also it is in the FDA's purview to grant periods of marketing exclusivity during which the agency will not accept a competitive filing. For new clinical entities, the first product approved under an NDA can receive a five-year period of marketing exclusivity, and an additional five years is added to the expiration date of any patents. New indications, formulations, or routes of administration requiring additional clinical trials (beyond bioequivalency studies) are granted a three-year period of marketing exclusivity and patent term extension. Under the Orphan Drug Act of 1983, drugs for rare disorders for which the target indication occurs in less than 200,000 individuals annually in the United States, are granted the maximum term of seven years exclusivity and patent extension. Pediatric indications can provide an extra six months of protection. No similar provisions are available for dietary supplements or conventional foods.

Finally, "new" drug approval following the demonstration of safety and efficacy through the IND/NDA process brings with it an added benefit of medical and scientific acceptance that can significantly boost the marketing message. For a drug, clinical results may be conveyed in more direct language for advertising and promotion, rather than the restrictive wording delineated for supplement "structure or function" or "health" claims.

Cost

The ongoing debate on U.S. drug development costs is another reason sponsors look to alternative development strategies for their products. At issue are recent estimates arrived at through a survey of 10 large pharmaceutical companies. Average development costs for an NCE were estimated at US $403 million (in 2000), and when the time between investment and marketing is added, costs totaled a mind-boggling US $802 million. The figures were based on new synthetic chemicals not previously tested in humans, reflecting costs from all NCE candidates tested, including those that had failed. From the tens of thousands of chemicals generated in the discovery process, only a few hundred made it through the screening process, leaving only a dozen or so to undergo animal safety testing. In one review, attrition rates were reportedly due to "safety issues" (20.2%), "toxicology concerns" (19.4%), and "disappointing clinical efficacy" (22.5%). Another 39% of candidates were terminated for business reasons and "other factors". Cost increases often begin in the laboratory: "What big pharmaceutical companies have done is tested a lot of existing materials. But now they've run out of those materials. Today, you have to create new compounds and then test them".

But botanical products do not have to be "created," and many have already been shown to produce potentially useful biological effects in humans. More importantly, documentation of safe use in the target species—humans—is a monumental step that can shorten the development time considerably.

Whether a particular botanical should be developed as a pharmaceutical depends on the product and the business objectives of the sponsor. Sponsors should be cognizant of the costs incurred in "Good Manufacturing Practices upgrades"—modifying the product's manufacturing standards either to meet U.S. drug standards or to move from a food to a pharmaceutical-grade product. Regardless of the extent of prior human use, a botanical drug will likely be required to undergo additional safety and efficacy testing. Undoubtedly, the majority of costs of drug development is incurred in the conduct of clinical trials. However, unlike NCEs, FDA may permit an initial study to be conducted with a product purchased "off-the-shelf" as a dietary supplement.

A randomized, controlled "pilot" study may be the initial trial for a botanical drug under an IND, with an agreement between the agency and the product sponsor that at least one other large multicenter trial with a pharmaceutical-grade product will be conducted for the NDA, if initial results are promising. Animal toxicology testing may also be required to address safety questions that cannot be easily assessed in humans. Although not a requirement for foods, interactions of the botanical drug with other drugs and with foods must also be evaluated, depending on the indication and the potential for interactions. Under the Prescription Drug User Fee Act, the FDA can levy fees for the review of applications containing clinical trial data, although waivers can be sought for nonprofit sponsors and small businesses.

Whole is Greater than the Parts

Whether a botanical should be pursued as a drug or whether it should be "mined" for its actives, depends on the botanical and its constituents. Isolation, purification, and synthesis of single active chemical moieties from natural products have produced a substantial number of the pharmaceuticals in use today. By some accounts, 62% of the current NCE anticancer drugs are nonsynthetic, and more than half of the antihypertensive drugs can be traced to natural product structures or mimics. Determining what is "active," however, is not always straightforward. Most botanical extracts yield legions of constituents with diverse biochemical profiles and pharmacologic effects. A constituent identified as "active" for one particular effect may be "inactive" for others. So-called "inactive" ingredients also may contribute to the biological effects of a product indirectly, through modulation of the actives.

To ensure lot-to-lot consistency, standardization of extracts often relies on constituents as "*biomarkers*" for plant identity and potency. SJW-(*Hypericum perforatum*), a perennial shrub traditionally used as a mood enhancer and mild antidepressant, has been tested in dozens of clinical trials, with mixed results for efficacy. Some of its purported bioactive constituents include naphthodianthrones, including hypericin; flavonoids; phloroglucinols, including hyperforin; and essential oils. For many years, hypericin was presumed to be the active component. As a result most extracts were standardized based on hypericin concentration. Recent data, however, support other components such as hyperforin and the flavanoids, that may also contribute to the therapeutic efficacy of the SJW extracts. Because these secondary components were previously unaccounted for in the standardization of the former clinical test articles, and because these constituents are chemically unrelated to and their content within the plant varies independently of hypericin, it has been argued that the potency of these constituents in any particular batch was unlikely to be similar to that of other batches. This variability between batches could explain the observed differences in the clinical trial results.

For many botanicals, the "whole is greater than the parts." Indeed, individual constituents of an extract may actually produce contradictory effects. Oriental ginseng (*Panax ginseng*) root, widely used in traditional Chinese and Korean medicine, contains over 28 different ginsenosides. Although chemically similar in structure, various ginsenosides have been shown experimentally to produce opposite effects: hypothermia or hyperthermia, hypotension or hypertension, and hemolysis or inhibition of hemolysis—depending on the type of ginsenoside. One must, therefore, use caution in determining what is "active" and be aware that the properties— both positive and negative—of any particular constituent may not represent the biological activity of the extract as a whole. In summary, botanicals are as diverse as nature itself. They bring a wealth of possibilities for innovative new drugs. As a result of the options available to botanical producers, a number of development approaches exist in the United States, but no single paradigm. While many botanicals are best sold as "foods," others will find a more promising future as pharmaceuticals. Those that are systematically studied in scientifically designed trials and are able to demonstrate consistent, clinically relevant biological activity may traverse the drug development process to achieve the status of "new" drugs—the "*botanical pharmaceuticals.*"

Chinese Plant Products

Many Asian communities throughout the world have used Chinese botanical products for centuries. Recently, the usage of these botanical products has also increased in Western societies. Although the use of Chinese botanical products is on the rise, the potential and significance of interaction with Western drugs is not widely recognized and well characterized. While there are very few adequate, well-controlled clinical studies designed to investigate the potential for interaction between Chinese botanical products and drugs, in the English literature, there are examples of documented interaction between commonly used Chinese botanical products and currently available Western drugs, and these case reports will be reviewed in this chapter. In addition, issues that are more pertinent to the evaluation of the importance and clinical relevance of Chinese botanical product–drug interactions will be discussed.

In contrast to theoretical, in vitro, or animal data, the reports reviewed in this chapter provide the clinicians more relevant information, including description of the time course, the magnitude of the suspected interaction, and clinical outcome of the patient. This not only allows an evaluation of the clinical significance, but also provides a basis for further evaluation with well-designed studies. Obviously, case reports have their own inherent limitations, including the existence of potential confounding variables and limited generalizability, which in view of the known product variability of active constituents or content, could be of particular importance in botanical product–drug interactions. Finally, it should be recognized that the occurrence of one or more case reports does not necessarily imply an absolute contraindication of concurrent use of the botanical product and prescription or over-the-counter drug.

Currently, most of the literature reports of Chinese botanical product- drug interaction in humans involve warfarin, likely a function of its narrow therapeutic index requiring close monitoring of therapy with international normalized ratio (INR) and the presence of coumarin derivatives in a number of Chinese botanical products rendering them with anticoagulant property. In addition, some Chinese botanical products also possess antiplatelet effects and have potential for adverse interactions with analgesic drugs such as aspirin or nonsteroidal anti-inflammatory drugs. Based on human, animal, and in vitro data, other Chinese botanical products such as hawthorn have also been reported to interact with a variety of drugs.

It should be noted that while the focus of most Chinese botanical product–drug interaction reports understandably is on the occurrence of adverse effects, not all interactions result in an undesirable effect. An example is *Salviae miltiorrhizae* (danshen), which has been reported by multiple clinicians to cause bleeding with the concurrent use of warfarin [section "*Salviae miltiorrhizae* (Danshen)"], whereas less is known about the potential benefits that might result from combining danshen with an aminoglycoside. Wang et al. had demonstrated in animals the potential usefulness of combining danshen with kanamycin to reduce aminoglycoside-induced free-radical generation in vitro and ototoxicity in vivo, without interfering with serum concentration or efficacy of kanamycin in mice. Other examples of potential beneficial botanical product–drug interaction that warrants further studies include the combined use of the Chinese medicinal plant *Tripterygium wilfordi* and cyclosporin, which is described elsewhere.

In addition to the more conventional nomenclature system of using the botanical name, e.g., *Angelica sinensis*, Chinese botanical products also can be identified by their pinyin name, e.g., dong quai for A. sinensis. Although most English literature refer to Chinese botanical products by their botanical names or pharmaceutical names, the corresponding pinyin names are often used instead in most Chinese herbal literature. Therefore, searching for literature information regarding Chinese botanical products should ideally include the pinyin names in the search strategies, especially if the source of information is primary Chinese herbal literature.

Chinese Plant Products and Warfarin

Angelica sinensis

Dong quai (dang gui, tang kuei) is the extract from the dried root of *Radix Angelicae sinensis*, which belongs to the family Umbelliferae. It has been used for many years as a Chinese botanical remedy for management of menstrual cramps, irregular menses, and menopausal symptoms, and the usual dosage range is 3 to 15 g per day of raw drug prepared as a hot water decoction or alcoholic infusion. Different preparations, including alcoholic extracts, tablets, and teas, are available to the consumer. Dong quai contains coumarins and also may inhibit platelet aggregation. Therefore, this Chinese botanical product could potentially enhance the pharmacologic effect of warfarin-like compounds.

Page and Lawrence reported a 46-year-old female patient with rheumatic heart disease and atrial fibrillation, who was referred to the anticoagulation clinic for warfarin therapy management. She was successfully managed with warfarin (Coumadin) 5 mg/day, which maintained her INR within the range of 2 to 3 for about two years. At a routine clinic visit, the patient was found to have an elevated INR of 4.05 compared to 1.89 a month earlier. The prothrombin time (PT) also increased over the same time period from 16.2 to 23.5 seconds. Because she did not show any evidence of clinical bleeding, and there were no readily identifiable sources for the increased laboratory values, including dosing error and abnormal liver function, she was instructed to withhold the warfarin dose for one day. The patient missed a follow-up clinic visit and only returned after another month had passed. At that time her PT and INR were further increased to 27 seconds and 4.9, respectively. The patient also disclosed that she had been taking dong quai at a dosage of 565 mg once to twice daily for four weeks to manage her perimenopausal symptoms. She was instructed to miss a day of warfarin dosing with no additional change of warfarin dosage, and also to discontinue consumption of dong quai. Two weeks after discontinuing the dong quai regimen, her PT and INR decreased to 21.6 seconds and 3.41, respectively, with further reduction to 18.5 seconds and 2.48 after an additional two weeks. Ellis and Stephens reported similar interaction in a brief case report describing a patient with a mitral valve replacement, who had been stabilized on warfarin (dosage regimen not reported) for 10 years. After taking an unknown quantity of dong quai for a month, she presented to the clinic with an INR of 10. Although details of the report were very few, significant bruising as a result of the interaction was shown in a photographic figure published with the case.

Although the exact mechanism is not known, the coumarin constituent of dong quai is likely responsible for the enhanced pharmacological effect. An animal study also suggested that the basis of the interaction is likely pharmacodynamic and not pharmacokinetic in nature. Nevertheless, it should be noted that dong quai belongs to the family Umbelliferae, and plants within this family contain furocoumarins, which have been reported to inhibit cytochrome P-450 (CYP) activity, especially CYP3A4. In this regard, it is of note that the extract of the dried root of *Radix Angelica dahurica*, another botanical product belonging to the Umbelliferae family, has been reported to increase the area under the plasma concentration–time curve (AUC) and to prolong the elimination half-life of tolbutamide in rats by 2.5- and 2.3-fold, respectively, which was likely a result of the inhibitory effect of its furocoumarin components on different CYP isoenzymes, including those belonging to the 2C subfamily. Based on in vitro studies, it has also been suggested that another dong quai component, sodium ferulate, might inhibit platelet aggregation and cyclooxygenase activity.

Salviae miltiorrhizae

Danshen, the dried root and rhizome of *S. miltiorrhizae*, is another Chinese botanical product used for its ability to alleviate menstrual irregularities, as well as for its vasodilative and hypotensive functions in a variety of cardiovascular conditions. The botanical product had also been shown to inhibit platelet aggregation in vitro. Danshen is widely available in different preparations for oral consumption, with usual dose range of 9 to 15 g per decoction. In addition, its increasing popularity is reflected by its availability even in Chinese cigarettes.

Clinicians from Hong Kong reported a case of potential danshen– warfarin interaction in a 48-year-old female with a history of rheumatic heart disease, atrial fibrillation, and mitral stenosis (11). The patient underwent successful transvenous mitral valvuloplasty for management of her medical conditions, and was discharged with 1 mg warfarin, as well as furosemide and digoxin. Since discharge the patient's warfarin dosage ranged from 2.5 to 3.5 mg daily with an INR of 1.5 to 3. Her last warfarin dose adjustment was an increase in dose to 4 mg daily in response to an INR of 1.35. Since then the patient also had intermittent influenza-like symptoms, for which she took botanical products with danshen as one of the main ingredients, every other day. When the patient presented to the emergency room several weeks later because of increased flu-like symptoms, her clotting profile was noted to be significantly abnormal with an INR exceeding 5.6 and PT above 60 seconds.

There was no other clinical source of clotting abnormality and the most likely cause of over-anticoagulation was believed to be an interaction between warfarin and danshen. Although the patient stopped taking both warfarin and all botanical products, and received fresh frozen plasma, her clotting abnormality persisted for more than five days. Nevertheless, the patient suffered no clinical evidence of bleeding and over the next four months, she was stable on a daily warfarin regimen of 3mg and an INR of 2.5. There were two additional reports of danshen–warfarin interaction in the literature. A 62-year-old man with rheumatic mitral regurgitation had been stabilized on warfarin 5mg with INR of about 3.0 over four weeks after discharge. His other medications included captopril, furosemide, and digoxin. The patient then started taking danshen daily to help his heart condition. Two weeks later, he was admitted to the hospital with an INR of 8.4. Both the warfarin and danshen regimens were stopped. Fresh frozen plasma and packed red blood cells were administered, eventually decreasing the INR to 2.0. Over the next two weeks, he was restarted on warfarin and the dose titrated back to the previous regimen of 5 mg/day, resulting in a stable INR of 3.

Another case involved a 66-year-old male patient who was stabilized on 2 to 2.5 mg of warfarin per day with INR of about 2. About nine days prior to admission to the hospital, the patient developed nonspecific chest wall pain, for which he self-treated with two to three topical applications of 15% methyl salicylate and two decoctions of danshen over the next few days. On the day of admission, his INR was found to be greater than 5.5, and his warfarin regimen was stopped, followed by administration of fresh frozen plasma and packed red blood cells. The INR was subsequently stabilized at 2.0 to 2.5.

These three cases suggested that danshen might potentiate the anticoagulant effect of warfarin, although information regarding consumption of other Chinese botanical products was not available for two of the three cases. In the report of Tam et al., the patient also self-medicated with topical application of methyl salicylate, which might have initially exaggerated the anticoagulant effect of danshen. In all three reports, the absence of identifiable precipitating factors and the temporal relationship between botanical product consumption and onset of exaggerated anticoagulation effect suggested an interaction between danshen and warfarin. In addition to inhibiting platelet aggregation and interfering with extrinsic blood coagulation, danshen was also shown to affect warfarin pharmacokinetics in an animal study. Chan et al. reported that single-dose administration of danshen in rats increased the AUC and maximal concentration of the R- and S-isomers of warfarin. In addition, concurrent administration of warfarin and danshen for three days also increased the steady-state *R*- and *S*-warfarin concentrations, with resultant increases in PT by 11 seconds.

Lycium barbarum

The dried fruit of *L. barbarum* L., a common Chinese botanical product belonging to the family of Solanacaea, is available in different tea formulations for its beneficial effects on the kidney and the liver. Lam et al. described a potential interaction between a concentrated Chinese herbal tea and warfarin in a 61-year-old Chinese woman. The patient had been stabilized on a weekly warfarin dosage regimen of 18 to 19 mg/week, with a therapeutic INR ranging between 2 and 3, for her recurring atrial fibrillation. There were no signs and symptoms of abnormal anticoagulation.

On a routine anticoagulation clinic evaluation, the patient's INR was elevated to 4.1 from 2.5 obtained at the prior monthly visit, albeit with no clinical evidence of bleeding. There was no reported change in any of her medication regimens, diet, or lifestyle. However, the patient indicated that she had been consuming one cup of a concentrated herbal tea made from dried fruits of *L. barbarum* L. several times a day, to manage blurred vision secondary to a sore eye. When she presented to the clinic, the vision problems had already resolved. The patient was advised to discontinue the herbal tea consumption, and the warfarin weekly dosage regimen was adjusted to 16mg with a resultant INR of 2.0, followed by 18 mg/week with a resultant INR of 2.2, before resumption of the original dose of 19 mg/ week with a resultant INR of 2.5.

This case suggested that the elevated INR might be related to the consumption of the herbal tea made from the dried fruits of *L. barbarum* L. The investigators further performed an experiment using human liver microsomes to investigate the effect of the tea on warfarin metabolism. Using method provided by the patient, the investigator produced the herbal tea by adding 5 g of the fruit to 100 mL of boiling water. The hot water decoction was eventually reduced in volume to about 30 mL. The extract was then filtered and the resulting filtrate used in microsomal incubation.

The investigators reported that the prepared tea inhibited the metabolism of the *S*-warfarin isomer by CYP2C9. Furthermore, based on the amount of tea ingested, the solids concentration of the prepared tea, and assumed values of bioavailability and volume of distribution, the plasma concentration of the inhibitory component was estimated to be much lower than the inhibitory concentrations calculated from the in vitro experiment. However, the investigators emphasized the lack of knowledge regarding actual measured inhibitory concentration at the active site of metabolism and the actual bioavailability and distribution volumes of the inhibitory component. In addition, whether *L. barbarum* also possesses an anticoagulant or antiplatelet effect is not known. Therefore, despite the time sequence of INR changes with the use of the herbal tea, it is not known whether the effect is related to altered CYP or non-CYP disposition variables or to an anticoagulant effect of the botanical product itself.

Chinese plant product quilinggao

It is not uncommon for Chinese botanical products to be combined in different preparations for a variety of uses. "*Quilinggao,*" also referred to as "Essence of Tortoise Shell," is a combination Chinese botanical product produced by different manufacturers and promoted for improving general health and reducing internal "*body heat.*" At times, consumers consider and take the product as a health food rather than an herbal medicine. Clinicians in Hong Kong recently reported a patient with clinical evidence of bleeding and over-anticoagulation after consuming different brands of quilinggao.

A 61-year-old man had been receiving warfarin for his atrial fibrillation and chronic rheumatic heart disease. With a warfarin regimen of 3 mg alternating with 3.5 mg every other day, his INR was mostly stabilized within the range of 1.6 to 2.8. On a routine clinic visit for INR monitoring, his INR was found to be greater than 6.0 and he had complained of gum bleeding and epistaxis over three days prior to the clinic visit. There were no reports of changes in medication adherence and dietary habit of vitamin K. Upon further questioning, the patient revealed that he had been taking the combination botanical product quilinggao daily for over three years with a change in the brand just one week prior to the clinic visit. Although he noticed bruising on his left leg five days after taking the new (second) brand of quilinggao product, he continued to consume one can per day until the clinic visit.

His warfarin therapy was withheld and his INR decreased to 2.9 and 1.9, three and five days later, respectively. His warfarin regimen was restarted at the same 3/3.5mg on alternate days as before. The patient was later discharged with an INR of 2.5. He was consulted regarding the possible adverse consequences of taking warfarin and quilinggao concurrently. However, immediately after discharge, he began drinking one can of another (third) brand of quilinggao product daily and three days later his INR was elevated to 5.2. The patient was readmitted to the hospital and warfarin therapy withheld, resulting in decreases of INR to 4.3 and 3.4, two and three days later, respectively. The warfarin therapy was eventually restarted after an INR of 1.9 was reached.

Among the different ingredients listed on the labels, from the first and the second brands of quilinggao products, Chuanbeimu (*Fritillaria cirrhosa*) in the first brand, as well as Beimu (*Fritillaria* spp.), Chishao (*Paeoniae rubra*, Chinese peony), Jinyinhua (*Lonicera japonica*), and Jishi (*Poncirus trifoliata*) in the second brand were constituents that had antiplatelet and/or antithrombotic effects. The potential interacting constituent(s) could not be identified with the third quilinggao product because the patient could not remember its brand name. There was no readily identifiable cause for over-anticoagulation during both hospitalizations, and the temporal relationship between consumption of the last two quilinggao products and the changes in the INR values suggested that an additive interaction between the botanical product and warfarin was the likely cause of the exaggerated pharmacologic effect. The difference in interaction outcome between the first and second quilinggao products could be related to the greater number of interacting botanical constituents present in the second brand product.

***Camellia sinensis* (Green tea)**

Consumption of green tea is a common practice in Asian countries such as China and Japan, and its use as a dietary supplement in the United States has also increased significantly over the years, perhaps reflecting a belief that it may prevent carcinogenesis. Although it is not usually considered as a botanical product, dry green tea leaves contain as much as 1.4 mg of vitamin K per 100 g of dry leaves . Dietary intake of vitamin K facilitates clotting factor synthesis and is well known to antagonize the anticoagulant effect of warfarin. The following report described a probable case of interaction between warfarin and green tea.

A 44-year-old Caucasian male had been treated with warfarin for more than a year for prophylaxis of thromboembolic complications associated with his St. Jude mechanical valve replacement in the aortic position. The therapeutic goal was to maintain his INR within the range of 2.5 to 3.5, and a review of the patient's medication history indicated that a decrease in his INR was always associated with a reduction in warfarin dose. One month prior to clinic visit, his warfarin regimen was 7.5 mg/day and the INR was 3.2. At the clinic, the patient's INR was found to be 3.79 with the same warfarin dosage regimen. However, he was asymptomatic and there was no obvious reason for the increased INR. He was counseled on the importance of a consistent intake of vitamin K-containing foods and instructed to continue on the same dosage regimen.

About three weeks later, the patient returned to the clinic for INR monitoring, and the value reported the next day was 1.37. Multiple attempts to contact the patient failed and he was lost to follow-up for another month, at which time he returned to clinic for a recheck of INR, which was reported as 1.14. The patient reported no change in compliance, diet, medications, or disease states. Nevertheless, on further questioning about his diet, the patient indicated that a week prior to his previous INR of 1.37, he had begun drinking about one-half to one gallon of green tea each day. The patient did not show any signs and symptoms associated with suboptimal anticoagulation, and he was instructed to continue his warfarin regimen and stop the green tea consumption. One week later, the patient's INR was 2.55, and subsequent values were mostly within the target range.

The time course of green tea consumption and discontinuance suggests that the tea could partially account for the changes in the patient's INR values. Although brewed green tea was reported to only contain 0.03 μg of vitamin K per 100 g of brewed tea, this patient's copious consumption of the green tea would obviously provide an exogenous amount of vitamin K that exceeds the usual recommended daily dietary intake of 0.5 to 1.0 μg/kg of vitamin K. In addition, the final concentration of vitamin K in any brewed tea would be affected not only by the amount of dry tea leaves used for brewing, but also by the volume of water used to prepare the tea for consumption. In summary, this case highlights the importance of consistent dietary intake of vitamin K for patients receiving warfarin therapy, and the fact that less well-known sources of exogenous vitamin K could provide an amount that greatly exceeds the recommended range of daily dietary intake.

Panax ginseng

Decreased INR associated with the use of *P. ginseng* was reported in a 47-year-old patient who had been stabilized on warfarin. Another case of inadequate anticoagulation with ginseng product resulting in thrombosis on a mechanical aortic valve prosthesis was reported in a 58-year-old patient.

Chinese Plant Products and Phenprocoumon

Zingiber officinale (ginger) has been used for centuries by traditional medical practitioners in East Asian countries to manage symptoms of common cold and rheumatic and digestive disorders, as well as for prophylaxis in the management of nausea and vomiting. For these different purposes, ginger has been used either as fresh or dried root, or in different preparations including capsules, liquid extracts, powders, tablets, or teas. In addition, aqueous extract of ginger has been shown to inhibit thromboxane synthase in a dose-dependent manner, thereby resulting in the reduction of platelet aggregation. This hemostasis effect could be related to gingerols, the active ingredients of ginger. Therefore, the potential exists for ginger to interact pharmacologically with coumarin derivatives. While to date there has been no report of interaction between ginger and warfarin, ginger has been recently reported to interact with phenprocoumon, a coumarin derivative commonly used in most European countries.

Kruth et al. reported that a 76-year-old woman who had been stabilized on long-term phenprocoumon therapy with therapeutic INR values was admitted to the hospital, secondary to elevated INR of greater than 10, prolonged partial thromboplastin time (PTT) of 84.4 seconds (normal <35 seconds), and epistaxis. Although the patient took several concurrent medications for her medical problems, which included atrial fibrillation, hypertension, chronic heart failure, and osteoporcsis, none of the drugs is known to interact with coumarin derivatives. More importantly, there have not been any changes in any of her drug regimens. However, for several weeks before the bleeding incident, the patient had regularly taken several ginger preparations, including dried ginger and tea prepared from ginger powder. Ginger intake was discontinued and with administration of several doses of vitamin K, the patient's INR and PTT eventually returned to baseline values, enabling resumption of her normal doses of phenprocoumon, with no further recurrence of bleeding episodes.

The time course of ginger administration and the absence of other potential interacting drugs suggest that ginger might be the cause of over-anticoagulation in this patient. In vitro evidence of CYP2C9 involvement in phenprocoumon metabolism is not supported by human pharmacokinetic data. The effect of ginger on CYP activity is not known and a possible pharmacokinetic basis cannot be established at this time. Although the literature evidence of ginger's effect on hemostasis is conflicting, this case suggests that caution needs to be exercised with ginger use in patients receiving anticoagulants. In this regard, it is noteworthy that even though abnormal clotting function as well as mild clinical bleeding in a 25-year-old woman was attributed to several natural coumarin constituents in a herbal tea product, the herbal tea also contains one whole ginger root that might exaggerate the anticoagulant effect of the coumarin constituents.

Chinese Plant Products and Aspirin

As discussed above, the pharmacological action of ginger has prompted suggestion that concurrent use of ginger and aspirin or nonsteroidal anti-inflammatory drugs may exaggerate bleeding potential, especially if the amount of ginger used is larger than that found in usual food items. The following case report indicates such potential, and there are three human studies in the literature, investigating the effect of ginger on platelets.

An unspecified but potentially large amount of marmalade containing 15% raw ginger was consumed by a patient, resulting in significant inhibition of platelet aggregation, although the patient was asymptomatic. One week after discontinuation of the ginger supplement, platelet function was found to be normal. The investigator also performed an in vitro study and reported that ground raw ginger has the potential to inhibit platelet aggregation.

To determine the relevance of in vitro results to clinical setting, Srivastava extended his previous in vitro study to seven healthy female volunteers, who received 5 g of fresh ginger daily for one week. The serum thromboxane activity (thromboxane B_2 formation) at baseline was not significantly different compared to that obtained after one week of ginger administration. There were also no evidence of ecchymosis or reports of unusual bleeding episodes. Eight healthy male volunteers received a single 2 g dose of dried ginger (Schwartz spice) or placebo in a randomized, double-blind, crossover study.

Three blood samples were obtained before, and at 3 and 24 hours after dose administration. Ginger intake resulted in no significant effect on bleeding time, platelet count, and platelet aggregation compared to administration of placebo capsules.

In another study, 18 healthy subjects (nine men and nine women) received an extemporaneous formulation of vanilla custard containing 15 g of raw Brazilian ginger root, 40 g of cooked stem ginger, or placebo once daily for 14 days in a randomized crossover manner. Blood sampling was performed on days 12 and 14 of each treatment for determination of platelet thromboxane B_2 production ex vivo. There were no significant changes with either of the ginger preparations when compared to placebo. In addition, no treatment order effects were noted, although there were no washout periods between the three treatment phases.

The effect of ginger on platelet aggregation and the potential for increased bleeding have been cited as reasons to exercise caution in the use of ginger in patients receiving aspirin and nonsteroidal anti-inflammatory drugs. Although the three clinical investigations reviewed above are associated with the usual study limitations, including extrapolation of observed effects from healthy volunteers to patients, relevance of negative findings in a small number of subjects, variable range of ginger doses and preparations used in the subjects, as well as whether the doses studied represent equivalent doses found in dietary supplements or botanical preparations, there is insufficient evidence at this time to conclude an unequivocal significant antiplatelet effect associated with the use of ginger. Additional human studies similar to those conducted for St. John's wort would clarify the interaction potential of ginger.

Angelica sinensis

In addition to the presence of natural coumarin derivatives, phytochemical analysis found that dong quai also contains ferulic acid and osthole as ingredients. Ferulic acid was reported to have antithrombotic activity. Similarly, study using the closely related *Angelica pubescens* also found osthole to be antithrombotic. These two chemical constituents exert their antithrombotic effects by interfering with different pathways responsible for platelet activation. Ferulic acid inhibits the release of serotonin and adenosine diphosphate from platelets, as well as reduces the thromboxane A_2 production, resulting in impaired platelet aggregation. Osthole directly inhibits the conversion of arachidonic acid to thromboxane A_2. Therefore, even though currently there is no report of an interaction available in the English literature, dong quai may potentiate the risk of bleeding if used concurrently with aspirin or nonsteroidal anti-inflammatory drugs.

Chinese Plant Products and Digoxin

Crataegus pinnatifida

Hawthorn has long been used as a medicinal substance, and an extract such as WS 1442, a formulation of hawthorn leaves with flowers, has been evaluated in different studies for treatment of heart failure. Patients with New York Heart Association class II heart failure participated in a placebo-controlled, randomized, multicenter trial. They received 30 drops of the extract three times daily for eight weeks. At the end of the study, heart failure condition was improved. A meta-analysis of available clinical trials suggests that the extract is useful as an adjunct treatment for patients with mild to moderate heart failure. Therefore, it is likely that hawthorn products would be administered together with digoxin in clinical management of patients.

Although a synergistic interaction between hawthorn and digoxin has been reported in Chinese herbal literature, until recently, there has been no case report or pharmacokinetic/pharmacodynamic data available in the English literature. A recent study evaluated the interaction potential between hawthorn and digoxin. Eight healthy volunteers participating in the study received, in a randomized crossover manner, digoxin 0.25 mg daily for 10 days and digoxin 0.25mg daily concurrent with 450 mg twice daily of Crataegus extract WS 1442 for 21 days, with a three-week wash-out period between the two treatment phases. Based on pharmacokinetic analysis of digoxin concentration–time profiles from both the treatment periods, administration of the hawthorn preparation produced a slight and statistically insignificant change in any of the pharmacokinetic parameters. There were also no statistically significant differences in blood pressure, heart rate, and PR interval. The pharmacological results from this study appear to contradict the Chinese literature of synergism between hawthorn fruit and cardiac glycoside. However, hawthorn may increase digoxin's effect on myocardial contractility, although that was not measured in the study. Future studies confirming the lack of pharmacokinetic interaction and adverse additive effect would provide additional evidence that hawthorn and digoxin can be administered safely together.

Chinese Plant Products and Digoxin-like Immunoreactivity

As discussed earlier, many patients use danshen for a variety of cardiovascular uses. Currently, there is no literature report of interaction between danshen and digoxin. However, Chinese botanical products can interfere with clinical laboratory monitoring of digoxin serum concentrations via their digoxin-like immunoreactive components. For example, danshen contains more than 20 diterpene quinines with chemical structures similar to digoxin. Depending on the type of immunoassay used, both falsely elevated and falsely decreased concentrations have been reported. Similarly, the bufadienolide constituents of the Chinese botanical product lu-shen-wan also bear structural similarity with digoxin, resulting in serum digoxin concentration of about 0.9 ng/mL in patients who took lu-shen-wan pills. Even though it is not necessarily considered to be a real botanical product–drug interaction, it would be prudent to check for potential interference by serum digoxin concentration determination, when these Chinese botanical products are used together with digoxin.

Limitations of Current Literature

Although literature publications on the use of herbal medicine have increased over the years, there are relatively few retrievable literature reports regarding concurrent use of Chinese botanical products and prescription and/or over-the-counter medications, when compared to drug interaction reports associated with concurrent use of two or more Western prescription drugs. While this may simply reflect a lack of reporting system for the consumers, another likely reason could be that pertinent information is not readily available in the English literature. Pharmacodynamic and pharmacokinetic interaction cases have been published in Chinese herbal literature, including Herb-Drug Interaction and Combined Medication, Chinese Herbal Medicine, and Pharmacology and Application of Herbal Medicine, and attempts are currently undertaken to provide this information in the mainstream literature.

Most of the Chinese botanical product–drug interaction cases involving warfarin and/or salicylate described above did not result in clinical bleeding episodes. Nevertheless, these and other botanical product–drug interaction reports discussed in this chapter underscore the limitation of available evidence based on case reports and extrapolation of relevance to other botanical products, which could be confounded by patient-specific variables, details of individual report, as well as variability in the content of active constituents among different botanical products. These limitations of interpretation and extrapolation are further challenged by unique ways of prescribing and preparing Chinese botanical products by Traditional Chinese Medicine (TCM) practitioners and patients, respectively. These will be discussed in the following sections.

Specific Issues Regarding Evaluation of Chinese Plant Product—Drug Interactions

Prescribing vs. Over-the-Counter Use of Chinese Plant Product

Using traditional and acceptable ways of reviewing and analyzing the drug- drug interaction literature, it is tempting for clinicians to report a case and/ or review the literature of botanical product–

drug interaction based on the available information for an individual botanical product. However, many herbal remedies used by consumers contain multiple herbs, e.g., the Chinese botanical product quilinggao reviewed above, Ping Wei San, the Chinese medicine used for the management of gastrointestinal disorders, and the different Kampo medicine (traditional Chinese botanical prescriptions) available in Japan. Different constituents within a botanical formula or remedy could have multiple effects on an individual constituent that range from augmenting to antagonizing its intended effect, thereby posing limitation on the usefulness of research or report pertaining to an individual botanical constituent.

In contrast to over-the-counter use by consumers, Chinese botanical products prescribed by TCM practitioners or herbalists are usually in the form of a formula combination, designed to enhance or reduce the effects of different botanical products. Indeed, it is a common knowledge that TCM practitioners and herbalists prefer prescribing Chinese botanical products in the form of "*raw herbs*" or raw plant materials rather than fixed-formula products, so that modification to a formula can be used to achieve the desirable therapeutic effect with minimal adverse outcome for a specific patient. TCM practitioners and herbalists have contended that by using a balanced combination of Chinese botanical products and by taking a therapeutic approach that tailor to a patient's holistic needs, i.e., his or her physical and psychological loss of balance, the Chinese botanical products have minimal potential to interact with Western drugs. Obviously, this knowledge of appropriate combination of Chinese botanical products would not play a role in the consumer's choice of botanical remedies purchased over the counter. In addition, the TCM practitioner usually assesses the patient on a regular basis, and adjustment is then made to the ingredient within the formulation. In this regard, it is not much different from warfarin dose adjustment by a clinician based on the patient's INR and clinical status.

By the same token, not all Chinese botanical products are compatible with each other. Classic Chinese herbal texts have mentioned 18 Incompatibles and 19 Counteractions. The 18 Incompatibles refer to a classic list of 18 botanical product–botanical product interactions, whereas the 19 Counteractions list 19 botanical product combinations in which the effect of one botanical product counteracts that of the other. Given this complexity of modified effect, self-administration of Chinese botanical products without consultation with health care providers or TCM practitioners likely poses more risk than benefit. In addition, for conventional drugs, the magnitude of interaction is mostly dose related or concentration related. Undoubtedly, the dosage of the interacting constituent, whether known or yet to be identified, could vary from one manufacturer to another. Therefore patients switching between different Chinese botanical products might have different outcomes, according to the botanical product– drug interaction, as discussed above for the patient who experienced an apparent interaction between quilinggao products and warfarin.

Preparation of Chinese Herbal Medicine for Consumption

After the prescription is filled and taken home, the Chinese botanical products or formula are usually prepared prior to consumption. In contrast to an oral dosage form of a synthetic drug taken orally in its entirety, the raw botanical products can be ground and taken directly. More commonly, the botanical product or formula of multiple botanical products can be prepared either as a hot water decoction (extraction) or as a 35% to 45% alcoholic infusion. The decoction method of preparation involves boiling the botanical products in about 500 to 600 mL of water until the volume is reduced to one-half and drinking the supernatant of the resulting concentrate or "soup." The infusion method of preparation involves immersing the botanical products in liquor (usually ethanol) for a period of time and then drinking the supernatant. Because it is known that allicin, the major component of garlic, is destroyed when garlic is cooked in oil, how the boiling process would affect the metabolic activity of major constituents has not been studied systematically. Interestingly, Guo et al. had shown that in vitro CYP3A4 inhibition by seven botanical products was consistently greater with the infusion method of preparation. This was true regardless of the lots or geographic locations of the source of the botanical products. Therefore, this represents an additional complexity in evaluating the botanical product–drug or botanical product–botanical product interaction and the need for inquiring the method of preparation during interview of patients regarding their use of botanical products.

Chinese Fixed-Botanical Formulations

Commercial Chinese fixed-botanical formulations are manufactured and marketed in various dosage forms. It is usually not known to what extent individual botanical constituent(s) would be chemically altered during the manufacturing process, regardless of whether the final formulation contains a standardized amount of an active constituent. In addition, commercially available products might differ in their formulation of constituents. The case report by Page and Lawrence listed different over-the-counter dong quai–containing botanical supplements that are available in the United States. Some of these supplements contain not only dong quai, but also multiple botanical products such as ginger, licorice root, or Siberian ginseng. The patient described in their report took Nature's Way PMS formula, which contains dong quai, cramping bark, chaste tree berry, licorice root, and ginger, in addition to folic acid and several vitamins.

Although specific ingredient information may not be easily available or apparent in case report or literature review, it is important to take into consideration the multiple ingredients within a commercially available product or a Chinese botanical formula, when reporting cases of botanical product–drug interaction, so that clinicians can come to appropriate conclusions regarding the significance of the interaction and/or extrapolation of the result to other products. Another good example of this attempt to report constituents within a botanical product or formulation is the case of the quilinggao–warfarin interaction discussed above.

The fact that most Chinese herbal medicines are complex mixtures of multiple active constituents further complicates the interpretation of study data, as well as extrapolation to other botanical products. Japanese Kampo (traditional Chinese herbal mixtures) prescriptions have been used for many years to treat different chronic conditions and are presently manufactured in Japan as drugs with standardized quantities and qualities of constituents. Homma et al. evaluated the effect of three commonly used Japanese Kampo prescriptions, Sho-saiko-to, Saiboku-to, and Sairei-to, on prednisolone pharmacokinetics in humans. All three botanical prescriptions contain glycyrrhizin, a strong inhibitor of 11-β-hydroxysteroid dehydrogenase. Chen et al. had shown that glycyrrhizin decreased plasma clearance and increased AUC and concentration of prednisolone.

However, even though glycyrrhizin was present in all three Kampo prescriptions, Homma et al. reported differential effect with respect to changes in prednisolone pharmacokinetics. Concurrent administration of Sho-saiko-to resulted in a 17% decrease in prednisolone AUC. On the other hand, coadministration of Saiboku-to resulted in a 15% increase in prednisolone AUC. Sairei-to administration resulted in no appreciable change in prednisolone pharmacokinetics. Similarly, Sho-saiko-to increased the prednisone to prednisolone ratio, which reflects 11-β-hydroxysteroid dehydrogenase activity, whereas the ratio was decreased in the presence of Saiboku-to and not changed by administration of Sairei-to. Sho-saiko-to contains seven botanical products with glycyrrhizin being one of them, whereas a total of 12 botanical products including glycyrrhizin are present in Sairei-to, although the relative amount of glycyrrhizin differs between these two botanical products.

These results suggest that botanical prescriptions containing higher glycyrrhizin content or constituents other than glycyrrhizin might be responsible for this differential effect on prednisolone pharmacokinetics and 11-β-hydroxysteroid dehydrogenase activity. The report by Wong and Chan on warfarin–quilinggao interaction also illustrates these two limitations: the presence of multiple active or interacting constituents and the often present variation in the composition of the constituents between different manufacturers. In this regard, although Sho-saiko-to and Sairei-to were shown to not alter the pharmacokinetics of the quinolone ofloxacin in seven healthy volunteers, it remains to be determined whether other Kampo prescriptions such as Saiboku-to would produce the same negligible effect.

With an increasing number of consumers using traditional Chinese herbal medicines, mostly without the advice of health professionals or TCM practitioners, the likelihood of Chinese botanical product–drug interactions is potentially high. To date, the number of interaction reports remain relatively low and, fortunately, few cases reported adverse clinical outcome in patients. However, the low prevalence of interaction simply might reflect a lack of recognition of the interaction potential, scant information from the primary Chinese literature, insufficient number of patients taking Chinese botanical products and potent Western drugs at the same time, or a combination of these factors. As demonstrated by the numerous interaction reports involving warfarin, it is important for clinicians to inquire patients specifically about their use of botanical products, which most do not necessarily disclose during patient interview or medication review. Likewise, to understand further the magnitude and clinical significance of potential or reported interactions, it is important to have more pharmacokinetic and pharmacodynamic studies conducted with quality botanical products in healthy volunteers and/or patients.

3

POSTMARKETING AERS

St. John's wort is a member of the genus *Hypericum*, which has 400 species worldwide in Europe, West Asia, North Africa, North America, and Australia. In the Western United States, the use of St. John's wort is especially prevalent in Northern California and Southern Oregon. The commercially available product contains hypericum dry extracts or their by-products prepared from flowers gathered during the time of blooming or from dried parts above ground.

In modern European medicine, St. John's wort extracts are included in many over-the-counter and prescription drugs for management of mild depression, and have clinical implications for bed-wetting and nightmares in children. The extracts are included in diuretic preparations and the oil is taken orally using a teaspoon to help heal gastritis, gastric ulcers, and inflammatory conditions of the colon. The oil is also used extensively externally in burn and wound remedies.

Recent reports in animal studies by Rolli et al. and Muller et al. show that clinically used hypericum extract inhibited the synaptic reuptake of 5-hydroxytriptamine (5-HT), noradrenaline, and dopamine with an inhibition concentration at 50% (IC_{50}) around 2 μg/mL. The bioactive substance responsible for the inhibition is identified as hyperforin, from a study by Muller et al. The effect of hypericin as an inhibitor of MAO-A has not been confirmed; however, other ingredients such as flavonoid aglycone, quercetin, and quercitrin have been shown to inhibit MAO-A.

Overall significant benefits of St. John's wort for mild depression compared to a placebo, or equivalent efficacy compared to tricyclic antidepressants (maprotiline, imipramine, and amitriptyline), in mild-to-moderate depression have been reported. However, cautious interpretation of these studies is warranted due to methodological weaknesses. Most tested preparations varied in several major ingredients. An advantage hypericum has over other antidepressants is its favorable side-effect profile. Hypericum has been shown to be well tolerated in patients with the incidence of adverse reactions similar to that of a placebo. The most common adverse effects reported after short-term therapy are gastrointestinal symptoms, dizziness/confusion, and tiredness/sedation.

DRUG INTERACTIONS WITH ST. JOHN'S WORT

There were multiple official regulatory warnings regarding the risk of increased drug levels of CYP3A4 substrates as a result of interactions with St. John's wort. For example, the U.S. Food and Drug Administration (FDA) published a Public Health Advisory in 2000, alerting about the risk of drug interaction with indinavir, antiretroviral agents, and other drugs used to treat heart disease, depression, seizure, certain cancers, transplant rejection, and oral contraceptives. The European Agency for the Evaluation of Medicinal Products (EMEA) issued a Public Statement in 2000, on the risk of drug interactions between *H. perforatum* (St. John's wort) and cyclosporine, digoxin, oral contraceptives, theophylline, warfarin, and antiretroviral medicinal products such as protease inhibitors (PIs) and non-nucleoside reverse transcriptase inhibitors such as zidovudine, didanosine, and zalcitabine. The Australia Therapeutic Goods Administration published a Media Release in 2000 on interactions with indinavir, cyclosporine, warfarin, digoxin, theophylline, PIs, HIV non-nucleoside reverse transcriptase inhibitors, anticonvulsants, oral contraceptives, nefazodone, selective serotonin-reuptake inhibitors (SSRIs) such as citalopram, fluoxetine, fluvoxamine, paroxetine, sertraline, and antimigraine drugs. The Canadians marketed St. John's wort products as food, without health claims. The Irish Medicines Board subjected St. John's wort to prescription control. New Zealand's Medsafe issued a media release statement for St. John's wort interactions with antiepileptic drugs, PIs, immunosuppressive agents, antidepressants, antimigraine drugs, and oral contraceptives.

The FDA's Adverse Event Reporting System (AERS) at the Center for Drug Evaluation and Research (CDER) is an electronic database that currently contains over three million reports of suspected drug-related adverse events, both serious and nonserious outcomes, from all marketed drugs since 1969, which have been submitted to the agency. The reports are initiated on a voluntary basis from both United States and foreign sources that include both health care professionals and consumers and submitted to manufacturers or directly to the FDA. It is important to note that AERS reports are usually of variable quality and completeness and do not necessarily imply a direct causal relationship between drug exposure and the adverse event(s). In some cases, an analysis of such reports may suggest that they are the consequence of the treated underlying disease, other concurrent medical conditions, and/or concomitant medical product treatment. In addition, due to the voluntary nature of reporting, it is not possible to determine the actual incidence of drug-related events or determine the actual degree of risk associated with drug usage. Moreover, due to differences in reporting of adverse events for different type of drugs and other factors affecting reporting, a quantitative comparison of risk between products is highly problematic.

Up to 2001, AERS indicated up to 39 case reports of possible drug interactions between St. John's wort and a prescription drug. In these case reports, the potential drug interactions occurred mostly with oral contraceptives, antidepressants, cyclosporine, and sildenafil. All cases were reported between 1997 and 2000. Most of the reported cases were in females, with an age range between 17 and 73 (mean 42.5) years of age. Four reported hospitalization as a serious outcome. Examples of reported drug interactions with St. John's wort are summarized below.

Cyclosporine

Coadministration of St. John's wort with cyclosporine has resulted in a significant reduction in cyclosporine concentrations, which has led to graft rejection. Decreased cyclosporine drug levels were reported in five cases. Two cases from the United States, one from Australia, and two from Switzerland reported decreased cyclosporine levels or decreased therapeutic response while on St. John's wort concomitantly. The age ranges and doses of cyclosporine used in these five patients, where the data was reported, were 26 to 62 and 200 to 250 mg, respectively. Dose of St. John's wort was 300mg in one case and 600 mg in another, but unspecified in three cases. Time to onset ranged from two to seven weeks after St. John's wort administration, and was unspecified in one case. The Australian case reported that cyclosporine levels returned to within normal range two weeks after stopping St. John's wort. The two Swiss cases documented endomyocardial rejection with concurrent St. John's wort therapy.

Oral Contraceptive Hormones

The metabolism of the components of oral contraceptives, ethinyl estradiol and norethindrone, is thought to be mediated at least in part by intestinal and hepatic CYP3A. St. John's wort significantly increased the oral clearance of norethindrone and decreased the peak serum concentration of norethindrone. Likewise, the elimination half-life of ethinyl estradiol was significantly reduced, therefore potentially reducing oral contraceptive efficacy or even failure. The most frequently reported hormones possibly interacting with St. John's wort were levonorgestrel in combination with estradiol through increased 3A4 metabolism. There were ten case reports of breakthrough bleeding while Alesse-28 and St. John's wort product were used concomitantly. The bleeding occurred from nine days to four months after Alesse-28 was started. The bleeding continued up to seven days while taking Alesse. Age ranged from 33 to 53 (n = 7, mean 41). Two patients were instructed to double the doses of Alesse-28 for an unspecified number of days and the bleeding stopped. One discontinued the use of Alesse-28. One patient became pregnant and had a miscarriage. This subject resumed taking St. John's wort and Alesse-28 and conceived again.

There were three reports of breakthrough bleeding while patients were on norgestimate and ethinyl estradiol (Ortho-Cyclen). A 29-year-old female took Ortho-Cyclen 28 tablets for a few months and experienced moderate breakthrough bleeding and some abdominal pain. She began taking two capsules of St. John's wort 10 days prior to her breakthrough bleeding. A 25-year-old female had been taking Ortho-Cyclen for years. She started taking St. John's wort for 30 days and experienced a lot of breakthrough bleeding. She is led to believe that St. John's wort decreased the efficacy of the oral contraceptive. A female of unknown age taking Ortho-Cyclen experienced breakthrough bleeding 17 days after starting St. John's wort.

There was one report in a 22-year-old female of irregular menses and unintended pregnancy while on levonorgestrel and St. John's wort with unspecified dose or indication. A 32-year-old female developed PMS symptoms, breakthrough bleeding, and unintended pregnancy while taking St. John's wort about the same time that she was taking levonorgestrel and ethinyl estradiol.

Antidepressants

For venlafaxine, fluvoxamine, and fluoxetine, the most frequently reported adverse events while on St. John's wort were hypertension and potential serotonin syndrome. There were no reports of lack of effect for these SSRIs, although St. John's wort may decrease the drug levels by inducing 3A4. Because St. John's wort inhibits reuptake of serotonin, noradrenaline, dopamine, and MAO, these events were likely associated with increased serotonin and/or adrenaline levels. Possibly under a similar mechanism, addition of St. John's wort to the MAOI phenelzine was associated with hypertensive crisis in one case, and with mild serotonin syndrome in another patient taking the tricyclic, doxepine. It is unclear whether sertraline had any drug interaction with St. John's wort, although four cases reported depression or intermittent ineffectiveness. According to the labeling, sertraline goes through extensive first-pass *N*-demethylation and the extent of 3A4 inhibition by sertraline is not likely to be of clinical significance.

One case from the United States and one from the United Kingdom reported hypertension and manic reaction, respectively, while on venlaflaxine and St. John's wort concomitantly. The case of hypertension from the United Kingdom was a 56-year-old male who had taken venlafaxine 300 mg daily for management of depression. Prior to consuming St. John's wort, the patient's blood pressure readings were 120/82 mmHg and five weeks after St. John's wort blood pressures were elevated at 180/115 mmHg and 165/112 mmHg. A 29-year-old male received Effexor 150mg for the treatment of dysrhythmia. He decreased the dose and started taking St. John's wort, three tablets daily or every other day, without his prescribing physician's knowledge. He experienced a hypomanic episode that was described as sleeping poorly and feeling "wired" for two days with a lot of "energy" and inability to relax or calm down. A literature report from France described "*serotonin syndrome*" experienced by a 32-year-old male patient as malaise with anxiety, excessive sweating, chills, and tachycardia four days after St. John's wort therapy while on venlafaxine. St. John's wort dose was interrupted on day 4, and the symptoms regressed in three days without modifying the dosage of the antidepressant.

There were two cases of hypertension from the United States, or possible serotonin syndrome reported with fluvoxamine while on St. John's wort concomitantly. A 44-year-old male with obsessive-compulsive disorder received fluvoxamine and experienced severe hypertensive crisis (160–170/120 mmHg) after two tablets of St. John's wort. The physician stated that the reaction was probably due to the combination of fluvoxamine and St. John's wort, which has MAOI activity. A 38-year-old male was on fluvoxamine for approximately two months and hypericum 600 mg daily for approximately two weeks before reporting possible serotonin syndrome with severe bitemporal headache. He was hospitalized to rule out myocardial infarction. There were no electrocardiogram (EKG) changes or apparent causative pathology. Symptoms resolved on discontinuation of both drugs.

A 73-year-old female was treated with fluoxetine for depression for a long period of time and had a history of hypertension managed with multiple concomitant drugs: digoxin, enalapril, aspirin, isosorbide, amlodipine, carvedilol, metformin, and furosemide. The patient was treated with hypericum extract 425 mg for one time. Half an hour to one hour after the first dose, the patient experienced a hypertensive crisis (270/130 mmHg) during her stay in a rehabilitation center. The event was treated with nifedipine and abated (with blood pressures decreasing to 160/96 mmHg).

Five cases (ages 36, 48, 48 and 60 and one unknown; three males and two females) reported intermittent ineffectiveness with sertraline, including complaints of "does not seem to be working," anxiety attack, or worsening depression. In four cases, symptoms occurred after sertraline was added to the continuing St. John's wort therapy. In contrast to reports with other antidepressants, these cases did not report hypertension or possible serotonin syndrome. It is uncertain if the occasional events were possibly associated with the patients' unstable psychiatric status following sertraline therapy, or due to potential sertraline-related adverse events.

Potential drug interaction between sertraline and St. John's wort cannot be ruled out in one case that experienced manic depressive disorder symptoms one to two weeks after St. John's wort was started into sertraline therapy. The patient was treated with an antipsychotic and has had no problems after discontinuing St. John's wort and decreasing the sertraline dose.

Sildenafil

Four cases of lack of effect or impotence were reported in patients using sildenafil while on St. John's wort and other concomitant drugs (what are they? Are any of them significant from the standpoint of drug interaction?). The age range of the four male patients was between 55 to 73 years. Viagra doses were all 50 mg p.r.n. The St. John's wort dose was 600 mg daily in one case but unspecified in the other three cases. One case reported that Viagra did not work, but provided no additional details. Another two cases experienced facial flushing, headache, and ineffective Viagra treatment. One case indicated that Viagra 50 mg was used several times with only partial erection. The dose was increased to 100 mg with similar results. The fourth case summarized below had no other concomitant drug listed and indicated that the Viagra worked without St. John's wort, but did not work when St. John's wort was taken.

A physician reported that a 60-year-old male started sildenafil 50 mg while he was also taking 600 mg of St. John's wort daily for depression. When the patient increased the dose of St. John's wort to 1200 to 1800 mg daily for unknown reasons, the sildenafil was reported to be partially effective. Patient increased the dose of sildenafil to 100mg but it was completely ineffective. The physician suspected that a drug interaction caused the adverse events. No other significant medical history was noted.

Anticonvulsants—Carbamazepine

There were two reported cases with carbamazepine. One case was that of a 17-year-old female who reported increased levels of carbamazepine following three months of St. John's wort and carbamazepine 200 mg b.i.d. with a baseline level of 4.7 μg/mL. She became nauseated with flu-like symptoms on 12/5/98. After experiencing a seizure, dizziness, and disorientation the next day, she was hospitalized with a carbamazepine level of 36 μg/mL.

Another case was a female who reported with complaints of increased incidence of "*muscle twitching*" episodes during daytime hours. These included "slapping leg and turning head to right." Patient was on valproic acid and carbamazepine and St. John's wort was started 50 days prior to the occurrence of adverse events. No carbamazepine levels were reported. Because carbamazepine is also a CYP450 3A4 inducer, the role of St. John's wort is not clear from these two cases because only one case reported increased carbamazepine levels.

The available case reports in the FDA AERS support the published literature that there are pharmacokinetic interactions between St. John's wort and CYP3A4 and/or *p*-glycoprotein substrates, such as cyclosporine, levonorgestrel/estradiol and sildenafil, and pharmacodynamic interactions with the SSRIs or MAOI. Subsequent clinical studies including those conducted via a CDER clinical pharmacology research cooperative agreement provided mechanistic basis of many of these interactions.

Postmarketing Reporting Systems

In the United States, the use of products, including botanicals, thought to fall within the realm of complementary and alternative medicine is very common. It is difficult to obtain reliable estimates of use or to compare many of the current publications in this area because of diverse definitions for categorizing these products (e.g., dietary supplement, food supplement, herbal medicine, natural remedy, traditional medicine, etc.) in both the United States and elsewhere. A recent report on the use of complementary and alternative medicine by U.S. adults in 2002 indicated that approximately 19% of the population used "nonvitamin, nonmineral, and natural products," 19% used folk medicine, and 3% used megavitamin therapy in the past 12 months. All of these types of products are collectively referred to as "complementary and alternative health products" (CAHP). The regulatory classification of individual products, even those containing the same or similar botanical ingredients, may be different and can influence the safety of the product as is briefly discussed below.

Regulatory Classification of Plant Products

Botanical products, including those containing herbs, may be marketed as foods, dietary supplements, or drugs in the United States. Claims made by the manufacturer, particularly on the product label and labeling (information accompanying the product), determine how a product is regulated in the United States, and not necessarily what ingredients the product contains, how the doctor prescribes it, or how the consumer uses it. A product's regulatory classification is important because it determines what safety and effectiveness standards apply, the types of data needed to make this determination, and who makes the determination.

Products that make claims on their labels or labeling that state or suggest that it can treat, cure, prevent, mitigate symptoms, or diagnose a disease are drugs [prescription and over-the-counter (OTC) drugs] in the United States. Drugs must be shown to be safe and effective prior to marketing, and the Food and Drug Administration (FDA) makes these determinations. There are very specific requirements for drug manufacture and marketing. These include factors such as the purity, potency, and formulation of the ingredients in the finished drug, and the kinds of information that can or must appear on the product label (e.g., product claims, safety information, or warnings). Conventionally, foods are items ingested for flavor, taste, aroma, or nutrition. The standards for foods primarily involve the safety and suitability of the food to meet nutritional needs, rather than safety and effectiveness as a form of treatment. Furthermore, the current standards for manufacturing or holding foods are mainly sanitation standards.

In the United States, dietary supplements are a special category of foods as defined under the Dietary Supplement Health and Education Act of 1994. Unlike prescription and OTC medicines, dietary supplements are not reviewed by the FDA before marketing. Manufacturers also do not need to register before producing or selling their products. Manufacturers of dietary supplements are legally responsible for assuring the safety of their marketed products, and the FDA has the responsibility to take action against unsafe dietary supplement products after they reach the market. Except in the case of a new dietary ingredient, where the law requires premarket review for safety data and other information, a firm does not have to provide the FDA with the evidence that shows that its product is safe and effective. The FDA intends to publish minimum standards for manufacturing dietary supplements, which will focus on practices that ensure the identity, purity, quality, strength, and composition of dietary supplements. Dietary supplements can make claims about the effect of a product on the structure or function of the body, but may not make "disease" claims.

Worldwide, the majority of commercially available finished medical botanical products are regulated as drugs, although the raw botanicals themselves may be commercially available and fall outside regulatory schemes. In contrast, in the United States, the majority of marketed botanical products with any type of health information are sold as dietary supplements. Despite being labeled as a dietary supplement, botanical products with disease claims are unapproved drugs, because their safety and efficacy for a particular indication have not been proven prior to marketing. Currently there are a few botanicals in OTC drug products, but no prescription drug products in the United States. This situation may ultimately change, because a number of new drug applications on botanical products have been submitted to the FDA.

Safety Concerns Related to Plants

As noted by numerous recent publications, the use of CAHP has increased dramatically in recent years, with echinacea, ginseng, ginkgo biloba, garlic, glucosamine, St. John's wort, peppermint, fish oils/omega fatty acids, ginger, and soy being the most commonly used products for health reasons. Safety concerns related to botanicals fall into two general areas—those related to populations using them and those related to the actual product or its ingredients.

There are a number of reasons to be concerned about the potential safety of such widespread use of CAHP. These products are frequently used by vulnerable populations, including older adults, those with chronic disorders, children, and women during pregnancy and lactation. These products are also used by patients to treat a variety of chronic disorders that are difficult to medically manage (e.g., anxiety, depression, dementia and memory impairment, headache, weight loss, back disorders, chronic pain, prostatic hypertrophy, and cancer). Choice of a particular product for a particular condition is usually based on the claims made for the product and anecdotes of "historical" use, rather than conclusive scientific evidence that establishes the safety and efficacy of a particular product for a particular condition.

Concurrent use of CAHP with prescription medicines is common, with reported frequencies ranging from about 20% to 43%. Less is known about potential interactions with OTC medications, but this too is of concern, particularly with the increasing switch of prescription drugs to OTC status. In addition, as with other types of CAHP, there are issues related to the recognition and monitoring of adverse events related to OTC drug products. Concurrent use of CAHP with OTC and prescription drug products can result in therapeutic failures or adverse events. Although many supplements are commonly advertised as being "natural," this does not make them automatically safer or better than drugs or synthetic ingredients. In many cases, there is much less credible information about the effects of particular natural products or their ingredients, and there is more product variability. Product quality and variability are known safety concerns. Natural products can contain anything found in our environment—including pesticides, bacteria, molds, heavy metals, and other poisons—as has been documented in the literature.

Identification and Evaluation of Potential Product Interactions

Consumers frequently do not tell their health providers about their use of CAHP, health providers often fail to ask about the use of such products, and most of the purchases of these products occur outside a pharmacy—all of these factors enhance the likelihood of adverse product interactions and make detection of such interactions much more difficult.

Identification and evaluation of potential interactions is also difficult because there is a paucity of reliable scientific information about the effects of ingredients in CAHP, and this difficulty is compounded by product- related factors: many of the products are multi-ingredient, and as noted above there can be wide variability in the quality and consistency of ingredients and products. A number of recent reviews have tried to evaluate the credibility of data as it relates to drug–CAHP interactions, but these are limited to the published literature and do not consider information available in various adverse event reporting systems (e.g., FDA systems, Poison Control Centers). Because adverse events are underreported, and even fewer will ever be published in the scientific literature, it is not possible to estimate the true magnitude or significance of the drug–CAPH interactions, which is likely far greater than any current published estimates. Consequently, the results from these studies should be used with caution because the lack of documented cases in the scientific literature does not mean that a particular CAHP is safe or that interactions with drugs have not occurred or will not occur. It is critical, therefore, that health professional be cognizant of the use of CAHP by their patients and be on the alert for potential interactions. Health professionals would also increase the knowledge in this area if they diligently reported suspected adverse events.

Adverse Event Reporting at FDA: Medwatch Program

MedWatch is an umbrella program developed by the FDA to enhance the reporting of serious adverse events by health professionals, which are suspected to be related to the use of FDA-regulated products. Within the FDA, there are many different systems at various levels in the agency, which deal with adverse event reports (AERs), including mandatory (active) and voluntary (passive) surveillance, which may have different infrastructure and system requirements. The particular system utilized depends upon the regulatory authority for the particular product. There is no central system based on the type of ingredients (i.e., botanical); the AER goes ultimately to the center with regulatory responsibility for the particular product. Consequently, more than one center in the FDA may have information about particular product interactions; for instance, an adverse event associated with a dietary supplement might be voluntarily reported by a consumer or the adverse event might be a mandatory report from a drug manufacturer where a CAHP is listed as a concurrent exposure.

The FDA considers postmarketing surveillance, which includes adverse event reporting, as one of the most useful indicators or signals of potential safety problems associated with a product. Although premarketing clinical studies can reveal certain safety problems, a major portion of the information concerning product safety becomes known only after marketing, with widespread use in "real life" situations. Postmarketing surveillance can either be active, such as in mandatory reporting by manufacturers of adverse events, or can utilize more passive systems, including voluntary reporting of adverse events, evaluation of consumer use data, etc. For certain drugs (those subject to the new drug approval process), it is mandatory that the manufacturers report adverse events to the FDA. Additionally, health professionals may voluntarily report adverse events associated with medical products. For other drugs, including many OTC drugs, reporting is currently voluntary.

In general, most systems used to evaluate adverse events associated with foods are passive or voluntary and are in their infancy when compared to the more formal and elaborate pharmaco-epidemiologic systems that exist for certain types of drugs. The FDA learns about problems with foods, including dietary supplements, through a wide variety of sources, including the FDA MedWatch program for health professionals' reporting of adverse events. Other reporters of adverse events include consumers, state and local health departments, professional societies, other federal agencies or groups, and industry representatives that contact the FDA via multiple mechanisms (written and electronic correspondence, telephone, etc.).

There have been increasing calls from health professionals and certain members of Congress to require dietary supplements manufacturers to report serious adverse events to the FDA. The recent Institute of Medicine Report on dietary supplement safety also recommended that Congress amend the Dietary Supplement Health and Education Act (DSHEA) to require manufacturers and distributors to report to the FDA in a timely manner any serious adverse events associated with the use of its marketed products.

Adverse Events and Risk Management

The FDA plays an important public health role in the identification and management of health risks associated with the use of products that it regulates. An important function of postmarketing surveillance systems is signal generation (i.e., the identification of new or emerging health risks). Signals from adverse event information become apparent in a variety of ways. These include the emergence of a specific pattern of signs and symptoms, which is occurring with the use of a particular product or ingredient, an increasing number of adverse events or a change in the pattern, seriousness, or severity of adverse events observed with the use of a particular product or ingredient, or the occurrence of an adverse event that is unexpected with the use of a particular product. These systems are important because they can provide data not found or available prior to marketing on adverse effects seen in special groups, adverse effects that occur with relative infrequency, and adverse effects that develop with chronic use or exhibit latency.

For all the recognized advantages of using adverse event reporting as a component of pharmacovigilance of drug interactions, including those occurring with botanical products, there are also well-recognized limitations to current reporting systems, which are generally "passive" in nature. These include substantial and unquantified underreporting, frequent incomplete or inaccurate information in submitted reports, lack of exposure data, inability to detect adverse events with a long latency period, and the absence of a control group for the specific exposure.

A number of variables influence the likelihood of an adverse event being reported. These include the length of time that a product has been marketed, the market share, experience and sophistication of the population using the product, and publicity about adverse events. Currently there is little incentive for health professional reporting of adverse events, which partially underlies the problem with underreporting. Lack of exposure data and the issue of underreporting preclude estimation of incidence rates. Causality assessment is difficult or impossible because of the quality of the data received and the lack of a comparator (control) group. Finally, comparisons of product safety cannot be directly obtained from adverse event data.

When signals become apparent from the routine review of data in an adverse event reporting, additional elements of risk assessment are implemented, generally on a case-by-case basis, to provide the agency with adequate information to appropriately manage any public health risks. These additional elements may include clinical or scientific evaluation of all adverse events reported as associated with a particular product or ingredient; market surveys to gather information on product use (directions for use, warnings, populations using product, etc.); sample analyses, where appropriate, to identify particular substances in a product, the amount of a substance, etc.; independent scientific and clinical reviews from scientists in other Centers, or outside the agency; and expert scientific advisory committees.

This information serves as the basis of any FDA actions to mitigate risk. These actions, depending on the nature and severity of the identified risks, may include changes in the product's warnings or directions for use, education of the public (consumer, health professional, industry), or withdrawal of the product from the market. Because of the very limited amount of information that is available to the FDA at premarketing or first marketing, the majority of the FDA's efforts related to dietary supplement safety are focused in the postmarketing period. Any efforts to improve the safe use of CAHP, therefore, will include mechanisms to improve the type, quality, and availability of data that are available on these products. Such efforts could include more centralized electronic databases for scientific data, including that obtained from postmarketing surveillance of adverse events. Because we are in an era of limited resources, such efforts will require the coordinated efforts of federal agencies, academia, other public health groups, and industry to be successful.

4

STANDARDIZATION IN PLANT PRODUCTS

The popularity of botanical products in the United States is reflected in a survey on complementary and alternative medicine that showed that American consumers had spent an estimated $5.1 billion on botanical products in 1997. In the same year, the global market for botanical medicinal products was estimated to be approximately $20 billion. It has been estimated that currently more than 1500 botanical products are available in the U.S. market alone. This popularity has been fueled, in part, by the perception that botanicals are naturally derived products, and hence are safe and devoid of adverse effects. This perception appeared to be justified by a paper summarizing the fatality of pharmaceutical drugs and botanical products in the 1981–1993 period, in which statistics compiled by the National Center for Health Statistics, the American Association of Poison Control Centers, Centers for Disease Control and Prevention, the Journal of the American Medical Association, and the U.S. Consumer Product Safety Commission showed an annual mortality rate of 100,000 deaths for pharmaceuticals and none for botanical products.

However, because the information covered was only to the end of 1993, this report did not take into consideration the subsequent fatalities attributed to *Ephedra* and ephedrine products. With the increase in the number of incidents of adverse reactions being reported, a database on adverse reactions of botanical products has been created as part of the World Health Organization (WHO) International Drug Monitoring System. In recent years, it has become increasingly apparent that even therapeutically safe botanical products can manifest toxic effects as a result of botanical product–drug interaction, when administered concomitantly with synthetic pharmaceutical agents. The best-documented examples have been cases involving grapefruit juice and St. John's wort with a variety of drugs. Grapefruit (*Citrus* × *paradisi* Macfad.) juice has been documented to interact with calcium channel blockers as well as to increase the level of cyclosporin in the blood of transplant patients.

St. John's wort (*Hypericum perforatum* L.), a botanical used in the management of mild to moderate depression, has been found to increase the effects of monoamine oxidase inhibitors or serotonin reuptake inhibitors; reduce the blood levels, and hence the pharmacological effects of anticonvulsants (carbamazepine and phenobarbitone), anticoagulants (warfarin and phenprocoumon), oral contraceptives, theophylline, digoxin, cyclosporin, HIV reverse transcriptase inhibitors (nevirapine and efavirenz), and protease inhibitors (indinavir); increase photosensitivity with other such drugs; prolong narcotic-induced sleeping time; and decrease the level of cyclosporin in organ transplant patients. The adverse effects recorded for these and some other botanical products are due to true pharmacological interactions. There are, however, botanical product–drug interactions reported for botanical products that may not be true pharmacological/physiological events, and that can be avoided if in-process quality control

(QC) is in place during the manufacturing process. Botanical products adulterated with synthetic drugs such as phenylbutazone, indomethacin, corticoid steroids, caffeine, acetaminophen, indomethacin, hydrochlorothiazide, ethoxybenzamide, theophylline, diazepam, chlorpheniramine maleate, ibuprofen, phenobarbital, mefenamic acid, prioxicam, salicylamide, diethylstilbestrol, and warfarin have led to botanical product–drug interactions. Multicomponent Chinese or Ayurvedic botanical remedies, known to contain heavy metals such as lead and mercury as active ingredients, can likewise lead to adverse events and/or botanical product–drug interactions.

On the other hand, a number of adverse event reports recorded in the literature are themselves erroneous in nature due to the quality of the assessment and reporting, with Siegel's report of the so-called "*ginseng-abuse-syndrome*" (GAS) being a prime example. In this report, the author simply recorded adverse reactions in patients who had ingested "ginseng" without reference to which of a number of plants having the same common name were actually ingested. Further, the author did not take into account the concomitant pharmaceutical drugs and drugs of abuse used by the patients being reported to have adverse drug reactions to "*ginseng.*"

In monitoring botanical product–drug interactions, the quality of the data obtained may be influenced by a number of factors. Among the important issues to be addressed include raw material source and sourcing practices; intrinsic and extrinsic factors affecting the occurrence and concentration of active or marker chemical constituents in both the starting and finished products; the meaning of the word "*standardization*"; the methods of chemical and biological analyses employed; the manufacturing practices employed; substitution; adulteration of botanical products with pharmaceutical drugs or contamination with foreign toxic substances; formulation of the dosage form; regulatory requirements; and clinical experimental design and data interpretation. In this chapter, the influence of these quality assurance (QA)/QC and standardization issues on botanical product safety will be examined.

Material Quality and Quality Control Issues

The quality of presently available botanical products varies from very high to very low. Our study on selected commercial ginseng products prepared from *Panax ginseng* C.A. Meyer, *P. quinquefolius* L., and *Eleutherococcus senticosus* Max. (Araliaceae) and marketed as botanical supplements in North America in the 1995–1998 period showed that 74% of these products met label claims, with the ginsenoside contents of the *P. ginseng* and *P. quinquefolius* products analyzed ranging from 0.00% to 13.54% and 0.009% to 8.00%, respectively. The eleutherosides B and E content of *E. senticosus* root powder and other formulated products also showed similarly large variations. Studies on the quality of St. John's wort products showed that hypericin content ranged from 22% to 165% and that silymarin content in milk thistle [*Silybum marianum* (L.) Gaertn.] products ranged from 58% to 116% of the labeled claims. These content variations not only will influence the efficacy, but also could affect the safety of botanical products, because chemically induced drug interactions may be active compound–concentration dependent. Why are there such wide variations in the content of active/marker compounds in these products? Are such variations intrinsic to botanical products or are they due to external factors, or both?

Intrinsic and Extrinsic Factors

It is well established that intrinsic and extrinsic factors including plant species differences, organ specificity, diurnal and seasonal variation, environment, field collection and cultivation methods, contamination, substitution, adulteration, processing, and manufacturing practices greatly affect botanical quality. Intrinsically, plants are dynamic living organisms, each of which is capable of being genetically influenced to be slightly different in its physical and chemical characters. For example, a study on the accumulation of hypericin in *H. perforatum* showed that narrow-leafed populations have greater concentrations than the broader-leafed variety; variations of phytochemicals are greater in wild than in domesticated populations of the same species, as exemplified by the results of studies on the content of artemisinin, an antimalarial agent, in *Artemisia annua* L.; on michellamine B, a compound with in vitro anti-HIV activity, in *Ancistrocladus korupensis* D.W. Thomas & R.E. Gereau; and on the essential oil composition of *Ocimum basilicum* L. Also, the secondary chemical constituents of medicinal plants differ qualitatively as well as quantitatively from species to species as demonstrated by the presence of structurally different alkylamides in the roots of *Echinacea angustifolia* D.C. and *E. purpurea* (L.) Moench, and by their total absence in *E. pallida* (Nutt.) Nutt.

Organ specificity is yet another intrinsic factor influencing chemical variation because the site of biosynthesis and the site of accumulation and storage are normally different. Chemical biosynthesis usually takes place in the leaves, and then the product synthesized is transported through the stems to the roots for storage, with the chemical profiles in these organs being different from each other. Accumulation and storage can also take place in the leaves, but to a much lower extent, and very infrequently in the stems. An example of site-specific accumulation, as well as species specificity, is that of the compounds considered responsible for the immunostimulant effect of *Echinacea* species. These compounds encompass five groups of chemicals: caffeic acid derivatives, alkylamides, polyacetylenes (ketodialkenes and ketodialkynes), glycoproteins, and polysaccharides. As indicated above, alkylamides are found in the roots of *E. angustifolia* and *E. purpurea*, but they are structurally different, and are totally absent in *E. pallida* roots. Polyacetylenes, on the other hand, are present abundantly in the roots of *E. pallida*, but are absent in *E. angustifolia* and *E. purpurea* roots. Whereas the glycoproteins and polysaccharides are present in the aerial parts of all three species, they occur only in minute quantities in the roots.

Diurnal variation and seasonal variation are other intrinsic factors affecting chemical accumulation in both wild and cultivated plants. Depending on the plant, the accumulation of chemical constituents can occur at any time during the various stages of growth. In a majority of cases, maximum chemical accumulation occurs at the time of flowering, followed by a decline beginning at the fruiting stage. The time of harvest or field collection can thus influence the quality, efficacy, and safety of the final botanical product.

With respect to extrinsic factors, there are many that can affect the quality of medicinal plants. It has been well established that environmental factors such as soil, light, water, temperature, and nutrients can affect phytochemical accumulation in plants. For example, alkaloid concentrations in *Atropa belladonna* L. have been found to vary from 0.3% to 1.3%, when grown in different areas of the world. Also, the silymarin content in milk thistle was found to be highest in the fruits of plants grown under 60% water/field capacity (1.39%) and nitrogen level of 100 (1.46%) per acre. The methods employed in field collection from the wild, as well as in commercial cultivation, harvest, postharvest processing, shipping, and storage can also influence the physical appearance and chemical quality of the botanical source materials. Contaminations by microbial and chemical agents (pesticides, herbicides and heavy metals) as well as by insects, animals, animal parts, and animal excreta during any of the stages of source plant material production and collection can lead to lower quality and/or unsafe source materials. Heavy-metal contamination can occur at the cultivation, postharvest treatment, or product-manufacturing stages. Lead and thallium contaminations have been reported in multicomponent botanical mixtures, and cases of lead, thallium, mercury, arsenic, gold, and cadmium poisoning from the consumption of such products have been documented.

Botanical source materials collected in the wild often include non- targeted species either by accidental substitution or by intentional adulteration. However, substitution and adulteration of cultivated botanicals can also occur. Substitution of *Periploca sepium* Bunge for *E. senticosus* (eleuthero) has been widely documented and is regarded as being responsible for the "*hairy baby*" case involving maternal/neonatal androgenization. Adverse reactions due to plantain (*Plantago ovata* Forskal) being contaminated by *Digitalis lanata* Ehr. during harvest is another example of accidental adulteration by human error.

Adulteration of botanical products with synthetic drugs represents another problem in product quality and botanical product–drug interactions. Foremost among the documented cases are multicomponent Chinese or Ayurvedic botanical remedies. Chemical analyses of some arthritis remedies have led to the finding that synthetic anti-inflammatory drugs such as phenylbutazone, indomethacin, and/or corticoid steroids have been added. In a classic study of chemical adulteration of traditional medicine in Taiwan, 23.7% (618 of 2609) of botanical remedy samples collected by eight major hospitals were found to contain one or more synthetic therapeutic agents, including caffeine, acetaminophen, indomethacin, hydrochlorothiazide, prednisolone, ethoxybenzamide, phenylbutazone, betamethasone, theophylline, dexamethasone, diazepam, bucetin, chlorpheniramine maleate, prednisone, oxyphenbutazone, diclofenac sodium, ibuprofen, cortisone, ketoprofen, phenobarbital, hydrocortisone acetate, niflumic acid, triamcinolone, diethylpropion, mefenamic acid, prioxicam, and salicylamide. The most frequent adulterants were caffeine, acetaminophen, indomethacin, hydrochlorothiazide, prednisone, and chloroxazone. Obviously, such adulterated botanical products are prime candidates for botanical product–drug interactions.

Besides the unintentional in-process adulteration of heavy metals, it is well established that Ayurvedic medicine and traditional Chinese medicine sometimes employ complex mixtures of plant, animal, and mineral substances, and it is not uncommon to find appreciable quantities of heavy metals such as lead, mercury, cadmium, arsenic, and gold in certain formulations.

With respect to the words/claims, "*active compound*," "*marker compounds*," "*standardization*," and "*standardized products*," the clinician should be vigilant about their meaning when monitoring botanical safety. In the case of prescription and over-the-counter (OTC) drugs, each product has a single, defined "active" chemical constituent, which is used to measure or standardize product quality and determine shelf life. The active principle(s) of botanical products/dietary supplements, on the other hand, are largely unknown. For example, there is no evidence that the marker compounds eleutherosides B and E are the active principles in eleuthero (*E. senticosus*). Presently, there is also considerable disagreement as to whether hypericin or hyperforin is the active antidepressant principle in St. John's wort, with the latter being the current leading candidate.

Further, even when the active principles of a medicinal plant have been identified, the compound may not be commercially available for use as a reference standard. Hence, major constituent(s) of the source plant, whether biologically active or not, are currently employed as marker compounds for the standardization of most of the botanical products marketed, so that one manufacturer may not use the same reference standard as another. Compounding the issue of standardizing is the meaning of a "*standardized extract*," which may refer to (i) an extract made to a consistent standard such as a ratio of the starting plant material to that of the dried extract, (ii) an extract manufactured to contain a specific concentration of a marker compound(s), or (iii) any one of a number of botanical, agricultural, and/or manufacturing process control measures in the production of a material of reasonable consistency. With these inconsistencies in the meaning of standardization and standardized products, variations in efficacy and adverse events/drug interactions can, and will, occur.

Regulatory Influence

Botanical product quality and safety can also be influenced by regulatory status, which varies from country to country. In some countries, botanical products are regulated as medicine and are subject to mandated standards of quality, whereas in the United States a majority of botanicals are marketed as dietary supplements. Good manufacturing practices (GMPs) are required in the production of prescription and OTC drugs, but the regulatory provisions under the Dietary Supplement Health and Education Act (DSHEA) of 1994 provide little assurance of identity, quality, or purity for botanical dietary supplements. Thus, botanical dietary supplement products have not been subjected to mandated QA/QC standards as in the case of prescription and OTC drugs. Although the Food and Drug Administration advanced a notice of proposed rulemaking on current good manufacturing practice in the labeling and manufacturing standards on dietary supplements in March 2003, such standards have not yet been implemented. Elsewhere in the world, e.g., in the European Union and in most of Asia and Southeast Asia, national policies exist, but in some countries, these products are totally unregulated. Consequently, product quality, efficacy, and safety differ internationally, nationally, and from product brand to product brand, and even from lot to lot within the same brand.

Quality Assurance and Quality Control

For effective monitoring of botanical product–drug interaction in clinical studies or application, the clinician must be aware that standards of quality for botanical products do not exist in many countries, including the United States. Therefore, the products being evaluated must be accurately defined as to the quality of botanicals employed, and information on the QC measures employed to ensure their quality must be taken into consideration. If such QC/QA information, including standardization and what is meant by the term, is lacking, it is not possible to attribute the drug interactions observed to the botanical product in the clinical study/use, and the data being published will be invalid and/or misleading.

Information on QC of the botanical product under investigation or in clinical use must be derived from measures taken, from the procurement of source material to the production of the final formulation. Whether by field collection from the wild or by cultivation, good agricultural and/or collection practices must be adhered to during the procurement process, because the quality of the finished botanical products is obviously directly related to the quality and safety of the raw materials. Hence, whether field-collected or produced by cultivation, the identification and authentication of plant species by a taxonomic botanist is critical to ensuring that the correct source material is acquired. It is essential that the plant materials are identified by their scientific names (Latin binomial), and a description of the macroscopic, microscopic, and organoleptic (sensory) characters be provided along with herbarium specimens, drawings, or photographs. In the field collection of medicinal plants, care must be exercised to avoid the acquisition of nontargeted species and to free the targeted source material of undesirable plant parts, soil, rock, insects, animals, animal excreta, and other contaminants. Postcollection treatments should mirror those accorded cultivated plant materials.

Due to their genetic and chemical content variations, the site and date should be recorded for each collection. The production of raw materials by cultivation should normally lead to more uniform botanical products due to greater genetic uniformity. The production of quality raw materials can only be assured by employing good agricultural practices such as those described in the recently published WHO Guidelines on Good Agriculture and Collection Practices. The harvested source materials must be processed to produce the finished products under GMPs. GMP procedures employed for the manufacture of botanical products involving, at the raw material production end, botanical taxonomic identification to assure species identification must be implemented. Otherwise the efficacy, safety, and botanical product–drug interaction reported for one medicinal plant may in fact be those caused by another botanical product. It should be noted that although common names are most frequently used by the source material producers/collectors, a common name may apply to more than one plant. For example, "ginseng" may refer to American ginseng [*P. quinquefolius* L. (Araliaceae)], Asian/Korean ginseng [*P. ginseng* C.A. Meyer (Araliaceae)], Russian/Siberian ginseng [*E. senticosus* (Rupr. & Maxim.)

Maxim. (Araliaceae)], Blue ginseng [*Caulophyllum thalictroides* L. Michx. (Berberidaceae)], Brazilian ginseng [*Pfaffia paniculata* Kuntz (Amaranthaceae)], Indian ginseng [*Withania somnifera* L. Dunal (Solanaceae)], or Wild Red American ginseng [*Rumex hymenosepalus* (Polygonaceae)]. Thus, the identification of the source material from which the botanical product is being monitored must be by its Latin binomial.

At the processing and manufacturing stage, macroscopic, microscopic, and organoleptic analyses and analytical procedures similar to those employed for the manufacture of conventional drugs to assure quality and purity by appropriate protocols must be used. Otherwise, the quality of the finished product under clinical investigation/use may be compromised, and this can lead to adverse events and/or botanical product–drug interactions. Microscopic and organoleptic examinations will help assure botanical identity and purity because each plant species possesses characteristic microscopic cellular features, and may have distinct sensory properties. Macroscopic examination will reveal the presence of deterioration and signs of contamination by molds, insects, rodents, and other animals, as well as by other plants.

As with pharmaceutical drugs, botanical products should be thoroughly evaluated biologically, employing not only in vitro methods, but also the more relevant in vivo animal studies, particularly with respect to acute and chronic toxicity.

Procedures for the QC analysis of active and/or marker chemical compounds in botanical products during the manufacturing and post- marketing surveillance processes can be accomplished by colorimetric, spectroscopic, and/or chromatographic methods. Colorimetric and direct spectroscopic methods are older analytical procedures that quantify the absorption of structurally related compounds at a specific wavelength of light, expressed as a concentration of a reference standard (marker), which is normally the active or major chemical constituent in that plant material. Because other plant constituents possessing the same absorbance are included in the measurement, a higher concentration is usually ascribed to the test material. The use of these procedures has recently been on the decline. Modern methods for the chemical analysis of secondary chemical constituent markers in botanical products involve some form of chromatography. Thin-layer chromatographic procedures have the advantages of being simple and rapid, and they can provide useful characteristic profile patterns and are inexpensive to use. However, their resolving power is limited and quantitative data for minor constituents is difficult to obtain. Gas chromatography can provide a high resolution of the more volatile complex mixtures, but is of limited value in the case of nonvolatile polar compounds, especially the polar polyhydroxylated and glycosidic compounds.

High-performance liquid chromatography (HPLC) is capable of resolving complex mixtures of polar and nonpolar compounds, and has become the chromatographic method of choice for the qualitative and quantitative analysis of botanical extracts and products. HPLC can be coupled with a range of analytical techniques including ultraviolet (UV) spectroscopy, mass spectrometry, nuclear magnetic resonance (NMR), and evaporative light- scattering detection (ELSD). Combined with HPLC, any of these techniques is capable of producing a "*fingerprint*" of the botanical product. However, some of these detection methods may be inappropriate for the quantitative determination of a specific active or marker compound. The literature is replete with HPLC methods for the analysis of specific compounds in more than 95% of the botanical extracts or products in the market. Detection by UV is readily available in most labs, and is carried out either with a single- or dual-wavelength, or a full spectrum (e.g., photodiode array) detector, and is the most appropriate technique for the routine analysis of compounds that contain a UV-active chromophore. Combined HPLC–mass spectrometry (LC–MS) and liquid chromatography–tandem mass spectrometry (LC–MS^n) is being used increasingly.

The advantage of these methods is that as each compound is being eluted, it is captured by the mass spectrometer and provides a molecular ion and/or major mass fragment, which can provide a specific identification of the eluting "peak." However, ionization techniques compatible with HPLC, such as electro-spray ionization, show a broad range of sensitivity to various compound classes. This technique is excellent for compounds such as alkaloids, phenols, and organic acids, but can be highly insensitive to others such as aliphatic hydrocarbons, sterols, and polysaccharides. All compounds containing protons, including virtually all medicinally significant phytochemicals, can be detected by NMR. This technique generally provides more structural information than any other single technique. However, LC–NMR is available in only a few labs worldwide, requires the use of deuterated solvents for chromatography, and will remain inaccessible and prohibitively expensive for routine use for some time. A vast majority of all plant secondary metabolites are detectable by ELSD, but this method provides no structural information. There can exist no standardization regime that would be universally applicable to all medicinal botanical products. Ideally, the formulated product should be chemically assayed for an active constituent, using an analytical method appropriate for the given compound class, and also biologically assayed for in vitro and/or in vivo activity, using assay(s) relevant to the intended use of the product.

Clinical Experimental Design and Data Interpretation

For effective botanical product–drug interaction monitoring, there is a most critical need for a well-designed clinical experiment that not only takes into account the aforementioned QC issues, but also includes a safety monitoring component that will enable the clinician to delineate between adverse reactions caused by botanical product–drug interactions and those by drug–drug interactions due to concomitant ingestions of multiple pharmaceutical drugs by the patient, or adverse events owing to idiosyncratic causes. A system designed for careful and rational interpretation of study data should be devised so as to avoid erroneous conclusions such as those reported on the so-called GAS. In monitoring botanical product–drug interactions, the quality of the data obtained may be influenced by a number of factors. Among the contributing factors are: raw material source and sourcing practices; intrinsic and extrinsic factors affecting the occurrence and concentration of active or marker chemical constituents in both the starting and the finished products; standardization and standardized products; the methods of chemical and biological analyses; manufacturing practices; substitution; adulteration of botanical products with pharmaceutical drugs or contamination with foreign toxic substances; regulatory requirements; and the quality of the clinical experimental design and data interpretation.

5

PHARMACOKINETICS OF PLANT PRODUCTS

A general disillusionment with conventional medicines, coupled with the desire for a "natural" lifestyle has resulted in an increasing utilization of herbal medicinal products (HMPs) across the developed world. Sales of botanical products in the United States have increased sharply in recent years, according to industry reports. An estimated $4 billion was spent in health food stores in 2000 for botanical products in bulk, as well as capsules, tablets, extracts, and teas. A similar trend is noted for European countries. Many consumers use HMPs in a holistic manner and mainly on the basis of their empirical and traditional applications. The use of HMPs in an evidence-based approach is known as "*rational phytotherapy*," which is in contrast to traditional medical herbalism. To obtain "*rationality*," HMPs must meet acceptable standards of quality, safety, and efficacy. Besides quality and safety issues, establishing the pharmacological basis for efficacy of HMPs is a constant challenge for researchers worldwide. In general, pharmacology can be defined as the study of the interaction of biologically active agents with living systems.

The study of pharmacology can be further divided into two main areas: pharmacodynamics and pharmacokinetics. Whereas in recent years the number of studies investigating the pharmacodynamic effects of HMPs has increased rapidly, there is still limited information available regarding herbal pharmacokinetics. This might be due to the following reasons. The study of herbal pharmacokinetics is extraordinarily complex because HMPs are multicomponent mixtures, which contain several chemical constituents. Therefore, concentrations of single compounds in the final product are in the lower milligram range per dose. The resulting plasma concentrations are often in the microgram per liter to picogram per liter range. As a consequence, analytical methods determining bioavailability and pharmacokinetics of HMPs have to be sufficiently sensitive. Advanced techniques such as gas chromatography–mass spectrometry (GC–MS)/MS or high-performance liquid chromatography–MS/MS can be used nowadays to accomplish these goals. For the majority of these multicomponent mixtures, the active constituents are often unknown. In other words, a substance that is detectable in body fluids is not necessarily the active compound of an extract. Further, the different compounds will have a different bioavailability, thereby complicating the design of pharmacokinetic studies with HMPs. Natural compounds are often prodrugs that are metabolized in the digestive tract. Moreover, HMPs can contain large polar molecules that might be expected to have poor and unpredictable bioavailability.

Bioavailability is defined as the rate and extent of active substances in the blood stream after oral doses. The bioavailability of a substance depends on several factors: the pharmaceutical preparation, the size of the molecule, the fat/water solubility of the compound, factors within the gut, first-pass effects, interaction with food, and individual factors in the patient, such as the influence of pathological factors. Bioavailability of compounds in the plant extract might also be influenced by other components in the mixture, which are not active themselves but can act to improve the stability, solubility, or the half-life time of the active compounds. Some authors divide their components into active and accompanying substances (so-called coeffectors). Coeffectors have an influence on the physicochemical properties of active compounds of an extract and, as a consequence, on their biopharmaceutical parameters.

There are several examples in the literature showing that such coeffectors improve not only the solubility but also the bioavailability of single compounds. Saponines were shown to significantly increase the absorption of corticosteroids, some antibiotics, flavones, phytosterols, and silicic acid. The concentration of kavain and yangonin in mouse brain samples is higher after administration of a Piper methysticum extract than after administration of the purified single compounds in the same amount. Similarly, the oral bioavailability of kavain from an extract of *P. methysticum* is 10 times higher than that of pure kavain. The improved bioavailability of ascorbic acid from a Citrus extract compared to pure ascorbic acid is explained by an increased absorption and an improved stability of vitamin C in presence of several flavonoids contained in the *Citrus* extract. List et al. showed that the transport of L-hyoscyamin from the mucosal to the serosal side of the rat's isolated ileum is increased when a native extract prepared from the leaves of Hyoscyamus niger is used instead of pure hyoscyamin; they suggest unidentified flavonoid glycosides as the responsible compounds.

Unfortunately, most investigations on this topic give few or no information about the mechanism of interaction and, in particular, about the compounds involved. One approach to identify the chemical structure of a coeffector was recently performed by Butterweck et al. Taken together, although the study of herbal pharmacokinetics appears to be difficult, the information derived from such investigations will become an important issue to link data from pharmacological assays and clinical effects. In particular, a better understanding of the pharmacokinetics and bioavailability of natural compounds can help in designing rational dosage regimen; and it can help to predict potential botanical product–drug interactions. In addition, those studies would provide supporting evidence for the synergistic nature of herbal medicines and would further help in optimizing the bioavailability and, hence, the efficacy of HMPs. In the following chapter, pharmacokinetic studies that have been conducted for some of the top-selling HMPs worldwide are listed, including SJW, ginkgo, garlic, willow bark, milk thistle, and horse chestnut.

GINKGO BILOBA

G. biloba L. is a member of the Ginkgoaceae family, a gymnosperm that has survived unchanged from the Triassic period. In traditional Chinese medicine, the seeds (nuts) of *G. biloba* were used as an antitussive, expectorant, and antiasthmatic, and in bladder infection. In China, the leaves of *G. biloba* were also used for the treatment of asthma and cardiovascular disorders. Today, standardized concentrated extracts prepared from the leaves of *G. biloba* are used for the treatment of peripheral circulatory insufficiency, cerebrovascular disorders, geriatric complaints, and for Alzheimer dementia.

Interestingly, no preclinical or clinical work has been done investigating the pharmacology, therapeutic efficacy, or safety of crude ginkgo leaf preparations. Almost all of the existing data focus on dry extracts characterized by 22% to 27% flavonol glycosides, 5% to 7% terpene trilactones, and less than 5ppm ginkgolic acids (EGb 761). Other chemicals present in the extracts are hydroxykynurenic acid, shikimic acid, protocatechuic acid, vanillic acid, and p-hydroxybenzoic acid. The monograph published by the Commission E of the German Health Authorities states that acceptable extracts should have an herb-to-extract ratio in the average range of 50:1. Extracts should be prepared with an acetone–water mixture and then be purified further. This standardization process eliminates unwanted components that might have toxic effects. In particular, it has been shown that adverse effects such as allergies were related to ginkgolic acids. Therefore, extracts that are used in drug manufacture are free of

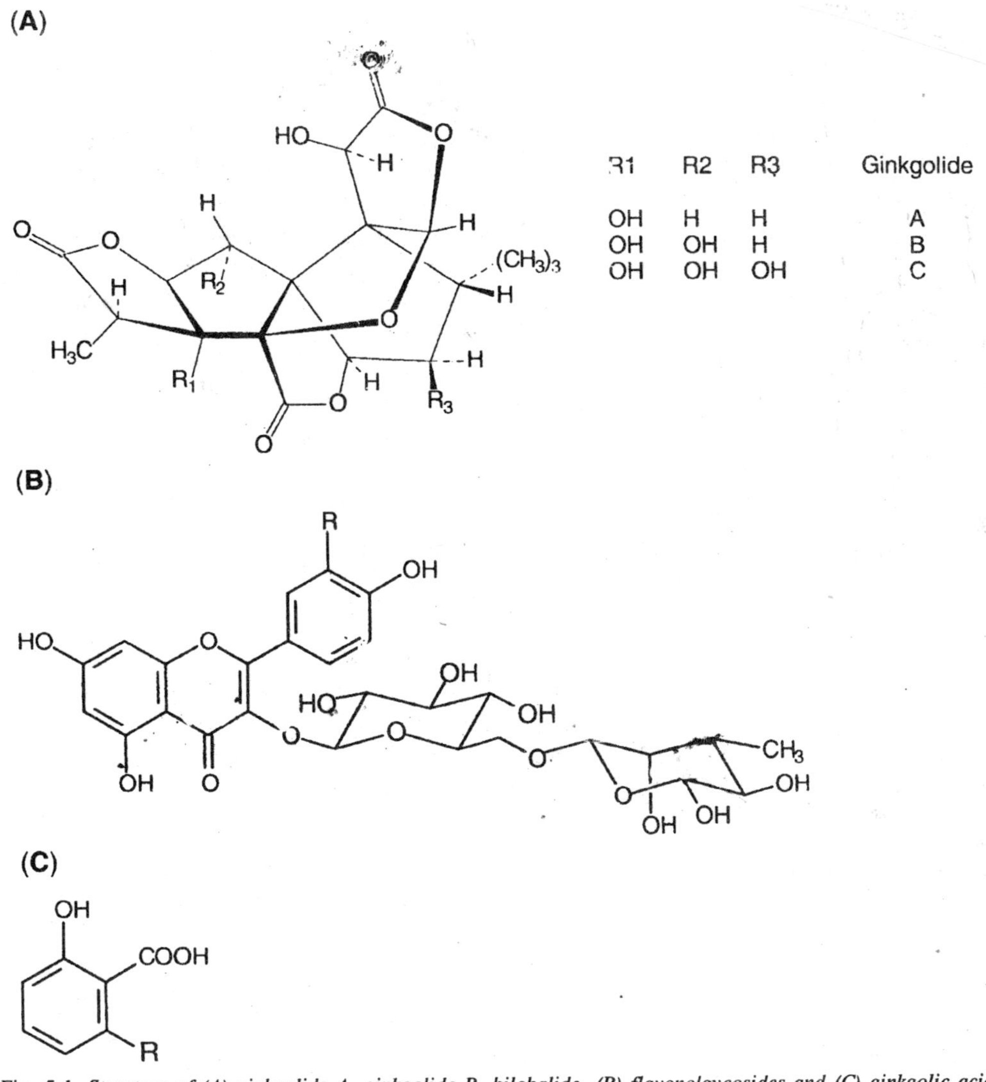

(A)

R1	R2	R3	Ginkgolide
OH	H	H	A
OH	OH	H	B
OH	OH	OH	C

(B)

(C)

Fig. 5.1. Structure of (A) ginkgolide A, ginkgolide B, bilobalide, (B) flavonolgycosides and (C) ginkgolic acids.

ginkgolic acids (less than 5 ppm). The question of whether ginkgolic acids possess allergenic potential or not is still discussed controversially, especially because it has been shown that leaf extracts, if taken orally, showed adverse effects even if they contained ginkgolic acids in a concentration of 1000 ppm, whereas a pure ginkgolic acid extract showed allergic effects.

Pharmacokinetics

Both human and animal pharmacokinetic studies have been done on ginkgo flavonol aglycones (quercetin, kaempferol, and isorhamnetin) and terpene rilactones (ginkgolide A and B and bilobalide).

Flavonol glycosides

Human clinical studies

In general, pharmacokinetic studies on flavonol glycosides are difficult to conduct because flavonoids are commonly present in the diet and their metabolites are numerous. An accurate pharmacokinetic assessment requires subjects to be maintained on a flavonoid-free diet for a period of time prior to dosing. This has been done in the study by Pietta et al. Six volunteers received the relatively high single oral dose of 4 g (equivalent to 1 g flavonol glycosides) of ginkgo leaf extract (EGb 761) following seven days of a flavonoid-free diet. The following flavonol metabolites were found in the urine over three days: 4-hydroxybenzoic acid conjugate, 4-hydroxyhippuric acid, 3-methoxy-4-hydroxyhippuric acid, 3,4-dihydroxybenzoic acid, 4-hydroxybenzoic acid, hippuric acid, and 3-methoxy-4-hydroxybenzoic acid, which represented less than 30% of the flavonols administered. The authors noted that the very high dose of extract administered to the subjects made it difficult to extrapolate the results to normal clinical dosages (40–240mg extract daily).

The oral pharmacokinetics of the flavonol aglycones quercetin, kaempferol, and isorhamnetin in two healthy volunteers were studied by Nieder. Subjects were given 50, 100, and 300mg of ginkgo leaf extract–coated tablets (LI 1370). Peak plasma concentrations (C_{max}) of 25 to 30, 65, and 130 ng/mL, respectively, were achieved within two to three hours with half-lives ($t_{1/2}$) of two to four hours. Values returned to baseline 24 hours after intake. There was a linear relationship between the dose administered and the peak plasma level. In the study by Wocjcicki et al., the bioavailabilities of the same aglycones were determined using three different single oral dosage forms (capsule, liquid, and tablet). Results were similar to those of Nieder. However, the t_{max} was longer with the capsules. Values were back to baseline 24 hours after intake. The area under the curve (AUC) for the evaluated flavonoids did not differ significantly among formulations. The researchers concluded that the three formulations could be modeled by a one-compartment model with zero-order absorption without lag time, indicating that the aglycones were rapidly absorbed, and that the preparations had similar bioavailability. That the dosage form might have an influence of the bioavailability of ginkgolides and bilobalide was studied by Kressmann et al.

Increasing doses of a commercial special extract of *G. biloba* (LI 1370) were administered to two healthy volunteers (50, 100, and 300 mg). The amounts of kaempferol and quercetin were significantly higher compared to baseline. The flavonoids were metabolized and excreted primarily as glucuronic acid conjugates in urine.

Animal studies

In the study by Pietta et al., a single dose of ginkgo leaf extract (EGb 761) was administered orally to rats. Metabolites found in the urine represented less than 40% of the flavonoids administered. The presence of phenylalkyl acids in the rat urine but not in the human urine indicates that the flavonols were more extensively metabolized in humans than in rats. In the study by W tanabe et al., mice received a diet containing ginkgo leaf extract (EGb761; 36mg/kg daily) or a standard diet without the extract for four weeks. Afterwards, plasma levels of quercetin (12.0 ng/mL vs. 4.8 ng/mL), kaempferol (7.0 ng/mL vs. 3.2 ng/ mL), and isorhamnetin (49.6 ng/mL vs. 0 ng/mL) in both treatment groups were determined. The study indicates that these compounds can be absorbed intact into the blood stream.

Triterpene lactones

Human clinical studies

Mauri et al. investigated the pharmacokinetics of ginkgolides A, B, and bilobalide, after administration of ginkgo leaf extract (160 mg oral single dose) to 15 healthy subjects. The product given contained either a phospholipid complex (Ginkgoselect Phytosome) or not (Ginkgoselect) (both products contained 24% flavonol glycosides and 6% terpene trilactones; Indena SpA). Administration with the phospholipids enhanced maximum absorption (C_{max}) of total ginkgolides and bilobalide two- to threefold (from 85.0 to 181.8 µg/mL), but delayed t_{max} 1.5- to 2-fold. The AUC increased two- to threefold when the phospholipid complex was administered. In this single-compartment model, the mean elimination half-life ($t_{1/2}$) was approximately 120 to 180 minutes for all of the terpene trilactones, regardless of the product administered. Fourtillan et al. studied the pharmacokinetics of terpene trilactones in 12 healthy volunteers after single-dose intravenous (i.v.) or oral administration of ginkgo leaf extract (EGb 761), given with or without a meal. The authors could show that the consumption of a standard meal along with the oral dose of EGb 761 did not affect pharmacokinetic parameters. In a recent study, Drago et al. focused on the pharmacokinetics of two different dosage regimens for orally administered ginkgo leaf extract (Egb 761) in healthy volunteers. The subjects received either 40 mg twice daily or 80 mg once daily, with an interval of 21 days between cycles. It could be shown that a dosage of 40 mg twice daily resulted in a significantly longer $t_{1/2}$ (11.6 ± 5.2 vs. 4.3 ± 0.5) and mean residence time (MRT) (13.1 ±0.3 vs. 7.3 ± 0.6) than a single 80 mg dose. t_{max} was reached two to three hours after administration with both dosages. The authors conclude that the twice-daily dosage regimen with the lower dose is superior to that of a higher single daily dose.

The influence of the type of extract, the formulation, and dosage form on the bioavailability and pharmacokinetics of ginkolide A and B and bilobalide was recently investigated by Kressmann et al. Twelve healthy volunteers received either Ginkgol (containing Egb 761 = reference) or *G. biloba* capsules

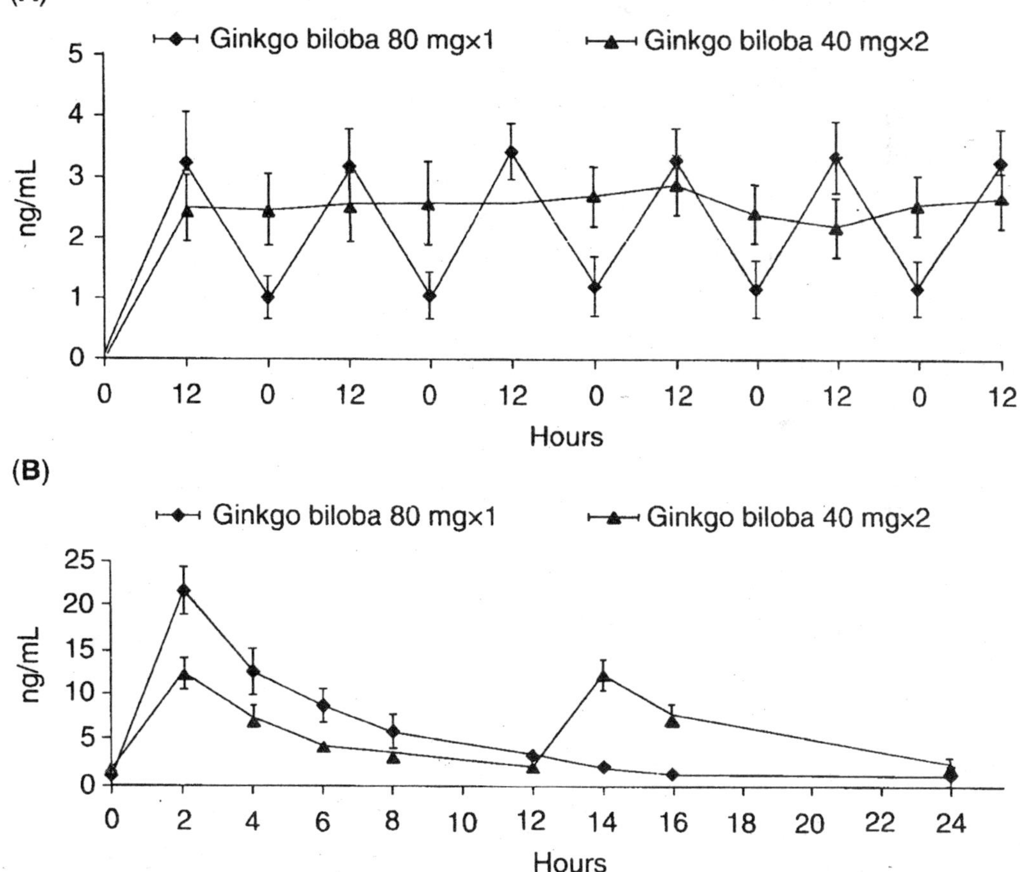

Fig. 5.2. Plasma concentrations of (ng/mL) of ginkgolide B (A) from day 1 to day 6 and (B) on day 7 after oral administration of 40 and 80 mg tablets of Ginkgo biloba extract.

(= test comp[illegible] containing another commercial dry extract in an open, single-dose crossover design study [illegible] subjects received an oral dose of 120 mg extract under fasting conditions. Pronounced differences could be detected between the test and reference formulations regarding the bioavailability of the investigated constituents, ginkgolide A, ginkgolide B, and bilobalide. The authors clearly could show that the type of extract, the formulation, and dosage form influence the pharmacokinetics and bioavailability of potential active *Ginkgo* ingredients.

Animal studies

The bioavailability of ginkgolides A and B and bilobalide was studied in rats after a single oral administration of 30, 55, and 100 mg/kg Ginkgo leaf extract (EGb 761). The pharmacokinetics of these compounds was found to be dose-linear. Maximum plasma levels of ginkgolides A and B and bilobalide were reached in 30 to 60 minutes, with $t_{1/2}$ of ginkgolides A and B and bilobalide equaling 1.7, 2.0, and 2.2 hours, respectively, at the 30-mg dose and 1.8, 2.0, and 3.0 hours, respectively, at the 100-mg dose. Li and Wong examined the pharmacokinetics of two *Ginkgo* leaf extracts in rabbits: one standardized to 27% flavonoids and 6% terpenoids and specially prepared to yield at least 80% higher levels of ginkgolide B compared to other standardized extracts (BioGinkgo; Pharmanex), the other containing EGb 761 and standardized to 24% flavonoids and 6% terpenoids (Ginkoba, Pharmaton). Plasma concentrations of ginkgolides from the BioGinkgo extract exhibited peaks at two and five hours post-treatment with the 40 mg/kg dose and at one and five hours with the 60mg/kg dose. Mean C_{max} for the 40 and 60 mg/kg doses of the BioGinkgo extract were 18.8 ± 1.97 and 25.1 ± 3.39 μg/mL, respectively, demonstrating dose dependency. With the Ginkoba preparation (40 mg/kg), a single peak in plasma concentration was observed at three hours with mean C_{max} of 17.8 ± 0.59 μg/mL, similar to that of the former extract at the same dose. Twelve hours after the 40 mg/kg treatment, plasma ginkgolide levels were 2.6 times greater for BioGinkgo than for Ginkoba. The prolonged residence time and greater bioavailability was attributed to two factors: the slightly higher terpenoid content of the BioGinkgo preparation and, more importantly, the fact that the extract was enriched with ginkgolide B, which has a longer half-life than ginkgolide A.

St. John's Wort

Hypericum perforatum (Clusiaceae), commonly known as SJW, is used in many countries for the treatment of mild-to-moderate forms of depression. Several clinical studies provide evidence that SJW is as effective as conventional synthetic antidepressants. From a phytochemical point of view, *H. perforatum* belongs to one of the best-investigated medicinal plants. A series of bioactive compounds have been detected in the crude material, namely phenylpropanes, flavonol derivatives, biflavones, proanthocyanidins, xanthones, phloroglucinols, some amino acids, naphthodianthrones, and essential oil constituents.

Recent reports have shown that the antidepressant activity of *Hypericum* extracts can be attributed to the phloroglucinol derivative hyperforin, to the naphthodianthrones hypericin and pseudohypericin, and to several flavonoids. The role and the mechanisms of action of these different compounds are still a matter of debate. But, taking these previous findings together, it is likely that several constituents are responsible for the clinically observed antidepressant efficacy of SJW.

Pharmacokinetics

Single- and multiple-dose pharmacokinetic studies with extracts of SJW were performed in rats and humans, which focused on the determination of plasma levels of the naphthodianthrones hypericin and pseudohypericin and the phloroglucinol derivative hyperforin. Results from pharmacokinetic studies investigating plasma levels of different flavonoids after intake of SJW preparations are presently not available.

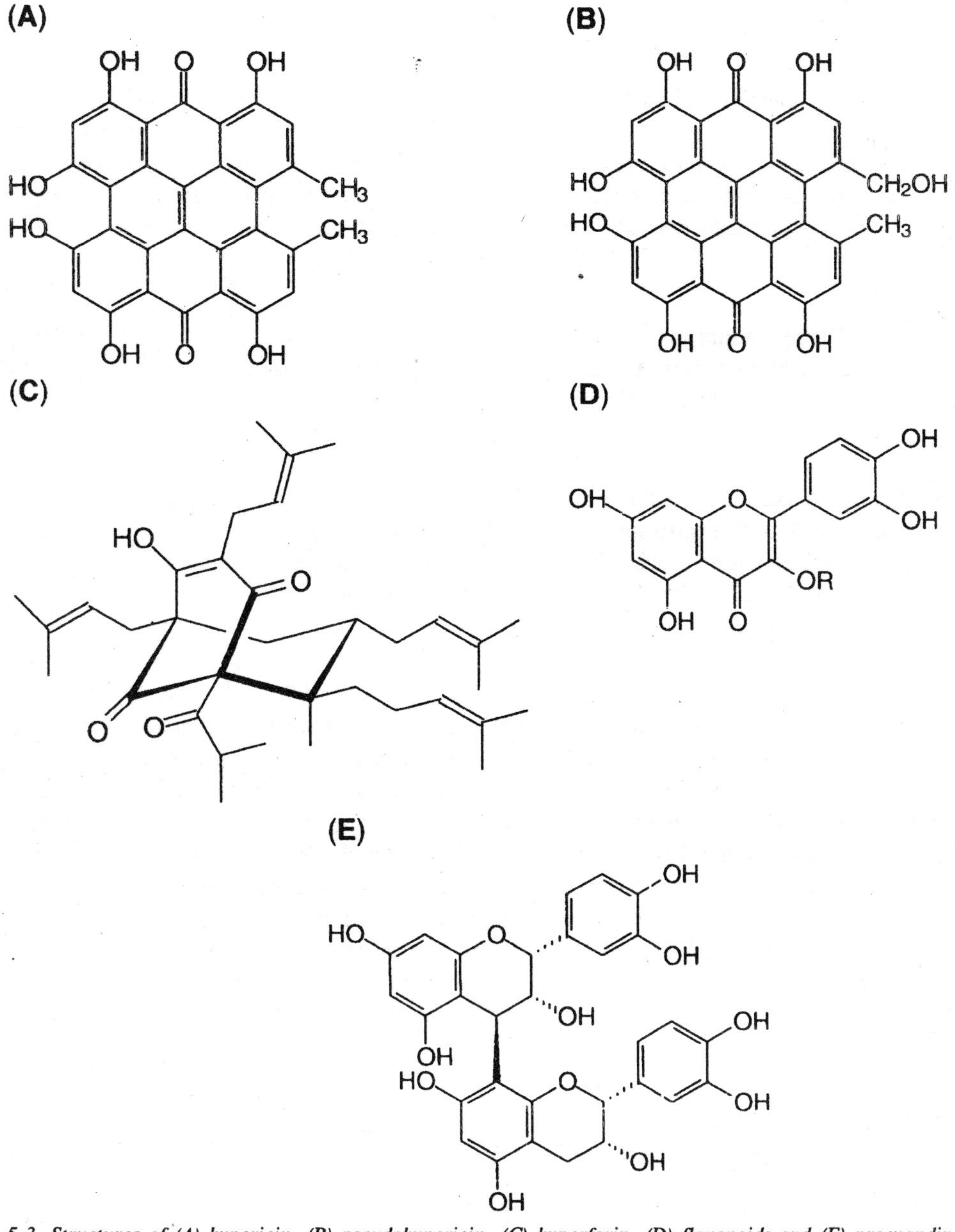

Fig. 5.3. Structures of (A) hypericin, (B) pseudohypericin, (C) hyperforin, (D) flavonoids and (E) procyandin B2.

Naphthodianthrones

Human clinical studies

Detailed pharmacokinetic studies have been carried out with the hypericin-standardized SJW extract LI 160. The preparation is reported to contain 300 mg of the dried extract of SJW, yielding 0.24% to 0.32% total hypericin. Administration of single oral doses of LI 160 (300, 900, and 1800 mg) to healthy male volunteers resulted in peak plasma hypericin concentrations of 1.5, 7.5, and 14.2 ng/mL for the three doses, respectively. Peak plasma concentrations were seen with hypericin between 2.0

and 2.6 hours and with pseudohypericin after 0.4 to 0.6 hours. The elimination half-life of hypericin was between 24.8 and 26.5 hours, and varied for pseudohypericin from 16.3 to 36.0 hours. The AUC showed a nonlinear increase on raising the dose—this effect was statistically significant for hypericin. Repeated doses of LI 160 (300 mg) three times daily resulted in steady-state concentrations after four days. Mean maximal plasma level during the steady-state treatment was 8.5 ng/mL for hypericin and 5.8 ng/mL for pseudohypericin. Kinetic parameters after i.v. administration of SJW extract (115 and 38 mg for hypericin and pseudohypericin, respectively) in two subjects correspond to those estimated after an oral dosage. Both hypericin and pseudohypericin were initially distributed into a central volume of 4.2 and 5.0 L, respectively. The mean distribution volumes at steady state were 19.7 L for hypericin and 39.3 L for pseudohypericin, and the mean total clearance rates were 9.2 mL/min for hypericin and 43.3 mL/min for pseudohypericin. The systemic availability of hypericin and pseudohypericin were roughly estimated to be 14% and 21%, respectively. In spite of their structural similarities, there were substantial pharmacokinetic differences between hypericin and pseudohypericin, which is not surprising considering the differences in the planarity of both molecules.

A placebo-controlled, randomized clinical trial with monitoring of hypericin and pseudohypericin plasma concentrations was performed to evaluate the increase in dermal photosensitivity in humans after application of high doses of SJW extract. The study was divided into a single-dose and a multiple-dose part. In the single dose crossover study, each of the 13 volunteers received either placebo or 900, 1800, or 3600 mg of the SJW extract LI 160. Maximum total hypericin plasma concentrations were observed about four hours after dosage and were 0, 28, 61, and 159 ng/mL, respectively. Pharmacokinetic parameters had a dose relationship that appeared to follow linear kinetics. In another study, the concentrations of hypericin and pseudohypericin in serum and skin blister fluid after oral intake (single and steady state) of relatively high doses of LI 160 were determined in 12 healthy volunteers. After a single oral administration of SJW extract (1800 mg), the mean serum level of total hypericin (hypericin þ pseudohypericin) was 43 ng/mL and the mean skin blister fluid level was 5.3 ng/mL. After steady-state administration (900 mg/day for seven days), the mean serum level of total hypericin was 12.5 ng/mL and the mean skin blister fluid level was 2.8 ng/mL. Serum levels of total hypericin were always higher than skin levels. However, the skin levels observed in this study are far below the hypericin skin levels that are estimated to be phototoxic (greater than 100 ng/mL).

Pharmacokinetics, safety, and antiviral effects of hypericin were studied in patients with chronic hepatitis C infection. The patients received an eight-weeks course of 0.05 and 0.10mg/kg hypericin orally once a day. The pharmacokinetic data revealed a long elimination half-life (mean values of 36.1 and 33.8 hours, respectively, for the doses of 0.05 and 0.10 mg/ kg) and mean AUC determinations of 1.5 and 3.1 μg/mL/hr, respectively. Because relatively high doses of 0.05 and 0.10 mg/kg/day were given, which will probably be not reached after oral intake of recommended doses of SJW extract preparations, it is not surprising that hypericin caused a considerable phototoxicity in this study.

Animal studies

Early pharmacokinetic studies in mice report that maximum plasma concentrations of hypericin and pseudohypericin were reached at six hours and were maintained for at least eight hours. The aqueous-ethanolic SJW extract used in this study contained 1.0 mg of hypericin. Pharmacokinetics and cerebrospinal fluid penetration of hypericin were studied after i.v. dose of 2mg/kg in monkeys. Mean peak plasma concentration of hypericin following this dose was 71.7 μg/mL (142 μM). Elimination of hypericin from plasma was biexponential, with an average terminal half-life of 26 $\pm$ 14 hours. The 2 mg/kg dose in nonhuman primates was sufficient to maintain plasma concentrations above 5.1 μg/mL (10 μM) for up to 12 hours (the in vitro concentration required for growth inhibition of human glioma cell lines is greater than 10 μM).

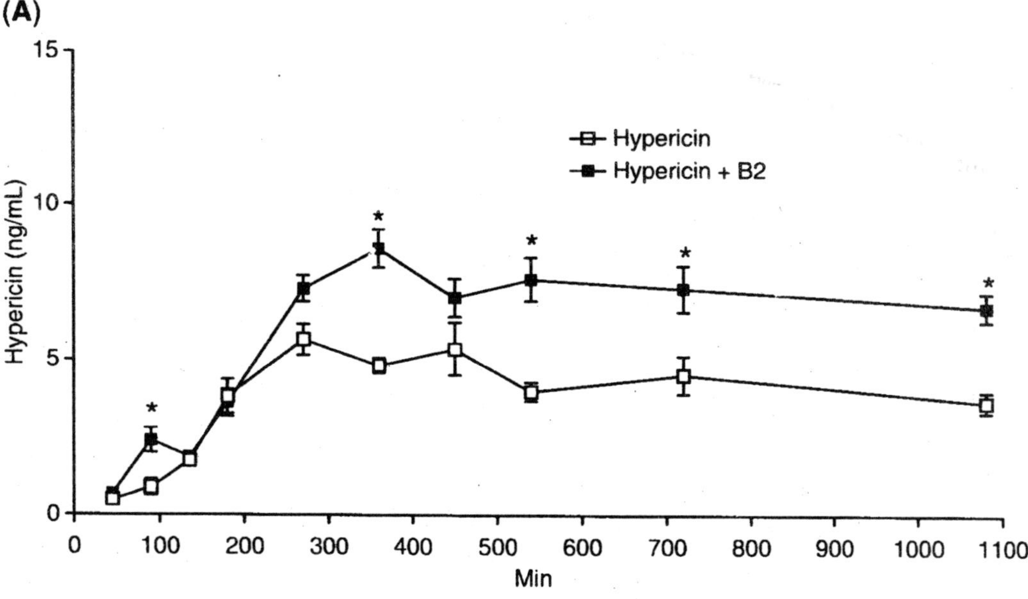

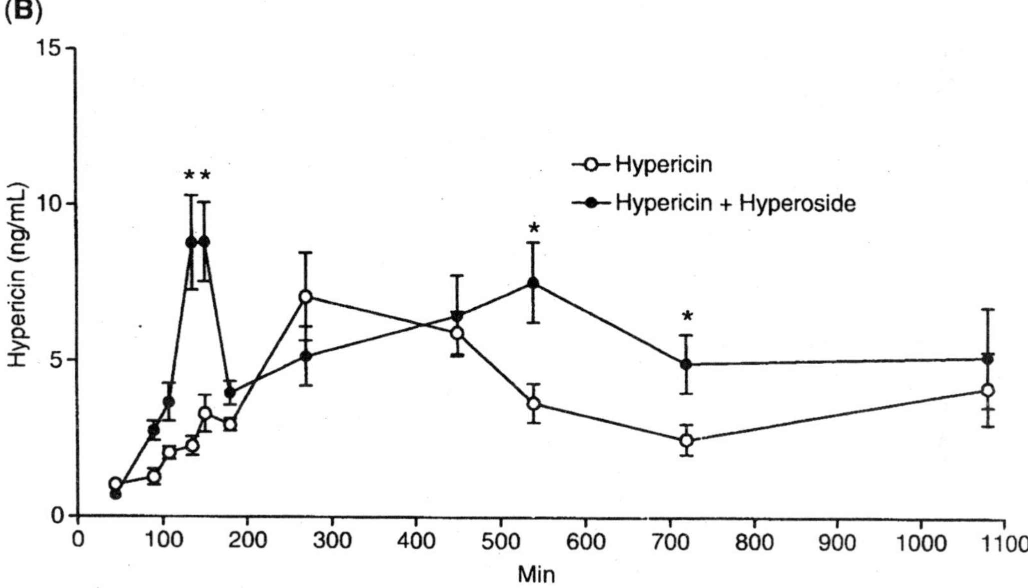

Fig. 5.4. (A) Plasma levels of hypericin in the presence and absence of procyanidin B2. (B) Plasma levels of hypericin in the presence and absence of hyperoside.

In general, the biological evaluation of hypericin in various test models is limited by its poor water solubility. It was shown in in vitro as well as in vivo studies that the water solubility of hypericin was remarkably enhanced in the presence of procyanidins or flavonol glycosides of SJW extract. In a recent pharmacokinetic study in rats, it was shown that procyanidin B2 as well as hyperoside increased the oral bioavailability of hypericin by approximately 58% (B2) and 34% (hyperoside). Procyanidin B2 and hyperoside had a different influence on the plasma kinetics of hypericin; median maximal plasma levels of hypericin were detected after 360 minutes (C_{max}: 8.6 ng/mL) for B2, and after 150

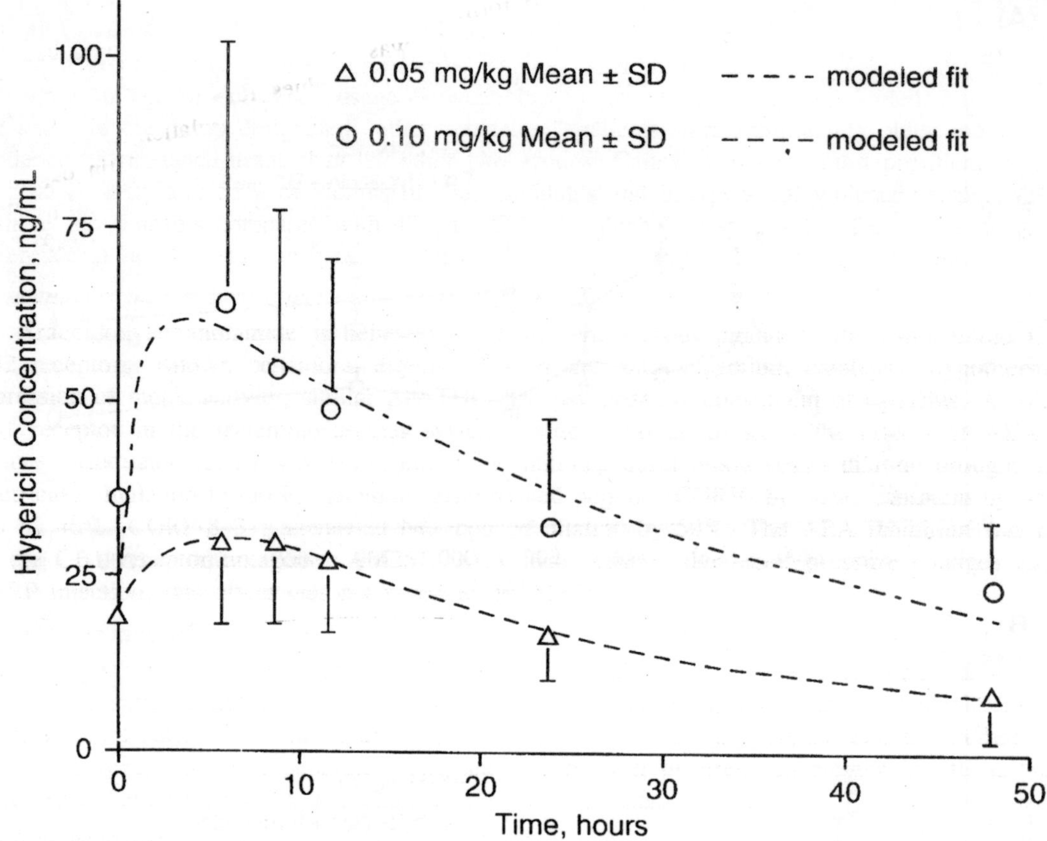

Fig. 5.5. Plasma concentrations of hypericin after oral administration of hypericin (0.05 and 1 mg/kg) to hepatitis C patients.

minutes (C_{max}: 8.8 ng/mL) for hyperoside. The authors suggest that treatment of patients with the entire SJW extract, depending on its composition, should be superior to the treatment with isolated compounds, because the extract provides not only different classes of active compounds, but also constituents that influence their bioavailability.

Hyperforin

Human clinical studies

Plasma levels of hyperforin were followed for 24 hours in two studies with healthy volunteers after administration of film-coated tablets containing 300 mg SJW extract representing 14.8 mg hyperforin. In the first crossover study, six male volunteers received 300, 600, or 1200 mg of a SJW extract preparation (WS 5572) after a 10-hour fasting time. Maximum plasma levels of 150 ng/mL (approximately 280 nM) were reached after 3.5 hours after intake of 300 mg SJW extract. Half-life and MRT were 9 and 12 hours, respectively. Hyperforin pharmacokinetics were linear up to 600 mg of the extract. Increasing the doses to 900 or 1200 mg resulted in lower C_{max} and AUC values than those expected from linear extrapolation of data from lower doses. In a repeated dose study with seven healthy volunteers, no accumulation of hyperforin in plasma was observed after intake of 900 mg/day SJW extract for seven days. The estimated steady-state plasma concentrations of hyperforin after intake of 3 × 300 mg/day was approximately 100 ng/mL (approximately 180 nM). The bioavailability of compounds of SJW was found to be influenced by the formulation characteristics.

An ethanolic SJW extract containing 5% hyperforin and 0.3% hypericin was administered as softgel capsules to 12 healthy volunteers. A second standard formulation in a two-piece hard gelatin capsule was also used for comparison purposes. C_{max} of hyperforin was 168.4ng/mL for the soft gelatin formulation and 84.3 ng/mL for the hard gelatin capsule. The t_{max} values for hyperforin were 2.5 hours for the soft gelatin capsule compared to 3.1 hours for the reference formulation, whereas the total AUCs were 1483 and 583.7 hr ng/mL, respectively. Taken together, the soft gelatin capsules exhibited a higher individual absorption when compared with the corresponding data for the hard gelatin capsule. This finding confirms former results, which show that the absorption from soft gelatin capsules is in general higher if compared to hard gelatin capsules.

Animal studies

Pharmacokinetics of hyperforin after administration of an ethanolic SJW extract (WS 5572) to rats were investigated by Biber et al. Maximum plasma levels of approximately 370 ng/mL (approximately 690 nM) were reached after three hours. Estimated half-life and clearance values were six hours and 70 mL/min/kg, respectively.

GARLIC

Garlic (*Allium sativum* L., Alliaceae) is a commonly used food and botanical supplement. Garlic is stated to possess diaphoretic, expectorant, antispasmodic, antiseptic, bacteriostatic, antiviral, hypotensive, and anthelmintic properties. Traditionally, it has been used to treat chronic bronchitis, respiratory catarrh, recurrent colds, bronchitic asthma, influenza, and chronic bronchitis. Modern use of garlic and garlic preparations is focused on their reputed antihypertensive, antiatherogenic, antithrombotic, antimicrobial, fibrinolytic, cancer preventive, and lipid-lowering effects. Garlic contains

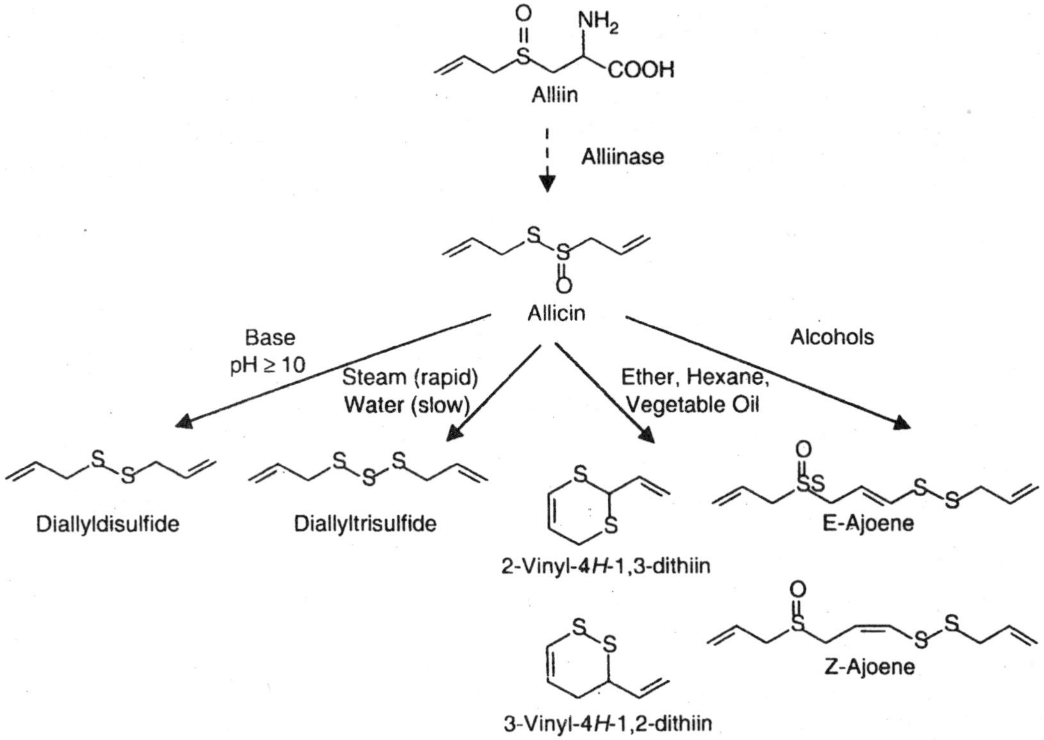

Fig. 5.6. Typical garlic compounds.

a large number of biologically active constituents. The constituents of garlic can be simply divided into two groups: sulfur-containing and non–sulfur-containing compounds. Most of the medicinal effects of garlic are referable to the sulfur compounds and the alliin-splitting enzyme alliinase, which converts alliin into allicin. This enzymatic reaction occurs when fresh garlic is chopped or crushed and alliin comes into contact with alliinase (enzyme and substrate are located in different·compartments in the garlic bulb). Allicin is responsible for the characteristic garlic odor but it is unstable in aqueous and oily solution, and within a few hours it degrades into vinyldithiins and ajoenes. Depending on the chemical nature of the solvent, the extract can contain a spectrum of different compounds. As a result, garlic is available in the form of different pharmaceutical preparations, such as dry powder products, oil-macerates, volatile garlic oil (obtained by water vapor distillation), or juices of fresh garlic. Most clinical studies have been mainly performed with the dry powder preparations and some volatile oil macerates.

Pharmacokinetics

There are only a few reports on the absorption, metabolism, and excretion of garlic's sulfur compounds available. Further, until now it is not known what metabolic form of allicin actually reaches the target cells, and it is still unknown how garlic compounds might function in the body.

Allicin

Human clinical studies

Allicin is well absorbed, as indicated by a persistent garlicky odor on the breath, skin, and amniotic fluid of persons after consumption of fresh garlic. Because oral comsumption of pure allicin has been shown to significantly increase overall body catabolism of triglycerides, a substantial absorption of allicin is assumed to occur. However, the metabolic fate of allicin in the body is not well understood. Neither allicin nor its common transformation products diallyl sulfides, vinyldithiins, or ajoene can be found in the blood or urine, nor can their odor be detected in the stool after consuming large amounts of garlic (up to 25 g) or pure allicin, indicating that it is rapidly metabolized to new compounds. In a recent study, Rosen et al. used GC–MS/MS as major techniques to determine various metabolites after consumption of dehydrated granular garlic and an enteric-coated garlic preparation, in breath and plasma. The authors found that methyl allyl sulfide is the main volatile metabolite on the consumption of dehydrated dry garlic and enteric-coated garlic formulations. Hydrogen sulfide was observed but not quantified due to its extremely low levels. The non–sulfur-containing compounds limonene and *p*-cymene were also observed in the breath in those consuming garlic preparations. S-Allylcysteine can be observed in the blood of those who consume aged garlic preparations (so-called "*Kyolic*").

Animal studies

The pharmacokinetic behavior of vinyldithiins, the main constituents of oily preparations of garlic, was investigated after oral administration of 27 mg 1,2-vinyldithiin and 9 mg 1,3-vinyldithiin to rats. In serum both forms of vinyldithiins could be detected. The serum concentration–time profile of 1,2-vinyldithiin can be characterized by an one-compartment model, whereas a two-compartment model is used as a best fit of the serum concentration of 1,3-vinyldithiin.

In rats, alliin and allicin were administered orally at doses of 8 mg/kg. Absorption of alliin and allicin was complete after 10 minutes and 30 to 60 minutes, respectively. The mean total urinary and fecal excretion of allicin after 72 hours was 85.5% of the dose. Pharmacokinetic studies of the garlic constituent S-allyl-L-cysteine administered orally in large doses to three different species (rat, mouse, and dog) showed that it is rapidly absorbed and is more abundant initially in several tissues, especially kidney, than it is in the blood. Its half-life in blood plasma (0.8–10.3 hours) and distribution among urinary metabolites varied greatly among the types of animals. The study showed that the bioavailability of S-allylcysteine decreased linearly with decreased dose, from 98% at 50 mg/kg body weight to 77% at 25 mg/kg and 64% at 12 mg/kg. Recently, Germain et al. studied the in vivo metabolism of diallyl disulfide (DADS), a garlic compound claimed to have anticarcinogenic effects. After oral administration of a single dose of 200 mg/kg, metabolites were measured in the stomach, liver, plasma, and urine by GC coupled with MS over 15 days. DADS was detected in almost all analyzed tissues within the first hours. In addition, the metabolites allylmercaptan (AM) and allyl methyl sulfide (AMS) were detected. The C_{max} of the metabolites were higher than that of DADS (1.46 μg/mL). The t_{max} for DADS was estimated to be less than one hour, whereas this time increased to 24 hours for AM and AMS.

Willow Bark

The willow family includes a number of different species of deciduous trees and shrubs native to Europe, Asia, and some parts of North America. Some of the more commonly known are white willow/European willow (*Salix alba*), black willow (*Salix nigra*), crack willow (*Salix fragilis*), purple willow (*Salix purpurea*), and weeping willow (*Salix babylonica*). The willow bark sold in Europe and the United States usually includes a combination of the bark from white, purple, and crack willows. Willow

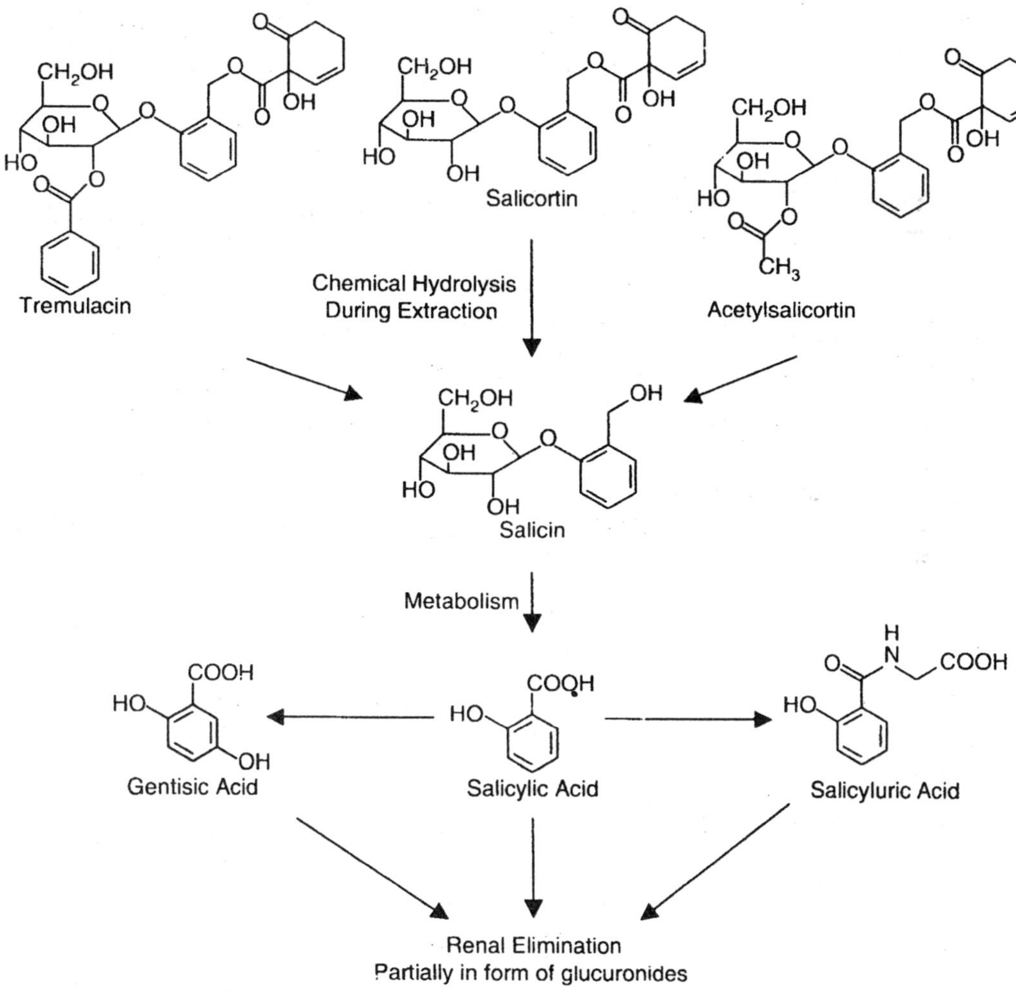

Fig. 5.7. Main constituents of willow bark and pharmacokinetics of salicin in humans.

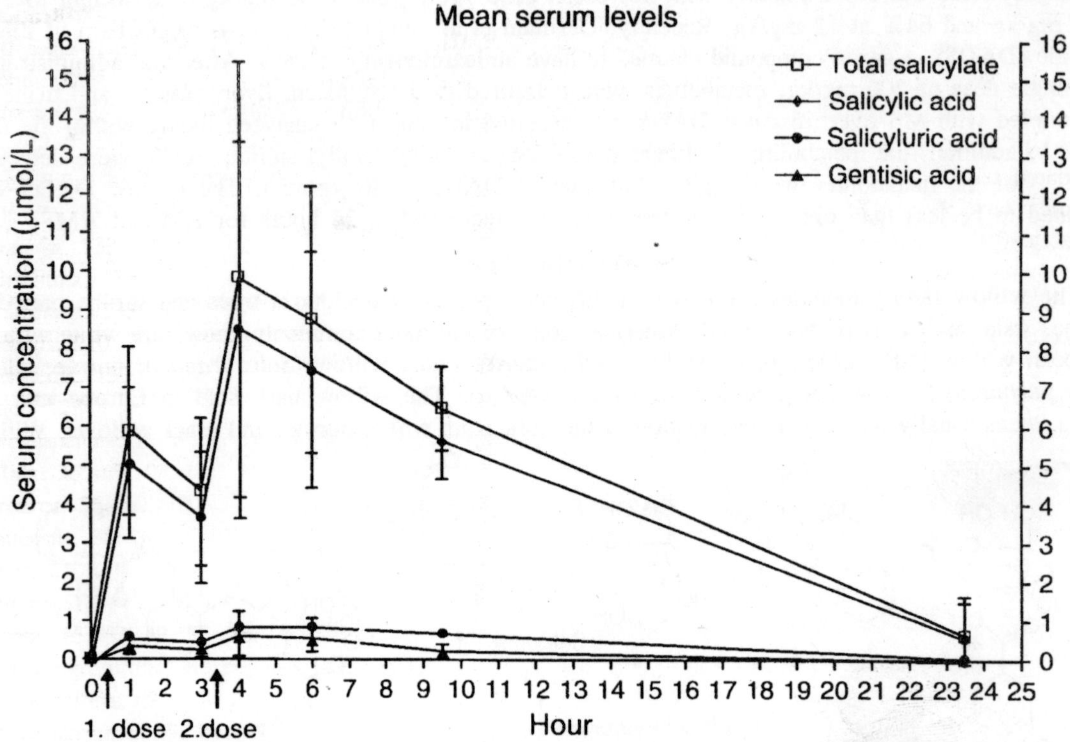

Fig. 5.8. Mean serum levels of salicylic acid, gentisic acid, and salicyluric acid of 10 volunteers. "Total salicylate" represents the sum of the three individual compounds.

bark's most important medicinal qualities are its ability to ease pain and reduce inflammation. Salicin is probably the most active anti-inflammatory compound in willow; it is metabolized to salicylic acid. The enzymatic degradation of salicin, salicortin, and tremulacin by β-glucosidase and by esterase has been investigated. Studies have identified several other components of willow bark that have antioxidant, fever-reducing, antiseptic, and immune-boosting effects. The pharmacological actions of salicylates in humans are well documented and are applicable to willow. In recent clinical studies, willow bark extract had moderate analgesic effects in osteoarthritis and low back pain.

Pharmacokinetics

There are only a limited number of studies available evaluating the pharmacokinetics of salicin and its major metabolites in humans after oral administration.

Salicin

Human clinical studies

Two early studies have been published on the oral bioavailability of salicin in humans, but they showed different results. Oral ingestion of 4000 mg (13.97 mmol) of pure salicin by a single volunteer resulted in high serum concentrations of salicylic acid, with a peak level of 110 µg/mL. The peak level of salicylic acid in the serum after ingestion of salicin was reached somewhat later than after ingestion of an equimolar dose of sodium salicylate, with the fact that salicin must be first metabolized to salicylic acid. Eighty-six percent of the total ingested salicin was found in the 24-hour urine in the form of the usual salicylic acid metabolites, indicating a good oral bioavailability of pure salicin. In contrast, oral administration of a willow bark extract showed a low bioavailability of salicin. After ingestion of commercial sugar-coated tablets containing willow bark extract corresponding to a total amount of 54.9 mg (0.192 mmol) salicin, the serum of 12 volunteers showed a peak concentration of only 0.13 μg/mL salicylic acid; this is only 5% of the serum level expected after oral intake of an equimolar amount of synthetic salicylates. In a recent pharmacokinetic study of willow bark, Schmid et al. carried out a pharmacokinetic study on the oral bioavailability of salicylates from willow bark extract in 10 healthy volunteers. A chemically standardized willow bark extract was used in the form of coated tablets. Willow bark extract was given in two equal doses corresponding to 240 mg salicin at times zero and three hours. Over a period of 24 hours, urine and serum levels of salicylic acid and its metabolites, gentisic acid and salicyluric acid, were determined. Peak plasma levels of salicylic acid were on average 1.2 μg/mL and were reached less than two hours after oral administration. Salicylic acid was the major metabolite of salicin in the serum (86% of total salicylates), besides salicyluric acid (10%) and gentisic acid (4%). After 24 hours, 15.8% of the orally ingested dose of salicin was detected in the urine on average. The AUC of salicylate obtained in this study was equivalent to that expected from an intake of 87 mg of acetylsalicylic acid. Taken together, in the study by Schmid et al., willow bark in the dosage of 240 mg led to much lower serum salicylate levels than observed after analgesic doses of synthetic salicylates. The authors conclude that the formation of salicylic acid alone is therefore unlikely to explain analgesic or antirheumatic effects of willow bark.

HORSE CHESTNUT

The horse chestnut, *Aesculus hippocastaneum* (Hippocastanaceae), was introduced into the northern Europe from the Near East in the 16th century. Extracts from horse chestnut seeds were already being used therapeutically in France in the early 1800s. Several French works published between 1896 and 1909 reported successful outcomes in the treatment of hemorrhoidal ailments. Traditionally, horse chestnut has been used for the treatment of varicose veins, hemorrhoids, phlebitis, diarrhea, fever, and

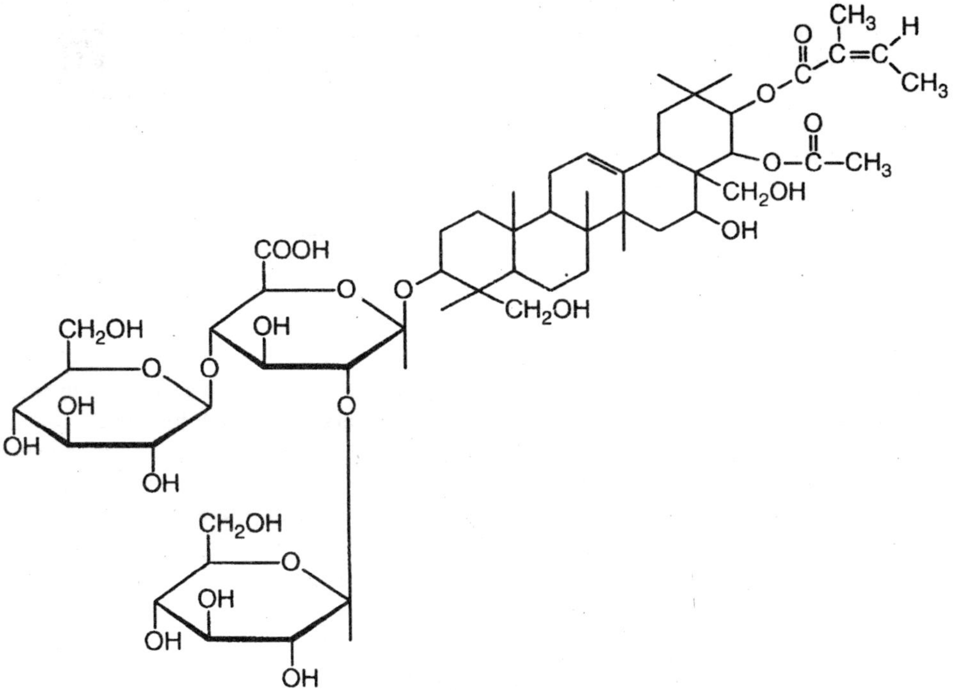

Fig. 5.9. Chemical structure of aescin.

enlargement of the prostate gland. The German Commission E approved its use in the treatment of chronic venous insufficiency in the legs. The seeds of horse chestnut contain mainly aescin, which is a complex mixture of various chemically very similar triterpene glycosides having saponifying activities. The aglycones of these saponins are barringtogenol C and protoescigenin. Former investigations of the saponin mixture differentiated between three aescin subtypes, including the slightly soluble β-aescin, a C-21 and C-22 diester, readily water soluble crypto-aescin, which is created by spontaneous migration of the acetyl group from C-22 to C-28, and α-aescin, an equilibrium mixture of these two isomer diesters. A number of other compounds have been isolated from the chestnut seeds, i.e., flavonols (kaempferol and quercetin), flavonol glycosides (astragalin, isoquercitrin, and rutin), and coumarins (aesculetin, fraxin, and scopolin). However, all of these compounds can be found in larger amounts from other sources and, furthermore, during 1960, Lorenz and Marek concluded that the antiedemigenous, antiexudative, and vasoprotective activities of horse chestnut extracts are mainly due to aescin.

Pharmacokinetics

Pharmacokinetic studies with horse chestnut focus on the absorption, metabolism, and excretion of the main constituent—β-aescin.

Aescin

Human clinical studies

The significant advances in understanding of bioavailability and kinetics of β-aescin should be attributed to the development of a highly specific radioimmunoassay (RIA) allowing the detection of concentrations in the nanogram per milliliter range. The relative oral bioavailability of beta-aescin from a sugar-coated tablet formulation was compared to a reference preparation available in capsule form to 18 healthy, male volunteers over a 48 h period. A large variation in absorption parameters for beta-aescin was measured. Maximum concentration (Cmax) after a dose containing 50 mg aescin varied from 0.19 to 45.1 ng/mL, time for maximum concentration (t_{max}) varied from 0.73 to 8.5 hours, and the AUC varied from 24.6 to 389 ng/hr/mL. The second study, also on two solid-dose preparations (one with sustained release), using 24 volunteers found more consistent results. Parameters of the sustained-release tablet were superior. For example, after a dose containing 50 mg aescin, C_{max} for the sustained-release tablet 9.81 ± 8.9 ng/mL, t_{max} was 2.23 ± 0.9 hours, and AUC averaged 187.1 ng/hr/mL.

The half-life time for both preparations was about 20 hours. However, the data of both studies have to be evaluated with care, because the RIA used for the determination is highly specific and its potential of cross-reactivity with different types of β-aescin is not known for the different extracts used in the different preparations. Thus, absolute plasma concentration values of β-aescin from a single preparation cannot be compared with other preparations. Further, saponins are large molecules containing highly polar groups and their intact bioavailability can be expected to be low after oral doses. This was confirmed in the above-mentioned studies, because the pharmacokinetic parameters indicate an absorption less than 10% of the administered dose. However, saponins can be hydrolyzed by intestinal flora, leaving the less polar aglycone or sapogenin available for absorption. These sapogenins, or their hepatic metabolites, may in fact be the main active form of aescin following oral doses. Further studies are needed to clarify this issue.

Animal studies

Pharmacokinetics and bioavailability of aescin was studied after oral and i.v. administration of tritiated aescin. About 66% and 33% of the dose was excreted in bile and urine, respectively, after i.v. administration. The oral bioavailability of aescin was about 12.5%. Percutaneous absorption of aescin was studied in mice and rats. The amounts of aescin in muscle were greater than in other organs. These results indicate that percutaneous administration of aescin could be beneficial.

GINSENG

Ginseng, a commonly used natural product, has a reputation as a "*herb of eternal life.*" A survey of herbal-based over-the-counter products indicates that 28% of them contain ginseng. It has been estimated that ginseng comprises 15% to 20% of the total annual sales of botanical products in the United States. Botanical remedies known as "ginseng" are based on the roots of several distinct species of plants, mainly Korean or Asian ginseng (*Panax ginseng*), Siberian ginseng (*Eleutherococcus senticosus*), and American ginseng (*Panax quinquefolius* and *Panax notoginseng*). All of these species belong to the Araliaceae family, but each of these different species has specific pharmacological effects. *P. ginseng* is the most commonly used and highly researched species of ginseng. This species, which is native to China, Korea, and Russia, has been an important botanical remedy in traditional Chinese medicine for thousands of years, where it has been used primarily as a treatment for weakness and fatigue. The main constituents of *P. ginseng* are the so-called ginsenosides, a complex mixture of saponins from the tetracyclic dammarane type (sapogenins protopanaxadiol and protopanaxatriol) and a pentacyclic triterpene from the oleanolic acid type. The ginsenosides can be divided into two classes: the protopanaxatriol class, consisting mainly of Rg_1, Rg_2, Rf, and Re, and the protopanaxadiol class, consisting mainly of Rc, Rd, Rb_1, and Rb_2. Further, ginseng constituents are polysaccharides, essential oil constituents, polyacetylenes, peptides, and other lipids. Ginseng is included in the pharmacopeias of several countries such as China, Germany, and the United Kingdom. Modern therapeutic claims refer to vitality, immune function, cancer, cardiovascular diseases, and sexual function.

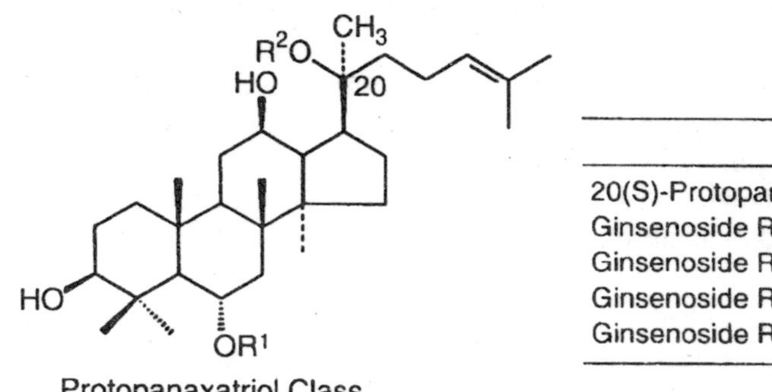

	R1	R2
20(S)-Protopanaxatriol	H	H
Ginsenoside Re	glc(2-1)rha	glc
Ginsenoside Rf	glc(2-1)glc	H
Ginsenoside Rg_1	glc	glc
Ginsenoside Rg_2	glc(2-1)rha	H

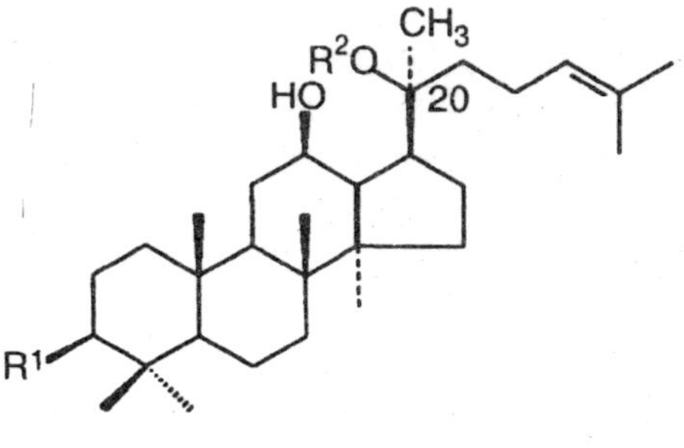

Protopanaxadiol Class

	R1	R2
20(S)-Protopanaxadiol	H	H
Ginsenoside Re	glc(2-1)glc	glc(6-1)glc
Ginsenoside Rf	glc(2-1)glc	glc(6-1)ara *p*
Ginsenoside Rg_1	glc(2-1)glc	glc(6-1)ara *f*
Ginsenoside Rg_2	glc(2-1)glc	glc

Fig. 5.10. Chemical structures of ginsenosides.

Pharmacokinetics

Although ginseng is commonly used as an adaptogenic and immunomodulatory drug, and its efficacy has been shown in pharmacologic assays as well as in clinical trials, the number of pharmacokinetic studies is limited. This might be due to the chemical nature of the ginsenosides—as saponins, they are large molecules containing highly polar groups. Thus, their intact bioavailability can be expected to be low after oral intake.

Ginsenoside

Human clinical studies

Analysis of urine samples from Swedish athletes who had consumed ginseng preparations within 10 days before urine collection showed that out of 65 samples analyzed, 60 were found to contain the sapogenin 20(S)-protopanaxatriol. The concentrations of 20(S)-protopanaxatriol varied from 2 to 35 ng/mL urine. The results after intake of oral doses of ginseng preparations demonstrated a linear relationship between the amounts of ginsenosides consumed and the 20(S)-protopanaxatriol glycosides excreted in the urine. About 1.2% of the dose was recovered in the glycosidic form over five days. The main metabolites of ginsenosides Rb_1, Rb_2, Rc, Re, and Rg_1 after anaerobic incubation with fecal flora were identified as prosapogenins and sapogenins, although the metabolic rate and mode were affected by fermentation media. Further, prosapogenins and sapogenins were detected in blood (0.3–5.1 μg/mL) and in urine (2.2– 96 μg/day) after the oral administration of ginseng extract (150 mg/day) to humans. One organism in the human fecal flora hydrolyzing ginsenosides was *Prevotella oris*.

Animal studies

Studies in rats focus on the pharmacokinetics of ginsenosides Rg_1, Rb_1, and Rb_2. Ginsenoside Rg_1 was absorbed rapidly from the upper parts of the digestive tract (accounting for 1.9–20.0% of the dose of Rg_1 administered orally, 100 mg/kg). The serum level of ginsenoside Rg_1 reached its peak at 30 minutes, and the maximum levels of ginsenosides Rg_1 in tissues were attained within 1.5 hours. However, Rg_1 was not found in the brain. About 80% of the dose of Rg_1 was excreted into urine and bile after i.v. administration to rats, showing that Rg_1 is hardly metabolized in rat liver. The authors could further show that degradation and/or metabolism of Rg_1 occurs in the stomach and large intestine of rats.

Only a small amount of Rb_1 was absorbed from the digestive tract after oral administration (100 mg/kg) to rats. The serum level of Rb_1 in rats after i.v. injection (5 mg/kg) declined biexponentially, a rapid decline (α-phase) followed by a slow decline (β-phase). The half-lives of Rb_1 were 11.6 minutes for the α-phase and 14.5 hours for the β-phase. The persistence of Rb_1 in serum and tissues in rats for long after i.v. administration was assumed to correlate with the high activity of plasma protein binding.

In one study, the degradation of ginsenoside Rg_1, Rb_1, and Rb_2 was studied in further detail. Rg_1 was decomposed to its prosapogenin in both the rat stomach and diluted hydrochloric acid, whereas Rb_1 and Rb_2 were little degraded in rat stomach but were easily converted to their prosapogenins by diluted hydrochloric acid. The ginsenosides were also metabolized to several prosapogenins by gut bacteria and enteric enzymes. The amount of Rg_1, Rb_1, and Rb_2 absorbed from the gastrointestinal tract (GI) of the rat were 1.9%, 0.1%, and 3.7%, respectively. Ginsenoside Rg_1 was excreted into rat urine bile in a ratio of 2:5. Rb_1 and Rb_2 were mainly excreted into the urine.

Milk Thistle

Milk thistle (*Silybum marianum*) is an annual to biennial plant of the Asteraceae family. It is native principally to southern Europe and northern Africa. The crude drug consists of the ripe fruits from which the pappus has been removed. Milk thistle fruits contain 15% to 30% proteins. The main

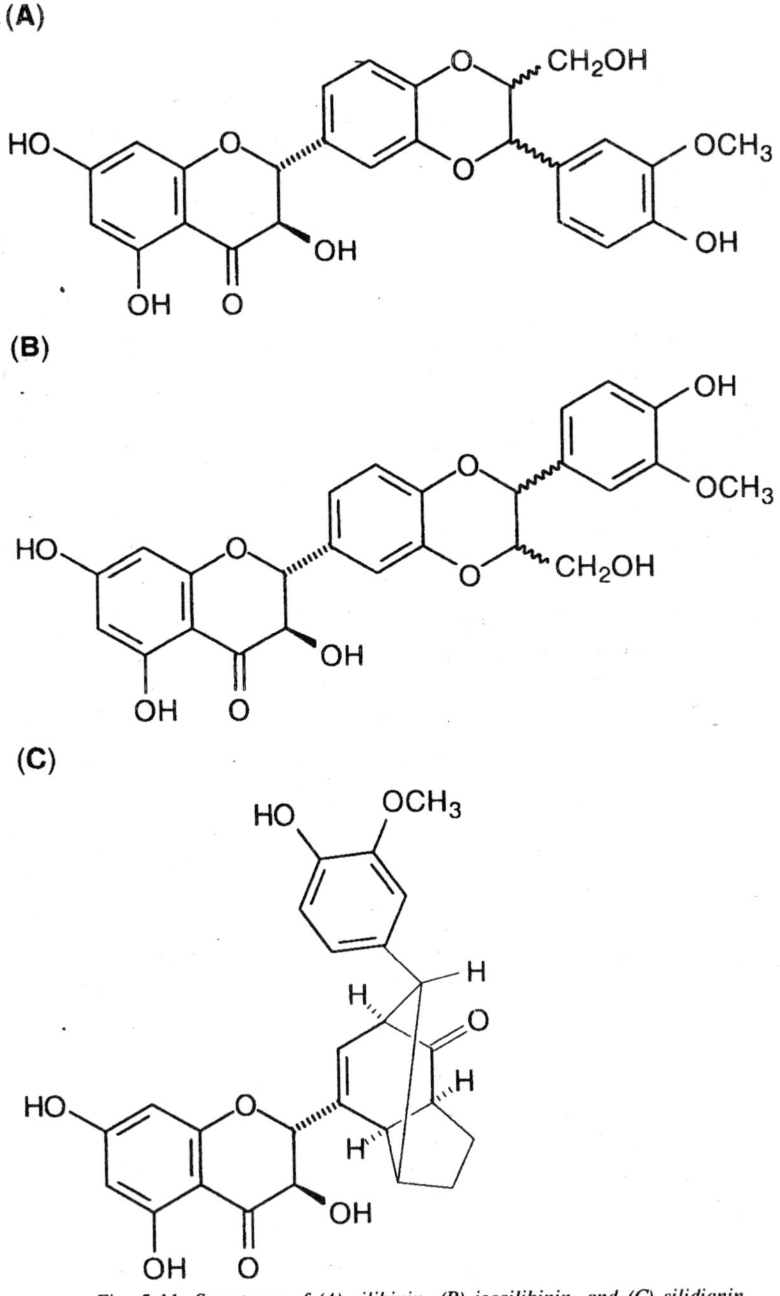

(A)

(B)

(C)

Fig. 5.11. Structures of (A) silibinin, (B) isosilibinin, and (C) silidianin.

active compounds constitute only about 2% to 3% of the dried fruits. The active principle is a mixture of flavolignans called silymarin. Silymarin, a polyphenolic extract isolated from the seeds of milk thistle, is composed mainly of silybin (50–70%), with small amounts of other silybin structural isomers, namely isosilybin, silydianin, and silychristin. The highest concentration of silymarin is found in the ripe fruits. Silibinin is the main compound, also considered to be the most active one in several paradigms. Traditionally, milk thistle fruits have been used for disorders of the liver, spleen, and gall bladder, such as jaundice and gall bladder colic. Milk thistle has also been used for nursing mothers for stimulating milk production, as a bitter tonic, for hemorrhoids, for dyspeptic complaints, and as a demulcent in catarrh and pleurisy. It is stated to possess hepatoprotective, antioxidant, and choleretic properties. Current interest is focused on the hepatoprotective activity of milk thistle and its use for the treatment of liver, spleen, and gall bladder disorders. Recently it has been shown that silibinin reduced prostate-specific antigen levels in prostate carcinoma cells lines, indicating a possible role of silibinin in human prostate cancer.

Pharmacokinetics

Studies of the pharmacokinetics of silymarin and of a silibinin–phosphatidylcholine complex preparation (IdB 1016; silipide) in humans as well as rodents have been performed. Because silibinin is the main compound, pharmacokinetic parameters of silymarin and the active principle of any silymarin-containing products are always referred to, and standardized, as silibinin.

The bioavailability of silibinin from the extract is low and seems to depend on several factors such as (i) the content of accompanying substances with a solubilizing character such as other flavonoids, phenol derivatives, aminoacids, proteins, tocopherol, fat, cholesterol, and others found in the extract and (ii) the concentration of the extract itself. The systemic bioavailability can be enhanced by adding solubilizing substances to the extract. The bioavailability of silibinin can also be enhanced by the complexation with phosphatidylcholine or β-cyclodextrin, and possibly by the choice of the capsule material. The variations in content, dissolution, and (oral) bioavailability of silibinin between different commercially available silymarin products—despite the same declaration of content—are significant.

Therefore, comparisons between studies should be carried out with caution and consider the differences between the analytical methods used and whether free, conjugated, or total silibinin is the object of measurement. Systemic plasma concentrations are usually measured, even though the site of action of silymarin is the liver, because they provide an estimate on the quantity of the drug being absorbed from the GI tract.

Silibinin

Human clinical studies

In male volunteers, after single oral administration of a standardized dose of silibinin 100 to 360 mg, plasma silibinin Cmax is reached after approximately two hours and ranges between 200 and 1400 ng/mL, of which approximately 75% is presented in the conjugated form. For total silibinin, an elimination half-life of approximately six hours is estimated. Between 3% and 8% of an oral dose is excreted in the urine, while 20% to 40% is recovered from the bile as glucuronide and sulfate conjugates. The remaining part is excreted via the feces (unchanged, not absorbed). Silibinin concentrations in bile reach approximately 100 times those found in serum, with peak concentrations reached within two to nine hours. Biliary excretion continues for 24 hours after a single dose. After multiple dose administration, no accumulation is observed. In patients with cirrhosis, the plasma C_{max} of silibinin after a single dose of silibinin 360 mg was lower (120 ng/mL) and time to C_{max} (t_{max}; 2.6 hours) slightly delayed compared with healthy volunteers.

Animal studies

The comparative pharmacokinetics of silipide (IdB 1016, a silybin–phosphatidylcholine complex) and silybin were investigated by measuring unconjugated and total plasma silybin levels as well as total biliary and urinary silybin excretion in rats following administration of a single dose (200 mg/kg as silybin). Mean peak levels of unconjugated and total silybin after IdB 1016 were 8.17 and 74.23 mg/mL, respectively. Mean AUC (0–6) values were 9.78 and 232.15 μg/hr/mL, indicating that about

94% of the plasma silybin is present in a conjugated form. Cumulative biliary (zero to two hours) and urinary (0 to 72 hours) excretion values after administration of IdB 1016 accounted for 3.73% and 3.26% of the administered dose, respectively. After silybin administration, the biliary and urinary excretion accounted for only 0.001% and 0.032% of the dose, respectively.

The use of HMPs, including their use in addition or instead of conventional drugs, is continuing to increase. Unfortunately, only limited information is available regarding the pharmacokinetics and bioavailability of herbal medicines but the awareness of this issue is increasing. In the present chapter, we focused on the bioavailability and pharmacokinetics of some of the top selling botanical products on the U.S. and European market. However, some of the most popular medicinal plants were not further discussed in this chapter, because pharmacokinetic data are not available yet (e.g., Chasteberry, Saw palmetto, or Feverfew). A reason for the lack of pharmacokinetic data could be that the active compounds of these plants are still unknown. This issue points to the fact that the determination of herbal pharmacokinetics is a unique field, which is extremely complex. Thus, the question arises— Is studying herbal pharmacokinetics of any value in the therapeutic use of the plant, especially when the drug has been used therapeutically without this information for centuries?

However, the information derived from a detailed pharmacokinetic study will help to anticipate potential botanical product-drug interactions, to optimize the bioavailability, the quality, and hence the efficacy of herbal medicines, to support evidence for the synergistic nature of herbal medicines, and to better appreciate the safety and toxicity of the plant. Because pharmacokinetic studies with herbal medicines are often complicated by their chemical complexity and by the fact that the active compounds are often unknown, it could be one future issue to assess bioavailability by measuring surrogate parameters in plasma or tissue instead of directly assaying putative active compounds in the blood. In summary, to use HMPs in an evidence-based approach and to achieve the status "*rational phytomedicine*," more experimental studies are needed to characterize the bioavailability and pharmacokinetics of botanical products.

Plant Products: Garlic, Ginkgo and Ginseng

Garlic, ginkgo, and ginseng are, respectively, the second, first, and fourth top-selling botanical supplements in U.S. retail outlets. Their retail sales are impressive, totalling US $35, $46, and $31 million, respectively. These 2002 figures look impressive but actually represent a substantial decline in comparison to those of 2001 (-17%, -35%, and -33%, respectively). Given this nevertheless huge popularity, it is important for health care professionals to advise patients responsibly about the proper use of these products.

Garlic (Allium sativum L.)

Fresh garlic bulb, dried and powdered extract, or oil extracted from the bulb have been used for medicinal purposes. The active constituents include alliin, allinase, diallyldisulfide, ajoens, and others. Alliin is enzymatically converted to allicin, the major garlic component, which is also responsible for its characteristic, sulfur-like smell. Although the best-researched pharmacological property of garlic is that of lowering total serum cholesterol levels, probably via inhibition of hepatic cholesterol synthesis, multiple additional pharmacological actions of garlic, including antibacterial, antiviral, antifungal, antihypertensive, hypoglycemic, antithrombotic, antimutagenic, and antiplatelet activities, have been described. The recommended dose is about 4 g of fresh garlic daily, which is equivalent to approximately 8mg garlic oil or 600 to 900 mg garlic powder preparations standardized to 1.3% alliin content. Adverse effects of garlic are usually mild and transient; they include breath and body odor, allergic reactions, nausea, heartburn, and flatulence. Garlic has been reported to inhibit platelet aggregation, and patients with bleeding abnormalities should be cautioned about the uncontrolled use of garlic supplements. It is recommended that garlic supplements be discontinued before major surgery. The following section describes the available evidence of pharmacodynamic and pharmacokinetic interaction between garlic and prescription drugs.

Interactions

Pharmacodynamic interaction

The primary garlic metabolite allicin has been shown to possess antiplatelet activity. Bordia showed that administration of essential oil of garlic 25 mg daily for five days resulted in significant inhibition of platelet aggregation. A case report of spontaneous epidural hematoma in an 87-year-old male was attributed to excessive garlic consumption. Because the patient was not taking any prescription medications at the time of the bleeding episode, and all laboratory parameters, including clotting factor profile, were normal, the clinicians believed that the only probable explanation for the occurrence of the hematoma was the patient's daily ingestion of four cloves (approximately 2 g) of garlic for an unspecified time period. Another case reporting bleeding disorders associated with garlic use described a 72-year-old male patient admitted to the hospital with acute urinary retention and scheduled to undergo a transurethral resection for benign prostrate hyperplasia. He was not taking any medications on admission except for years of garlic tablets consumption for "*medicinal purposes.*" However, no information regarding the strength and amount of garlic was provided. The patient experienced hemostasis and hemorrhage at the site of resection during and after surgery. The patient had a full recovery with four units of blood transfusion.

Platelet aggregation test was not done during the hospitalization. However, three months after resumption of garlic use, the patient returned to clinic and blood tests were reported to show abnormal platelet aggregation. Therefore, this pharmacological effect suggests that use of garlic could potentially increase the effect of anticoagulants. Two brief cases described that patients who had been stabilized on warfarin experienced a doubling of international normalized ratio (INR) after they took garlic products, but there were no information provided regarding the strength of garlic preparation and the duration of use, the INR values, description of symptoms, and clinical outcomes. Other than these two anecdotal cases, there are no literature reports of interaction between garlic and anticoagulants such as warfarin. Despite this lack of clinical data, especially from pharmacokinetic studies, the potential for irreversible platelet function inhibition has prompted the suggestion to discontinue garlic use at least one week prior to surgery, so as to minimize the risk of postoperative bleeding.

Garlic, as a component of curry, had also been suggested to enhance the hypoglycemic effects of the oral hypoglycemic agent chlorpropamide in a 40-year-old Pakistani woman. The estimated amount of garlic consumed by the patient was not provided. In addition, because the food product also contains karela, another ingredient reported to also possess hypoglycemic effect, it is impossible to conclude from this brief report that a cause–effect relationship exists for garlic. Since the publication of this report there have been no additional evidence to confirm the clinical observation or formal study to evaluate the likely mechanism.

Pharmacokinetic interaction

Garlic is one of the most common botanical remedies used by patients with human immunodeficiency virus (HIV), probably because of to the antiviral claim associated with its consumption, as well as the possibility of lowering total serum cholesterol, which could counteract the common side effect of hypercholesterolemia associated with the use of antiretroviral drug regimens. Conflicting results have been reported in vitro and in animals regarding the effect of garlic on drug metabolism. Piscitelli et al. investigated in human volunteers the effect of garlic supplements on the pharmacokinetics of saquinavir. Because saquinavir has negligible inhibitory or induction effect on drug-metabolizing enzymes, its use as a study drug by the investigators would minimize the potential of confounding the effect of garlic. Ten healthy volunteers participated in a three-period, single-sequence interaction study. In period 1, they received 1200mg of saquinavir three times daily for three days, with blood sampling over eight hours after administration of the 10th dose on day 4. All subjects then entered phase 2 of the study, in which they received garlic caplets twice daily for 20 days (days 5–24). In addition, saquinavir was administered concurrently for three days (days 22–24), with blood sampling over eight hours after administration of the 10th saquinavir and 25th garlic dose on day 25. Both garlic and saquinavir were discontinued for 10 days, after which saquinavir was administered in period 3 for 10 doses with blood sampling as in period 1. Adherence assessment was based on interview at each study visit and dosing calendars kept by the subjects.

Compared to baseline saquinavir pharmacokinetic parameters obtained in period 1, the use of garlic reduced the mean saquinavir area under the concentration–time curve (AUC) by 51%, and the maximum (C_{max}) and minimum (C_{min}) saquinavir concentrations by 54% and 49%, respectively. After a 10-day washout, the AUC, C_{max}, and C_{min} values were within a range of 60% to 70% of baseline values. The magnitude of the decline in concentration might result in therapeutic failure and viral rebound in patients with HIV. Based on the pharmacokinetic parameters obtained in period 3, it also appears that garlic might have a prolonged, albeit lesser, effect on saquinavir exposure. The effects of combined treatment with other protease inhibitors that are also potent cytochrome P-450 (CYP) enzymes modulators need to be further evaluated.

Although this study was not designed to address the mechanism of the interaction, the use of garlic clearly resulted in reduction of saquinavir bioavailability, possibly via induction of CYP enzymes, specifically the CYP3A4 isoform that is primarily responsible for metabolism of saquinavir. Therefore, it is likely that other drugs with significant CYP3A4-mediated metabolism could also be affected. Other mechanisms could include induction of P-glycoprotein and/or impairment of absorption. The results from this study also highlight several problems associated with interpretation of botanical product–drug interaction data from different studies. First, the study results were consistent with that of Dalvi, who showed a significant increase in CYP enzyme activity after five days administration of garlic in rats, and provided further evidence that in vivo studies employing short-term or single-dose administration and in vitro microsomal studies could provide contradictory results that might not be observed with prolonged use in clinical setting.

On the other hand, Gurley et al. showed that a four-week administration of 500mg garlic oil three times daily resulted in no significant change in phenotypic ratios of probe drugs for several CYP enzymes, including CYP3A4. While the specific constituent(s) responsible for the effect on drug metabolism is not known, Borek suggested that allicin is converted to an intermediate by-product that induces production of CYP enzymes. To minimize product variability in content, investigators from both studies used single lot of the supplement from the same manufacturer. The study of Piscitelli et al. used garlic preparation that is supposedly standardized according to allicin content, whereas product information regarding allicin content were not provided by Gurley et al. If allicin is responsible for garlic's effect on metabolism, garlic preparations that contain minimal or no allicin content might have a different metabolic effect compared to one with maximum allicin content.

Finally, even if all garlic preparations were standardized to allicin content, currently the "standardization" practices and therefore the standardized content can vary significantly from one manufacturer to another, while product inconsistency has not been demonstrated for garlic preparations, there is literature data on the disparity of constituent content among different *echinacea* products and ginseng products. As such, the choice of a specific botanical product or preparation may make a difference in the presence and magnitude of a botanical product–drug interaction.

Ginkgo (Ginkgo biloba L.)

Medicinal ginkgo products are made from the leaves of the plant, the main pharmacological constituents of which include ginkgolides A, B, C, J, bilobalide, and flavonoids. Ginkgo leads to an increase in microcirculatory blood flow, inhibition of erythrocyte aggregation, platelet-activating factor antagonism, free radical scavenging, and edema protection. These actions suggest that there is no single mechanism of action but that a complex interaction of a multitude of effects could be responsible for its many therapeutic claims, including intermittent claudication, dementia, and tinnitus. The recommended dosages of an oral standardized dry extract of ginkgo (24% ginkgo flavonol glycosides and 6% terpene lactones) are 120 to 240 mg daily for dementia and memory impairment, and 120 to 160mg daily for intermittent claudication and tinnitus. Adverse effects include gastrointestinal disturbances, diarrhea, vomiting, allergic reactions, pruritus, headache, dizziness, and nose bleeds.

Interactions

Pharmacodynamic interaction

The most frequently cited potential interaction associated with the use of ginkgo is the potentiation of anticoagulants. This is biologically plausible considering the well-documented antiplatelet effects of the various ginkgolides of ginkgo, which have been associated with cases of postoperative bleeding, spontaneous hyphema, and spontaneous intracranial bleeding.

While it is not known whether these case reports are just coincidence or actually have a cause–effect relationship, it does establish the bleeding potential of ginkgo and therefore the caution regarding additive pharmacodynamic effect with concurrent use of aspirin or anticoagulants, although currently there is little supporting data. A 78-year-old female patient who had been stabilized on warfarin for five years experienced an intracerebral hemorrhage after taking an unknown regimen of ginkgo for two months. The prothrombin time and partial thromboplastin time were 16.9 and 35.5 seconds, respectively, when the hemorrhage was discovered. Discontinuance of both warfarin and ginkgo resulted in no further bleeding episode and no vitamin K administration was required.

A 70-year-old man developed a spontaneous bleeding of the iris into the anterior chamber of the eye (hyphema) after ingesting concentrated ginkgo extract 40mg twice daily for one week. His only other medication was aspirin taken for three years at a dosage of 325 mg without any adverse bleeding event. After the bleeding episode, the patient continued the aspirin regimen but not the ginkgo supplement, and there were no additional bleeding events over the next three months. The clinicians attributed the bleeding event to an interaction between aspirin and ginkgo. Based on these and reports of spontaneous bleeding with ginkgo alone, ginkgo has also been recommended to be discontinued before major surgery. In addition, concurrent use of ginkgo with aspirin or other nonsteroidal anti-inflammatory drugs might pose an additive risk of bleeding. Further studies are necessary to confirm the potential of interaction between ginkgo and warfarin or aspirin.

An interaction between *G. biloba* administered as 80 mg leaf extract twice a day and low-dose trazodone (20 mg twice daily) was suspected in a patient with Alzheimer's disease, who took the two products together. It is postulated that a pharmacodynamic (increased gamma-aminobutyric acid-ergic activity) and pharmacokinetic mechanisms [increased metabolism of trazodone to *m*-chlorophenyl-piperazine (*m*-CPP), which acts on the benzodiazepine-binding sites and releases gamma-aminobutyric acid] contribute to the observed effect.

Pharmacokinetic interaction

Gurley et al. evaluated the effect of *G. biloba* standardized to contain 24% of flavone glycosides and 6% terpene lactones on phenotypic markers of CYP1A2, 2D6, 3A4 and 2E1. Twelve healthy individuals (six males and six females) received 60 mg of the standardized G. biloba preparation four times per day for 28 days. The four CYP phenotypes were assessed before and at the end of the 28-day study period. Although there was a trend of increased CYP2E1 activity by 23%, the effect was not statistically significant. *G. biloba* produced no significant changes in phenotypic ratios of the other three CYP isoforms. The results from this study suggested that standardized *G. biloba* preparation containing 24% of flavone glycosides and 6% terpene lactones have minimal effect on the activity of the four CYP isoforms, and therefore the metabolism of drugs mediated by these enzymes.

In general, the study results also are consistent with that of Duche et al., who reported that administration of a 13-day regimen of *G. biloba* in healthy volunteers did not affect the pharmacokinetics of antipyrine, a nonspecific marker of overall CYP enzyme activity. However, there was no evaluation of CYP2C9 activity in both studies, so it remains unknown whether any reports or concerns of interaction with warfarin could have a pharmacokinetic basis as well. Separately, Smith et al. reported in an abstract that *G. biloba* administered over an 18-day period produced a 53% increase in concentration of nifedipine, a CYP3A4 substrate. However, the amount of flavone glycosides and terpene lactones in the botanical supplement were not known, and nifedipine might not reflect CYP3A4 activity in a manner similar to that with midazolam, which is a well-recognized, specific marker for CYP3A4. In another study, 14 patients with Alzheimer's disease received the acetycholinesterase inhibitor donepezil 5 mg per day for at least 20 weeks with steady-state donepezil concentrations of 22.7 ± 10.3 ng/mL and a Mini-Mental Scale Examination (MMSE) score of 9.0 ± 7.8. Concurrent administration of 90 mg/day of *G. biloba* for 30 days did not alter the concentration (24.4 ± 12.6 ng/mL) and MMSE score (8.7 ± 7.7), suggesting that there is no adverse interaction between the *G. biloba* and donepezil when used together in patients with Alzheimer's disease. However, the amount of flavone glycosides and terpene lactones in the botanical supplement were also not known.

Asian Ginseng (Panax ginseng)

There is considerable confusion about terminology for the different species known collectively to the consumer as ginseng; Asian ginseng is also sometimes called Chinese ginseng, Korean ginseng, ninjin (Japanese), or true ginseng. It is often confused with Siberian ginseng (*Eleutherococcus senticosus* Maxim), which belongs to the same family (*Araliaceae*) but is a different genus. Another popular ginseng product is American ginseng or Canadian ginseng (*Panax quinquefolius* L.)

The dried roots of Asian ginseng are used for medicinal purposes and its main constituents are triterpene saponins known as ginsenosides or panaxosides. The pharmacologic actions of ginseng include immunomodulatory, anti-inflammatory, antitumor, smooth muscle relaxation, stimulant, and hypoglycemic effects. The recommended dosage is 200 mg daily of standardized extract (4% total ginsenosides). Reported adverse effects include insomnia, diarrhea, vaginal bleeding, mastalgia, swollen tender breasts, increased libido, manic episodes, and a possible cause of Stevens–Johnson syndrome. A "*Ginseng abuse syndrome*" (consumed dose approximately 3 g daily) has been described with symptoms such as hypertension, sleeplessness, skin eruptions, morning diarrhoea, and agitation. Doses of 15 g daily and over were associated with depersonalization, confusion, and depression.

Interactions

Pharmacodynamic interactions

The most frequently reported interactions are those with monoamine oxidase inhibitors (MAOIs). There were reports in the literature of a potential interaction between ginseng and the MAOI phenelzine. The symptoms described included insomnia, headache and tremulousness in a 64-year-old woman when ginseng was added to her phenelzine regimen. Jones and Runikis reported that the use of ginseng in a 42-year-old woman treated with phenelzine was associated with manic-like symptoms, irritability, tension headache, and occasional vague visual hallucinations. After discontinuing the ginseng, the patient's symptoms resolved with only a few headache episodes thereafter. The clinicians considered that her other medications including lorazepam and triazolam were not contributory factors and the symptoms were mostly likely associated with ginseng–phenelzine interaction. However, ginseng is a stimulant and one of the common side effects of the use of ginseng is insomnia, and MAOI can also cause insomnia and headache; it is difficult to determine whether the described symptoms in these two reports are related to the use of each product alone or are attributed to botanical product–drug interaction.

Ginseng has the potential to interfere with the coagulation cascade and therefore interact with warfarin. However, there is no literature report of increased INR with concurrent use of both drugs. Interestingly, the use of ginseng has been associated with decreased INR. Janetzky and Morreale described a 47-year-old man with a mechanical heart valve, who was stabilized on warfarin with therapeutic INR within the range of 3.0 to 4.0. Two weeks after the patient took an unknown strength of ginger (*P. ginseng*) three times daily, his INR decreased to 1.5. Upon discontinuance of the ginger preparation, his INR returned to 3.3 two weeks later. Fortunately, there were no adverse effects during the two-week period of subtherapeutic INR. On the other hand, a thrombosis of a prosthetic aortic valve was attributed to the use of ginseng in a patient who had been stabilized on warfarin regimen (dosage regimen and INR values not reported). Because there is no human pharmacokinetic study evaluating this potential interaction or metabolic study data showing an effect of ginseng on CYP2C9, the primary CYP isoenzyme responsible for metabolism of the pharmacologically more potent S-isomer of warfarin, the reported paradoxical decrease in INR associated with ginger use is difficult to explain and evaluate. An animal study in rats demonstrated no effect of ginseng on either absorption or elimination of a single dose of warfarin. There were also no changes in prothrombin time after steady-state dosing of warfarin. The confusion about ginseng terminology mentioned above extends to case reports of ginseng–drug interactions, and it is not sure that all of these pharmacodynamic interactions are related to *P. ginseng*. In particular, the intake of concomitant drugs is a potentially significant confounding factor. Any conclusions about causality seem premature at this time.

Pharmacokinetic interactions

Anderson et al. evaluated the effect of *P. ginseng* on the 6-β-hydroxycortisol to cortisol ratio, a marker of CYP3A4 activity. Ten male and 10 female healthy subjects were given 100 mg of *P. ginseng* standardized to contain 4% ginsenosides (Ginsana) twice daily for 14 days. Comparing the 6-β-hydroxycortisol-to-cortisol ratio before and after the 14-day regimen of *P. ginseng* showed no appreciable difference, suggesting that there is no enzyme induction effect on CYP3A4. The result from this study confirms the data of Gurley et al. who administered 500 mg of *P. ginseng* standardized to contain 5% ginsenosides. It is of note that both Asian and Siberian ginsengs contain glycosides with structural similarities to digoxin, and both ginseng products have been reported to interfere with fluorescent polarization immunoassay determination of digoxin concentrations. Even though not an in vivo interaction per se, the digoxin-like immunoreactive substances associated with the use of ginseng cause false elevation of digoxin concentrations and could result in inappropriate dosage adjustment. There is little doubt about the therapeutic potential of some of the herbal medicines. Their safety profile is equally encouraging. The scope for botanical product–drug interactions, however, seems considerable. This is sharply contrasted by the paucity of actual clinical reports of such interactions occurring in practice. There are at least two explanations for this overt discrepancy. Firstly, interactions could indeed be rare. Secondly, the paucity of reports could be the result of underreporting. Under-reporting of adverse effects is significant and, in the realm of herbal medicine, it is likely to be even larger than with conventional drugs. In the absence of sufficient data it is impossible to decide which explanation is correct. What we can say, however, is that the subject of botanical product–drug interactions is potentially important and grossly under-researched. Thus it warrants further systematic study.

6

In Vitro Inhibition with Plant Products

The nature of plants having secondary metabolites as defensive agents greatly increases the expectation that there will be interactions with other botanical products and drugs. If well-established traditional botanical products are used according to directions, they are likely a "low risk." Risk increases when botanical products are combined with conventional drug therapies and lies in the possibility of unknown natural product–drug interactions. Other risks include product deviation due to misidentification of species, the lack of standardization, or adulteration. Most of the interactions have been reported with cytochrome P-450 (CYP) 3A4, but there are interactions with other metabolism enzymes and transport proteins.

The intent of this review is to provide an understanding of what constitutes a representative product, experimental test conditions, and the presence of contaminants that can affect the interpretation of these interactions using an in vitro assay system. Zou et al. evaluated the effects of 25 purified components of commonly used botanical products and found that many significantly inhibited one or more of the cDNA human P450 isoforms at concentrations of less than 10 μM. These findings are consistent with that of many other botanical components and suggest that there may be a potential for botanical products to affect drug disposition. However, negative findings with such purified biomarkers do not preclude the possibility that the combined total of the plant constituents could have an effect on drug safety and efficacy.

Natural Product Variation

Unlike conventional drugs, botanical products are complex mixtures that have inherent variation due to environmental and genetic factors affecting the fresh product, processing and manufacturing conditions, and the possible presence of nonactive components, which need to be converted to the active moiety. In addition, there are individual variations in the amount taken, form, manner of preparation, length of use, combination with other products, genetic characteristics, and health status of the user. Botanical products can be used either fresh or as a formulated single entity or in the blended dosage form. These forms include powder or soft gel liquid–filled capsules, cosmetics, liquids, ointments, tablets, tinctures, or suppositories. Exposure to botanical products may be intentional or fortuitous through their use in beverages, cosmetics, and foodstuffs.

Botanical bulk products may be sourced from several regions or countries and may have unique genotypic and phenotypic characteristics, which can confound interpretation of adverse event reports and product selection for clinical examination. The examination of one or even a few samples may inadvertently lead to the testing of a single chemotype. A chemotype is a variety or population of plants belonging to one particular species, which differ chemically from others of that species. These differences are genetic not phenotypic. Examples include *Melaleuca alternifolia*, volatile oils from single plants of *Thymus serpylloides* ssp. *gadorensis*, and peel and leaf oils of 43 taxa of lemons and limes obtained from fruits and leaves collected from trees under the same climatic and cultural conditions where there are multiple chemotypes. Together, these factors can compromise the testing process.

An interesting example is the report from Fukuda et al. who determined the amounts of three furanocoumarins in 28 white grapefruit juices, and orange, apple, lemon, grape, and tangerine beverages. Considerable differences were observed on the contents among commercial brands and also batches. The contents were determined to be 321.4 ± 95.2 ng/mL GF-I-1, 5641.2 ± 1538.1 ng/mL GF-I-2, and 296.3 ± 84.9 ng/mL GF-I-4 in white grapefruit juices. None was detected in beverages from orange, apple, grape, and tangerine, although trace amounts of GF-I-2 and GF-I-4 were found in lemon juice. The average levels of these furanocoumarins were lower in the juice from red grapefruit than in that from white fruit. This variation may reflect both genetic chemotype and phenotypic differences. The highest level of these components was found in the fruit meat. Sources of variation include the distribution of the constituents into various compartments within the fruit and procedures used in extracting juice from the whole fruit. Grapefruits exposed to freezing temperatures produce more naringin and less limonin.

It was reported that even under stable conditions, temperature and humidity could modulate naringin concentrations. Naringin, limonin, and nomolin reach peak levels in the early development stage of the fruit and decline as the fruit matures. Processing factors can include the pressure used to extract the juice, removal of bitter components, and the balancing of the final juice product by adding back the volatile essential oils and pulp. The clinical effects of the products containing any of the above chemotypes may vary; hence, it is difficult to attribute an effect without additional studies or set limitations on how the data can be extrapolated.

Labeling Information

Currently, there is little consistency in the information provided on botanical product labels in Canada. Some labels are clear as to the amount of botanical product and excipients, stated indications, contraindications, and warnings. In some cases, the information is confusing or difficult to understand, confounding the comparison of products. Examples of confusing or potentially misleading information on some valerian, milk thistle, St. John's wort (SJW), and echinacea product labels are provided. Three of these examples demonstrate the confusion created by or within the industry on chemical names. Information printed on some valerian root product labels stated that the products were standardized to valerenic acid and valeric acid. Although the names are similar, valeric acid is a five-carbon molecule that is not related chemically or pharmacologically to the larger C15 valerenic acids.

Silymarin is considered the active constituent of the milk thistle seed, but it is not a single compound but a descriptive term for several flavonolignans. Constituent analysis of five milk thistle products identified six constituents (representative amount): taxifolin (3.3%), silichristin (23.6%), silidianin (5.3%), silybin A (20%), silybin B (30.7%), and isosilybin (17.3%). The total amounts of silybin A and B in the five different products analyzed ranged from 45.7% to 61%. The biological effect of each constituent is not known; hence, spectrophotometric analysis would not provide sufficient information for a critical comparison of these products.

Many SJW products are standardized to either 0.3% hypericin or 4% hyperforin. Some product labels stated standardization to hypericins. Together hypericin and pseudohypericin have been referred to as total hypericins. Other biosynthetic precursors such as isohypericin, protohypericin, and protopseudohypericin may also be present, which are indistinguishable when analyzed spectrophotometrically.

The perceived message from this standardization is that the remaining 96% to 99.7% of the botanical material has no pharmacological effect. This is particularly disturbing with regard to SJW where pharmacological activity has been attributed to at least two dozen constituents or groups of compounds present in *Hypericum* extracts (8,9), including quinones such as hypericin and pseudohypericin, flavonoids such as hyperoside, and phloroglucinols such as hyperforin (about 8%), and water-soluble components such as organic acids.

Hence, standardization to one or two SJW constituents and testing of one to two products should be viewed as a starting point but not the end of the comparative process. In the end, simple unit weight was used to prepare solutions to determine the potential of each sample to inhibit metabolism of the test substrate. There are confounding issues with such an approach, but it does provide a simple quantitative basis for comparison of products. Hypericin, pseudohypericin, and hyperforin levels in the products examined varied widely within and between products. The results obtained from this study showed wide variation in inhibitory potential of teas and tablets, which does not correlate with the constituent levels. The final example of potentially misleading or confusing product labels is *Echinacea* (Asteraceae). The taxonomy has been revised by morphometric analysis to four species with distinct varieties. Two *Echinacea* species are widely used as botanical medicines: *Echinacea angustifolia* (syn *Echinacea pallida* var. *angustifolia*) and *Echinacea purpurea*. A third species, *E. pallida* (*E. pallida* var. *pallida*), has been widely used in Europe. Over 70 compounds were identified in the headspace volatile components of roots, stems, leaves, and flowers of *E. angustifolia*, *E. pallida*, and *E. purpurea* analyzed by gas chromatography/mass spectrometry (MS).

The constituents of echinacea include alkamides, caffeic acid, glycoproteins/ polysaccharides, and ketoalkenynes. In our study, label information indicated that two products contained 4% phenols and three products (NRP 70, 71, 73) were standardized to contain 4% echinacoside. Echinacoside is not, however, a good marker for the genus Echinacea. This is also indicative of the confusion in the botanical product industry, because echinacoside is a marker only for *E. angustifolia*. Echinacoside was not detected in a number of products. Where detectable, the level ranged from above detection up to 32.4 mg/g. Echinacea Special tea is an example of a blended tea, which is not readily evident from the label. The Special tea tested contained multiple ingredients such as lemon grass, peppermint leaf, spearmint leaf, triple echinacea root (*E. angustifolia*, *E. purpurea*, and *E. pallida*), liquorice root, ginger root, wild cherry bark, cinnamon bark, fennel seed, astragalus root, cardamom seed, rose hips, elder berry, burdock root, mullein leaf, clove bud, black pepper, and standardized E. purpurea root extract (4% phenols). All echinacea extracts markedly inhibited CYP-mediated metabolism. The findings with aliquots of the soft gel product extracts were variable. Inhibition was moderate to high toward CYP2D6 and 3A4, but only NRP 69 and 72 had an inhibitory effect against CYP2C9. In addition, NRP 71 did not inhibit CYP2C19-mediated metabolism.

Manufacturing and Storage

Echinacea products provide an example of the large variation in manufactured products. The whole plant has been used for therapeutic purposes, but single-entity product can consist of *E. purpurea* herb extracts, combination root and herb extracts, and teas, or they could be blended as root extracts of the three species, herbal teas with other botanicals, and blends of *E. purpurea* and *E. angustifolia* leaves, stems, and flowers plus a dry extract of *E. purpurea* root. The relative amounts of aerial and root stock materials in formulated products vary widely in composition. All plant tissues, irrespective of the species, contained acetaldehyde, dimethyl sulfide, camphene, hexanal, β-pinene, and limonene (12). The main headspace constituents of the aerial parts of the plant are β-myrcene, α-pinene, limonene, camphene, β-pinene, *trans*-ocimene, 3-hexen-1-ol, and 2-methyl-4-pentenal. The major headspace components of the root tissue are α-phellandrene (present only in the roots of *E. purpurea* and *E.*

angustifolia), dimethyl sulfide, 2-methylbutanal, 3-methylbutanal, 2-methylpropanal, acetaldehyde, camphene, 2-propanal, and limonene. Aldehydes, particularly butanals and propanals, make up 41% to 57% of the headspace of the root tissue, 19% to 29% of the headspace of the leaf tissue, and only 6% to 14% of the headspace of flower and stem tissues. Terpenoids including α- and β-pinene, β-myrcene, ocimene, limonene, camphene, and terpinene make up 81% to 91% of the headspace of flowers and stems, 46% to 58% of the headspace of the leaf tissue, and only 6% to 21% of the roots. The relative amounts of these products will vary greatly in the manufactured and fresh product making it difficult to choose a representative product.

A second example is garlic products. As with other botanicals, garlic can be processed by different procedures including drying or dehydration without enzyme deactivation, aqueous or oil extraction, distillation, and heating, including frying and boiling, processes that contribute to the variability of the extracts and complex nature of these products. These garlic preparations can then be formulated into single and blended products as oils of steam-distilled garlic, aged garlic, garlic macerated in vegetable oils, garlic powder, and gelatinous suspensions. Lawson et al. conducted an extensive phytochemical analysis of organic sulfur compounds of representative fresh and commercially available garlic products and found a wide variation in composition and chemical profile of sulfur compounds. Garlic powders suspended in a gel did not contain detectable amounts of nonionic sulfur compounds. Thiosulfinates were only recovered from garlic cloves and powders. Vinyldithiins and ajoenes were only detected in garlic macerated in vegetable oil. Diallyl, methyl allyl, and dimethyl sulfides were exclusively found in oil of steam-distilled garlic.

Typical steam-distilled garlic oil products contained similar amounts of total sulfur compounds as the total thiosulfinates released from freshly homogenized cloves; however, oil-macerated products contained about 20% whereas the garlic powders varied from 0% to 100%. Garlic is aged to reduce the content of sulfur compounds, such as alliin and the odor commonly associated with garlic. Gel and aged garlic in aqueous ethanol products did not have detectable levels of these nonionic sulfur compounds. Analysis of thiosulfinates from various *Allium* sp. revealed a threefold order of magnitude variation among species. Common garlic (*Allium sativum*) and wild garlic had the highest levels, while Chinese chives and the leek known as elephant garlic (*Allium ampeloprasum*) had intermediary levels. Environmental conditions were also found to influence the total thiosulfinate levels. As would be expected, storage conditions affect constituent content.

Fresh garlic stored at 4EC for two months was found to have decreased levels of γ-glutamly-S-allylcysteine with increased levels of alliin and allicin. Lawson et al. considered the increase in alliin and allicin contents in stored garlic to be a result of sprouting. In a study considering four product classes, there were marked differences in how the various extracts inhibited CYP-mediated metabolism. The effect was lowest against CYP2D6. Extracts from common garlic exhibited a similar inhibitory effect on all CYP3A isoforms. Chinese and elephant garlic had a lesser inhibitory effect on 3A7; Chinese garlic extracts also had a lesser inhibitory effect on CYP3A5-mediated metabolism. These findings were confirmed in a broader study with more products.

Extracts from three fresh garlic varieties were screened for their effect on CYP 2C9*1–, 2C9*2–, 2C19–, 2D6–, and 3A4–mediated metabolism. All three varieties had a slight inhibitory effect on 2C9* 1-mediated metabolism, but highly stimulated metabolism of the marker substrate with the 2C9*2 isoform. The extracts had negligible to no effect on 2C19- and 2D6-mediated metabolism. However, all extracts strongly inhibited 3A4-mediated metabolism. The effects of aqueous extracts from aged garlic capsules and the three fresh varieties were examined for their ability to interact with human P-glycoprotein membranes. Relative to 20 μM verapamil as the positive control, the aged, common, and Chinese phosphate buffer extracts had moderate levels of product-stimulated, vanadate-sensitive adenosine triphosphatase activity. Elephant garlic was inactive. Spices were analyzed for their capacity to inhibit in vitro metabolism of drug marker substrates by human CYP isoforms. Aliquots and infusions of all natural product categories inhibited 3A4 metabolism to some extent. Of the spices tested with 2C9, 2C19, and 2D6, most demonstrated significant inhibitory activity. Spices showed species-specific isoform inhibition with cloves, sage, and thyme having the highest activity against the four isoforms examined.

Blended and single-entity herbal teas, and some bulk spices were analyzed for their capacity to inhibit in vitro metabolism of marker substrates. Aliquots and infusions of all natural product categories inhibited 3A4 metabolism to some extent. Of the aliquots tested with 2C9, 2C19, and 2D6, many demonstrated significant inhibitory activity on the metabolism mediated by these isoforms. Herbal tea mixtures were generally more inhibitory than single-entity herbal teas. Single-entity herbal teas showed species-specific isoform inhibition with SJW and goldenseal having the highest activity against several isoforms.

Traditional Chinese medicine (TCM) includes both crude Chinese medicinal materials (plants, animal parts, and minerals) and Chinese proprietary medicine (CPM). The quality of TCM, as with other products, can vary emphasizing that there can be broad differences in these products. In a study undertaken with 12 purported TCM products, one was found to be a CPM containing three drugs. Extracts from most products inhibited at least three of the four CYP450 isozymes examined in a range from 25% to 100%. All liquid samples markedly inhibited the metabolism of all four isozymes. De le ke chuan kang and Rensheng dao were the strongest CYP450 inhibitors. These in vitro findings helped demonstrate that TCMs can inhibit CYP450 2C9–, 2C19–, 2D6–, and 3A4–mediated metabolism. TCMs need to be examined further under clinical settings to determine if potential interactions occur, which affect the safety and efficacy of conventional therapeutic products.

Experimental Factors

Many of the reported interaction studies with botanical products have used a single aqueous or organic extract. However, botanical products contain several major classes of biologically active constituents, with differing chemical characteristics that can directly or indirectly affect drug disposition. A series of solvents ranging from hexane, with high lipophilicity, down to water have been used to sequentially extract different botanical products. In this representative example, capsule material from aged garlic extract, and the two fresh varieties of garlic and one leek were extracted sequentially. Extracts were reduced to dryness and reconstituted into methanol prior to testing for their effect on 3A4-mediated metabolism. Most extract fractions exhibited a high inhibitory activity against the isoforms studied. There was varietal variation. Inhibition results with hexane (136%) and chloroform (116%) extracts suggest the presence of botanical fluorescent quenching substances. This observation is consistent with the concerns for intrinsic fluorescence and quenching as confounding variables in these assays noted by Zou et al.

As was determined with other botanical products, several 100% inhibitions were evident with this simple extraction sequence. A series of nonsequential extracts with these solvents (data not reported) also revealed high inhibitory activity in all extracts. Selective pH extraction of the Chinese garlic bulb showed significant (50–80%) inhibitory activity in the strong acid, weak acid, neutral, and basic fractions against CYP3A4. Because differences in the inhibitory effects of aqueous and methanolic extracts of fresh and aged garlic cloves on CYP3A4-mediated metabolism were previously noted, the three varieties were extracted under four different conditions. Results varied with variety, but in general, the distilled water and phosphate buffer extracts gave the strongest overall inhibitory effect on CYP450-mediated metabolism of the marker substrates.

Many plant constituents are conjugates, the main form being glucosides. Seven soybean varieties were analyzed by high-performance liquid chromatography (HPLC) for the isoflavones, daidzein and genistein, and their respective glycoside derivatives to determine if the amounts of these compounds could reliably predict the activity of the variety or year of harvest. Genistein levels ranged from 5.8 to 28.7μg/g and daidzein levels from 0 to 42.6 μg/g. The glycosides daidzin and genistin were present in much larger amounts ranging from 198 to 792 μg/g and from 458 to 1261 μg/g, respectively. The free aglycones accounted for less than 7% of the total in these samples. Neither the concentration of the individual compounds nor their total correlated with the inhibition of CYP3A4-mediated metabolism across genotypes and years. In a comparative inhibition test, the glycones were inactive relative to the corresponding aglycones.

Dissolution

As with formulated pharmaceuticals, dissolution of constituents from teas is an important consideration. Visual examination of the contents from tea bags from several botanical products showed that there were inter- and intraproduct differences in particulate size. Particle sizes ranged from fine powder to substantially intact leaves and stems. Under controlled tea-brewing conditions, there were marked differences in the dissolution of constituents relative to the amount and temperature of the water, degree of agitation, and time. Many of these factors are individualistic, so one individual may be exposed to different amounts of constituents relative to another person. In a representative study, several botanical products were examined as tea bag infusions at different temperatures. In this example, three different patterns were noted. The initial 10-minute values for the echinacea special tea were markedly higher than that for the other botanical products, but the inhibition curve only increased slightly with time. Two products, goldenseal herb, and echinacea and goldenseal, had low initial values, which nearly doubled after a second 10-minute incubation. The third pattern with feverfew showed a linear increase throughout the incubation period.

Westerhoff et al. studied the dissolution characteristics of several SJW products under biorelevant conditions. Components of SJW have a broad spectrum of polarity and solubility, and representative compounds from each group were examined. Although labelling indicates that several of the products studied should be pharmaceutically equivalent, dissolution under biorelevant conditions revealed that they have quite different release profiles and cannot be considered interchangeable. It was concluded that biorelevant dissolution testing can be a powerful tool for comparing botanical products as well as synthetically produced drug products. Jurgenliemk and Nahrstedt examined the dissolution of water-soluble phenolic constituents of Hypericum perforatum from a medicinal tea and a coated tablet formulation and found different dissolution profiles.

In general, the flavonoid glycosides were well dissolved, followed by flavonoid aglycones and hypericin, while hyperforin was only detectable at a very low level. Interestingly, hypericin exhibited much better extraction and dissolution rates than the similarly lipophilic hyperforin. When determining the octanol- water partition coefficient, it became obvious that the solubility of pure hypericin in water increased upon addition of some phenolic constituents typical for Hypericum extracts. Most effective in solubilizing hypericin was hyperoside, which increased the concentration of hypericin in the water phase up to 400-fold in this model.

Stability

As with drugs and purified biomarkers, thermal- and photostability of botanical products are the factors that must be considered. Commercial dried extract and capsules of SJW were evaluated under harmonized test conditions. Photostability testing showed all the constituents to be photosensitive in the tested conditions. However, different opacity agents and pigments influenced the stability of the constituents. Amber containers had little effect on the photostability of the investigated constituents. Long-term thermal stability testing showed a shelf life of less than four months for hyperforins and hypericins, even when ascorbic and citric acids were added to the formulation.

Photostability affected several botanical products. To overcome this confounding factor, samples of all products were extracted and tested under reduced lighting conditions, frequently under F40 gold fluorescence lighting.

Marked variations in the stability of 21 tinctures and 13 related single- entity plant compounds were noted. Bilia et al. investigated the stability of 40% and 60% v/v tinctures of artichoke, SJW, calendula flower, milk thistle fruit, and passionflower. The investigation showed a very low thermal stability of the constituents from accelerated and long-term testing as determined by HPLC–diode array detector and -MS analyses. Stability was related both to the class of flavonoids and water content of the investigated tinctures. Shelf life at 25°C of the most stable tincture (passion-flower 60% v/v) was about six months, whereas that of the milk thistle tinctures was only about three months. The stability of artichoke and SJW tinctures also were shown to be variable and seem to be related to the water content of the preparations.

Test Conditions

The first step with all botanical products is authentication to confirm identity. Bulk single-entity products can occasionally be inspected visually and authenticated by comparison to reference materials. However, most products require authentication through phytochemical analysis with comparison against authentic marker substances, preferably with a chromatographic stage to separate constituents for individual assessment. Authentication generally confirms the presence of a botanical product but does not exclude the possibility of the presence of other botanical products, adulterants, or contaminants. In some cases, historical information may suggest that samples be examined in depth for potential contaminants. Ideally, test samples of a product should be prepared from a minimum of five units mixed together to provide a representative sample of a particular product or lot. Test samples should be reduced to a consistent size using a mortar and pestle, ball mill, or blender. In our studies, we routinely begin with either a 100 mg/mL aqueous suspension or a 25 mg/mL ethanolic suspension that is then reduced further to constant particle size in a polytron to facilitate reproducible extraction for one minute. Standardization of this phase of testing is critical to ensure intra-and interday reproducibility in testing. Soft liquid-filled gel capsules are cut open, and the contents emptied into a 1.5 mL microfuge tube and extracted. The mixtures are centrifuged for 18 minutes in a microcentrifuge at a high setting to give a particulate-free stock solution.

Aliquots of aqueous or organic extracts are screened for their ability to inhibit the major human cDNA-metabolizing CYP isozyme CYP 2C9, 2C19, 2D6, and 3A marker substrates using an in vitro fluorometric micro- titer plate assay (4), modified from the one reported by Crespi et al., with balanced amounts of specific activity and protein content. Despite the inherent limitations of these test substrates, these probes provide a quantitative basis for additional studies. Briefly, assays are performed with either a 2 to 4 μL of an organic extract or up to 10 μL of an aqueous extract in a total volume of 200 μL in 96-well, clear-bottom, opaque-walled microtiter plates. The complex nature of the extracts requires blank and test controls to evaluate the effects of intrinsic fluorescence and quenching as confounding variables in these assays. We include controls for both the blank and test product using denatured enzyme with the extraction solvent. Where possible, studies should include one or more test substrates representative of the isozyme as positive control(s).

The effect of botanical products on the expression of drug-metabolizing enzymes or transport proteins can be examined in cell culture with established cell lines or primary human hepatocytes. The cells are incubated under standard conditions and treated with the blank, positive, or negative controls and the botanical extracts. Vehicle use should be consistent in all cultures. Multiple time points should examine the immediate and prolonged effect of these treatments. After treatment, total RNA and/or microsomes are prepared from the harvested cells using standard methodologies.

All assays should be performed under reduced or F40 gold fluorescence lighting to minimize the potential for photodecomposition or activation. Assays are run in triplicate to determine percent inhibition. The tests are repeated at least once with a freshly prepared sample. If there is greater than 15% coefficiency of variation, the samples are run at least one additional time. When the reaction mixture is incubated within the plate reader, readings are taken immediately and at set times throughout the prescribed incubation period as established by the microsome supplier. For assays incubated outside of the plate reader, reactions were stopped in accordance with the product test procedure.

In studies where either intrinsic fluorescence or quenching is a confounding variable, the botanical product should be examined in an assay using a chromatographic separation step with a representative probe substance for the isozyme being examined.

Product Selection for Clinical Studies

In vitro testing with cell-free systems can provide only qualitative information on the inhibitory potential of the particular extract from a specific sample to affect the isozyme-mediated metabolism of a test substrate. There is no a priori basis to extrapolate either positive or negative in vitro inhibitory results to acute or chronic clinical exposure. Despite this caveat, there were, however, clinical reports with echinacea, garlic, and SJW that these botanical products can affect drug pharmacokinetics. The explanation being that in some cases, prolonged exposure to an inhibitory product led to reduced plasma levels of a probe substance presumably due to induction of a transport protein or metabolic enzyme. Negative in vitro findings are limited to the extract and the inherent weakness of these probes' substrates; only further testing with additional extracts and test products can truly demonstrate the potential of these botanical products to cause interactions. In addition, there is no a priori basis to extrapolate in vitro findings from an single active ingredient (SAI) to the complex botanical product.

The number of fresh varieties, dosage forms, and formulations in combination with the variability in botanical material make it impossible to evaluate all of these products in animal models or clinical trials. As a minimum, several products used by the patient community should be obtained and authenticated. The testing and selection criteria should include multiple-lot testing, cost, and product availability, and take into consideration how these products are used. Drug combinations are being examined increasingly in comparative clinical trials with a goal of enhancing efficacy with the same or fewer adverse events. In many instances, the amount of drug exposure, the total drug load, is a major contributing factor to the safety of the combinations.

Four SJW products with similar CYP3A-inhibitory activity were evaluated for their effects on cell viability, the potential of such preparations to modulate induction of nitric oxide and CYP1A1/2-mediated ethoxyresorufin *O*-deethylase (EROD) activity in glial cell cultures. SJW A, B, and D had little effect on EROD activity. SJW C had the highest inductive effect on EROD activity. SJW B and C treatment resulted in the highest nitric oxide levels, raising concern for potential central nervous system toxicity. SJW A and D produced significant lactic dehydrogenase–released cell toxicity. Which product should be studied? The difficult decision is whether to choose an average or a superior product because the results of the study will subsequently be viewed as representative of all related products.

Synergistic interactions are of vital importance in phytomedicines and under-pin the philosophy of herbal medicine. Spinella emphasizes that, in addition to searching for more potent mechanisms, one must consider the additive and supra-additive effects of a plant's multiple constituents. Synergy may occur through pharmacokinetic and/or pharmacodynamic interactions. Synergistic interactions are documented for constituents within a total extract of a single botanical product, as well as between different botanical products in a formulation. Thus interactions with pharmacologically active secondary metabolites are not unexpected because these constituents are part of the plant defensive mechanisms.

In vitro studies can help determine the potential for adverse effects associated with botanical product–drug interactions. Accumulated findings from many studies have confirmed our earlier observations that there is seldom a direct correlation between levels of the purported active ingredient biomarkers and the potential for these extracts to affect P450-mediated metabolism. At best, in vitro studies with an inhibitory finding in these cell-free extracts can only provide a qualitative basis for further studies. A negative finding, particularly with an SAI, can only be interpreted to mean that there is no activity under the stated test conditions. Unfortunately, some negative findings have been erroneously taken to mean that related botanical products containing this SAI would not affect drug disposition. The dilemma for all health care professionals and consumers is that what is apparently safe with one botanical product and pharmaceutical, or another botanical product, may be neither safe nor effective in another combination or patient population.

7

Drug Interactions with Plant Products

The use of botanicals by consumers in North American and European countries has significantly increased over the last decade, with one survey showing an almost 10% increase in usage from 1990 to 1997. Although the efficacy of some botanicals has been documented, there is concern regarding the perceived safety of these products, particularly with respect to the lack of research and knowledge on botanical–drug interaction potential and significance. As more consumers use botanicals for various purposes, the likelihood of concurrent use of botanicals with prescription and/or over-the-counter medications, as well as the potential of pharmacokinetic and/or pharmacodynamic botanical–drug interactions will increase. The survey conducted by Eisenberg et al. reported that as many as 15 million adults in 1997 took botanical supplements concurrently with prescription drugs. Over the subsequent years, there has been no change in this usage pattern, with as many as 16% of consumers surveyed indicating concurrent use of botanical dietary supplements and prescription drugs. This continued trend of concurrent use of drug and botanical supplements, together with an underreporting of such use and a general lack of knowledge of the interaction potential, poses a challenge for the health care professionals and a safety concern for patients and/or consumers. Indeed, several clinically important botanical–drug interactions have been reported and some have resulted in altered efficacy and/or toxicity of the drug. The purpose of this chapter is to present an overview of common mechanisms of botanical–drug interactions, and using specific literature examples, discuss challenges associated with the interpretation of available study data or reports, and the of prediction of botanical–drug interactions.

Mechanism of Plant-drug Interactions

In essence, interactions between pharmacologically active botanicals and drugs involve the same pharmacokinetic and pharmacodynamic mechanisms as drug–drug interactions. Pharmacokinetic interactions may involve alteration in absorption, distribution, metabolism, or excretion of the affected drug or botanical. Pharmacodynamic interactions, on the other hand, alter the relationship between the drug concentration and the pharmacological response for a drug or botanical. Although most pharmacodynamic interactions reported in the literature and reviewed in this chapter focus on adverse effects as an outcome, not all pharmacodynamic botanical–drug interactions result in an undesirable effect. Animal studies have shown that the combination of an extract of the Chinese medicinal plant, *Tripterygium wilfordi*, and cyclosporine significantly increased the heart and kidney allograft survival compared to cyclosporine administered alone.

The effective cyclosporine dose required for 100% kidney allograft survival was reduced by 50% to 75% in the presence of the botanical extract. The immunosuppressive activity associated with the use of the botanical extract needs to be studied further in humans in order to explore the clinical potential of their combined use, perhaps by a mechanism similar to that for the ketoconazole and cyclosporine interaction. Most pharmacokinetic and pharmacodynamic botanical–drug interaction studies and clinical cases in the literature evaluated the quantitative effect or reported the consequence of adding a specific botanical to a drug regimen, and not the other way around. This likely represents the challenge of not knowing the identify and constitution of the botanical or botanical product, the difficulty of measuring concentration of a specific botanical or its active ingredient(s), and the more common scenario of patients using botanical preparations on a sporadic basis, while being stabilized on a drug regimen. Nevertheless, the pharmacokinetic profiles of different botanical products are currently being investigated. A better understanding of botanical pharmacokinetics in humans is needed if the prediction of botanical–drug interactions is to be successful.

Altered Pharmacokinetics

Drug Absorption

While reduction in the extent of drug absorption can potentially occur as a result of increased intestinal transit time, secondary to the use of botanicals containing anthranoid laxatives (e.g., aloe; *Aloe* spp.) or as a result of complex formation between botanical constituents (e.g., polyphenols in green tea), clinical cases of these types of interaction have not been reported. Nevertheless, based on the well-documented chelation of fluoroquinolones by different divalent and trivalent cations (e.g., sucralfate and didanosine) with the resultant significant decrease in fluoroquinolone concentrations and potential treatment failure, there remains the possibility that natural product supplements containing cations might also exert the same undesirable effect. Indeed, concurrent administration of an aqueous extract of fennel, the fruit of *Foeniculum vulgare*, in rats was shown to reduce maximum blood concentration, area under the concentration time curve (AUC), and urinary recovery of ciprofloxacin by 83%, 48%, and 43%, respectively. None of the phenolic or terpene constituents were reported to have an interacting effect, and the most likely mechanism is chelation of ciprofloxacin by metal cations present in the extract. The dose of the extract employed (2 g/kg) is unlikely to be consumed by humans, but the potential of impaired absorption of ciprofloxacin and other fluoroquinolones needs to be considered when patients take concurrent botanical products containing large amount of inorganic materials; staggering administration times of the two products should be considered when such physical interactions are possible.

Interestingly, there was a report of an interaction between aspirin and tamarind, an Asian fruit used not only as an Ayurvedic medicine, but also as a flavoring ingredient for cooking. In six healthy volunteers, tamarind significantly increased the extent of absorption of a single 600mg dose of aspirin, which might result in toxicity if a large amount of acetylsalicylate was ingested concurrently with tamarind. The more significant botanical–drug interaction resulting in altered extent of drug absorption involves modulation of P-glycoprotein within the gastrointestinal tract. Originally discovered by Juliano and Ling, P-glycoprotein has been primarily known for its association with drug resistance to chemotherapeutic agents. However, P-glycoprotein also possesses a physiological protective role by transporting toxic xenobiotics or metabolites out of normal cells. In humans, P-glycoprotein is also expressed in several tissues including the gastrointestinal tract, liver, and blood–brain barrier. The presence of this efflux transporter on the luminal surface of the intestinal mucosa suggests a possible role in limiting drug bioavailability after oral administration.

In early 2000, several reports publicized the now well-recognized interaction between St. John's wort (*Hypericum perforatum*) and commonly used drugs such as cyclosporine, some with significant clinical consequences, e.g., organ transplant rejection. Because cyclosporine is primarily metabolized by cytochrome P-450 3A4 (CYP3A4), induction of CYP3A4 was originally thought to be the primary mechanism of the interaction. However, there is substantial overlapping drug selectivity between CYP3A4 and P-glycoprotein, and it has been demonstrated that St. John's wort is an inducer of P-glycoprotein. P-glycoprotein induction results in reduced oral absorption and at least partially accounts for the reduced systemic concentration of cyclosporine when St. John's wort is coadministered. Indeed, demonstration of correlation between pharmacokinetic parameters of cyclosporine and intestinal P-glycoprotein level in kidney transplant recipients suggests a significant role of P-glycoprotein in reducing cyclosporine absorption after oral administration. St. John's wort has also been reported to reduce concentration of other P-glycoprotein substrates such as digoxin. Current evidence strongly indicates that long-term administration of St. John's wort (longer than 14 days) induces both intestinal CYP3A4 and P-glycoprotein, secondary to activation of the nuclear factor pregnane X receptor (PXR) by the hyperforin component of St. John's wort.

Based on the same principle of modulation of drug absorption, other less known botanicals could produce similar or different effects compared to St. John's wort. Rosemary (*Rosemarinus officinalis* Labiatae) is a commonly used dietary botanical that has been found to have a chemopreventive effect. Furthermore, in drug-resistant MCF-7 human breast cancer cells expressing P-glycoprotein, methanol extracts of Rosemary at two concentrations (16.5 and 85 μg/mL) inhibited the efflux and increased intracellular accumulation of doxorubicin and vinblastine, two chemotherapeutic drugs that are known substrates of P-glycoprotein. Treatment of drug-resistant cells with the extracts also increased the cytotoxic effects of doxorubicin. On the other hand, in wild-type MCF-7 cells that do not express P-glycoprotein, the extracts did not affect accumulation or efflux of doxorubicin. Binding of azidopine, an analog of vinblastine, to P-glycoprotein was also reduced by the extract. The investigators concluded that Rosemary extracts appear to exert an inhibitory effect on P-glycoprotein activity via inhibition of drug binding to P-glycoprotein, with the responsible constituent(s) yet to be identified. Therefore, despite no reported interaction with cyclosporine, this botanical has the potential to increase plasma concentration of cyclosporine via an increase in its oral bioavailability.

Similarly, green tea (*Camellia sinensis*), a commonly consumed dietary supplement in many Asian countries, contains catechins, which have been shown to inhibit the activity of P-glycoprotein and the efflux of doxorubicin by a carcinoma cell line. Although currently there is no literature report of an interaction between green tea and prescription or over-the-counter drug based on modulation of P-glycoprotein, a potential interaction between green tea and warfarin was reported.

Drug Distribution

Changes in distribution of drugs resulting from altered protein binding of highly protein-bound drugs have been studied intensively. However, the clinical significance of interactions based on this mechanism is usually minor and transient, unless accompanied by impaired metabolism and/or excretion that almost always result in persistently elevated blood concentrations of the affected drug. Examples of botanical–drug interactions involving changes in drug distribution and/or protein binding have not been reported in the literature.

Drug Metabolism

Inhibition

More than half of the drugs in current use or in development are eliminated primarily by metabolism, and the most common cause of clinically significant drug–drug interaction is a result of drug-metabolizing enzyme inhibition or induction. Botanicals can have similar effects on drug-metabolizing enzymes, and therefore it is not surprising that most of the reports of botanical–drug pharmacokinetic interactions involve altered drug metabolism. The most common pathway of drug metabolism is oxidation by the cytochrome P-450 (CYP) super family of enzymes located in the endoplasmic reticulum of the hepatocytes. Although there are many subfamilies in the human CYP superfamily, only three are responsible for the majority of drug oxidations in humans, namely CYP1, CYP2, and CYP3. Nine individual CYPs make contributions to drug oxidation in humans: CYP1A2, CYP2B6, CYP2C8, CYP2C9, CYP2C19, CYP2D6, CYP2E1, CYP3A4, and CYP3A5. However, a simpler outlook is often useful because the majority of drug interactions are seen with substrates of just four enzymes. CYP2C9, CYP2D6, and CYP3A4/5 metabolize 15%, 20%, and 60%, respectively, of the drugs that are principally eliminated by metabolism.

Considerable effort has been focused on understanding and predicting the inhibition of CYPs in vivo. Over the past decade, an impressive arsenal of gene- and protein-based tools has been brought to bear on this issue and significant advances have been made in the use of in vitro data to identify the specific CYPs involved in a given biotransformation and to predict clinically important drug interactions. These techniques have recently been extended to characterize botanical–drug interactions. All new drugs are required by the Food and Drug Administration to have the extent of metabolism defined, the CYPs responsible for major metabolite formation to be identified, and the potency of CYP inhibition to be quantified. These regulatory requirements are in part a response to the need to withdraw several drugs from the marketplace due to an unacceptable level of adverse events that stemmed from drug interactions. Whenever two substrates are cometabolized, there is the potential for a metabolic drug interaction, but in most cases a clinically important event does not occur because sufficient systemic blood concentrations of inhibitor are not achieved.

In some cases, drug interactions occur in the wall of the small intestine as well as in the liver. To date, this has only been described for drugs metabolized by CYP3A4/5, because these are the only enzymes expressed at a high level in the gut wall. The balance between the rates of absorption through the intestinal epithelium and the rates of metabolism will determine the net availability at the gut wall. Thus a CYP3A substrate that is either rapidly absorbed or not efficiently metabolized will not experience significant gut wall metabolism, e.g., alprazolam. For a drug such as midazolam, the complete inhibition of intestinal CYP3A4/5 alone could increase the oral AUC of midazolam by 2.5-fold. However, it has been speculated that the remarkable sensitivity of some CYP3A substrates, such as lovastatin, simvastatin, and buspirone, to drug interactions reflects a very low gut wall availability. The clinically important inhibitors of CYP3A4/5 share the capability to completely inhibit the enzymes in the intestinal wall, as illustrated by the high intestinal wall availability of oral midazolam in the presence of clarithromycin and ketoconazole. This is not unexpected because there are high concentrations of inhibitor at the gut wall during absorption. A similar pattern should be anticipated for botanical products that contain strong inhibitors of CYP3A enzymes.

We often rationalize drug interactions as reflecting the reversible competition of two substrates for an active site. However, it is becoming increasingly clear that other mechanisms of inhibition are operational in vivo. For example, some mechanism-based inhibitors are activated during metabolism and form a complex with the heme of CYP3A, known as a metabolite intermediate complex, or make a covalent modification of enzymes and result in irreversible loss of enzyme activity. These irreversible mechanisms appear to contribute to the inhibition of CYPs that occurs following exposure to bergamottins (in grapefruit juice), capsaicin (in chili peppers), glabridin (in licorice root), isothiocyanates (from cruciferous vegetables), oleuropein (from olive oil), diallyl sulfone (from garlic), and resveratrol, a red wine constituent. An important consequence of this irreversible inhibition is that interactions take one to two weeks to resolve on termination of the drug because this is how long the CYP3A takes to resume its predrug steady state. This is one reason why a good medical history should include questions about drugs and botanical products that have been discontinued in the past two weeks, when addressing possible botanical–drug interactions.

Induction

The term "*induction*" has evolved to include any mechanism that results in increased tissue concentration of catalytically active protein involved in drug metabolism. This increased enzyme activity results in greater systemic clearance and lower bioavailability of extensively metabolized drugs. The resulting lower drug concentrations often result in therapeutic failure. For example, it is well known that oral contraceptive pills become ineffective when rifampin is coprescribed. In general, induction may result from enhanced gene transcription rates, increased mRNA stability or translational efficiency, and protein stabilization induced by substrate binding or posttranslational modifications. However, the most common mechanism of induction is binding to and activation of discrete nuclear factors that act in the form of protein heteromers to enhance rates of gene transcription. It is clear that a single nuclear factor may modulate the expression of numerous genes and this mechanism of induction most likely applies to all drug-metabolizing enzymes but the extent of induction, tissue selectivity, and ligand selectivity vary widely between genes. Some degree of predictability has arisen from the discovery of the nuclear factors primarily responsible for the effects of the clinically important inducers. It is worth noting that some inducers, such as ritonavir for CYP3A4, are also potent inhibitors of at least some of the enzymes induced. Therefore, despite greater concentrations of enzyme, the net interaction maybe inhibition prior to full induction, followed by induction or even no effect.

The transcriptional regulation of drug-metabolizing enzymes is commonly cell-type and tissue selective. Thus, tissues that express low concentrations of nuclear factors do not experience significant induction. In contrast, both liver and intestines express significant concentrations of nuclear factors such as the PXR and experience profound induction in the presence of its ligands. The best example of a botanical product altering drug metabolism efficiency is that of St. John's wort, which is a potent inducer of CYP3A4 and causes accelerated metabolism of cyclosporine and indinavir. Of equal importance but less studied is the effect of botanicals on oral contraceptive disposition, which can potentially affect a large number of subjects. Recently, Hall et al. reported that St. John's wort induced the metabolism of both ethynyl estradiol and norethindrone in 12 healthy women via enhanced CYP3A4 activity.

The incidence of breakthrough bleeding was higher with concurrent use of St. John's wort (seven subjects) than without (two subjects), and subjects with breakthrough bleeding had a higher CYP3A4 activity, as measured by midazolam clearance. Therefore, this study provides supportive evidence and explanation for case reports of unexpected menstrual bleedings in women taking concurrent oral contraceptive and St. John's wort. Although Hall et al. did not find evidence of loss of oral contraceptive efficacy or ovulation, breakthrough bleeding is well known as a contributory factor for discontinuance of oral contraceptive use that may lead to a higher incidence of pregnancy. Schwartz et al. reported the loss of contraceptive efficacy associated with the use of St. John's wort with resultant unwanted pregnancies. This issue of oral contraceptive–botanical interaction requires further studies.

The effect of garlic (*Allium sativum*)–containing botanicals on drug metabolism has also been studied in vitro, and in vivo in both animal and human studies. Using human liver microsome as an in vitro drug- metabolism model, Foster et al. showed that raw garlic constituents inhibit CYP3A4-mediated drug metabolism. In rats, acute administration of a single dose of garlic oil produced significant reduction in the activity of several enzymes, including CYPs. However, chronic administration for five days produced the opposite effect—a significant increase in CYP activity. Gurley et al. reported that chronic administration of garlic oil for 28 days in humans reduced CYP2E1 activity by 39%, possibly a result of inhibition of the CYP by diallyl sulfone, a metabolic product of alliin, the major component of garlic. A pharmacokinetic study in healthy volunteers showed that a three-week course of garlic tablets taken twice daily resulted in a 51% reduction in AUC of the protease inhibitor saquinavir, a CYP3A4 substrate. In view of the multiplicity of CYPs and the many possible botanical–drug interactions, highly efficient clinical study designs using CYP probe cocktails have been explored. Following successful application to St. John's wort, other botanicals that have been evaluated in this fashion include echinacea, saw palmetto, garlic, peppermint oil, and ascorbyl palmitate. Curbicin, a botanical remedy taken by patients for the management of prostate enlargement, contains saw palmetto as one of the ingredients. Elevated international normalized ratio (INR) values were reported in two patients taking curbicin, and one of the patients also took warfarin. Cheema et al. also reported a patient who suffered from severe intraoperative hemorrhage with doubling of the bleeding time value after taking saw palmetto. The prolonged bleeding times were normalized after the botanical use was discontinued.

Although the effect of saw palmetto on CYP2C9, the enzyme responsible for metabolism of the active S-isomer of warfarin, has not been studied, it is of note that the prothrombin time (PT) and activated partial thromblastin time were both within normal limits before, during, and after the surgical procedure. It is also not known whether the bleeding abnormality observed in the patient might be related to the reported inhibitory effect of the botanical on cyclooxygenase in animal studies. The differential effect of echinacea on CYP3A4 will be discussed later in this chapter. With the exception of garlic, at present there are no reported drug interactions with the other three botanicals, but based on available data, potential interaction, especially with drugs metabolized by CYP3A4, could be expected.

Drug Excretion

While theoretically it is possible that botanicals with diuretic effects can increase drug excretion, most botanical diuretics are not as potent as furosemide and are unlikely to result in significant interactions. Most botanicals also do not affect urinary pH significantly, and hence are unlikely to affect renal tubular reabsorption of drugs. Nevertheless, lithium toxicity was thought to be related to the use of a botanical diuretic mixture in a patient. If the toxicity indeed is related to the use of the botanical diuretic, the mechanism of action or the responsible constituent(s) is not known.

Altered Pharmacodynamics

In addition to pharmacokinetic botanical–drug interaction, pharmacodynamic interactions can also occur, resulting in either an augmented or attenuated response. These effects can occur without any significant changes in either the systemic or tissue concentrations of the affected drug or botanical, and generally are more difficult to predict. In addition, unlike pharmacokinetic botanical–drug interactions, most pharmacodynamic interactions reported in the literature are mostly based on patient cases or clinicians' experience and seldom involve clinical or experimental study. For example, combining St. John's wort and selective serotonin reuptake inhibitors have been reported to result in an additive pharmacological effect and possibly serotonin syndrome, but there were no clinical studies or literature reports of changes in the pharmacokinetics of the selective serotonin reuptake inhibitors when combined with St. John's wort. The most commonly reported pharmacodynamic botanical–drug interactions primarily involve anticoagulants and antiplatelet agents.

Augmented Pharmacological Effect

Warfarin

Most literature reports of pharmacodynamic botanical–drug interaction involve the anticoagulant warfarin, likely because it has therapeutic end points such as the INR and PT, which are routinely closely monitored. In addition, most botanicals possess anticoagulant and/or antiplatelet activities, and their combined use with warfarin provides a good example of pharmacodynamic interaction with additive pharmacological effect. Botanicals such as garlic can inhibit platelet aggregation, likely accounting for episodes of spontaneous spinal epidural hematoma and postoperative bleeding reported in the literature. Currently, there are no reports of an interaction between garlic and warfarin, but based on the inhibitory effect of garlic on platelet aggregation, one would expect that there is at least a risk of additive pharmacological response to warfarin when the two compounds are taken concurrently. In fact, such interactions have been reported with other botanicals that also inhibit platelet aggregation, including ginkgo and the traditional Chinese medicines, dong quai (*Angelica sinensis*) and dan shen (*Salvia miltiorrhiza*).

In a patient who had been stabilized on warfarin for five years, recent use of ginkgo was reported to result in intracerebral hemorrhage. In an in vitro model using human liver microsomes, the activity of CYP2C9, which metabolizes the active S-isomer of warfarin, was inhibited by commercial ginkgo extracts. Therefore, the interaction between ginkgo and warfarin potentially involves both pharmacokinetic and pharmacodynamic mechanisms. Dong quai also inhibits platelet aggregation, and there have been several reports of increased INR in patients taking concurrent warfarin and dong quai. Despite the elevated INR, the patient did not experience any bleeding episodes. It is not known whether the lack of clinical consequence in this report is a result of intersubject variability in the magnitude of interaction or the absence of a pharmacokinetic component, as an animal study demonstrated that warfarin pharmacokinetics was unchanged by dong quai.

Antiplatelet drugs

Although no pharmacokinetic antiplatelet drug–botanical interactions have been reported in the literature, there is the potential of an additive pharmacodynamic effect with concurrent use of antiplatelet drugs or botanicals that possess antiplatelet activity or contain salicylates, such as willow bark (*Salix* spp.) and meadowsweet (*Filipendula ulmaria*). The ginkgolide constituents, found in ginkgo, are known to exhibit platelet-activating factor antagonistic activity. In an elderly patient who was prescribed aspirin therapy after a coronary bypass surgery, self-initiation of ginkgo use resulted in spontaneous bleeding within the eye and blurred vision. On cessation of ginkgo use, the bleeding stopped and the visual changes resolved.

Drugs Acting on the Central Nervous System

Selective serotonin reuptake inhibitors

The similar pharmacological profile of selective serotonin reuptake inhibitors and St. John's wort would suggest the potential of a pharmacodynamic interaction due to an additive effect. A case of concurrent use of sertraline and St. John's wort, resulting in mania, was reported for a patient with a history of depression who was prescribed sertraline and who also took St. John's wort against medical advice. A similar potentiation of serotonergic effect was reported by Gordon.

Benzodiazepines

Kava (*Piper methysticum*) is a popular botanical product used for management of anxiety and insomnia. Almeida and Grimsley reported a case of potentiation of the central nervous system (CNS)-depressant effect of alprazolam by kava extract and/or kavalactones in a 54-year-old, male patient who became lethargic and disoriented after taking kava for three days. Kava ingestion was concurrent with his usual medications, including alprazolam, cimetidine, and terazosin, but the patient denied overdose of any of his medications. The physicians attributed the patient's mental state to a kava–alprazolam interaction. Both kava extract and kavalactones have been shown in vitro to inhibit several CYPs, including CYP3A4. However, it is possible that in this case, the enhanced effect involves not just a pharmacokinetic component but also a pharmacodynamic basis secondary to synergistic activity at the gamma-aminobutyric acid (GABA) receptor.

Miscellaneous central nervous system acting drugs

Ephedra (ma huang) is a popular botanical incorporated into a variety of formulations for weight loss, "energy" or "performance" enhancement, and symptomatic control of asthma. A pharmacodynamic interaction leading to a fatality has been reported with concurrent use of caffeine and ephedra, possibly as a result of additive adrenergic agonist effect of the ephedrine alkaloids and caffeine on the cardiovascular system and the CNS. Ephedra was recently withdrawn from the market. A botanical–drug interaction postulated to have both pharmacokinetic and pharmacodynamic mechanisms was reported in an elderly Alzheimer's patient, who developed coma likely as a result of concurrent use of ginkgo leaf extract 80mg twice daily and the antidepressant trazodone 20 mg twice a day. The pharmacodynamic mechanism was suggested because the coma was reversed by flumazenil, indicating increased activity at GABA-activated receptors; ginkgo flavonoids possess GABA agonist activity on the benzodiazepine receptor. A pharmacokinetic basis of the interaction was also proposed to be a result of CYP3A4 induction, and subsequent increased conversion of trazodone, to *m*-chlorophenylpiperazine, an active metabolite with GABA agonist activity.

Digoxin

The use of botanicals containing laxatives has not been reported to result in altered drug absorption to date. However, excessive use of laxative-containing botanicals such as cascara (*Rhamnus purshiana*), senna leaves, and/or pods from *Cassia senna* can potentially decrease serum potassium and other electrolyte concentrations, and therefore enhance toxicity of digoxin. To date, no clinical interactions have been reported between digoxin and these botanicals, but given the narrow therapeutic range of digoxin, it would be prudent to monitor for signs and symptoms of digitalis toxicity with long-term, excessive use of these botanical laxatives. The concurrent administration of these botanicals with prescription diuretics should be approached with caution.

The narrow therapeutic index of digoxin necessitates the monitoring of serum digoxin concentration as an aid for optimizing drug therapy in patients, and an in vitro laboratory interaction between digoxin and several botanicals such as danshen and ginseng products have been reported in the literature. These "*cardioactive*" botanicals possess active constituents with structures similar to digoxin, and therefore can demonstrate digoxin-like immunoreactivity. Chow et al. reported that small amounts (2–5 mL) of aqueous extracts of these "*cardioactive*" botanicals interfered with immunoassays used to determine digoxin concentration, both in vitro and ex vivo. Patients taking digoxin might also take these "*cardioactive*" botanicals and this laboratory interference could result in falsely elevated digoxin concentrations in patients. McRae reported a 74-year-old man who had been stabilized on digoxin for about 10 years with therapeutic concentrations between 0.9 and 2.2 ng/mL. Ingestion of Siberian ginseng resulted in a serum concentration of 5.2 ng/mL, even though the patient was asymptomatic with no electrocardiographic changes. The digoxin concentration returned to normal after the patient stopped taking the ginseng product.

Oral Hypoglycemic Agents

In a brief report, a potential interaction between curry and chlorpropamide, leading to reduction in chlorpropamide dose in a 40-year-old woman was attributed to the garlic and karela components of this complex mixture. Garlic reportedly can lower blood glucose. However, there was no information provided regarding the estimated amount of garlic intake in this patient. To date, there are no formal studies that confirm the initial clinical observation or evaluate the likely mechanism.

Antagonistic Pharmacodynamic Effect

While dong quai and possibly garlic have an additive effect on the pharmacological action of warfarin, an antagonistic interaction between warfarin and coenzyme Q_{10} had been reported. Spigset reported three elderly patients who were all stabilized on different warfarin dosage regimens. All experienced a decrease in INR to values below 2 after taking ubidecarenone (coenzyme Q_{10}). The dose of coenzyme Q_{10} was documented as 30 mg/day in two of the patients. In both patients, the warfarin dose was temporarily increased and coenzyme Q_{10} discontinued. The INR returned to the patients' previous stabilized values prior to taking the coenzyme Q_{10}. Because coenzyme Q_{10} is structurally similar to vitamin K_2, the authors suggested that one potential mechanism might be related to the enhanced coagulation effect of coenzyme Q_{10}. Animal data showed that antagonism of coenzyme Q_{10} resulted in increased PT, suggesting that coenzyme Q_{10} might have an opposite pharmacological effect to that of warfarin.

Two patients stabilized on a phenytoin regimen suffered a loss of seizure control after taking shankhapushpi, an Ayurvedic antiepileptic medicine, three times a day. There was also a significant decrease in serum phenytoin concentration from 9.6 to 5.1 mg/L. To investigate the possible mechanisms, multiple doses of shankhapushpi were administered to rats and resulted in decreased plasma phenytoin concentrations, whereas single-dose administration was reported to interfere with the antiplatelet effect of phenytoin, thereby implying both a pharmacokinetic and pharmacodynamic basis for the interaction.

There are several botanicals that have purported immunostimulating effects. These include *Panax ginseng* and *Echinacea purpurea*, which have both been used as an immune stimulant. Any potential adverse effect on the pharmacological activity of immunosuppressants has not been reported in patients or evaluated in clinical studies. Given the lack of data, it would be prudent to advise against concurrent intake of these botanicals, and closely monitor changes in efficacy in patients who self-administer these botanicals.

Evaluating Plant-Drug Interaction

Overall, an accurate assessment of the reliability of reported botanical–drug interactions with a pharmacodynamic basis or mechanism is usually more difficult than the assessment of those with a pharmacokinetic basis. This likely reflects the fact that the former reports are usually case reports, whereas the later reports are often accompanied with objectively measured end points. Also, despite a common belief that botanical–drug interactions are underreported, the overall incidence of this phenomenon is difficult to define. This partly reflects the lack of a mechanism for reporting the interactions, and difficulty in obtaining reliable information to assess clinical relevance or to establish a definitive causality relationship. For example, even with the evidence of St. John's wort increasing the metabolism of oral contraceptive hormone and possibly contributing to reports of break-through bleeding and pregnancy, it is well established that pregnancy can occur with oral contraceptive used alone or with other drugs, and a definitive causality relationship has not been established. Nevertheless, there is sufficient clinical evidence that interaction involving commonly used drugs such as cyclosporine and protease inhibitors with St. John's wort can be serious and sometimes life threatening. In addition, the lack of fatalities resulting from the various reports of botanical–anticoagulant interaction likely reflects close clinical and laboratory monitoring with appropriate dosage adjustment, if necessary, in the patients.

Challenges of Predicting Botanical–Drug Interaction

While defining the overall pharmacokinetic or pharmacodynamic basis of botanical–drug interactions may be relatively straightforward, attempts to explain the underlying mechanism of altered drug concentrations or to predict the magnitude and significance of the interaction is certainly not easy. There are several factors that contribute to this difficulty, and they are briefly discussed below.

Lack of Definition of Active Constituents

First and foremost, it must be emphasized that botanicals or botanical preparations are not pure synthetic molecules but are composed of many constituents, sometimes from multiple botanicals, and some or many of them can be biologically active. Although altered drug concentration can be caused by induction or inhibition of intestinal and hepatic drug-metabolizing enzymes as well as P-glycoprotein, the identity of the biologically active constituent(s) that is responsible for these effects is usually not known. Without this knowledge, most investigations are restricted to studying the commercially available products containing multiple constituents with potentially different modulating effects on these proteins. Commercial preparations of St. John's wort used in most clinical and interaction studies are usually standardized to contain specific amounts of hypericin, but it is another constituent, hyperforin, which was shown to be responsible for induction of CYP3A4. Similarly, although administration of milk thistle 175 mg (containing 153 mg of silymarin) three times a day for three weeks resulted in 9% and 25% reduction in AUC and trough concentration, respectively, of indinavir, its differential effect on CYP3A4 and P-glycoprotein needs to be further studied. In addition, while the overall study result suggested a minimal clinical consequence for AIDS patients receiving indinavir, whether botanical constituents other than silymarin would have a greater modulating effect remains unknown.

In addition, very few studies provide information on the content of important constituents of the botanical or botanical preparation. This obviously poses a problem of general applicability in terms of predicting interaction across different preparations with variable content of constituents, or extrapolating the result of one study to the overall interaction potential. For example, one of the active constituents in garlic is allicin, which gives garlic its specific, well-known odor. Although allicin has been suggested to enhance production of CYP, there is no data to confirm or refute the possibility, let alone the identity of the specific enzyme that is induced. It is clear, however, that commercial garlic preparations have highly variable contents ranging from no allicin to maximum standardized allicin content used in the garlic-saquinavir study described above. In the study by Gurley et al. garlic oil 500 mg did not result in appreciable differences in the 1-hydroxymidazolam/midazolam phenotypic ratio for CYP3A4, the enzyme that mediates the metabolism of saquinavir. Both studies administered the garlic preparations for at least three weeks, and therefore it is unlikely that the duration of therapy would account for the difference between studies. On the other hand, if allicin content is a critical issue, it may be that one of the reasons for the conflicting results between the two studies is potential variability in this active constituent in the two garlic preparations used.

Lack of Standardization of Known Active Constituents

Even though the active constituent responsible for the interaction has been identified, conflict in study results can still occur due to variable content of the known active constituent(s). In the study by Piscitelli et al., the investigators took extra effort in analyzing the allicin and allin content of the commercial garlic caplets administered to the subjects. They reported that the allicin and allin contents were 4.64 and 11.2 mg per caplet, which were different from the labeled content. This study highlights the challenge associated with evaluating any aspect of pharmacology or therapeutic use of dietary supplement, including botanicals. While consumers increasingly are aware of the fact that dietary supplements and botanical products do not have to be proven to be efficacious or to be safe, they are less aware of the lack of standardization among products.

Although dietary supplements and botanical products are required to state exactly the content of active ingredients and their amounts on the label, the manufacturers do not necessarily comply. More importantly, the labels are not routinely checked for compliance by any government agency. In addition, unlike prescription drugs, dietary supplement and botanical products are not required to be manufactured under standardized conditions. This has led to substantial variability in the amount of active constituent(s) between batches. Prime examples of this include *echinacea* and ginseng products. Gilroy analyzed different single botanical *echinacea* preparations purchased from retail stores and reported that only 10 of 19 preparations (53%), labeled as standardized, had an assayed content consistent with the labeled content. There were only weak correlations between labeled milligram content of *echinacea* versus measured milligram for the standardized preparations ($r = 0.49$, $p = 0.02$) and the correlation was even lower for nonstandardized preparations ($r = 0.21$, $p = 0.28$). Similar discrepancies in content were reported in a study conducted by the Consumer Unions, in which they tested the content of 10 marketed ginseng preparations, and found significant differences in the amount of the active constituent ginsenosides (range: 0.4–23.2 mg). Of particular concern is that this inconsistency in product and active constituent occurs even within the same batch. As part of a clinical study with St. John's wort, Hall et al. analyzed 10 capsules of St. John's wort from the same lot and found the mean total weight to be 444 mg (4.6% CV) versus 300 mg as stated on the label. In addition, the dosage form was supposed to be standardized to contain 900 mg of hypericin, but the mean content was found to be 840 mg (6.6% CV). There was also variability of the hyperforin content (mean 11 mg and 5.7% CV), which was not stated on the label. Our experience with two random capsules from one batch of kava-kava also showed the same extent of undesirable variance: the total content of the pharmacologically active kavalactone was 47.3 mg in one capsule and 39.4 mg in the second one.

Confounding Issue Related to Study Design

Extrapolation of Result from In Vitro Study

Similar to evaluation of potential inhibitory effect of different drugs on the CYPs, in vitro preparations such as human liver microsomes have also been used to evaluate the potential of a botanical to cause interaction. Nevertheless, there are numerous reasons why in vitro results based on human liver microsomes do not necessarily agree with in vivo study results. One reason is the inability of human liver microsomes to evaluate and predict enzyme induction. St. John's wort serves as an excellent example to illustrate this limitation. In vitro, St. John's wort has been shown to inhibit CYP2C9, CYP2D6, and CYP3A4. However, as discussed above, St. John's wort has been shown in numerous human studies to induce CYP3A4. This may be due to the finding of hyperforin, a constituent of St. John's wort, binding to the PXR and upregulating CYP3A4 gene expression. Importantly, microsomal preparations lack the capability to synthesize new protein and cannot be expected to provide any insight into the potential for induction to occur in vivo.

Differential Effect on Intestinal and Hepatic CYP3A4

Another confounding issue specific to CYP3A4 would be the potential differential effect of a specific botanical or botanical constituent on intestinal and hepatic CYP3A4. The clinical study by Gorski et al. elegantly showed that, consistent with in vitro inhibition of CYP3A4 by *echinacea* tinctures, administration of echinacea 400 mg four times a day for eight days in healthy volunteers inhibited intestinal CYP3A4 and resulted in an 85% increase in systemic bioavailability. However, hepatic CYP3A4 activity, as measured by systemic clearance of midazolam after intravenous administration, was increased by 34%. Therefore predicting potential interaction between *echinacea* and CYP3A4 substrate would depend on whether the substrate has high oral bioavailability, in which case the likely pharmacokinetic and clinical outcome would be increased clearance secondary to hepatic CYP3A4 induction and lower serum drug concentration versus substrate with a low bioavailability secondary to extensive intestinal first-pass effect, in which case the likely pharmacokinetic and clinical outcome would be decreased oral clearance secondary to intestinal CYP3A4 inhibition and increased serum drug concentration. One can only imagine the difficulty of predicting the potential and extent of interaction between echinacea and CYP3A4 substrates if a patient who is receiving CYP3A4 substrate for medical conditions also treats a cold at the same time by taking *echinacea* and drinking grapefruit juice, which potently inhibit intestinal CYP3A4.

Single-Dose Administration vs. Multiple Dosing

Results from single-dose studies could be different from chronic dose administration. Although St. John's wort administered as a single 900mg dose to healthy volunteers was found to increase the maximum plasma concentration and decrease the oral clearance by 45% and 20%, respectively, of the P-glycoprotein substrate fexofenadine, the opposite effects (35% decrease in maximum plasma concentration and 47% increase in oral clearance) were observed after daily administration of the same dose of St. John's wort for two weeks. Similar differential effects between single versus chronic dose administration have been shown before with CYP3A4: single-dose ritonavir caused inhibition of CYP3A4 and chronic administration resulted in CYP3A4 induction.

Drug Interaction with St. John's Wort

Botanical use is prevalent throughout the world with between 10% and 30% of individuals residing in the United States using complementary and alternative medicines routinely. Of particular concern is the finding that up to 30% of individuals taking prescription medicines have also used botanical remedies concurrently within the past year. The number of individuals consuming St. John's wort on a daily basis has been estimated at more than 11 million and approximately one-third of these are using St. John's wort to treat self-diagnosed depression. In the United States, St. John's wort is one of the top-selling botanical preparations with sales ranking second in 1999 and seventh in 2002. Although botanical preparations are widely considered by the public to be without adverse effect or a source of drug interactions, this is not the case. The report of Ruschitzka et al. clearly illustrates the danger of coadministering botanical products (i.e., St. John's wort) with prescription products and demonstrates that, despite popular belief, the indiscriminant use of botanical products does involve risk. This chapter will review the historical indications, formulations, pharmacology, and interactions between St. John's wort, echinacea, and other medicines.

Indications

St. John's wort (*Hypericum perforatum*) is a perennial wildflower indigenous to Europe, North Africa, and western Asia and has been used for medicinal purposes for over two millennia. As far back as the early 16th century, St. John's wort was used primarily to treat anxiety, depression, and sleep disorders. In the late 20th and early 21st century, St. John's wort has been recommended for the treatment of mild to moderate depression. In support of its use for the treatment of mild to moderate depression, a number of clinical trials have demonstrated that St. John's wort has comparable efficacy to the tricyclic antidepressants (i.e., imipramine) and selective serotonin reuptake inhibitors (e.g., fluoxetine and paroxetine). It should be noted that these clinical trials are typically conducted within a short time period and thus may not reflect long-term outcomes. The utility of St. John's wort in the treatment of moderate to severe depression has been investigated in large randomized placebo-controlled multi-institutional studies. Some such studies demonstrated efficacy, but others failed to detect a clinically significant effect on the symptoms of the moderate to severely depressed individuals. Gelenberg et al. demonstrated a relapse rate of approximately 30% in moderate to severely depressed individuals who initially responded to St. John's wort therapy as would be expected from experience with prescription antidepressants. Other conditions in which St. John's wort has been advocated include neuralgia, anxiety, neurosis, dyspepsia, and external treatment of wounds, bruises, sprains, myalgia, and first-degree burns. In vitro studies conducted in the late 1 980s and early 1990s suggested that components of St. John's wort (e.g., hypericin) may have antiviral properties. However, an open- label clinical trial demonstrated that the intravenous or oral administration of the St. John's wort constituent, hypericin, provided no clinical benefit, as reflected by increasing CD4 counts or decreasing viral load in a group of HIV-infected individuals and resulted in significant adverse events necessitating discontinuation of therapy.

Dosage Forms

St. John's wort and some individual constituents of the preparations have been administered orally, topically, and intravenously in various pharmaceutical formulations, including tinctures, teas, capsules,

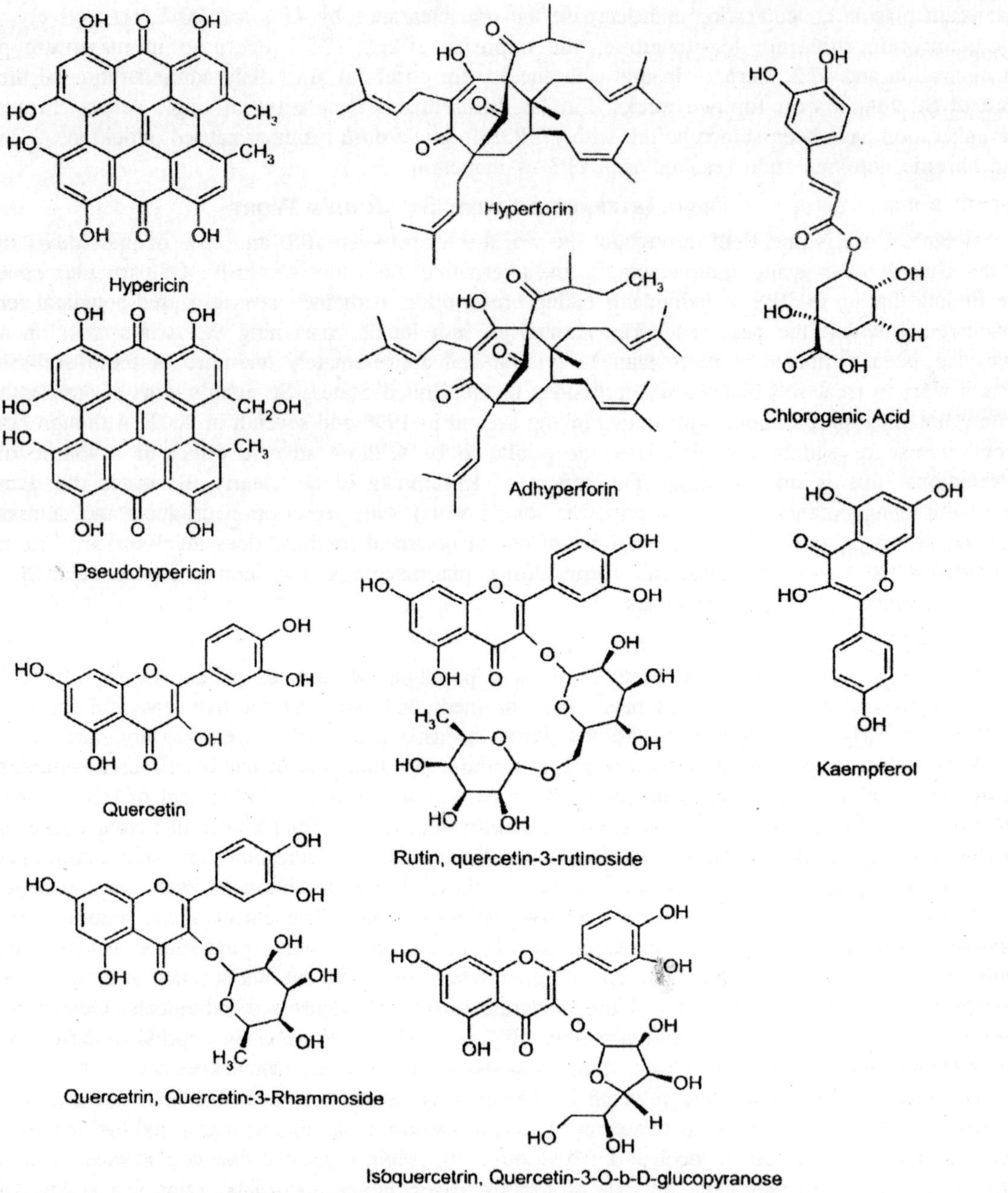

Fig. 7.1. Chemical structures of common phytochemicals found in SJW.

purified components, and tablets. These botanical preparations of St. John's wort are prepared from plant components (i.e., flowers, buds, and stalk) whose content of the wide array of structurally diverse bioactive constituents may differ. Many commercial tablet and capsule formulations of St. John's wort are standardized using the ultraviolet absorbance of the naphthodianthrones, hypericin, and pseudohypericin, to contain 0.3% "*hypericin*" content. Thus, a 300 mg dose of St. John's wort contains approximately 900 μg "*hypericin*" per dose.

Despite the standardization of dosage forms on hypericin content, the principal active ingredient is thought to be a phloroglucinol, hyperforin. As a result of inappropriate standardization on an ingredient that has limited pharmacological activity, the concentration of hyperforin varies greatly among commercial preparations. Draves and Walker assessed the hypericin and pseudohypericin (naphthodianthrones) content in 54 commercially available St. John's wort products and determined that only two of the products were within 10% of the labeled claims for "*hypericin*" content. Likewise, Wurglics et al. assessed hypericin and hyperforin content and inter-batch variability in eight German St. John's wort products. Pronounced interbatch variability was observed for some products whereas others demonstrated consistent hyperforin and hypericin content. In addition, the expected naphthodianthrone (*hypericin*) content in the preparations also demonstrated considerable variability. It is clear from the reports of a number of investigators that there is wide inter- and intraproduct variability in hyperforin and hypericin content. The lack of consistent phytomedicinal (hypericin and hyperforin) content across and within products is not limited to St. John's wort preparations but is seen with many other botanical medicines. The administration of St. John's wort via tea is no longer recommended because the efficacy of this preparation is questionable; however, the drug interaction potential of St. John's wort in this formulation appears to be maintained.

The preparation used in many of the described interactions between St. John's wort and conventional pharmaceutical products is the product manufactured by Lichtwer Pharma GmbH. This product is marketed under the trade name, Jarsin (LI 160) in Germany and marketed in the United States under the trade name Kira. St. John's wort may also be sold in combination products with vitamins and other botanical preparations. The drug interaction potential between these combination products and cytochrome P450 (CYP) 3A and P-glycoprotein substrates has not been investigated, but should be assumed to be no different than single-agent St. John's wort products.

Adverse Effects and Pharmacodynamic Interactions

It is a reasonable expectation that, as observed with other pharmacotherapies, the administration of St. John's wort will result in adverse effects. In a study examining the efficacy of St. John's wort for mild to moderate depression, dry mouth was the most common adverse effect occurring in 8% of patients (13/157), and other adverse events including headache, sweating, asthenia, and nausea occurred in 3% or less of the participants. In addition, only four individuals withdrew from the trial compared to 26 individuals who withdrew while taking the comparator drug, imipramine. Likewise, Woelk et al. reported a low incidence of adverse events in a group of 3250 (76% women) patients receiving St. John's wort three times daily (LI 160) for the treatment of depression (33). The most frequently recorded adverse events were gastrointestinal irritation (0.6%), allergic reactions (0.5%), tiredness (0.4%), and restlessness (0.3%). Other adverse effects associated with St. John's wort intake include sedation, anxiety, and dizziness. It is clear from these reports that St. John's wort is well tolerated.

Dean et al. described a 58-year-old postmenopausal woman who experienced nausea, anorexia, retching, dry mouth, dizziness, thirst, cold chills, weight loss, and extreme fatigue following the discontinuation of St. John's wort (1800 mg three times daily for 32 days). The symptoms peaked three days after cessation of St. John's wort for suspected photosensitivity reaction and resolved within eight days. The reported symptoms and the temporal relationship to the discontinuation of the St. John's wort dosing were considered by Dean et al. to be consistent with "*withdrawal syndrome.*" Additionally, the high dose of St. John's wort administered was considered to be a contributing factor in the patient adverse-event profiles.

In studies examining the antiviral activity of synthetic hypericin following oral and intravenous administration for the treatment of HIV infection, a dose-limiting toxicity was moderate to severe photosensitivity, including the erythema, numbness, pain, and temperature sensitivity. There is a case report of hypertensive crisis in a 41-year-old male, following the ingestion of St. John's wort for approximately one week, and the consumption of tyramine-rich foods (aged cheese and red wine). Although the interaction between monoamine oxidase inhibitors and the eating of tyramine-rich foods is well recognized, alcoholic extracts of St. John's wort have been shown to weakly interact with monoamine oxidase receptors A and B. Thus, the mechanism of the observed hypertensive crisis is unclear. Other serious adverse effects attributed to St. John's wort due to drug–drug pharmacokinetic or pharmacodynamic interactions include cardiovascular collapse, mania in patients with bipolar depression, and photosensitivity.

Mechanisms of St. John's Wort–Mediated Drug Interactions

In vitro

Using crude extracts and isolated constituents, Obach demonstrated that St. John's wort was capable of inhibiting cDNA-expressed CYP-mediated metabolism. cDNA-expressed CYP2C9-, CYP2D6-, and CYP3A4-mediated biotransformations were inhibited by purified hyperforin. Likewise, I3, II8 biapigenin was shown to competitively inhibit CYP1A2-, CYP2C9-, and CYP3A4-mediated phenacetin *O*-deethylation, diclofenac 4-hydroxylation, and testosterone 6β-hydroxylation, respectively. The results demonstrated that constituents of *H. perforatum* were capable of inhibiting biotransformations mediated by both CYPs, CYP2D6 and CYP3A. Likewise, Budzinski et al. demonstrated that commercial tinctures of St. John's wort and hypericin, a principal component of these tinctures, were capable of inhibiting cDNA-expressed CYP3A4- mediated metabolism of 7-benzyloxyresorufin. Although the crude extracts and purified constituents of St. John's wort were relatively good inhibitors of CYP3A in vitro, the subsequent in vivo studies failed to confirm these observations. It is clear from the current body of literature that the coadministration of St. John's wort with many therapeutic agents, especially those that are CYP3A substrates, results in reduced serum concentration and diminished drug efficacy. These observations are consistent with increased drug elimination.

CYP3A4 and P-glycoprotein are transcriptionally regulated by an orphan nuclear receptor designated as the pregnane X receptor (PXR). Small molecule ligands such as rifampicin bind to PXR and encourage heterodimerization of PXR with the retinoid X receptor. mRNA synthesis of numerous target genes is stimulated after this complex undergoes trans- location to complimentary sequences in the regulatory region of the genes. Moore et al. examined the effect of extracts of commercial St. John's wort preparations on CYP3A4 mRNA expression in cultures of human hepatocytes. CYP3A4 mRNA expression was induced in human hepatocytes treated for 30 hours with either extracts of commercial St. John's wort preparations or purified hyperforin. Additional experiments conducted by this group employing CV-1 cells transiently transfected with both a PXR expression vector and a human chloramphenicol acetyltransferase reporter system containing a PXR-binding site demonstrated that hypericum extract and hyperforin, but not hypericin, induced CYP3A4 mRNA expression via activation of the PXR. Hyperforin has an EC_{50} for the activation of PXR of around 20 nM and is one of the most potent inducers discovered to date.

In vitro studies indicate that other constituents of St. John's wort, such as hypericin, kampferol, pseudohypericin, and hyperoside, are not PXR ligands and thus do not contribute to the enhanced CYP3A4 mRNA expression. Likewise, Wentworth et al., using a reporter gene construct containing the ligand-binding domain of the CYP3A promoter, determined that hyperforin but not hypericin was capable of activating CYP3A transcription when coexpressed with the steroid X receptor, which is synonymous with PXR. Hyperforin but not hypericin interacts directly with the receptor ligand–binding domain of PXR and contributes to the recruitment of steroid receptor coactivator-1 with an efficiency that is comparable to that of rifampicin. In addition, hyperforin has been shown to induce other PXR-responsive genes, such as CYP2C9, CYP2C19, CYP2B6, and p-glycoprotein (MDR-1), by mechanisms that may involve both the PXR- and the constitutive androstane receptor (CAR)-responsive elements, but the extent of induction of these genes is modest compared to that of CYP3A. In the case of the CYP2C9 gene, a PXR-responsive element was identified –1839/–1 824 base pairs upstream from translation start site at the same location as the CAR-responsive element. Komoroski et al. reported increased mRNA and protein expression and catalytic activity following exposure of human hepatocytes to hyperforin, confirming the in vivo observations (*vide infra*) concerning CYP2C9 and CYP3A4 induction by St. John's wort. The treatment of human hepatocytes with hyperforin did not alter CYP1A2 expression (mRNA and protein) or catalytic activity. In vitro, studies using LS-180 cells have demonstrated that hyperforin was capable of inducing the PXR-dependent expression of P-glycoprotein by western blot analysis, and functionally reduced the cellular uptake of the P-glycoprotein substrate, rhodamine 123.

Role of CYP3A in Drug Interactions

The most abundant CYPs in humans belong to the CYP3A subfamily, which accounts for up to 60% of total hepatic and up to 90% of total intestinal CYP. Like other CYPs, CYP3A family members are heme-containing proteins that along with the conjugating enzymes, such as the sulfotransferases (SULTs) and glucuronosyltransferases (UGTs), are instrumental in metabolizing a wide variety of endogenous and exogenous agents. The human CYP3A subfamily includes four members, namely CYP3A4, CYP3A5, CYP3A7, and CYP3A43. CYP3A4 is abundantly expressed in all adults and is responsible for the metabolism of a wide variety of structurally diverse chemicals including macrolide antibiotics, 3-hydroxy-3-methylgluatryl coenzyme A (HMG-CoA)–reductase inhibitors, HIV protease inhibitors, benzodiazepines, and immunosuppressants. It has been estimated that approximately 40% to 50% of drugs requiring metabolism for elimination undergo biotransformation by CYP3A4. The CYP3A5*1 gene product is detected in about 30% of Caucasian and 70% of African-American human livers and intestines and has comparable catalytic activity and substrate selectivity to CYP3A4, although there are important exceptions to this generalization. CYP3A7 is expressed only in fetal tissue and the level of expression and catalytic activity of CYP3A43 are extremely low and consequently, an important role for these enzymes in drug metabolism is not anticipated.

The expression of CYP3A4 and CYP3A5 at both the intestine and liver results in a greater first-pass removal of CYP3A substrates than would be predicted if the liver was the sole organ of removal. For example, the CYP3A substrates cyclosporine, nifedipine, midazolam, and verapamil exhibit low oral bioavailability because of the substantial contribution of both intestinal wall and hepatic metabolism to their first-pass elimination in man. In view of the broad substrate selectivity, along with expression in both the enterocyte and hepatocyte, it is not surprising that modulation of CYP3A expression and activity by environment, disease, and other drugs, such as St. John's wort, is a significant public health issue with implications in regard to drug safety and efficacy. The remaining portion of the chapter will review the reported interactions between St. John's wort and prescription medications.

Interactions with CYP3A Substrates

Anticancer agents

Irinotecan is a topoisomerase-I inhibitor, which is used in the treatment of colorectal and non-small cell lung cancer. Individuals diagnosed with cancer routinely become depressed and may require pharmacotherapy with prescription or botanical antidepressants. Mathijssen et al. reported that the disposition of 7-ethyl-10-hydroxycamptothecin (SN-38), the active metabolite of irinotecan, was altered following coadministration of St. John's wort to five individuals. SN-38 levels were reduced 43%, while plasma concentrations of irinotecan remained unaltered. The formation of a CYP3A-mediated metabolite of SN-38, 7-ethyl-10-[4-N-(5-aminopentanoic acid)-1-piperidino]-carbonyl-oxy-camptothecin

(APC), did not appear to be significantly altered, although the APC/irinotecan serum ratio was reduced by 28%. Likewise, SN-38 glucuronidation was not altered by St. John's wort. The investigators concluded that St. John's wort and irinotecan should not be coadministered.

Imatinib is an inhibitor of the protein tyrosine kinase involved with platelet-derived growth factor (Bcr-ABL). A loss of cellular control of this tyrosine kinase has been identified as a key mechanism for malignant cell growth. The ability of imatinib to inhibit Bcr-ABL provides a rationale for its use in the treatment of human cancers such as Philadelphia chromosome–positive chronic myologenous leukemia. CYP3A4 plays a principal role in the biotransformation of imatinib. The effect of St. John's wort on imatinib disposition was investigated in 12 healthy volunteers using a two-period, open-labeled, fixed-sequence study by Frye et al. Imatinib (400 mg) was administered before and after the administration of St. John's wort [300 mg; Kira (LI 160), Lichtwer Pharma AG, Berlin, Germany] three times a day for 14 days. The administration of St. John's wort resulted in 30% reduction in imatinib exposure from 34.5 ± 9.5 to 24.2 ± 7.0 μg hr/mL. A corresponding 43% increase in the oral clearance of imatinib was observed following St. John's wort dosing. Frye et al. concluded that the imatinib–St. John's wort (drug–botanical product) interaction is clinically significant and may result in a loss of imatinib efficacy.

Anticonvulsants

Carbamazepine is a dibenzazepine carboxamide derivative that is used to treat epilepsy and other neurologic conditions. A substrate of CYP3A, carbamazepine, is also recognized as a potent in vivo and in vitro inducer of CYP3A4 (74–77). Induction of CYP3A4 by carbamazepine is mediated at least in part through activation of PXR, although other mechanisms such as glucorticoid receptor–activation have been proposed. The effect of St. John's wort administration (300 mg t.i.d. × 14 days) on carbamazepine disposition at steady state was examined in eight healthy adults. The oral clearance of carbamazepine (2.8 ± 0.3 L/hr) was not significantly altered by St. John's wort (2.9 ± 0.6 L/hr) administration. Likewise, the area under the plasma concentration–time curve (AUC) at steady state of the CYP3A4-mediated metabolite carbamazepine 10,11-epoxide was not altered by St. John's wort dosing (37.5 ±7.4 vs. 41.9 ± 10.9 mg hr/L). These data indicate that a 14-day course of therapy with St. John's wort does not enhance the elimination of carbamazepine. This may reflect a lack of influence of intestinal CYP3A4 on carbamazepine disposition, given that the oral availability of carbamazepine approaches unity. In addition, the product used in this study may have lacked sufficient quantities of hyperforin to induce hepatic CYP3A4 activity. Also, many anticonvulsants (phenobarbital, carbamazepine, and phenytoin) are CYP3A inducers and modulate their own pharmacokinetics via enzyme induction. The lack of effect of St. John's wort on carbamazepine disposition may therefore reflect the possibility that the enzyme system (CYP3A4) is already close to maximal induction.

Antihypertensives

Nifedipine is a dihydropyridine calcium channel modulator, often used in the treatment of hypertension and angina. CYP3A4, with a minor contribution from CYP3A5, is the principal enzyme involved in the metabolism of nifedipine. Smith et al. examined the effect of St. John's wort (900 mg/day for 18 days) on nifedipine disposition by examining changes in C_{MAX} in 22 healthy volunteers. St. John's wort coadministration reduced the maximum nifedipine plasma concentration obtained by approximately 50%, following a 10 mg oral dose. It is to be expected that other dihydropyridine calcium channel blockers that rely on CYP3A for their metabolism (e.g., isradapine and nimodipine) will be similarly affected by St. John's wort administration.

Verapamil is a diphenylalkylamine calcium channel modulator that is widely used in the treatment of hypertension, angina, and cardiac arrhythmias. Verapamil is extensively metabolized by the CYP3A enzymes. Tannergren et al. examined the effect of St. John's wort on the jejunal transport and presystemic extraction of single-dose verapamil in eight healthy male volunteers using a fixed-order design (control–treatment). St. John's wort 300 mg was administered three times daily for 14 days. The administration of St. John's wort did not alter the cellular permeability of verapamil, but did increase the excretion of the CYP3A-mediated metabolite norverapamil into the intestine. Furthermore, jejunal transport of the verapamil enantiomers was not altered by St. John's wort pretreatment. St. John's wort administration resulted in an 89% reduction in R- and S-verapamil plasma concentrations. Verapamil has also been shown to inactivate CYP3A4 through the formation of a metabolic intermediate complex and is also a modest inducer of CYP3A4. The effect of St. John's wort on the disposition of verapamil at steady state has not been assessed and is not readily predictable from single-dose data. Unless proven otherwise, it would be prudent to expect that the coadministration of St. John's wort with verapamil will result in decreased verapamil concentrations and possibly efficacy.

Antiretroviral agents

Indinavir is a protease inhibitor used in the management of HIV infection. CYP3A4 mediates the biotransformation of indinavir in vitro, and in vivo, indinavir has been shown to be a potent competitive and mechanism-based inhibitor of CYP3A4. Piscitelli and coworkers examined the effect of St. John's wort (300 mg t.i.d. × 14 days) administration on indinavir (800 mg q.i.d. × 8 hr × four doses) exposure in eight healthy volunteers (two females). The administration of St. John's wort for 14 days resulted in a significant 54% reduction in the indinavir eight- hour area under the concentration–time curve, from 35.8 ± 13.0 to 15.6 ± 5.8 μg × hr/mL. The authors conclude that the magnitude in the reduction in indinavir concentrations may result in the development of antiretroviral resistance and subsequent treatment failure.

Nevirapine is a non-nucleoside reverse transcriptase inhibitor used in the treatment of AIDS. Elimination of nevirapine from the body occurs via P-glycoprotein, and it is extensively metabolized by the CYPs. In addition, nevirapine dosing is known to increase CYP3A and CYP2B6 enzymes by approximately 25%. This induction appears to be mediated by the orphan nuclear factor PXR. de Maat et al. reported data from five HIV-1-infected individuals who were treated with nevirapine and coadministered St. John's wort for several months. The median oral clearance of nevirapine for all patients (n = 171) was 3.2 L/hr (range 2.7–3.9); for the five individuals taking St. John's wort, the median oral clearance of nevirapine on St. John's wort was 4.3 (range 3.8–4.7 L/hr), whereas the median oral clearance without St. John's wort coadministration was 3.3 L/hr (range 3.2–4.2 L/hr). The authors concluded that the coadministration of St. John's wort resulted in a 35% increase in median oral clearance of nevirapine and that dose adjustment is indicated.

Benzodiazepines

Midazolam

Midazolam is a 1,4-imidazobenzodiazepine that is widely employed therapeutically as a sedative/hypnotic in major and minor surgical procedures. In humans, midazolam is primarily eliminated from the body by CYP3A-mediated metabolism to the major primary metabolite, 1-hydroxymidazolam, and to a much lesser extent to 4-hydroxymidazolam. Midazolam is widely used as a selective metabolic probe for assessing CYP3A activity in vivo, because it is not a substrate for the P-glycoprotein efflux transporter. Following intravenous administration, less than 1% of the dose is excreted unchanged in the urine. Consequently, the clearance of midazolam following intravenous administration has proven to be an effective index of hepatic CYP3A activity in vivo. Up to 75% of the first-pass loss of midazolam following oral administration occurs in the intestinal wall using the simultaneous administration of oral and intravenous drug. Additionally, approximately 90% of the variability in oral availability was accounted for by variations in intestinal availability alone.

Wang et al. demonstrated that multiple-dose St. John's wort dosing resulted in a 50% reduction in the midazolam oral AUC and maximum serum drug concentration and a corresponding doubling of the oral clearance, from 122 ± 71 to 255 ± 128 L/hr. In contrast, the systemic clearance of midazolam increased from 34.3 ± 10.8 to 43.6 ± 15.8 L/hr, but this change was not significant. The oral bioavailability demonstrated a significant decrease from 0.28 ± 0.15 to 0.17 ± 0.06, but changes in hepatic and intestinal availability were not significant. Similar results were observed following St. John's wort administration for eight weeks in a group of 12 women. These changes are in good agreement with the observation of Du¨rr et al. who reported a 1.5-fold increase in intestinal CYP3A4 expression and a 1.4-fold increase in erythromycin breath test.

Dresser et al. administered St. John's wort (LI 160 300 mg t.i.d.) to 20 ethnically diverse individuals and observed a 44% increase in the systemic clearance of midazolam. In contrast, the oral clearance of midazolam was increased 1.7-fold. The combined changes in midazolam disposition resulted in a significant reduction in the oral bioavailability of midazolam. Gurley et al. examined the one-hour 1-hydroxymidazolam-to-midazolam serum ratio and concluded that St. John's wort administration for 28 days resulted in a significant increase in the ratio, which is indicative of CYP3A4 induction.

Alprazolam

Markowitz et al. initially reported that St. John's wort administration did not alter the disposition of alprazolam following oral dosing. It was subsequently determined that the duration of St. John's wort administration (three days) was insufficient to demonstrate the inductive effects of this botanical medicine on CYP3A4. In a follow-up study in which St. John's wort was administered for 14 days, there was more than a doubling of the oral clearance of alprazolam, from 3.7 ± 0.9 to 8.4 ± 3.2 L/hr. There was also a corresponding reduction in the elimination half-life by approximately 50%, from 12 ± 4 to 6.0 ± 2.0 hours. However, the maximum plasma concentration and the time to maximum concentration were not significantly different before and after St. John's wort dosing. The change in oral clearance is consistent with a change in the systemic elimination but not first- pass elimination of alprazolam, because the maximum serum alprazolam concentration achieved was not significantly different before and after St. John's wort administration. This is to be expected, considering that the oral bioavailability of alprazolam is high (>0.8), which is consistent with alprazolam being a low-affinity substrate for CYP3A4.

HMG-CoA–reductase inhibitors

Sugimoto et al. examined the effect of St. John's wort administration (300 mg three times a day for 14 days) on the disposition of simvastatin and pravastatin in 16 healthy male Japanese subjects in a double-blind crossover study. The administration of St. John's wort significantly reduced the mean maximum plasma concentration from 3.6 ± 1.0 to 2.5 ± 0.7 after oral simvastatin (10 mg) dosing and a corresponding 48% reduction in the mean systemic exposure to simvastatin, from 11.1 ± 3.7 to 5.8 ± 1.8 ng hr/mL. The authors reported similar results for the active metabolite (simvastatin hydroxy acid) of simvastatin. In contrast to the significant changes observed with simvastatin, St. John's wort administration (300 mg three times a day for 14 days) did not significantly alter the mean maximum plasma concentration achieved following pravastatin (20 mg) administration (36.5 ± 5.7 ng/mL before vs. 30.8 ± 5.2 ng/mL after). Likewise, significant differences in the mean systemic exposure to pravastatin were not observed following placebo (109.4 ± 17.4 ng hr/mL) and St. John's wort (96.6 ± 13.4 ng hr/mL) dosing. The differences reflect the fact that simvastatin is a substrate for CYP3A4 and P-glycoprotein, whereas pravastatin is not a substrate for either CYP3A or P-glycoprotein (MDR1). Similar effects are expected for other HMG-CoA–reductase inhibitors, such as lovastatin, cerivastatin, and atorvastatin, which rely on CYP3A4 and P-glycoprotein for their distribution and elimination. In the case of the CYP2C9 substrate, fluvastatin, a drug interaction between St. John's wort and fluvastatin is expected to be at most modest, even though there is evidence that St. John's wort alters CYP2C9 expression in vitro. This is because Wang et al. did not observe an alteration in the disposition of the prototypic CYP2C9 probe drug, tolbutamide, in a group of 12 healthy volunteers.

Immunosuppressants

Cyclosporine is a calcineurin-inhibitor immunosuppressant that is in part metabolized by CYP3A4/5 and transported by P-glycoprotein (MDR1). Coadministration of St. John's wort with cyclosporine has resulted in significant reduction in circulating cyclosporine concentrations, which has led to graft rejection. Breidenbach et al. reported a series of 30 renal transplant recipients who were stabilized on cyclosporine and subsequently administered St. John's wort. Following initiation of St. John's wort therapy, blood cyclosporine concentrations were reduced 47% (range: 33–62%) and the corresponding cyclosporine doses were increased on average 47% (15–115%), to maintain therapeutic cyclosporine blood concentrations. Cessation of St. John's wort dosing resulted in a 187% (84–292%) rise in blood cyclosporine concentration, which required subsequent cyclosporine dose adjustment. These changes

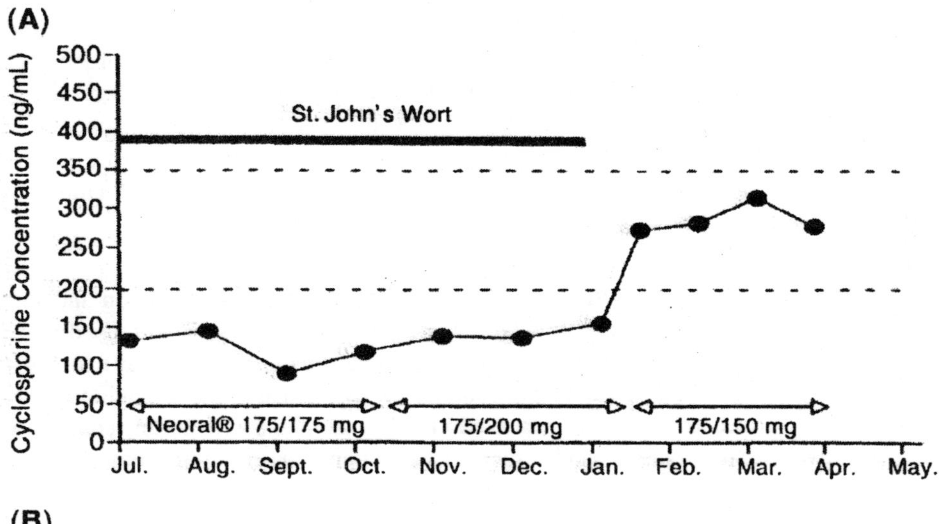

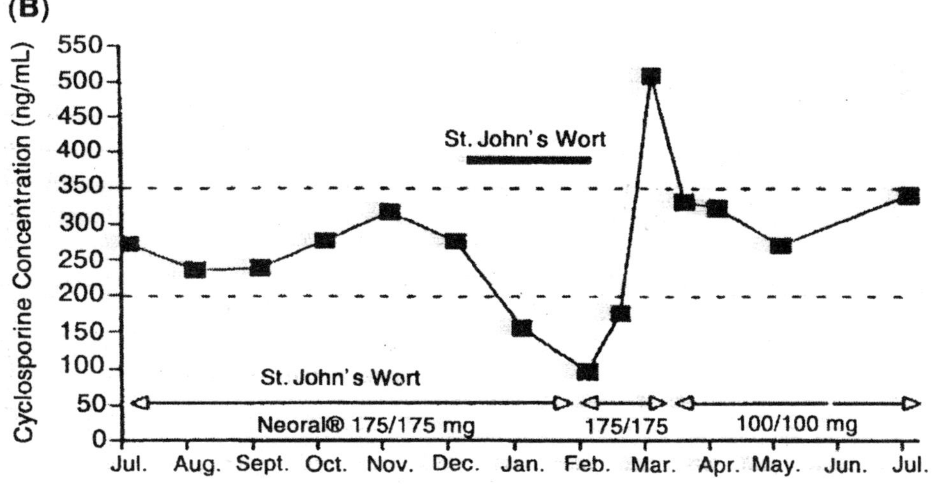

Fig. 7.2. A–Chronology of CSA through concentrations in patient 1 self-mediating with SJW (dotted lines). B–Chronology of CSA trough concentration in patient 2 self-medicating with SJW (dotted lines)

have been confirmed by others. Barone et al. reported the occurrence of acute graft rejection in two kidney transplant patients and Ruschitzka et al. reported a similar loss of immunosuppression in cardiac transplant patients. Bauer et al. also examined the effect of St. John's wort administration on the disposition of cyclosporine and its metabolites in 11 renal allograft recipients. St. John's wort was administered for 15 days and cyclosporine plasma concentrations were adjusted every four days by assessing trough concentrations. The investigators demonstrated that St. John's wort administration resulted in a 45% decrease in cyclosporine exposure compared to baseline. Likewise, metabolite exposure was altered significantly following St. John's wort administration with metabolites AM1c and AM1, demonstrating a 60% decrease after dose correction, but exposure to the metabolites AM9 and AM19 was not affected. In addition, the interaction between cyclosporine and St. John's wort was confirmed by Dresser et al., with the oral clearance increasing 63% from 728 ± 195 to 1155 ± 236 mL/min.

Tacrolimus is a calcineurin-inhibitor immunosuppressive used to prevent organ rejection following kidney and liver transplantation. The disposition of tacrolimus, like cyclosporine, is dependent on both CYP3A activity and P-glycoprotein activity. Circulating tacrolimus concentrations were reduced following the administration of St. John's wort. Hebert et al. examined the effect of St. John's wort (300 mg t.i.d. × 18 days) coadministration on the oral disposition of tacrolimus. The oral clearance of tacrolimus increased from 349 ± 126 to 586 ± 275 mL/hr/kg and a corresponding 35% decrease in the AUC from 307 ± 176 to 199 ± 140 μg hr/L was observed. The disposition pharmacokinetics of the adjunct agent, mycophenolic acid, was not altered following coadministration with St. John's wort. It is clear from these reports that individuals who require immunosuppressive therapy to maintain transplanted organ function should not receive St. John's wort.

Opioids

Methadone is a long-acting opiate that is used in the treatment of opiate addiction and for analgesia. Eich-Hochli et al. described four addicts in whom St. John's wort (Jarsin) was coadministered with three daily doses of methadone. The administration of St. John's wort (900 mg/day) for 14 to 47 days (median 31 days) resulted in trough methadone concentrations, which were a median of 47% (range 19–60%) of the original concentration. The observed changes in methadone serum concentrations were not enantiomer selective, because both R- and S-methadone trough concentrations demonstrated reductions of similar magnitude. Two female patients reported symptoms suggestive of withdrawal and requested increases in their methadone dose.

Oral contraceptives

Oral contraceptives are combination products that are typically used to prevent pregnancy. The combination of an estrogen (17-alphaethinylestradiol) and a progestin (e.g., norethindrone) is used to prevent the release of the oocyte (egg) and to alter the cervical mucous and lining of the uterus. Drugs that induce CYP3A enzymes have been associated with reduced oral contraceptive efficacy or even failure. The metabolism of the components of oral contraceptives, ethinylestradiol and norethindrone, is thought to be catalyzed at least in part by intestinal and hepatic CYP3A. A number of reports have indicated that St. John's wort may be responsible for the occurrence of breakthrough bleeding in women formerly stabilized on oral contraceptives.

In addition, "*miracle babies*" have been identified in the lay press to be a result of St. John's wort consumption. Furthermore, Schwarz et al. reported oral contraceptive failure in four women after St. John's wort coadministration, which resulted in the termination of the unwanted pregnancies. Subsequently, Hall et al. examined the effect of St. John's wort administration on the disposition and efficacy of the oral contraceptive components, ethinylestradiol and norethindrone (Ortho-Novum 1/35), in 12 healthy females. St. John's wort (Sundown Herbals) was administered three times a day for eight weeks. The pharmacokinetics of ethinylestradiol and norethindrone (CYP3A substrates) were assessed before and six weeks after the start of the St. John's wort dosing. St. John's wort significantly ($P \leq 0.05$) increased the oral clearance of norethindrone from 8.2 ± 2.7 to 9.5 ± 2.4 L/hr, with a corresponding decrease in the peak serum concentration of norethindrone (from 17.4 ± 5.1 to 16.4 ±5.2 ng/mL; $P < 0.05$). Likewise, the elimination half-life of ethinylestradiol was significantly reduced from 23 ±20 to 12 ±7 hours.

Furthermore, the incidence of breakthrough bleeding increased with the duration of St. John's wort administration with 7 of 12 individuals having breakthrough bleeding compared to two individuals prior to initiation of St. John's wort dosing. In good agreement with the observation of Hall et al., Pfrunder et al. reported that St. John's wort given twice daily or three times a day resulted in a greater incidence in break-through bleeding, 13/17 or 15/17, respectively, compared to oral contraceptive (20 μg ethinylestradiol and 150 μg desogestrel) dosing alone. Although, pharmacokinetic changes were not observed for ethinylestradiol, the maximum plasma concentration and the AUC of 3-ketodesogestrel decreased 18% and 44%, respectively, during twice-daily dosing of St. John's wort. It is clear that the combination of St. John's wort with oral contraceptive has resulted in the induction of norethindrone clearance, increased incidence of breakthrough bleeding, and reports of unplanned pregnancy and resultant termination. Thus, the coadministration of St. John's wort in women taking oral contraceptives is contraindicated and should be discouraged. To prevent this interaction, it is the author's opinion that all St. John's wort products must clearly carry warning labels concerning the potential for St. John's wort to alter the efficacy of oral contraceptives and of many other prescription products.

Interactions with Substrates of Other P450s

Theophylline

Theophylline is a bronchodilator that is commonly used to treat the symptoms of chronic asthma. The principal enzyme involved in the biotransformation of theophylline is CYP1A2. In a case report, Nebel et al. described an individual who required theophylline dosage adjustment following the initiation and cessation of St. John's wort pharmacotherapy. The dose of theophylline (Theodur) was increased from 300 mg twice daily to 800 mg twice daily following the initiation of St. John's wort intake. The resultant steady-state theophylline concentration was 9.2 μg/mL. Subsequently, termination of St. John's wort resulted in a twofold increase in serum theophylline concentration and necessitated dose reduction. Preliminary in vitro experiments conducted suggested that hypericin and pseudohypericin were capable of activating the xenobiotic response element, which is responsible in part for CYP1A2 induction. However, it should be noted the individual described in the case report by Nebel et al. was a smoker taking a multitude of other medications, including furosemide, morphine, zolpidem, valproic acid, ibuprofen, amitriptyline, albuterol, prednisone, and zafirlukast. Zafirlukast has been shown to be an inhibitor of theophylline both in vitro and in vivo.

Thus, the observed changes in theophylline disposition may be a result of St. John's wort altering the disposition of one of the many concurrent medications. In addition, a study by Morimoto et al. failed to confirm the observation of Nebel et al. Briefly, Morimoto et al. examined the potential for St. John's wort to alter the disposition of theophylline in vivo by conducting a randomized open-label crossover study. The oral clearance of theophylline was determined in 12 healthy Japanese men before and after 15 days of St. John's wort administration (300mg three times daily). St. John's wort did not alter the oral clearance of theophylline (2.3 ± 0.6 L/hr vs. 2.4 ± 0.6 L/hr).

Caffeine

Caffeine is a methylxanthine that is a central nervous system stimulant found in a number of beverages such as coffee, tea, soda (Pepsi, Coke, Mountain Dew, etc.), and over-the-counter products (Vivarin, NoDoz, etc.). Caffeine is principally metabolized to paraxanthine by CYP1A2 and the six-hour plasma ratio (paraxanthine to caffeine) has been used as an index of in vivo CYP1A2 activity. The administration of St. John's wort (300 mg three times daily) for two weeks did not alter the disposition of caffeine. In the same study, Wang et al. reported that a single dose of St. John's wort (900 mg) did not affect the oral clearance of caffeine. Likewise, Wenk et al. examined the effect of 14 days of St. John's wort administration (300 mg t.i.d., $n = 16$) on the in vivo activities of CYP3A4, CYP1A2, and CYP2D6 using 6β-hydroxycortisol-to-cortisol urinary ratio, paraxanthine-to-caffeine salivary ratio, and dextromethorphan-to-dextrorphan urinary metabolic ratio, respectively. The mean values for the salivary estimates of CYP1A2 were not significantly altered by treatment with St. John's wort. This observation is in good agreement with the observation of Morimoto et al. with St. John's wort and theophylline (*supra vide*). In addition, Komoroski et al. noted that hyperforin did not alter the mRNA expression, protein expression, or catalytic activity of CYP1A2 in human hepatocytes. These observations taken together suggest that interactions between CYP1A2 substrates and St. John's wort are unlikely.

Omeprazole

H. perforatum II 300 mg was used in assessing the effect of St. John's wort on the pharmacokinetics of a single dose of omeprazole. A placebo-controlled randomized crossover study was conducted over a five-week period in 12 individuals. Six individuals had CYP2C19 * 1/ *1 and six individuals had either *2/*2 ($n = 4$) or *2/*3 ($n = 2$) genotypes. The sulfoxidation of omeprazole is mediated primarily by CYP3A4 and the 5-hydroxylation of omeprazole is mediated principally by CYP2C19. Administration of St. John's wort 300 mg three times a day for 14 days resulted in a significant reduction in the AUC of omeprazole in both homozygous wild-type individuals and homozygous variant individuals. A corresponding increase in the principal metabolites for both CYP2C19 (5-hydroxyomeprazole) and CYP3A4 (omeprazole sulfone)-mediated biotransformations demonstrated increased AUCs following St. John's wort administration. The authors suggest that the study provides evidence for in vivo CYP2C19 induction by St. John's wort.

Warfarin

Warfarin is an anticoagulant that is administered as a racemic mixture with the S-enantiomer having most of the pharmacologic activity. Warfarin is extensively metabolized in the liver by CYP2C9 with 7-hydroxylation being the principal route of metabolism for the S-enantiomer. R-warfarin is 8-hydroxylated, 6-hydroxylated, and 10-hydroxylated by CYP2C19, CYP1A2, and CYP3A4, respectively. Likewise, additional enzymes are involved in the metabolism of the S-warfarin, namely CYP3A4 and CYP1A2. In light of the overlap between the P450s involved in warfarin metabolism and those affected by St. John's wort, namely CYP2C9, CYP2C19, and CYP3A4, it is clear that an interaction between St. John's wort and warfarin is possible. To determine the potential for interaction, Jiang et al. examined the effect of St. John's wort administration on the pharmacokinetics and pharmacodynamics of warfarin (25 mg) administered to 12 healthy male volunteers.

The oral clearance of S- and R-warfarin was increased 36% and 29%, from 198 ± 38 to 270 ± 44 mL/min and from 110 ± 25 to 142 ± 29 mL/min, respectively. A corresponding reduction in the pharmacodynamic effect was observed with St. John's wort (one tablet three times a day for two weeks) dosing, significantly reducing the area under the effect curve of the international normalized ratio of pro- thrombin time by approximately 20% from 111 ± 49.3 to 88.3 ± 30.7. Although the data quite clearly indicate that St. John's wort and warfarin should not be coadministered, the enzyme(s) responsible for the increased clearance of S- and R-warfarin in vivo cannot be determined, because changes in metabolite formation were not assessed. Thus, it is possible that the observed changes in S- and R-warfarin clearance were a result of a St. John's wort–mediated induction of CYP2C9, CYP2C19, CYP3A4, or some combination of these enzymes.

Role of P-Glycoprotein in St. Johns's Wort Interaction

Fexofenadine

Fexofenadine is a nonsedating antihistamine that has been shown to be transported by P-glycoprotein (MDR1) and organic anion transport poly- peptide in vitro using cell culture models and MDR1 knockout animals. Wang et al. demonstrated that the administration of St. John's wort for 14 days resulted in a significant increase in the oral clearance of fexofenadine observed after a single 900mg dose of St. John's wort, from 62 ± 26 L/hr to 91 ± 32 L/hr. In good agreement with the observations of Wang et al., Dresser et al. observed a significant reduction in the maximum plasma concentration and a 94% increase in the oral clearance of fexofenadine following the administration of St. John's wort (Jarsin 300 three times daily for two weeks). The increase in the oral clearance of fexofenadine reported by these two groups is consistent with PXR-mediated induction of P-glycoprotein (MDR1) by St. John's wort.

Digoxin

Digoxin is a cardiac glycoside that is used traditionally in the treatment of congestive heart failure and is a substrate of the transporter P-glycoprotein. Johne et al. conducted a single-blind, placebo-controlled parallel study in 25 healthy volunteers (12 women). Volunteers were given a 0.25 mg loading dose of digoxin followed by 0.125 mg daily for 10 days. On day 6 of digoxin dosing, a single 900 mg (three tablet) dose of St. John's wort (LI 160) or placebo was administered and on day 15 of digoxin dosing (10 days of St. John's wort or placebo), the pharmacokinetic study was repeated. Single dose of St. John's wort had no effect on the pharmacokinetics of digoxin. In contrast, 10 days of St. John's wort dosing resulted in significant 25% decrease in the AUC from 0 to 24 hours and a corresponding 24% decrease in the maximum plasma concentration. Treatment with placebo did not alter the pharmacokinetic parameters of digoxin.

Likewise, Dürr et al. demonstrated an 18% reduction in digoxin exposure with a corresponding increase in intestinal P-glycoprotein/MDR1 and CYP3A4. In agreement with the above results, Mueller et al. reported that hyperforin-rich St. John's wort products (i.e., LI 160) resulted in a significant 25% reduction in the 24-hour area under the digoxin concentration–time curve. The observation with fexofenadine and digoxin are in good agreement. It is clear that P-glycoprotein, along with CYP3A4, provides a competent barrier to the absorption of xenobiotics. The administration of St. John's wort for a period of two weeks results in a reduction in drug exposure due to the increased efflux activity of P-glycoprotein at the brush border membrane of enterocytes. For drugs that are not substrates of CYP3A, the increased expression of P-glycoprotein results in a reduced bioavailability but no change in the elimination half-life. This pattern of interaction is suggestive of an alteration in first-pass elimination but not systemic clearance.

Echinacea

Echinacea is a widely available over-the-counter botanical remedy used for the treatment of the common cold, coughs, bronchitis, "flu," and inflammation of the mouth and pharynx. It is one of the more popular botanical remedies with a sales ranking of 5 and sales of US $70 million. About 10% to 20% of the adult and child botanical users consume echinacea routinely. Three species of *echinacea* (*Echinacea purpurea*, *E. angustinfolia*, and *E. pallida*) have been used medicinally. However, only the aboveground parts of *E. purpura* and the root of *E. pallida* have been approved for oral administration by the German E Commission.

The beneficial effect of *echinacea* in the treatment of infections appears to be a result of its ability to stimulate the host's immune system. Following exposure to *echinacea*, macrophages and T-lymphocytes demonstrate increased phagocytic activity and release of immunomodulators such as tumor necrosis factor-a and interferons. Although the exact mechanism of echinacea immunostimulatory effect is unknown, controlled studies suggest that the oral administration of echinacea is beneficial in the early treatment of upper respiratory infections. However, this observation is still controversial and the usefulness of long-term echinacea administration to prevent illness appears to be limited. Although echinacea appears to be well tolerated following acute and chronic dosing, the unsupervised self-medication by patients in an effort to cure, ameliorate, and/or prevent sickness provides the potential for a multitude of drug–botanical product interactions.

Budzinski et al. examined the capability of 5% to 10% (v/v) dilutions of marketed *echinacea* tinctures to inhibit the metabolism of 7-benzyloxyresorufin by cDNA-expressed CYP3A4. The relative inhibitory concentration, in relation to the full-strength product for *E. angustifolia* roots, *E. purpurea* roots, *E. angustifolia/purpurea* mixture (1:1), and *E. purpurea* tops was 1.1%, 4.0%, 6.7%, and 8.6%, respectively. The effect of these echinacea extracts on the in vitro catalytic activity of other drug-metabolizing enzymes (e.g., CYP1A2, CYP2C9, and CYP2D6) has not been assessed. However, extracts of teas prepared from combination products containing echinacea plus other botanical products (e.g., goldenseal, lemon grass leaf, spearmint leaf, and wild cherry bark) have inhibited drug metabolism mediated by cDNA-expressed CYP2C9, CYP2C19, and CYP2D6. The effect of extracts of *E. purpurea* on other hepatic and intestinal enzyme systems such as UGTs and SULTs has not been reported.

Although in vitro data suggest that echinacea products may be inhibitory, Gorski et al. observed a mixed effect in vivo. The effect of *E. purpurea* on the in vivo activity of CYP1A2, CYP2C9, CYP2D6, and CYP3A4 was investigated in 12 healthy volunteers (six males). This two-period, open-label, fixed-order study involved the administration of a cocktail of probes (caffeine, dextromethorphan, tolbutamide, and intravenous and oral midazolam) that were administered before and after eight days of *echinacea* (400 mg four times daily) dosing. Briefly, echinacea reduced the oral clearance of caffeine and tolbutamide by 27% and 11%, respectively. Although the change in tolbutamide clearance was statistically significant, the clinical relevance of the observed change is unclear. It appears from this study that echinacea does not alter the in vivo catalytic activity of CYP2D6, as reflected by the absence of change in the oral clearance of dextromethorphan. In contrast to the activity of these enzymes, hepatic and intestinal CYP3A alterations are a little less clear.

The systemic clearance of midazolam, a reflection of hepatic CYP3A activity, was increased significantly. In light of the enhanced systemic elimination of midazolam and considering the "well-stirred" model of hepatic elimination, it is predicted that the oral clearance of midazolam should be increased and midazolam exposure reduced. Or in other words, the oral clearance reflects the contribution of both intestinal and hepatic CYP3A to first-pass elimination and hepatic CYP3A to the systemic elimination of midazolam. However, the oral clearance of midazolam was not significantly altered by *echinacea* dosing. In addition, the oral availability of midazolam (F_{PO}) was significantly increased from 0.23 ± 0.06 to 0.33 ± 0.13. Given the relationship between hepatic (F_H) and intestinal (F_G) availabilities and oral bioavailability ($F_{PO} = F_H \times F_G$), it is possible to examine the effect of *echinacea* on these independent sites of CYP3A expression.

As expected from the change in the systemic clearance, the hepatic availability was reduced significantly from 0.72 ± 0.08 to 0.61 ± 0.016. In contrast to the observed enhanced hepatic extraction ($F = 1 - E$) of midazolam caused by echinacea dosing, the intestinal availability of midazolam was enhanced 85% from 0.33 ± 0.11 to 0.61 ± 38, resulting in an unchanged midazolam exposure (AUC) following oral midazolam administration. This observation suggests that intestinal CYP3A is inhibited. The mechanism(s) of the differential effects of echinacea on intestinal and hepatic CYP3A could be due to one or more of the following: (i) intestinal and hepatic CYP3A induction is mediated by tissue-specific activators; (ii) the inducing component is rapidly absorbed and thus the intestine has limited exposure; (iii) hepatic and intestinal CYP3A are induced, but there is a potent inhibitor of CYP3A which is not systemically available; and (iv) a metabolite of a constituent of the echinacea preparation is responsible for the induction of hepatic CYP3A but not intestinal CYP3A. It is interesting that Gurley et al. reported no effect of echinacea on CYP3A; however, midazolam was only administered as an oral dose. The differential effect of echinacea on intestinal and hepatic CYP3A complicates the predication of drug interactions with other CYP3A substrates. For instance, drugs that undergo minimal first-pass elimination by the intestine and liver may demonstrate an increased oral clearance as expected due to the induction of hepatic CYP3A. However, substrates that undergo high first-pass elimination by the intestine may demonstrate increased serum concentrations due to the inhibitory effect of echinacea on intestinal CYP3A. It is clear from the data presented that caution should be used when echinacea and CYP3A substrates are coadministered.

8

DRUGS AND POISONS FROM PLANTS

In the previous chapter, we discussed drugs that are used medicinally to releive pain or control disease. A large number of same drugs can effect an individual's sense of perception by producing feelings of transquality, invigoration, or otherworldiness. Sometimes people want to escape from, or "alter," reality and thus seek out these drugs, but in excessive quantities, most are toxic. This chapter focuses on plant substances used because of their psychoactive properties, and on the overlapping group of poisons obtained from plants. The psychoactive drugs can be classified on the basis of the chemical nature of the compounds involved, the effects they produce, or thesource from which they are obtained. None of these classification schemes is perfect. The psychological effects of the compounds involved sometimes differ between chemically very similar substances, and a classification based on chemical structure is rather difficult for a nonchemist to remember.

It is difficult to categorises the psychoactive drugs into stimultants or depressants, hallucinogens or narcotics because many drugs can act in a combination of ways. For example, many of the so-called depressants, like the narcotic analgesics (opiates) and the solanaceous alkaloids, can also act as hallucinogens. Stimulants such as nitotine and cocaine will likewise cause vision if taken in sufficient quantities. The word narcotic itself a dangerous and filled with problems because some people use it to refer strictly to those drugs obtained from the opium poppy (as here), while others employ it for any habit-forming drug or even for any drug used illicity. One way of grouping psychoactive drugs by their primary effects, but since this is a botany text, we will follow yet another system and discuss drugs taxonomically in terms of the species from which they are obtained. Caffeine and alcohol these are wildly used. Psychoactive drugs are discussed in next chapter. These are obtined from a variety of plant sources and are economically and culturally important.

CHEMISTRY AND PHARMACOLOGY OF PSYCHOACTIVE DRUGS

Almost all chemicals thathave psychoactive properties contain nitrogen, and most belong to one of the classes of alkaloids. The most notable chemical exception is the active compound of marijuana, Δ-*trans-tetrahydrocannabinol* (THC). Some other alcohols (including ethanol) and terpenes have psychoactive effects and have been designated as hallucinogenic agents. First of all the psychoactive drugs absorbed into the blood stream and transported via circulation to sites where they can exert their effects. Like medicinal drugs, psychoactive drugs can be taken orally, injected into the body, or absorbed through membranes such as those lining the nose, rectum, vagina, or lungs. Once the active compounds enter the bloodstream, they are transported to all parts of the body. A drug may exert its influence in only one place in the the body, but it is still present (at least initially) throughout the bloodstream because blood and the products it carries continuously circulate around the body. As the blood passes through the liver on its cycle, some drugs are degraded in the places where they act, and the breakdown products are picked up by the blood and transported to the kidneys for excretion. In this process of circulation, ending in degradation and excretion, that accounts for the initial "rush" followed by an enventual "wearing off" of a drug's effect.

Most of the psychoactive drugs acts on cell of the central nervous system (the brain and spinal column) and affect very badly as the blood flow to the brain is 10 times that to other tissues. Therefore drugs reach the brain more quickly than tissues. However, blood capillaries around the brain are more tightly packed that those elsewhere and are covered by sheaths that make passage of compounds from them into the brain difficult. Thus the actual amounts of drugs that enter the brain are less than the blood flow to it might suggest. Once they have reached the central nervous system. Psychoactive drugs disturbed the natural interactions between nervous, or sensory cells. These cells transmit information by chemical signals.

Neurons release chemical substances called *neurotransmitters* in response to stimulation. Once released, these transmitters flow across the space, or *synapse*, between a transmitting neurons and a receiving neuron. Specific sites on the receptor recognize the transmitted compound and bind briefly with it. Once the compound has been accepted, it triggers a response in the receptor neuron. Among the receptor neurons involved in psychological reactions are those responsible for our perception of pain and emotion, as well as interpretations of audio and visual stimuli. Psychoactive drugs, for the most part, alter or mimic the behaviour of four kinds of natural neurotransmitters: acetylcholine, norepinephrine, serotonin, and neuropeptides. The way in which THC works is still unclear.

Caffeine appears to act as a stimulant by activating intracellular metabolism,and alcohol is a general central nervous system depressant. Acetylchonine is released by neurons of the brain and the peripheral nervous system. It is a neutral transmitting chemicals. It causes muscle contractions and also speed up the heart beat. The compund is synthesized within the transmitting neuron and stored until the neuron is triggered. Once stimulated, the neuron releases acetylcholine into the synaptic region. After a neighbouring neuron has received the chemical at specific places on its dendrite and reacted, the acetylcholine is broken down by an enzyme so that it can no longer produce an effect.

Drugs can effect this sequence by blocking the transmission of acetylcholine (atropine and scopolamine), preventing the breakdown of the chemical, or by mimicking its action (nitotine). The drugs prevent the action of acetylcholine or neurotransmitter, prevent rapid muscle reaction and thus produce a relaxed sensation.

Compounds that prevent acetylcholine breakdown, or mimic its effects, act as stimulants because they cause the receptor neurons to fire at an increased or continuous rate. Norepinephrine is another of the brain's endogenous (made within the body) neurotransmitters. Synthesis of norepinephrine takes place in transmitting neurons and released ofter receiving stimulus. However, after it exerts its effect, norepinephrine is reabsorbed, not broken down. Apparently, the same molecules are reused over and over. Some drugs (e.g., reserpine) deplete norepinephrine. Others such as cocaine prevent reabsorption of norepinephrine or mimic its action (mescaline, myristicine, and elemicin).

Serotonin is a brain neurotransmitter and it acts on the cells regulating body temperature, sensory perceptin, and sleep. Some psychoactive drugs such as the LSD-type compounds appear to alter the functioning of the neurons that transmit serotonin, thereby producing illusions of strange images. Finally, a recently didsovered group of neurotransmitter are peptides, polymers of amino acids. These include enkephalin, beta endorphin, and oxytocin. These chemicals are produced in minute quqntities and are received by very specific receptors. Some of these appear to act like the body's own pain killers. It is believed that opiates effect the same receptor sites as these endogenous pain killers and thus produce a dull, relaxed sensation. The evidence for this hypothesis isi that opiates are very specific in their effects, effective in low concentrations, and blocked by antagonistic agents. Opiates influence receptor cells in the brainstem, the medial thalamus, and at several places in the spinal cord.

History of Drug Use

We tend to think of our society as "the drug culture," but the use of mindaltering drugs is very ancient. What perhaps distinguishes our culture from previous ones is the modern dissociation of drugs from formal cultural or religious customs. It is easy to understand why humans would appreciate a substance that alleviated pain or reduced hunger and fagigue. At this stage the psychoactive properties of drugs merge into medicinal usage. Nevertheless, many drugs have always been taken in excessive quantities when ther was no physical need for them. These doese led to audio and visual hallucinations. The original appeal of these kinds of psychological effects was quite different from the modern enjoyment of the sensations as recreational experiences. Primitive peoples were unknown about hte natural phenomena and other events that was going around them and they used to call the action of supernatural agents.

Under normal conditions, people cannot see or speak with such powers, but under th einfluence of psychoactive agents, they could be transported to another world where communication with gods, demons, or even the dead was possible. In most cultures, only specific individuals were allowed to ingest psychedelic substances. Such people, usually men, were variously called healers, medicine men, witches, or shamans. Shaman, originally a Siberian word, has been adopted by anthropologists for this group of diviners because it lacks the connotations attached to most of the other designations. The initiation of an individual into the role of shaman was often painful and dangerous. Initiation rites sometimes involved starvation, some form of self-mutation, and consumption pf psychoactive drugs.

The combined effect produced a physical condition that enhanced the illusion of visiting the supernatural world and acquiring the insights necessary to serve as the intermediary between the earthly and spiritual worlds. The shaman took the drugs repeatedly whenever he needed the advice of ancestors or divine guidence to solve a problem. Anthropologists and botanists who have studied psychoactive drug use have found that New World peoples employed many more species of plants for their psychoactive properties than their counterparts in the Old World (40 versus 6 species).

It is assumed that the distribution of psychoactive drug plants is uniform in the two hemispheres, some authors have suggested that the explanation for the use of few plants in the Old World lies in the cultural superiority of Eurasian civilizations. This explanation assumes that shamanism is a primitive trait and that the cultural environments of the ancient European and Asian civilizations provided a milieu that replaced the need for spiritual intermediaries. Such authors forget, however, the localized distributions of many of the plants used by New World peoples and the overwhelming dominance of two psychoactive drug plants, the opium poppy and marijuana, in the Old World.

Cannabaceae

According to a Neolithic Chinese legend, the gods gave humans once plant to fulfill all needs. The plant was *Cannabis sativa*, ma, marijuana, or hemp. This assertion is not so far-fetched. *Cannabis* assuredly ranks among the world's most remarkable plants. It produces highly durable fibres that can be turned into ropes, fish nets, and clothing, its peeds are highly nutritious, and oil obtained from it, used in lamp or in paints and varnishes. Ten-thousand-year-old pot shards imprinted with twisted hempen fibers are part of the evidence that *Cannabis* was among the oldest cultivated plants. Today, the species is best known for the psychoactive chemicals it produces. Marijuana rivals alcohol, caffeine, and nicotine as the most widely used nonmedical drugs. It is said to be the most profitable of California's agricultural commodities and perhaps the second most lucrative crop in the United States. How it came to occupy this position is a fascinating story, involving cultures spanning almost every continent.

Cannabis, native to central Asia, the disperson of the seeds of *Cannabis* takes place by means of water, wind, birds or animals. Still, it is humans who have spread the species worldwide, often without knowledge of its psychoactive properties. The first to use *Cannabis* were the Chinese, who had such high respect for the plant that they referred to their country as the "land of mulberry and hemp." The first true paper was made by the hemp fibre the T'si Lun in 105 A.D. The ancient Chinese *Book of Rites* instructed that mourners wear hempen clothes to show respect for the dead. The Chinese apparently knew of hemp's psychoactive properties, but they were primarily interested in its medicinal virtues.

The legendary Shen Nung (ca, 3000 B.C.) observed that th female plants contained a greater proportion of the creative (yin) principles than the male (yang), and recommended cultivation of the former and its use in correcting spiritual imbalances. The ancient Hindu texts, the Vedas, describe Siva, the Lod of Bhang, bringing *Cannabis* down from the Himalays for the enjoyment of the Indian people. India was the country in which the hallucinogenic properties of *Cannabis* were first exploited. Chinese grew their plants very closely in order to reduce the branching and in this way they improve their fibre production, the Bengalese (from "Bhangland") developed a cultivation strategy that maximized production of the psychoactive compounds. The Indians also realized that marijuana was dioecious and that female plant swere more potent than males.

The resins exuded on the upper leaves and bracts of the female inflorescences are particularly rich in intoxiating substances. Resins protect the vulnerable part of the plant from desiccation, they are produced in greatest abundance when the plants are exposed to heat and sun. By growing the plants widely spaced and removing the male plants (to prevent fertilization and prolong female flowering) resin producton is enhanced. The stimulation of resin production by dry conditions is the reason why plants grown in semiarid climates are more potent than those from cool temperate regions.

Likewise, sinsemilla (unfertilized, or without seeds) marijuana is one of the strongest forms. In India *Cannabis* is taken in the form of bhang, a milk-based beverage concocted with ground *Cannabis* leaves, sugar, and an assortment of spices. Bhang is widely drunk and is commonly offered as a gesture of hospitality. Indians classify *Cannabis* products into ganja, consisting of the potent female flowers and upper leaves, and hashish (charas), which is relatively pure resin. There are many colourful stories about traditional hashish collection. In Nepal, naked men used to run through the fields of flowering female plants and then scraped off the clinging resin globules. In Persia, the plants were beaten on rugs which wer subsequently washed to dislodge the resins.

Marijuana may have also had a role in Western civilizations, but it is generally believed that the species had not spread farther west than Turkey in ancien ttimes. The history of Arab use of hashish is not documented, but many legends exist to fill this gap. One of them credits an ascetic monk with finding Cannabis growing wild on the hillsides and sharing it with the poor (Sufis). The monk Haydar was so delighted with the plant that he ate nothing else until his death 10 years later in 1221 A.D. The Sufis used hashish to comfort the pain of their cheerless existence. When Marco Polo returned from his travels to the east in 1297 A.D., he brought back a story that was destined to become a classic. He recounted that there was a terrorist, Hasan-ibn-Sabah, the "Old Man of the Mountain," who had a large band of followers willing to do anything, even commit murder or sucide, for their leader. This blind loyalty was attributed to a very clever recruitment strategy. Political candidates were drugged and brought unconscious into an exquisite mountain garden. There, among the exotic flowers and water works, beautiful women were ready to minister to every need.

After experiencing the pleasures of this paradise, the recruit was drugged once again and, upon awakening, told that he could return to the garden in this life or after death only if he swore complete allegiance to the Old Man. The technique was apparently very successful, and the band of loyal followers became known as assassins, a name purportedly derived from hashish, the drug they were supposed to have been given.

There is no evidence to substantiate this story, and much to refute it, but it was compelling enough to be retold countless times and has been misinterpreted even in recent history by antimarijuana zealots who imply that the hashish produced violence rather than to ensure loyalty to the assassins. In the fifteenth and sixteenth centuries, Arab traders introduced marijuana to Africa where its use quickly spread. The drug was commonly given to women in childbirth and fed to babies when they were weaned. The Kafirs called the plant daga, a name later applied to a culture that made widespread use of *Cannabis*. The dried plant part was mixed into beverages which was taken by Africans. The technique of smoking became popular only after the Dutch colonized the continent. By the time of the Crusades, when European contact with the Arabs was reestablished, marijuana use was common throughout Africa and Asia.

The *Tales of the Arabian Nights* (written sometime between 1000 and 1700 A.D.) was widely read in Europe and provided a romantic introduction for many to hashish. "The Tale of the Hashish Eater," in particular, described the effects of the drug ona degenerate who used it to delude himself that he was wealthy and handsome. When Napoleon's army was stationed in Egypt in 1798, recrutis experimented with the local intoxicant and returned to France with stories and samples. The French student visited the northern Africa and returned back with glowing youthful reports of marijuana use. A frecnch psychiarist, Dr. Jacques Joseph Moreau de Tours, read the medicinal uses of hashish in combinating plague and dysentery and decided to test the drug himself. Because he had read that the drug produced drastic change in perception, he thought that he might be able to administer it to sane individuals in order to reproduce the symptoms of psychosis and thereby learn about the causes of mental illness. He asked an artist friend, Theophilie Gautier, to try the experiment of the drug and report his reaction.

Gautier was impressed with the effect of hashish on hsi artistic senses, and he recommended it to his frient, the painter Boissard. Eventually the group expanded, meeting monthly in Boissard's hotel suite where they consumed hashish while being observed by Dr. Moreau. The 'Club des Hachichins' named after the story of the Old Man of the mountains by themselves. The club eventually became a meeting place of the great French artists and writers of the day: Alexander Dumas, Victor Hugo, Eugene Delacroix, and Charles Baudelaire.

Not surprisingly, much of the art and literature of this period reflects the preoccupation with the newly discovered drug. Despite Moreau's eventual conclusions published in "On Hashish and Mental Alienation" (1845) that hashish use had overall deleterious effects on mental health, the use of the drug continued to spread. The fascination with hashish travelled across the English Channel, from the French to the British intellectual community, where W.B. Yeats, Oscar Wilde, and Ernest Dawson experimented with it to see if it enhanced creativity. After introduction of Marijuana into the Americans it was scattered all over the country The first introduction of cannabis to the New World was done by the Spaniards during hemp cultivation in Chile in 1545.

The British, hoping to produce a lucrative attempts failed, *Cannabis* managed to escape cultivation and spread around the island. When African slaves were brought to Jamaica in the middle of the century to harvest sugar cane, they found a local source of their familiar drug already established. Before 1800, the British had sent formal orders for the colonists in North America to produce hemp. Even Thomas Jafferson and George Washington realized the military need for rope-making fibers and started hemp cultivation. An appreciation of the other uses of *Cannabis* did not develop in the United States unti the 1800s. The introduction of hemp's psychedelic effects followed the same pattern as in France and England.

First there was tremendous curiosity, primarily by intellecturals and artists, a rash of drug-inspired art, and then a general spread of marijuana use. In fact, the 1876 Centennial Exposition had a Turkish bazaar which featured hashish smoking as a special attraction. Despite the sensatinalized stories that soon began to appear about decadent hashish dens and violent consumption by the poor in such manner the use of the drug spread. During prohibition, marijuana smoke floated up and down the Mississippi to the tunes of Dixieland. Jazz musicians found "moota" a pleasurable way to enhance their music without experiencing the stupefying effects of alcohol. They expressed their appreciation of the drug with such songs as Benny Goodman's "Sweet Mrijuana Brown," Cab Calloway's "That Funny Feefer Man," "Texas Tea Party," the "Mary Jane Polka," and others. It has been suggested that the desire to suppress the increasing popularity of black and Latin-inspired music began the movement that eventually led to the criminalization of marijuana. However, racism would have been only one of many factors that countered marijuans use.

Harry Anslinger was trying to justify the existence of the newly created Narcotics Bureau of the Government. He also carried out the most effective antimarijuana campaign. He publicized stories of the horrors of marijuana "addiction" and depicted the put smoker as a savage fiend whose aroused sexual desires and violent tendencies led to criminal activities and the use of stronger drugs. The story of the "Old Man of Mountain" was revived by Anslinger but the story was twisted a little so that the drug iteself was the cause of irrational violence. Marijuana was tried by the press and condemned by an emotional, ill-informed public. In the late 1920s and 1930s, marijuana use was banned in Louisiana, Texas, and Illinois.

Other states soon followed, and in 1937 the use of cannabis came under federal jurisdiction withe the passage of the 1937 Marijuana Tax Law which actually heavily taxed, but did not prohibit, the drug. Other countries had previously taken hard step to prevent Cannabis use. In this field South Africa passed the first anti-Cannabis law in 1870, and by 1925, the League of Nations agreed to an international statute against its use. All of these legal sanctions against *Cannabis* had two things in common, they were not based on any substantial medical evidence of severe effects of marijuana use, and they universally failed to halt its spread. Most medical studies beginning in 1893 with the Indian Commission's through report failed to find any detrimental effects of moderate use. Sanctions against marijuana only seem to increase its popularity.

In the 1960s the explosive spread of pot smoking provides the drastic demonstration of such kind of effect. Young people throughout the world, disillusioned with the ways in which the older generation was handling affairs, made marijuana smoking a symbol of their rebellion. While attention was focused on marijuana in the 1960s, the suggested medical virtues as well as the possible detrimental effects were investigated. Once THC was finally isolated in 1965 and measured quantities could be used for testing, it was discovered that the active principal is effective in reducing the pressure exerted against the eyes of glaucoma patients. Cancer patients undergoing radiation or chemotherapy treatment when used such compound, the nausea problem reduced. Since THC dilates the bronchial vessels, it provides relief for asthma sufferers. Because of the useful medicinal qualities, marijuana cigarettes or concentrated THC in the form of pills can now be prescribed by physicians when appropriate. In 1972, a federal government study on the effects of marijuana was released. The report suggested decriminalization of marijuana because there was no evidence of medical or mentla damage from use of the drug and because the drug was so widely used that laws against it were unforceable.

In 1981, the results of another study made by the National Academy of Sciences were released. The academy panel observed the use of marijuana very carefully and came to conclusion that the low or moderate use weakened the sense, sensibility and sensitivity of users. They could find no evidence of addiction or permanent deleterious medical effects with low or moderate use, but heavy use was correlated with several psychological and physiological problems. The use of marijuana is directly linked with low sperm count in males. Since marijuana is usually smoked, heavy and regular user suffers lung disorders similar to those incurred by cigarette smoking. Finally, the Academy found that ther was a high probability that heavy users would turn to "hard drugs." The panel did conclude, however, that marijuana was safer thanits legal, more widespread counterparts, alcohol and tobacco, and suggested that the present legal sanctions against possession and trade be removed.

Papaveraceae

In United States poppies are well known as garden ornamentals or for their culinary seeds, but they rose to fame because of opium. The capsules of the fruits from which the seeds are obtained are rich in an alkaloid-containing latex. The latex has medicinal use but opium and morphine these are the most abundant of the opium alkaloids and are used as mind-altering drugs. The collection of opium from fruits of the opium poppy (*Papaver somniferum*) extends back to at least 3000 B.C. Sumerian tablets from 2500 B.C. refer to opium as the "joy plant" and describe the ingestion of smal balls of the latex to induce sleep and relieve pain. Opium is mentioned in every medical treatise written during ancient Greek and Roman times. The name opium comes from the Greek "opion" for poppy "juice."

The early Greeks realized that the driniking of wine in which latex had been dissolved led to trancelike state, and they therefore associated poppies with several divinities such as Hypnos, the God of Sleep, Morpheus, the God of Dreams, and Thanatos, the God of Death. It is commonly known that Chinese was responsible for introducing opium to the rest of the world, but China was ignorant of the drug until the seventh century A.D. when Arab traders first brought samples to the Orient. In the East, it is used to cure dysentory in some manner that paragoric (tincture of opium) is used for diarrhea today.

In the seventeenth century, the Dutch introduced tobacco smoking to Formosa and began to mix tobacco with opium in their pipes as a treatment for malaria. The practice of smoking opium spread to the mainland where it was rapidly adopted throughout the country. Soon, tobacco disappeared from the mixture, and smokers inhaled vapours from heated balls of latex that were droped into the bowl of a pipe. Opium smoking became so popular that Chinese officials thaught to ban the sale of opium. Their antiopium edicts, issued as early as 1729, were ignored by both the Chinese populace and th Portuguese suppliers. In 1800, the British gained a monopoly over trade rights with China. Since China had little use for of opium dealing because it was one of the few commodities for which the Chinese would exchange coveted products such as silk and spices. Eventually, England even established opium plantations in her Indian colonies to provide opium for trade.

Importation of opium into England was, however, illegal at this time, but distance and the need to maintain international trade seems to have exonerated the practice elsewhere. The Chinese lords tried again and again to halt the drug trafficking because they could see the debilitating effects on their people, but without the support of the British, their efforts failed. The situation came to a head in 1839 when the Chinese confiscated and destroyed British opium supplies in Canton. England retaliated by invading China, touching off the first Opium War. The war ended wiht a treaty that ceded Hong Kong to the British.

A second Opium War broke out in 1865 and the Chinese were again defeated. This time they were forced to agree to British opium importation. Naturally, opium consumption among the Chinese continued to escalate. Trafficking in the drug was finally reduced in 1906 when the last emperor of China managed to get the British to agree to a reduction in importation. Still, use did not drastically drop until the revolution and the establishment of the People's Republic of China in 1949. Opium trading and use are now strictly forbidden. Opium consumption was not common in Europe until 1525 when Paracelsus discovered, or rediscovered, a way to dissolve it inalcohol.

The opium is dissolved in alcohol to obtained the tincture was known as laudanum. At that time laudanum was the most popular drug due to its meaningful medical benefits of the case with which it could be consumed. In 1803, morphine was isolated form opium, producing a purified alkaloid that could be given in measured doses. On a per weight basis, morphine is 10 times as strong as opium (which contains at least 24 other alkaloids andnumerous other compounds). Purified morphin can be administred intravenously to releaf the pain. When the hypodermic syringe was developed in 1853, it presented doctors with a rapid method of introducing this potent pain killer into the bloodstream and morphine use rose. Morphine's effectiveness was both a blessing and a curse. In many cases, the speed with which a drug enters the bloodstream (and thus the intensity of the "rush") is correlated with the level of addiction it can produce.

Only after 45,000 soldiers returned home from the Civil War addicted to thepain killer were the dangers of morphine use recognized. In an attempt to develop a nonaddicting pain killer, scientiets discovered that morphine could be chemically altered by the addiction of two acetyl groups. The end product is a semisynthetic compound known as *heroin*. Heroin is an even more powerful analgesic than morphine, and it, like morphine, was initially explained that heroin contain less addicting qualities of its parent drug. While mark of this idea persisted untill 1905, but very soon become apparent that heroin was even more dangerous than morphine because it crosses the cell membranes very easily and rapidly than its natural counterpart. Because of this fast absorption (and hence cycling around the bloodstream), heroin must be more frequently administed than other opiates. In addition to the effects produced by heroin itself, users of the drug suffer from disruption of the blood flow, infections, diseases such as hepatitis, and collapsed blood veins.

Heroin is very physically addicting and produces pronounced withdrwal symptoms once the habit has become established. Two to three weeks of injecting 30 mg per day is considered enough to create a tenacious habit. The main cause of death for heroin addicts is by overdose. Because of the common usage of adulterantnts in heroin and the use of heroin in combination with other drugs, "overdose" levels for an individual ar enot constant and therfore cannot be adequately gauged. The lifestyle of the heroin addict who no longer seeks the drug for pleasure, but because he or she desperately needs it to avoid withdrawal, tends eventually to lead to overall physical problems. The death rate for heroin users is more than twice the normal rate. In 1914, a law was passed prohibiting the possession of opiates for nonmedical purposes. In 1924, the production of heroin was proved illegal in the United States and in 1956 existing legal supplies of the drug were destroyed completely. Because of its addictive properties, even morphine is seldom used in its pure form as a modern-day medicine.

In contrat, the use of heroin, all illegal, has dramatically increased during the last 30 years. Since heroin is made from morphine, the total production of opium has correspondingly increased. In 1972 most of the opium production ended up in the United States but still grow in Turkey. When Turkey and the U.S. government reached an agreement to limit opium poppy cultivation, th ecenter of productio shifted to southeast Asia. Economically, opium is an extremely lucrative crop. In 1972 10 kg of crude opium which sold for $250 where it was grown, would eventually gross $200,000 when sold on the street. With profits such as these, people are willing to risk the penalties if caught.

Fabaceae

A large number of new wrold Indian tribes used the species of the bean family which is rich in alkaloids, as hallucinogenic agents. Snuff made from powdered pods of cohoba (*Anadenanthera peregrina*) was first reported form Hispaniola in 1496 and was much later found to be used by the Indians of the Orinoco region of Venezuela. In South America, the snuff is called "yopo," and it is often mixed with lime (Calcium carbonate) when taken. The snuffs can be inhaled througha number of devices, one of which is a long, hollow pole. One end of the pole is placed in a nostril and the other inot a pile of snuff on the ground. Mescal, or red bean (*Sophora secundiflora*), a common ornamental shrub or small tree of the American southwest, was used by native proples of this region to induce trances. The plant has received some recent publicity because mescal beans have been confused with mescaline and unknowing youths have been tempted to try them. However, *Sophora* contains cytisine, a much more dangerous alkaloid than mescaline, and one that can easily cause death due to respiratory failure if slight overdoses are taken.

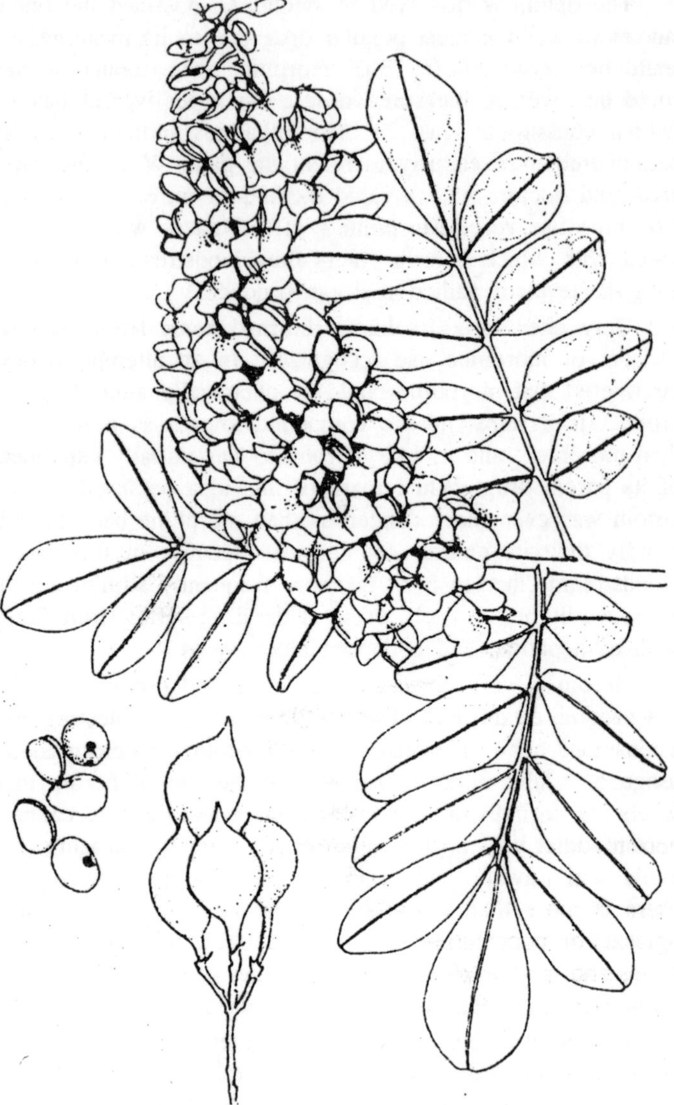

Fig. 8.1. Sophora secundiflora is valued as an ornamental plant because of its fragrant purple flowers and glossy green foliage.

Celastraceae

As Americans, we are accustomed to take a cup of coffee, tea, or other caffeine-containing beverage when we need a lift or freshness, but in other parts of the world the same effect is produced by consuming parts with different but equally effective stimulatory alkaloids. Among these is kat (*Catha edulis*), a native of Arabia but now most widely grown along the eastern edge of Africa. The alkaloids are ingested by chewing wads of freshly cut leaves usually mixed with small amounts of lime. Each lump, or quid, is masticated for about 10 min until all of the juice has been expressed. The remaining cellulose mass is than swalloed.

Erythroxylaceae

The stimulatory alkaloids are extracted by chewing the coca just like kat (varieties of either *Erythroxylum coca* or *E. novogranatense*). Coca is native to the north-central Andes. Discoveries of bags of coca leaves and utensils in 3,000 year old Andean burial sites indicate that it was used by natives of this region long before Europeans discovered South America. By the time Pizarro conqured Peru, coca was an integral part of Inca life and was considered to be a sacred plant. The preparation of coca involves very simple method the leaves are collected, dryed and sometimes allowed to sweet (lightly ferment) in order to render them pliable rather than crisp. Indians normally dip the leaves into lime that they carry in a small bag before chewing them.

As in the case of its use with kat, lime aids in the extraction and absorptin of alkaloids. The masticated residue is either expelled or swallowed. Cocaine, the active principle in coca, affect directly on the central nervous system by blocking reasorbtion of norepinephrine in the brain. This blockage has the result of making the coca chewer feel invigorated and relatively immune to fatigue and hunger, peasants of the Inca Empire depended on coa, as do an estimated 90 percent of their modern descendants, to mitigate the harsh environment of the high elevations of the Peruvian and Bolivian Andes.

The Spanish conquerors tried to prohibit coca use until they realized that the Indians they enslaved would work harder if allowed to chew it. Coca was taken back to Europe by the Spanish, but in leaf form it never received much attention. In 1860, cocaine was isolated and, unlike the homely leaes, it soon became extraordinarily popular. Sigmund Freud publicized the drug in his treatise *Uber Coca.* Among other things, Freud recommended coca as a treatment for alcoholism and morphine addiction. He also lauded it as a local anesthetic and praised its use in psychotherapy to relieve depression. In both Europe and the United States, doctors began to prescribe its use.

An enterprising Italian, Angelo Mariani, developed a coca wine beverage in 1860 which was soon the rage of Europe. Mariani's wine earned commendations from scores of celebrities including Jules Verne, Ulysses S. Grant, President McKinley, Emile Zola, Henrik Ibsen, and Thomas Edison. Coca cola; which originally consist both caffine-rich extracts from Cola nitida and coca txtracts, was first marketed in 1880 as a headache remedy. Since 1904, however, federal law has prohibited the inclusion of cocaine in nay beverage. Ironically enough, after the Coca Cola Company complied with the federal law, it was sued for misleading advertising on the groudns that the name implied that the beverage contained coca products.

As a result, coca leaves, with the cocaine removed, are now used to flavour the syrup from which the soda is made. As more and more reports of cocaine-induced violence and other unsubstantiated effects of the drug circulated after the turn of the century, the government took steps to curb its use. In 1914, the drug was formally declared illegal by the Harrison Narcotic Act. As a result, cocaine costs escalated, but despite illegality and high costs, its use continues to increase. Status seekers appear delighted to pay exorbitant prices for a brief experience. Indulgers usually chop or grind crystals of cocaine hydrochloride before sniffing ("snorting") a line of the fine powder. Cocaine may also be smoked or injected.

The conversion of cocaine from the salt form to the base form is termed 'Free basing', which alters its solubility (increasing the drug's potency), has proved to be particularly more harmful. Both these latter methods of ingestion produce stronger sensations but are much more dangerous to the user than sniffing. Just how dangerous is cocaine? While researchers have not been able to find any organic damage from prolonged coca use per se among Andean Indians, their findings do nto mean that cocaine is a harmless drug.

Indians used to chew coca leaves and so they absorbs only limited quantities of the drug because the leaves contains alkoloides in relatively small amount (0.65 to 1.25 percent on a dry weight basis). An average native user might consumes 2 oz of leaves per day or about 0.7 grains of cocaine. A person who "snorts" or injects cocaine could be consuming as much as 6–8 grains per day of the drug plus adulterants. 1.2 grams of cocaine is considered as a lethal dose. Cocaine is not physically addiciting, but its use can become a pronounced habit as indicated by the burgeoning number of treatment centers for cocaine abusers.

After becoming accustomed to the elevated feelings it produces, habitual users suffer from depression when denied the drug. While occasional use produces feelings of mood elevation, vitality, mental clarity, sexual stimulation, and reduction in appetite in many users, chronic users can suffer from anxiety, conofusion, insomnia, and impotence. Paranoid psychosis can develop from longterm heavy use. Cocaine ingestion of pregnant animals is harmful to fetal development. This is concluded by recent experiments. As more reserach is conducted, other harmful effects may be discovered.

Malpighiaceae

One of the most important groups of plants used by South American Amazonian tribes as a source of hallucinogenic compounds are members of the genus *Banisteriopsis*, primarily *B. caapi*. Depending on the tribe, this species is called caapi, ayahuasca, yaje, or cipo. Infusions of mashed bark or stems are usually prepared, but stems can also simply be chewed in order to release the active alkaloid. People using ayahuasca describe the perceptions produced as feelings of having experienced death or of experiencing a separation of spirit and body. Sometimes the hallucinations are pleasant, other times apparently terrifying with vivid apparitions of jaguars or snakes. Like many other alkaloid-rich preparations, mixtures of ayahuasca often cause vomiting and diarrhea. Unlike the use of many other psychoactive drugs by native peoples, ayahuasca is often taken in communal rituals.

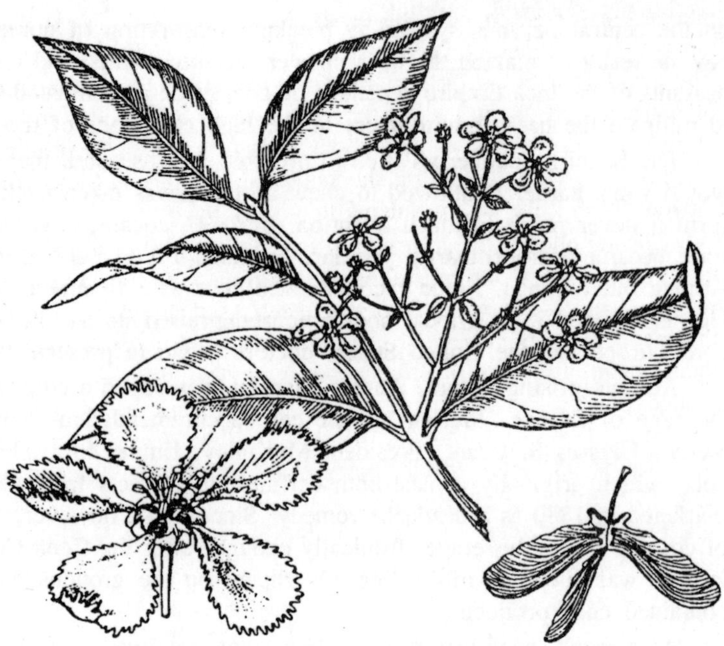

Fig. 8.2. Banisteriopsis caapi is a tropical vine with stems tha contain the alkaloid hormone, a psychoactive substance known as yaje or ayahuasca by the Amazonian Indians who use it in rituals.

It is thought that this practice of communal ingestion enhances feelings of clairovoyance or telepathy. The group, under the supervision of a yaquero, is led through chants to experience shared hallucinations. This effect was reflected in the name "telepathine" given to the mixture of active chemicals first isolated from *Banisteriopsis caapi*. Since this initial chemical work, the active compounds have been further purified and named harmine and harmaline. In some tribes, the rituals commemorae an act of incest by a deity. In almost all cases, the ceremonies are filled with sexual symbolism, but there is no sexual gratification during the experience.

Cactaceae

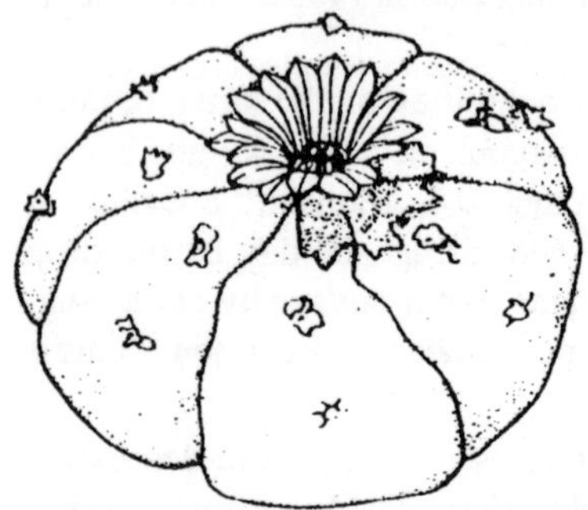

Fig. 8.3. Mescaline is the psychoactive compound in the gray-green peyote buttons that grow natively in southwestern U.S. and adjacent Mexico.

A large number of species of the Cactaces family are good source of hallucinogenic compounds. The best known is peyote, *Lophophora williamsii*, a small, globose, gray-green cactus native to the Rio Grande Valley bordering the United States and Mexico. Native American Indians appear to have extended its distribution to Arizona and New Mexico centuries ago. No one is sure when peyote was first used, but sixteenth century reports by European explorers describe its use by the Aztecs as a divinatory plant. These accounts refer to peyote as the "diabolic root," because the Spanish observed the Aztecs using the plants ritualistically.

After the collapse of the Aztec Empire, use of peyote survived among a few Mexican Indian tries such as the Huichol, Cora, and Taramara. Inthe United States, the Plains Indians began to use it as late as the 1880s. In India harvesting is done by cutting off the top of the stems and leavign the sturdy taproot for regeneration. The stem tips, or buttons,were eaten fresh, or dried for later consumption. The dried buttons can be swallowed by softening and mastication. The initial reaction after swallowing in nausea. One to two hours later, quesiness disappears and is replaced by kaleidoscopic illusions of vivid colours, sensual hallucinations, and distorted perceptions of time. During this last period, which can last from 5 to 12 hours, the faithful report hearing the voices of their ancestors who help them to diagnose and cure any problems they may have.

Consumption of peyote means ingestion of 30 to 40 different alkaloids and several chemicals at a time, mescaline is one of the most active compound present in the alkaloids. Isolated in 1896, mescaline was the basis for research into psychedelic compounds for the next 50 years. While there is no evidence that peyote or pure mescaline is addicting, repeatrd use may permanently affect the mind. Because of their potentially harmful effects, both the plnat and the compound are illegal to possess or sell in the United States. However, one religious sect, the Native American Church, uses peyote as an integral part of its services. In a case that went before the Supreme Court, the church received an exemption from the Prohibition against peyote use. Originally founded by natives in northern Mexico, the sect holds Christian services modified by the use of peyote and espouses as doctrine, brotherly love, abstinence from alcohol, and high standards of moral conduct. Today, there are over a quarter million members of the church within the United States. Other cacti such as the San Pedro cacti have been widely used by native peoples in their native regions of Peru and Chile. All of these species used mostly contain mescaline and are used to produce hallucinations.

Apocynaceae

While fewer drug plants were used by native Africans than by South and Central American natives, one, iboga (*Tabernathe iboga*) was important as an hallucinogen. Iboga is, in fact, one of the very few psychoactive drugs in the entire periwinkle family. Although th species of the family are rich in alkaloids, most of them are toxic. A few species such as *Rauwolfia serpentina* and *Catharanthus roseus* are used medicinally, but there is no indication that they were used in rituals. In preparing iboga, the bark or roots of the shrubs are powdered or chewed, often with other plant species. Ingestion of the alkaloids, one of which is ibogamine, is said to lead to frightening visions and in large doses can produce severe convulsions, respiratoty arrest, and death.

Convolvulaceae

No species of morning glory family were known by scientists before 1903, which could be used for psychoactive purposes. In 1955, Humphrey Osmond described the use of *Rivea corymbosa* by Mexican natives, and, in 1960. T. MacDougall detailed the use of another member of the family, *Ipomoea tricolor* for altering perceptions. Still more startling was the discovery in 1960 that the sees of these plants contained D-lysergic acid amide. Prior to this time, lysergic acid

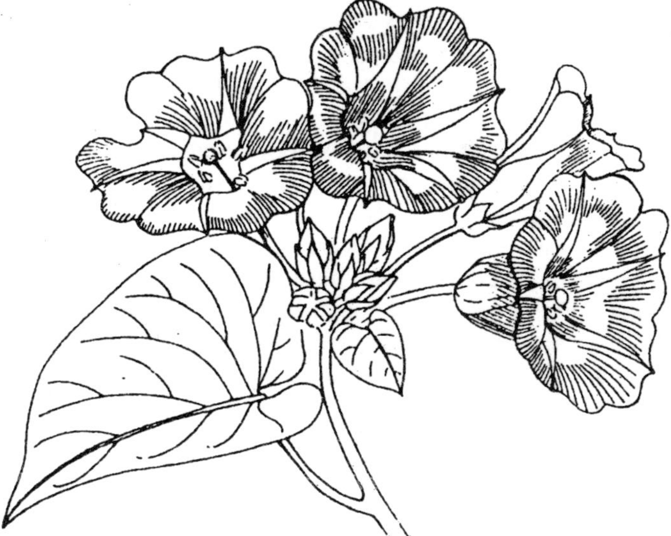

Fig. 8.4. Rivea corymbosa, or ololiuqui a white-flowered vine of the morning glory family contains the psychoactive compound, D-lysergic acid amide.

alkaloids were thought to be restricted in nature to ergot (*Claviceps purpurea*), a rust that infests grains, and to a few other fungi. Synthetically produced LSD had become a part of the Americna counterculture in the 1960s and was regarded as something very modrn and exciting.

Osmond's and MacDougall's discoveries showed that the effects of these kinds of compounds had been recognized and utilized by native peoples, perhaps for thousands of years. Both of the convolvulaceous species now known to be used are called *ololiqui* (pronounced o-low-lee-oo-key) by the peoples that use them. The carefully measured quantities of seeds should be ingested especially by experienced individual because there is a little difference between the quantities seeds that produced vivid hallucinations and the quantities that produce death, there has been little lay experimentation with the seeds, despite the fact that one of the species is a commonly cultivated ornamental plant.

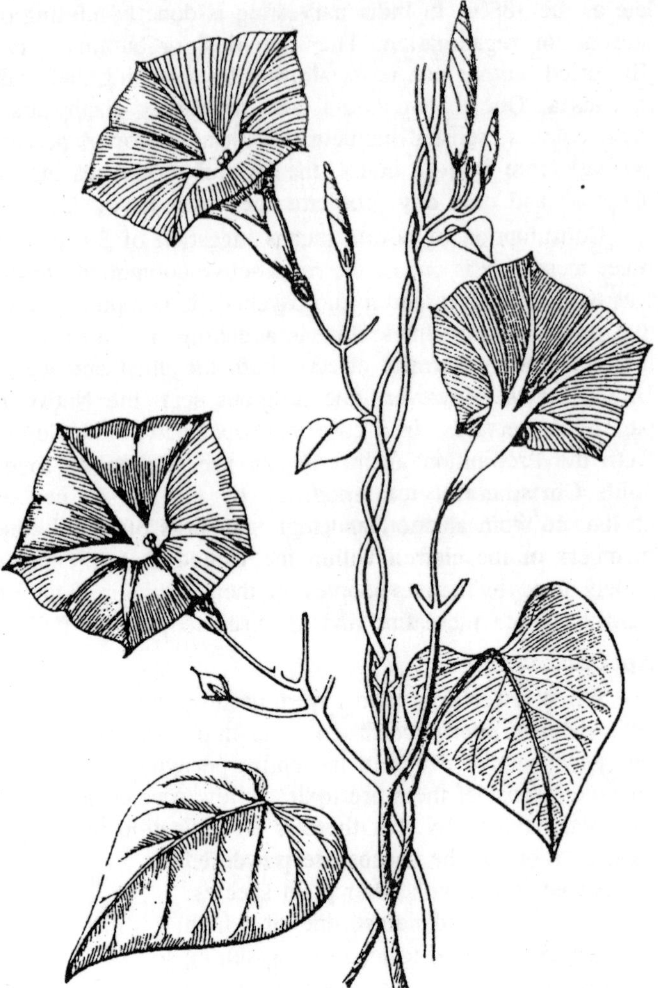

Fig. 8.5. *Because of the extremely fine line between effective and lethal doses, the seeds of hallucinogenic morning glories have rarely been used even by primitive peoples.*

Solanaceae

The plants of the Solanaceae is highly toxic therefore their use is restricted outside of some Central and South American people rarely used today as source of mind-altering drugs. Undoubtedly, the major reason for their restricted use is their toxicity. At one time, however, various species were used in both Eurasia and the Americas as sources of hallucinogenic compounds. Historically, the most important of these were species of *Datura*, *Hyoscyamus*, *Atropa belladonna*, and *Mandragora officinarum*. Many of these were also used medicinally, and a few have become important modern sources of pharmaceutical compounds. The tropane alkaloids (atropine, scopolamine, and hyoscyamine) which these species contain are effective in controlling smooth muscle action. It is careful measured amount is useful in the treatment of heart irregularities. In larger, but sublethal, doses, the same alkaloids produce hallucinations. Of the plants in this group, only datura is native to the New World.

Datura is particularly rich in scopolamine, which is considered to be the most hallucinogenic of the solanaceous alkaloids. Seeds or roots of various species provides vision upon eating. So it is widely used in Central and South America, but even among people that use datura, it is considered dangerous and too strong for general use. Usually datura was ingested only by boys during puberty rites or by trained shamans. In South America, alcoholic beverages made from datura fruts were given to women and slaves of dead warriors to stupefy them before they were buried alive with their deceased masters.

Infusions of bark and leaves were also used by various tribes. Congeneric species is widely used in the New World while the species of datura native to Europe and Asia were less widely used, but belladonna, mandrake, and henbane assumed great importance in Europe during the Middle Ages.

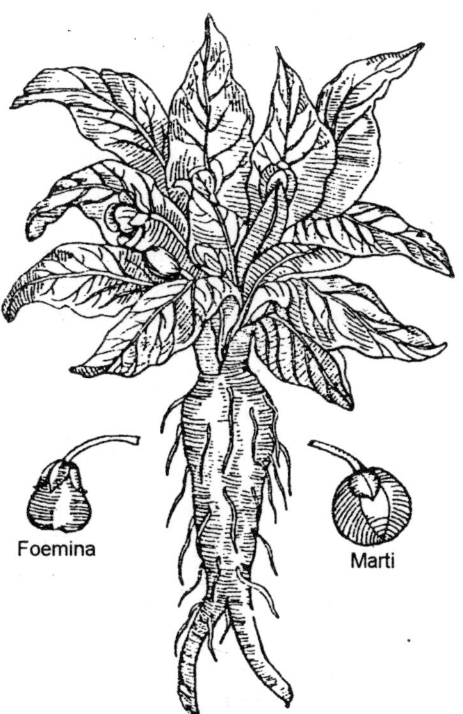

Fig. 8.6. Mandrake, or Mandragora was long thought to be an aphrodisiac because of the human shape of its root.

The ancient use of solanaceous alkaloids in witchcraft and folk medicine led European scientists after the Renaissance to investigate their actionand eventually to the discovery of their medicinal properties. Likewise, their uses as hallucinogens and poisons prompted writers and artists to include them in the writtings and paintings of the time. Belladonna or henbane are the source of Atropine. Atropine is directly absorbed by skin, and during the Middle Ages, witches rubbed ointments containing it on their bodies. The psychological sensations produced give one the feeling of flying. While under the influence of atropine, witches were supposed to be transported to rendezvous with spirits of demons. These meetings, called sabats, are often figured in European art of the period. Our modern portrayal of a witch riding a broom may stem from these ancient rites.

The depiction of the flying comes from the hallucinogenic sensations of being transported, and the broom purportedly represents the stick used to apply atropine-impregnated ointements to vaginal membranes for absorption. Another figure commonly attributed to visions seen while under the influence of solanaceous alkaloids is the werewolf. Similar to the visions of jaguars and snakes produced when South American natives use caapi, wolves were associated with trances induced by henbane, belladonna, and related species. A quite different member of the Solanaceae, however, has had the greates tworldwide impact. N. rustica is believed to be the relative of Nicotiana tabacum. Both of them become important commercial items in almost every country of the world. The genus *Nicotiana* is thought to be native to the New World, but at least one species, *N. suavolens*, which occurs in Australia, was independently domesticated.

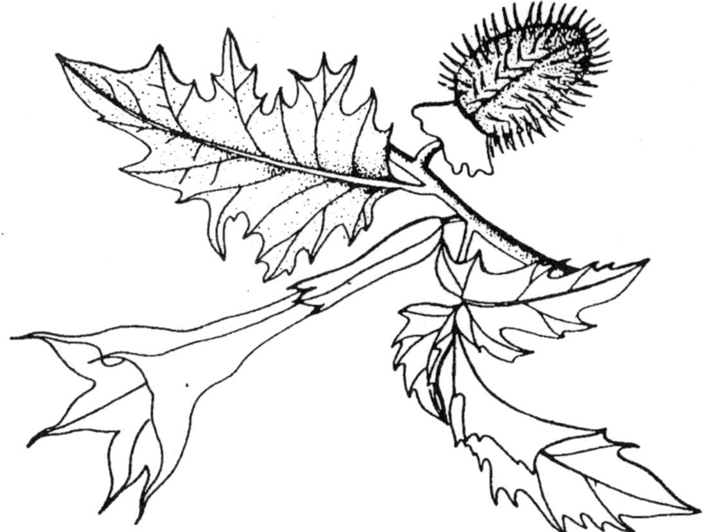

Fig. 8.7. Datura acquired its common name jimsonweed in 1705.

At least 1,000 years before Columbus landed in the West Indies, tobacco was smoked, eaten, and snuffed by native peoples throughout the New World. Among American Indians, tobacco was used medicinally to ease childbirth pains and stave off hunger on long hunts. The dried leaves of tobacco become so valuable that it becomes the source of money and incorporated into ritualistic and symbolistic practices such as the smoking of a peacepipe. Tobacco was considered sacred by many American tribes. Mayan priests thought that smoke rising from their pipes carried messages to the gods. Recent studies of Amazonian tribes have shown that the use of tobacco in divination rites continues today.

Shamans of the Warao tribe of Venezuela, for example, fast almost to starvation during their initiation rites and then eat and smoke large quantities of tobacco. The resultant hallucinations produce the sensation of being transported to another world for mettings with the spirits that govern the lives of the people. Later in their careers, shamans frequently turn to tobacco to help them solve tribal problems. Although Columbus brought "cigars" to Queen Isabella after his first voyage, it was not until Andre Thevet brought seeds of Nicotiana tabbacum from Brazil to France in 1556 that tobacco cultivation started in Europe. Linnaeus named the genus after Jean Nicot, the French ambassador to Portugal who made a fortunate importing and popularizing the use of the plant in Paris.

Tobacco spread across Europe and Asia and gained a special place because its medicinal virtues as a remed for several female problems, a snakebite antidote, lung strengthener ulcer remedy, cure for the plague and potent aphrodiasiae. Tobacco use became so widespread that King James I was alarmed to find that purchases of tobacco were depleting England's silve supply. Neither the high cost of the leaves nor King James's blistering attack in his *Counterblaste to Tobacco* (1604) checked the spread of smokingor sniffing. In other countries as well, leader tried to discourage tobacco use. So many hard step and stricked rule were formed in order to prohibit the smoking as one Chinese emperor ordered smokers to be decapitated and Russian Tsar ordered the nostrils of snuffers to be split so that they could no longer practice the habit. Still, tobacco continued to attract followers. Eventually, the British promoted tobacco cultivation in their colonies to ensure a national supply. Virginians started growing tobacco in 1612. Since an acre planted in tobacco yielded four times the revenue of an acre planted to corn, colonists turned more and more exclusively to tobacco farming. The Virginia monopoly on tobacco production granted by the Queen was broken when settlers in Maryland began to cultivate the crop.

Soon, much of the eastern seaborad of the United States was engated in tobacco production. For many years, tobacco was the most important item of trade between England and North America. Primitive method of cultivation of tobacco consisted simply of saving seeds of the previous year's crop and sowing them in a cleared area. After maturity plants are harvested and the leaves dried in the sun. In contrast, modern tobacco farming is quite elaborate and employs various cultivation techniques for the many different cultivars and the types of of tobacco being produced. On modern U.S. farms, tobacco is usually first sown in seed beds and the seedlings transplanted into fields after 2 months of growth. The spacing of plants and fertilizer regime varies with the final type of tobacco to be produced.

Nitrogen-rich fertilizers are applied to encourage the development of large, pliable leaves suitable for cigar wrappers, while the small, more brittle leaves favoured for cigarettes are produced by limiting nitrogen and supplyign phosphorus and potassium at critical stages. While it is growing, the flower stalks and the side shoots are usually removed to prevent the plants from diverting resources to seeds and low branch development. Leaves used for cigar wrappers should be large so the plants are generally grown under cheesecloth where the high humidity and protection from sunscald also promote formation of large, thin, blemish-free leaves.

Two to 4 months after planting, the crop is considered mature Good grades can be picked a leaf at a time, or whole stalks can be harvested. In either case, the leaves or stalks are tied into bunches called "hogsheads" for curing. During the curing process, themoisture content in the leaves is reduced from about 80 to 20 percent. Starches are converted to sugars, and some proteins are broken down enzymatically. Slow drying permits aerobic fermentation to take place but prevents the growht of molds or fungi. Curing can be done by circulating air or by smoking. Occasinally, bundles of leaves are sun-dried. Following curing, the leaves are aged for periods varying between a few months and a year. The tobacco used for the cigarette and cigar filling is remoistered before marketing and the veins and petioles removed. The softened leaves are then cut by machines into strips. Depending on the ultimate tobacco product, are then cut by machines into strips. Depending on the ultimate tobacco product, various materials can be added.

Mositure-retaining substances such as glycerin, cider concentrate, and diethyl glycol are common additives, but honey or sugar, oil of hops, licorice, coumarin, rum, or menthol can be added for flavouring. Additives have been increasingly used in tobacco mixtures since the middle 1970s to compensate for the flavour and aroma lost when manufacturers produce cigarettes with low tar and nicotine. While most of these are drawn from the FDA list of "Additives Generally Recognized as Safe," there is concern that, when burned, many may constitue health hazards. Coumarin, a compound used as additives removed from the FDA list of safe drugs because it has been shown to be carcinogenic, is stull being purchased in large quantities by cigarette manufacturers.

Locorice, likewise, produces carcinogenic compounds when burned. Even the sugars added produce tars when burned. Ironically, the federal government exempts tobacco manufacturers from the labeling requirements that other food and drug producers must observe. While tobacco smoking was widely enjoyed before 1880 change in the curing process make the tobacco smoking more popular after this year. Before 1880, most tobacco was cured by direclty placing it over the hot smoke of a charcoal fire. After 1880, farmers began to use hot air brought to the drying rooms by flues. This indirect drying produced a milder form of tobacco than that produced by smoke drying.

Mild tobaccos were perfect for cigarettes, a relatively "general" way of smoking. However, thee light tobaccos produce an acidsmoke when they are burned. Tobacco cured directly tends to produce an alkaline smoke. Acid tobacco smoke has little physiological effect on the body if it is simply puffed. Consequently, it must be inhaled in orde rto produce an exhilarating effect. The surface of the lungs neutrilized the inhaled smoke and the lung membrane absorbed the nicotine carried in the smoke. Smokers who inhale tend to become addicted to tobacco because they become physiologically dependent on the strong sensory reaction produced when nicotine is absorbed. Pipe and cigar smokers can become accustomed to smoking and dearly miss their habit if they quit smoking, but, in general, there is little physical reaction to the absence of nicotine in their blood since they normally do not inhale.

Nicotine acts as stimulant of the central nervous system as it is a major alkaloid in tobacco. It causes nausea, dizziness, and hallucinations in large doses. It is physiologically addicting, and withdrawal symptoms appear when it is kept from habituates. In pure form, nicotine is a poison and is often used, after treatment with sulfuric acid, as an insecticide. In addition to nicotine, smoking leads to the inhalation of tars. These tars are known carcinogens, and cigarette comapnies have therefore tried to manufacture cigarettes that reduce the intake of tars. However, none of the various filtering or extraction devices is perfect, and some tars are drawn in by smokers who inhale. There is a direct correlations between smoking and lung cancer and heart disease all these are dut to toxicity of nicotine and tars. Smokers age prematurely, die at a younger age than nonsmokers, and tend to be susceptible to emphysema, bronchitis, and other respiratory ailments. Smoking during pregnancy increases the risk of miscarriage and problesm in early infancy. Infants born to mothers who smoke can emerge into the world underweight and addicted to nicotine. Despite the warning of the Surgeon General that smoking is bad for your health, tobacco smoking is a legal form of drugs ingestion. In direct contrast to its stance concerning many less harmful drugs, the government continues to subsidize nicotine drug addiction by providing price supports for tobacco farmers. Cigarette companies also blissfully ignore the effects of tobacco smoking and continue to lure people into smoking with advertisements that portray smokers as healthy, particularly masculine, independent, and/or beautiful.

PLANT POISONS

A large number of plants are poisonous to varying degree that an enumeration would be futile. Regional agricultural stations usually publish lists of local plants that are dangerous to humans or livestock, and many horticulture books indicate which ornamental plants can be toxic if eaten. Some of these plants have been used by humans for their poisonous compounds. These are the ones in which we are interested here. As we explain earlier, a large number of plants used for their physiological effects are poisonous if used in large quantities.

It is difficult to know exactly how humans discovered which plants were or were not toxic and the quantities that could be ingested relatively safely. Ancient Greek and Roman medical rocords attest to an early interes in documenting the occurrence and usefulness of plant toxins. Administration of plant poisons as a form of capital punishment is well known from the story of the death of Socrates, after being sentenced to drink the juice of poison "hemlock" (*Conium maculatum*, Apiaceae). In the Middle Ages, "succession powders" were deviously employed to eliminate potential heirs to the throne. The employment of these powders became so common that th wealthy and powerful hired tasters as protection against sudden death from "food poisoning."

Today, scientists often seek out plants known by natives to be poisonous. Many poisonous plants are the sources of drugs or commercial poisons for use as insecticides, herbicides, or fungicides because all these poisons are either alkaloids or steroids. Some modern primitive tribes in the tropics use arrow or fish poisons such as curare or barbasco. Curare is made from extracts of the bark and stems of *Chondodendron tomentosum* (Menispermaceae) and from seeds of species of *Strychnos*, particularly *S. nux-vomica* (Loganiaceae). *Chondodendron*, a vine native to South America, contains tubocurarine. Species of Strychnos occur natively in South America, southeast Asia, and Indonesia and many yield the potent alkaloids curarine, strychnine, and toucine.

Curare alkaloids, primarily tubocurarine chloride, have had limited applications in medicine because they block neuromuscular activity and thus help relax muscles that remain contracted under anesthesia. Initially Strychnine was used medicinally as a central nervous system stimulant but has now been replaced by safer compounds. Barbasco and tuba are fish poisons used by Amazonian peoples. The first is prepared from various species of *Derris*, such as *Derris elliptica*, and the second from *Lonchocarpus nicou* (both Fabaceae).

Recently, species of both these genera have been shown to be effective insecticides because they contain rotenone. This isoflavanoid compound is fatal to insects but comparatively harmless to humans because it leaves no residue. Pyrethrum (*Chrysanthemum coccineum*, *C. cinerariifolium*, and *C. marschallii*) and tobacco acts as the sources of natural insecticides. Insecticidal compounds form species of *Chrysanthemum* are sold as Persian insect powder or Dalmation. Pyrethrins, the active compounds, are esters that break down into acids and alcohols. Since they stun insects, but do not instantly kill them, pyrethrins are usually mixed with other substances that ensure death of the insect. In some regions, notably Kenya, Tanzania, and parts of northeastern South America, pyrethrum is grown commercially for natural compound extraction. Approximately 1,200 plants are use as sources of insecticides. Yet, the fact that these would be natural insecticides does not mean that they are, or would be, less harmful than synthetic compounds. In fact, nicotine sulfate, a commercially available, natural insecticide is one of the most toxic pesticides on the market today.

9

Implications of Interaction

Serious drug–drug interactions have contributed to recent U.S. market withdrawals and nonapprovals of new molecular entities (NMEs). In addition to coadministration of other drugs, concomitant ingestion of dietary supplement or citrus fruit or fruit juice could also alter systemic exposure, leading to adverse drug reactions or loss of drug efficacy.

Metabolism of New Molecular Entities and Interactions with Other Drugs

The interactions of concern can be divided into two types. First, other drugs can affect the blood levels of the NME by inhibiting or inducing its absorption, distribution, metabolism, or excretion pathways. Second, the NME can affect the blood levels of other drugs by inhibiting or inducing their absorption, distribution, metabolism, or excretion pathways. Of particular interest is the role of hepatic and intestinal cytochrome P450 (CYP) enzymes. Thus, "Is the drug a substrate for CYP enzymes?" and "Is the drug an inhibitor and/or an inducer of CYP enzymes?" are among the critical questions that need to be addressed when evaluating clinical pharmacology data of NMEs in new drug applications. Recognizing the importance of addressing these questions early in drug development, pharmaceutical companies routinely assess a NME's clearance pathways, including in vitro evaluation of a drug's metabolic pathways and its modulating effects on CYP1A2, CYP2C9, CYP2C19, CYP2D6, and CYP3A activities and subsequent clinical interaction studies based on in vitro data. In addition to CYP enzymes, other enzymes such as glucuronosyl transferases and various transporters also play important roles in drug interactions and changes in systemic exposure.

The clinical significance of altered systemic exposure of coadministered drugs depends on the concentration–response relationships for clinical effects, both effectiveness and toxicity. If the concentration– response relationship is well described, knowledge of the effects of interactions can lead to rational adjustment of dose or dosing interval, or to appropriate warnings and precautions.

Labeling descriptions of drug–drug interactions can be based on interactions observed in clinical studies or projected interactions extrapolated from other studies. If a drug is shown not to inhibit a particular CYP enzyme based on in vitro data, labeling will indicate no interaction with substrates of that CYP. For example, the current ABILIFY labeling states that "aripiprazole and dehydro-aripiprazole did not show potential for altering CYP1A2-mediated metabolism in vitro".

If a drug has been determined to be a sensitive CYP3A substrate (e.g., budesonide, buspirone, eletriptan, eplerenone, felodipine, lovastatin, midazolam, saquinavir, sildenafil, simvastatin, triazolam, and vardenafil) or a CYP3A substrate with a narrow therapeutic range (e.g., alfentanil, astemizole, cisapride, cyclosporine, diergotamine, ergotamine, fentanyl, pimozide, quinidine, sirolimus, tacrolimus, and terfenadine), it does not need to be tested with all strong or moderate inhibitors of CYP3A, to

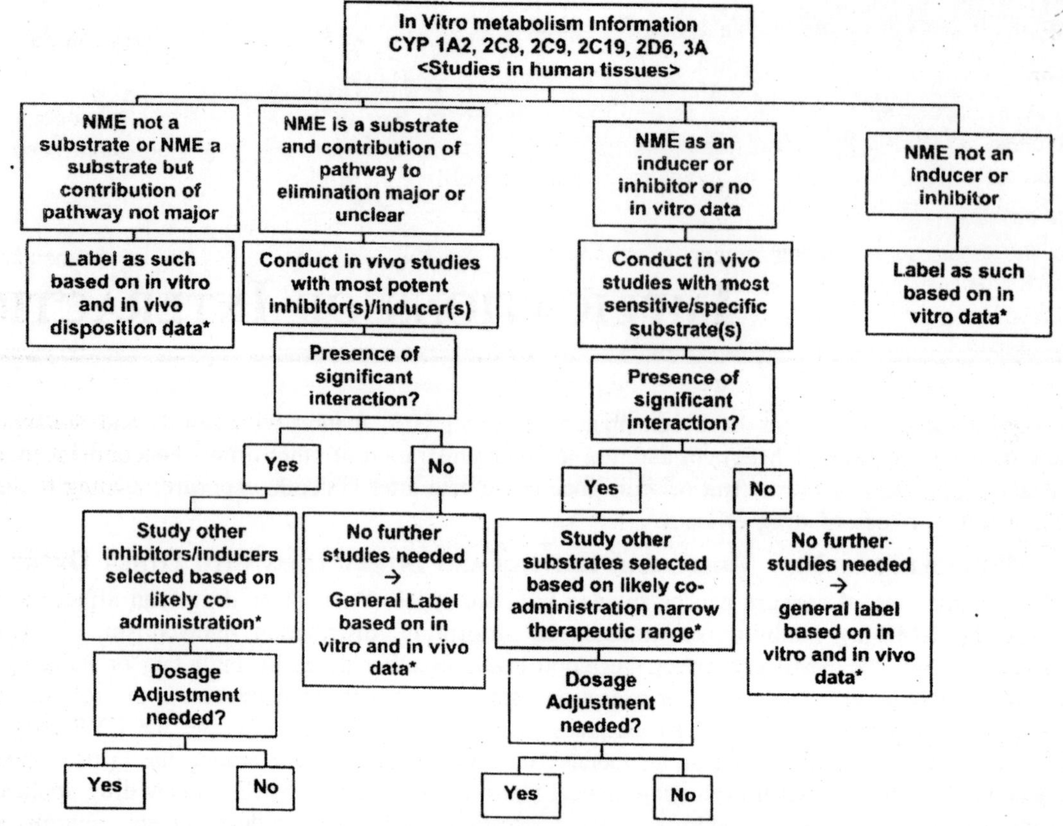

Fig. 9.1. CYP-based drug-drug interaction studies decision tree.

warn about an interaction with "strong" or "moderate" CYP3A inhibitors. For example, the labeling of RELPAX indicates that it should not be taken with strong CYP3A inhibitors such as ketoconazole, itraconazole, nefazodone, troleandomycin, clarithromycin, ritonavir, and nelfinavir. The interactions with itraconazole, nefazodone, troleandomycin, clarithromycin, ritonavir, and nelfinavir have not been evaluated; the warnings are based on data from a clinical interaction study conducted with ketoconazole and on other relevant in vitro data.

Labeling of drugs as "strong" or "potent" CYP3A inhibitors can facilitate, for example, the projection of its interaction with other sensitive substrates. Examples of "strong CYP3A inhibitors" include atanazavir, clarithromycin, indinavir, itraconazole, ketoconazole, nefazodone, nelfinavir, ritonavir, saquinavir, telithromycin, etc. These are drugs that increase the area under the plasma concentration-time curve (AUC) of either orally administered midazolam or other CYP3A substrates by five-fold or greater. Examples of "*moderate CYP3A inhibitors*" include amprenavir, aprepitant, diltiazem, erythromycin, fluconazole, fosaprenavir, (grapefruit juice), verapamil, etc. These are drugs that increase the AUC of orally administered midazolam or other sensitive CYP3A substrates by two-fold or greater, but less than five-fold. The labeling of KETEK indicates that telithromycin is a strong inhibitor of CYP3A, tha its concomitant use with simvastatin, lovastatin, or atorvastatin should be avoided, and that its use is contraindicated with cisapride and pimozide. Note that the warnings in the labeling about interactions with lovastatin, atorvastatin, and pimozide are based on extrapolation from clinical studies with simvastatin and cisapride.

Effect of Dietary Supplements on New Molecular Entities and Interactions

St. John's Wort

FDA has received adverse-event reports that suggested a role of St. John's wort in reducing the effectiveness of a number of drugs, such as cyclosporine (e.g., transplant rejection), oral contraceptives (e.g., breakthrough bleedings and pregnancy), and sildenafil (e.g., loss of efficacy).

Impact on drug labeling

As the effect of an enzyme inducer is reasonably predictable, the current labeling recommendation is that, for drugs that are substrates of CYP3A or P-gp, and when the products' effectiveness would be reduced upon coadministration of St. John's wort, St. John's wort should be listed along with other known inducers, such as rifampin, rifabutin, rifapentin, dexamethasone, phenytoin, carbamazepine, phenobarbital, etc., in the labeling as possibly decreasing the plasma levels. Of these 55 labels, only two labels, CRIXIVAN and INSPRA, are based on actual clinical studies on these drug products. The others either indicate that there are reports of interactions (e.g., NEORAL and TRIPHASIL) or that there are mechanistic reasons and there is the potential for interactions (e.g., AGENERASE, ALESSE, and UNIPHIL).

Several products with teratogenic potential (e.g., ACCUTANE and THALOMID) list interactions not directly related to the drug products, but to the oral contraceptives that need to be taken. Except for ACCUTANE, whose warning about the interaction with St. John's wort is in the "Contraindications" section, all current labelings on St. John's wort appear either in the "Warnings" or the "Precautions" sections, the two sections that will be combined in one section "Warnings/Precautions" under the new labeling rule. A recently published guidance for industry entitled "Labeling for combined oral contraceptives" includes labeling language on drug interactions between oral contraceptives and St. John's wort, such as "Herbal products containing St. John's wort (*Hypericum perforatum*) may induce hepatic enzymes (cytochrome P450) and P-glycoprotein transporter and may reduce the effectiveness of contraceptive steroids. This may also result in breakthrough bleeding". Several St. John's wort products also carry warning language about potential interactions with various drug products.

Effect of Citrus Fruit/Fruit Juice on New Molecular Entities

Grapefruit Juice Effects on CYP3A

FDA has received adverse-event reports that implicated grapefruit juice in the observed exaggeration of pharmacological effects or adverse drug reactions for calcium channel blockers (e.g., resulting in hypotension), statins (e.g., leading to muscle pain), antihistamines (e.g., QT prolongation and arrhythmias), and others. Clinical pharmacology studies have also clearly shown that concomitant grapefruit juice ingestion increased the systemic exposure of orally administered drugs that are CYP3A substrates and have low oral bioavailability due to extensive presystemic extraction contributed by enteric CYP3A.

Impact on drug labeling

The current labeling recommendation is that, for drugs that are primarily substrates of CYP3A with low oral bioavailability due to extensive presystemic extraction, grapefruit juice should be listed along with other CYP3A inhibitors in the labeling as possibly increasing the plasma levels of coadministered drugs. Table 4 lists 28 labeling examples of grapefruit juice–drug interactions. Of these labels, half of them contain actual clinical data (e.g., ADALAT, ADVICOR, BILTRICIDE, CLARINEX, CONERA, CRIXIVAN, INSPRA, KETEK, NOR VASC, PACERONE, LETAL, PROGRAF, SULAR, and ZOCOR). All relevant literature data on grapefruit juice interactions with a particular drug product may be considered in the labeling of the drug product. For example, the latest package inserts for lovastatin and simvastatin include data from two clinical studies; one conducted by the sponsor and the other by an independent researcher.

The results of the two studies differ widely, possibly because of the different study designs (timing and frequency of coadministration), and also because of variables that are difficult to control, such as the source, brand, lot-to-lot variation of the same brand, and the preparation procedure (including the extent of dilution by the consumers when using frozen concentrates) of the grapefruit juice. For both drug products, both sets of data have been included in the labeling. Other labels include those based on theoretical interaction potential (e.g., CENESTIN). Grapefruit juice has been considered as a "*moderate CYP3A inhibitor*" that can be included with other moderate CYP3A inhibitors, such as erythromycin and diltiazem, as appropriate. Unlike most other CYP3A inhibitors, which affect both enteric and hepatic CYP3A, grapefruit juice appears to affect only enteric CYP3A; it would therefore be listed in the labeling only for drug products for oral administration and with low oral bioavailability.

Grapefruit Juice, Apple Juice, and Orange Juice Effects on Transporters

Grapefruit juice has been shown to inhibit P-gp transporter, resulting in increases in plasma levels of drugs that are substrates of P-gp transporter. Limited data have shown that grapefruit juice, as well as apple juice and orange juice, may inhibit organic anion transporting peptides (OATP), leading to decreased systemic exposure of drugs that are substrates of OATP. The overall effect of fruit juices on drugs that are substrates for both transporters may depend not only on the contribution of either transporter and other clearance pathways to the drugs' overall clearance, but also on other variables, including the amount, the type, and frequency of juices being consumed. Until more data are available, current labeling for known substrates of both transporters that are not substrates of CYP3A is to recommend taking these drug products with "water".

Calcium-Fortified Orange Juice Effect on Bioavailability

Chemical complexation of the fluoroquinolones with the calcium ion may play a major role in the reduced absorption and decreased plasma levels when calcium-fortified orange juice was coadministered with ciprofloxacin. The current labeling for Cipro (ciprofloxacin) tablets has warnings against the use of these products with calcium-fortified orange juice.

Future Prospectives

Drug–drug interactions have been a significant cause of adverse drug reactions. Various guidance documents for industry and for reviewers have stressed the importance of evaluating drug–drug interactions during drug development.

With increased understanding of how certain dietary supplements (e.g., St. John's wort) and juices (e.g., grapefruit juice) affect the systemic exposure of drug products, it is possible to anticipate an interaction with a drug based on the drug's clearance pathway and label the drug products accordingly. But while the potential for an interaction can be understood, it is much harder to describe the effect quantitatively or recommend dose modifications or usage. Dietary supplements or juices have multiple unknown components that are not well defined and vary from product to product and are used at very different doses and in a very variable time with relationship to drug use. Current labeling recommendations therefore urge avoidance of the coadministration of a drug and a dietary supplement or food that interacts with it in a clinically significant way, rather than adjustment of the drug dose or dosing interval, a recommendation that is common for dealing with drug–drug interactions.

Despite the increased understanding and documentation of drug interactions in the labeling and in letters to "*dear health care professionals*," adverse reactions resulting from well-recognized drug–drug interactions continue to be reported. The increased use of dietary supplements with significant drug interaction potential increases the propensity for adverse drug reactions.

To better translate information into practice, Center for Drug Evaluation and Research (CDER) has published a final rule on the physician's labeling format. When drug interactions that are significant, or their absence when they are expected to occur, would appear in labeling "Highlights," in addition to being included in the main body of the labeling. In addition, a proposed revision of the 1999 drug interaction guidance includes a proposal to use a classification system for CYP3A inhibitors (including grapefruit juice) in the labeling, in an effort to improve the consistency of labeling language and to highlight key drug interactions. Additional risk management tools have been proposed for particularly serious situations, including use of medication guides and restricted distribution.

With continued improvement in our understanding of the mechanisms of interactions and contributions of additional patient factors (e.g., genetics and gender), the risks associated with these interactions can be better predicted, assessed, and managed to reduce the frequency of clinically significant adverse drug reactions.

10

UTILIZATION OF PLANT MEDICINE

Comprehending the use and safety of botanical dietary supplements is challenging largely owing to the lack of regulation and the paucity of data on their utilization, effectiveness, and safety. The literature describing the utilization of botanical products tends to be poorly documented and incomplete and evidence in the form of clinical trials is sparse; safety data are largely derived from anecdotal case reports. Medications from botanical sources have been described as far back as 60 millennia and most of the medications used throughout the world were derived from plants until the early 1900s. It is estimated that 35,000 to 70,000 plants have been used for medical purposes. For example, opium and willow bark have long been used for the treatment of pain. It was not uncommon for over-the-counter medications to contain opium without warnings or legal restrictions. Willow bark may still be purchased over the counter as an extract to relieve pain and many other prescriptions medications are currently derived from botanical sources.

HISTORICAL OVERVIEW

Prescriptions Derived from Plant Sources

Today, it is estimated that 25% of the Western pharmacopoeia contains chemical entities that were first isolated from plants and another 25% are derived from chemical entities modified from plant sources. In 1999, 121 prescription medicines worldwide came directly from plant extracts and it is now a $10 billion-a-year industry. These medicines are not dietary supplements but rather are botanical products that have passed the more rigorous process of approval to be used as a prescription drug. The World Health Organization estimates that 75% to 80% of the developing world continues to rely heavily on botanicals for medication. However, most products available are considered dietary supplements in the United States.

Plant Dietary Supplements

The use of botanicals in the industrialized world is growing. In the United States, it has been estimated that about 20,000 products are in use, with the top ten botanical products comprising 50% of the commercial botanical market. In China, approximately 80% of medications are obtained from between 5000 and 30,000 types of plants. In the era of increased globalization, many botanical products are available to people all over the world through the Internet, imported for sale by botanical shops catering to high-use ethnic populations, or imported (often illegally) by individuals returning from global travel. Utilization of these products has dramatically increased in the past decade. In 1991, the U.S. Congress passed legislation to establish the National Institutes of Health Office of Alternative Medicine, which later became the National Center for Complementary and Alternative Medicine, to better understand how Americans are embracing the use of unconventional therapies.

Utilization of Plant Dietary Supplements

Although physicians in the United States infrequently prescribe botanicals, they receive little formal training on the benefits and risks of these and other complementary and alternative medications (CAM). This is disturbing because a significant proportion of patients take botanical dietary supplements. More than 37 million Americans utilize botanical remedies and some estimates put forth a much higher. Since the Dietary Supplement Health and Education Act (DSHEA) of 1994, growth of the botanical market has been dramatic. However, the industry is fragmented, with a few large corporations manufacturing the bulk of botanical products and many smaller companies targeting specific herbs. Market research organizations have traditionally avoided analyzing botanical products because the market was too small, but this has changed recently because botanicals are now profitable to analyze. As a result of DSHEA, the public now has many botanical dietary supplements from which to choose. With the increasing number of products competing against one another, corporations have taken action to distinguish their products from one another. As such, dietary supplement manufacturers have taken a page from the pharmaceutical industry and have begun branding botanical products to develop a market following for their product.

Many products also consist of combinations of dietary supplements and at least one of them also uses a nonprescription medication in combination with the botanical dietary supplement. At least one pharmaceutical manufacturer has also entered the branded botanical market. Direct-to-consumer advertising of branded botanical dietary supplements appears to be quite effective, judging from the number of advertisements appearing in the print and electronic media. Many of these products claim to improve conditions that are refractory to conventional medical treatment or they are touted to be natural and, as such, purported to be safer than conventional pharmaceuticals and free of side effects. The public is well aware of dietary supplements, because many of these have appeared on late-night infomercials. Some examples of branded products touted for weight loss include Metabolife, Leptoprin, and Cortislim. Most weight loss products in the United States contained ephedra before the Food and Drug Administration (FDA) banned ephedra-containing dietary supplements. It appears that weight loss products are now being reformulated with other stimulants that have not received the intense scrutiny of the FDA, such as bitter orange (synephrine), green tea extract (caffeine), and guarana (methylxanthines: caffeine, theobromine, and theophylline).

Other branded combination botanical products such as Enzyte and Avlimil are touted for treatment of sexual dysfunction and are advertised in a manner similar to sexual dysfunction pharmaceuticals. Still other formulations are advertised for breast enhancement—Bloussant, hair loss—Avacor, depression—Amoryn, nourishing the brain—Focus Factor, and sleep—Alluna Sleep. All of these contain one or more botanical constituents and are sold under the auspices of DSHEA, and therefore are not regulated by the FDA and the Federal Trade Commission as rigorously as prescription pharmaceuticals or food additives. Sizing up the economics of the botanical dietary supplements market in the United States is challenging because the market is prodigiously dynamic. The market has been estimated to represent a demand between $0.6 and $5.1 billion. It is important to note that each study sampled a different population. Growth in the market occurred rapidly between 1991 and 1998, but recent sales appear to have reached a plateau. Americans usually pay for botanical dietary supplements as well as other CAM therapies out of their own pockets because most health insurance programs do not cover CAM therapies.

In 1997, total CAM out-of-pocket expenses exceeded $27 billion, with the expenditure on botanical products estimated at greater than $5 billion. Insurance coverage that covered CAM therapies would also likely result in growth in the botanical industry. One study found that full insurance coverage for botanical dietary supplements predicted an increase in usage of five-fold and partial insurance coverage

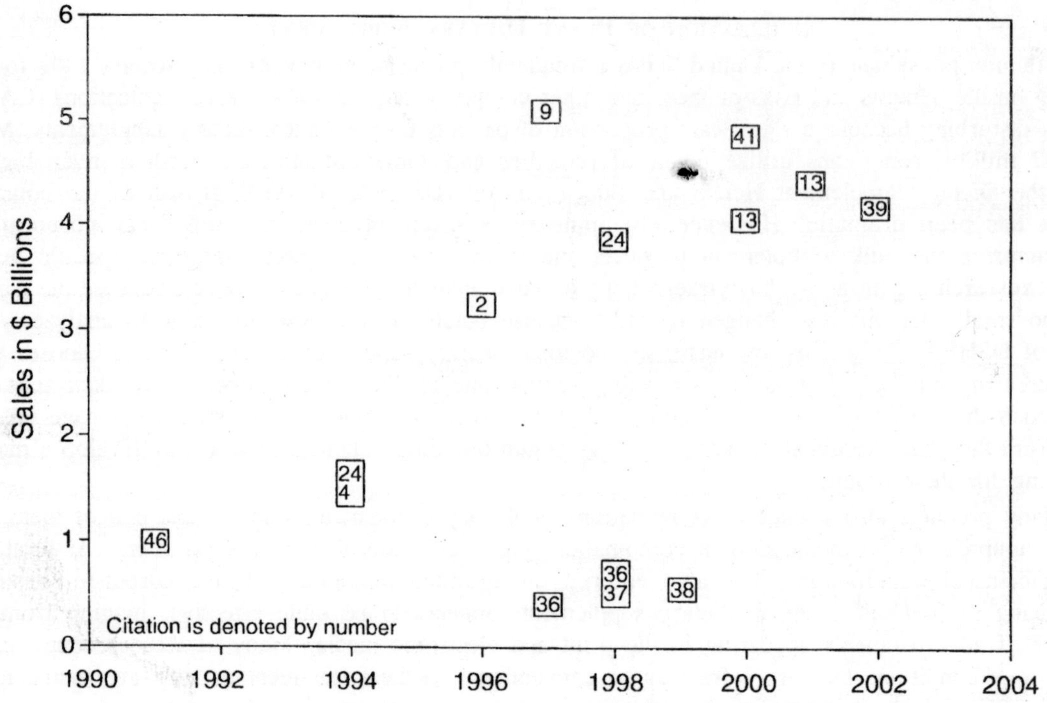

Fig. 10.1. Estimates of retail botanical sales in billions of dollars by year from multiple citations.

predicted a threefold increase in botanical utilization. Rapid growth in the botanical dietary supplement industry occurred within the first four years of DSHEA and there was also a concurrent growth spurt in the U.S. economy in the mid-1990s. DSHEA relaxed regulatory restrictions on dietary supplements, thus lowering the barrier to enter the market. As a result, growth in CAM likely is a result of deregulation by DSHEA and may reflect the disposable income available. This would explain the rapid growth in the mid-1990s and leveling of spending on botanical products at the turn of the century. Also, Eisenberg et al. found that the increase in botanical product utilization between 1990 and 1997 was likely due to an increase in the proportion of the population using botanicals rather than an increase in per patient utilization. In contrast to the growth of botanical products in the mid-1990s reported by Eisenberg et al., growth of the botanical market in early 2000 was reported to be from patients already using sundry botanical products according to the Natural Marketing Institute (NMI). This indicates that botanical dietary supplement market expansion among new patients has moderated.

Market Analyses

Several major surveys of dietary supplement utilization have been conducted recently. The Saskatchewan Nutriceutical Network (SNN), National Nutritional Food Association (NNFA), Consumer Healthcare Products Association (CHPA), Landmark Healthcare, Inc., The NMI, individual investigators, Centers for Disease Control and Prevention (CDC), and FDA have all recently either conducted or contracted market analyses of CAM utilization in the United States, which included botanicals. Each survey is presented individually because the data are so heterogeneous among studies.

Saskatchewan nutriceutical network

The SSN estimated U.S. botanical sales in 1999 to be $4 billion. The network further quantified where consumers buy their botanical products. Forty-seven percent are sold in retail stores, 30% are sold in multilevel distribution systems, 8% are sold by mail order or practitioners, 6% was sold by

Asian herbal shops, and only 1% was purchased on the Internet. Notwithstanding these findings, it is important to note that the Internet was the fastest growing sales market for botanical products, at 150% per year.

National nutritional food association

The NNFA commissioned a telephone survey of 736 adults in October of 2001. The key finding was that women (25%) were more likely to take botanical products than men (15%). The survey emphasizes the importance of accurate labeling. Seventy percent agreed with the statement "*Labels on supplements*' bottles or packages are carefully read by most: they help the majority of older adults choose the right supplement and to determine the correct dosage." Only 22% disagreed with that statement. Fifty-five percent of respondents agreed with this statement: "Labels on dietary supplements help me understand if this is the right supplement for me," while 64% agreed with the following statement: "Labels on dietary supplements help me determine the dosage I need to take." The more educated patients were less likely to agree with this statement.

Consumer healthcare products association

The CHPA commissioned a study entitled "Self-Care in the New Millenium: American Attitudes Toward Maintaining Personal Health and Treatment." They conducted 1505 telephone interviews in January of 2001, using random telephone numbers. African-Americans and Hispanics were over- sampled to conduct in-depth subgroup analysis. Of particular interest is the finding that 96% of respondents felt confident that they could take care of their own health. This might explain why so many people want access to pharmacologically active botanicals. These products do not require a prescription and thus allow patients to treat themselves.

Many of these products are being used for specific medical conditions. The top five conditions, in many cases are refractory to conventional medicine, namely menopausal symptoms, colds, allergies/ sinus, muscle/joint/back pain, and premenstrual/menstrual symptoms.

The demographics of utilization in the past six months were reported. Thirty percent of women reported using a dietary supplement and 23% of men used a dietary supplement in the six-month period. Results for the effect of age on utilization have been mixed across studies. Patients who were between 50 and 64 years old had the highest reported use of dietary supplements, and 59% and those who were 18 to 34 years old had the lowest use at 48%. Income may be reflected in the utilization-by-age category. Utilization of dietary supplements by ethnicity was characteristic of other studies. Forty-four percent of African-Americans and 42% of Hispanics reportedly used dietary supplements, as compared to 53% of the general population. Although the study did not report Caucasian dietary supplement utilization rates, we can infer that Caucasians increased the overall utilization rate for the population. Health insurance status was associated with greater dietary supplement use, 56% versus 45%. This likely reflected the fact that patients who had health insurance also had more income. Those with some college education reported the highest utilization rate of 60%. People with college degrees used dietary supplements slightly less, 57%, but those with high school education or lesser educational qualification reported 48% utilization of dietary supplements in the past six months.

Landmark healthcare inc.

In 1997, Landmark Healthcare Inc. commissioned a report entitled "The Landmark Report on Public Perceptions of Alternative Care." They conducted 1500 telephone interviews in November 1997, using random digit selection. The survey included a representative sample of minority patients—85% Caucasian, 8% African-Americans, and 3% Hispanic. The survey found that 17% of the U.S. population used botanical dietary supplements in the past year and even more striking, 75% of the U.S. population was most likely to use botanical products. Eighty-five percent of those reported to have taken a botanical supplement self-prescribed and self-administered the products. Three-fourths of patients who used alternative forms of care did so in conjunction with conventional medicine, yet 15% of patients replaced their conventional treatment with alternative care.

Natural marketing institute

The NMI surveyed by mail 2002 households, July through August 2001. Only 53% of botanical supplement users were satisfied with botanical supplements. Despite the low satisfaction for botanical products, supplement users accounted for most of the increase in the previous year: 46% of botanical users increased utilization while only 10% of the general population increased utilization of botanical dietary supplements. Consumers took botanical supplements primarily for general health benefits, 59% versus 40% for a specific condition. Only 6% took botanicals products for short- term benefits, whereas 80% took them for daily or long-term benefit. Many have recently started, with only 50% having used an herb for more than three years.

Independent investigators

Eisenberg et al. surveyed 1539 adults in 1990 and 2055 adults in 1997. Botanical use in the prior 12 months increased from 2.5% in 1990 to 12.1% in 1997—a 4.8-fold increase. They estimated, in 1997, that 15 million adults took a botanical product or high-dose vitamins with other medications, which represented approximately 18.4% of those taking medications in the United States. Growth in botanicals was found to be from an increase in the percentage of the population taking botanicals and not due to an increase in utilization per patient. More than 60% of patients did not discuss CAM use with their doctor. Patients spent an estimated $5.1 billion on botanical medications. Kaufman surveyed 2590 patients, February 1998 through December 1999. Fourteen percent of the U.S. population reported using botanical supplements. Concurrent use with medication was highest with patients on fluoxetine, 22%; overall, 16% of those taking medication reported using botanical medications.

Centers for disease control and prevention

The Division of Health Interview Statistics, National Center for Health Statistics, CDC conducted a survey entitled "Utilization of Complementary and Alternative Medicine by United States Adults" in 1999. The survey attempted to obtain a representative sample of minorities and also patients without telephones. This is important because these demographic groups tend to report lower utilization of botanicals products than Caucasians and those of higher socioeconomic status. The CDC found that 9.6% of the population took botanical medicines. Hispanics reported the lowest use of CAM followed by African-Americans, and then Caucasians: 19.9%, 24.1%, and 30.8%, respectively. The western part of the United States reported the highest use of CAM.

Food and drug administration

FDA commissioned a study of dietary supplement sales in the United States in 1999. Samples of products were purchased from a representative sample of retail establishments, catalogs, and the Internet. The authors looked at the consistency of botanical products purchased. Forty percent to 46% of botanicals and botanical products were consistent with the ingredients listed on the label. Botanical extracts were even less consistent with the label, only 12% to 24% (depending on where purchased) were found to be consistent with the label. They also gave the mean, minimum, and maximum price paid for dietary supplements by source of purchase. Interestingly, the mean purchased price on the Internet was the most expensive at $23.34, followed by the mean catalog price, $16.40. The mean retail price was less than half the cost of the mean Internet price, at $11.62.

Utilization Summary

Patients who use botanicals tend to have attained higher education, be female, be older persons, have higher incomes, and have a recalcitrant chronic disease unresponsive to conventional medicine.

There is also evidence that cultural differences have a strong impact on the use of botanicals. Certain subpopulations may defy these generalizations to the U.S. population. Asian-Americans have a long history of using botanicals as medication and often consider botanicals a conventional form of treatment. Southern rural poor are also reported to have a higher utilization profile of plant-derived products. Rural poor may treat illness with botanical products while the U.S. population as a whole tends to use botanical products for general health benefits rather than to treat a specific illness.

Safety of Plant Products

As a result of DSHEA, the majority of botanical drug products are used in the United States without medical supervision. Only 8% of those who use botanicals do so under medical supervision and 85% of those who treat themselves with herbs do not seek professional guidance or advice. Even if patients utilizing botanical dietary supplements were medically supervised, adulteration and misbranding are prevalent and so little is known about the supplements that many untoward events could not be prevented or recognized in a timely fashion. Despite the widespread acceptance of CAM by the lay public, clinicians possess little scientific information about the practices of CAM relative to conventional western medicine. This is particularly unsettling because it is estimated that 16% to 18% of prescription medication users took botanical and supplements coincidentally. Medication–botanical interactions are largely unknown. Even more alarming is a report that 14.5% of women used botanical products during pregnancy and 23.5% of children under 16 may be taking botanical products. Neonatal heart failure has been attributed to the use of Blue cohosh during pregnancy.

Up to 60% of patients using alternative therapies are reported to have never informed their physician of their botanical or CAM use. Furthermore, only 40% of physicians ask their patients about alternative therapy. The 60% of physicians who do not ask about the use of botanical supplements and other CAM are unlikely be informed of alternative therapies their patients are using. Clearly, there is a lack of communication between patients and providers. Some patients may fear disapproval by physicians and wish to give socially desirable answers. However, the majority of patients express a lack of concern about their physician's approval, rather they were more concerned with their physician's inability to understand and incorporate CAM into their medical management. Patients are not using alternative therapy because they are dissatisfied with conventional medicine but instead because they value both types of therapy.

Many botanical dietary supplements are potentially unsafe because of adulteration and misbranding. Thirty-two percent of botanical medications collected in California contained an undeclared pharmaceutical or heavy metal. Pharmaceuticals adulterating botanical products are one of the most frequent reasons botanical dietary supplements are placed on the FDA MedWatch site, and this is undoubtedly a small fraction of what actually occurs. Many of these adulterants are not detected until patient illnesses are first detected. Consumers often do not recognize that many imported products, purported to be traditional medications, are actually recognized pharmaceuticals. For example, a "*Mexican asthma cure*" had a claim on the label that said it contained no corticosteroids and was free of adverse effects, but the product was found to contain triamcinolone, a moderately potent corticosteroid with well-documented systemic adverse effects common to all glucocorticoids. In another example, a patient used an illegally imported Chinese medicine; it was reported to last much longer than the medication the physician had prescribed. The label on the Chinese medicine said it contained astemizole, a long-acting antihistamine with-drawn from the United States as a result of its effect of prolonging the cardiac QTc interval. In many cases, patients may not recognize pharmaceuticals that are sold as traditional medicines. In the past, consumers have had difficulty distinguishing between vitamins and botanical products. It is likely no different for botanicals and pharmaceuticals. This may be problematic because corporations are creating proprietary botanical blends and branding them for use in specific medical conditions. Patients could inadvertently assume they are treating themselves with a medication that has undergone the same rigorous clinical testing as other FDA-approved medications. Patients readily read and trust the directions on labels of dietary supplements. In fact 59% of the public incorrectly thought a government body reviewed and approved botanical supplements before they are sold.

There are other risks of contamination to botanical and botanical supplements. Due to stress on the supply of cultivars for botanical supplements, products may vary greatly in their active content. In the era of limited resources, with increasing utilization and decreasing wild production, there is pressure to produce a product. Raw material costs may override the quality and purity of the product. There are few barriers to bringing new products to the market and many newer entrants may lack expertise to prevent quality issues and contamination in their product. This creates the potential for inadvertent poisoning as a result of overdosing or contamination as well as treatment failure through under-dosing. Indeed, a study of botanical consistency found that only 43% of the products tested were consistent for ingredients and dose with the benchmark or recommended daily dose. Twenty percent had the correct ingredient but not the stated dose and 37% were not consistent with either ingredients; dose or the labeling was too vague to draw conclusions. The FDA also found that many botanical products were inconsistent with the ingredients listed on the label and estimated that only 12% to 24% of botanical extracts and 40% to 46% of botanical products contained what was on the label.

Adulteration was found to be a problem in another dietary supplement containing androstenedione; although not strictly a botanical, it is regulated in a similar fashion under the auspices of DSHEA. Ingestion of androstenedione contaminated with trace amounts of 19-norandrosterone resulted in a positive test for 19-norandrosterone, a metabolite used to detect nandrolone. Other samples were also found to be contaminated with testosterone. The FDA has been cautious in its enforcement of DSHEA after its experience with the passage of The Nutritional Labeling and Education Act of 1990. This act severely restricted unproven claims on foods and dietary supplements. Fearful of the loss of the ability to conduct business as usual, the dietary supplement industry responded with forceful lobbying to the Congress, which responded with DSHEA, exempting dietary supplements from the earlier law.

DSHEA severely limited when the FDA could take action to protect the public and what actions could be taken. The burden of proof to show harm is now placed on the FDA. Moreover, dietary supplement manufacturers are not required to report adverse dietary supplement events. In fact, between 1994 and 1999 fewer than 10 of the 2500 adverse events associated with dietary supplements and reported to the FDA were reported by the manufacturer. The Office of Inspector General concluded the spontaneous adverse event reporting "system has difficulty generating signals of possible public health concern" due to "limited medical information, product information, manufacturer information, consumer information, and ability to analyze trends". One weight loss supplement manufacturer is reported to have withheld from the FDA 14,684 complaints of adverse events regarding ephedra, which included heart attacks, strokes, seizures, and deaths.

Recently, the FDA has begun to enforce DSHEA more assertively. Ephedra was banned as a dietary supplement in April of 2004 because ephedra presented an "*unreasonable risk*." However, this ban does not include foods containing ephedra, approved drugs, or Asian medicines, which are allowed to contain ephedra under the final rule. It appears that FDA may address androstenedione in the near future. In March of 2004, FDA sent warning letters to 23 manufactures or distributors of androstenedione threatening enforcement if they do not immediately cease distribution of androstenedione and within 15 days advise the FDA, in writing, of actions taken. The FDA did this on the grounds that androstene dione was not marketed on October 15, 1994 and as such is not presumed safe under DSHEA. Furthermore, the FDA has stated that androstenedione consumption would be considered an unreasonable risk, given what is now known.

Other botanical products are receiving FDA attention. The acting commissioner of the FDA, Lester Crawford, told members at the American Society for Pharmacology and Experimental Therapeutics in April 2004 that the FDA was compiling data on other botanical products that have been associated with safety issues (64). Kava, used as an anxiolytic, and usnic acid, used for weight loss, have both been associated with liver disease; bitter orange is used as a sympathomimetic in weight loss products to replace ephedra; all the pyrrolizidine alkaloids have the eye of the FDA. There are other products that could receive scrutiny of the FDA in the future. Examples profiled in Consumer Reports include a list of what they call "the dirty dozen herbs listed by risk."

The botanicals are broken down as follows: "*definitively hazardous*": aristolochic acid; "*very likely hazardous*": comfrey, androstenedione, chaparral, germander, and kava; and "*likely hazardous*": bitter orange, organ/glandular extracts, lobelia, pennyroyal oil, skullcap, and yohimbe. These are products with potent pharmacological actions and poorly documented toxicities, and as long as they are available safety will clearly be an issue. As a result of DSHEA, botanical supplements are presumed safe by virtue of being "grandfathered" by the FDA if the product was marketed before October 15, 1994. Products brought to market after that date only require 75-day pre-market notification to the FDA with information that substantiates that the ingredients will reasonably be expected to be safe. FDA cannot take action until patients are injured but it is increasingly clear relatively rare adverse events may not be detected until a significant number of patients are killed or injured.

Safety

With little knowledge of dietary supplements, many physicians do not ask patients about botanical products and patients are also not disclosing the consumption of these products. Some of these products also have substantial pharmacologic activity that interacts with prescription medications and disease states while other are devoid of any biological activity. Many patients may actually think they are taking something that is rigorously tested and regulated by the FDA when in fact some have been reported have serious issues with contaminants. Safety has been presumed as a result of DSHEA despite common misbranding, and adulteration. Several dietary supplements have been linked to cancer, renal and liver failure, and even death.

The vast majority of products are probably safe but many likely have low level undocumented adverse effects. This leaves the possibility most adverse events likely go unrecognized and untreated. Under current practices, the situation is unlikely to change. The profile of the patient who uses a botanical product will likely be someone with higher education, be female, have higher socioeconomic status, have more disposable income, and be older. The market is estimated to be in excess of $5 billion in the United States with an estimated 10% to 20% of the population using botanicals. Utilization of botanical dietary supplements will continue to grow under the deregulation of DSHEA and as they gain acceptance by the public and medical establishment. With increasing stress on the harvesting of wild foliage, corporations must resort to harvesting domestically grown botanical dietary supplements to meet the demand. This should result in a more consistent product base.

By increasing direct-to-consumer marketing and branding of specific products, there will likely be an acceleration of market growth. New ads for branded botanicals have already appeared as this chapter was being published. Products will continue to be imported and Internet sales will continue to grow. As more patients use these products and regulatory issues remain, safety will continue to be a concern and the market will likely be difficult to define. Drug–botanical interactions and disease–botanical interactions are only now beginning to be recognized by health care professionals as a potential source of harm, as the prevalence of botanical dietary supplement utilization increases.

11

Ephedra Alkaloids

Ephedra, and other medicinal plants have been identified at European neanderthal burial sites dating from 60,000 BCE. Thousands of years later, Pliny accurately described the medicinal uses of ephedra. But thousands of years before Pliny, traditional Chinese healers used ephedra extracts. Chinese texts from the 15th century recommended ephedra as an antipyretic and antitussive. In Russia, around the same time, extracts of ephedra were used to treat joint pain; and though recent laboratory studies confirm that ephedra might be useful for that purpose, additional trials and studies have not been forthcoming. In the 1600s, Indians and Spaniards in the American South-west used ephedra as a treatment for venereal disease. That idea might also have had some merit, as some studies show that ephedra contains compounds with antibiotic activity called *transtorines*. Whether the transtorines will prove to be clinically useful has not been determined.

In 1885, Nagayoshi Nagi, a German-trained, Japanese-born chemist, isolated and synthesized ephedrine. Nagi's original observations were confirmed by Merck chemists 40 years later. Merck's attempts at commercializing ephedrine were unsuccessful, at least until 1930, when Chen and Schmidt published a monograph recommending ephedrine as the treatment of choice for asthma. During the 1920s and 1930s, epinephrine was the only effective oral agent for treating asthma. Epinephrine, which had been available since the early 1900s was (and still is) an effective bronchodilator, but it has to be given by injection, or administered with special nebulizers. Ephedrine was nearly as effective as epinephrine, and could be taken orally.

As a result, ephedrine became the first-line drug against asthma. It was displaced from that front during the late 1970s and early 1980s, when aerosolized synthetic β-agonists were introduced. Unlike most of the other alkaloids contained in ephedra (methylephedrine and cathinone are both psychoactive, but the amount contained in unadulterated ephedra is too low to be of clinical significance), ephedrine is also a potent *central nervous system* (CNS) stimulant. Injections of ephedrine, called *philopon* (which means "love of work") were given to Japanese kamikaze pilots during World War II. A major epidemic of ephedrine abuse occurred in postwar Japan, when stockpiles of ephedrine accumulated for use by the Army were dumped on the black market. Abusers in Tokyo, and other large Japanese cities, injected themselves with ephedrine (then referred to as hirapon), in much the same way that methamphetamine is injected today.

In the Philippines, a mixture of ephedrine and caffeine called *shabu* was traditionally smoked for its stimulating effect. In the late 1980s, shabu smoking gave way to the practice of smoking methamphetamine ("ice"). In what is perhaps a tribute to the past, some "ice" is sold under the philopon name. The chemistry and nomenclature of these compounds are somewhat confusing, and are best understood by reference to the synthetic route used by plants to make ephedrine. All ephedra plants contain phenylalanine-derived alkaloids. Plants use phenylalanine as a precursor, but incorporate only seven of its carbon atoms. Phenylalanine is metabolized to benzoic acid, which is then acetylated and decarboxylated to form pyruvic acid. Transamination, results in the formation of forms (–)-cathinone.

Reduction of one carbonlyl group leads to the formation of either (–)- norephedrine (phenylpropanolamine is the name used to refer to the synthetic mixture of ± norephedrine), or norpseudoephedrine (called *cathine*). N-methylation of (–)-norephedrine results in the formation of (+)-ephedrine. N-methylation of cathine leads to the formation of (+)-pseudoephedrine.

Current Promoted Uses

Physicians routinely used intravenous ephedrine for the prophylaxis and treatment of hypotension caused by spinal anesthesia particularly during caesarean section. In the past, ephedrine was used to treat Stokes–Adams attacks (complete heart block), and was also recommended as a treatment for narcolepsy. Over the years, ephedrine has been replaced by other, more effective agents, and the advent of highly selective β-agonists has mostly eliminated the need to use ephedrine in treating asthma.

European medical researchers have, for several years, used ephedrine to help promote weight loss, at least in the morbidly obese, and nutritional supplements containing naturally occurring ephedra alkaloids are sold in the United States for the same purpose. Clinical trials confirm that, taken as directed, use of these supplements does result in weight loss, though whether such losses are sustained has not been determined.

Prior to its banning by the Food and Drug Administration (FDA) in 2004, ephedra was found in many "*food supplements*," used by bodybuilders. Generally, it was compounded with other ingredients such as vitamins, minerals, and amino acids in products, which are said to increase muscle mass and enhance endurance. Performance improvement secondary to ephedrine ingestion has been established in a controlled clinical trials, and use of ephedrine has been prohibited by the International Olympic Committee.

Ephedra was also sold in combination with many other herbs in obscure combinations. Labels frequently listed 10 or 15 different herbs, but, analysis usually disclosed only the ephedra alkaloids and caffeine as present in sufficient quantities to be physiologically active. After several well-publicized accidental deaths, products clearly intended for abuse, such as "*herbal ecstasy*," and other "look-alike drugs" (products usually containing ephedrine or phenylpropanolamine designed to look like illicit methamphetamine, but in concentrations higher than recommended by industry or the FDA) were withdrawn from the market. Labels on these products were frequently misleading. For example, one might suppose that a product called "Ephedrine 60" contained 60 mg of ephedrine when, in fact, the actual ephedrine content was 25 mg.

Sources and Chemical Composition

Ephedra is a small perennial shrub with thin stems. It rarely grows to more than a foot in height, and at first glance, the plant looks very much like a small broom. Different, closely related species are found in Western Europe, southeastern Europe, Asia, and even the Americas. Some of the better known species include *Ephedra sinica* and *E. equisentina* from China (collectively known as ma haung), as well as *E. geriardiana*, *E. intermedia*, and *E. major*, which grow in India and Pakistan, and countless other members of the family Ephedraceae that grow in Europe and the United States (*E. distachya*, *E. vulgaris*).

Ephedra species vary widely in their ephedrine content. One of the most common Chinese cultivars, known as "China 3," contains 1.39% ephedrine, 0.361% pseudoephedrine, and 0.069% methyl-ephedrine. This mix is fairly typical for commercially grown ephedra plants. Noncommercial varieties of ephedra may contain no ephedrine at all, while others may contain more pseudoephedrine than ephedrine. Depending on the variety, trace amounts of phenylpropanolamine, (-) norephedrine, and methylephedrine may also be present, however (+) norephedrine does not occur naturally, and its presence is proof of adulteration.

Labels on herbal supplements listed total ephedra alkaloid content, usually 10 or 11 mg per serving. Depending on the raw materials used, different production runs of the same product contained ephedrine and pseudoephedrine in varying proportions. Occasionally, supplement makers were accused of adulterating their product by adding synthetic ephedrine or pseudoephedrine. Unlike with (+)-norephedrine, these compounds occur naturally and product adulteration should not have been alleged just because alkaloids other than ephedrine were detected in trace amounts, or because the ratio of ephedrine to pseudoephedrine was close to, or even greater than, 1:1. Of course, if one of the minor alkaloids, such as methylephedrine, were found to be present in concentrations approaching those of ephedrine, the ratio could only be explained by adulteration.

Products Available

Prior to its ban in 2004, no one government agency was tasked with tracking production of ephedrine-containing products. Nor were these products indexed by any industry or trade organization. Ephedrine-containing supplement products were mostly purchased at health food stores or over the Internet. Claims made by some of the Internet vendors were quite outrageous and totally unsupported by any scientific research.

The large supplement makers, of course, had web pages, many of which contained, or had links to, the most recent peer review studies. But in addition to the established names, hundreds of other, smaller manufacturers also advertised and sold over the Internet. These companies came into and went out of existence so rapidly that a detailed listing of their web sites would likely be outdated before the links were published. Even today, a simple search using the word "*ephedrine*," will disclosed numerous off-shore vendors, along with numbers of attorneys soliciting for ephedra-related class action legal cases.

In addition to selling their own proprietary mixture, many of these same web sites sold the same popular products as the herbal and general retail outlets, such as a previous Twin Labs best seller "Ripped Fuel," which contained ephedrine in the form of ma huang, combined with guarana, L-carnitine, and chromium picolinate. Metabolife 356TM contained guarana (40 mg caffeine), 12 mg ephedrine as ma huang, chromium picolinate 75 mg, and several other ingredients. Ever since ephedrine became the precursor of choice for making methamphetamine, federal regulators have severely restricted bulk sales of ephedrine, but these restrictions have been bypassed in some cases by illegally ordering from a foreign web site.

In most products, ephedrine content ranged anywhere from 12 to 80 mg per serving, with the majority of products falling into the lower range. Industry standards called for a total dose of ephedrine of less than 100 mg/day. The FDA, however, allowed a maximum daily dose of 150 mg/day of synthetic ephedrine. Unless fortified, the expected ephedrine content of ma huang capsules was generally less than 10%. Thus, a capsule said to contain 1000 g of ephedra would probably have contained no more than 80 mg of ephedrine.

In the United States, (+)-norpseudoephedrine, in its pure form, is considered a Schedule IV controlled substance. However, because of the small amounts of this alkaloid in ephedra plants or extracts, the Drug Enforcement Administration (DEA) had never stated or proposed that ephedra products were subject to the scheduling requirements of the Controlled Substances Act. Quite the contrary, DEA published a proposed rule in 1998 that stated DEA's intent to exempt legitimate ephedra products in finished form from regulation even as "chemical mixtures." Other regulatory sanctions and actions on ephedra rendered action on this regulation moot.

Pharmacological Effects

Studies have shown that resultant effects are similar, regardless of whether pure synthetic ephedrine or naturally occurring ephedra is ingested. There are, however, significant enantioselective differences between the enantomers in both pharmacokinetic and pharmacodynamic effects. All of the ephedra alkaloids have important effects on the cardiovascular and respiratory systems, but not to the same degree.

Ephedrine, the predominant alkaloid in ephedra, is both an α and β stimulant. It directly stimulates α_2 and β_1; receptors and, because it also causes the release of norepinephrine from nerve endings, it also acts as a β_2 stimulant. The resultant physiological changes are variable, depending on receptor distribution and receptor regulation. Tolerance to ephedrine's β agonist actions emerges rapidly, which is why ephedrine is no longer the preferred agent for treating asthma; receptor downregulation quickly occurs and the bronchodilator effects are lost.

Receptor distribution probably explains why ephedrine has no effect on diastolic pressure, and only minimal effect on systolic. β_2 Stimulation of vessels in peripheral muscles results in peripheral vasodilation and "*diastolic runoff*," which more than cancels ephedrine's other inotropic effects. The absence of any significant effect on blood pressure was firmly established during the late 1970s and early 1980s in dozens of double-blind, placebo-controlled studies performed to compare the effectiveness of ephedrine with that of newly synthesized adrenergic agents. The pharmacokinetic and toxicokinetic behavior of any isomer cannot be used to predict that of any other ephedrine isomer. The (+) isomer of methamphetamine, for example, is a potent CNS stimulant, but the (-)-isomer is merely a decongestant. There is a tendency in the literature to lump together all "*ephedrine alkaloids*" and use the term "*class effect*" to assume that all the different drugs in that class exert the same effects on the same biological targets. In fact, some of the drugs in the class will be similar in some regards and different in others.

The affinity of the various ephedrine isomers for human β-receptors has been measured and compared (as indicated by the amount of cyclic adenosine monophosphate produced compared to that of isoproterenol) in tissue culture. Activity of the different isomers is highly stereoselective, i.e., the different isomers had very different receptor-binding characteristics. For β_1-receptors, maximal response (relative to isoproterenol = 100%) was greatest for ephedrine (68% for 1R, 2S-ephedrine and 66% for the 1S, 2R-ephedrine isomer). Both of the pseudoephedrine isomers had much lower affinities (53%). When binding to 32-receptors was measured, the rank order of potency for 1R, 2S-ephedrine was 78%, followed by 1R, 2R-pseudoephedrine (50%), followed by 1S, 2S-pseudoephedrine (47%). The 1S, 2R-ephedrine isomer had only 22% of the activity exerted by isoproterenol, but was the only isomer that showed any significant agonist activity on human β_3-receptors (31%). Stimulation of β_3-receptors, which are thought to be located only in fat cells, may account for ephedrine's ability to cause weight loss.

Ephedrine is also an α agonist and, as such, is capable of stimulating bladder smooth muscle. At one time, it was used to promote urinary continence. In animal models, when compared to norepinephrine, ephedrine is a relatively weak α-adrenergic agonist, possessing less than one-third the activity of norepinephrine. Ephedrine's usefulness as a bronchodilator is limited by the number of β-receptors on the bronchi. The number of β-receptors located on human lymphocytes (which correlates with the number found in the lungs) decreases rapidly after the administration of ephedrine; the density of binding sites drops to 50% after 8 days of treatment and returns to normal 5 to 7 days after the drug has been withdrawn.

Clinical Studies

Bronchodilation

Banner et al. summarized studies where the effects of ephedrine and ephedra were compared to placebo in controlled studies in humans. None of the controlled trials disclosed any evidence of cardiovascular toxicity when ephedrine was given in doses as high as 1 mg/kg, even when it was administered to severe asthmatics with known cardiac arrhythmias. The trial reported by Banner et al. studied the respiratory and circulatory effects of orally administered ephedrine sulfate, 25 mg, aminophylline, 400 mg, terbutaline sulfate, 5 mg, and placebo in 20 patients with ventricular arrhythmia by a double-blind crossover method. The study was comprised of 20 patients, with an average age of 60 years and a preexisting history of both asthma and heart disease (as evidence by the presence of frequent premature ventricular contractions). The bronchodilator effect of terbutaline was similar to that of aminophylline over 4 hours but superior to ephedrine at hour 4. Both terbutaline and ephedrine exhibited chronotropic effects, with the effect of terbutaline greater than that of ephedrine at hour 4. The effect of aminophylline on heart rate (HR) did not differ from placebo. Only terbutaline was associated with an increase in ventricular ectopic beats. Ventricular tachycardia occurred in three patients treated with terbutaline and in one patient with ephedrine (which occurred before he was given ephedrine). There were no significant changes in blood pressure. Orally administered terbutaline should not be regarded as safer than orally administered ephedrine or aminophylline in patients with arrhythmias.

In 1992, Astrup studied the effects of ephedrine and caffeine in a group of obese patients. In a randomized, placebo-controlled, double-blind study, 180 obese patients were treated by diet (4.2 mJ/day) and either an ephedrine/caffeine combination (20 mg/200 mg), ephedrine (20 mg), caffeine (200 mg), or placebo three times a day for 24 weeks. Withdrawals were distributed equally in the four groups, and 141 patients completed the trial. Mean weight losses was significantly greater with the combination than with placebo from week 8 to week 24 (ephedrine/caffeine, 16.6 ± 6.8 kg vs placebo, 13.2 ± 6.6 kg [mean ± standard deviation {SD}], $P = 0.0015$). Weight loss in both the ephedrine and the caffeine groups was similar to that of the placebo group. Side effects (tremor, insomnia, and dizziness) were transient and after 8 weeks of treatment they had reached placebo levels. Systolic and diastolic blood pressure fell similarly in all four groups.

Weight Loss

The most recent of the studies examining weight control were designed to address concerns about long-term safety and efficacy for weight loss using a mixture containing 90 mg of ephedrine (from ephedra) and 192 mg of caffeine, derived from cola nuts. A 6-month randomized, double-blind, placebo-controlled trial was performed, in which a total of 167 subjects (body mass index 31.8 ± 4.1 kg/m^2) were randomized to receive either placebo ($n = 84$) or herbal treatment ($n = 83$). The primary outcome measurements were changes in blood pressure, heart function, and body weight. Secondary variables included body composition and metabolic changes. It was found that herbal vs placebo treatment decreased body weight (–5.3 ± 5.0 vs –2.6 ± 3.2 kg, $P < 0.001$), body fat (–4.3 ± 3.3 vs –2.7 ± 2.8 kg, $P = 0.020$), and low- density lipoprotein cholesterol (–8 ± 20 vs 0 ± 17 mg/dL, $P = 0.013$), and increased high-density lipoprotein cholesterol (+2.7 ± 5.7 vs –0.3 ± 6.7 mg/ dL, $P = 0.004$). Herbal treatment produced small changes in blood pressure variables (+3 to –5 mmHg, $P \sim 0.05$), and increased HR (4 ± 9 vs –3 ± 9 beats per minute, $P < 0.001$), but cardiac arrhythmias were not increased ($P > 0.05$). By self-report, dry mouth ($P < 0.01$), heartburn ($P < 0.05$), and insomnia ($P < 0.01$) were increased and diarrhea decreased ($P < 0.05$). Irritability, nausea, chest pain, and palpitations did not differ, nor did numbers of subjects who withdrew. *Conclusions*: In this 6-month placebo-controlled trial, herbal ephedra/caffeine (90/192 mg/day) promoted body-weight and body-fat reduction and improved blood lipids without significant adverse events.

Athletic Performance

In a series of studies, Bell et al. assessed the effects of ephedrine mixtures on performance, and found measurable improvement. One and one-half hours after ingesting a placebo (P), caffeine (C) (4 mg/kg), ephedrine (E) (0.8 mg/kg), or caffeine and ephedrine, 12 subjects performed a 10-km run while wearing a helmet and backpack weighing 11 kg. The trials were performed in a climatic suite at 12–13°C, on a treadmill where the speed was regulated by the subject. VO_2, VCO_2, V(E), HR, and rating of perceived exertion were measured during the run at 15 and 30 minutes, and again when the individual reached 9 km.

Blood was sampled at 15 and 30 minutes and again at the end of the run and assayed for lactate, glucose, and catecholamines. Run times (mean ± SD), in minutes, were for C (46.0 ± 2.8), E (45.5 ± 2.9), C + E (45.7 ± 3.3), and P (46.8 ± 3.2). The run times for the E trials (E and C + E) were significantly reduced compared with the non-E trials (C and P). Pace was increased for the E trials compared with the non-E trials over the last 5 km of the run. VO_2 was not affected by drug ingestion. HR was elevated for the ephedrine trials (E and C + E), but the respiratory exchange ratio (a measure of maximal exertion) remained similar for all trails. Caffeine increased the epinephrine and norepinephrine response associated with exercise and also increased blood lactate, glucose, and glycerol levels. Ephedrine reduced the epinephrine response but increased dopamine and free fatty acid levels. Bell concluded previously that the effects of caffeine, when taken with ephedrine, were not additive, and that all of the observed improvement could be accounted for by the presence of ephedrine.

Pharmacokinetics

Phenylpropanolamine is readily and completely absorbed, but pseudoephedrine, with a bioavailability of only approx 38%, is subject to gut wall metabolism, and absorption may be erratic. Pure ephedrine is well absorbed from the stomach, but absorption is much slower when it is given as a component of ma huang, rather than in its pure form. Ephedrine ingested in the form of ma huang has a t_{max} of nearly 4 hours, compared to only 2 hours when pure ephedrine is given. Like its enantiomers, ephedrine is eliminated in the urine largely as unchanged drug, with a half-life of approx 3–6 hours.

The rate at which any of the enantiomers is eliminated depends upon the urinary pH. At high pHs, excretion time is prolonged. At low pH ranges, excretion is accelerated. In controlled laboratory studies, where volunteer subjects were given either bicarbonate or ammonium chloride, the higher the urine pH, the more slowly the ephedrine and pseudoephedrine were excreted. Conversely, when the urine pH is low, excretion is accelerated. The importance of these observations is hard to assess, because without the addition of bicarbonate, urine pH values in the general population rarely approach 8.0. A study of pseudoephedrine pharmacokinetics in 33 volunteers who were not treated with drugs to alter urine pH found that these parameters could not be correlated to urine pH, mainly because there was little difference in pH between the different participants. Excretion patterns may be much more rapid in children, and a greater dosage may be required to achieve therapeutic effects. Patients with renal impairment are at special risk for toxicity.

Peak concentrations for the other enantiomers, specifically phenylpropanolamine and pseudoephedrine, occur earlier (0.5 and 2 hours, respectively) than for ephedrine, but all three drugs are extensively distributed into extravascular sites (apparent volume of distribution between 2.6 and 5.0 L/kg). No protein-binding data in humans are available. Peak ephedrine levels after ingestion of 400 mg of ma huang, containing 20 mg of ephedrine, resulted in blood concentrations of 81 ng/mL—essentially no different than the peak ephedrine levels observed after giving an equivalent amount of pure ephedrine. In another study, 50 mg of ephedrine given orally to six healthy, 21-year-old women produced mean peak plasma concentrations of 168 ng/mL, 127 min after ingestion, with a half-life of slightly more than 9 hours. The results are comparable to those obtained in studies done nearly 30 years earlier. Very high levels of methylephedrine have been observed in Japanese polydrug abusers taking a cough medication called BRON. Concentrations of methylephedrine less than 0.3 mg/L, the range generally observed in individuals taking BRON for therapeutic rather than recreational purposes, appear to be nontoxic and devoid of measurable effects. Methylephedrine is a minor component of most ephedra plants, but in Japan (where, unlike in the United States, methylephedrine is legally sold) it is produced synthetically, and is used in cough and cold remedies, especially BRON. In terms of catecholamine stimulation, methylephedrine appears comparable to ephedrine; however, it does not react with most standard urine screening tests for ephedrine. This can be a cause of some forensic confusion, because 10–15% of a given dose of methylephedrine is converted to ephedrine.

Although the issue has been raised in litigation, the amounts of methylephedrine and norephedrine contained in naturally occurring ephedra are so low as to be of no clinical consequence. For example, the study by Gurley et al. found that most of the commercial products tested had no methylephedrine whatsoever, but when it was present, it was usually in quantities of less than 1 mg per serving (range 0.2 to 2.2 mg). If the volume of distriution (Vd) of methylephedrine is assumed to be 3.5, approximately the same as ephedrine, then a 70-kg man ingesting a 2-mg serving of methylephedrine would produce a blood concentration of (dose = kg weight × blood concentration × Vd) 0–0.06 mg, undoubtedly below most laboratories' minimum level of detection, and a clinically insignificant finding. Similar considerations apply to the small amounts of norephedrine found in these products.

Adverse Effects and Toxicity

Two journal articles analyzing *adverse event reporters* (AERs) have been published in the peer-reviewed literature, and both reports have received wide publicity. The reports are, however, of limited use in assessing toxicity, because they are comprised of passively collected anecdotal data, which is often incomplete and unreliably reported. For example, one of the FDA ephedrine AERs "analyzed" in an article published in the *New England Journal of Medicine* described the sudden death of a teenage girl who had been born with a lethal cardiac malformation who died while playing volleyball. Postmortem blood and tissue tested negative for ephedrine, and the article failed to mention the existence of the cardiac malformation. In other AERs, massive doses of ephedrine were consumed (as with products intended for abuse, such as "*herbal ecstasy*," now withdrawn from the market). Toxicology testing was rarely performed in any of these cases, and it is not known with any certainty whether ephedrine was even taken. Even the authors of the two papers concede that anecdotal reports cannot be used to prove causality, stating that "Our report does not prove causation, nor does it provide quantitative information with regard to risk". There is little point in reviewing material that cannot be used to prove causality, and it is not included in the summaries that follow, which are comprised only of published, peer-review case reports, epidemiological surveys, and controlled clinical trials. An additional review of the utility of spontaneously reported adverse events involving supplements and, more specifically, ephedra was published by Kingston et al.. The review discussed the limitations of spontaneously reported data in assessing supplement safety and determining causality between exposure and adverse effects.

Despite conflicting data regarding the safety of ephedra from clinical studies and conclusions drawn from spontaneously reported adverse events, FDA banned the sale of ephedra-containing supplements in 2004.

Neurological Disorders

Many strokes attributed to ephedrine have actually been caused by the ingestion of ephedrine enantiomers, pseudoephedrine, phenylpropanolamine, and even methylephedrine. Two cases of ischemic stroke have been reported, but in neither case was their any toxicological testing to confirm the use of ephedrine. A decade-old report described the autopsy findings in three individuals with intracerebral hemorrhage and positive toxicology testing for ephedrine; however, one had hypertensive cerbrovasular disease and the other had a demonstrable ruptured aneurysm.

Intracerebral hemorrhage has also been described in suicide and attempted suicide victims who took overdoses of pseudoephedrine. There is also a report describing a patient who developed described arteritis following the intravenous administration of ephedrine during a surgical procedure. On the other hand, a large study to assess risk factors for stroke in young people (age 20–49) over a 1-year period was carried out in Poland, a country where ephedra-based products are widely used. Nearly one-half the cases of stroke were associated with preexisting hypertension, another 15% had hyperlipidemia, and 6% were diabetic. None of the individuals were ephedrine users.

Sometimes, especially in Japan and the Philippines, ephedrine is taken specifically as a psychostimulant. In Japan, BRON, the OTC cough medication containing methylephedrine, dihydrocodeine, caffeine, and chlorpheniramine, is very widely abused, and transient psychosis commonly results. Reports of ephedrine-related psychosis following prolonged, heavy use are fairly common. In general, psychosis is only seen in ephedrine users ingesting more than 1000 mg/day, and it resolves rapidly once the drug is withdrawn.

Ephedrine psychosis closely resembles psychosis induced by amphetamines: paranoia with delusions of persecution and auditory and visual hallucinations, even though consciousness remains unclouded. Typically, patients with ephedrine psychosis will have ingested more than 1000 mg/day. Recovery is rapid after the drug is withdrawn. The ephedrine content per serving of most food supplements is on the order of 10–20 mg, making it extremely unlikely that, in recommended doses, use of any of the products would lead to neurological symptoms.

Renal Disorders

Reports, particularly in the European literature, have described the occurrence of renal calculi in chronic ephedrine users. A review of cases from a large commercial laboratory specializing in the analysis of kidney stones found that 200 out of 166,466, or 0.064%, of stones analyzed by that laboratory, contained either ephedrine or pseudoephedrine. Unfortunately, the analytic technique used could not distinguish ephedrine from pseudoephedrine, and because pseudoephedrine is used so much more widely than ephedrine, it seems that the risk of renal calculus associated with ephedrine use must be quite small. There have been no new reports of ephedrine-related nephrolithiasis since 1999. Direct toxicity, with altered renal function and demonstrable kidney lesions related to ephedrine use, has never been demonstrated. Urinary retention, occurring as a consequence of drug overdose, was occasionally reported, but additional cases have not been described in more than a decade. The FDA and Commission E both warn against the possibility of urinary retention in patients with prostatic enlargement, but the theoretical basis for this concern is unclear, and, in any case, retention in patients with prostate disease has not been reported.

Small amounts of ephedrine are oxidized in to norephedrine and norpseudoephedrine in the liver. In patients with diminished renal function, these drugs may accumulate and have the potential to cause serious toxicity. None of the ephedrine enantiomers are easily removed by dialysis, and treatment of overdose remains supportive, using pharmacological antagonists to counter the α- and β-adrenergic effects of these drugs. Because excretion is pH-dependent, patients with renal tubular acidosis are also at risk. The FDA reports having received a number of accounts of hematuria after use of ephedra-based products, but no such cases have ever appeared in the peer-reviewed literature, and review of the reports published by the FDA shows that all of the affected individuals were taking multiple remedies, some capable of causing interstitial nephritis.

Cardiovascular Diseases

Ephedrine and pseudoephedrine share properties with cocaine and with the amphetamines because they: (1) stimulate β-receptors directly, and (2) also cause the increased release of norepinephrine. Chronic exposure to abnormally high levels of circulating catecholamines can damage the heart. This is certainly the case with cocaine and methamphetamine, but ephedrine-related cardiomyopathy is an extremely rare occurrence, occurring only in individuals who take massive amounts of drug for prolonged periods of time. Only two papers have ever been published on the subject. The two existing reports are uninterpretable, because histological findings were not described in either report, and angiography was not performed, thereby making it impossible to actually establish the diagnosis of cardiomyopathy.

Similar considerations apply to the relationship (if any) between myocardial infarction and ephedrine use. The report by Cockings and Brown described a 25-year-old drug abuser who injected himself with an unknown amount of cocaine intravenously. The only other published reports involved a woman in labor who was receiving other vasoactive drugs; and two pseudoephedrine users, one of whom was also taking bupropion, who developed coronary artery spasm.

Three cases of ephedra-related coronary spasm in anesthetized patients have also been reported, but multiple agents were administred in all three cases, and the normal innervation of the coronary arteries was disrupted in two of the cases where a high spinal anesthetic had been administered. One case of alleged ephedrine-related hypersensitivity myocarditis has been reported, but the patient was taking many other herbal supplements, and the responsible agent is not known with certainty. Although there are no reasons why ephedra alkaloids should not cause allergic reactions, the incidence appears to be extremely low.

Although clinical trials or epidemiological studies are lacking, it has been suggested that maternal use of OTC cold medication may result in fetal arrhythmias, but linkage between ephedrine and isomers and arrhythmia has never been demonstrated. The literature contains one case report describing arrhythmias occurring in a 14-year-old who overdosed on cold medications. The child had taken a total of 3300 mg of caffeine, 825 mg of phenylpropanolamine, and 412 mg of ephedrine. Clearly, large doses of ephedrine, and its enantiomers, are capable of exerting toxicity.

The paucity of peer-reviewed studies describing cardiovascular complication with ephedra alkaloids suggests that few such cases are occurring. This notion is support by the studies of Porta et al., who performed a follow-up study of more than 100,000 persons below age 65 years who filled a total of 243,286 prescriptions for pseudoephedrine. No hospitalizations could be attributed to the drug. There were no admissions within 15 days of filling a prescription for pseudoephedrine for cerebral hemorrhage, thrombotic stroke, or hypertensive crisis. There were a small number of hospitalizations for myocardial infarction, seizures, and neuropsychiatric disorders, but the rate of such admissions among the pseudoephedrine users was close to the expected rate in the population at large.

Workplace Drug Testing

Ephedra alkaloids, even when used in the recommended amounts, can cause positive urine screening tests for methamphetamine, sometimes yielding surprisingly high concentrations.

Postmortem Toxicology

Very few fatalities have ever been reported (or studied), but it appears that the therapeutic index for ephedrine is very great. A 1997 case report described a 28-year-old woman with two prior suicide attempts, who died after ingesting amitriptyline and ephedrine. The blood ephedrine concentration was 11,000 ng/mL, and the liver concentration was twice that value (kidney, 14 mg/kg; brain, 8.9 mg/kg). The amitriptyline concentration was 0.33 mg/kg in blood and 7.8 mg/kg in liver. Values in a second case report (where methylephedrine concentrations were nearly 6000 ng/mL) may or may not be relevant to the problem of ephedrine toxicity, as the individual in question took massive quantities of a calcium channel blocker, and it is not known whether methylephedrine exerts all the same effects as ephedrine. Baselt and Cravey mention the case of a young woman who died several hours after ingesting 2.1 g of ephedrine combined with 7.0 g of caffeine, but tissue findings were not described. Her blood ephedrine level was 5 mg/L, whereas the concentration in the liver was 15 mg/kg.

A report from the European literature describes the findings in a 19- year-old woman who committed suicide by taking 40 Letigen tablets (200 mg of caffeine and 20 mg of ephedrine) amounting to 10 g of caffeine and 1 g of ephedrine. She developed severe toxic manifestations from the heart, CNS, muscles, liver, and kidneys leading to several cardiac arrests, and died subsequently of cerebral edema and incarceration on the fourth day of hospitalization. Postmortem blood concentrations were not given.

Pseudoephedrine concentrations, but not measurements for ephedrine or any of the other enantiomers, have been published by the National Association of Medical Examiners in their Annual Registry report. In 15 children diagnosed with sudden infant death syndrome, the mean blood pseudoephedrine concentration was 3.55 mg/L, the median 2.3 mg/L, with a range of 0.07–13.0 mg/L (SD = 3.36 mg/L). The authors of the study take pains to point out that "The data do not allow definitive statements about the toxicity of pseudoephedrine at a given concentration".

In the only autopsy study yet published, all autopsies in the San Francisco Medical Examiner's jurisdiction from 1994 to 2001 where ephedrine or any its isomers (E+) were detected were reviewed. Cases where ephedrine or its isomers were detected were compared with those in a control group of drug-free trauma victims. Of 127 ephedrine-positive cases identified, 33 were the result of trauma. Decedents were mostly male (80.3%) and mostly Caucasian (59%). Blood ephedrine concentrations were less than 0.49 mg/L in 50% of the cases, with a range of 0.07–11.73 mg/L in trauma victims, and 0.02–12.35 mg/L in nontrauma cases. Norephedrine was present in the blood of only 22.8% (mean concentration of 1.81 mg/L, SD=3.14 mg/L) and in the urine of 36.2% of the urine specimens, with a mean concentration of 15.6 mg/L, SD=21.50 mg/L). Pseudoephedrine (PE) was detected in the blood of 6.3%. More than 88% of the decedents who tested positive for ephedrine or one of its isomers also tested positive for other drugs, the most common being cocaine (or its metabolites) and morphine. The most frequent pathological diagnoses were hepatic steatosis and nephrosclerosis. Left ventricular hypertrophy was common, and coronary artery disease was detected in nearly one-third of the cases. The most common findings in the ephedrine-positive deaths reviwed were those generally associated with chronic stimulant abuse. There were no cases of heat stroke and no cases of rhabdomyolysis.

Methamphetamine Manufacture

Either (–)-ephedrine or (+)-pseudoephedrine can be used to make meth- amphetamine by reductive dehalogenation using red phosphorus as a catalyst. If (–)-ephedrine is used as the starting material, the process will generate (+)-methamphetamine. If psuedoephedrine is used, the result will be dextromethamphetamine. As this synthetic route has become nearly universal, both state and federal governments have enacted laws limiting the amount of pure ephedrine or pseudoephedrine that can be purchased.

Drug Interactions

The ephedra alkaloids are all sympathomimetic amines, which means that a host of drug interactions are theoretically possible. In fact, only a handful of adverse drug interactions have been reported in the peer-reviewed literature. The most important of these involve the monoamine oxidase inhibitors (MAOI). Irreversible, nonselective MAOIs have been reported to adversely interact with indirectly acting sympathomimetic amines present in many cough and cold medicine. In controlled trials with individuals taking moclobemide, ephedrine's effects on pulse and blood pressure were potentiated, but only at higher doses than those currently provided in health supplements. Ephedrine-MAOI interaction may, on occasion, be severe enough to mimic pheo-chromocytoma. In addition, there is decreased metabolic clearance of pseudoephedrine when MAOIs are administered concurrently. At least one case report suggests that selective serotonin reuptake inhibitor antidepressants can react with pseudoephedrine, leading to the occurrence of "*serotonin syndrome*". Bromocriptine, the ergot-derived dopamine agonist can interact with pseudoephedrine, and would presumably interact with ephedrine as well. Surgical patients being treated with clonidine have an enhanced pressor response to ephedrine, apparently a result of clonidineinduced potentiation of α_1-adrenoceptor-mediated vasoconstriction. In some clinical trials, the coadministration of ephedrine with morphine has been shown to increase analgesia, but this approach to pain relief remains somewhat controversial.

Reproduction

Use of ephedra-containing products is likely unsafe during pregnancy because of reports of psychoses and cardiovascular effects.

Regulatory Status

In 2004, the FDA issued a final rule prohibiting the sale of dietary supplements containing ephedrine alkaloids (ephedra), citing concerns over safety and potential risk of illness or injury. The FDA reviewed evidence about ephedra' s pharmacology: peer-reviewed scientific literature on ephedra' s safety and effectiveness, adverse event reports, and a seminal report by the RAND Corporation, an independent scientific institute. Spontaneously reported adverse effects with high-profile sports figures and others raised public awareness and fueled the debate over safety. Subsequent to the ban, various trade groups and supplement companies have criticized the ban, and an appeal of the decision with temporary suspension of sanctions in some jurisdictions, pending further review, has occurred. Regardless of the regulatory outcome, reintroduction of OTC ephedra-containing supplements is not likely to occur. Although banned in the United States, use of ephedra in other countries is likely to continue.

12

GRAPEFRUIT AND OTHER CITRUS

The first report of grapefruit juice (GFJ) interacting with a drug, altering its bioavailability, was published in 1991. This accidental discovery was made in a study on ethanol–drug interactions—the bioavailability of felodipine was increased when subjects were consuming GFJ concomitantly with felodipine, associated with a lower dehydrofelodipine/felodipine area under the curve (AUC) ratio, decreased diastolic blood pressure, and an increased heart rate (1). Subsequent research in the area of fruit–drug interactions focused on grapefruit and grapefruit compounds of which several were found to affect the absorption or metabolism of certain drugs. GFJ was shown to alter the pharmacokinetics of several drugs such as statins, calcium channel blockers, antibiotics, and others. Other fruits, vegetables, and dietary supplements also have the potential to cause an adverse interaction with conventional drugs. Over 16% of all prescription drug users reported that they concurrently use at least one plant-based dietary supplement, including grapefruit and citrus products.

Many consumers have become more aware of the health benefits of antioxidants, phytochemical-rich fruits and vegetables, and products that contain these. In 1997, GFJ was purchased by 21% of all households as a popular antioxidant breakfast juice, predominantly preferred by the elderly. By-products from the citrus-processing industry, such as grapefruit seed extract, flavonoids, essential oils from the peel, and pectins may be added to other food products to improve taste, consistency, or overall quality. These by-products also may be used in the production of dietary supplements. Consequently, citrus compounds that have a potential for an interaction with drugs may find their way into other food products.

Hence, increased availability and consumption of drugs, dietary supplements, and phytochemical-containing antioxidant foods may increase the likelihood of an adverse interaction between foods and certain drugs. Absorption and metabolism of a drug may be adversely affected, shifting the administered dose outside of the therapeutic range, which may lead to a lower effectiveness of the drug or to an overdose associated with undesired or even dangerous side effects.

Based on our current knowledge, grapefruit compounds interact with drugs that are metabolized by cytochrome P450 3A4 (CYP3A4) and also have a low or variable oral bioavailability. The major mechanism leading to a grapefruit–drug interaction appears to be the reduction of the *"pre-systemic"* metabolism through the inhibition of intestinal CYP3A4. Some hydroxymethylglutaryl-coenzyme A (HMG-CoA) reductase inhibitors and calcium channel antagonists are among the affected drugs.

Other mechanisms of interaction have also been reported, such as altered activity of other enzymes within the CYP450 family. Moreover, GFJ may also inhibit the intestinal P-glycoprotein (P-gp)-mediated efflux transport of drugs such as cyclosporine to increase its oral bioavailability. GFJ and other fruit juices have recently been shown to be potent in vitro inhibitors of a number of organic anion-transporting polypeptides (OATPs).

Grapefruits and GFJ have a potential to interact with several oral medications when consumed in moderate amounts, such as one or two servings of GFJ. The concern that the concomitant administration of grapefruit products with certain drugs may lessen the effect of a drug or cause a toxic effect based on the increases in oral drug bioavailability has lead to the recommendation to avoid the consumption of grapefruit products in combination with these drugs of concern. The Food and Drug Administration (FDA) requires some drugs such as cyclosporine, sirolimus, simvastatin, lovastatin, and felodipine to carry a warning label regarding the possibility of an interaction. For example, Neoral, an immunosuppressant drug, carries a label stating"... Grapefruit and GFJ affect metabolism, increasing blood concentrations of cyclosporine, thus should be avoided". Procardia is labeled "... Co-administration of nifedipine with GFJ resulted in approximately a 2-fold increase in nifedipine AUC and C_{max} with no change in half-life. The increased plasma concentrations are most likely due to inhibition of CYP3A4 related first-pass metabolism. Co-administration of nifedipine with GFJ is to be avoided". In addition to GFJ, interactions with certain medications also have been shown for Seville orange juice, although Seville oranges are usually not processed to juice.

For most drugs in question, definitive recommendations regarding their concomitant administration with GFJ are not available, because conclusions regarding the clinical significance of the observed or predicted grapefruit–drug interactions are still limited and most of the data available are derived from in vitro experiments. Furthermore, the determination of the clinical relevance of observed interactions in human intervention trials is complicated by interindividual variability. Whereas the attention of patients and health care professionals is currently focused mainly on interactions of drugs with grapefruit products, other fruits and vegetables and dietary supplements, such as St. John's wort, green tea, and ginseng are an additional potential source for drug interactions. On the other hand, it should be noted that almost all drugs that show an interaction with grapefruit can be replaced by another drug within the same drug class that is without a known potential for an interaction.

Phenolic Compounds in Grapefruit and Citrus with Potential Drug Interactions

A major group of citrus compounds interacting with drugs are phenolics, which include hydroxycinnamic acids, flavonoids such as flavanones, flavones, and flavonols, and anthocyanins, as well as coumarins. Many of these phenolic compounds have been shown to have antioxidant and anticancer properties that may play an important role in cancer prevention, but also in prevention of other chronic diseases such as coronary heart disease, gout, and arthritis.

Interactions with numerous drugs have been demonstrated for furanocoumarins, especially for bergamottin (BG) and 6'7'-dihydroxybergamottin (DHBG). Overall, furanocoumarins appear to interact with susceptible drugs through CYP3A4 and P-gp, but also were shown to influence OATP. In in vitro studies, BG and DHBG have been demonstrated to inhibit the activity of CYP3A4 by reversible and irreversible mechanism-based inhibition. Several studies report an inhibitory effect of BG on the activity of CYP3A4, which leads to an increased C_{max} and AUC of diazepam in dogs, of nifedipine in rats, and of felodipine in humans. BG and DHBG inhibited CYP3A4 in human liver microsomes in vitro, leading to a decreased metabolism of saquinavir, whereas naringin and DHBG decreased the ratio of basolateral-to-apical to apical-to-basolateral (BA/AB) transport of saquinavir. BG, DHBG, bergaptol, and bergapten increased the steady-state uptake of [^{3}H]-vinblastine sulfate by Caco-2 cells, and BG and DHBG decreased the OATP-B–mediated uptake of estrone-3-sulfate into human embryonic kidney cells.

Several human intervention studies confirm the contribution of BG and DHBG to drug interactions with GFJ. After previous reports had been inconsistent regarding the potency of BG and DHBG, Paine

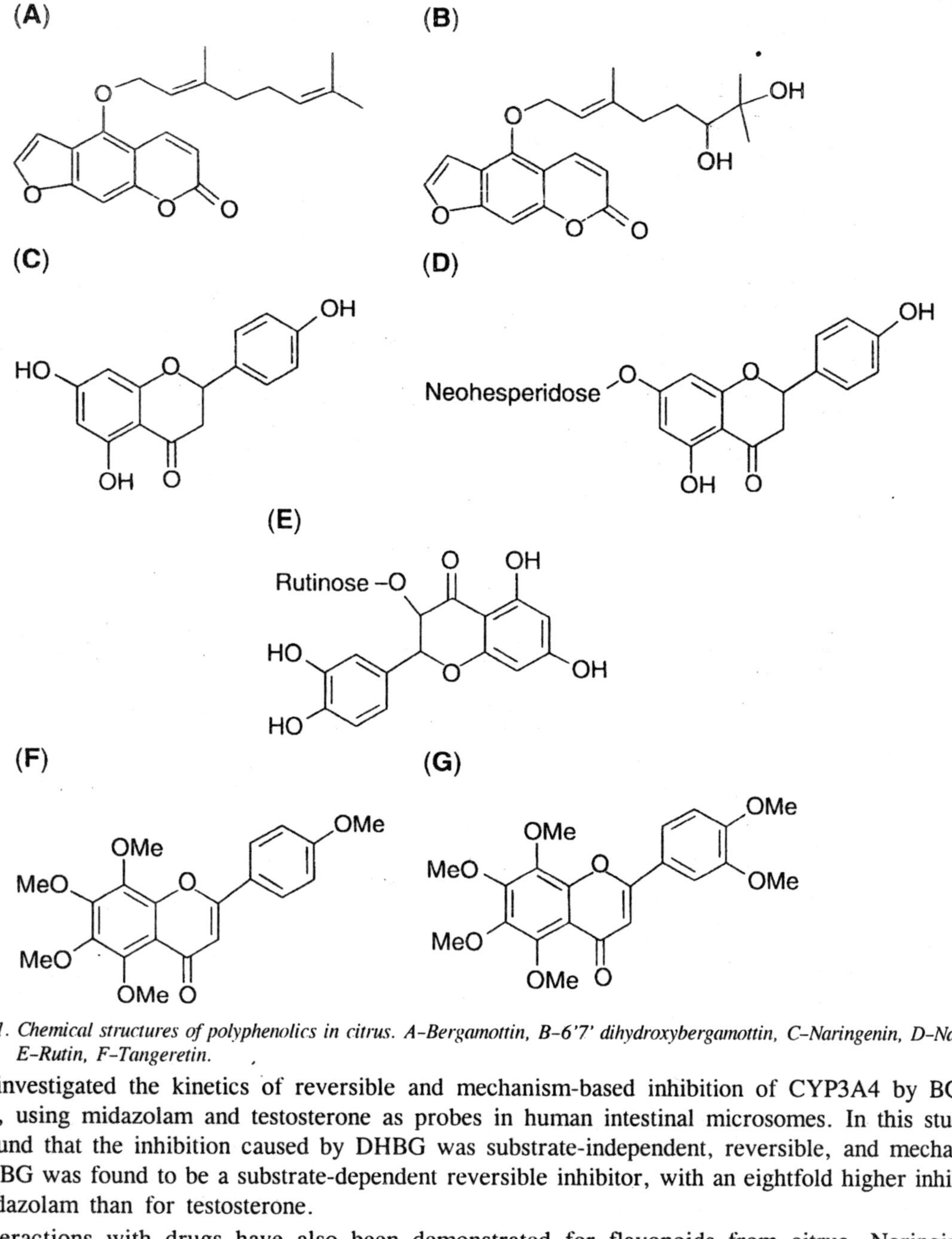

(A) (B) (C) (D) (E) (F) (G)

Fig. 12.1. Chemical structures of polyphenolics in citrus. A-Bergamottin, B-6'7' dihydroxybergamottin, C-Naringenin, D-Naringin, E-Rutin, F-Tangeretin.

et al. investigated the kinetics of reversible and mechanism-based inhibition of CYP3A4 by BG and DHBG, using midazolam and testosterone as probes in human intestinal microsomes. In this study, it was found that the inhibition caused by DHBG was substrate-independent, reversible, and mechanism-based. BG was found to be a substrate-dependent reversible inhibitor, with an eightfold higher inhibition for midazolam than for testosterone.

Interactions with drugs have also been demonstrated for flavonoids from .citrus. Naringin and naringenin were shown to interact with simvastatin and saquinavir in in vitro experiments and caused alterations in the pharmacokinetics of quinine in rats. Moreover, naringenin and naringin were found to inhibit the OATP-B–mediated uptake of estrone-3-sulfate into human embryonic kidney cells.

Quercetin has been found to inhibit P-gp–mediated efflux of ritonavir in Caco-2 cells, to reduce the oxidation of acetaminophen in rat liver micro somes and HepG2 cells, and to inhibit the metabolism of midazolam and quinidine in human liver microsomes. It did not have an effect on CYP3A4-mediated metabolism and P-gp–mediated transport of saquinavir. Rutin was demonstrated to moderately increase the uptake of idarubicin in an isolated perfused rat lung model, and also the outflow recovery of the major metabolite idarubicinol, possibly by affecting P-gp. Nobelitin and tangeretin were shown to inhibit OATP-B–mediated uptake of estrone-3-sulfate into human embryonic kidney cells. For several phenolics from citrus, such as eriocitrin, poncirin, and sinapic acid and anthocyanins, which occur in red grapefruit varieties and blood oranges, no specific drug interactions and also no interactions with CYP3A4 and P-gp are reported.

The clinical relevance of data obtained from studies with single compounds is questionable, because most studies were performed in in vitro systems, limiting the predictability of the effects of the examined compounds in vivo. Moreover, some polyphenolics, such as quercetin, were shown to interact with the absorption or metabolism of drugs only at very high concentrations (50–100 μmol/L), which are likely to exceed the expected in vivo concentration after the consumption of a moderate amount of a grapefruit/citrus product. Also, flavonoids have been demonstrated to potentially induce apoptosis in cell lines at concentrations comparable to those used for some in vitro drug interaction studies. This potentially could have impaired the investigation of enzyme and transporter activities. In summary, studies with single compounds demonstrate that furanocoumarins and their dimers are primarily responsible for the interactions of GFJ and drugs.

In conclusion, grapefruit, sour orange (Seville), and also limes, which contain BG seem to have the highest potential among the citrus species for interacting with drugs, whereas other citrus varieties such as sweet orange seem to have an overall low potential for interfering with medications. However, in studies using juices rather than single compounds, orange juice has also been shown to interact with drugs in some studies. A more recent study in rats demonstrated that orange juice (and apple juice) decreased the oral exposure of fexofenadine, possibly through an inhibition of the influx transporter OATP. The interaction of orange juice and fexofenadine has also been demonstrated in HeLa cells, where orange juice at 5% strength inhibited the uptake of fexofenadine in a concentration- dependent manner by an array of human and rat OATPs. Also, orange juice inhibited the uptake of estrone-3-sulfate into human embryonic kidney 293 cells, probably mediated through OATP-B. Overall it can be concluded that orange juice has a minor potential for drug interactions.

Possible Mechanisms of Interaction

A food–drug interaction can be defined as the alteration of absorption, metabolism, or effects of a drug by food. The underlying mechanisms can be classified into two broad categories. The first category is pharmacokinetics, which includes alterations in absorption, distribution, metabolism, and excretion. The second category is pharmacodynamics, which describes alterations in the drug concentration–effect relationship. Changes in the pharmacokinetics of drugs are the more common consequences of citrus–drug interactions, which may shift the effect of the drug outside of its therapeutic window, possibly leading either to loss of effect or undesired side effects, or even toxicity. Originally, the liver was expected to be the major site of grapefruit–drug interactions. However, for felodipine, it was shown that the interaction only occurred when drugs are administered orally, but not intravenously, which indicated that the interaction may take place during the gastrointestinal absorption phase.

For several other drugs such as cyclosporine, midazolam, and nifedipine, the gastrointestinal mucosa has been demonstrated to be a major metabolic organ, where an inhibition of CYP3A4 caused an increase in oral bioavailability. Because most drugs exhibiting an interaction with GFJ are metabolized primarily by CYP3A4, it has been suggested that the effect of GFJ may be due to the inhibition of CYP3A4 activity. This effect may be particularly important for orally administered drugs, because CYP3A4 is located not only in the hepatocytes, but also in the epithelial cells of the intestine, where major interactions occur. In addition to CYP3A4, enterocyte efflux transport proteins such as P-gp, and enterocyte uptake proteins, such as OATPs also appear to be involved in grapefruit–drug interactions. The activity of P-gp has been reported to be altered by GFJ and orange juice in in vitro experiments, whereas the clinical relevance currently seems unclear, as demonstrated by inconsistent results from human clinical trials.

Regarding interactions between citrus and OATP, data from in vitro, animal and also human clinical studies are available. These studies demonstrated the inhibition of OATP-A in HeLa cells and of OATP-B–mediated uptake of estrone-3-sulfate in human embryonic kidney cells and also in the oral intake of fexofenadine in rats by fruit juices, including GFJ and orange juice. Human clinical trials suggest a potential role of OATP in grapefruit- drug interactions using fexofenadine as substrate.

Cytochrome P450 Family

The cytochrome P450 (CYP) enzyme family is the major catalyst of phase I drug biotransformation reactions. CYP enzymes are bound to membranes of the endoplasmatic reticulum and are predominantly expressed in the liver, although they are also present in extrahepatic tissues such as the gut mucosa. In humans, 16 gene families and 29 subfamilies have been identified to date. CYP3A4 is the most abundantly expressed isoform and represents approximately 30% to 40% of the total CYP protein in human adult liver. CYP3A4 is located mainly in the liver and in apical enterocytes of the small intestine. The high expression levels in the intestinal mucosa and the broad substrate specificity may contribute to the high susceptibility of CYP3A4 for citrus–drug interactions. Many drugs for which interactions with citrus have been demonstrated are metabolized by CYP3A4. Grapefruit inhibits the activity of intestinal CYP3A4, which can lead to an interaction with drugs during their first passage from the intestinal lumen into the systemic circulation.

The alteration of intestinal CYP3A4 by GFJ includes reversible and mechanism-based inhibition and also destruction of the CYP3A4 protein, whereas mRNA levels remain unaltered, indicating an accelerated degradation after mechanism-based inhibition. A moderate consumption does not appear to lead to an inhibition of hepatic CYP3A4 activity. Several drug classes such as dihydropyridine calcium antagonists and HMG-CoA-reductase inhibitors are affected by grapefruit-induced inhibition of CYP3A4. GFJ increased the AUC and maximal plasma concentration (C_{max}) for these calcium antagonists within an approximated range of 1.5- to 2.5-fold on average in a single-dose study design. For the HMG-CoA reductase inhibitor atorvastatin, double-strength GFJ increased the AUC 2.5-fold but not the C_{max}, when the GFJ was administered over three days and the drug was given on day three. In a very similar study design performed by the same group with simvastatin, double-strength GFJ increased the AUC 16-fold and C_{max} ninefold. The same group demonstrated that one glass of GFJ caused an increase of plasma triazolam concentrations, and the repeated consumption of GFJ induced a higher increase in triazolam concentrations and a prolonged half-life of triazolam.

The repeated consumption may cause an inhibition of hepatic CYP3A4. In a three day study, GFJ increased the AUC of simvastatin 3.6-fold and that of simvastatin acid 3.3-fold. C_{max} of simvastatin and simvastatin acid were increased 3.9-fold and 4.3-fold, respectively, when the GFJ was administered for three days and simvastatin on day three. In an in vitro study performed with several grapefruit compounds, it was shown that BG, DHBG, and the furanocoumarin dimers GF-I-1 and GF-I-4 inhibited CYP3A4-catalyzed nifedipine oxidation in a concentration-and time-dependent manner, which is consistent with the mechanism-based inhibition. DHBG was more potent than BG, while the dimers were more potent than the monomers. Not only CYP3A4 but also CYP2C9, CYP2C19, and CYP2D6 seem to be affected by citrus compounds. In the same study, the inhibitory effect of BG was stronger on CYP1A2, CYP2C9, CYP2C19, and CYP2D6 than on CYP3A4. In an intervention trial with healthy volunteers, GFJ (twice daily) decreased the activity of CYP1A2, as determined with caffeine as a probe. In another human study, GFJ and naringenin caused a minor reduction of the activity of CYP1A2. Overall, the inhibition of CYP enzymes other than CYP3A4 does not appear to be of great magnitude and may clinically be relevant only for drugs with a narrow therapeutic range.

Not much information is available regarding the reversible and mechanism-based inhibition kinetics for grapefruit compounds. In a study conducted with human intestinal microsomes by Paine and coworkers, DHB induced a substrate-independent reversible and mechanism-based inhibition on CYP3A4. In contrast, BG, being more lipophilic, was a substrate- dependent reversible inhibitor and a substrate-independent mechanism-based inhibitor. Similar trends resulted with cDNA-expressed CYP3A4. For BG, the inhibition for testosterone was more potent than for midazolam, possibly due to the higher affinity of BG for the testosterone-binding site than for the midazolam-binding site. As mechanism-based inhibitors, BG and DHBG are substrates for CYP3A4, but the binding sites are not known. The authors conclude that both furanocoumarins inactivate CYP3A4 by the binding of the furanoepoxide to the apoprotein, presumably at or near their respective substrate domains. The same group determined the onset time of inhibition by both compounds.

It was found that DHBG inhibited 85% of CYP3A4 activity independent of substrate within 30 minutes, whereas the onset for BG-induced inhibition was much later—a 70% inhibition was reached after three hours. The substrate-dependent inhibition caused by BG was more than 50% after 0.5 to 3 hours for testosterone 6-hydroxylation, while midazolam 1'-hydroxylation was unaffected, or activated, within one hour. Both furanocoumarins caused 40% to 50% reduction of CYP3A4 protein, probably due to intracellular degradation of the enzyme caused by mechanism-based inactivation. These data imply that, after the consumption of GFJ, DHBG causes the enzyme inhibition earlier than BG. Greenblatt et al. determined, in a human intervention trial, the time of recovery of intestinal CYP3A4 after the consumption of 300 mL of regular-strength GFJ and a single dose of midazolam at 2, 26, 50, or 74 hours after administering the juice. After two hours, the AUC was 1.65-fold increased and after 26, 50, and 74hours, the AUC was 1.29-, 1.21-, and 1.06-fold increased, respectively, in comparison to the control. The recovery half-life was estimated at 23 hours. These results indicate that a single dose of GFJ was able to impair the intestinal presystemic metabolism of midazolam when administered orally, which appeared to recover after 74 hours, consistent with a mechanism-based inhibition.

In summary, the presented in vitro studies confirm the inhibitory effects of grapefruit compounds on CYP-enzymes, with major effects on CYP3A4 with both, mechanism-based and reversible inhibition. Overall, DHBG appears to be more potent than BG; however, coumarin dimers seem to be more effective than monomers in the inhibition of CYP3A4. The human intervention trials examining the pharmacokinetic interaction of GFJ revealed a great interindividual variability, where subjects with the highest content of CYP3A4 showed the largest reduction of this enzyme after the consumption of grapefruit. Overall, GFJ seems to interact with orally administered drugs, not with intravenously administered drugs.

P-Glycoprotein

The interest in transporters as mediators of interactions between grapefruit and drugs is increasing. One of the most studied drug transporters is P-gp. P-gp is a 170 kDa plasma glycoprotein, which is encoded by the multidrug resistance (MDR) 1 gene and belongs to the family of ATP-binding cassette transporters. P-gp was first characterized in tumor cells, where it contributes to the MDR. P-gp is expressed constitutively at high levels on the apical surface of the small intestines, liver, pancreas, kidney, colon, and adrenal glands, but also can be found at the blood–brain barrier and blood–cerebrospinal fluid barriers. Striking overlaps of substrates and inhibitors between CYP3A4 and P-gp were reported by Wacher et al. Consequently, the inhibition of P-gp function may also play a role in the effects of GFJ.

Earlier studies demonstrated that GFJ did not influence the activity of P-gp; Lown and coworkers found that 8 oz of GFJ (three times per day for six days) did not alter P-gp concentrations in healthy volunteers. Eagling et al. confirmed these findings in their in vitro study in Caco-2 cells, where compounds from grapefruit were not found to modulate P-gp. In 1999, it was reported that GFJ increased P-gp–mediated transport in Madin-Darby canine kidney epithelial cells (MDCK)–MDR1 cells. However, this finding is controversial to the later findings and was attributed to an equipment-generated artifact by the authors. Takanaga et al. were the first group to demonstrate the inhibition of P-gp by GFJ in Caco-2 cells with vinblastine as probe. Vinblastine also is a substrate of CYP3A4, which limits the conclusions regarding the inhibition of P-gp. Therefore, the same group showed that GFJ and phenolic compounds from orange, such as tangeretin, nobiletin, and heptamethoxyflavone, which have been demonstrated not to alter CYP3A4 activity, increased the net influx of vincristine into adriamycin-resistant human myelogenous leukemia cells conclusively, through the inhibition of P-gp.

Clinical studies that compare the effects of orange juice with GFJ on drug bioavailability confirm the involvement of P-gp in grapefruit-induced alterations in drug absorption. A clinical intervention study conducted by Edwards et al. in the same year indicated that GFJ may interact with P-gp activity. In this study, AUC and peak concentrations of cyclosporine, a P-gp substrate, were increased by GFJ, whereas Seville orange juice did not have an influence on cyclosporine, while it reduced enterocyte concentrations of CYP3A4. DHBG did not inhibit P-gp in vitro. These data imply that the inhibition of P-gp activity by other compounds in GFJ may be responsible for the increased bioavailability of cyclosporine.

These results were confirmed by Malhotra et al. in a randomized three-way crossover intervention study in healthy volunteers who received felodipine with Seville orange juice, dilute GFJ (normalized to equivalent total concentration of BG and DHBG), and sweet orange juice. Seville orange juice and GFJ increase the AUC of felodipine. While Seville orange juice and GFJ probably interact with felodipine through inactivation of intestinal CYP3A4, the lack of interaction between Seville orange juice and cyclosporine indicates that grapefruit may cause interactions also through the inhibition of intestinal P-gp. Several in vitro studies with different probes (talinolol, digoxin, and vinblastine) also confirm the findings that GFJ inhibits the efflux of P-gp substrates. In addition to GFJ, orange juice and pomelo juice also have been shown to inhibit the activity of P-gp in vitro. Flavones from orange juice have been shown to be more potent than compounds from grapefruit in the inhibition of P-gp.

The pharmacokinetics of several drugs that are known P-gp substrates were not altered by GFJ in several clinical studies that investigated the effect of GFJ on the bioavailability of digoxin, amlodipine, and indinavir. Possible other unknown mechanisms and factors such as strength of the administered juices and length of consumption are relevant for the interactions of citrus with drugs.

Overall, it can be stated that grapefruit and other citrus may interact with several drugs through the combined inhibition of CYP3A4 and P-gp. The magnitude of interactions may strongly depend on variations in the polyphenolic profile of the GFJs and study design. The clinical significance of P-gp–related interactions between drugs and GFJ needs to be clarified in further clinical studies.

Organic Anion Transporting Polypeptides

The family of OATPs consists of membrane carriers that mediate the transport of anionic molecules, although not exclusively, and more recently, transport of nonanionic molecules has been observed. OATPs are located in the small intestines on luminal membranes of enterocytes, where they mediate the uptake of drugs. In the liver, OATPs facilitate the uptake of drugs into the hepatocytes. Whereas OATP-A is predominantly located in the brain, OATP-B has been found to be expressed on the membranes of intestinal epithelial cells. The inhibition of drug uptake mediated by OATP may alter the plasma concentration of OATP substrates.

In a more recent work, GFJ and orange juice have been reported to reduce the availability of fexofenadine and celiprolol. Both drugs are substrates for P-gp and OATP, but not CYP3A4. If P-gp had played a major role in the observed interactions, the bioavailability would have been increased instead of decreased. This led to the conclusion that a mechanism other than P-gp was involved. In theory, the inhibition of OATP could lead to a decreased absorption of OATP substrates into intestinal enterocytes. This hypothesis was tested by several in vitro studies.

Dresser et al. determined that GFJ and orange juice decreased OATP-A–mediated fexofenadine uptake into HeLa cells, and that this inhibition of OATP was more potent than the inhibition of P-gp. In a corresponding human trial, the same authors found that GFJ and orange juice decreased the bioavailability of fexofenadine in healthy volunteers. These results imply that citrus juices may be able to inhibit both forms of OATP, namely OATP-A, which occurs in the brain and was used in the in vitro experiments, and OATP-B, which occurs in the intestine and may be responsible for the reduction of the availability of fexofenadine in the human trial. The authors also considered that the apparent decreased bioavailability of fexofenadine in human subjects may have been caused indirectly by an increased drug intake when the drug was administered with water, due to the lower osmolarity of water. Therefore a nonpolar fraction of GFJ was tested in a clinical trial. This nonpolar fraction also significantly reduced the bioavailability of fexofenadine. In a study with human embryonic kidney 293 cells expressing OATP-B, different citrus juices were tested in their effect on the uptake of estrone-3-sulfate. GFJ, orange juice, BG, DHBG, quercetin, naringin, and naringenin significantly inhibited OATP-B–mediated uptake of estrone-3-sulfate.

The citrus compounds DHBG and tangeretin significantly inhibited OATP-B–mediated influx of the probe ibenclamide The effects of fruit juices on the oral availability of fexofenadine also have been tested in rats. In this study, orange juice decreased the oral bioavailability of the drug to a lesser extent than that observed in humans. The clinical relevance of this study for the situation in humans is not clear, because fexofenadine mainly is substrate for OATP-A, which in humans predominantly occurs in the brain, whereas OATP-B occurs in the intestines. Overall, it has to be considered that genetic differences in the OATPs between humans and other species may contribute to differences in the susceptibility to grapefruit-induced inhibition, which also is true for other transporters and enzymes.

Two reports of human clinical trials discuss the potential role of OATP in grapefruit-drug interactions using fexofenadine as substrate. These studies in human healthy volunteers revealed that consumption of GFJ reduced the rate and extent of absorption of fexofenadine, an OATP substrate. The C_{max} and AUC was decreased by a range of 30% to 60% compared to when the drug was taken with water. Both studies suggested an inhibition of the influx mediated drug transporter OATP by GFJ. A recent report evaluates the effect of GFJ on disposition of talinolol in healthy human volunteers. A single glass of GFJ decreased the talinolol area under the serum concentration-time curve (AUC), peak serum drug concentration (C_{max}) and urinary excretion values to around 55%, compared with water. In addition repeated ingestion of GFJ had a similar effect. Because both single and repeated ingestion of GFJ lowered rather than increased talinolol AUC, the findings suggest that constituents present in GFJ preferentially inhibit an intestinal uptake process such as OATP rather than P-glycoprotein. In summary, OATPs appear to play an important role in the influx of a number of drugs into enterocytes and hepatocytes. The inhibition of OATP activity has been demonstrated for orange and GFJ in in vitro experiments. The clinical relevance of this mechanism remains to be investigated in further human intervention trials.

Classes of Drugs Interacting with GFJ

The major drug classes for which grapefruit or other citrus interactions have been reported are described below and the interactions are summarized. Predicting the clinical significance of pharmacokinetic drug interactions is sometimes difficult especially for drugs where there are no robust methods to quantify effects or side effects. There has been recent effort in the United States by the FDA and the Pharmaceutical Research and Manufacturers of America (PhRMA) to establish some general guidelines to help drug companies, prescribers, and patients interpret the clinical significance of drug interactions.

These are based on the clinical experience gained from some well-known drug interactions, such as the inhibition of CYP3A4. For this interaction, it could be shown that the benzodiazepine midazolam is a reproducible probe that allows quantitative determination of the interaction potential of an enzyme inhibitor. The degree of interaction can be measured in the form of an increase in the AUC of the midazolam serum concentrations. It was recently proposed to classify changes of midazolam AUC being less than twofold as "weak," which is the case observed on midazolam coadministration with ranitidine, relatively small volumes of GFJ, roxithromycin, fentanyl, or azithromycin. AUC changes that range from two- to five-fold, which occur on midazolam coadministration with erythromycin, diltiazem, fluconazole, verapamil, relatively large volumes of GFJ, and cimetidine are classified as "moderate." Changes that exceed a fivefold increase in midazolam AUC are labeled as "strong." Examples of drugs demonstrating strong midazolam interactions include: ketoconazole, itraconazole, mibefradil, clarithromycin, and nefazodone.

Strong drug interactions are considered clinically significant and result in contraindications or strong warnings on the product label. The clinical significance of moderate inhibitors may include decisions about dose adjustments that should be based on the concentration–effect relationship. Where applicable, the clinical relevance of GFJ interactions in the present paper was assessed according to the PhRMA classification. If not otherwise stated studies are performed with human subjects.

Antiallergics

Interaction studies were performed for the antiallergic drugs desloratadine, fexofenadine, and terfenadine. When taken with GFJ, the mean exposure for desloratadine was not altered, whereas for fexofenadine it was decreased. In one of the terfenadine interaction studies, the concentrations of the control group could not be quantified. Three other studies demonstrated a significant increase in exposure to terfenadine. The maximum difference in exposure to terfenadine of 2.4-fold was shown by Clifford et al. No significant changes were observed in electrocardiogram (ECG) parameters for desloratadine and fexofenadine. A statistically significant increase in rate-corrected QT (QTc) intervals was reported for terfenadine when administered with GFJ and this drug was taken off the market. The mean effect of GFJ on desloratadine pharmacokinetics seems to be unlikely to be clinically relevant.

Antibiotics

The effects of GFJ were studied for clarithromycin and erythromycin. A decrease in the time to reach the maximal plasma concentration (T_{max}) was found for clarithromycin. The exposure of erythromycin was mildly increased when administered concomitantly with GFJ. It seems unlikely that the reported interactions with the above drugs would be relevant in a clinical setting.

Anticoagulants

Data derived from studies performed with coumarin are inconsistent. In one study, the percentage of 7-hydroxycoumarin excreted in urine was decreased; in a second study the appearance of the metabolite was delayed when 300 mL GFJ were given concomitantly, but the recovery in urine was unchanged, whereas four times 250 mL juice in 30-minute intervals increased the recovery by 100%. The delay in appearance of the metabolite could also be confirmed in a third study. A study performed with warfarin did not assess any pharmacokinetic parameters. However, when patients were pretreated with 8 oz GFJ three times a day for one week, no change in prothrombin time or International Normalized Ratio could be observed. More conclusive clinical studies are necessary to assess the overall effect of GFJ on these anticoagulants.

Antimalaria Drugs

GFJ increases the exposure of artemether, chloroquine in chicken and mice, and halofantrine. No signs of bradycardia or changes in the QTc interval were observed when artemether was administered with GFJ. No overt signs of toxicity of chloroquine were observed in the chicken study. Furthermore, it was reported that GFJ increased the QTc interval when administered concomitantly with halofantrine. No changes in pharmacokinetic parameters were observed when quinidine or quinine was coadministered with GFJ. However, one study assessing the interaction with quinidine reported a significant change in QTc interval prolongation, although this change was only seen at one hour after drug administration. According to the classification of Bjornsson et al. the interactions of quinidine and quinine would be considered weak and unlikely to be clinically relevant. However, a further evaluation of the pharmacodynamic parameters would be desirable. Artemether showed a moderate interaction and halofantrine exhibited a strong interaction. GFJ should be avoided with halofantrine and should be consumed only after a cautious risk and benefit assessment with artemether.

Antiparasitic Drugs

The interactions of GFJ with albendazole and praziquantel can be considered moderate and weak, respectively. GFJ increases the AUC of albendazole 3.1-fold and the C_{max} 3.2-fold. A concomitant consumption should only be considered after a cautious risk and benefit assessment. Regarding the pharmacokinetic parameters, an interaction of GFJ with praziquantel seems unlikely to be clinically relevant (AUC increases 1.62-fold and C_{max} increases 1.9-fold).

Anxiolytics

Alprazolam did not exhibit any changes in pharmacokinetic parameters when administered concomitantly with GFJ in a single dose experiment. When predosing existed, GFJ increased the exposure of alprazolam only in smokers. However, this interaction seems unlikely to be clinically relevant. In both parts of this study psychomotor function remained unchanged; however, there was a small decrease in cognitive speed in the single dose part at one and two hours after dosing. Midazolam and triazolam exposure increased when administered concomitantly with GFJ, but these increases fall into the category of weak interactions. However, changes in psychomotor function have been reported. On the other hand, one study showed a 2.06-fold increase in exposure in patients with liver cirrhosis. These results would be considered a moderate interaction and cannot easily be extrapolated to healthy patients. Diazepam plasma concentrations in dogs were increased by GFJ. Buspirone plasma concentrations also were increased, as was the overall subjective effect. No changes in psychomotor function were observed. Patients should not consume buspirone concomitantly with GFJ, because they may exhibit a strong pharmacokinetic interaction.

Calcium Channel Blockers

Amlodipine, diltiazem, nimodipine, nifedipine, pranidipine, and verapamil exhibit a weak interaction with GFJ with regard to their mean exposure. However, only for amlodipine, diltiazem, nimodipine, and verapamil, no changes in the pharmacodynamic parameters heart rate and blood pressure were reported. Blood pressure was increased after verapamil and GFJ administration only at eight hours after drug administration. No pharmacodynamic parameters were recorded in the studies performed with nifedipine and GFJ. Heart rate was increased after pranidipine administration with GFJ, however the blood pressure remained constant. Felodipine, nicardipine, nisoldipine, and nitrendipine exhibit a moderate interaction with GFJ. However, blood pressure decreased in one study with nisoldipine and no change in pharmacodynamic parameters were observed in the study examining nitrendipine. The heart rates after concomitant nicardipine and GFJ administration changed only at two hours. Changes in pharmacodynamic parameters were reported after GFJ was administered with felodipine. Felodipine-, nicardipine-, nisoldipine-, and nitrendipine-containing products should only be consumed with GFJ after a cautious risk and benefit assessment.

HIV Protease Inhibitors

Amprenavir and indinavir showed no changes in pharmacokinetic parameters when administered concomitantly with GFJ. Even 180 mL double-strength GFJ had no effect on indinavir pharmacokinetics. The AUC of saquinavir was increased after predosing with GFJ. The mean increase was 1.5-fold. In a study performed with one subject, a 5-fold increase was reported. The reported interactions can be considered weak and are unlikely to be clinically relevant.

HMG-CoA Reductase Inhibitors

Increases in exposure were reported for atorvastatin, lovastatin, and simvastatin. GFJ was shown not to have an effect on the pharmacokinetics of pravastatin. Atorvastatin exhibited a moderate interaction with GFJ regarding the overall exposure. Lovastatin and simvastatin exhibited a strong interaction. Pravastatin could be chosen as an alternative drug if patients want to ensure a lack of interaction.

Hormones

No effect of GFJ was observed on 17-beta estradiol or prednisone pharmacokinetics. AUCs were increased for ethinyl-estradiol and methylprednisolone. The increases in exposure can be considered weak and seem to be unlikely to be clinically relevant. It has to be mentioned that a decrease in morning cortisol plasma concentrations has been observed after administration of methylprednisolone with GFJ.

Immunosupressants

An increase in cyclosporine exposure was reported by 11 out of a total of 13 studies. Two studies reported no change in AUC induced by GFJ. Even administration of a large amount of GFJ was shown to increase the AUC only by 7%. Regarding the exposure to cyclosporine, the reported interactions seem unlikely to be clinically relevant.

Antitumor Drugs

GFJ was demonstrated to decrease the mean AUC of etoposide when administered concomitantly. However, there was no indication of whether the results were statistically significant. Furthermore, an increased uptake has been shown for vinblastine in Caco-2 cells. These results can only serve as an estimate. Further research will have to be conducted to develop recommendations for this drug class.

Over-the-Counter Drugs

Contradicting results were reported for GFJ when administered with caffeine. One study reported no changes in AUC, blood pressure, and heart rate. A second study reported increases in AUC and half-life. However, no assessment of pharmacodynamic parameters was performed. Furthermore, GFJ increased the fraction absorbed and the percentage of excreted dextromethorphan. The above-mentioned interactions can be considered weak regarding the overall exposure. Furthermore, dextromethorphan has a broad therapeutic window. The interactions of GFJ with caffeine and dextromethorphan do not seem to be of clinical relevance. Hence, no clinically significant interactions of an over-the-counter drug with GFJ have been reported.

Beta-Blockers

When celiprolol was administered concomitantly with GFJ, AUC and Cmax of celiprolol decreased by 95%; however, heart rate and blood pressure remained the same. The authors of this study conclude the observed interactions to be clinically relevant. In an animal study, talinolol exposure has been reported to increase after GFJ administration. Further human studies will have to be conducted to derive reliable conclusions.

Other Drugs

GFJ has been shown to increase the exposure of carbamazepine, cisapride, fluvoxamine, losartan, methadone, scopolamine, and sertraline. However, only the interaction of GFJ with carbamazepine and cisapride seems to be clinically relevant. No alteration in exposure was observed for clozapine, heophylline, haloperidol, and omeprazole. Reports of increased pharmacokinetic parameters of clozapine, theophylline, and haloperidol suggest that an interaction is unlikely to be clinically relevant. Contradicting results were reported for itraconazole, digoxin, and sildenafil. An increased effect on concomitant use of diclofenac and GFJ was observed in rats. Overall, the clinical relevance for this drug class appears to be low.

Citrus-based products, and grapefruit in particular, can interact with several orally administered medications. In most cases, the expected interactions will be minor and of little clinical relevance. However, the overall observation that a single serving of GFJ can induce a long-lasting increase in oral bioavailability of some drugs, which may lead to potential drug toxicity, does call for caution. In situations where toxicity can be expected, GFJ and other citrus products with a known interaction should be avoided during the whole period of drug treatment. For those patients who want to consume GFJ while they are being medicated, many of the drugs showing an interaction could be replaced by other drugs that have been shown to not interact with GFJ. It also should be considered that, for patients who regularly consumed GFJ before the dose of their medication was adjusted and continued with a constant consumption of GFJ during their medication, a potential toxicity appears relatively unlikely, because the dose for these patients would be lower than for those not consuming GFJ.

There are a few situations in which toxicity could potentially occur: (i) in patients taking unusually high doses of a susceptible drug, who then consume GFJ for the first time, where the GFJ may lead to a sudden decrease of intestinal CYP3A4 activity, (ii) in patients with severe liver disease, the exposure to the drug would be expected to be higher with the intestines being the major site of metabolism. Also in these patients a sudden decrease in CYP activity in the intestines may lead to an increase of drug concentration, and (iii) patients susceptible to toxic effects from drugs are likely to exhibit drug toxicity when the bioavailability is increased.

Additionally, it has to be considered that patients consuming GFJ are also prone to consume other fruits and vegetables and dietary supplements, which may cause an interaction. Sales of dietary supplements containing phytochemicals have been expanding, in part driven by increased health awareness. In particular, patients with chronic diseases have a high propensity to consume prescription drugs and concomitant dietary supplements. Between 1990 and 1995, the use of alternative medicines, including dietary supplements, increased from 34% to 42%, leading to an expenditure of $27 billion for patients. Worldwide, up to 75% of cancer patients use alternative medicine. In a survey conducted in 2002, 54.9% of all users of alternative medicines, including dietary supplements, thought that the natural remedy would help when consumed in combination with the conventional drug. Although GFJ can cause a drug interaction by itself, it should not be taken out of the context of the complete diet, which may also contribute to drug interactions.

The extent of the grapefruit–drug interaction in the case of CYP3A4 appears to be dependent on the patient intestinal enzyme activity. Subjects with a high activity of CYP3A4 appear to show a higher inhibition by GFJ, whereas the inhibition of CYP was lower for subjects with a low initial CYP activity. Theoretically, the concomitant administration of GFJ with a susceptible drug would cause the highest increase in AUC in subjects with a high intestinal CYP3A4 activity; however unexpectedly, these subjects tend to have a low AUC after intake of a standard dose of drugs without the administration of

GFJ. More studies will have to be performed, especially in the area of P-gp and OATP-mediated drug interactions, before sound recommendations for the concomitant intake of citrus with certain drugs can be given.

Future Directives

According to the current, still limited knowledge, responsible recommendations should be communicated effectively to health care personnel and patients. Here care must be taken to avoid careless prescription of susceptible drugs without unnecessary overreaction leading to complete avoidance of citrus products, because these contain significant amounts of antioxidant phytochemicals with significant health benefits. It also appears possible to develop grapefruit furanocoumarins as additives to certain drugs in order to improve their oral bioavailability and reduce the variability. On the other hand, citrus juice manufacturers could develop GFJs without furanocoumarins, which would reduce the potential for a drug interaction. Citrus fruits, other than grapefruit, and other food products, in general, will have to be investigated further in their potential to induce a drug interaction. Further clinical research will have to be conducted to conclusively determine the mechanisms and clinical relevance of these interactions.

Grapefruit Juice Interaction

Communication to the public of medical product risks, such as drug–grapefruit juice interaction, is an important aspect of public health agency work. Health Canada, for example, advised the public in 2002 not to consume grapefruit products with medications used for certain medical conditions, such as anxiety, depression, and others. In the United States, the Food and Drug Administration (FDA) includes documented information on drug-grapefruit juice interaction in individual product labeling [also known as the package insert (PI)]. Information in the PI is typically based on the studies submitted by a drug's manufacturer. The FDA has also utilized spontaneous adverse event case reports as a tool in the evaluation of drug–grapefruit juice interaction labeling. Other sources of data that contribute to labeled information include studies or case reports from the medical literature.

Spontaneous Adverse Event Case Reports

To identify case reports containing information on drug and grapefruit juice interaction, the Adverse Event Reporting System (AERS) database was searched in April 2004 for any mention of a grapefruit-containing product (e.g., grapefruit, grapefruit juice, grapefruit seed) as either a "suspect" (the product that is suspected by the reporter to have caused the event) or a "*concomitant*" (other medical products that the patient was receiving at the same time) product. It must be understood that the FDA does not receive all reports of adverse events and product interactions that occur in medical practice. This is particularly true for a product such as grapefruit juice. First, there is no regulatory requirement to submit food (such as grapefruit juice)–related adverse events to the FDA. Further, grapefruit juice is not generally considered a "*medical product*," so it is possible that a reporter describing a "drug" adverse event report concerning such an interaction may not list "*grapefruit juice*" in either of the "*medical product*" blocks on the MedWatch form. Thus, all reports that mention grapefruit juice in the AERS database might not have been located. The grapefruit juice search described above identified 186 cases in the AERS database. At that point, we had a group of cases that could describe drug–grapefruit juice interaction. However, as with all searches in AERS for spontaneous case reports, each patient case must be scrutinized further, using either a case definition or a set of criteria to better focus on the safety concern of interest. The following criteria were chosen to better identify reports that were more likely to describe an interaction between a drug product and grapefruit juice:

1. The patient was documented to be stable on the drug product prior to receiving grapefruit juice, and,

2. The adverse event occurred after the initiation of grapefruit juice, is a known effect of the drug, and is usually dose-related. Allergic reaction events, lack of drug effect, and events describing gastrointestinal upset after grapefruit juice consumption were not included.

or,

1. The patient was documented to be consuming grapefruit juice each day prior to starting drug therapy, or started grapefruit juice and the drug product at the same time, and,
2. The adverse event occurred upon initiation of drug therapy, and,
3. The adverse event resolved upon retention of same dose of drug with discontinuation of grapefruit juice.

Among the original 186, forty case reports were identified that met the criteria. Thirty-three were from the United States, and seven were reported from foreign countries. Three case reports are presented in table 12.1.

Case 1

A 60-year-old male patient with hypertension, chronic lower extremity venous stasis/edema, renal insufficiency, non–insulin dependent diabetes mellitus, and a familial history of hyperlipidemia had been receiving lovastatin, 40mg tablet, twice a day for 5 to 10 years. Other therapy included gemfibrozil (600 mg b.i.d.), amlodipine, and an oral hypoglycemic agent. Early in the year, the patient's creatinine was 3.5 mg/dL. In October, the patient began drinking grapefruit juice in the morning for the first time in his life. During this time, the patient denied any strenuous exercise. Two weeks later, the patient was in so much pain that he went to an emergency room where his creatine phosphokinase was greater than 40,000 U/L. He was admitted to the hospital with a diagnosis of rhabdomyolysis. Therapy with lovastatin and gemfibrozil was discontinued. During that time, his creatinine increased to about 5.0 mg/dL. The patient was discharged from the hospital after approximately one week and was considered to be recovering. The physician felt that the patient's rhabdomyolysis was caused by the interaction of the grapefruit juice with lovastatin and gemfibrozil.

Case 2

A 92-year-old female with hypertension had been taking nifedipine 30mg daily for four years. While traveling in Florida, she took her nifedipine with grapefruit juice and experienced extreme fatigue, dizziness, vertigo, decreased appetite, and disorientation. She was hospitalized for three to four days, the grapefruit juice was stopped, and she recovered. After returning home from Florida, she took her nifedipine with grapefruit juice again and experienced a similar but milder reaction. Her pharmacist suspected an interaction between nifedipine and grapefruit juice.

Case 3

A 62-year-old female with a history of systemic lupus erythematosis, osteoporisis, angina pectoris, and renal failure began taking amlodipine. She had also been taking lisinopril and spironolactone for an unknown duration. A year later, she started eating grapefruit every day. She fell down after developing disturbance of consciousness for a few minutes. Four days later, she developed generalized fatigue and was admitted the next day to the hospital for shock symptoms consisting of decreased blood pressure, clouded consciousness, and vomiting. Her medications were discontinued, and she was treated for the shock symptoms. The patient recovered. Her physician suspected an interaction between amlodipine and grapefruit.

Case Reports Compared to Labeling

The next step in the assessment was to check the current status of product labeling for drug-grapefruit juice interaction. The Physicians' Desk Reference (PDR) was utilized as a tool for this

Table 12.1. Cases of possible drug–grapefruit interaction

Drug	*Events*
Amlodipine	Peripheral edema, asthenia, hypotension
Amlodipine	Dyspnea, anxiety, hypertension
Amlodipine	Dizziness
Amlodipine	Hypotension
Amlodipine	Head "fullness," strange sensations
Amlodipine	Hypotension, asthenia (feeling of tiredness)
Amlodipine	Dizziness, tachycardia, lightheadedness
Amlodipine	Near syncope
Amlodipine	Atrial fibrillation, ventricular tachycardia
Amlodipine	Increased LFTs and bilirubin
Amlodipine	Dizziness, asthenia
Amlodipine	Hypotension, syncope
Astemizole	Syncope, atrioventricular block
Atorvastatin	Anxiety
Atorvastatin	Epistaxis
Atorvastatin	Gingival bleeding
Atorvastatin	Myalgia, asthenia
Atorvastatin	Dizziness, nausea
Atorvastatin	Myalgia, myasthenia
Atorvastatin	Arm/shoulder pain
Atorvastatin	Paresthesia
Atorvastatin/azithromycin	Increased LFTs and bilirubin
Bupropion	Hypertensive crisis
Doxazosin	Near syncope
Estrogens, conjugated	Fluid retention
Gabapentin	Dizziness, syncope, slurred speech
Lisinopril	Headache, nausea, dizziness
Lisinopril	Dizziness, syncope, seizure
Lovastatin	Rhabdomyolysis
Nifedipine	Pedal edema
Nifedipine	Hypotension, gait abnormal
Nifedipine	Eye swelling, foggy feeling, headache
Nifedipine	Tiredness, asthenia
Nifedipine	Tachycardia
Nifedipine	Dizziness, asthenia, gingivitis
Nifedipine	Asthenia, dizziness, vertigo, disorientation
Risperidone/fluoxetine	Somnolence, fatigue
Sertraline	Sweating
Sibutramine	Insomnia
Verapamil	Palpitations, flushing, malaise, facial redness

purpose. An online query in April 2004 for "grapefruit" was performed, which identified relevant labeling. An important limitation of this strategy is that not all products are included in the PDR, so this search was not expected to identify 100% of drug product labeling containing information on grapefruit. There were 24 ingredients identified in the PDR online search, which described documented or theoretical effects of grapefruit consumption; these are listed in Table 2. The information was contained in a variety of labeling sections: "Clinical Pharmacology," "Warnings," "Precautions,"and "Dosage and Administration." For most drugs, placement of the information was in the Precautions/Drug Interactions section. The following three labeling examples were chosen to illustrate the range of information on drug–grapefruit interaction available.

Lovastatin (Mevacor)

Clinical pharmacology

Lovastatin is a substrate for cytochrome P450 isoform 3A4 (CYP3A4). Grapefruit juice contains one or more components that inhibit CYP3A4 and can increase the plasma concentrations of drugs metabolized by CYP3A4. In one study, 10 subjects consumed 200 mL of double-strength grapefruit juice (one can of frozen concentrate diluted with one rather than three cans of water) three times daily for two days and an additional 200 mL double-strength grapefruit juice together with and 30 and 90 minutes following a single dose of 80 mg lovastatin on the third day. This regimen of grapefruit juice resulted in a mean increase in the serum concentration of lovastatin and its (beta)-hydroxyacid metabolite (as measured by the area under the concentration–time curve) of 15-fold and 5-fold, respectively (as measured using a chemical assay—high performance liquid chromatography). In a second study, 15 subjects consumed one 8 oz glass of single-strength grapefruit juice (one can of frozen concentrate diluted with three cans of water) with breakfast for three consecutive days and a single dose of 40mg lovastatin in the evening of the third day. This regimen of grapefruit juice resulted in a mean increase in the plasma concentration (as measured by the area under the concentration–time curve) of active and total hydroxymethylglutaryl coenzyme A (HMG-CoA) reductase inhibitory activity [using an enzyme inhibition assay both before (for active inhibitors) and after (for total inhibitors) base hydrolysis] of 1.34-fold and 1.36-fold, respectively, and of lovastatin and its (beta)-hydroxyacid metabolite (measured using a chemical assay—liquid chromatography/tandem mass spectrometry—different from that used in the first study) of 1.94-fold and 1.57-fold, respectively. The effect of the difference in amounts of grapefruit juice in these two studies of lovastatin pharmacokinetics has not been studied.

Warnings

Myopathy caused by drug interactions

The incidence and severity of myopathy are increased by concomitant administration of HMG-CoA reductase inhibitors with drugs that can cause myopathy when given alone, such as gemfibrozil and other fibrates, and lipid-lowering doses (greater than or equal to 1 g/day) of niacin (nicotonic acid). In addition, the risk of myopathy may be increased by high levels of HMG-CoA reductase inhibitory activity in plasma. Lovastatin is metabolized by the CYP3A4. Potent inhibitors of this metabolic pathway can raise the plasma levels of HMG-CoA reductase inhibitory activity and may increase the risk of myopathy. These include cyclosporine; the azole antifungals itraconazole and ketoconazole; the macrolide antibiotics erythromycin and clarithromycin; HIV protease inhibitors; the antidepressant nefazodone; and large quantities of grapefruit juice (greater than 1 quart daily).

Precautions/Drug interactions

CYP3A4 interactions

Lovastatin has no CYP3A4 inhibitory activity; therefore, it is not expected to affect the plasma concentrations of other drugs metabolized by CYP3A4. However, lovastatin itself is a substrate for

CYP3A4. Potent inhibitors of CYP3A4 may increase the risk of myopathy by increasing the plasma concentration of HMG-CoA reductase inhibitory activity during lovastatin therapy. These inhibitors include cyclosporine, itraconazole, ketoconazole, erythromycin, clarithromycin, HIV protease inhibitors, nefazodone, and large quantities of grapefruit juice (greater than 1 quart daily).

Grapefruit juice contains one or more components that inhibit CYP3A4 and can increase the plasma concentrations of drugs metabolized by CYP3A4. Large quantities of grapefruit juice (greater than 1 quart daily) significantly increase the serum concentrations of lovastatin and its (beta)- hydroxyacid metabolite during lovastatin therapy and should be avoided.

Nifedipine (Procardia)

Clinical pharmacology

Coadministration of nifedipine and grapefruit juice resulted in an approximately twofold increase in nifedipine area under the curve (AUC) and Cmax with no change in half-life. The increased plasma concentrations are most likely due to the inhibition of CYP3A4-related first-pass metabolism.

Precautions/Other interactions

Grapefruit juice: Coadministration of nifedipine and grapefruit juice resulted in an approximately twofold increase in nifedipine AUC and C_{max} with no change in half-life. The increased plasma concentrations are most likely due to the inhibition of CYP3A4-related first-pass metabolism. Coadministration of nifedipine and grapefruit juice is to be avoided.

Dosage and administration

Coadministration of nifedipine and grapefruit juice is to be avoided.

Aripiprazole (Abilify)

Precautions/Drug interactions

Other strong inhibitors of CYP3A4 (itraconazole) would be expected to have similar effects and need similar dose reductions; weaker inhibitors (erythromycin and grapefruit juice) have not been studied.

Plausibility of Drug-Grapefruit Juice Interaction

When assessing cases identified in AERS, the plausibility of the drug–grapefruit juice interaction is also considered, based on the current knowledge of the mechanism of this interaction. Drugs that are likely to interact with grapefruit juice would have to be given orally, be a substrate for metabolism by CYP3A4, and have a relatively low bioavailability due to extensive presystemic extraction (first-pass metabolism) by CYP3A4.

The next step would be to compare the drugs identified in the AERS search with current labeling to check for potential drug–grapefruit juice interactions meriting further investigation and the possible need for labeling updates. One of the drugs is no longer marketed (astemizole). The following list categorizes the remaining drugs identified in the AERS cases in relation to product labeling.

1. Appropriate information on grapefruit juice interaction appears in product labeling: estrogens, lovastatin, nifedipine, and verapamil.
2. No information in product labeling, but low plausibility of grapefruit juice interaction: bupropion, doxazosin, gabapentin, lisinopril, risperidone, sertraline, and sibutramine.
3. Product labeling indicates lack of grapefruit juice interaction, but plausibility of interaction: amlodipine.
4. No information in product labeling, but plausibility of grapefruit interaction: atorvastatin.

This screening process indicated that the majority of drugs identified in the AERS cases contain appropriate information in their product labeling with the exception of the two drugs in categories 3 and 4. Other available resources, such as the literature and drug interaction studies submitted by manufacturers, will be sought to evaluate the need for labeling revisions for these two products. This process illustrates how the FDA continuously works with drug manufacturers to determine which drug products need revisions to their labeling to reflect accurate and clinically relevant information on drug–grapefruit juice interactions. This process has resulted in a number of changes to drug product labeling addressing grapefruit juice interaction in recent years.

Drugs that are already labeled for grapefruit juice interaction can also be reviewed to evaluate labeling for similar products, such as those that have a similar pharmacokinetic profile and are in the same drug class. For example, current labeling for tadalafil states that it is likely that grapefruit juice would increase tadalafil exposure. Two other drugs in this class, vardenafil and sildenafil, also appear to be sensitive substrates of CYP3A. This is suggested by high (10–49-fold) increases in AUC for these two drugs compared to a 2.2-fold increase with tadalafil after coadministration of strong CYP3A inhibitors such as ketoconazole and ritonavir. In addition, both have low oral bioavailability. There was one case of sildenafil–grapefruit juice interaction among the original 186 AERS cases that did not meet the specific criteria described above; however, the report was suggestive of an interaction. The FDA is evaluating the labeling for these two products to ensure that proper grapefruit interaction information is included.

A 52-year-old male with impotence experienced hypotension several hours after taking sildenafil 100 mg. The patient took sildenafil with grapefruit juice. He was also taking a mixture of dietary flavinoids and triamterene/hydrochlorothiazide. The reporting pharmacist did not state if the patient took sildenafil alone without problems before this episode. Spontaneous case reports have been an important addition to literature reports and manufacturer-submitted clinical studies to help the FDA continuously evaluate product labeling for drug–grapefruit interaction.

13

PHARMACEUTICAL PRODUCTS

Plants are amazing chemical factories! Provided only with the simplest and most inexpensive inputs of carbon dioxide, sunlight, water and minerals, plants produce thousands of sophisticated chemical molecules with different structures. A team of organic chemists starting with the same raw materials could never accomplish the same results in their lifetimes. Some of the chemicals that plants produce for their basic metabolic processes are the same ones found in all living organisms; amino acids, sugars, nucleic acids, and lipids are very similar or identical throughout the plant, animal, and microbial worlds. However, plants differ from other organisms in the vast diversity of additional products they produce. At least 50,000 different chemical structures have been characterized so far within the plant kingdom, and even the majority of plant species have not yet been closely analyzed! A single plant species produces only a fraction of this number of chemicals, but there are hundreds of thousands of different plant species, many of which produce chemicals that are unique to each one.

These so-called secondary metabolites apparently are not essential to the life of the cell, and are often produced only in certain cell types or at certain times. They can be classified into broad molecular types based on their distinguishing structural features. Why do plants produce these thousands of different chemical structures? For the vast majority of secondary products their specific function is unknown. In many cases, scientists have good evidence that they act as defense molecules or as deterrents against feeding by animals or microorganisms. Another possibility is that some compounds have no real function and represent the results of randomness in the evolutionary divergence of traits that are neutral for survival. There may be little or no negative impact on evolutionary fitness if a plant species uses some of its carbon and energy to produce additional structures.

Table 13.1. Diversity of chemical structures produced by plants

Molecular Class	*Number of Known Structures*	*Examples*
Isoprenoids	>25,000	Menthol, turpentine, rubber
Alkaloids	>12,000	Caffeine, nicotine
Phenolics	>8,000	Vanillin, anthocyanins
Fatty acids and derivatives	>500	Castor oil, urushiol (poison ivy toxin)
Miscellaneous	>5,000	Sorbitol, guar gum

In many cases, plants produce only small amounts of a secondary metabolite, but these metabolites can have extremely potent biological activities. Products that represent less than 1 % of the weight of a leaf or root can make the organ toxic to a potential grazer. In other cases, plants produce secondary metabolites that accumulate to very high levels often in specific cell types. The plant secretory glands found in specialized epidermal hairs of species such as mint represent a cell type able to produce large amounts of relatively pure organic compounds (such as menthol). Interestingly, epidermal hairs of other plant species also represent some amazing chemical factories. For example, hairs of some tomato species secrete sticky glucose fatty-acid esters that can represent 25% of the leaf dry weight, and cotton fibers represent specialized cellulose fiber factories that derive from epidermal hairs.

Harvesting Biochemical Diversity: Can (Green) Plants Replace (Chemical) Plants?

One of the major goals of 21st-century society will be to develop renewable and sustainable resources to replace limited petrochemical reserves. This goal is schematically illustrated and the following discussion outlines some factors that will affect the development of a more bio-based chemical industry.

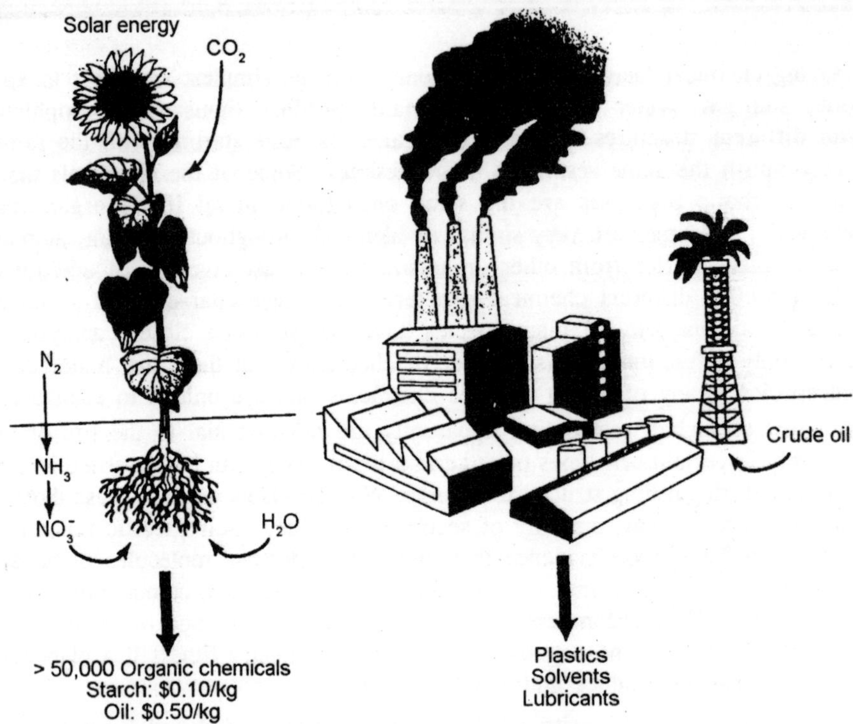

Fig. 13.1. Can plants replace plants? In green plants the inputs are carbon dioxide and solar energy, in chemical plants the input is petroleum.

Today people think of agriculture largely as a source of food for human consumption and feed for animals. There are of course many other uses for crops, such as the production of cotton, linen, or jojoba oil, but these represent only a small fraction of overall agricultural production. In the United States, nonfood and nonfeed uses of field crops account for only 10 to 20% of the total value of field crops. Thus, despite the amazing potential of plants, the agricultural products that humans now use are much more limited in chemical variety and in human applications. Seeds, harvested for their food value, constitute the economic value of most crops. Therefore, agricultural crop production largely takes the form of the starch, proteins, and oils that are the major constituents of field crop seeds.

For most of human civilization, plants provided a much wider range of products. Many ancient civilizations had highly evolved uses of plants to provide medicines, dyes, and other chemicals. One hundred years ago, a major proportion of human clothing, fuel, dyes, medicines, construction materials, and industrial chemicals was still derived from plants, and these products represented very substantial aspects of the agricultural economy. This situation changed dramatically over the past 50 to 100 years. Synthetic rubber and synthetic fibers for clothing (nylon, polyesters, and so on) are just two examples of petroleum derived products that were developed to replace products once obtained exclusively from agriculture. Over a 30-year period—between 1930 and 1960—the sources of industrial chemicals changed from coal and plants as the dominant raw materials to petroleum as the new feedstock. As of 2000, over 95% of organic chemicals that society uses are derived from petroleum, not from plants.

Why has the chemical industry switched to petroleum as the almost exclusive source of starting raw materials? Two major factors brought this about. First, the development of the automobile, which led to enormous demand for inexpensive liquid fuel, coincided with the discovery of vast petroleum reserves. Second, the chemical industry invented new processes that permitted the inexpensive conversion of oil into more valuable chemicals that replaced many products that society had long derived from agriculture. Furthermore, during the time the chemical industry was rapidly expanding, petroleum was a much less expensive raw material than agricultural products. For example, in the 1940s and 1950s, a kilogram of maize cost four to five times more than a kilo of crude oil. The development of the chemical industry, and in particular the plastics industry, is an amazing scientific and industrial success story that has led to the creation of an industry that produces US$ 110 billion in products per year in the United States, compared to US$ 90-100 billion for major U.S. field crops.

Technological advances and economic factors during the 20th century led people to replace many nonfood agricultural products with petroleum-derived products. Many believe this trend will be partially reversed in the 21st century by genetic engineering of plants and the continuing decline in the price of agricultural products. Over the past 50 years agricultural products have become less expensive because of the increased productivity of crops and decreased labor input, whereas the price of crude oil, even if one ignores the sharp peak in the 1980s, has been steadily rising. Relatively speaking, plants are a bargain. Additional factors that could bring about a switch from oil to plants may be the environmental, political, and social benefits that could accompany such a changeover. Petroleum is a limited commodity produced in a relatively small number of countries, and production at present levels cannot be sustained. Therefore, its cost is expected to continue to rise in the future and known supplies will likely be exhausted within the next 75-100 years, unless automobiles use a different source of energy. In contrast, over the past 50 years, agricultural production has continued to increase slightly faster than demand and crop prices have generally declined. Whether this trend continues, it seems almost certain that for the next 50 years or more agricultural raw materials will be less expensive than petroleum, a very different situation from when the chemical industry began its major expansion.

Table 13.2. Approximate cost of phyto- versus petrochemicals

Phytochemical	*US$/kg*	*Petrochemical*	*US$/kg*
Corn	0.10	Crude oil	0.12
Starch	0.11	Gasoline	0.2
Vegetable oil	0.55	Benzene	0.5
Glucose	0.22	Plastic	1.0
Ethanol	0.30		

If plant material is now less expensive than petroleum, why has the chemical industry not switched back to plants? A major reason is that the industry has over 50 years of experience using petroleum as its raw material and has invested huge sums in chemical plants that convert fossil hydrocarbons into plastics and other consumer goods. Additional comparisons of the advantages and disadvantages of fossil fuels versus plants as sources of raw material for the chemical industry are shown in Table 13.3.

Table 13.3 Industrial chemicals from fossil versus plant sources

Petroleum-based raw material	*Plant-based row material*
50-100 years of chemical experience in industry	Less chemical experience
Raw material is imported, and cost have increased	Raw material is domestic, and cost have declined
Petrochemical industry is major source of pollution	Less pollution
Chemical diversity is limited: Primarily highly reduced carbon	Chemical diversity is almost unlimited

Gene Manipulation will let Crop Plants Produce Specialty Chemicals and Permit Production of Biologically Based Plastics

The surplus capacity for agricultural production in industrialized countries and the innovation of plant genetic engineering are leading to new ideas about how people might use agriculture to benefit society. A recent coalition of government, industry, and academic groups suggested that the United States should attempt to use biological sources such as crops to supply 10% of industrial chemical needs by the year 2020 and to increase this to 50% by 2050. Can these ambitious goals be achieved? Ultimately, agriculture will produce almost all biological resources, and plant genetic engineering will be an essential tool for increasing use of renewable resources. An underlying concept of plant genetic engineering is that limitations to large-scale production and use of valuable plant chemicals can be overcome by transferring the genes for their biosynthesis from wild plants into crop species. In this way, much previously untapped chemical biodiversity can be harnessed for society. What are the prospects that biotechnology can create new uses for crops, and could this affect the cost of food?

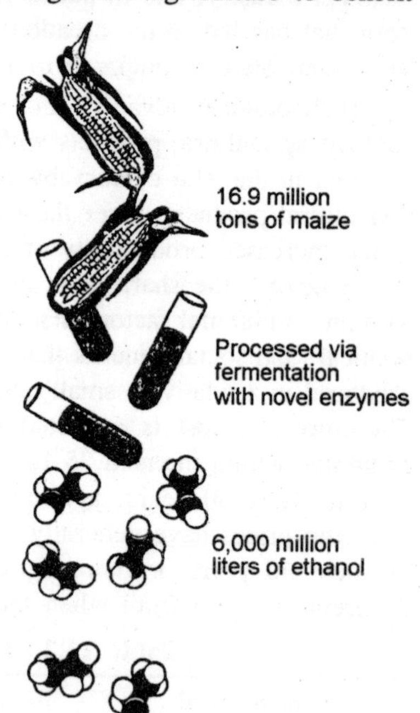

Fig. 13.2. Conversion of maize to ethanol by large-scale fermentation.

Currently, the major process for producing chemicals biologically is microbial fermentation. Worldwide, approximately 15 million tons of products such as ethanol, citric acid, lactic acid, and others are now produced by fungi or bacteria grown in huge 10,000-liter (or larger) stainless steel fermentors. The energy (carbon) source for growing the microorganisms in these fermentors is almost always derived from plant material, usually from maize starch. The microbes are always very highly selected or have been genetically engineered so that they efficiently convert feedstock (glucose) into end product (ethanol or other). Maize is the number one U.S. field crop, and the ability to produce maize starch at a price of less than 15 cents per kg has led to many uses of starch other than as food. Roughly 8% of the U.S. maize crop, or 14 million tons, is used in fermentation processes. Approximately 1 billion U.S gallons of ethanol are produced in this way for automobile fuel (compared to 130 billion gallons of gasoline used per year in the United States). By increasing demand for maize, production of fuel ethanol raises the price of maize (about 1 cent per kg of grain) and helps provide additional markets for excess U.S. agricultural capacity. Improvements over the past 10 years in ethanol yields and recovery have converted the overall ethanol production process from a net energy consumer to a positive energy balance. However, ethanol's ability to compete with low-cost petroleum still requires tax advantages to be practical.

The production of millions of tons of ethanol from maize has demonstrated the feasibility of large-scale conversion of crops into new products. In addition to ethanol, some new fermentation products are now becoming available; this will lead to higher-value products from agriculture that can fully compete with petroleum. Large-scale production facilities have recently been established for two precursor molecules that can be polymerized to make plastics. A plastic with the trade name NatureWorks is produced by CargillDow Polymers. The NatureWorks process is based on the fact that bacteria that are fed glucose derived from starch can produce very high yields of lactic acid. After recovery from the fermentor, technicians polymerize the lactic acid to polylactic acid (PLA), a biodegradable plastic with many attractive properties for products such as carpet fibers and thin films. By using a biologically produced feedstock (glucose), PLA uses 30 to 50% less fossil fuel than is required to produce conventional plastic resins. In 2001, a large-scale facility began production of 150 thousand tons per year. Analysts expect that up to 1 million tons of this plastic may be produced in 2004 at a cost comparable to most petroleum-derived plastics.

For another example, fermentation of glucose can produce 1-3 propane diol, which after combining with terephthalic acid can be polymerized to produce a plastic useful for fiber production. DuPont will market this bio-based plastic under the name Sorona. One key to economic production of both of these bio-based plastics has been genetic engineering of bacterial strains to achieve very high yield of the precursors for polymerization. In the case of PLA, almost 70% of the carbon from the plant glucose feedstock ends up in the final plastic.

An excellent application of PLA plastic films would be as a replacement for the polyethylene films now used to solarize soil for vegetable production. Covering the soil with plastic film reduces water evaporation, prevents weeds from growing, and, most importantly, kills harmful nematodes that accumulate when the same land is used year after year. This new method to prevent damage from nematodes could replace chemical fumigation of soils with methyl bromide, a potent pesticide that kills harmful and beneficial insects alike. If these films were made from a biodegradable plastic, the farmer could simply plow them under at the end of the growing season while preparing the new planting bed.

Chemical Production within a Plant may Offer Economic Advantages over Fermentation

Although fermentation can produce some chemicals at a relatively low cost, the expense of building and maintaining large fermentors increases the cost of the products. For this reason, most products sell for several-fold higher prices than starch or glucose. An ideal process would produce the desired chemical in the plant, where the major energy input is sunlight, and would require only minimal further processing after extraction from the plant. The production of the biodegradable plastic polyhydroxyalkanoate (PHA) in plants represents one effort to reach this goal. Many species of bacteria synthesize and accumulate biodegradable plastics called *polyhydroxyalkanoates* at levels up to 80% of their dry weight. One such PHA, called *polyhydroxybutyrate* (PHB), is produced commercially by fermentation with the bacterium *Alcaligenes eutrophus*. PHB combines biodegradability with water resistance, making it a suitable polymer for a wide variety of uses. The major drawback of bacterial PHB is its high production cost, making it substantially more expensive than synthetic plastics and thereby restricting its large-scale use. Could large-scale production of such plastics in plants rather than in bacteria lower their cost? In 1992, scientists at Michigan State University demonstrated that expression in the plant *Arabidopsis* of genes from the bacterium *Alcaligenes eutrophus* could lead to production of the plastic polyhydroxybutyrate (PHB) in plants. This landmark advance demonstrated that plants can be engineered to produce entirely new chemical products using genes from distant organisms. However, growth of the plants was stunted. In a 1994 study, three genes from this bacterium were engineered so that the proteins they encode would end up in the chloroplasts. The genetically engineered *Arabidopsis* plants produced PHB inclusions exclusively in their chloroplasts. The amount of PHB detected in fully expanded leaves of the plants was up to 10 mg/g fresh weight (about 14% of dry weight). No significant deleterious effect on growth or seed yield was detected in these plants. In response to these discoveries, industry has begun to explore production in plants of polyhydroxyalkanoate polymers that have physical properties superior to those of PHB.

Extraction, Purification, and Energy Costs can Greatly Influence the Success of Plant-produced Chemicals

Although at first it seemed that producing plastics directly in plants could offer the best approach toward a renewable, "green," chemical industry, many factors determine the balance of costs and benefits. To recover plastic from plants will require new extraction facilities that use organic solvents to extract the plastic. Calculations of the energy inputs needed to grow and harvest the crops, to operate the extraction facilities, and to recover the solvents suggest that the amount of fossil fuel consumed may actually be higher than if the same plastic were produced from petroleum. Such calculations require a number of assumptions that depend on future energy costs. If the energy used to run the extractions were derived from plant material, such as the crop residues after the plastic is extracted, the balance could again swing in favour of the plant-based production system. These considerations emphasize the complexities in judging the balance of costs and benefits for each chemical production system.

Plastic production via fermentation offers one useful comparison of how extraction and purification costs impact the cost of two biodegradable plastics produced biologically. PHA plastic (biopol) produced in bacteria at a level of 80% of their dry weight costs US$4- 5/kg. In contrast, polylactic acid (PLA) plastic is produced by chemical polymerization from lactic acid that is first produced by bacteria.

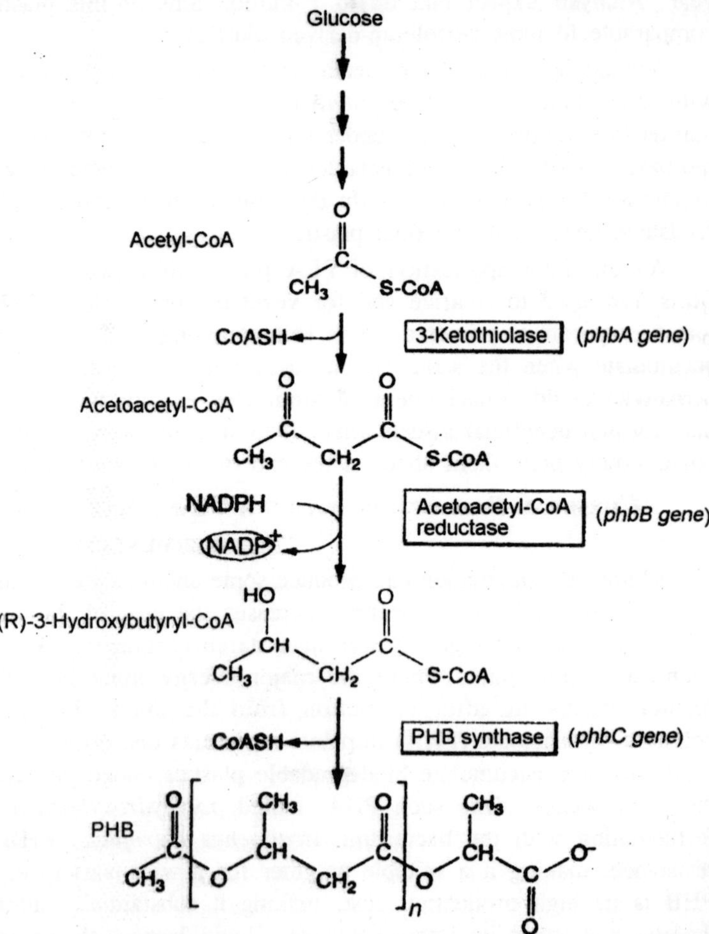

Fig. 13.3. Pathway of polyhydroxybutyrate (PHB) synthesis in chloroplasts of genetically modified plants.

PLA plastic can be produced for US$1-2/kg. This substantial price difference is in large part caused by the extraction and purification costs associated with recovering PHA polymer from bacterial cells, whereas the precursor of PLA is soluble and can be recovered from the fermentor at low cost. Thus, although all steps of PHA synthesis occur biologically, the extraction/recovery costs raise the final cost of the product above that of PLA, which requires two biological production steps (in plants and in bacteria), followed by a chemical polymerization. In many cases, producing a monomer or precursor in plants that is easily recovered, rather than producing a complex polymer, will lower overall costs. If the desired product can be recovered using existing plant-processing technology (such as oil extraction or wet milling), the economics of chemical production in plants may be even more favourable.

Plant Oils can be Engineered for New Industrial Uses

Different plant species use different polymers, usually oil or starch, to store energy needed for seedling growth. In oilseeds, up to 50% of the seed dry weight is in the form of oil. Some plants also produce large amounts of oil in other organs. For example, olive, avocado, and oil palm fruits contain high levels of oil. Here oil probably serves as an animal attractant, to aid in seed dispersal. Plant oils are triacylglycerols, also called *triglycerides* and consist of three fatty acids attached to glycerol that accumulate in discrete subcellular organelles called oil *bodies*. Oil bodies are droplets of vegetable oil surrounded by a monolayer of phospholipids.

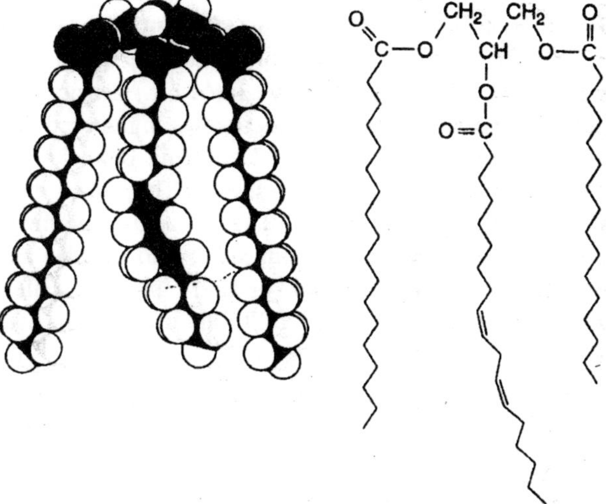

Fig. 13.4. Space-filling and conformational models of the structure of triacylglycerol, the major form of carbon and energy storage in oilseeds.

Vegetable oils are a major commodity, with a well-developed commercial infrastructure for production and use, supplying both food and industrial needs. World vegetable oil production, from soybean, palm, rapeseed (canola), and other crops is over 100 million metric tons per year and is valued at approximately US$50 billion in annual oil sales. The primary use for vegetable oils today is in the food industry and includes salad oils, margarine, and oils used in frying and baking. In most plants, the same five or six fatty acid structures that are also found in the phospholipids in the cell membranes occur in the triacylglycerols found in seeds. These 16- and 18-carbon fatty acids (primarily palmitic, oleic, and linoleic acids) are the major constituents of the vegetable oils that are consumed as foods.

In addition to food uses, about 30% of vegetable oils that are produced today are used by the oleo chemical industry for hundreds of products such as soaps, detergents, paints, lubricants, and polymers. In many cases, the fatty acid composition of the oils used for these applications differs from that found in edible oils, and these different structures lead to special applications. For example, the tropical oils from coconut and palm kernel are rich in lauric acid, which is a 12carbon saturated fatty acid. The properties of lauric acid lead to a balanced solubility in water and oil, which makes it ideal for production of soaps and detergents. As a result, the United States imports up to US$400 million of these tropical oils for use largely in soap and detergents. Thus, although these oils are edible, their major use is not for food.

Although most plant species store oils with the same five or six fatty acid structures in their seeds, analysis of seeds from more than 10,000 different plant species has revealed several hundred fatty acid structures that are considered "unusual." The chain lengths vary from 8 to 24 carbons and the number of unsaturated double bonds varies from zero to 4, or more. In addition, hydroxy, epoxy, acetylenic, cyclic, and conjugated unsaturated groups occur. As with lauric acid, the unique properties of these fatty acids have led to a number of industrial applications.

For over 100 years, chemists have explored plant fatty acid structures as interesting alternatives to petroleum. Thus, the chemical industry has a rich knowledge about the properties and chemical potential of plant oils. However, in most cases these unusual fatty acids are not available in large quantities and at a low enough cost to compete with petroleum alternatives in large-scale uses. The desirable fatty acid structures are generally produced only in wild plant species that produce low yields if planted in fields. Although efforts to domesticate some of these species are under way, this may take decades and may meet insurmountable barriers. Plant gene technology offers the potential to move genes that control production of these high-value fatty acids into high-yielding and well-developed oilseed crops such as canola.

High-Lauric Canola:Oil A Success Story in Genetic Engineering of Oils

The first commercial product to result from changing the composition of a plant seed via genetic engineering is high-lauric-acid canola oil. Lauric acid is found at a very high level in tropical oils, but could temperate crops be genetically engineered to produce the same high level of this short fatty acid? Scientists at Calgene, a California biotechnology company, discovered the biochemical pathway responsible for lauric acid synthesis. They used extracts of seeds from the California bay tree; these seeds accumulate high levels of lauric acid-containing oils. The scientists cloned the gene for the critical enzyme in the pathway, introduced it into canola, and dramatically changed the spectrum of fatty acids produced in the canola seeds. In 1995, industry achieved the first commercial production of a genetically engineered oil by extracting 500 tons of oil from canola seeds engineered to produce an oil with 40 to 50% lauric acid.

High-Oleic Soybean Oil has been Genetically Engineered with Improvements for both Food and Nonfood Uses

Soybeans are the largest source of vegetable oils in the world, and in the United States soybean oil accounts for about 70% of vegetable oil consumed. Most soybean varieties produce an oil rich in polyunsaturated fatty acids (about 50% linoleic acid or 18:2 and 10% linolenic acid or 18:3), and these fatty acids make the oil unstable and easily oxidized so that it becomes rancid. When heated, the oil develops objectionable flavors and odors. Thus unprocessed soybean oil is unsuitable for many applications, so it is chemically hydrogenated. This process adds to the cost of the oil and also introduces side reactions such as conversion of double bonds from the *cis* to *trans* configuration creating *trans*-fatty acids.

The biosynthesis of polyunsaturated fatty acids in plants is catalyzed by a series of enzymes; in the first step, an enzyme converts oleic acid (18:1) to linoleic acid (18:2). After the gene for this enzyme was isolated, molecular biologists succeeded in suppressing the expression of the gene in soybean. This decrease of the 18:1 fatty acid to 18:2 conversion step almost completely eliminated polyunsaturated fatty acids in the soybean oil.

The new transgenic soybean oil has 85% oleic acid, one of the highest oleic acid contents found in nature. The absence of polyunsaturated fatty acids eliminates the need for hydrogenation to stabilize the oil. Furthermore, an unanticipated benefit of the oleic increase was that the saturated fatty acid content of the oil fell from approximately 15% to less than 8%. The new soybean oil has a composition similar to olive and other high-oleic oils, which are considered to provide greater health benefits, compared to other plant and animal oils. The fatty acid trait was stable in field trials, and the oil yield of the crop was identical to the control lines. Thus, neither the transformation process nor the major change in fatty acid composition was detrimental to the high yield of the soybean line. This example is also instructive because it demonstrates how quickly some discoveries can be translated into new crops. With the resources of a major corporation, genetic engineers needed only five years from gene isolation to a field-tested transgenic soybean crop ready for commercialization of an industrial product. Marketing a food product would require additional safety tests mandated by U.S. regulatory agencies.

Vegetable oils have long been known to have useful properties as lubricants, and because they are biodegradable are ideal for applications where harm to the environment must be avoided. However, the tendency of the oils to break down or polymerize as a result of oxidation limits their use. With its very low polyunsaturated fatty acids, high-oleic soybean oil has an oxidative stability more than 10 times greater than most vegetable oils. As a result, it can substitute for mineral oil in many applications such as marine engines, chain saw lubricants, and other applications where oil spills are particularly damaging. A number of other industrial applications may also become possible, because chemical additions to the double bond can lead to polymers and other products that have desirable properties for certain plastics.

The Challenge of High-Level Production

In the two cases of high-lauric acid canola oil and high-oleic acid soybean oil, manipulation of only one gene produced a new commercial product in transgenic plants. However, these two cases may not be representative of the types of metabolic engineering that will be needed for most new products. A number of other attempts to engineer oilseed fatty acid composition have been less successful, because the amount of the desired product was too low. Although the genes were isolated from plants or other organisms that accumulate the unusual fatty acids at levels of 50 to 90% in their oils, when engineers transformed the genes into a crop plant, accumulation was much less. The activity of the introduced enzyme has generally not been limiting, so other factors probably limit product accumulation. In at least one case, the new fatty acid induces its own breakdown. Thus, it is clear that plant metabolic engineering will be technically challenging.

Table 13.4. The challenge of unusual fatty acid production in transgenic oilseeds. Specialty fatty acids are found at high levels in nature, but are produced at low levels in transgenic plants

Fatty Acid	*Level in Native plant*	*Level in Transgenic plant*
18: 1^{D6} (petroselinic)	85%	<10%
16:1^{D6}	85%	<10%
Cyclopropane	50%	<5%
Ricinoleic	90%	17%
Acetylenic	70%	25%
Epoxy	60%	15%
Conjugated	65%	17%
Lauric (+ 10:0)	65%(+25%)	50-60%

Furthermore, even if high-level production of a chemical is achieved, the costs of producing a new product in plants may be higher than production by existing methods. Such costs fall into several categories: First, the costs of crop breeding approximately doubles for each independently segregating gene that must be maintained in the breeding population. Second, any yield penalty associated with the transgene will add to the cost of the end product. Third, identity preservation of a GM crop adds to storage, transport, and processing costs. And fourth, perhaps most importantly, the cost of special extraction or processing of a new product can substantially increase the price of an end product. Plant metabolic engineering will be most successful if industry can recover the products at low cost and high yield.

Potential Impact of Large-scale Chemical Production in Temperate and Tropical Crops

If biotechnology can overcome the problems just discussed and many new chemicals are produced in plants, what will be the impact on agriculture? It could be huge, because of the area of land needed. Producing a chemical such as ricinoleic acid in a crop, rather than importing it, could be easily accommodated in the United States with little impact on land use or commodity prices. In contrast, producing the bulk of adipic acid for nylon manufacture could require 10 million hectares of canola. In comparison, only 2 million hectares of maize are needed to produce 1 billion gallons of ethanol. Large-scale production in plants of plastics or their monomers could greatly exceed the use of crops for ethanol production.

At present, genetic engineering of oilseeds is largely confined to temperate crops such as canola and soybean. The immediate goal is to expand the range of fatty acids available from crop species so that the commercial uses of plant fatty acids can be expanded. In the future, genetic engineering of perennial tropical species such as oil palm will increase in importance. Oil palm, which can grow year round, is capable of producing up to 100 barrels of oil per hectare per year. This production capacity is 3- to 10-fold higher than yields obtained from most annual temperate crops.

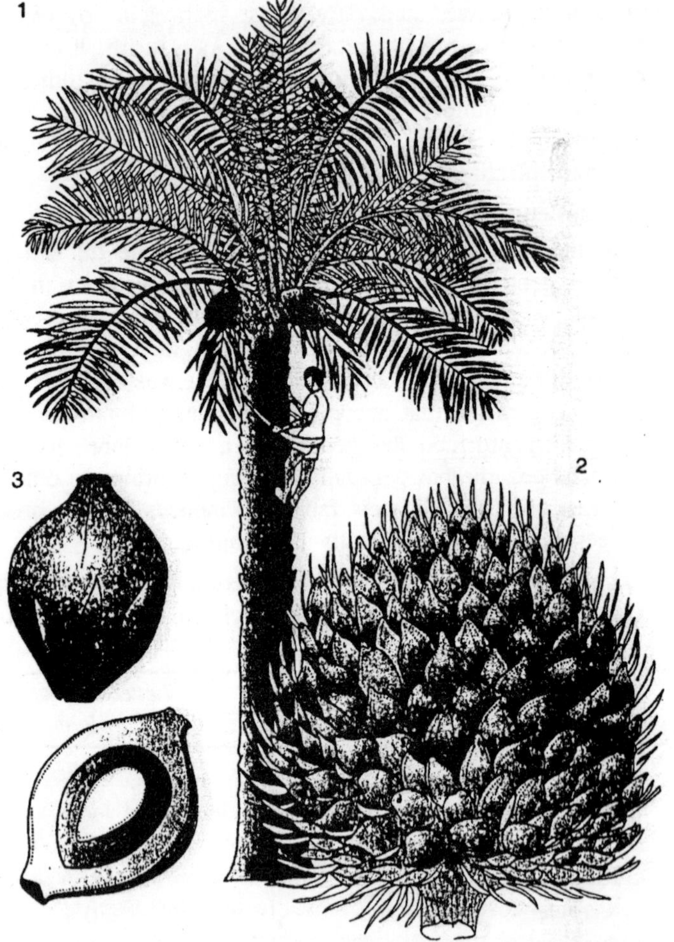

Fig. 13.5. Oil palm produces 3- to 10-fold more vegetable oil per hectare than oilseed crops grown in temperate climates.

Palm oil is currently the second largest type of vegetable oil worldwide, mostly coming from Malaysia, Indonesia, and the Philippines. However, in a number of tropical areas in Africa and South America oil palm production could be expanded. As genetic engineering of oil palm advances, this tree may produce a wide range of chemicals at a cost competitive with petroleum. Because oil palm can be grown in several less developed countries, such expansion could have important social benefits by bringing new agricultural income and exports to these areas. However, the governments will have to weigh the benefits of such cash crops against the need for food production.

Will "Plants as Factories" Biotechnology Hurt the Economies of Developing Countries?

Experts such as the Kenyan economist Calestous Juma warn that transferring production of high-value plant metabolites from farms in developing countries to biotech crops in developed countries will have a negative impact on the economies of the developing countries. They will lose an important source of foreign exchange, and many farmers will lose their livelihoods. In his book *The Gene Hunters: Biotechnology and the Scramble for Seeds* (1989, Princeton, N: Princeton University), Juma writes,

"The direction of this research is aimed at reducing dependence on imported raw materials. The impact on the countries exporting this product will be profound and irreversible. Over the years, large sections of the population have organized their lifestyles around the production of these crops. This is going to be changed by current developments in biotechnology. The impacts will not be only economic, but will have long-run political implications and the attempt by communities to reorganize themselves in response to the changed conditions. It is, therefore, in the interest of raw material exporters to closely monitor current trends in biotechnology and the use of genetic resources and modify their internal policies in anticipation of potential long-term effects."

One possible impact of biotechnology is illustrated by the present production of vanilla. Although the plant *Vanilla planifolia* is indigenous to Central and South America, commercial production of vanilla occurs largely in Madagascar, the Comoro Islands, and Reunion. Madagascar alone accounts for 75% of the world market (about US$80 million) and earns more than US$50 million in foreign exchange. Vanilla beans account for 10% of Madagascar's export earnings. The production of vanilla involves over 70,000 small landholders (owners of small farms) whose incomes depend on vanilla exports. The current price of vanilla is about US$70-75 per kg. By the two criteria mentioned in the previous section—price per kilogram and size of the market—vanilla is presently not threatened by genetically engineered crops. Yet research to try to change this is tempting, because the structure of vanilla is simple and may require modification of only one or two genes to produce vanilla in seeds.

Another example of the potential relocation of production from developing countries to developed countries is provided by the newly discovered sweet proteins such as thaumatin. Certain tropical fruits and leaves of tropical shrubs contain small proteins that are 1,500-3,000 times sweeter (based on weight) than sucrose. Some companies have established plantations in the tropics to produce these proteins. They can be used as sugar substitutes and advertised as "natural" sweeteners that are possibly safer than synthetic products such as saccharin and aspartame. Because they are proteins, each is encoded by a single gene, and such genes can easily be isolated and introduced into bacteria, yeast, or plants, which will then produce the sweet protein. Work on the genes of sweet proteins has attracted capital from some of the world's biggest companies, indicating the importance they attach to this emerging technology. Tate and Lyle, the British company that established plantations in Liberia, Ghana, and Malaysia to produce thaumatin, has also introduced the thaumatin gene into yeast by genetic engineering, allowing the company to manufacture the sweetener in large fermentors. The cheaper process will eventually displace the more expensive one.

It is important to note that the relocation of industries and production processes from one country to another has been going on for hundreds of years. The development of new chemical technology for producing synthetic rubber had an immense impact on the economics of rubber tree plantations in countries such as Malaysia. In some cases, the economy of a country can accommodate such changes, particularly if soil and climate conditions are favourable. In Malaysia, oil palm plantations replaced many of the rubber tree plantations and the agricultural economy remained strong. Many countries that were industrial leaders in the 20th century have seen their manufacturing industries move production facilities to locations with the lowest cost of labor and raw materials. Many products (such as electronics) once primarily produced in North America and Europe are now predominantly produced in (other) Pacific Rim countries. Thus the biotechnology industry is not unique or particularly to blame for long-standing trends where economic and political forces, rather than social considerations, drive relocation of production systems. Although in the short term the most developed countries may be the first to benefit from agricultural biotechnology, in the long term all countries with good climate, soil, and water will derive increased income and economic growth from the production of chemicals in plants.

Starch and Other Plant Carbohydrates have a Wide Range of Industrial Uses

Maize, wheat, rice, and other grains consist of 50 to 70% starch by dry weight. Potato and some other root crops are even richer in starch. Starch can be recovered at very low cost and in high purity by wet milling of grains. In this process maize is soaked 30 to 40 hours in water and then starch, gluten (protein), fiber, and the germ are physically separated. Very large-scale processing plants can recover starch at a price of less than 20 cents per kg. The other parts of the grain can be used as food or animal feed. This price for a complex organic polymer is substantially lower than for plastic polymers derived from petroleum (such as nylon or polystyrene), and the price comparison emphasizes the inherent efficiency of photosynthesis and large-scale agriculture. This low price has stimulated decades of research to find new uses for starch. For example, in the food industry starch is used as a thickening or gelling agent. The conversion of starch to high-fructose syrup is another important application. In the United States, more of this sweetener is now used as compared to sucrose (sugar beet or cane sugar), primarily because it is cheaper to produce. Starches are also used in hundreds of nonfood applications such as paper manufacture and adhesives and have been incorporated into plastic films to increase their breakdown in landfills. Chemical modifications of starch have led to dozens of other uses, such as absorbents. For example, Superslurper is a starch/acrylonitrile copolymer capable of absorbing 1,500 times its own weight in water and is used in diapers, bandages, and seed coatings. However, the major industrial use of starch has been for fermentation to produce ethanol and other chemicals described earlier.

Starch is a mixture of two glucose polymers: amylose, which is linear, and amylopectin, which is highly branched. The different properties of these two polymers and their relative proportions in starch determine the physical properties and uses of starch. A relatively small number of enzymes are involved in producing starch from glucose, and the relative activities of these enzymes determine the ratio between amylose and amylopectin. Genetic engineering of these enzymes might allow starches to be designed for specific end uses. However, almost all mutants in starch biosynthetic enzymes, although often providing useful starch properties, also lead to reductions in overall starch content and crop yields. Therefore, to date, genetic engineering of starch composition has not reached commercial success.

A number of bacterial and fungal carbohydrate polymers have important applications, and if plants could produce these in high yield the costs of production might be less than from fermentation. For example, xanthan gum—a glucose polymer produced by the bacterium *Xanthomonas campestris*—is used as a thickener and for other food and nonfood applications. Each year 20 million kg of xanthan gum are produced, with a price of US$6 to US$8/kg. This market size is sufficient to stimulate efforts to engineer plants to produce xanthan gum rather than starch.

Specialty Chemicals and Pharmaceuticals can be Produced in Plants

Most chemicals and products discussed so far can be considered "commodities." Such products are characterized by large market volume and low price. Both the agriculture and the petrochemical industries have excelled at producing low-cost commodity products and in some cases these two sectors compete with each other to capture markets. In such raw material markets, profit margins are small, and manufacturers often choose one supply source over another based on a price difference of 1 % or less. Specialty chemicals represent a different situation. These chemicals are more expensive to produce and almost always have a smaller volume of sales. Many thousands of chemicals fall into this category. For example, the Aldrich Chemical Company lists over 25,000 chemicals in its catalog and collectively these specialty chemicals have annual sales of many billions of dollars. Many flavors and fragrances, both synthetic and biologically produced, fall into this class.

What are the prospects that biotechnology will lead to alternative or improved plant sources for such compounds? Although scientists can envision schemes where plants are engineered to produce thousands of specialty chemicals, you have seen that metabolic engineering is not always as straightforward as expected. Despite much research in the past 10 years focused on new products, only a few processes have been commercialized. This is both because of complexities in engineering biochemical pathways and because of economic considerations. Economists estimate that research and development for a new product requires at least a la-year investment and that this investment can only be recovered if the product has an annual market of at least US$100 million. Only a small subset of new plant products falls into this category. For example, both jasmine and ajmalicine, components of perfume, are quite expensive (jasmine costs US$5,000 per kg and ajmalicine costs US$1,500 per kg), but the total market for jasmine is estimated to be only US$500,000 and for ajmalicine, US$5 million. Spearmint oil, in contrast, has a substantial market (US$100 million), but the relatively low price (US$30 per kg) means that new plant production systems must produce high yields. Currently, these considerations limit industry investments in research to products with very large market values. However, in the future, as more experience is gained in biotechnology, the process of rational plant metabolic engineering will become more cost effective and will be extended to a wider range of products.

Pharmaceuticals represent a type of specialty chemicals. As much as 25% of the pharmaceutical drugs that people use are either produced in plants or originated in plants. For example, morphine and codeine (and opium) are alkaloids derived from the opium poppy. Other legal and illegal plant-derived drugs consumed in large quantities include caffeine, nicotine, heroin, and tetrahydrocannabinol (from marijuana). Some medically important structures once isolated from plants are now produced synthetically, because synthesis provides a more reliable supply and sometimes at lower cost. However, some structures are so complex—taxol, for example—that chemical synthesis, although possible, is prohibitively expensive. However, in some cases, the complex structure makes chemical synthesis difficult. The anticancer drug, taxol, can be made from a precursor isolated from the European yew tree.

Can genetic engineering of plants result in increased yields of products such as taxol? In many cases, the biosynthetic pathways of these complex structures are still not completely understood. In addition, geneticists have not yet identified the genes that encode the enzymes that carry out the various synthetic steps. Over expression of the first enzyme in a pathway sometimes results in higher levels of the desired end product. However, even in some well-characterized pathways efforts to engineer higher flux (in both plants and microorganisms) have been disappointing. A promising strategy may be to discover global regulators, such as transcription factors that can regulate many steps in a biosynthetic pathway.

Fermentation and In-plant Production Systems are Complementary Technologies; both Depend on Agriculture

Microorganisms are often the preferred production system for producing small water-soluble molecules such as organic acids, because during fermentation the compounds are released into the growth medium, where they can be easily recovered. Citric acid, used in both food and nonfood applications is one example. In 1998, 200 million kg, with a value of US$500 million, were produced by fermentation in the United States. Although this is a large and attractive market, producing high concentrations of citric acid or other small molecules in a plant might be difficult, because if the compound accumulates to high levels in the cells the metabolic and osmotic consequences could be disastrous for the plant. Similarly, production of industrial enzymes now takes place largely by fungal or bacterial fermentation, with the enzymes being secreted into the medium. Tons of enzymes such as proteases, lipases, glucose isomerase, and pectinases can be produced at costs as low as US$3 to US$10 per kg. Subtilisin, a protease produced by bacteria, is added to laundry detergents, where it constitutes the largest single use of industrial enzymes. The detergent industry uses over 80 million kg of subtilisin worth US$500 million per year. At first glance it seems that large-scale production of these proteins in crops would be even cheaper than by fermentation. For example, soybean meal, which is 48% protein, sells for US$0.21 per kg and one hectare of soybeans can produce >1,000 kg of protein. If an industrial enzyme such as subtilisin could be produced at a level of 20% of the soy meal protein, then a single 100-hectare farm could produce 20,000 kg of enzyme. However, the crucial cost consideration in this example is purification of the product. Separating the desired enzyme from other proteins in the seed can be expensive, and therefore the fermentation process, although it requires more expensive inputs, often produces at a lower cost, a sufficiently pure enzyme, because the proteins are easily extracted from the medium.

A group of Canadian scientists has developed one ingenious solution that may help reduce the costs of purifying some proteins from plants. The gene of the desired protein is engineered by fusing it to the gene that encodes oleosin. Oleosin is an oil body surface protein with a long hydrophobic anchor and a cytoplasmic terminus found in the seeds of canola and other oil crops. The protein to which oleosin is fused will be firmly attached to the oil bodies. When oil is extracted from the seeds, the protein is recovered with the oil, where it is separated from the bulk of other proteins. The desired protein product can then be cleaved from its target sequence and recovered in relatively high purity.

There are other situations where producing industrial proteins in plants is likely to be cost effective. In some cases, the desired use of the enzyme does not require purification. For example, cell wall polymers cannot be digested by monogastric animals and therefore have no nutritive value. Adding enzymes that help break down cellulose or hemicellulose can free up more calories and increase feed efficiency. For example, a thermostable endoglucanase has been expressed in transgenic potato at levels up to 25% of leaf-soluble protein. A small amount of crop containing this enzyme could be mixed with other animal feed to partially digest cellulose, thereby enhancing feed use.

Plants are Ideal Production Stems for Diagnostic or Therapeutic Human Proteins Needed in Large Amounts

Mammalian genes can readily be expressed in plants, and plants are likely to become the production systems of choice for some mammalian proteins that are needed as diagnostics for detecting human diseases or as therapeutics for treating human and animal diseases. Research in "biopharming" is aimed at producing monoclonal antibodies, blood plasma proteins, peptide hormones, and cytokines in plants. The reasons that plants are emerging as the system of choice are purity and cost. Small amounts of human recombinant proteins can now be produced in cultured mammalian or insect cells, but many medical applications of monoclonal antibodies or plasma proteins require the production of as much as 1,000 kg of pure protein per year. Scaling up the production of antibodies by mammalian cells would require a capital investment of US$100 million, and the antibodies would cost thousands of dollars per gram. Extraction from crop plants, in contrast, can be done in a factory that costs US$10 million, and the antibodies will cost US$200 per gram. About 20 companies worldwide are now doing research to eventually produce recombinant human proteins in plants. Likely production systems are the leaves of tobacco plants, the endosperm of maize seeds, potato tubers, or the stems of sugar cane. The targets could include not only therapeutic proteins but also proteins such as collagen that are used in the cosmetics industry. Factories where human proteins made in plants will be purified have already been built.

Proteins could be produced after stable transformation of a plant or by transient expression after infecting the leaves with a virus that carries the gene of interest. One important aspect that scientists must consider is that if human proteins are made in seeds, the crops must be grown in relative isolation so that the human genes do not show up in maize used for human or animal consumption. Although the proteins might be harmless, their consumption could have unintended consequences. Genes could spread if, for example, pollen from maize plants that are producing the human proteins were to be blown to other fields. The fields therefore need to be isolated, so that there is no chance that pollen from the transgenic plants may cause the genes to spread to other fields. An advantage of using a vegetatively propagated crop such as sugar cane is that it eliminates the possibility of pollen spreading genes.

The problem of gene spread can also be circumvented with transient expression systems based on plant viruses that infect leaves. Transient expression means that the proteins are made for only a few days, but the goal is to have very high levels of expression during that short period. Viruses have small genomes consisting of only a few genes. It is sometimes possible to replace some of the viral genome with a segment of nucleic acid that carries the information to make the active fragment of an antibody molecule. When this is done, the virus may still be able to replicate and reproduce itself when it infects a plant. Whether or not this is possible depends on the type of virus. Thus, when a leaf of a plant is infected with a genetically engineered RNA virus that carries the active segment of a human gene, the virus will spread throughout the plant, making billions of copies of itself. If viral infection is done before the plant flowers, then the virus does not spread to the pollen. The plant cells will translate the messenger RNA and produce the antibody fragment. Engineering the virus and allowing the plants to make the protein can all be accomplished in two months. Such a rapid production system can be used to create antibodies that are customized for a particular patient—a requirement for treating non-Hodgkin's lymphoma, a type of cancer that attacks certain white blood cells.

The body uses antibodies to fight diseases (see later discussion), but antibodies also have many other uses in medicine. They can be used therapeutically, to deliver a killer drug specifically to cancer cells, for example, and also to diagnose diseases. Antibodies are directed at antigenic determinants (or epitopes) at the surfaces of proteins or other molecules. For example, an antigenic determinant could be a few amino acid side chains displayed on the surface of a protein. Antibodies directed at antigenic determinants displayed on the surface of cancer cells specifically bind to those cancer cells. Different antibodies will home in on different types of cancer cells. Such specific binding can be used to image the cancer, or to target the cancer cells for destruction. Antibodies produced in plants could also provide protection against intestinal pathogens such as hepatitis viruses, *Helicobacter pylori*, or toxic *E. coli*. They could target respiratory pathogens (rhinoviruses and influenza), sexually transmitted diseases, and dental caries, and could be used as contraceptives. Clinical trials with antibodies produced in plants are already under way, and these novel plant-derived pharmaceuticals may be in the marketplace by 2005.

Plants can be Used to Deliver Edible Vaccines for Serious Diseases of Humans and Domestic Animals

In humans and other warm-blooded animals, the primary task of the immune system is to defend against invading organisms—particularly against pathogenic bacteria and viruses. Most infections are initiated in the mucosal surfaces that line the digestive tract, the respiratory tract, and the urino-reproductive tract; these surfaces also contain the first line of defense—the mucosal immune system. Killing the invaders by engulfment is the function of phagocytic cells such as the macro phages in the bloodstream. Engulfment can occur after the pathogens have been covered with antibodies—proteins produced by the immune system—that are directed at specific antigenic determinants on the surface of the invaders. Producing antibodies is the function of specialized cells of the immune system. The unique features of antibodies are that they recognize a single molecular structure (often a protein) and bind to it with very high affinity. A common type of antibody is the immunoglobulin G (IgG) protein, consisting of two heavy (large) polypeptide chains and two light (small) polypeptide chains.

When a foreign invader comes calling the first time, the body's response in terms of antibody production has a considerable lag time and may not be strong enough to overpower the invader, so the animal may get very sick or even die. If the immune system has been exposed to the antigenic determinants on the invader's surface in the past, and now faces a second invasion, then the response is faster and more powerful. That is the basis of vaccination. Because detection of an invader can occur in the mucosal membranes or in the bloodstream, vaccines can be effective whether taken orally or injected. For example, there are effective oral and injected vaccines against the polio virus. Vaccination makes people immune because it triggers the immune system to produce antibodies by simulating that first invasion, not with virulent pathogens, but with a greatly attenuated strain of bacteria or viruses. Alternatively, immunity through vaccination can be achieved by injecting or ingesting only the antigenic determinants (often parts of proteins that are the antigens) that are displayed on the surface of the invading organisms.

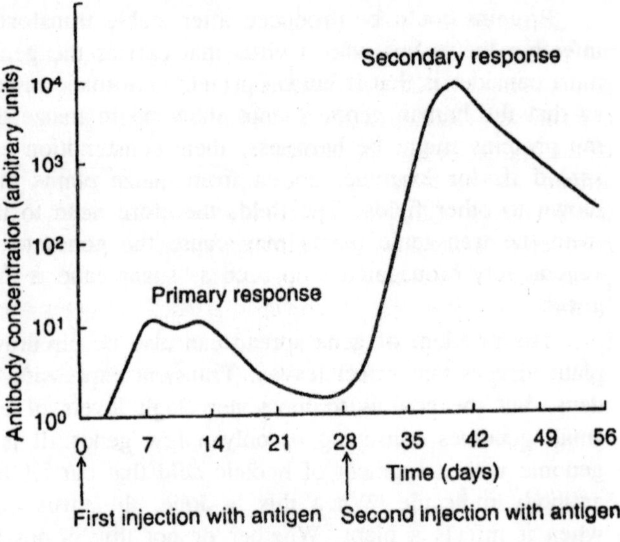

Fig. 13.6. Responses to initial and later injections of an antigen.

Such vaccines are called subunit vaccines. The use of subunit vaccines increases vaccine safety by circumventing the need to use live bacteria and viruses. However, subunit vaccines are not as stable and need to be refrigerated, increasing their cost. Safe vaccines for many important diseases such as cholera and hepatitis are well beyond the reach of the health care system in many developing countries. Scientists realized that plant genetic engineering could solve the problem of providing low-cost vaccinations to people in developing countries, a realization that prompted the idea of expressing the antigens in plants and creating edible plant vaccines. Various pharmaceutical companies are targeting quite a few diseases for vaccine production in plants.

Table 13.5. Production of vaccines in plants

Potential Application	*Protein Expressed in Plants*
Dental caries	*Streptococcus mutans* surface protein
Cholera and *E. coli* diarrhea	*E. coli* heat-labile enterotoxin
Hepatitis B	Hepatitis B antigen
Hoof-and-mouth disease	Hoof-and-mouth viral antigen
Malaria	Malarial B-cell epitope
Influenza	Hemagglutinin
Rabies	Rabies virus glycoprotein
HIV	HIV epitopes gp41 and gp 120

Some of the antigenic determinants on the surface of viruses and bacteria are proteins made by the pathogen. The genes encoding these antigens can be isolated from the pathogens and expressed in plants using standard recombinant DNA technology. In addition, it is possible to incorporate an antigenic determinant (usually a short stretch of amino acids) into an existing plant protein or into a plant virus. If the plant makes the antigenic determinant, then eating the plant (under the right conditions) will amount to vaccination. If the antigenic determinant is incorporated into a plant virus and expressed at the surface of the viral particle, the plant virus can be used as a vaccine (plant viruses are quite harmless to humans and animals; when eating vegetables, people consume large numbers of various plant viruses). Researchers conducted the first human clinical trials with transgenic plant-derived vaccines in the late 1990s. They showed that such vaccines are protected from digestion in the human intestinal tract and stimulate both the mucosal and systemic immune responses. Vaccinating people against cholera by feeding them bananas, or vaccinating animals against foot- or hoof-and mouth disease by feeding them sugar beets could well be a reality by 2010.

14

Phytotoxicology

At the subcellular level, plants and animals display more similarities than differences. Consider the processes of replication of information, genetic recombination, development of subcellular structures, and respiration. Attention should be focused on the fact that, although plants and animals are different, they are evolving branches of a common origin. The study of phytotoxicology, then, is an examination of those products characteristic of one major part of the biota that produce or evoke a specific deleterious reaction when they interact with systems characteristic of the other. This view emphasizes the differences that have evolved between plants and animals despite their common beginnings.

In every plant poisoning case it should be possible to identify precisely the plant product and the animal system involved, the route by which they are brought together, and the specific subsequent events that occur until the animal either dies or recovers. However, according to a recent authoritative statement on this subject, "Probably no field of scientific endeavor exists in which it is more difficult to separate fact from fiction than in the study of poisonous plants. Examination of the pertinent literature will reveal considerable confusion tending to mask an even greater amount of ignorance.... Unbelievable chaos reigns in the area of plant identification and nomenclature as applied by the nonspecialist".

This chapter is directed toward three main topics: (i) the importance of poisonous plants to man and animals, (ii) an assessment of current knowledge of poisonous plants, and (iii) a discussion of the effects of toxic principles elaborated by plants.

Importance of Poisonous Plants to Man and Animals

Although incomplete, the best figures on incidence of human poisoning by plants are those collected from individual poison control centers and analyzed by the National Clearinghouse for Poison Control Centers. Ingestions are grouped by categories in the annual summaries. Plants as a category have consistently ranked in the top seven, accounting for about 4 percent of the reported ingestions until the 1970s. In 1970, plants (excluding mushrooms and toadstools) accounted for 4,059 reported ingestions, representing 4.8 percent of all reported ingestions for that year. This was greater than the number of disinfectant, tranquilizer, insecticide, hormone, acid and alkali, antiseptic, polish, or paint ingestions and was exceeded only by the incidence of ingestion of aspirin and soap-detergents-cleaners. Since the, however, plants as a category has come to the top of the list of "products" most frequently implicated in poisoning of children under 5 years of age. Now, about one out of every ten cases reported by poison control centers is related to plants. This conspicuous rise in importance of plants since 1965 is related to the equally dramatic decrease in cases of poisoning from aspirin. These have fallen from greater than 25 percent of reported incidents in 1965 to just 4.1 percent in 1976. Safety packaging, limited quantities per package, and increased public awareness of hazards—the result of governmental and private compaigns—have been the main contributing factors in reducing the importance of aspirin. Only the latter method of decreasing incidents is easily applicable to the unnecessarily high volume of ingestions involving plants now being experienced at poison control centers. According to reported figures there are approximately 75,000 human ingestions of poisonous plants in the United States each year. According to Canadian figures, ingestions of nonfood plants are more than ten times greater than the number of reported incidents involving venomous bites or stings.

The above figures need to be viewed with a certain amount of caution. First, the majority of the ingestions were of materials, or in amounts, that would not have proved capable of eliciting a toxic response, or else treatment, usually emesis, intervened before such a response occurred. These, strictly speaking, are better defined as ingestions than as poisonings, without implying whether a toxic reaction was or was not possible. Second, many incidents are treated by private physicians who do not report to a poison control center. In addition, some poison control centers fail to report to the National Clearinghouse. Thus, the precise number of toxic responses that occur from plants annually in the human population cannot be determined from these data.

Poisoning of pets and livestock is even more extensive than is poisoning of man. No reliable figures exist, but estimates as to loss of range livestock in western states consistently place the annual figure at more than one million dollars per state or region. Certainly, well-documented instances in which more than 1,500 animals have been killed at a single time, such as losses of sheep to *Halogeton glomeratus*, represent considerable economic impact and do not need to be multiplied by many such events or by many similar plants to assume major importance to the livestock industry. The resulting economic loss includes not only the value of the animals but also the diminution in real value of the range acreage following its infestation with a poisonous weed. Looses of pets and wild animals are so poorly documented that no useful generalizations are possible.

Current Knowledge of Poisonous Plants

Effective consideration of phytotoxicology requires a synthesis across wide academic boundaries and is thus difficult. This, and the diversity of natural phenomena dealt with, perhaps more than other factors, have inhibited a more rapid, rigorous, development of the subject. Comparison of the principal current references dealing with North American poisonous plants shows immediately that fundamental input and analysis are required from botany, physiology, and pathology. In all cases, full development of a particular topic also requires the attention of one or more academic or practical specialists, such as physician, veterinarian, toxicologist, clinician, organic chemist or biochemist, plant physiologist, pharmacologist, pharmacognosist, agronomist, horticulturist, geneticist, and animal husbandman. Consideration must be given to identification and description of a toxic reaction; practical understanding of the history, to aid in diagnosis and in formulating control; secure determination of the etiology; identification and perhaps isolation of a toxic principle; specific description of tis action; the seasonal, ecologic, and genetic control of production of the toxic principle by the plant; and the way in which man or animals were or may be exposed. The latter involves agricultural practices in the case of livestock. In man, a plethora of possibilities exist, from overuse of plant-derived drugs by adults to accidental or experimental ingestions of drugs or whole plant parts by children.

Approximately 700 species of North American plants are considered to be poisonous on the basis of case histories, experimental investigations, or other specific reasons. More will be discovered. This is only a small fraction of the perhaps 30,000 species of plants in the wild and cultivated floras of North America. Nevertheless, it is a large number, and no generalization emerges from a review of their botany, ecology, or management by man to allow systematizing them for easier comprehension. Poisonous species are scattered throughout the plant kingdom from algae, to ferns, to gymnosperms, to angiosperms, and in the latter large groups they appear almost randomly among the plant families.

One sometimes hears that certain groups such as the nightshade or potato family (Solanaceae) are particularly dangerous, but such statements are not entirely valid. Such families are the larger ones, and certain poisonous species more or less in relation to their size.

Toxicity usually exists at the level of the genus. If one species of a genus is toxic, some or all others in that genus usually display similar toxicity. This is why species names are sometimes omitted in general discussion of toxicity. This is a mistake. First, exceptions to the generalization are numerous and important. Second, even when similar species display similar toxicity, they may have other important differences. For example, most species of the genus *Asclepias* (milkweeds) are toxic, but the most toxic species (*A. labriformis*) is found only in a limited area of Utah. However, the most troublesome milkweeds (*A. subverticillata*, *A. eriocarpa*) differs in appearance from the former and have significantly less toxicity on a weight basis, but are much more widely distributed geographically. Important distinctions such as these are lost when species names are not used.

In some cases, groups of genera within a single family display similar toxicity. This is true, for example, of the laurel group of the heath family (Ericaceae). At the other extreme, however, are those instances in which closely related species differ in toxicity. *Eupatorium rugosum* is closely related to the numerous other species of *Eupatorium*, but only the former is known to be toxic. Occasionally the same toxic principle is found in plants of great botanical or habitat difference. For example, the only other plant known to contain the same poisonous principle as *Eupatorium rugosum* is *Aplopappus heterophyllus*. These two are in the same plant family (Compositae), but the former is found in woodlands of eastern North America while the latter is limited to the dry ranges of the Southwest. Nicotine, as another example, can be isolated from plants as botanically distant as tobacco (*Nicotiana tabacum*) of the nightshade or potato family of angiosperms, and from club moss (*Lycopodium* spp.) of the primitive, spore-bearing lycopods.

The content of a given poisonous principle, and even to some extent its molecular structure, can vary widely in some species with the environmental conditions under which the plant grew. This is particularly true of many glycosides. In other cases, certain alkaloids for instance, elaboration of the poisonous principle in a given species in under reasonably tight genetic control and varies little with growing conditions. Even when under strict genetic control, the content of a poisonous principle in a given plant may vary with stage of growth; it may concentrate in particular parts of the plant, or it may vary with the particular variety or strain of plant.

Exemplifying the last point, one of the nightshades exists in two distinct populations, which fortunately do not normally interbreed. The botanic distinctions between them are so small that the two populations were originally recognized as a single species (*Solanum nigrum*). One kind, however, is quite toxic. The other, now set off taxonomically as *Solanum intrusum*, is not known to be toxic. In fact, *S. intrusum* has entered trade as "garden huckleberry" or "wonderberry" and is sometimes recommended to home gardeners for its edible fruits. Poinsettia (*Euphorbia pulcherrima*) may represent a similar example. Its listing as toxic was found originally on a reported case of human mortality in Hawaii in 1919. Recent feeding experiments, prompted by the belief of horticulturists that the poinsettia is really not poisonous, showed no toxic effect in rodents fed large quantities of the red bracts. However, poison control centers continue to report instances of gastric distress in children after ingestion of poinsettia. A possible explanation for the apparent conflict in these several observations is the very great horticultural manipulation that has in recent years been devoted to breeding showier, longer-lasting, and differently colored poinsettias. It is reasonable to suppose that the ability to form a toxic principle may have been consciously selected against at the same time that desirable floral characteristics were sought. If this is the case, older varieties of poinsettia, or ones distinctly different from those experimentally fed to the rodents, may still be capable of eliciting a toxic reaction. These examples could be extended to demonstrate that toxicity can vary not only with species, sex, age, and even individuality of plants and animals but also with environmental factors. The examples quoted above should suffice to convey an idea of the complexity of phytotoxicology.

A major factor in much of the present confusion regarding poisonous plants is the problem of adequate identification of the plant material involved. A physician or veterinarian faced with a case of plant poisoning is, in a sense, like a chemist conducting experiments by guesswork from a stockroom of unlabeled reagents. Accurate identification of the plant is prerequisite to making use of existing pertinent toxicologic information.

The layman rarely appreciates the difficulties involved in the accurate identification of plant materials. Not only are the reagents unknown, but some of them may not be identifiable with the material and tests at hand. Botanic identification often requires a particular part of the plant—usually the mature reproductive parts (which evolve most slowly and hence show relationships best). This means the flower, and the flower is often a very transitory event in the life of a plant. Flowers often are not present when the berries of a plant attract children. Also, flowers do not generally survive well in the gut, so that examination of vomitus or of ruminal or stomach contents will rarely yield identifiable flowering stages, even if initially present.

Most actual cases of poisoning of man and livestock involve the identification of plant material by common name alone. This can be disastrous. Serious errors in reputable reports in the medical and veterinary literature can be traced to erroneous use of common names or failure to appreciate the lac of precision in such usage. All plant materials involved in toxicologic examinations of any kind should be identified by genus and species. If this requires the help of a taxonomic botanist, it should be obtained. If experimental work resulting in a published report is done with plant materials, voucher specimens should be prepared and deposited in a major herbarium, and the fact should be noted in the publication. One or more such herbaria exist in every state, usually at the department of botany in the state university, but sometimes at the state museum or at a major private university. Herbaria function, somewhat like libraries, as depositories of materials that can be recalled in good condition at a later date if it prove necessary to reassess the botanic materials involved in a particular investigation. Despite the obvious benefit of such a practice and its relative simplicity, it is rarely done.

The foregoing discussion presents reasons why current practices make it difficult to deal with poisonous plants. There are historic reasons as well. At the risk of oversimplification, they may be summarized as follows.

The Greeks and Romans were astute and recorded, in some detail and with commendable accuracy, their conclusions concerning the useful, medicinal, or toxic characteristics of the natural world. For most areas of knowledge, these collected observations went into eclipse during the Dark Ages, surviving largely as manuscripts copied from generation to generation without significant addition or modification. This was not the case with poisonous materials, for the practice of poisoning to obtain succession of royalty or ecclesiastic authority, inheritance of wealth, or defeat of armies became a highly developed art. Persons able to get results commanded high fees. In order to protect their hard-won trade secrets, these artisans compounded recipes with many esoteric ingredients, thereby obscuring the identity of the actual active principle. A perhaps overdrawn, but nonetheless illuminating example is the several-stanza list of ingredients that went into the witches' cauldron in Shakespeare's *Macbeth*; only two could be expected to do the job.

With the Renaissance, it became necessary to separate fact from fiction, something that was only imperfectly accomplished. Further confusion resulted from an innocent attempt to relate the reports of the classic authors, who dealt mainly with Mediterranean plants, to the flora of central and northern Europe. Keep in mind that the science of naming plants originated with Linneaus' *Species Plantarum* of 1753; before that time all names applied to plants had no more authority than the common names used today.

Herbals supplanted classic manuscripts around 1470; floras and tomes on materia medica supplanted herbals around 1670; all contained frequent reference to toxic capacities of plants. Monographs devoted solely to poisonous plants began to appear shortly before 1700. All of these works were European, and interested educated persons were expected to know the literature of their subject well enough so that citation of authority for particular statements was not deemed necessary. Hence, for the most part, the first books dealing with poisonous plants do not say where the information came from. Most later writers on poisonous plants have apparently been reluctant to eliminate anything that sounds reasonable, in spite of their inability to verify the information. Some patently unreasonable things are also perpetuated. Even today, books may appear in which medieval error is repeated unconsciously but with devastating effect if taken as scientifically accurate documents.

In 1814 M.J.B. Orfila published the first edition of his substantial work on toxicology, to which the use of an experimental approach in toxicology is generally traced. Orfila experimented with a number of plants, describing their effects and attempting to trace the distribution of the poisonous principle in the body. His chief experimental animal was the dog, an animal that vomits readily, and Orfila frequently found it necessary to excise and tie off the esophagus to ensure absorption when dealing with plants or plant materials administered orally. Although Orfila recognized the difficulties this caused in interpreting his results, it remains problematic to separate the effects of the toxic principle from the effects of this relatively drastic procedure.

The flora of North America east of the Mississippi is essentially similar to that of Europe, while west of that river it becomes increasingly foreign. Thus, the early settlers of the United States were able to bring with them not only their livestock but also their practical experience in dealing with the plants they found here. The few persons interested in pursuing investigations of poisonous plants could look up appropriate information in European compendia and apply it with some usefulness to local conditions. The dawn of scientific agriculture in North America can be traced to events a score of years apart: the founding of the Department of Agriculture and the passage of the Morrill Land Grant Act in support of agricultural experimentation and experiment stations in 1887.

These events meant, in practical terms, that as settler moved their livestock west into an increasingly foreign flora and began to put pressure on it, they could no longer turn to experience or to European knowledge to cope with the poisonings that occurred. On the other hand, as each state organized it took advantage of federal programs to establish a college of agriculture and an experiment station, and it was to these agencies that the problems were referred. Increasingly sophisticated experimentation ensured, and by 1900 all but three states west of the Mississippi had published work dealing in a practical way with poisonous plants. At the same time, reports of experimental work from eastern states remained almost nonexistent. Looking at the results of these influence at the present time, one sees that about a third of thee existing body of information derives from case histories in man and animals, about a third derives from experimental investigation, mostly from a veterinary point of view, and about one third entered our literature from European source. At the same time, the excellence of mush of the recent experimental work with poisonous plants, and the continuous long-term record of productivity of such laboratories as the federal poisonous plants investigational program at Logan, Utah, contrast sharply with the fact that apparently current information being used to treat human poisonings today may in fact be traced to experiments of Orfila and even to Dioscorides.

Given so many potentially harmful plants and the variety of syndromes they may provoke under particular circumstances, a common first reaction of those who must learn to deal practically with the problem of plant poisoning in man is to seek a list of the few most dangerous or troublesome ones.

The National Clearinghouse for Poison Control Centers published a detailed review of the collected reports of plant ingestions for 1965 that were treated as poisoning emergencies. If reporting were accurate, this list should contain the most troublesome plants of the United States. It is not difficult, however, to show that the clearinghouse list is actually of little value for this purpose. Assuming that the personnel of most poison control centers are competent, concerned, conscientious, and medically trained, this list represents a summation of their frustrations in obtaining useful histories, identifying plants, finding or interpreting appropriate literature, discovering that useful or recent experimental results do not exist for the plant in question, or finding that no tested treatments have been recommended for particular circumstances, as was suggested earlier in this chapter.

Taking the plants in order as named:

Standard botanical manuals for the United States list at least three different genera to which the name "pokeweed" or "pokeroot" is commonly applied. All three (*Phytolacca americana* [=*P. decandra*], *Veratrum viride*, and *Symplocarpus foetidus*) have histories of toxicity, but the syndromes differ greatly, as would appropriate treatments. All three are discussed later in this chapter. (*Symplocarpus foetidus*, also called skunk cabbage, is an aroid or member of the plant family Araceae.)

"Yew" is another common name that can cause trouble. It normally refers to a species of *Taxus*. One of these species, *T. canadensis*, is more commonly called "ground hemlock" in some areas. Thus, it is easy for the uninitiated to transfer inadvertently in the literature from "yew" to "hemlock," especially since the latter is a well-known name associated with toxic plants. However, "hemlock" is applied as a common name to at least four genera of plant, only one of which is not lethal. Again the syndromes and appropriate treatments vary.

"Philodendron" is both a scientific name and a common name. As the later, it is applied by the public, and nearly as loosely by many florists, to almost any viny, leafy, nondeciduous (not shedding) potted plant, with or without holes in the leaf blade. A survey of plants with these characteristics, made with the help of the staff at Cornell's Hortorium, resulted in a tally or several score species of plants in nine genera. Only a plant specialist could accurately identify the plant involved when a call comes to a poison control center that a child has eaten "philodendron," and then probably only by seeing the actual plant.

The name "bittersweet" is commonly applied to two entirely different plant genera, one of which has only an ancient European record of putative toxicity. The other is a species of *Solanum* (*dulcamara*), thus a "nightshade." "Nightshade" is perhaps the worst possible designation for a poisonous plant. Usually it refers to one of the multitude of species of *Solanum*. However, it can apply to more than one genus (for example, *Atropa belladonna* is commonly called "nightshade") and is also regularly used to designate the family that contains these plants, the Solanaceae. This is one of the larger plant families and contains such useful plants as potato (*Solanum tuberosum*) and tomato (*Lycopersicon esculentum*). Any member of the family can be called a "nightshade") in a general way, and many are poisonous ("deadly nightshade") under some circumstances including potato and tomato, despite their widespread daily use as food. The last plant named is also a nightshade (Jerusalem cherry = *Solanum pseudocapsicum*), but is at worst only mildly poisonous according to the available information. In conclusion, "nightshade" and "deadly nightshade" are words many parents know. They are likely to come up when a child has eaten a wild plant whose identity is not known by the distraught mother. Under these circumstances, the usefulness of "nightshade" for indicating the identity of a species of plant is virtually nil.

"Holly" is applied to a dozen species of the genus *Ilex*. Many are native American plants and have no record to toxicity. English holly (*I. opaca*) figures in a wealth of Middle Ages mythology. The only definite published reference to the toxicity of *Ilex* is in a second-hand French report from

1889, with authority not stated. Although this has been carried forward in texts to the present, and may even have some validity to it, the present-day physician would be unwise to base his treatment on this kind of information.

"Honeysuckle" refers to more than a score of species of plants in eight genera belonging to four different plant families. The plant commonly referred to in the East as "honeysuckle" is not known to be toxic.

"Pyracantha" is a scientific name and, although several common names are available for this shrub. Without a species name this particular plant is identified only partially, although probably better than with only a common name. The berries of *Pyracantha*, however, have been shown by experiments to be nontoxic in four species of laboratory animals. At present there is no reason to assume that *Pyracantha* berries are poisonous to man.

"Castor bean" is a satisfactory (i.e. unambiguous) common name designation for a single plant species. *Ricinus communis*. The seeds of this plant are well known to be lethal if ingested in small to moderate amount. However, the plant has been subjected to horticultural manipulation so that two main commercial selections now exist. One is grown for production of oil; the other, as a showy, ornamental hedge or garden plant. The unselected native type grows wild in Florida. Whether these three types have equivalent toxicity is not known.

Greater impetus for detailed experimentation with poisonous plants might develop if more investigators realized the important discoveries that have come from such research in the past. Some, such as ergot, digitalis, belladonna, and morphine, are classic. The discovery of dicoumarol as an anticoagulant and the development of warfarin as a rodenticide came directly from an experiment station investigation of why cattle fed moldy sweetclover hay (*Melilotus* spp.) bled to death. More recently investigation of the toxicity of cyads (*Cycas* spp.) has yielded important information about carcinogenesis of bracken fern (*Pteridium aquilinum*), about avitaminosis B_1 in nonruminants; of pokeweed (*Phytolacca americana*), about mitogenesis in leukocytes of hellebore (*Veratrum californicum*) and lupine (*Lupinus sericeus*), about teratogenesis; and of groundsels (*Senecio* spp.) about liver function.

Other sources of sophisticated information on the effects of plants on animals are the pharmaceutical industry and feed manufacturers, or academic laboratories functioning in these areas. The pertinence of investigations of natural drug products is obvious. Less obvious, perhaps, is the work that has been done to analyze and determine nutritional insufficiencies or minor toxicities associated with utilizing large amounts of particular crops for feedstuffs. A good example is the detailed analysis of gossypol, the toxic component of cottonseed (*Gossypium* spp.) that makes cottonseed meal potentially poisonous to livestock.

Effects of Toxic Principles Elaborated by Plants

Poisonous principles of plants range from single elements or simple salts accumulated by some species under certain circumstances (e.g., selenium in cereal crops or oxalates in *Halogeton glomeratus*) to the elaboration of complex molecules of high toxicity (the phytotoxin abrin, a protein, in *Abrus precatorius*, the infamous Rosary pea or Jequirity bean). The specific action of a toxic principle in an animal as presently understood may range from simple irritation of mucous tissues to disruption of an enzymatic process at the microsomal or mitochondrial level. Thus, it is difficult to organize the available information along lines of either molecular structure or fundamental physiology. This difficulty is compounded by the fact that precise knowledge of the toxicity of the 700 species of plants known to be toxic is lacking for more than half. Different authors use various more or less successful schemes based on physiology, pathology, chemistry, or some combination. Any attempt to categorize poisonous principles of plants on chemical grounds suffers not only from the fact that the exact chemistry is rarely known but also that the common categories employed for such purposes (alkaloids, glycosides, saponins, etc.) are not parallel and therefore not mutually exclusive.

Information on poisonous principles and actions is organized below according to observed responses to average toxicologic exposures, and this in turn is considered in sequence of major target organ or tissue as the poison passes through the body, assuming initial exposure by ingestion. Poisons and responses they elicit are so numerous and varied that what follows is more of a summary than a discussion. Only one example is given for each situation, although numerous examples may exist, and subsidiary effects or consequences in additional organs or tissues are ignored, although they are often clinically important. The discussion is also limited to effects of plants ingested as such, not to overdoses of drugs of plant origin, and does not include consideration of differential diagnosis, clinical signs, pathology, or treatment, except as specially important to the point singled out for attention.

External Structure and Mouth

The sap of some plants is acrid and irritating to skin and mucous membranes. The mown stubble of a field of spurge (*Euphorbia esula*) has caused inflammation and loss of hair on the legs of horses used to mow it. Some plants taken into the mouth cause intense stomatitis by direct irritation. The foliage or berries of the ornamental shrub daphne (*Daphne mezereum*), for example, cause corrosive lesions of the mouth, if chewed or eaten. Animals will taken such distasteful materials into the mouth out of curiosity, and most poisonings occur when prunings or clippings are thrown into a pasture or stall. Children exhibit similar curiosity and will swallow distasteful material as readily as they spit it out, just to get it out of the mouth. Either of these plants, and many others of course, will produce intense irritation of the esophagus and, if swallowed, the gut. The exact nature of the irritant is usually unknown. Many aroids (members of the plant family Araceae) cause a similar intense burning sensation in the mouth. Perhaps the most notorious is dumbcane (*Dieffenbachia* spp.) These plants contain needle-like crystals of calcium oxalate that may cause some mechanical as well as chemical irritation. The severity of the reaction has been traced, however, to the presence of a proteolytic enzyme in the plant that attacks the oral tissues. This reaction is often accompanied by swelling and glottic edema and has been fatal in man when the breathing passages have been blocked as a consequence.

Degree of mastication of seeds and fleshy or thick plant parts may determine the severity of the subsequent reaction, or whether it takes place at all. Seeds of precatory bean (*Abrus precatorius*), for example, are highly toxic if chewed, but will pass through the gut undigested if the seed coat is left intact.

Rumen, or Foregut

Ruminants may react to plant poisons quite differently from nonruminants due to differences in digestive structure and function between these two major groups of animals. Ability to vomit effectively is one difference. Some plants stimulate a strong vomit reflex. The vomiting disease of swine, for example, requires ingestion of only a very small amount of barley grain parasitized by a mold fungus (*Gibberella* sp.). Cardioactive glycosides such as those in foxglove (*Digitalis purpurea*) similarly provoke vomiting in most species of animals, even when administered parenterally. Many simple-stomached animals (e.g., man and dog) vomit easily. Ruminants can vomit, but the reflex is not as easily stimulated and the degree to which vomiting is effective in removing poisonous material from the gut is much less than in nonruminants. Vomiting in ruminants is not equivalent to normal eructation. Horses can vomit, but the structure of the oral cavity leads to complications if vomiting occurs. In horses, vomitus is directed into the trachea. Pneumonitis is a common result, and this can develop into pneumonia and result in death. In severe cases, death may result directly from asphyxiation after vomiting. Many glycosides, as they exist in plants, are not toxic to animals. Toxicity comes from breakdown of the glycoside to release a toxic component. Breakdown often occurs more readily or more rapidly in the rumen than in the digestive tract of monogastric animals. Also, small molecules can be absorbed at the rumen and thus enter the circulation rapidly. Breakdown of cyanogenic glycosides, such as amygdalin, from members of the rose family (Rosaceae) is an example. The ruminant is more likely to achieve toxic levels of cyanide in the blood in the balance between breakdown of the glycoside, absorption of cyanide, and its detoxification and excretion, than is the nonruminant. Occasionally, unexpected events occur. Sheep on dry range pasture may die of cyanide poisoning shortly after drinking water. The loss of life from ingestion of poison suckleya (*Suckleyea suckleyana*) is an example. It is hypothesized that the ruminal contents are too dry for effective breakdown of the glycoside until the animal drinks, whereupon the reaction is intense. Sometimes such instances are erroneously diagnosed as poisoning from the water itself. Many of the symptoms are similar to those of nitrate poisoning.

Ingestion of abnormally large amounts of various forages or grains, or sudden massive change in diet, can provoke unusual reactions in the rumen that have toxicologic consequences. These can range from a simple pH shift to the elaboration of specific highly toxic molecules. For example, it has been suggested that, under unusual circumstances, silage of high nitrate content can undergo a reaction in the rumen that yields nitrogen oxide gases. Taken into the lungs, small amounts of nitrogen oxides cause severe, irreversible pulmonary emphysema. The same thing happens when nitrogen oxides are formed in silage made from forage (usually corn, *Zea mays*) of high nitrate concentration. Being heavier than air, the nitrogen oxides accumulate around the base of the silo. Breathed by man, they cause a similar syndrome, which is called "silo-filler's disease."

A syndrome of cattle, associated clinically with reduced levels of magnesium in the blood, is characterized by staggering that develops shortly after they are placed on lush pasturage. It has been postulated that, under these pasturage conditions, sufficient ammonia is formed in the rumen to react with, and tie up enough, magnesium (as hydroxide) to produce dietary insufficiency.

Some plants cause ruminal stasis. When this happens, a low-grade toxemia commences that becomes more severe with time. Also, signs of starvation appear. Mesquite bean (*Prosopis juliflora*) poisoning, recognized on southwestern ranges in cattle, is an example. Stasis is complete or nearly so. Mesquite beans have been found in the rumen on postmortem examination of animals that had not had access to this plant for as long as nine months. Under these conditions, the seeds have sometimes sprouted and begun to grow in the rumen.

Ruminants are more susceptible to bloat (the foamy entrapment of gases) than are monogastric animals. Bloat, if unrelieved, can have lethal consequences. Some plants promote bloat. These include some common leguminous forage crops and certain wild plants. Among the latter is the wild larkspur (*Delphinium* spp.) of western ranges. Under range conditions bloat may not be observed in time to be treated effectively.

Just as the rumen can promote the release of a toxic compound from an innocuous precursor, so can it sometimes aid in the detoxification of an initially poisonous compound. Sheep fed high-calcium alfalfa hay, for example, are protected to some degree against the toxic effects of halogeton (*Halogeton glomeratus*), which contains soluble oxalates. It is postulated that calcium is precipitated by the oxalate ions in the rumen, thus making the oxalate unavailable for absorption from the gut.

Another situation in which the ruminant has the advantage over the nonruminant occurs in the case of ingestion of plants containing a thiaminase, such as field horsetail (*Equisetum arvense*). In the horse, continued exposure to such plants causes destruction of the thiamine in the diet and the development of a definite and eventually lethal B_1 deficiency with classic signs of polyneuritis. This is one of the few instances where the ultimate biochemical lesion, disruption of carboxylation in the Krebs cycle, is known. In a ruminant, the microflora of the rumen manufacture copious quantities of thiamine, which apparently is carried intact in the bacterial cell to a point in the gut beyond which the thiaminase is inactivated or destroyed. There it is released by digestion of the bacterial cell and absorbed by the ruminant. In any event, ruminants do not suffer from thiamine deficiency despite having a level of thiaminase in the diet that would kill a horse.

The initial distribution of ingested materials in the ruminant is determined partly by density. Seeds tend to pass quickly through the rumen and to concentrate in the abomasum. Here irritant substances may be released from seeds in concentrated form and promote irritation and hemorrhage of the abomasal wall seeds of members of the mustard family (Cruciferae) are examples.

Lower Gut

Two important actions, irritation and absorption, may occur in the stomach and intestines. Many plants cause irritation, varying in severity from mild to ulcerative, and the principal signs or symptoms in many cases of poisoning are simply those of gastroenteritis. Pokeroot (*Phytolacca americana*), for example, experimentally produces hemorrhagic gastritis, and ulcers are found in postmortem examination at locations where pieces of root lie against the mucosa of the gut. Pokeweed poisoning in cattle results in copious, almost explosive diarrhea that may contain signs of hemorrhage. In contrast, although blood-tinged feces are characteristic of oak (*Quercus* spp.) poisoning of cattle, the gastroenteritis is usually accompanied by constipation.

Absorption of toxins into the bloodstream normally takes place in the lower gut. Some toxic principles are large molecules, not readily absorbed. Saponins, such as those of the cockles (*Saponaria* spp.), are examples. As irritants, however, they promote their own absorption. Cardioactive glycosides are saponic in physical properties. It has been shown that the nature of the sugar portion of the intact glycoside is important in determining the solubility of these molecules and, therefore, their physiologic availability.

Liver

Poisonous principles absorbed into the circulatory system pass first to the liver. Here many different things can happen. A number of plant substances are severely poisonous to hepatic tissue, causing rapid destruction and necrosis where contact is made. A common finding on necropsy is a pathologic liver, but the exact pathology varies considerably. In many cases, the assault is somewhat chronic, and the appearance and function of the liver represent whatever current balance exists between destructive and regenerative changes.

A great deal of recent work has gone into elucidation of the exact hepatotoxic effects of pyrrolizidine alkaloids. Alkaloids of this configuration are found in a number of genera of higher plants (such as *Senecio* spp.). The primary lesion is a characteristic megalocytosis accompanied by venous obstruction or occlusion. Some plants. (e.g., *Trifolium subterraneum*, subterranean clover) accumulate copper from soils of high copper content. Copper then accumulates in and produces degenerative changes of the liver. In akee (*Blighia sapida*) poisoning of man, a hypoglycemic poisonous principle in the plant reduces the glycogen content of the liver to nearly zero.

One of the types of liver dysfunction that commonly occurs in plant poisonings is the reduced ability to eliminate certain pigmented molecules in the bile. These, instead, enter general circulation. When they reach the capillaries of the skin, they react with light and cause the capillaries to leak serum. This reaction and its consequences constitute the syndrome of photosensitization. If edematous swelling is severe, the involved tissues die and are sloughed off. Thus, in range sheep, the disease known as bighead is characterized initially by erythema, then by edematous swelling, and ultimately by necrosis of portions of the ears, cheeks, and lips, if severe Animals that have lost the lips are unable to forage effectively and die of starvation. The identity of all pigments involved in photosensitization is not yet known, but several have been established. One or more are breakdown products of chlorophyll and are normally present in the hepatic portal circulation. In other cases, the photosensitizing pigment is contained in the plant itself and passes unchanged through digestion, absorption, and the normal liver. Photosensitization caused by the first type of pigment, always accompanied by signs of liver damage, and usually by icterus, is termed secondary. Photosensitization involving a normal liver and lacking any signs of liver dysfunction is termed primary. A range plant commonly provoking secondary photosensitization (bighead) is horsebrush (*Tetradymia* spp.). Primary photosensitization is less common, but can be caused by ingestion of St. Johnswort (*Hypericum perforatum*).

Circulatory System

The discussion of photosensitization has taken us from the liver to the general circulation. A number of other disease syndromes may occur in the circulatory system or involve the blood itself. The toxic principle of sweet pea (*Lathyrus odoratus*), β-aminopropionitrile, causes dissecting aneurysm of the aorta in small animals. A number of plants contain toxins that provoke lysis of red blood cells and consequent hemolytic anemia. Among them are cultivated onion (*Allium cepa*) and rape forage (*Brassica napus*). Saponins and phytotoxins cause lysis of red blood cells *in vitro*. Their role *in vivo* is less clear.

Coumarin, contained in sweetclover hay (*Melilotus* spp.), is converted to dicoumarin by molds under certain conditions. This compound interferes with prothrombin synthesis and results in a hemorrhagic disease when molded sweetclover hay is ingested over a period of time. Animals bleed to death from minor injuries or, in advanced cases, bleed to death internally. Large subdermal hemorrhages are usually found in these cases. Soluble oxalates in the diet can result in the precipitation of calcium ions in the circulating blood. The resulting ionic imbalance has neurologic consequences. Hypomagnesemia and its consequences have already been mentioned.

Kidney

Once a toxin is in the blood, all organs are exposed to its effect unless a membrane barrier intervenes. Many plant toxins are destructive to parenchymatous organs in general. Digenerative effects are seen primarily in liver and kidneys on postmortem examination. In some cases described above, the liver is the primary target organ. In a few others, the kidney shows the major pathology. The latter includes the effects of tannins in oak (*Quercus* spp.) poisoning, and the crystallization of oxalates in kidney tubules in oxalate poisoning as by halogeton (*Halogeton glomeratus*).

Heart

In many lethal poisonings, the immediate cause of death is heart failure. Heart dysfunction can be brought about by malfunction of innervation or of the heart's conducting tissues, or it may be a result of a more direct effect on the heart musculature. Ingestion of foxglove (*Digitalis purpurea*) is similar to an overdose of the drug digitalis, which acts by stimulating the vagus center. At toxic levels, cardioactive glycosides produce cardiac irregularities and heart block. The alkaloid of yew (*Taxus cuspidata*) depresses the conducting tissue of the heart and stops it, often very quickly, in diastole. Hypotensive alkaloids, such as in false hellebore (*Veratrum viride*), cause a marked slowing of the heart rate.

Bone

Bracken fern (*Pteridium aquilinum*) contains two toxins. One is a thiaminase. The other, more slowly acting, has its target the bone marrow. Thus, ruminants exposed to a steady diet of bracken for many weeks develop a blood dyscrasia, characterized particularly by diminished counts of leukocytes and platelets, which may be traced in origin to severe destruction of bone marrow. Clinical signs of this disease are unusual for a poisoning and consist chiefly of hemorrhaging throughout the body due to thrombocytopenia, and invasion of the body by ordinarily nonpathogenic bacteria due to leukocytopenia, and the concomitant development of an elevated temperature. This disease is basically indistinguishable from radiation poisoning.

Pokeweed (*Phytolacca americana*), in contrast, contains an active principle that promotes the division of white blood cells. The pokeweed mitogen is also associated with the stimulation of production of interferon. Some unusual plant toxins act on the skeletal structure itself. Sweet pea (*Lathyrus odoratus*) poisoning in laboratory animals consists primarily of disturbance of the normal deposition and resorption of bone in such a way that cartilage proliferates. The gross effect includes a twisting of the vertebral column. The poisonous principle is the same as that causing dissecting aneurysms in other animals. "Crooked-calf disease" is associated with lupines (*Lupinus sericeus*).

Lung

Under some circumstances, ingestion of rape (*Brassica napus*) forage results in lesions of the lung. Edematous swelling and emphysema are followed by rupture of the alveoli and passage of air from the lungs to collect subdermally on either side of the backbone, where it may be palpated. Somewhat similar lesions are produced by nitrogen gases, as described above.

Thyroid

Many members of the cabbage family (Cruciferae) contain glycosides that release goitrogenic factors (thiocyanates and thiooxazolidone) when digested. The thyroid responds to these compounds by enlarging, and other signs of goiter appear. These goitrogens are iodine responsive.

Eye

The eyes are sometimes involved in signs of poisoning. Severe mydriasis that may provoke visual disturbance is a common sign of poisoning by alkaloids of the tropane configuration, such as atropine found in jimsonweed (*Datura stramonium*). Blindness accompanies a number of poisonings in which other signs may be primary. Often the eye appears normal in structure and function, and blindness may be ascribed to malfunction in the central nervous system. An example of a plant that causes functional blindness is tansy mustard (*Descurainia pinnata*). In man, ingestion of poppy (isoquinoline) alkaloids as from prickly poppy (*Argemone mexicana*) often causes generalized edema and has been held responsible for producing glaucoma.

Nervous System

Nervous signs are perhaps second in frequency only to gastroenteric signs in case of plant poisoning. Nervous involvement and the consequent specific signs are extremely varied and may depend as much on species of animal as on the poisonous principle itself. When nervous tissue is the principal target, lesions are usually absent. There are exceptions. Cerebral demyelination has been reported in lambs born to ewes fed heavily on seaweeds. Liquefactive necrosis of cerebellar areas has been associated with molded forage and with ingestion of sensitive fern (*Onoclea sensibilis*) by horses. More recently, focal necrosis in the anterior globus pallidus of the cerebrum and substantia nigra of the mesencephalon has been described as the primary lesion in "chewing disease" of horses fed on yellow star thistle (*Centaurea solstitialis*). Pigs born to sows that have fed heavily on white clover (*Trifolium repens*) may under some circumstances display demyelination of the spinal cord and be unable to suckle . The exact signs associated with lesions of cranial and spinal nervous tissue vary widely and depend on exactly what areas are involved. An example of a type of poisoning in which obvious lesions of the nervous tissue do not occur is the convulsive syndrome characteristic of water hemlock (*Cicuta maculata*) poisoning.

In many cases a nervous syndrome may be characterized grossly as excitatory or depressive: An example of the former is the hyperexcitable condition produced in animals after ingestion of Dallis grass (*Paspalum dilatatum*) parasitized by an ergot (*Claviceps paspali*). In contrast, weakness and paralysis are characteristic of the effect of poisons that interfere with the normal action of the voluntary musculature through its innervation. For example, guajillo (*Acacia berlandieri*) provokes a classic syndrome of ascending posterior paralysis. In this case, the identity of the poisonous principle, N-methyl-β-phenylalanine, has been worked out. Coniine, the alkaloid of poison hemlock (*Conium maculatum*), the first alkaloid to be synthesized, has an action that is essentially similar in gross effect. Sleepy grass (*Stipa robusta*), found in a limited area of the American Southwest, provokes drowsiness in horses in small amounts and deep sleep in larger doses. The active principle is unknown.

Additional nervous symptoms can be described in man. Paresthesias and hallucinations are associated with particular types of poisoning. The alkaloid aconitine (e.g., from monkshood, *Aconitum napellus*) causes the former, and jimsonweed (*Datura stramonium*) in moderate amount gives rise to the latter.

In gangrenous ergotism, chronic ingestion of ergot (usually *Claviceps purpurea* on rye—*Secale cereale*) causes constriction of the musculature of arterioles. This results in a predisposition to thromboses or other occlusions of the circulation, particularly in the extremities where blood pressure is minimal. The tissue distal to the occlusion dies, becomes septic, and eventually is lost.

Respiratory System

Respiration can be inhibited or prevented at any level, from the mouth to the respiring cells themselves. Cases involving the oral cavity, the lungs, and the cardiovascular system have already been mentioned. In addition to these, respiration can be blocked by the inability of blood to carry oxygen, as in nitrate poisoning, or of the cells to use it, as in cyanide poisoning. Many plants can take up dangerously high levels of nitrogen under conditions of heavy fertilization; a few (such as corn—*Zea mays*) are predisposed to do so. Treatment of crops with 2,4-D can upset nitrogen metabolism with similar results. Nitrate in plants is largely converted to nitrite in the gut. This reacts with hemoglobin to form methemoglobin. The ability of the blood to carry oxygen is impaired in proportion to conversion. Cyanide, released from cyanogenetic glycosides of various kinds elaborated in a large number of plants (e.g., wild cherries—*Prunus* spp.), blocks the action of cytochrome oxidase and thereby interferes with the uptake of oxygen into cellular respiration. In both cases the general signs are those associated with asphyxiation.

Reproductive System

Some plants can elaborate estrogenic factors under certain conditions. Certain forage legumes are known to do so. Corn (*Zea mays*) molded by an unknown fungus has provoked a similar syndrome. Poisoning is characterized by vaginal swelling and prolapse in female animals. Some effects may also be observed in male animals.

Some plants, ingested by pregnant animals, have a pronounced teratogenic effect on the developing embryo. Perhaps the best example is the cycloptic lambs born to ewes that have been exposed to ingestion of hellebore (*Veratrum californicum*) on the fourteenth day of gestation. At that time the embryo is sensitive in development of facial structure. A massive exposure to the plant results in severely inhibited facial development. While the lower jaw remains more or less normal, the upper jaw disappears nearly entirely, and both eyes occupy a single orbit in the center of the forehead, or there may be but one central eye.

Some poisonous principles (fortunately few) are readily excreted in milk. These include especially those of high fat solubility, which may be concentrated in the butterfat. While excretion of toxic principles is beneficial to the animal doing so, the consumption of milk from poisoned animals can induce poisoning in man or nursing animals. The secondary poisoning can be more severe than that in the lactating animal because of the concentration of the poison and the lesser ability of the nonlactating consumer to eliminate it. Perhaps the best example is given by white snakeroot (*Eupatorium rugosum*). The poisonous principle (tremetol) it contains provokes a disease in cattle called trembles. Ingestion of milk from poisoned cattle causes a serious debilitating disease, "milksickness," in man. Farmers commonly associate abortion in livestock with ingestion of weeds. The actual causes of abortion are many. Some plants in toxic amounts (e.g., broomweed—*Gutierrezia microcephala*) undoubtedly can lead to abortion in pregnant animals, but the mechanism is undetermined.

Hair and Skin

The effect of photosensitization on the skin has been mentioned above. Thickening of the skin (hyperkeratosis), usually accompanied by loss of hair, can result from a variety of causes but is often related to a deficiency of vitamin A. It has been shown that some isolates of the imperfect fungus *Aspergillus* can induce the formation of a factor in the substrate that produces well-developed cases of hyperkeratosis in experimental animals. Some forage plants, particularly legumes, grown on high molybdenum soils accumulate enough molybdenum to become toxic to grazing animals. One of the chief signs of poisoning is depigmentation of the hair. The incidence of this disease in cattle at pasture can be mapped by airplane. Depigmentation, which develops slowly, is ascribed to the inability of tyrosinase to mediate the formation of melanin in the absence of copper, the availability of which in the body is reciprocally related to the bodily concentration of molybdenum. Loss of long hair and hoof deformity accompany one type of selenium poisoning. On certain seleniferous soils, grain crops may develop concentrations of selenium, in organic combination, of 5 ppm or more. At this level, continued ingestion of grain or forage produces the syndrome known as "alkali disease." It appears that selenium substitutes for sulfur in amino acids. Hoof deformity and sloughing will become severe enough in time that affected animals will graze from a kneeling position and eventually starve to death. The amino acid mimosine (as in koa haole, *Leucaena glauca*) is held responsible for causing a similar syndrome when ingested.

Poisonous plants are numerous, ubiquitous, troublesome, and poorly studied. No general botanic, ecologic, or geographic relationship exists among them to bring order to an understanding of the diversity of toxic principles contained in plants, viewed either chemically or physiologically, and in the syndromes provoked by them in man and animals. Syndromes in which a plant poison is the prime etiologic factor may involve the integument and hair, the mouth and any portion of the digestive system (with a major distinction possible between ruminant and simple-stomached animals), the parenchymatous organs (especially the liver and kidney), the circulatory system (including the heart, vascularization, and blood itself), the skeletal system, the lungs and respiratory system (including cellular respiration), various glands (especially the thyroid), the central and autonomic nervous systems, the eye, and the reproductive system. Full elucidation of a poisonous plant syndrome usually requires the efforts of a team of research specialists. Some past investigations have yielded results of great medical or economic importance. Results are needed even more urgently so that reaction to poisoning by plants, its treatment, and prevention can be more intelligently founded than at present.

15

Valerian

Valerian is a perennial herb comprised of grooved hollow stems and saw-toothed green leaves. White, pale pink, or reddish flowers appear from June to August. Valerian grows to heights of 3–5 feet in the temperate climates of North America, western Asia, and Europe, often in moist soil along riverbanks. The vertical rhizome and attached roots of valerian are parts used medicinally, and are best harvested in the autumn of the second year. Although the fresh drug has no distinctive odor, over time hydrolysis of compounds present in the volatile oil produces isovaleric acid, which has an offensive, somewhat putrid odor. Fortunately, the smell can be removed from the skin and utensils by washing with sodium bicarbonate. Even though valerian has a disagreeable odor, people in the 16th century considered it a fragrant perfume. Traditional uses include treatment of insomnia, migraine headache, anxiety, fatigue, and seizures. It has also been applied externally on cuts, sores, and acne. Traditional Chinese uses include treatment of headache, numbness caused by rheumatic conditions, colds, menstrual difficulties, and bruises. The pharmacological effects of valerian have been attributed to the constituents of volatile oils, monoterpenes, valepotriates, and sesquiterpenes (valerenic acid). Some of these constituents have been shown to have a direct action on the brain, and valerenic acid inhibits enzyme-induced breakdown of γ-amino butyric acid (GABA) in the brain resulting in sedation.

Current Promoted Uses

Valerian is promoted in the United States primarily as a sedative-hypnotic for treatment of insomnia, and as an anxiolytic for restlessness and sleeping disorders associated with anxiety.

Sources and Chemical Composition

Also referred to as: *Valeriana officinalis* (L.), *Valeriana wallichii* DC. (Indian valerian), *Valeriana alliariifolia Vahl*, *Valeriana sambucifolia Mik*, *Radix valerianae*, red valerian (*Centranthus ruber* [L.] DC), valerian root, *Valerianae radix*, garden heliotrope, all heal, amantilla, and setwall.

Products Available

Crude valerian root, rhizome, or stolon is dried and used either "as is" or to prepare an extract. Valerian is available as a capsule, tablet, oral solution, or tea. Valerian is also administered externally as a bath additive.

Pharmacological/Toxicological Effects

Insomnia

Several studies have examined the effects of valerian on sleep. Donath and colleagues performed a randomized, double-blind, placebo- controlled, cross-over study assessing the short-term (single dose) and long-term (14-day multiple dosage) effects of valerian extract on sleep structure and sleep quality. There were significant differences between valerian and placebo for parameters describing *slow-wave sleep* (SWS) and shorter sleep latency, with very low adverse events. Leathwood and colleagues demonstrated valerian's effect on sleep quality. A freeze-dried aqueous extract of valerian root (*Rhizomå valeriana officinalis* [L.]) 400 mg was compared to two Hova (valerian 60 mg and hop flower extract 30 mg per tablet) tablets and placebo (finely ground brown sugar) in this crossover study involving 128 volunteers. Study participants took the study medication 1 hour before retiring, and filled out a questionnaire the following morning. This was repeated on nonconsecutive nights, such that each of the three treatments, identified only by a code number, was administered in random order three times to each patient. Valerian caused a significant improvement in subjectively evaluated sleep quality and a significant decrease in perceived sleep latency. The self-reported improvement in sleep quality was especially notable in smokers, those patients who considered themselves poor or irregular sleepers, and those who reported having difficulty falling asleep on a prestudy questionnaire. Hova did not demonstrate any beneficial effect, but it was reported to cause a "*hangover effect*" the next morning. Because subjective sleep questionnaires may not correlate with sleep *electroencephalogram* (EEG) results, a parallel EEG sleep study was performed comparing valerian to placebo in 10 young men. There was not a statistically significant difference between valerian and placebo in this small study. The authors hypothesized that the results of this experiment might have differed from the questionnaire-assessed study because of small sample size and differences in study populations. The larger study involved young and older individuals, men and women, and good and poor sleepers, whereas the EEG study involved young men with no reported sleep abnormalities. Rather than place more credence on the objective study, the investigators concluded that the questionnaire provides a more sensitive means of detecting mild sedative effects.

A double-blind, placebo-controlled study was performed in eight volunteers recruited from among the research staff at Nestle Products and their families who reported that they "usually have problems getting to sleep." Sleep latency was measured using an activity monitor and questionnaire. The investigators documented a small (7 minute) but statistically significant decrease in sleep latency with 450 mg of an extract of valerian (*V. officinalis* [L.]). No further improvement was demonstrated with a 900-mg valerian dose; however, patients receiving the higher dose were more likely to feel sleepy the next morning. Sleep quality, sleep latency, and sleep depth also improved according to a nine-point subjective rating scale. However, the appropriateness of the statistical analysis used to interpret the results of the subjective portion of the study is unclear.

A more objective double-blind, placebo-controlled trial evaluated the effect of 450- and 900-mg doses of an aqueous valerian extract (*V. officinalis* [L.]) on two groups of healthy, young (21–44 years of age) volunteers at home and in a laboratory setting. The effect of valerian on sleep was measured using a questionnaire and night-time motor activity recordings in both settings. The effects of valerian on the volunteers in the sleep laboratory were also measured using polysomnography and spectral analysis of the sleep EEG. Both groups demonstrated the mild hypnotic effects of valerian; however, the benefits of valerian were statistically significant only under home conditions.

Another double-blind, placebo-controlled crossover study evaluated Valerina Natt, a preparation equivalent to 400 mg of valerian root composed mainly of sesquiterpenes from *V. officinalis* [L.], on subjective sleep quality assessed using a three-point rating scale. Study subjects were 27 consecutive patients seen in a medical clinic for evaluation of sleep difficulty and fatigue who were willing to participate in the investigation. Statistically significant improvement in sleep quality was noted with the valerian preparation. Valerian was rated as better than placebo by 21 subjects, two rated the preparations equally, and four preferred placebo. No adverse effects were reported. Although some study subjects had experienced nightmares when using conventional hypnotics, nightmares were not reported in the study. The effects of repeated doses (three tablets three times daily) for 8 days of Valdispert Forte (135 mg of dried extract of *V. officinalis* [L.]) in 14 elderly women with sleeping difficulties was assessed using polysomnography in a particularly well-designed study. Inclusion criteria were well defined: sleep latency longer than 30 minutes, more than three nocturnal awakenings per night with inability to go back to sleep within 5 minutes, and total sleep time less than 5 hours. Subjects could not have medical, psychological, or weight-related causes of sleep difficulty, and had to have normal health status for their age. Sedatives, hypnotics, and other *central nervous system* (CNS)-active drugs were discontinued 2 weeks prior to the study, and drug screening for morphine, benzodiazepines, barbiturates, and amphetamine was done prior to study commencement. Results showed an increase in SWS, and a decrease in sleep stage 1. There was no effect on *rapid eye movement* (REM) sleep, sleep latency, time awake after sleep onset, or self-rated sleep quality.

In aggregate, the results of these clinical studies suggest that at doses of approx 450 mg of the aqueous extract, valerian has mild hypnotic effects, possibly by affecting non-REM sleep in patients with reduced SWS. Unlike benzodiazepines, valerian appears not to adversely affect SWS or REM sleep, and does not appear to cause nightmares or hangover. Further well-designed studies are needed to objectively evaluate valerian. Results of animal studies reflect the clinical data. Sedative properties of Valdispert (dried aqueous extract of *V. officinalis* [L.]) in mice were documented based on reduced spontaneous movement and an increase in thiopental-induced sleep time; however, these effects were slightly less than those of diazepam and chlorpromazine. No significant anticonvulsant effect was observed.

Hendriks and colleagues tested several components of the volatile oil, obtained by steam distillation of *V. officinalis* [L.], on mice. The essential oil, its hydrocarbon fraction, its oxygen fraction, valeranone, valerenal, valerenic acid, and isoeugenyl-isovalerate were injected intraperitoneally at various doses ranging from 50 to 1600 mg/kg, with three mice receiving each dose. The mice were observed between 15 and 30 minutes post-injection for various symptoms suggestive of CNS stimulation or depression, analgesia, sympathomimetic or sympatholytic activity, vasodilation, or vasoconstriction. It was concluded that components of the essential oil, particularly valerenic acid and valerenal, which are present in the oxygen fraction, have a sedative and/or muscle relaxant effect. The authors tested the effect of intraperitoneal valerenic acid compared to diazepam, chlorpromazine, and pentobarbital on ability to walk on a rotating rod and grip strength in mice. The effects of valerinic acid on spontaneous motor activity and on pentobarbital-induced sleeping time were also assessed. Diazepam, a muscle relaxant, affected the grip test but not the rotarod test, whereas chlorpromazine, a neuroleptic, affected the rotarod test but not the grip test. Valerenic acid, like pentobarbital, decreased performance in both the rotarod and grip tests. The authors concluded that valerenic acid, like pentobarbital, has general CNS depressant activity. Valerenic acid also decreased spontaneous motor activity and prolonged pentobarbital-induced sleeping time. Dose–response effects of valerenic acid were also observed by the investigators. At a dose of 50 mg/kg, a decrease in spontaneous motor activity occurred. At 100 mg/kg, mice exhibited ataxia, then remained motionless. Muscle spasms occurred at 150–200 mg/kg and convulsions at 400 mg/kg, followed by death in six of seven mice within 24 hours.

Sedation is mediated predominantly through the inhibitory neurotransmitter GAB A. Although the mechanism of action of valerian as a sleep aid is not fully understood, it may involve inhibition of the enzyme that breaks down GABA. Dihydrovaltrate, hydroxyvalerenic acid, a hydroalcoholic extract containing 0.8% valerenic acid; a lipid extract; an aqueous extract of the hydroalcoholic extract, and another aqueous extract of *V. officinalis* (L.) were assessed for in vitro binding to rat GABA, benzodiazepine, and barbiturate receptors. The results indicated that an interaction of some component of the hydroalcoholic extract, the aqueous extract derived from the hydroalcoholic extract, and the other aqueous extract had affinity for the $GABA_A$ receptor. Because hydroxyvalerenic acid (a volatile oil sesquiterpene) and dihydrovaltrate (a valepotriate) did not show any notable activity, the investigators could not identify the specific constituents responsible for this activity. The lipophilic extract derived from the hydroalcoholic extract, as well as dihydrovaltrate, showed affinity for barbiturate receptors, and some affinity for peripheral benzodiazepine receptors.

Other in vitro studies have also yielded results that suggest GABA-mediated activity; however, the active constituent was unidentified. Cavadas and colleagues verified that valerenic acid (0.1 mmol/L) was not able to displace [^{3}H] muscimol from the $GABA_A$ receptor, although both an aqueous and a hydroalcoholic extract were able to do so. The investigators then attempted to identify other compounds in the extracts capable of displacing [^{3}H] muscinol. Both glutamate and glutamine, amino acids present in the aqueous extract, had little inhibitory effect on [^{3}H] muscinol binding. However, glutamine can cross the blood-brain barrier (BBB) and can be taken up by nerve terminals and converted to GABA inside GABA-nergic neurons. Thus, glutamine could be responsible for the sedative effect of the aqueous extract, but not the hydroalcoholic extract, in which it is not present. GABA is found in both extracts, but GABA itself cannot explain the sedative effects of valerian because it is unlikely to cross the BBB in amounts significant enough to cause sedation. However, the amount of GABA present in the aqueous extract is sufficient to have effects on peripheral GABA receptors, perhaps resulting in muscle relaxation. Another study suggests a different mechanism of action involving inhibition of neuronal GABA uptake and stimulation of GABA release from synaptosomes. These investigators did not attempt to elucidate which constituent of the aqueous extract was responsible for these effects.

The CNS-depressant component of valerian is still unknown. Thus far, three major constituents of valerian have been identified: the volatile or essential oil, containing sesquiterpenes and monoterpenes, nonglycosidic iridoid esters (valepotriates), and a small number of alkaloids. Valepotriates are unstable compounds and are easily hydrolyzed by heat and moisture. In addition, valepotriates are not water soluble, and aqueous extracts contain small amounts. For example, the aqueous extract used in the study by Balderer and Borbely, described previously was analyzed using thin-layer chromatography, and no valepotriates were detectable. Furthermore, valepotriates are not well absorbed orally. Therefore, the likelihood that valepotriates are a major contributor to valerian's effects is questionable. Because of the low amount of alkaloid present in preparations, their contribution is also questionable. It is postulated that a combination of volatile oils, valepotriates, and possibly certain water-soluble constituents that have not yet been identified are responsible for valerian's sedative effects.

Antidepressant effects of valerian were identified by Oshima and associates using a methanol extract of *V. fauriei* roots. They found a strong antidepressant activity in mice as measured by the forced swimming test. One active component isolated was α-kessyl alcohol, a volatile oil component. At 30 mg/kg intraperitoneally, α-kessyl alcohol exhibited an effect similar to imipramine, a commonly used antidepressant. Kessanol and cyclokessyl acetate, guaiane-type sesquiterpenoids, also exhibited antidepressant activity. Kanokonol, kessyl glycol, and kessyl glycol diacetate, valerane-type sesquiterpenoids, did not exhibit an effect. A 30% ethanol extract of the Japanese valerian root extract (4.1 g/kg and 5.7 g/kg) and imipramine (20 mg/kg) also demonstrated statistically significant antidepressant effects compared to placebo as measured by the forced swimming test in rats. As in the Oshima study, kessyl glycol diacetate exhibited no antidepressant activity in the forced swimming test. Because the forced swimming test can be affected by stimulants, anticholinergics, and antihistamines as well as antidepressants, the effect of the valerian extract on reserpine-induced hypothermia, a test for antidepressant activity and inhibition of neuronal reuptake of monoamines, was measured. Both valerian (11.2 g/kg) and imipramine (20 mg/kg) reversed reserpine-induced hypothermia, suggesting that the antidepressant effect of valerian is caused by reuptake of monoamine neurotransmitters, as with conventional antidepressants. More evidence is needed to evaluate the use of valerian in children. One study using a combination product of valerian root extract and lemon balm leaf extract found that symptoms of dyssomnia or pathological restlessness might decrease in children under age 12.

Anxiety

A few studies have examined the effects of valerian on anxiety. Cropley and colleagues investigated whether kava or valerian could moderate physiological stress induced under laboratory conditions in healthy volunteers. Subject (*n* = 18-kava, and *n* = 18-valerian) and comparison group (*n* = 36) volunteers performed a standardized mental stress task 1 week apart. Cases had their blood pressure, heart rate, and subjective ratings of pressure assessed at rest and during the mental stress task (time 1 = *T1*). The valerian subjects took a standard dose for 7 days (time 2 = *T2*). In the valerian group, heart rate reaction to mental stress was found to decline, systolic blood pressure decreased significantly, and subjects reported less pressure during mental stress test tasks at *T2* relative to *T1*. Behavioral performance on the standardized mental stress test task did not change between the groups over the two time points. There were no significant differences in blood pressure, heart rate, or subjective reports of pressure between *T1* and *T2* in the control group. Kohnen and Oswald conducted a study on the effects of valerian, propranolol, and combinations on activation, performance, and mood of healthy volunteers under social stressor conditions. The results of this study were equivocal and published over 15 years ago; however, it is mentioned here for historical reference.

Andreatini and colleagues examined the effect of valerian extract (valepotriates) using a randomized, parallel, double-blind placebo-controlled pilot study design in patients with generalized anxiety disorder (GAD). After a 2-week wash-out period, 36 patients with GAD as defined by the *Diagnostic and Statistical Manual of Mental Disorders,* were randomized to one of the following three treatment groups for 4 weeks: valepotriates, mean daily dose of 81.3 mg; diazepam, mean daily dose of 6.5 mg; or placebo. There was a significant reduction in the psychic factor of the Hamilton anxiety scale in the valepotriates group; however, the principal study analysis using between group comparisons on total Hamilton anxiety scale scores found negative results. The conclusion of this study suggests that there may be a potential anxiolytic effect of valepotriates on the psychic symptoms of anxiety, but the total number of subjects per group (*n* = 12) was very small and results must be viewed as preliminary.

Musculoskeletal Relaxation

Isovaltrate and valtrate (valepotriates) and valeronone, an essential oil component, isolated from *V. edulis* ssp. procera Meyer (Valeriana "mexicana") caused suppression of rhythmic contractions in guinea pig ileum in vivo at a dose of 20 mg/kg administered intravenously via the jugular vein. The investigators also demonstrated that the same compounds as well as dihydrovaltrate isolated from the same valerian species produced relaxation of carbachol-stimulated guinea pig ileum preparations in vitro. They concluded that these compounds have a musculotropic action in concentrations from 10^{-5} to 10^{-4} *M*.

Pharmacokinetics

One study has evaluated the pharmacokinetics of valerian following administration to humans. Following administration of a single 600-mg dose of valerian, the pharmacokinetics of valerenic acid were measured. The T_{max} occurred between 1 and 2 hours and the C_{max} was between 0.9 and 2.3 ng/mL. Concentrations of valerenic acid were measurable for at least 5 hours following the dose. The elimination half-life was approx 1 hour. The authors suggest that based on the expected use of valerian (sedative effects), dosing 30 minutes to 2 hours prior to bedtime would be appropriate based on the previously mentioned pharmacokinetics.

Adverse Effects and Toxicity

Reproductive System

There has been a theoretical concern with regard to pregnant women taking valerian because of possible effects on uterine contractions, but no problems were noted in three cases of intentional overdose with 2–5 g of valerian during weeks 3–10 of pregnancy. A mentally retarded child was born to a woman who overdosed on valerian 3 g, phenobarbital, glutethamide, amobarbital, and promethazine at 20 weeks of gestation, but this same woman delivered a mentally retarded child 2 years later after an overdose attempt with glutethamide, amobarbital, and promethazine.

V. officinalis (L.) was tested on rats and their offspring. A mixture, containing three valepotriates (80% dihydrovaltrate, 15% valtrate, and 5% acevaltrate), was orally administered to female rats for 30 days at 6-, 12-, and 24-mg/kg doses. Each dose was given to 10 rats, and placebo was given to another 10. No changes were noted in the average length of the estrus cycle, or the number of estrus phases during the 30-day observation period. The valepotriate mixture or placebo were also administered to 40 pregnant rats in the manner described previously from the day 1 through day 19 of pregnancy. Valerian did not increase the risk of fetotoxicity or external malformation. However, internal examination revealed a significant increase in the number of fetuses with retarded ossification with the 12- and 24-mg/kg doses. No developmental changes were detected in the offspring after treatment during pregnancy.

Cardiovascular System

Pharmacological investigations using a particular valepotriate fraction called Vpt2 extracted from the roots of *V. officinalis* (L.) have shown antiarrhythmic activity and ability to dilate coronary arteries in experimental animals. Moderate positive inotropic and a negative chronotropic effect were also observed. Vpt2 contains valtratum (50%), valeridine (25%), and valechlorin (3%), with trace amounts of acevaltrate, dihydrovaltratum, and epi-7-desacetyl-isovaltrate.

Alcoholic extracts of *V. officinalis* (L.) root (labeled V103 and V115) demonstrated hypotensive effects in rats, cats, and dogs. The V115 fraction showed greater potency and was extracted by a countercurrent distribution to yield three fractions. The first two fractions demonstrated hypotensive effects in rats, with the first fraction showing a hypotensive effect at 30 mg/kg. The third fraction produced hypertensive effects at a dose of 200 mg/kg. The authors noted that, apparently, with each succeeding extraction, less of the hypotensive principle was extracted. The hypotensive effect of the V103 fraction in rats was demonstrated at a dose of 500 mg/kg, and was hypothesized to act via a parasympathomimetic effect, blockade of the carotid sinus reflex, and CNS depression.

Cytotoxicity

The valepotriates valtrate/isovaltrate and dihydrovaltrate were isolated from *V. mexicana* and *V. wallichii*, respectively. The valepotriates tested were cytotoxic to granulocyte/macrophage colony-forming units (GM-CFCUs), lymphocytes, and erythrocyte colony-forming units (E-CFCUs). Valtrate was found to be a more potent inhibitor of GM-CFCUs (ID50 $\sim 3.7 \times 10^{-6}$ *M* vs $\sim 1.7 \times 10^{-5}$ *M*) and T-lymphocytes (ID50 $\sim 2.8 \times 10^{-6}$ *M* vs $\sim 3 \times 10^{-5}$ *M*) than dihydrovaltrate. Valtrate and dihydrovaltrate were similar in their activity against E-CFCUs (ID50 $\sim 2.3 \times 10^{-8}$ *M* vs $\sim 4.2 \times 10^{-8}$ *M*). Because pharmaceutical products containing valepotriates are orally administered, their cytotoxicity to gastrointestinal mucosal cells is of concern.

The effects of valtrate, dihydrovaltrate, and deoxido-dihydrovaltrate, valepotriates extracted from *V. wallichii* (DC.), on cultured rat hepatoma cells have been studied. Valtrate killed 50% of the cell population at a concentration of 5 μM, Deoxido-dihydrovaltrate and dihydrovaltae demonstrated this same toxicity at double the dose. Valtrate was also the most potent inhibitor of DNA and protein synthesis. These results suggest a mechanism by which valerian may cause hepatotoxicity.

Case Reports of Toxicity

Four cases of women who sustained liver damage after taking valerian-containing herbal medicines to relieve stress have been described. In addition, valerian was used by a patient who exhibited hepatotoxicity attributed to Chaparral.

Hospitals admitted 23 patients for treatment of intentional overdose with Sleep-Qik (75 mg of valerian dry extract, 0.25 mg of hyoscine hydrobromide 2 mg of cyproheptadine hydrochloride) between 1988 and 1991. Of these 23, 9 were men and 14 were women, with a mean age of 23.8 years (range 15–37 years). They were previously healthy, except for two patients with histories of psychiatric illness. The mean number of Sleep-Qik tablets taken per patient history was 33 (range 6–166), for an average of 2.5 g (range 0.5–12 g) of valerian. Four patients were asymptomatic. The other 19 patients reported drowsiness (n = 11), dilated pupils (n = 11), tachycardia (n = 6), nausea (n = 4), confusion (n = 3), urinary retention (n = 3), visual hallucination (n = 2), flushing (n = 2), dry mouth (n = 1), and dizziness (n = 1). Coingestants were alcohol (n = 2), a pesticide (n = 1), and Pansedan (n = 1) (*Passiflora* extract, *Viscum album* extract, *Uncariarhyncophylla* extract, and *Humulus lupulus*). One patient who was drowsy had also taken Panseden, and one who was confused had ingested alcohol.

Most patients received gastric lavage (n = 14), and one received syrup of ipecac. The patient who took 60 tablets of Sleep-Qik required ventilatory support. Liver function tests were performed on 12 patients approx 6–12 hours after ingestion with normal results. Drowsiness and confusion resolved within 24 hours. All patients recovered completely and were discharged after an average of 1.7 days (range 1–6 days). At an average of 43 months (range 27–65 months) after presentation, 10 patients were contacted by telephone. They had all remained well after discharge and none continued taking Sleep-Qik. Delayed onset of severe liver damage was ruled out via telephone interview, but subclinical disease could not be ruled out.

Subsequently, Chan reported on 24 cases of overdose of a product containing valerian dry extract 75 mg, hyoscine hydrobromide 0.25 mg, and cyproheptadine hydrochloride 2 mg. Six patients developed vomiting, and 15 underwent gastric lavage. Co-ingestants included alcohol (n = 10), cold products (n = 3), hypnotics (n = 2), unknown drugs (n = 2), and gasoline (n = 1). Symptoms were mainly CNS depression and anticholinergic symptoms. One patient required ventilatory support. Liver function tests were performed in 17 cases, and all were normal. Over the next 22–48 months postingestion, none of the patients returned to the hospital or clinic for any reason, suggesting that serious hepatotoxicity did not occur. The author points out that gastric lavage and spontaneous vomiting may have limited the amount of valerian absorbed in these patients, thus decreasing the risk of any delayed adverse effects. Other adverse effects attributed to overdose or chronic use of valerian include headaches, excitability, restlessness, uneasiness, blurred vision, and cardiac disturbances.

In another reported suicide attempt, an 18-year-old female ingested between 40 and 50, 470-mg capsules (18.8–23.5 g valerian) of 100% powered valerian root. The patient complained of fatigue, crampy abdominal pain, chest tightness, tremor of the hands and feet, and lightheadedness 30 minutes after ingestion. She presented to the emergency room 3 hours postingestion. Her vital signs were: blood pressure 111/64 mmHg, pulse 72 beats/minute, respiratory rate 14 breaths/minute, and temperature 37.6°C. Physical exam was unremark-able except for mydriasis (6 mm bilaterally). Electrocardiograph, complete blood count, and chemistry profile including liver function tests were normal. Toxicology screen was positive for marijuana, which she admitted using 2 weeks previously. She denied ingesting anything else. After two doses of activated charcoal, her symptoms resolved within 24 hours.

A withdrawal syndrome was described after abrupt discontinuation of valerian root extract in a 58-year-old man who had taken 530–2000 mg/dose five times daily as an anxiolytic and hypnotic for many years. Withdrawal symptoms included sinus tachycardia of up to 150 beats/minute, tremulousness, and delirium after recovery from general anesthesia (propofol, nitrous oxide, isoflurane, and thiopental) for open biopsy of a lung nodule. Medical history included coronary artery disease, hypertension, and congestive heart failure with an ejection fraction of 30–35%. Medications included isosorbide dinitrate, digoxin, furosemide, benazepril, aspirin, lovastatin, ibuprofen, potassium, zinc supplement, and vitamins.

The biopsy was complicated by multiple episodes of oxygen desaturation, and after extubation, the patient experienced tacycardia, oliguria, and increasing oxygen requirement. Despite naloxone administration, symptoms worsened. Swan-Ganz catheterization revealed high-output heart failure. At this time, interview with family members revealed the patient's long-standing valerian use. Because valerian withdrawal was suspected, midazolam 1 mg/hour (total dose 11 mg in 17 hours) was administered. Signs and symptoms improved, and stabilized by the third postoperative day. He was switched to lorazepam 1 mg/hour as needed (total dose 5 mg in 24 hours), and then to a tapering dose of clonazepam. He was discharged on postoperative day 7, and was stable at 5-month follow-up. Other causes of high-output heart failure were ruled out, but because of the patient's multiple medical problems, postsurgical status, and medications administered, the cause of the patient's symptoms is unclear. The authors of this case report note that valerian has been reported to attenuate benzodiazepine withdrawal in rats.

Interactions

Two alcoholic valerian extracts were found to potentiate pentobarbital sleeping time in mice, and Valdispert, an aqueous extract prepared from *V. officinalis* (L.), increased the thiopental sleeping time in a dose-dependent manner in rats. Based on these animal studies, in vitro studies of valerian's effect on GABAnergic transmission, as well as the case series reported by Chan and colleagues, valerian would be expected to have at least an additive effect with barbiturates, alcohol, benzodiazepines, and other CNS depressants. Valerian may have the potential to increase the level of drugs metabolized by the cytochrome P-450 3A4 (CYP3A4) enzyme. In vitro studies have found that valerian may have an inhibitory effect on CYP3A4. A clinical research study suggested that low to moderate doses of valerian did not significantly inhibit CYP3A4, although taking valerian extract 1000 mg/day increased alprazolam levels by 19%. Therefore, it may be wise to use valerian cautiously in patients taking medications that are CYP3A4 substrates such as lovastatin, ketoconazole, itraconazole, fexofenadine, alprazolam, triazolam, and various chemotherapeutic agents.

Reproduction

No information is available concerning any potential effects of valerian on female reproductive function. However, Mkrtchyan and colleagues reported that valerian had no effect on human male sterility.

Regulatory Status

Valerian was included as an official drug in the US Pharmacopeia until 1936 and in the National Formulary until 1946. Currently, the USP advisory panel does not recommend valerian's use owing to lack of adequate scientific evidence and conflicting study results. They encourage further research. Valerian is generally recognized as safe as a food and beverage flavoring by the FDA. The German Commission Monograph E has approved valerian as a sleep-promoting and calmative agent to be used in the treatment of unrest and sleep disturbances caused by anxiety. In Australia, valerian is acceptable as an active ingredient in the "listed products" category of the Therapeutic Goods Administration. In Belgium, subterranean parts, powder extract, and tincture are allowed for use as traditional tranquilizers. The Health Protection Branch of Health Canada allows products containing valerian as a single agent in the form of crude dried root in tablets, capsules, powders, extracts, tinctures, drops, or tea bags intended for use as sleeping aids and sedatives.

16

VITEX AGNUS-CASTUS

Vitex agnus-castus is a botanical plant that has the following National Oceanographic Data Center Taxonomic Code: Kingdom, Plantae; Phylum, Tracheobionta; Class, Magnoliopsida; Order, Lamiales; Family, Verbenaceae; Genus, *Vitex* L.; Species, *Vitex agnus-castus* L. The genus name *Vitex* is a Latin derivation for plaiting or weaving. The species name *agnus-castus* combines two Latin word origins: "*agnus*," which means lamb, and "*castitas*," which means chastity. *V. agnus-castus* is a large deciduous shrub, native to Mediterranean countries and central Asia, and is also used in America as an ornamental plant. *V. agnus-castus* has long, finger-shaped leaves and displays fragrant blue-violet flowers in midsummer. Its fruit is a very dark-purple berry that is yellowish inside, resembles a peppercorn, and has an aromatic odor. Upon ripening, the berry is picked and allowed to dry. The twigs of this shrub are very flexible and were used for furniture in ancient times.

References to *V. agnus-castus* go back more than 2000 years, describing it as a healing herb. Ancient Egyptians, Greeks, and Romans used it for a variety of health problems. In 400 BCE, Hippocrates recommended chaste tree for injuries and inflammation. Four centuries later, Greek botanist Dioscorides recommended *V. agnus-castus* specifically for inflammation of the womb and lactation. Use of *V. agnus-castus* continued into the Middle Ages, where folklore persists that medieval monks chewed *V. agnus-castus* tree parts to maintain their celibacy, used the dried berries in their food, or placed the berries in the pockets of their robes in order to reduce sexual desire; thus, the synonym of Monk's pepper. Use of *V. agnus-castus* has persisted to modern times. Though its use was initially concentrated in the Mediterranean area, its popularity has increased in England and America since the mid-1900s.

Traditional medicinal uses of *V. agnus-castus* lie predominantly around the oral ingestion of the shrub's fruit; however, other plant parts such as leaves and flowers have been used in some preparations. The dry or liquid extract of, or oils from, the berry have been used for a variety of symptoms, most commonly related to the female reproductive system. Other uses include the treatment of hangovers, flatulence, fevers, benign prostatic hyperplasia, nervousness, dementia, rheumatic conditions, colds, dyspepsia, spleen disorders, constipation, and promoting urination. Traditional topical medicinal uses of *V. agnus-castus* include acne, body inflammation, and insect bites and stings. Use of *V. agnus-castus* is not commonly employed in traditional Chinese medicine or traditional Indian medicine (Ayurveda); however, other *Vitex* species (*negundo*, *trifoliata*) are used in these therapies.

CURRENT PROMOTED USES

Current promoted uses of *V. agnus-castus* relate to treatment of disorders of the female reproductive system such as short menstrual cycles, *premenstrual syndrome* (PMS), and breast swelling and pain (mastodynia/ mastalgia). The Commission E has approved the use of *V. agnus-castus* for irregularities of the menstrual cycle, premenstrual complaints, and mastalgia. Recent randomized, placebo-controlled studies have been conducted and found *V. agnus-castus* to be effective and well-tolerated for the relief of PMS symptoms, especially the physical symptoms of breast tenderness/fullness, edema, and headache. *V. agnus-castus* is not considered effective for PMS-related symptoms of abdominal bloating, craving sweets, sweating, palpitations, or dizziness.

V. agnus-castus is not used in foods and is not recommended for use in children, adolescents, pregnant women, or women who are breast- feeding. *V. agnus-castus* should be avoided in patients receiving exogenous sex hormones, including oral contraceptives, as *V. agnus-castus* may counteract the effectiveness of birth control pills by its effect on prolactin.

Sources and Chemical Composition

V. agnus-castus (L.), Agnolyt, arbre chaste, chaste berry, chasteberry, chaste tree, chaste tree fruit, chastetree, chastetree berry, Cloister Pepper, *Fructus Agni Casti*, Fruit de Gattilier, Gattilier, Hemp Tree, Keuschlamm, Mönchspfeffer, Monk's Pepper, *V. agnus castus*, *V. agnus castus fructus*, Vitex. The major constituents of *V. agnus-castus* include the following. Flavonoids: flavonol (kaempferol, quercetagetin) derivatives, the major constituent being casticin. Additional flavonoids found include penduletin, orientin, chrysophanol D, and apigenin. Water-soluble flavones: vitexin and isovitexin. Alkaloids: viticin. Diterpenes: rotundifuran (labdane-type); vitexilactone; 6-β,7-β-diacetoxy-13-hydroxy-labda-8,14-diene; 8,13-dihydroxy-14-labden; X-hydroxy-y-keto-15,16-epoxy-13, 14-labdadien;X-acetonxy-13-hydroxylabda-y,14-dien; cleroda-x,14-dien-13-ol; cleroda-x,y, 14-trien- 13-ol. Iridoid glycosides: In the leaf: 0.3% aucubin, 0.6% agnuside (the *p*-hydroxybenzoyl derivative of aucubin), and 0.07% unidentified glycosides. In the flowering stem (6'-O-foliamenthoyl-mussaenosidic acid [agnucastoside A], 6'O (6,7- dihydrofoliamenthoyl) mussaenosidic acid [agnucastoside B], and 7-O-trans-*p*-coumaroyl-'-O-trans-caffeoyl-8-epiloganic acid [agnucastoside C], aucubin, agnuside, mussaenosidic acid, 62-O--hydroxybenzoylmussaenosidic acid, and phenylbutanone glucoside [myzodendrone]. Essential oil of leaves and flowers: monoterpenes (major chemicals found: limonene, cineole, sabinene, and α-terpineol, linalool, citronellol, camphene, myrcene) and sesquiterpenes (major chemicals found: β-caryophyllene, -gurjunene, cuparene, and globulol). Depending on the maturity of the fruits used and the distillation processes, the components of the essential oil can vary greatly. Other constituents: fatty acids (including stearic, oleic, linoleic, and palmitic acids), amino acids (glycine, alanine, valine, leucine), castine (a bitter principle), vitamin C and carotene, and trace amounts of hormones from leaves and flowers (progesterone and 17 α-hydroxyprogesterone). Main components of the volatile oil 0.5%: mixtures of monoterpenes and sesquiterpenes, cineol, and pinene.

Products Available

V. agnus-castus is available as bulk berries, bulk powder, crushed fresh or dried berry, tea (loose or in tea bags), extract, tonic, elixir, or tincture. Chasteberry products may consist of the herb alone or in combination with other herbs and vitamins. Topically, it is used primarily as the essential oil, mixed in combination with other products in cream form.

A proprietary preparation (Agnolyt) containing an alcoholic extract of *V. agnus-castus* (0.2% w/v) has been available in Germany since the 1950s. Other products using *V. agnus-castus* synonyms in their nomenclature are available by a myriad of manufacturers. Some single-entity brand names include Agnofem, Agno-Sabona, Agnucaston, Agnufemil, Agnuside, Agnumens, Agnurell, Antimast N, Antimast N, Gynocastus, Mastodynon, and Vitex Extract. Many combination products also contain *V. agnus-castus* and include, but are not limited to, the following: Herbal Premens, Herbal Support For Women Over 45, Dong Quai Complex, Emoton, Feminine Herbal Complex (FM), Menosan, Mulimen,

Phytoestrin, Virilis-Gastreu SR41, Femisana, Lifesystem Herbal Formula 4 Women's Formula (FM), PMT Complex (FM), Presselin Dysmen Olin 3 N (FM), Women's Formula Herbal Formula 3 (FM), and others. The amount of *V. agnus-castus* contained in oral tablets or capsules varies depending on whether the product contains crushed fruit or extract of the berry. For example, tablet or capsule formulations have included the following: Chaste Berry 450 mg/Chase Berry Extract 50 mg, Chastetree fruit 500 mg, Chaste Berry Dried Extract 1.6–3.0 mg corresponding to 20 mg *Vitex*, Chaste Tree Berry Extract (0.5% agnuside) 225 mg. Commercial extract forms of chasteberry are usually standardized to contain 6% agnuside constituent. Chasteberry liquid extract may or may not contain alcohol.

Dosage

Generally, the Expanded Commission E Monographs reports the following total daily dosages:

- 30 to 40 mg of dry or fluid extracts of crushed fruit
- 0.03 to 0.04 mL of fluid extract 1:1 (g/mL), 50–70% alcohol (v/v)
- 0.15 to 0.2 mL of tincture 1:5 (g/mL), 50–70% alcohol (v/v)
- 2.6 to 4.2 mg of dry native extract (9.5–11.5:1 (w/w)

Other references have reported total daily dosages ranging from 20 to 1800 mg/day of crude *V. agnus-castus* extracts. *V. agnus-castus* is considered safe when used orally and appropriately.

Pharmacological/Toxicological Effects

Prolactin Secretion

Evidence of varying levels of discrimination exists that demonstrate *V. agnus-castus* inhibits the secretion of prolactin by the pituitary gland. In a randomized, placebo-controlled, double-blind study, Milewicz et al. examined whether *V. agnus-castus* affected elevated pituitary prolactin reserve. Participants were 52 women with luteal phase defects caused by latent hyperprolactinemia. Intervention was *V. agnus-castus* 20 mg daily or placebo, for 3 months. Only 37 women (20 = placebo, 17 = *V. agnus-castus*) completed the study. Outcome measures were pre- and posthormonal analysis (blood draws taken on days 5–8 and day 20 of menstrual cycle) 1 month prior to treatment and after 3 months of treatment and latent hyperprolactinemia analysis (monitoring prolactin release 15 and 30 minutes after intravenous injection of 200 μg *thyrotropin-releasing hormone* (TRH). Results from this study showed that compared to preintervention, the *V. agnu-scastus* group had statistically significant reduced prolactin release after 3 months, whereas the control group did not. The study's information came from an English abstract of a German publication. Information about inclusion/exclusion criteria, study specifics, study funding, or author disclosures were not available.

In an open and intraindividual comparison study, Merz et al. conducted a clinical study of tolerance and prolactin secretion of *V. agnus-castus* using 20 healthy male subjects between the ages of 18 and 40 years. Placebo and three doses of *V. agnus-castus* (total daily dosages of 120, 240, and 480 mg were divided into 8-hour administration times) were given in an increasing sequence. Prolactin concentration profile after TRH stimulation was assessed by determining the maximum concentrations (C_{max}) and the area under the curve over a period of one hour ($AUC_{0\text{-}1h}$). These procedures were identical in all four study phases. Results for the $AUC_{0\text{-}24h}$ showed that as daily doses increased, prolactin levels decreased ([$AUC_{0\text{-}24h}$ {μIU · hour}/μΛ ± standard deviation]; placebo: 6182 ± 1827; 120 mg: 6874 ± 1790; 240 mg: 5750 ± 1594; 480 mg: 5998 ± 1664), with statistically significant findings for the 120-mg dosage only.

Wuttke reported in a 1996 abstract the results of experiments demonstrating that 3 months of *V. agnus-castus* therapy (double-blind clinical study vs placebo) significantly reduced basal prolactin levels in patients. However, details of the experiments and study subjects were not outlined or referenced.

Follicle-Stimulating Hormone, Luteinizing Hormone

There are a limited number of human studies regarding how *V. agnus-castus* directly effects *luteinizing hormone* (LH) or follicle-stimulating hormone (FSH). In a 1994 case report by Cahill et al., a 32-year-old woman undergoing unstimulated in vitro fertilization (IVF) treatment took *V. agnus-castus* for one cycle without consulting her physician. During this cycle, she had symptoms of mild ovarian hyperstimulation in the luteal phase. Her FSH and LH levels prior to day 13, the predicted day of LH surge in the IVF cycle, were reviewed and found to be much higher than normal. Reviewing five other cycles of this patient and finding normal pituitary gonadotrophin file and normal follicular ovarian responses, the authors suggest that *V. agnus-castus* was the causative agent.

In the 1996 study by Merz et al. that primarily examined prolactin secretion in male subjects, initial hormone levels of FSH and LH were measured on days 1 and 13 (beginning and near-end of placebo phase) and from blood samples taken during the prolactin secretion profiling. The authors state that *V. agnus-castus* had no effect on FSH or LH levels, but no other details were provided.

Progesterone/Testosterone Synthesis

In a randomized, placebo-controlled, double-blind study, Milewicz et al. examined the effect of *V. agnus-castus* on prolactin reserve and luteal phase progesterone synthesis in 52 women. The intervention was *V. agnus-astus* 20 mg daily or placebo, for 3 months. Results from the 37 women (20 = placebo, 17 = *agnus-castus*) who completed the study showed that compared to preintervention, the *V. agnus-castus group* had statistically significant increases in luteal phase progesterone synthesis. The study information came from a German publication with an English abstract. Information about inclusion/exclusion criteria, study specifics, study funding, or author disclosures were not available.

In the 1996 study by Merz et al. that primarily examined prolactin secretion in male subjects, initial hormone level of testosterone was measured on days 1 and 13 (beginning and near-end of placebo phase), and from blood samples taken during the prolactin secretion profiling. The authors state that *V. agnus-castus* had no effect on testosterone levels, but no other details were provided.

Infertility

Gerhard et al. studied the influence of a commercially available preparation of *V. agnus-castus* on infertility. Using a randomized, placebo-controlled, double-blind design, 96 women with fertility disorders (31 with luteal insufficiency; 38 with secondary amenorrhea; 27 with idiopathic infertility) received either *V. agnus-castus* or placebo twice a day for 3 months. The dose of *V. agnus-castus* was 30 drops of Mastodynon twice a day (*agnus-castus* or casticin-standardization not mentioned). The outcome measures were: (i) pregnancy or spontaneous menstruation for women with secondary amenorrhea, and (ii) pregnancy or improved luteal hormone levels in women with luteal insufficiency or idiopathic infertility. A total of 66 women were suitable for evaluation. No differences were noted between the placebo and *V. agnus-castus* groups with respect to effect.

PMS and Menopausal Symptoms

In a 1997 multicenter, randomized, double-blind, controlled trial, Lauritzen et al. examined the efficacy and tolerability of a commercially available capsule formulation of *V. agnus-castus* (Agnolyt) compared with pyridoxine in women with PMS. Inclusion criteria were females aged 18 to 45 years, PMS symptoms in luteal phase of menstrual cycle, PMS symptoms with each cycle, PMS symptoms affecting quality of life, and no drug therapy for PMS in 3 months preceding the study. Of 175 participants, 85 were in the *V. agnus-castus* group (took one capsule twice a day, with one capsule containing 3.5 to 4.2 mg of *V. agnus-castus*, the second capsule containing placebo), and 90 were in the pyridoxine group (days 1–15, took one capsule twice a day, each capsule containing placebo; days 16–35, took one capsule twice a day, each capsule containing 100 mg of pyridoxine). Women in both treatment groups had equal reductions in PMS scores (*V. agnus-castus*: 15.2 to 5.1; pyridoxine: 11.9 to 5.1; $p = 0.37$), suggesting no differences in effect.

In 2000, Loch et al. conducted an open label, uncontrolled study examining the efficacy and safety of a new oral *V. agnus-castus* treatment for PMS complaints. Suffering from PMS was the only inclusion criterion and pregnancy was the only exclusion criterion. A questionnaire on mental and somatic PMS symptoms was completed by 857 gynecologists after interviewing 1634 females at the start of Femicur therapy (20 mg daily), and after a period of three menstrual cycles under therapy. Physicians reported that 42% of women reported that they had no more PMS symptoms, 51% showed a decrease in symptoms ($p < 0.001$), and 1% had an increase in number of symptoms. After 3 months of treatment, both psychic and somatic complaints were dramatically lowered. Although 30% of the women still complained about mastodynia after *V. agnus-castus* treatment, most reported complaints of lower intensity. Physicians described the patients' tolerance of this *V. agnus-castus* product as good or very good in 94% of women. Although one of the authors works for the pharmaceutical company that makes Femicur, the article did not contain funding disclosure statements.

In 2000, Berger et al., using a prospective, multicenter trial design, examined the efficacy of an oral, casticin-standardized *V. agnus-castus* therapy on 43 women diagnosed with PMS. Treatment phases consisted of baseline (two cycles, pretreatment), treatment (three cycles), posttreatment (three cycles, no treatment). The dose was 20 mg, but no placebo control was included. At the end of the trial, Moos' menstrual distress questionnaire (MMDQ) scores were reduced by 43% compared with start (statistically significant, $p < 0.001$), but that improvement decreased gradually in the post-treatment phase. At the end of the posttreatment phase, patients had improved compared to the start of therapy ($p < 0.001$) and for up to three cycles thereafter. A group of 20 women had baseline MMDQ scores that were reduced by at least 50% at the end of treatment phase. *Visual analogue scale* (VAS) and global efficacy scales showed similar findings ($p < 0.001$ and global efficacy rated excellent by 38 women). Areas of improvement included symptoms related to pain, behavior, negativity, and fluid retention. The most frequent adverse events were acne, headaches, and menstrual spotting.

In 2001, using a prospective, randomized, double-blind, placebo-controlled, parallel-group comparison design, Schellenberg studied the efficacy and tolerability of *V. agnus-castus* extract on PMS. Participants were female outpatients, 18 years of age or older, of six general medicine clinics and had a PMS diagnosis according to the *Diagnostic and Statistical Manual of Mental Disorders*. Dose of *V. agnus-castus* was 20 mg daily for 3 months. Results showed that the group receiving *V. agnus-castus* had significant improvements ($p < 0.001$) in all symptoms except bloating compared to the placebo group. Sensitivity analyses removing women taking contraceptives did not alter results. Tolerability was good with acne, itching, and mid-cycle bleeding as the adverse events noted.

An uncontrolled study in 2002 by Lucks examined the effects of 3-month dermal application of *V. agnus-castus* essential oil (oil distilled at some point in the shrubs' development of the fruit but while some leaves were still on the plant) on menopausal and perimenopausal symptoms. A 1.5% solution of the essential oil was incorporated in a bland cream or lotion and applied once a day, 5 to 7 days/week, for 3 months. Descriptive outcome measures were self-report via a survey of symptomatic relief (major, moderate, mild, none, worse) and side effects. A total of 33% of women reported major improvement in symptoms, with the most often area of improvement being hot flashes/night sweats. Both improvement and worsening occurred in the areas of emotions and menstruation flow. Subjects who were also on progesterone supplementation reported breakthrough bleeding.

Mastodynia

In a 1987, Kubista et al. reported results from a placebo-controlled study comparing the effects of lynestrenol, *V. agnus-castus* (Mastodynon), and placebo therapy in women with severe mastopathy with cyclic mastalgia. More women in the lynestrenol and *V. agnus-castus* groups than placebo group reported good relief of PMS symptoms (82, 54, 37%, respectively).

In 1998, Halaska and colleagues examined the tolerability and efficacy of *V. agnus-castus* extract on mastodynia/mastalgia (breast pain, breast tenderness). The study was a double-blind, placebo-controlled, parallel-group (50 women each) design. Length of treatment (*V. agnus-castus* [60 drops daily dose] or placebo) was 3 months. Efficacy was determined using a VAS. Results of study showed that the intensity of mastodynia diminished more quickly in the *V. agnus-castus* group with low incidence of side effects.

Luteal Phase Length

In the 1993 randomized, placebo-controlled, double-blind study where Milewicz et al. examined the effect of *V. agnus-castus* on pituitary prolactin reserve, they also examined luteal phase length. Of the 37 women (20 = placebo, 17 = *V. agnus-castus*) who completed the study (1 month prior to, and 3 months treatment), the shortened luteal phases of the *agnus-castus* group became normal. The study information came from a German publication with an English abstract. Information about inclusion/exclusion criteria and study specifics were not available.

Premenstrual Dysphoric Disorder

Premenstrual dysphoric disorder (PMDD) is characterized by markedly depressed mood, anxiety, affective lability, and decreased interest in daily activities during the last week of luteal phase in menstrual cycles of the last year. In 2002, Atmaca et al. conducted an 8-week, randomized, single-blind, rater-blinded, prospective- and parallel-group, flexible-dosing trial to compare the efficacy of fluoxetine with *V. agnus-castus* for the treatment of PMDD in 42 females. Both fluoxetine and *V. agnus-castus* had dose ranges from 20 to 40 mg. Outcome measures included the Penn daily symptom report, Hamilton depression rating scale, clinical global impression (CGI)-severity of illness scale, and CGI-improvement scale. Both drugs were well tolerated. No statistically significant differences between groups were found. The authors concluded that fluoxetine was more effective (a decrease of more than 50% in rating symptoms) for psychological symptoms (depression, irritability, insomnia, nervousness), whereas *V. agnus-castus* helped with physical symptoms (irritability, breast tenderness, swelling, cramps). Lack of placebo-control and short duration of treatment were significant limitations.

Toxicological Effects

No systematic toxicological studies have been conducted, according to the Expanded Commission E Mongraphs.

Adverse Effects and Toxicity

Throughout years of use, *V. agnus-castus* has shown only mild adverse effects. Pruritus, rash (unspecified), urticaria, increased menstrual blood flow, persistent headaches, and gastrointestinal discomfort have been reported. Few adverse events related to chasteberry have been reported to the Food and Drug Administration.

Case Reports of Toxicity Caused by Commercially Available Products

An extensive search of all standard references, as well as reports of studies in humans, shows that there have been no case reports of toxic exposure to *V. agnus-castus* use. However, one case of nocturnal seizures, possibly attributed to *V. agnus-castus,* has been reported. The patient was taking concomitantly black cohosh root (*Cimicifuga racemosa*), *V. agnus-castus*, and evening primrose as well. Thus, attribution of effect to a specific agent was not possible. In animals, an adverse influence on nursing (lactation) performance has been observed; *V. agnus-castus* could potentially interfere with proper lactation.

Interactions

According to the German Commission E Monographs, drug interactions with *V. agnus-castus* are unknown. However, with animal experiments showing evidence of a "*dopaminergic effect*," it is generally recommended that the effect of *V. agnus-castus* can be diminished in cases when there is concurrent ingestion of dopamine-receptor antagonists (e.g., haloperidol). Similarly, because *V. agnus-castus* inhibits the secretion of prolactin via a dopamine-agonist action, drug interactions may occur with the D_2 family of dopamine-receptor agonists (bromocriptine, pergolide, pramipexole, ropinirole, cabergoline).

Some liquid formulations contain large percentages of alcohol (≥50% vol); health risks from ethanol may exist, and in certain populations, use of the dried extract formulations instead would be advisable.

Reproduction

Although there are no known case reports of toxicity in human reproduction, because of possible endocrine effects, *V. agnus-castus* could disrupt fetal development or proper gestation. A case of ovarian hyperstimulation syndrome and multiple follicular development resulting in no pregnancy occurred in a woman who took *V. agnus-castus* prior to one of her IVF protocol cycles. Tests showed that her serum gonadotropin and hormone evels were out of the desired range.

Regulatory Status

V. agnus-castus is available for use without a prescription in all Member States of the European Union and the United States. In the United States, *V. agnus-castus* is categorized as a dietary supplement. Throughout the world, *V. agnus-castus* is available through pharmacies, health-food shops, mail order companies, supermarkets, and department stores.

17

MEDICINAL PLANTS

Medicinal plants were known to the early civilization. As a matter of fact the history of the durg plants is as old as the hisotory of these civilizations. The Chines have used drug plants quite earlier in 5,000 to 4,000 B.C. The Assyrians, Babylonians, Herbrews and Egyptians knew many drug plants in about 1600 B.C. The works of Greeks, viz., Aristotle (384-322 B.C.), Hippocrates (460-370 B.C.), Pythagoras and Theophrastus (370-287 B.C.) have numerous references of many of the present day drugs. In 77 B.C., a Roma physician Dioscordies wrote 'De Materia Medicia' which described the nature and properties of all the 500 medicinal plants known at that time. His book was was considered to be the most authentic work on medicinal plants for the next 16 centuries or so. There was no advancement in the knowledge of durg plants during the Dark Ages.

After the introduction of printing in Europe in the fifteenth century many persons published 'herbalts' which contained many true and and false informations. Some people advanced the 'Doctrine of Signs of Signatures' which meant that the appearance of a plant or its organs indicated its utility, the sign being placed there by the Creator. Superstition about one such plant Mandrake (*Mandragora officinarum*) to be useful in

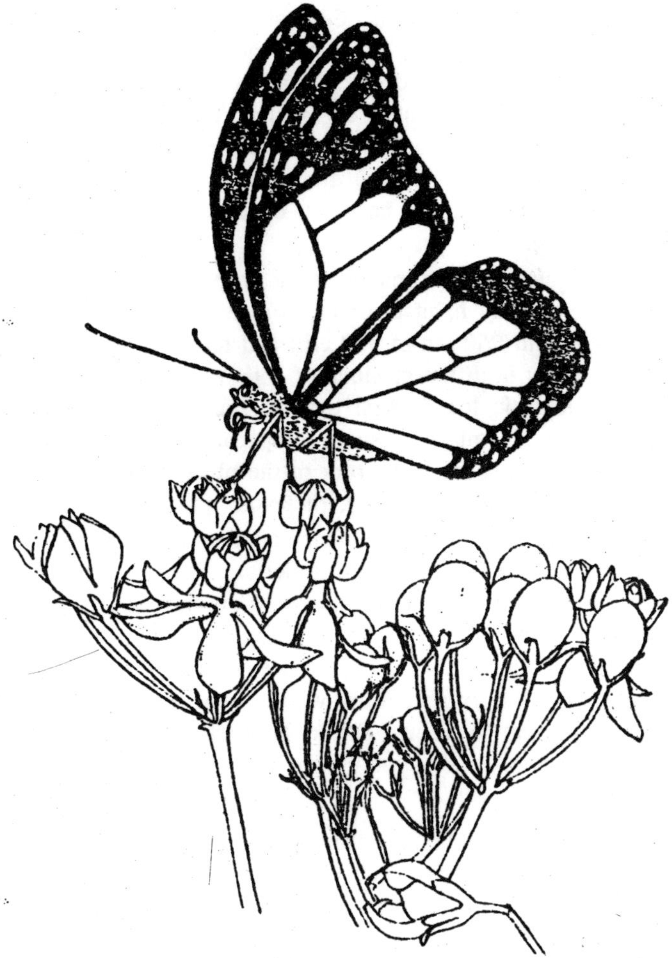

Fig. 17.1. Glycosides ingested by the caterpillar of this butterfly while feeding on milkweed are stored in the body and after metamorphosis, appear in the adult monarch's body.

treatment of human disease as due to its human body like appearance. In the present times medicinal science has paid great attention to the study of drug plants. The branch of medical science which deals with the drug plant is called *pharmoacognosy*, whereas the study of the action of drugs is called *pharmacology*. Usually the morphology of drug yielding plant is the main basis of drugs' classification.

DRUGS OBTAINED FROM ROOTS

Rauwolfia

The drug Rauwolfia is obtained from the roots of *Rauwolfia serpentina* of *Apocynaceae*. It is native of India. The genus is found growing in the tropical regions of Asia, Africa and America. The Asian countries are India, Bangla Desh, Sri Lanka, Burma, Malaysia, Thailand and Indonesia. Five species of *Rauwolfia* grow in India. *R. Serpentina*, the most important of the five species is found in the sub-Himalayan tract from Punjab through Nepal, Sikkim, Bhutan to Assam, eastern and western ghats, Central India and the Andamans. The plant is grown commercially in Uttar Pradesh, Bihar, Orissa, West Bengal, Assam, Andhra Pradesh, Tamil Nadu, Karnataka, Keralan and Maharashtra. The plant is an erect perennial shrub. It is of a height of ½ ft. to 1½ ft. and may sometimes attain a height of 3 ft. The plant is evergreen. Leaves are in whorls of three. Flowers are small white or pink and are borne in cyme in large number. The fruit is a drupe.

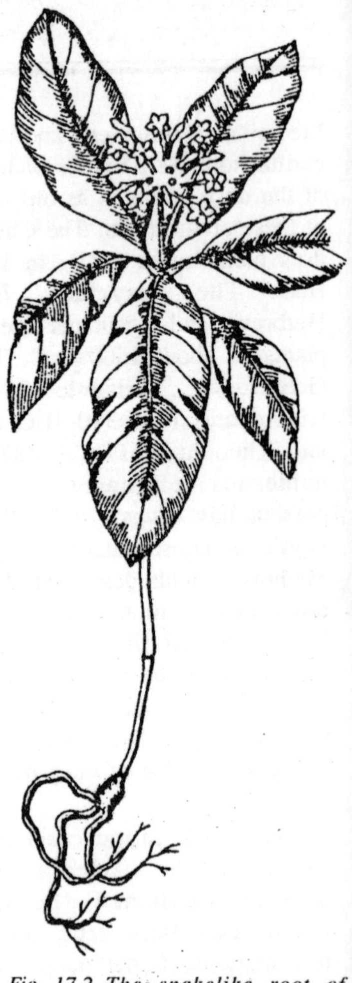

Hot and humid climates of the tropics is best suited for its growth. It prefers shady habitats of the forests. It grows well in areas of very high rainfall (250 cm to 500 cm) and temperature range of 10 to 38°C. It can grow in different kinds of soils ranging from sandy alluvial loam to red lateritic loam. Well drained humus rich clayey soil is best for its growth. The plant is usually propagated by means of seeds. Rauwolfia drug is obtained from the root of the plant. The bark of the roots yields several alkaloids (about 80), the most important of which is *reserpine*.

Reserpine is extracted from another two species—*R. vomitoria* of Africa and *R. tetraphylla* of America. Reserpine is of great medicinal use in treatment of violent kinds of insanity and high blood pressure. It acts as a sedative and depressant in hypertension and chronic psychoses. It is also used for treatment of insect bites, fevers and dysentery. Reserpine is now widely used by research workers to study physiological systems. Other important alkaloids are *deserpidine*, *rescinnamine*, *reserpinine*, *serpentine*, *serpentinine*, *ajmaline*, etc.

Fig. 17.2. The snakelike root of Rauwalfia contains an alkaloid used in the treatment of hypertension and schizophrenia.

Aconite

The drug is obtained from the tuberous roots of *Aconitum napellus* of the *Ranunculaceae*. The plant is a perennial herb. The plant is also known as monk's hood or wolfbane. It is indigenous to the mountains of Europe (Alps, Pyrenees, etc.and western Asia.) It is also cultivated as an ornamental plant is most of the countries. Several alkaloids are obtained from the roots. Aconite, the most important alkaloid, is poisonous. Aconite is usually used externally for the treatment of neuralgia and rheumatism. Internally it is taken to relieve pain and fever.

Drugs obtained from Barks

Quinine

Quinine is obtained from the bark of several species of *Cinchona* of the *Rubiaceae*. The plant is native to Andean highlands of tropical America. It still grows in Peru and Bolivia at altitudes of 3,000 feet to 9,000 feet. The medicinal properties of the bark of the tree were discovered in 1638 when it cured the malarial fever of the wife of the Viceroy of Peru, the Countess of Cinchon. She carried it to Spain in 1639. The plant was named *Cinchona* by Linnaeus in the eighteenth century after her name.

The bark of the plant called Jesuit's bark or Peruvian bark and it has got the attention of the people throughout the world. From mid-seventeenth to the mid-nineteenth century the wild trees in south America were ruthlessly cut down to get the bark. The British and the Dutch secured the seeds from South America and started large plantations in India and Java respectively. The Britishers had collected seeds from *Cinchona succirubra*. The Dutch plantations of Java were established from the seeds of *Cinchona ledgeriana* named after a British resident of Bolivia, Charles Ledger, who had collected the seeds. About 90 percent of the world export trade in quinine is carried on by Java. Other species of Cinchona used for the drug are *C. officinalis* and *C. calisaya*. The tea plantation has replaced the plant in Sri Lanka because the drug has quite uneconomic price.

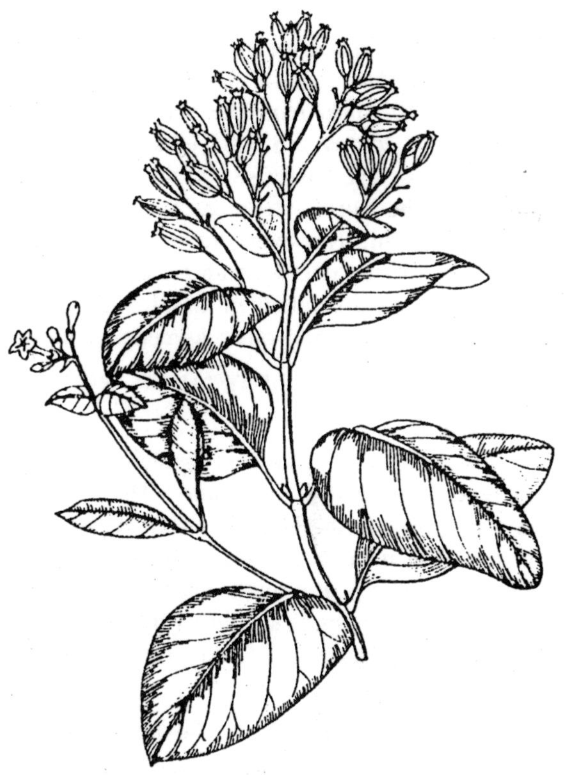

Fig. 17.3. A flowering and fruiting branch of Cinchona officinalis, of which yields quinine, a remedy for malaria.

The other *Cinchona*-growing regions are Burma and Tanganyika (Tanzania). *Cincona* plant is a fairly large tree and may attain a height of fifty feet or more. Depending upon the species of plant, the bark covering the stem can be light coloured, pale, brown or dark brown. The leaves are opposite. Yellow or pink coloured flowers are borne in terminal panicles. They are produed from the third or fourth year of growth. Cross pollination takes place. The plants are limited in distribution. They grow in the topics between 10° north and 20° south of the Equator at altitudes more than 1,000 feet. They grow well in regions of very high temperature and high rainfall (60 inches or more). Good porous soils are good for their growth.

Cinchona is propagated by seeds. Mixing of characters and consequent variation in plant is attained as a result of natural hybridization. It is now usually propagated by means of graftings and cuttings. The trees are usually felled down after they are 10 years old since the bark develops maximum alkaloid content by that time. The bark is removed from the stems, branches and roots and is slowly dried at not very high temperature. The dried bark is sent to the factory where the alkaloids are extracted by solvent extraction.

Cinchona bark has four important alkaloids (totaquine) which are quinine, quinidine, cinchonine and cinchonidine. Quinine is the most important of the alkaloides. *C. ledgeriana* has the maximum percentage of quinine in relation to the other alkaloids. Quinine is a antimalarial drug and is very bitter and white granular in appearance. It is also useful as a tonic and anti-septic. Some synthetic antimalarial drugs are also manufactured these days.

Drugs obtained from Stems

Ephedrine

The drug ephedrine is an alkaloid. It is obtained from several species of *Ephedra* of the *Gnetaceae*. Two important species are *E. sinica* and *E. equisetina*. The plant is native of Asia. In China it has been in use for over 5,000 years. The plant is leafless shrub with green stems. The plant is woody and xerophytic and grows in arid regions of the world. The plant is dioecious. Entire plant is the source of the alkoloid. However, its importance as a source of ephedrine has been reduced due to synthetic manufacture of the drug. The drug is used in the treatment of nasal and bronchial congestion, colds, asthma, hay fever and other ailments. It also acts as a stimulant.

Drugs obtained from Leaves

Eucalyptus

Eucalyptus oil is used in medicine. It is obtained from the leaves of several species of *Eucalyptus*. The plant is native to Australia. It is also grown in the Mediterranean region. U. S. A. and many other places. The plant is a tall tree which attains a height of 200 to 300 feet. The leaves are scythe-shaped in *E. globulus* and of different shapes in other species. Eucalyptus oil is used in the treatment of cold, malaria, nose and throat troubles and fevers.

Cocaine

Cocaine obtained from the leaves of a South American plant, *Erythroxylon coca* of the *Erythroxyllaceae*. The plant is indigenous to the Andean regions of Peru and Bolivia. The plant is now widely cultivated in the tropical regions of South America, Java, Sri Lanka and Taiwan (Formosa). The plant grows are higher altitudes. The plant is a small, much branched shrub or tree. Small, sessile, elliptical leaves are alternately arranged. The flowers are borne is small axillary groups. The leaves are harvested by hand when the trees are two to three years old. The leaves are picked three or four times in a year. Dried leaves are immediately exported in boxes. The alkaloid cocaine ($C_{17}H_{21}O_4N$) is ususlly extracted in the importing countries by solvent process. The drug is chiefly used as a local anesthetic. It is also used as a tonic for the digestive and nervous symptoms. The leaves are chewed by the natives of South America for stimulating physical and mental activities. The coca is 'de-alkaoidized' in U. S. A. to be used as 'cola' flavourings.

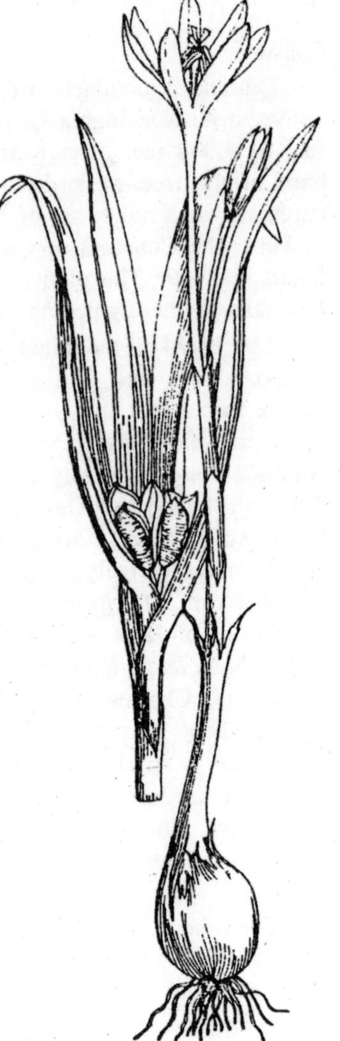

Fig. 17.4. The autumn crocus yields colchicine used to treat gout and cell malignancies.

Digitalis

Digitalis is obtained from the dried leaves of foxglove (*Digitalis purpurea*) of the *Scrophulairceae*. The plant is a native of Southern and Central Europe, which continues to be its chief grower. However it is grown as beautiful ornamental plant in other parts of world. The plant is a pubescent biennial or pernnial herb. The plant stem can attain a height of 5 feet but leaves are crowded in lower portion of stem. The stem bears purplish flowers in a terminal spike. The leaves are dried in shaded conditions. The active glycosides are extracted fron the dried leaves by solvent (alcohol) process. The glycosides are digitoxin, digitaline and digitalein and digiton. They are very important as stimulants of heart and as diuretics. Digitalis tone up the circulatory system by inducing the heart to make powerful and complete contraction.

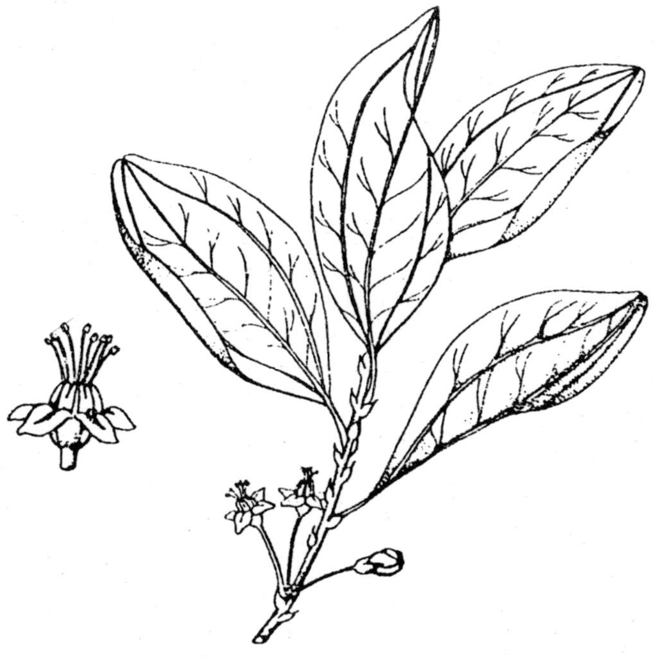

Fig. 17.5. A branch and flower of a coca plant, which yields the alkaloid cocoine.

Belladona

The drug is obtained mainly form the dried leaves of the deadly nightshade, *Atropa belladona* of the *Solanaceae*. The plant is indigenous to Europe and Asia Minor. It is widely grown in Europe, U.S.A. and India. The plant is a perennial herb with a creeping root stock. It bears alternately arranged ovate leaves. The stem is hollow. The flowers are purplish. The plant bears brownish or blackish berry. The leaves are harvested at the flowering time (May-June). The leaves are then dried at low temperature for a period of 2 to 15 weeks. The alkaloids present in the plant are extracted with the help of solvents.

The plant yields several alkaloids–atropine ($C_{17}H_{22}O_3N$) hyoscyamine, scopolamine, apoatropine, belladonine, norhyocyamine noratropine, hyoscine, tropacocaine and meteloidine out of which the first three are of greater importance. They are used as a stimulant to the sympathetic nervous system, as diuretics, in dilating the pupil of the eye and in the treatment of palsy. Externally it is used in ointment to relieve pain. Dilation of eye, to check the excessive perspiration, stimulation of circulation, local pain releaf and counteracting the muscle sperm are the various purposes for which Atropine or hyoscyamine is used. Scopolamine is used as a narcotic anti-insomniac and anesthesia.

Drugs Obtained from Flowers, Fruits and Seeds

Opium

Immature capsules of opium poppu (*Papaver somniforvm*) of the *Papaveraceae* are source of opium. The plant is indigenous to Asia Minor and India. It is also grown in China, West Asia and the Mediterranean region. The plant is an annual herb of a height of 2 to 4 feet.

Plant leaves are alternate and white, pink or reddish flowers are borne. The fruit is a globular pale green capsule. A number of fine parallel slits are made into the unripe capsules in the evening and in dry weather. The exuding latex is collected in the moring. It is rolled into balls which are covered by dried petals. Whereas the 'alba' varietes are grown in India and China for getting commercial opium, the 'glabra' varieties are used for exraction of the alkaloids to be used in medicines. There are about 30 alkaloids out of which the important ones are morphine, codeine, narcotine and papaverine. Morphine and codeine are widely used as sedatives to relieve pain and cause sleep. They are usually taken orally, rectally or by injections to cause local insensitiveness. Morphine is also used in the treatment of cough.

While opium is a very valuable, it is also a dangerous drug. Opium has narotic effects. It is eaten and smoked by millions of people for deriving pleasant feelings of exhilaration and peace. However, physical and mental degradation debility, delirium and even death can be caused as a result of addition of opium, morphine codeine, heroine (artificial derivative of morphine) etc. The drug should be used in very limited quantities and under strict supervision of physician.

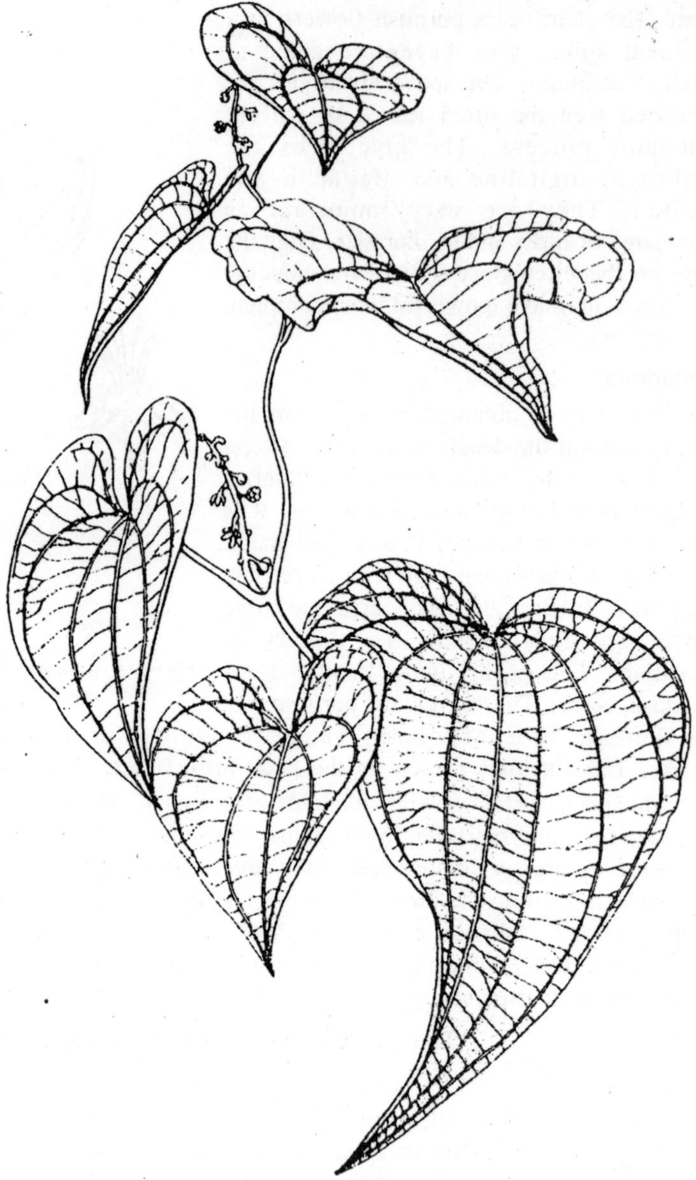

Fig. 17.6. The roots of yam vines are the principal sources of steroid precursors used to produce active compounds in oral contraceptives, and to treat hormone imbalances and heart.

Strychnine

The drug is obtained from the seeds of *Strychnos Nuxvomica* of the *Loganiaceae*. The plant is indigenous to Australia, India, Sri Lanka and Cochin China. The plant also grows widely in South America and Europe. It was introduced in Europe in the 16th century. The plant is a woody vine of the tropical forests. The stem bears ovate leaves in opposite manner. The plant bears small flowers and large indehiscent fruits. A fruit of *Strychnos* contains 3 to 5 hard and greyish seeds.

The alkaloids present in the seeds are strychnine ($C_{21}H_{22}N_2O_2$) and brucine ($C_{23}H_{26}N_2O_4$). They are expressed from the seed with boiling sulphuric acid. The alkaloids are first precipitated and are then purified. *Strychnine* is a very poisonous substance. It is of medicinal uses in the treatment of nervous disorders and paralysis It stimulates the central nervous system and acts as a tonic. It is famous as arrow poison (curare).

Drugs Obtained from Various Plants

Hordeum vulgare

Hordeum vulgare is grass that may be either a winter or a spring annual of the Poaceae (Graminae) family. It forms a rosette type of growth in fall and winter, developing elongated stems and flower heads in early summer. Winter varieties form branched stems or tillers at the base, so several stems rise from a single plant. The stems of both winter and spring varieties may vary in length from 30 to

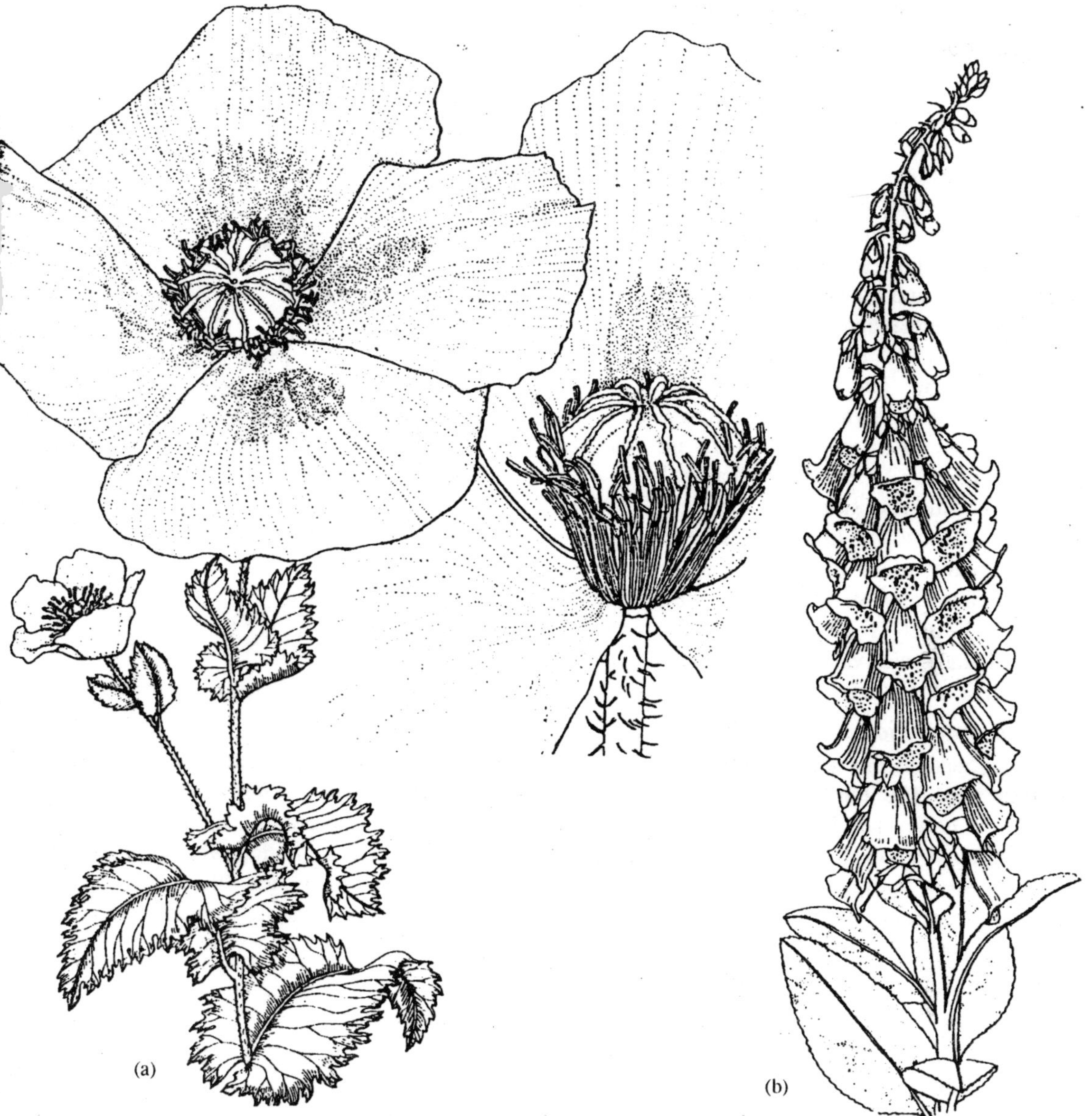

g. 17.7. *(a) The opium poppy is the source of morphine, papaverine, and codeine. (b) The leaves of the garden ornamental foxglove which yields digitoxin, a steroidal glycoside effective in stabilizing the heart's action.*

20 cm, depending on variety and growing conditions. Stems are round, hollow between nodes, and evelop five to seven nodes below the head. At each node, a clasping leaf develops. In most varieties, e leaves are coated with a waxy chalk-like deposit. Shape and size of leaves vary with variety, owing conditions, and position on the plant. The spike contains the flowers and consists of spike-ts attached to the central stem or rachis. Stem intervals between spikelets are 2 mm or less in dense-eaded varieties and up to 4–5 mm in lax or open-headed kinds. Three spikelets develop at each node the rachis. *Hordeum vulgare* is six-row variety, where all three of the spikelets at each node develop seed. Each spikelet has two linear to lanceolate glumes rising from near the base and flat and terminates

in an awn. The glumes, minus the awn, are approximately half the length of the kernel in most varieties, but this varies from less than half to equal to the kernel in length. Glumes may be covered with hairs, weakly haired, or hairless. The awns on the glumes may be shorter than the gume, equal in length, or longer. The barley kernel consists of the caryopsis, or internal seed, the lemma, and palea. In most barley varieties, the lemma and palea adhere to the caryopsis and are a part of the grain following threshing. The lemmas in barley are usually awned. Awns vary in length from very short up to as much as 12 in. Edges of awns may be rough or "barbed" (bearded) or nearly smooth. Awnless varieties are also known. In six-row barley, awns are usually more developed on the central spikelets than on the lateral ones. The barley kernel is generally spindle shaped. In commercial varieties, the length ranges from 7 to 12 mm.

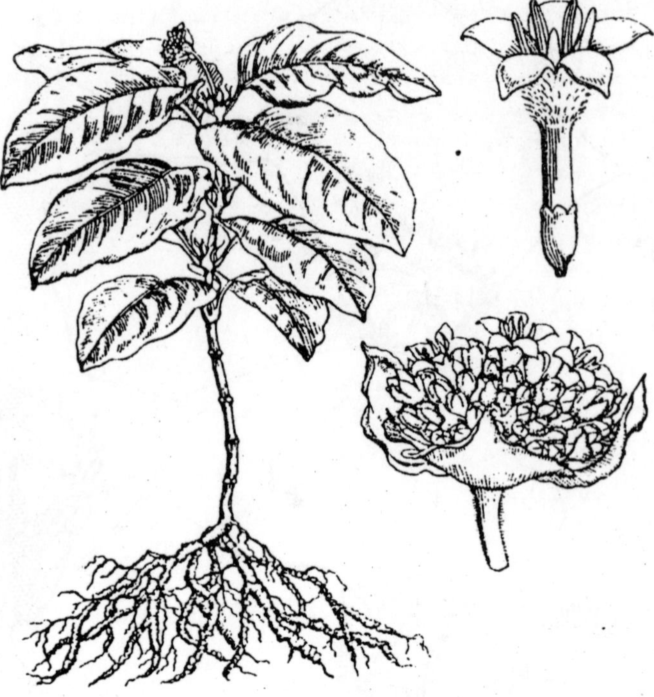

Fig. 17.8. Cephaelis, from which ipecac is obtained.

Origin and distribution

Grains found in pits and pyramids in Egypt indicated that barley was cultivated there more than 5000 years ago. The most ancient glyph or pictograph found for barley is dated approx 3000 BC. References to barley and beer are found in the earliest Egyptian and Sumerian writings. The origin of barley is still not known. There are differing views among researchers regarding whether the original wild forms were indigenous to Eastern Asia, particularly Tibet, or to the Near East, Eastern Mediterranean area, or both. Varieties are constantly changing as new ones are developed and tested while others pass out of cultivation.

Traditional uses

Afghanistan. Flowers are taken orally by females for contraception.

Argentina. Decoction of the dried fruit is taken orally for diarrhea and to treat respiratory and urinary tract infections.

Egypt. Dried fruits are smoked as a treatment for schistosomiasis. The fruit is used intravaginally as a contraceptive before and after coitus. Fifty-three percent of 1200 puerperal women interviewed practiced this method, of whom 47% depended on indigenous method and/or prolonged lactation.

Guatemala. Hot water extract of the dried seed is taken orally for renal inflammation and kidney disease. Hot water extract of the dried seed is used externally for dermatitis, inflammations, erysipelas, and skin eruptions.

India. Powdered flowers of *Calotropis procera*, fruits of *Piper nigrum*, seed ash of *Hordeum vulgare*, and rose water are taken orally for cholera.

Iran. Flour is used as a food. A decoction of the dried seed is used externally as an emollient and applied on hemorrhoids and infected ulcers. A decoction of the dried seed is taken orally as a diuretic and antipyretic and used for hepatitis, diarrhea, scorbutism, nephritis, bladder inflammation, gout, enema, and its tonic effect. Decoction of the dried seed is applied to the nose to reduce internasal inflammation.

Italy. Seeds are eaten as a urinary antiseptic. Compresses of boiled seeds are used to soothe rheumatic and joint pains. Infusion of the dried seed is used as a galactogogue.

Korea. Hot water extract of the dried entire plant is taken orally for beriberi, coughs, influenza, measles, syphilis, nephritis, jaundice, dysentery, and ancylostomiasis; for thrush in infants; and as a diuretic. Extract of the dried entire plant is used externally for prickly heat.

Peru. Hot water extract of dried fruits is used externally for measles and as an emollient and taken orally as a diuretic.

South Korea. Hot water extracts of the fruit and dried seeds are taken orally by pregnant women to induce abortion. Hot water extracts of the fruits taken orally by females as a contraceptive.

Turkey. Decoction of the fruit is taken orally for common colds.

United States. Infusion of the dried seed is taken orally for dysentery, diarrhea, and colic and for digestive and gastrointestinal disorders.

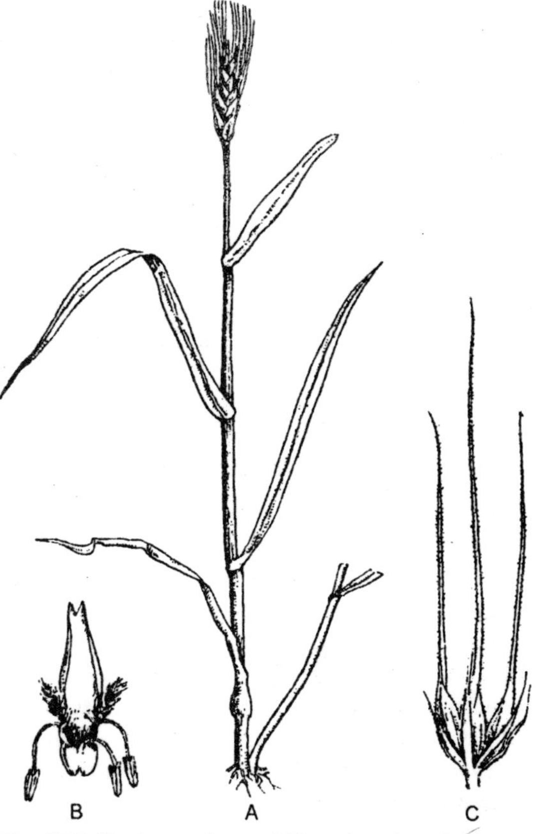

Fig. 17.9. Hordeum vulgare. A–Flowering plant, B–Flower, C–Spikelet.

Medicinal uses

Acquired immune deficiency syndrome therapeutic effect

Hot water extract of the dried fruit, administered orally to patients with acquired immuodeficiency syndrome (AIDS) four to five doses/week for a year for the purpose of in clearing heat and detoxifying the blood, produced an improvement in the patient's health.

Allergenic activity

Extract of the dried seed, administered externally to male adults at a concentration of 10%, was active. Allergens, administered by ingestion or inhalation to 40 children aged 3–6 months who suffered from diarrhea, vomiting, eczema, or weight loss after the introduction of the cereal in the diet and to 18 food-allergic adults and eight patients with Baker's asthma, produced strong effect in children. Protein Z(4), administered to four patients with beer allergy, provoked weak positive response to skin testing in two of the patients and was recognized by the four individual sera tested. Lipid transfer protein 1 showed reactivity with three of four individual sera and induced strong positive skin prick test responses in all four of the patients tested. Two cases of severe systemic reactions resulted from beer ingestion: one case of anaphylaxis requiring emergency care and one of generalized urticaria and angioedema were reported. Barley was recognized as the specific ingredient responsible for the observed allergic reaction. Beer and malt allergens were found in three patients with urticaria. Urticaria from beer was an immunoglobulin E (IgE)-mediated hypersensitivity reaction induced by a protein component of approx 10 kDa deriving from barley. A 50-year-old man, who developed bronchial asthma after exposure to barley flour, was confirmed by skin prick test and serum-specific IgE. Bronchial challenge test with every allergen showed no response, except for an immediate response to barley flour. The most relevant clinical feature was an immediate asthmatic response developed after oral provocation with either barley-made beer or barley flour itself that indicated IgE-mediated food-induced bronchial asthma. A 32-year-old storeman developed occupational asthma resulting from barley grain dust in the packaging of flour, barley, and peanuts. He developed immediate symptoms of sneezing, cough, and dyspnea on exposure to barley only. Bronchial provocation test to the barley confirmed the diagnosis.

Anti-atherogenic activity

β-Glucan in barley cellulose, administered to Syrian golden F(1)B hamsters at doses of 2, 4, or 8 g/100 g in a semipurified hyper-cholesterolemic diet of 0.15 g/g cholesterol, 20 g/100 g of hydrogenated coconut oil and 15 g/100 g of cellulose, produced cholesterol-lowering effect. Compared with control hamsters, dose-dependent decreases that were similar in magnitude in plasma total and low-density lipoprotein cholesterol concentrations were observed in hamsters fed the β-glucan diet at weeks 3,6, and 9. Liver cholesterol concentrations were also reduced significantly in hamsters consuming 8 g/100 g β-glucan.

Antibacterial activity

Decoction of the dried fruit, on agar plate, was inactive on *Pseudomonas aeruginosa*. Ethanol (95%) and water extracts of the dried fruit, on agar plate at a concentration of 50 μL/plate, were inactive on *Staphylococcus aureus*. Water extract of the dried fruit, on agar plate, at a concentration of 1 mg/mL, was inactive on *Salmonella typhi*. Hot water extract of the dried fruit, on agar plate at a concentration of 62.5 mg/mL, was inactive on *Escherichia coli* and *Staphylococcus aureus*. Tincture of the dried seed, on agar plate at a concentration of 30 μL/disc, was inactive on *Escherichia coli*, *Pseudomonas aeruginosa*, and *Staphylococcus aureus*. Extract of 10 g plant material in 100 mL ethanol was used.

Anticoagulation activity

Serpin BSZx (an inhibitor of trypsin and chemotrypsin) inhibited thrombin, plasma kallikrein, factor VIIa/tissue factor, and factor Xa at heparin-independent association rates. Only factor Xa turned a significant fraction of BSZx over as substrate. Activated protein C and leukocyte elastase were slowly inhibited by BSZx, whereas factor XIIa, urokinase and tissue type plasminogen activator, plasmin and pancreas kallikrein, and elastase were not or only weakly affected. Trypsin from *Fusarium* was not inhibited, while interaction with subtilisin Carlsberg and Novo was rapid, but most BSZx was cleaved as a substrate.

Antidiabetic activity

The plant, administered to diabetic rats, produced a decrease of blood glucose concentration, water consumption, and weight loss. No differences were found in healthy animals.

Antidiarrheal activity

Extract of the germinating seeds, administered in the ration of male rats, was active vs cecocolectomy-induced diarrhea. Germinated barley and scutellum fraction of germinated barley, administered to rats, prevented diarrhea caused by cecocolectomy and increased the protein content and sucrose activity of small intestinal mucosa. The aleurone and scutellum fractions of barley grains before and after germination, administered to rats with diarrhea, were active. The addition of fractions of germinated barley and not barley collected before germination increased the fecal output and jejunal mucosal protein content. The effect of malted barley was similar to that of germinated barley foodstuff.

Antifungal activity

Dried stem, on agar plate, was active on *Sphacelia segetum*. Hot water extract of the dried fruit, on agar plate at a concentration of 62.5 mg/mL, was inactive on *Aspergillus niger*. Water extract of the seed, on agar plate at a concentration of 5 mg/mL, was inactive on *Helicobacter pylori*. Protein fraction of the seed without seed coat, on agar plate at a concentration of 2 μg/disc, was active on *Neurospora crassa* and *Trichoderma* sp. Protein fraction of the seed without seed coat, on agar plate at a concentration of 2 μg/disc, was active on *Neurospora crassa*.

Antihepatotoxic activity

Methanol extract of the dried fruit, administered by gastric intubation to rabbits at a dose of 0.5 g/kg, was active vs CCl_4-induced hepatotoxicity. A mixture of *Machilus* sp., *Alisma* sp., *Amomum xanthioides*, *Bulboschoenus maritimus*, *Artemisia iwaymogis*, *Atractylodes japonica*, *Crataegus cuneata*, *Hordeum vulgare*, *Citrus sinensis*, *Polyporus umbellatus*, *Agastache rugosa*, *Raphanus sativus*, *Poncirus trifoliatus*, *Curcuma zeodaria*, *Citrus aurantium*, *Saussurea lappa*, *Glycyrrhiza glabra*, and *Zingiber officinale* was used.

Antihypercholesterolemic activity

Dried bran, administered in ration of male rats, was active. Methanol extract of the dried fruit, administered by gastric intubation to rabbits at a dose of 500 mg/kg, was active vs CCl_4-induced hepatotoxicity. A mixture of *Machilus* sp., *Alisma* sp., *Amomum xanthioides*, *Bulboschoenus maritimus*, *Artemisia iwaymogis*, *Atractylodes japonica*, *C. cuneata*, *Hordeum vulgare*, *Citrus sinensis*, *Polyporus umbellatus*, *Agastache rugosa*, *Raphanus sativus*, *Poncirus trifoliatus*, *Curcuma zeodaria*, *Citrus aurantium*, *Saussurea lappa*, *Glycyrrhiza glabra*, and *Zingiber officinale* was used. Results were significant at $p < 0.01$ level. Gum, administered orally to male rats for 4 weeks, was active. Biological activity reported had been patented. Chromatographic fraction of the green leaf juice, administered to rats at a dose of 1% of diet, was active vs cholesterol-loaded animals. The results were significant at $p < 0.005$ level. Seeds, administered to 20 men with hypercholesterolemia aged 41 ± 5 years, resulted in significant fall in serum total cholesterol, LDL cholesterol, and phospholipids, and LDL and very low-density lipoprotein (VLDL). A dose of 50/50 w/w mix with rice, administered to seven women with mild hypercholesterolemia aged 56.± 7 years twice daily for 2–4 weeks, produced a significant improvement of serum lipid profiles. In the normolipemic subjects, serum lipids were unaffected. Bran flour and oil extract, administered to 79 patients with hypercholesterolemia, aged 48.2 years at a dose of 3 g oil extract or 30 g flour for 30 days, significantly decreased total serum cholesterol. LDL cholesterol was decreased 6.5% with addition of bran flour and 9.2% with oil. High-density lipoprotein (HDL) cholesterol decreased significantly in the bran flour group but not in the oil group. Fiber (nonstarch polysaccharides), administered to 21 men with mild hypercholesterolemia aged 30–59 years for 4 weeks, produced a significant fall in plasma total cholesterol and LDL cholesterol. The triglyceride and glucose concentrations did not change significantly.

Antihyperglycemic activity

Dried seeds, administered orally to six patients with noninsulin-dependent diabetes mellitus at a dose of 50 g/person, was active. A single dose resulted in a glycemic index of 53.4. Water extract of the dried fruit, administered intragastrically to rats at a dose of 150 mg/kg, produced weak activity on blood vs streptozotocin-induced hyperglycemia. Dried seeds, administered orally to eight adults with normal glucose tolerance at a dose of 50 g/person, were active. Flour, administered in the ration of male rats, was active vs streptozotocin- induced hyperglycemia. Barley gum, administered to 4-week-old male Sprague–Dawley rats as a 2% dietary supplement for 14 days, lowered serum cholesterol concentration and suppressed the elevation of serum and liver triglyceride concentrations. Thick and thin rolled oat made from raw or preheated kernel, administered to healthy subjects, produced high glucose, insulin, and metabolic responses. Barley flour naturally high in β-glucan and β-glucan-enriched flour, administered to 11 healthy men, resulted in a decrease of the insulin response. Plasma glucose and insulin concentrations increased significantly. Cholesterol concentration dropped below the fasting concentration 4 hours after the meal and was significantly lower than after low-fiber meal. The cholecystokinin remained elevated for a long time after the barley-containing meals. Boiled intact and milled kernels with different amylase-amylopectin ratios, administered to healthy subjects, produced lower metabolic responses and higher satiety scores when compared to white wheat bread. The boiled flours produced higher glucose and insulin responses than did the corresponding boiled kernels. The impact of amylase to amylopectin on the metabolic responses was marginal. The intact kernels, administered to healthy subjects at concentrations of 40 and 80% (SCB-40 and SCB-80), produced the glycemic and insulinemic indices 39 and 33 for SCB-80, compared to pumpernickel bread 69 and 61, respectively. The glycemic index for SCB-40 was 66.

Anti-inflammatory activity

Germinated barley foodstuff, administered to mice with DSS-induced colitis, prevented disease activity and loss of body weight after induction of colitis. Serum interleukin (IL)-6 level, mucosal STAT3 expression, necrosis factor-κB activity, and mucosal damages were decreased and cecal butyrate content increased. The germinated barley foodstuff-fed mice had lower bile acid concentration than the control group. Green barley extract, in LPS-activated human monocytes cell line culture (THP-1), was active.

Antioxidant activity

Water extract of the roasted seed, at a concentration of 1 mg/mL, produced strong activity vs a liposome model system. A concentration of 25 mg/mL was active vs 2,2-diphenyl-1-picryl-hydrazyl-hydrate-induced radical. A concentration of 5 mg/mL was inactive vs linoleic acid system. Ethanol (80%) extract of the freeze- dried leaf, at a concentration of 60 μg/mL, was active vs oxidation of ethyl linoleate by Fenton's reagent. Young leaf extract, administered orally to 36 patients with type 2 diabetes at a dose of 15 g daily for 4 weeks, enhanced the scavenging of oxygen free radicals, saved the LDL-vitamin E content, and inhibited LDL oxidation. Purified green barley extract, in human mononuclear culture of cells isolated from perithelial blood and synovial fluid of patients with rheumatoid arthritis, was active. Leaf essence, administered to atherosclerotic New Zealand White male rabbits at a dose of 1% of diet, produced a decrease of plasma total cholesterol, triacylglycerol, lucigenin-chemiluminescence, and luminal-chemiluminescence levels. The value of T_{50} of red blood cell hemolysis and the lag phase of LDL oxidation increased in barley- treated group compared with the control. Ninety percent of the intimal surface of the thoracic aorta was covered with atherosclerotic lesions in the control group, but only 60% of the surface was covered in the barley group. This inhibition was associated with a decrease in plasma lipids and an increase in antioxidative abilities.

Anti-tumor activity

Commercial barley bran (13% dietary fiber) from the aleurone/ subaleurone layer; outer-layer barley bran, including the germ (25.5% dietary fiber); and spent barley grain bran (product of the brewery including the hull) (47.7% dietary fiber) were administered to male Sprague–Dawley rats as a 5% dietary supplement for 7 months. Commercial barley bran was most effective in reducing tumor incidence and burden. Tumor burden and tumor mass index were reduced significantly by outer-layer barley bran and spent barley grain bran. Commercial barley bran and spent barley grain bran, administered to rats with 1,2-dimethylhydrazine-induced intestinal tumor, produced a higher incidence and burden of tumor. Fiber was administered to 4-week-old male Sprague–Dawley rats with dimethylhydrazine-induced tumors at a dose of 5% of diet. The insoluble fiber-rich fraction (spent barley grain) was significantly more effective at preventing induced tumors than the soluble commercial barley bran. The incidence of rats affected, tumor mass index, and plasma cholesterol concentration were reduced by spent barley grain. Outer-layer barley bran was moderately effective in cancer prevention. The crude and partially purified lunasin, in stably *ras*-transfected mouse fibroblast cell culture, suppressed colony formation induced with isopropylthiogalactoside. This fraction also inhibited histone acetylation in mouse fibroblast (NIH 3T3) and human breast (MCF-7) cells in the presence of the histone deacetylase inhibitor sodium butyrate.

Anti-ulcer activity

Water extract of the green leaf juice, administered by gastric intubation to rats at a dose of 500 mg/kg, was active vs stress-induced (restraint) ulcers. The results were significant at $p < 0.001$ level. Water extract was active vs acetic acid-induced and aspirin-induced ulcers. The results were significant at $p < 0.01$ and $p < 0.005$ levels, respectively. Water extract was inactive vs pylorus ligation-induced ulcers. Extract of the dried seedling, administered orally to adults at a dose of 30 g/person, was active. Germinated barley foodstuff, administered orally to male Sprague–Dawley rats on day 6 after initiation of colitis, was active vs dextran sodium sulfate-induced colitis. Germinated barley foodstuff treatment reduced colonic inflammation with an increase in cecal butyrate levels. Fiber and protein factions of germinated barley foodstuff, administered to dextran sodium sulfate-induced colitis Sprague–Dawley rats, significantly attenuated the clinical signs of colitis and decreased serum α1-acid glycoprotein levels, with an increase in cecal butyrate production, whereas germinated barley foodstuff- protein did not. Germinated barley foodstuff with or without salazosulfapyridine, administered to rats after the onset of colitis, accelerated colonic epithelial repair and improved clinical signs. Germinated barley foodstuff, administered orally to patients with mild to moderate active ulcerative colitis at a dose of 30 g/person daily for 4 weeks, produced a significant clinical and endoscopic improvement independent of disease extent.

The improvement was associated with an increase in stool butyrate concentrations and in luminal *Bifidobacterium* and *Eubacterium* levels. After the end of treatment, the patients had an exacerbation of the disease. Germinated barley foodstuff with or without *Clostridium butyricum*, administered to 3% dextran sodium sulfate-induced colitis in Sprague–Dawley rats for 8 days, prevented bloody diarrhea and mucosal damage and increased the fecal short-chain fatty acid levels. Germinated barley foodstuff, administered to Sprague–Dawley rats for 5 days, prevented bloody diarrhea and mucosal damage, elevated fecal acetic acid and *N*-butyric acid levels, and tended to increase the number of *Eubacteria* and *Bifidobacteria*. The number of *Enterobacteriaceae*, the total number of aerobes and *Bacteroidaceae*, were lowered by germinated barley foodstuff treatment. Germinated barley foodstuff, administered to HLA-B27 transgenic rats for 13 weeks, produced an increase of bacterial butyrate production and the decrease of cecal occult blood, colonic mucosal hyperplasia, colonic mucosal necrosis factor-κB-DNA binding activity, and the production of IL-8. Butyrate from germinated barley foodstuff, administered orally or intracecally to Sprague–Dawley rats, produced reduction of mucosal damage only by intrathecal administration. Bacterial butyrate production and reduction of mucosal damage depended on the dose of germinated barley foodstuff in the diet.

Germinated barley foodstuff and scutellum fraction of germinated barley, administered to Sprague–Dawley rats with colitis induced by 3% dextran sodium sulfate, prevented bloody diarrhea and mucosal damage in colitis. The germinated samples did not produce a protective effect. Germinated barley foodstuff increased mucosal protein and RNA content in the colitis model. Germinated barley foodstuff, administered to 18 patients with mildly to moderately active ulcerative colitis at a dose of 20–30 g germinated barley foodstuff daily for 4 weeks, produced a significant decrease in clinical activity index scores compared to the control group. No side effects related to germinated barley foodstuff were observed. Germinated barley foodstuff therapy increased fecal concentrations of *Bifidobacterium* and *Eubacterium limosum*. Germinated barley foodstuff, administered to patients with mild to moderate active ulcerative colitis, irresponsible to or intolerant of standard treatment at a dose of 20–30 g germinated barley foodstuff daily for 4 weeks, resulted in a significant clinical and endoscopic improvement associated with an increase in stool butyrate concentrations.

Cardiovascular activity

β-glucan, administered to 18 men with mild hypercholesterolemia with a mean body weight index of 27.4 ± 4.6 at a dose of 8.1–11.9 g β-glucan per day, produced no significant change in total, LDL and HDL cholesterol, triacylglycerol, fasting glucose, and postprandial glucose.

Cholesterol biosynthesis inhibition

The inhibitor I from oily nonpolar fraction of flour, administered to chicken at a dose of 2.5–20 ppm, produced a significant decrease in hepatic cholesterogenesis and serum total and LDL cholesterol and an increase in lipogenic activity.

Cholesterol-7-α-hydroxylase inhibition

Petroleum ether extract of the fresh fruit, administered to pigs at a concentration of 3.5 g/kg of diet for 29 days, produced 40% inhibition of the hepatic enzyme activity.

Cytotoxic activity

Water extract of the dried fruit, in cell culture at a concentration of 500 μg/mL, produced weak activity on CA-mammary-microalveolar. Ethanol (50%) extract of the seed, in cell culture, was inactive on CA-9KB, ED_{50} greater than 20 μg/mL. Methanol extract of the dried seed, in cell culture, was inactive on SNU-1 human cells, IC_{50} greater than 0.3 mg/mL, and on SNU-C4 human cells, IC_{50} greater than 0.3 mg/mL. Protein fraction of the seed without seed coat, in cell culture at a concentration of 2 μg/disc, was active on CA-Ehrlich ascites. Methanol extract of the aerial parts, in cell culture at a concentration of 50 mg/mL, was equivocal on CA-9KB.

Gastrointestinal activity

Water extract of the green leaf juice, administered by gastric intubation to rats at a dose of 500 mg/kg, was inactive vs pylorus ligation-induced ulcers. Fiber, administered orally to young male Wistar rats at a dose of 500 g extrudates/kg of diet for 6 weeks, produced a higher concentration of neutral sterols in the intestinal content of the barley-fed group than in the control group ($p < 0.005$) and affected indirectly the amount of formed secondary bile acids. Fiber, administered orally to young male Wistar rats at a dose of 50 g/100 g extrudates or mixtures for 6 weeks, produced greater food intake in the last 2 weeks and increased ceca and colon masses, cecal and colon contents, concentration of resistant starch in cecal, most of colon contents, and β-glucan level in the small intestine, cecum, and colon. The numbers of coliforms and *Bacteroides* were lower and those of *Lactobacillus* were higher than in the control group. The dose increased weight gain in the sixth week. Short-chain fatty acids were higher in the cecal, colon, and feces content of the test group. The proportion of secondary bile acids was lower and the amount of neutral sterol was higher in feces of fiber-treated animals. The concentrations of excreted bile acids increased up to 30% during the feeding period. Germinated barley food-stuff, administered to Sprague–Dawley rats fed on various diets with the same protein and dietary fiber levels, produced an increase fecal output compared with commercial water-soluble and insoluble dietary fibers.

The dietary fiber from germinated barley foodstuff increased the fecal output and mucosal protein content. The protein fraction of germinated barley foodstuff degraded to the peptide form did not increase the fecal output or mucosal protein content[HV152]. Germinated barley foodstuff from aleurone and scutellum fractions of germinated barley, administrated to healthy volunteers at a dose of 9 g daily for 14 days, significantly increased fecal butyrate content and fecal *Bifidobacterium* and *Eubacterium*. Ten anaerobic microorganisms selected from intestinal microflora were cultured in vitro in germinated barley foodstuff medium. After 3 days of incubation, seven strains (*Bifidobacterium breve*, *Bifidobacterium longum*, *Lactobacillus acidophilus*, *Lactobacillus casei* ssp. *casei*, *Bacteroides ovatus*, *Clostridium butyricum*, and *Eubacterium limosum*) lowered the medium pH producing short-chain fatty acid. Germinated barley foodstuff changed the intestinal microflora and increased probiotics such as *Bifidobacterium*. Butyrate was produced by the mutual action of *Eubacterium* and *Bifidobacterium*. Germinated barley foodstuff from aleurone layer, scutellum, and germ, administered to 10 healthy volunteers at a dose of 30 g/day/person for 28 days, produced an increased fecal butyrate content, fecal weight, and water content.

There were no significant changes in body weight and major abnormalities in hematologic and urinary analysis. Fiber, administered to nine patients with ileostomies at a dose of 35 g/day, increased the ileal excretion of starch. Flaked and finely milled barley, eaten by patients with ileostomies, showed that only 2 ± 1% of starch remained undigested after the consumption of finely milled barley and 17 ± 1% resisted digestion, partly as oligosaccharides but largely as intact unpitted starch granules bound by intact cell walls. The energy excretion from the stoma was three times higher after flaked that after milled barley. Nonstarch polysaccharide, starch, and fat made almost equal contributions to the higher energy excretion. Bran flour, administered to 44 volunteers at a dose of 30 g/day, decreased the transit time by 8.02 hours from baseline and increased daily fecal weight by 48.6. Groats were administered to volunteers at a dose of 1 g carbohydrate/kg body weight, three times or at three different doses of 0.75, 1, and 1.5 g carbohydrate/kg body weight. After consumption of 1 g carbohydrate/kg body weight, produced a mean mouth to cecum transit time of 8.4 ± 0.4 hour. After consumption of the high dose, a mean mouth-to-cecum transit time of 9.0 ± 0.5 hours was produced. Particle size did not significantly affect the mouth-to-caecum transit time.

Germinated barley food-stuff, administered to Sprague–Dawley rats, prevented diarrhea and mucosal damages; increased mucosal protein, DNA, and RNA content; and depressed bacterial translocation and elevation of myeloperoxidase activity induced by methotrexate. β-glucan-rich barley fraction, administered to ileostomy subjects at a dose of 13.0 g β-glucan/day for 2 days, increased the cholesterol excretion higher than with the oat bran with β-glucanase and wheat flour diets. Bile acid excretion was 755 (133–1187) mg/day. Carbohydrates, administered to healthy subjects at a dose of 90 g for dinner in random order 1 week apart, significantly increased the breath hydrogen and improved glucose tolerance. No difference in the rates of glucose disappearance or gut glucose absorption was observed. Serum-free fatty acid concentrations were significantly reduced the morning after the barley meal. Germinated barley foodstuff, administered to Sprague–Dawley rats with constipation induced by loperamide, produced an increase of bowel movements, fecal water content, and concentration of short-chain fatty acids in cecal content, especially butyrate.

Glucose tolerance effect

Fiber, administered orally to type 2 diabetic Goto– Kakizaki male rats for 9 months, improved the area under the plasma glucose concentration time curves, lowered the fasting plasma glucose and glycosylated hemoglobin levels, and decreased plasma total cholesterol, triglycerides, and free fatty acid levels. Fiber, administered orally to 8- week-old male Goto–Kakizaki strain rats, at a dose of 1.79 g/day/rat for 3 months, improved glucose tolerance and lowered the plasma cholesterol and triglyceride levels. The fasting plasma glucose level was significantly lower in comparison to rice and corn starch-fed rats. High barley (high-fiber diet), administered to 10 women (20.4 ± 1.3 year-old,

19.2 ± 2 kg/m²) for 4 weeks with a 1-month interval, resulted in lowering plasma total and LDL cholesterol concentrations and reduced plasma triacylglycerol concentration. The barley diet increased stool volume. There was no significant difference in glucose tolerance between diet regimens. Barley bread containing lactic acid and reference barley bread, administered in the morning to 10 healthy men and women, produced a significant lowering of the incremental glycemic area and of the glucose response at 95 minutes after ingestion of the bread with lactic acid. At 45 minutes after the meal, the insulin level was significantly lower after the lactic acid bread, compared with reference barley bread.

Glucose-6-phosphate dehydrogenase inhibition

Petroleum ether extract of the fresh fruit, administered to pigs at a concentration of 3.5 g/kg of diet for 29 days, was active on hepatic enzymes.

Glutamate–oxaloacetate–transaminase inhibition

Methanol extract of the dried fruit, administered by gastric intubation to rabbits at a dose of 500 mg/kg, was active vs CCl_4-induced hepatotoxicity. A mixture of *Machilus* sp., *Alisma* sp., *Amomum xanthioides*, *Bulboschoenus maritimus*, *Artemisia iwaymogis*, *Atractylodes japonica*, *Crataegus cuneata*, *Hordeum vulgare*, *Citrus sinensis*, *Polyporus umbellatus*, *Agastache rugosa*, *Raphanus sativus*, *Poncirus trifoliatus*, *Curcuma zeodaria*, *Citrus aurantium*, *Saussurea lappa*, *Glycyrrhiza glabra*, and *Zingiber officinale* was used. Results were significant at $p < 0.01$ level.

Glutamate–pyruvate–transaminase inhibition

Methanol extract of the dried fruit, administered by gastric intubation to rabbits at a dose of 500 mg/kg, was active vs carbon tetrachloride (CCl_4)-induced hepatotoxicity. A mixture of *Machilus* sp., *Alisma* sp., *Amomum xanthioides*, *Bulboschoenus maritimus*, *Artemisia iwaymogis*, *Atractylodes japonica*, *Crataegus cuneata*, *Hordeum vulgare*, *Citrus sinensis*, *Polyporus umbellatus*, *Agastache rugosa*, *Raphanus sativus*, *Poncirus trifoliatus*, *Curcuma zeodaria*, *Citrus aurantium*, *Saussurea lappa*, *Glycyrrhiza glabra*, and *Zingiber officinale* was used. Result was significant at $p < 0.01$ level.

Hypocholesterolemic activity

Fixed oil of the bran, administered orally to adults of both sexes at a dose of 30 mg/day, was active. Flour bran, administered orally to adults at a dose of 3 g/day, was active. Dried bran, administered in the ration of male rats, was active. Petroleum ether extract of the fresh fruit, administered to pigs at a concentration of 3.5 g/kg of diet, produced a decrease of serum total cholesterol, LDL cholesterol, and HDL cholesterol after 29 days of feeding. Flour, administered orally to adults with hypercholesterolemia at a dose of 44 g/day, produced a decrease of total and LDL cholesterol levels.

Hypoglycemic activity

Water extract of the fermented root, administered intravenously to rabbits, was active. The dried seed, administered orally to eight healthy volunteers at a dose of 50 g/person, was active. A single dose resulted in a glycemic index of 68.7 and an insulinemic index of 71.1.

Hypolipemic activity

Fiber, administered orally to nine adults with ileostomies at a dose of 13 g/day, increased the excretion of cholesterol. Petroleum ether extract of the fresh fruit, administered to pigs at a concentration of 3.5 g/kg of diet, was inactive. Purified green barley extract, in human mononuclear culture of cells isolated from perithelial blood and synovial fluid of patients with rheumatoid arthritis, was active. Leaf essence, administered to atherosclerotic New Zealand White male rabbits at a dose of 1% of diet, produced a decrease of plasma total cholesterol, triacylglycerol, lucigenin–chemiluminescence, and luminal–chemiluminescence levels. The value of T_{50} of red blood cell hemolysis and the lag phase of LDL oxidation increased in barley-treated group compared with the control. Ninety percent of the intimal surface of the thoracic aorta was covered with atherosclerotic lesions in the control group, but only 60% of the surface was covered in the barley group. This inhibition was associated with a decrease in plasma lipids and an increase in antioxidative abilities.

Hypotriglyceridemic activity

Fixed oil of the bran, administered orally to adults of both sexes at a dose of 30 mg/day, was active. Flour bran, administered orally to adults at a dose of 3 g/day, was inactive.

Laxative effect

Powdered dried bran, administered orally to 44 adults at a dose of 30 g/person, was active on gastrointestinal motility. Transit time decreased by 8 hours, and fecal mass increased by 48.6 g/day.

Lipid metabolism

Fiber, administered orally to male type 2 diabetic Goto– Kakizaki rats for 9 months, improved the area under the plasma glucose concentration time curves, lowered the fasting plasma glucose and glycosylated hemoglobin levels, and decreased plasma total cholesterol, triglycerides and free fatty acid levels.

Lipolytic effect

Ethanol (95%) extract of the dried entire plant in combination with *Rhizoma zingiberis*, *Ligustrum chuanxiong*, *Lilium brownii*, *Nephelium longa*, and *Polygonum multiflorum*, administered in drinking water to C57BL/6J obese mice at a concentration of 5%, was active.

Lung function

Exposure of six men to barley dust for 2 days decreased ventilatory capacity. Five volunteers not previously exposed to barley dust, when exposed to the dust for 2 hours, decreased the ventilatory capacity ranging from 200 mL to 800 mL, with recovery taking up to 72 hours. All of the subjects had decreases in flow at 50% vital capacity but little or no change in flow at 75% vital capacity. In three subjects, there was a drop in specific conductance that lasted for less than 24 hours. Sixty-ine of 80 dockworkers handling grains reported evening feverish episodes/symptoms not related to smoking or atopic status. No gross deficits in lung function were detected.

Malic enzyme inhibition

Petroleum ether extract of the fresh fruit, administered to pigs at a concentration of 3.5 g/kg of diet for 29 days, was active on hepatic enzymes.

Mineral utilization

Germinated barley foodstuff, administered orally to 5-week-old Sprague–Dawley rats for 14 days, promoted the absorption of calcium (Ca) and magnesium (Mg) by the gastrointestinal tract. The absorption of iron and potassium was not attenuated and mineral absorption was not inhibited. Barley husk, administered to 5- and 9-week-old rats at different doses, produced a lowering of zinc (Zn) and Ca absorption already at dose 20 g dietary fiber/kg dry matter and had a small negative effect on potassium absorption. Phytate did not appear as a major factor affecting mineral absorption in barley husk. All of the diets containing barley husk had very low molar ratios (phytate:Zn was 4). Processed or unprocessed barley was administered to healthy subjects in two single meals containing porridge or breakfast (60 g) cereals for 2 months. Zn absorption from hydrothermally-treated barley porridge was significantly higher than from the control porridge; Ca absorption did not differ. Zn absorption from breakfast cereals of malted barley with phytase activity was significantly higher than from flakes of barley without phytase activity; Ca absorption was not significantly different. Standard barley and β-glucan-enriched barley dehulled grains was administered to 10 healthy hydrogen-producing adults at a dose of 35 g. The percentage of the ^{13}C dose oxidized was greater after standard barley than after enriched barley consumption. The area under the curve for H_2 was greater after enriched barley intake. There was no difference in CO_2 production. Hull fiber extract, in Caco-2 cell culture, produced no effect on the rate of transepithelial ^{45}Ca transport across Caco-2 cell monolayers and the uptake of ^{45}Ca into Caco-2 cells. A low-phytate barley-fiber concentrate was administered to young women at a dose of 15 g barley fiber (high-fiber, high-protein diet) and 15 g barley fiber (high-fiber, low-protein diet). The mean daily intake of the cations was 25.4 and 22.9 mmol Ca, 10.1 and 10 mmol Mg, 166.8 and 119.3 μmol Zn, and 186.2 and 154 μmol Fe, respectively. Mean balances were 1.9 and -0.8 mmol Ca, -0.2 and -0.5 mmol Mg, -4.6, and -18.4 imol Zn, respectively. The mean apparent iron absorption was 5.4 and -23.2 μmol.

Monocytic differentiation

Prodelphinidin B-3, T1, T2, and T3 from bran polyphenol extract, in HL60 human myeloid leukemia cell culture, induced 26–40% nitro blue tetrazolium positive cells and 22–32% α-naphthyl-butyrate esterase-positive cells. Proanthocyanidins potentiated all-*trans*-retinoic acid-induced granulocytic and sodium butyrate-induced monocytic differentiation in HL60 cells.

Mutagenic activity

Ethanol (70%) extract of the dried seed, on agar plate at a concentration of 50 mg/mL, was inactive on *Escherichia coli* PQ 37. The water and chloroform extracts of the ethanol (70%) extract were inactive. Metabolic activation had no effect on the results.

Oxidative effect

Ethanol (95%) extract of the dried entire plant, administered in drinking water to C57BL/6J obese mice at a concentration of 5%, increased glucose oxidation in epididymal fat pads. Extract of mixture of following plants: *Hordeum vulgare*, *Rhizoma zingiberis*, *Ligustrum chuanxiong*, *Lilium brownii*, *Nephelium longa*, and *Polygonum multiflorum* was used.

Pepsin inhibition

Water extract of the green leaf juice, administered by gastric intubation to rats at a dose of 500 mg/kg, was inactive vs pylorus ligation-induced ulcers.

Phosphogluconate dehydrogenase inhibition

Petroleum ether extract of the fresh fruit, administered to pigs at a concentration of 3.5 g/kg of diet for 29 days, was active on hepatic enzymes.

Proteinemic effect

Methanol extract of the dried fruit, administered by gastric intubation to rabbits at a dose of 500 mg/kg, produced an increase in serum albumin and protein content vs CCl_4-induced hepatotoxicity. A mixture of *Machilus* sp., *Alisma* sp., *Amomum xanthioides*, *Bulboschoenus maritimus*, *Artemisia iwaymogis*, *Atractylodes japonica*, *Crataegus cuneata*, *Hordeum vulgare*, *Citrus sinensis*, *Polyporus umbellatus*, *Agastache rugosa*, *Raphanus sativus*, *Poncirus trifoliatus*, *Curcuma zeodaria*, *Citrus aurantium*, *Saussurea lappa*, *Glycyrrhiza glabra*, and *Zingiber officinale* was used. Results were significant at $p < 0.01$ level.

Respiratory effect

Barley ear inhaled by a 2.5-year-old child produced fever, dyspnea, right paracardiac infiltrate with pleural reaction on X-rays, and normal bronchoscopy after 8 days. On day 11, extensive right pneumothorax, and on day 20, right axillary inflammatory lesion were observed. On day 28, the ear of barley was expulsed and there was complete recovery. Barley spike, inhaled into the tracheobronchial tree of 18 children under the age of 5 years, produced coughing and choking in 14 of the children. The spikes were removed by laryngoscopy in 12 patients and by rigid bronchoscopy in two. Four patients with history of cough, dyspnea, fever, and serious respiratory diseases, such as pneumothorax, lobar pneumonia, and pleural empyema, required surgical intervention. All of the children made satisfactory recoveries. Dust extract of barley, in cell culture on nonsensitized guinea pig tracheal smooth muscle pretreated with drugs, produced constrictor effect that was significantly inhibited by atropine indicating an interaction of the extracts with parasympathetic nerves. Inhibition of contraction of other mediators was less effective and varied with the dust extract.

Toxic effect

β-glucan-enriched soluble barley fiber, administered orally to Wistar rats at concentrations of 0.7, 3.5, and 7.0% β-glucan for 28 days, increased the number of circulating lymphocytes in males. The increase was not dose-dependent and was not observed in females. A dose-dependent increase in full and empty cecum weight was observed. There were no adverse effects on general condition and behavior, growth, feed and water consumption, feed conversion efficiency, red blood cell and clotting potential parameters, clinical chemistry values, and organ weight. Necropsy and histopathology findings revealed no treatment-related changes in any organ evaluated. β-glucan (64%) preparation (barley β-fiber), administered to CD-1 mice at concentrations of 1,5, or 10% of diet (0.7, 3.5, and 7% β-glucan) for 28 days, produced no adverse effect in hematological or clinical chemistry measurements, in organ weights and immunopathology in either sex after treatment or after the recovery period. Azidoalanine and the azide-treated extracts, in Chinese hamster and normal human skin fibroblast cell cultures, significantly increased the frequency of sister chromatid exchanges observed in both cultures. This increase was approximately twofold, as compared with the control.

Toxicity assessment

Ethanol (50%) extract of the seed, administered intraperitoneally to mice, produced a maximum tolerated dose of 1 g/kg. Hexane extract of the green leaf juice, administered in ration of rats, produced lethal $dose_{50}$ greater than 10 g/kg.

Weight gain inhibition

Ethanol (95%) extract of the dried entire plant, administered in drinking water to C57BL/6J obese mice at a concentration of 5%, was active. The extract also contained *Rhizoma zingiberis*, *Ligustrum chuangxiong*, *Lilium brownii*, *Nephelium longa*, and *Polygonum multiflorum*.

Camellia sinensis

Camellia sinensis is an evergreen tree or shrub of the *Theaceae* family that grows to 10–15 m high in the wild, and 0.6–1.5 m under cultivation. The leaves are short- stalked, light green, coriaceous, alternate, elliptic-obovate or lanceolate, with serrate margin, glabrous, or sometimes pubescent beneath, varying in length from 5 to 30 cm, and about 4 cm wide. Young leaves are pubescent. Mature leaves are bright green in color, leathery, and smooth.

Flowers are white, fragrant, 2.5–4 cm in diameter, solitary or in clusters of two to four. They have numerous stamens with yellow anthers and produces brownish-red, one- to four-lobed capsules. Each lobe contains one to three spherical or flattened brown seeds. There are numerous varieties and races of tea. There are three main groups of the cultivated forms: China, Assam, and hybrid tea, differing in form. *Camellia sinensis assamica*, the source of much of the commercial tea crop of Ceylon is a tree that, unpruned, may attain a height of 15 m and has proportionally longer, thinner leaves than typical species.

Origin and distribution

The cultivation and enjoyment of tea are recorded in Chinese literature of 2700 BC and in Japan about 1100. Through the Arabs, tea reached Europe about 1550. Native to Assam, Burma, and the

Chinese province of Yunnan, it is highly regarded in southern Asia and planted in India, southern Russia, East Africa, Java, Ceylon, Sumatra, Argentina, and Turkey. China, India, Indonesia, and Japan produced about a half of the total world production.

Traditional uses

India. Decoctions of the dried and fresh buds and leaves are taken orally for headache and fever. Powder or decoction of the dried leaf is applied to teeth to prevent tooth decay. Fresh leaf juice is taken orally for abortion, and as a contraceptive and hemostatic.

Mexico. Hot water extract of the leaf is taken orally by nursing mothers to increase milk production.

Turkey. Leaves are taken orally to treat diarrhea.

China. Hot water extract of the dried leaf is taken orally as a sedative, an antihypertensive, and anti-inflammatory.

Guatemala. Hot water extract of the dried leaf is used as eyewash for conjunctivitis.

Kenya. Water extract of the dried leaf is applied ophthalmically to treat corneal opacities. The infusion is used for chalzion and conjunctivitis.

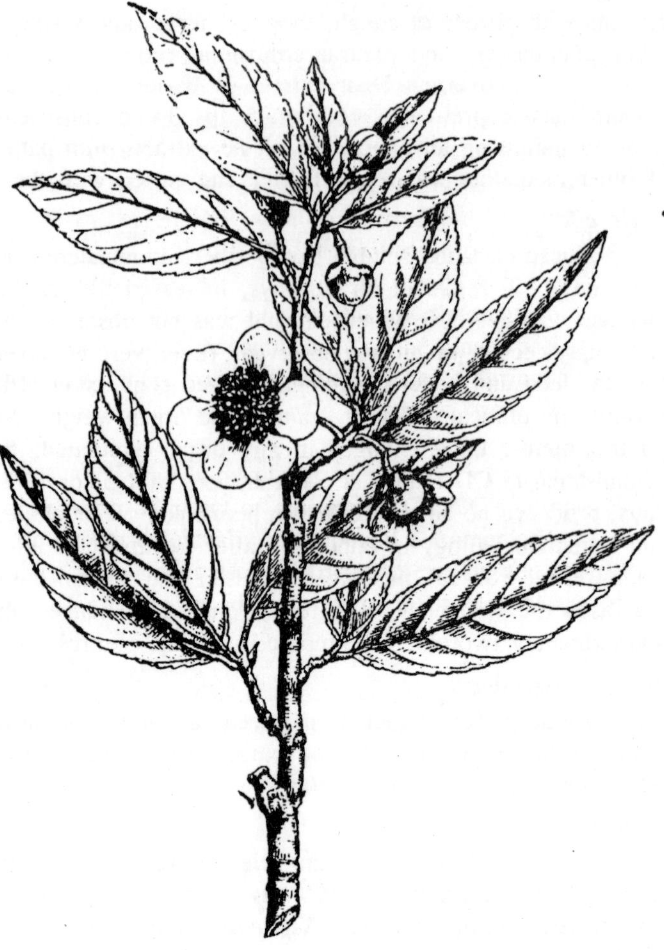

Fig. 17.10. Camellia sinensis – flowering branch.

Thailand. Hot water extract of the dried leaf is taken orally as a cardiotonic and neurotonic. Hot water extract of the dried seed is taken orally as an antifungal.

Medicinal values

Antibacterial activity

Alcohol extract of black tea, assayed on *Salmonella typhi* and *Salmonella paratyphi* A, was active on all strains of Salmonella paratyphi A, and only 42.19% of Salmonella typhi strains were inhibited by the extract. Hot water extract of the dried entire plant and the tannin fraction, on agar plate, were active on *Escherichia coli*, *Pseudomonas aeruginosa*, and *Staphylococcus aureus*.

Anticancer activity

Catechin, administered to pheochromocytoma cells in cell culture, was active. The cells were incubated with different concentrations of catechin at short-term (2 days) and long-term (7 days) in Dulbecco's modified Eagle medium. The activity of superoxide dismutase was measured and its mRNA assayed by Northern blotting. After incubation for 2 days, catechin significantly increased the activity of copper/zinc superoxide dismutase. However, it did not produce significant effect at 7 days. The magnesium superoxide dismutase activity produced significant changes in both short- and long-term treatment groups. The amount of mRNA also showed similar changes.

Anticarcinogenic activity

The anti-carcinogenic activity of tea phenols has been demonstrated in rats and mice transplantable tumors, carcinogen-induced tumors in digestive organs, mammary glands, hepatocarcinomas, lung cancers, skin tumors, leukemia, tumor promotion, and metastasis. The mechanisms of this effect indicated that the inhibition of tumors may be the result of both extracellular and intracellular mechanisms indicating the modulation of metabolism, blocking or suppression, modulation of DNA replication and repair effects, promotion, inhibition of invasion and metastasis, and induction of novel mechanisms. The association of green tea and cancer has been investigated in 8552 Japanese women 40 years of age. After 9 years of follow-up study, 384 cases of cancer were identified. There was a negative association between cancer incidence and green tea consumption, especially among females consuming more than 10 cups of tea a day. A slow down in increases of cancer incidence with age was observed among females who consumed more than 10 cups daily. Tea, taken by lung cancer patients at a dose of two or more cups per day, reduced the risk by 95%. The protected effect was more evident among Kreyberg I tumors (squamous cell and small cells) and among light smokers. The green tea polyphenols, epigallocatechin-*3*-gallate, applied topically to human skin, prevented penetration of ultraviolet (UV) radiation. This was demonstrated by the absence of immunostaining for cyclobutane pyrimidine dimers in the reticular dermis. Topical administration to the skin of mice inhibited UVB-induced infiltration of $CDIIb^{+}$ cells. The treatment also results in reduction of the UVB-induced immuno-regulatory cytokine interleukin (IL)-10 in the skin and draining lymph nodes, and an elevated amount of IL- 12 in draining lymph nodes. Green tea extract, in human umbilical vein endothelial cells, did not affect cell viability but significantly reduced cell proliferation dose-dependently and produced a dose-dependent accumulation of cells in the gastrointestinal phase. The decrease of the expression of vascular endothelial growth factor receptors fms-like tyrosine kinase and fetal liver kinase-I/kinase insert domain containing receptor in the cell culture by the extract was detected with immunohistochemical and Western blotting methods. Green and black tea, administered orally to hairless mice in the absence of any chemical initiators or promoters, resulted in significantly fewer skin papillomas and tumors induced by UVA and UVB light. Black tea however, provided better protection against UVB-induced tumors than green tea. Black tea consumption was associated with a reduction in the number of sunburn cells in the epidermis of mice 24 hours after irradiation, although there was no effect of green tea. Other indices of early damage such as necrotic cells or mitotic figures were not affected. Neutrophil infiltration as a measure of skin redness was slightly lowered by tea consumption in the UVB group. Epigallocatechin-3-gallate, in cell culture, activated proMMP-2 in U-87 glioblastoma cells in the presence of concanavalin A or cytochalasin D, two potent activators of MT1-MMP, resulted in proMMP-2 activation that was correlated with the cell surface proteolytic processing of Mt1-MMP to it's inactive 43 kDa form. Addition of epigallocatechin-3-gallate strongly inhibited the MT1-MMP-driven migration in the cells. The treatment of cells with non-cytotoxic doses of epigallocatechin-3-gallate significantly reduced the amount of secreted pro MMP-2, and led to a concomitant increase in intracellular levels of that protein. The effect was similar to that observed using well-characterized secretion inhibitors such as brefeldin A and manumycin, indicative that epigallocatechin could also potentially act on intracellular secretory pathways. Green tea polyphenols, at a dose of 30 mg/mL, inhibited the photolabeling of P-glycoprotein (P-gp) by 75% and increased the accumulation of rhodamine-123 in the multidrug-resistant cell line CH(R)C5. This result indicated that green tea polyphenols interact with P-gp and inhibited its transport activity. The modulation of P-gp was a reversible process. Epigallocatechin-3-gallate potentiates the cytotoxicity of vinblastine in CH(R)C5 cells. The inhibitory effect on P-gp was also observed in human Caco-2 cells.

Anticataract activity

Tea, administered in culture to enucleated rat lens, reduced the incidence of selenite cataract in vivo. The rat lenses were randomly divided into normal, control and treated groups and incubated for 24 hours at 37°C. Oxidative stress was induced by sodium selenite in the culture medium of the two groups (except the normal group). The medium of the treated group was additionally supplemented with tea extract. After incubation, lenses were subjected to glutathione and malondialdehyde estimation. Enzyme activity of superoxide dismutase, catalase, and glutathione peroxidase were also measured in different sets of the experiment. In vivo cataract was induced in 9-day-old rat pups of both control and treated groups by a single subcutaneous injection of sodium selenite. The treated pups were injected with tea extract intraperitoneally prior to selenite challenge and continued for 2 consecutive days thereafter. Cataract incidence was evaluated on 16 postnatal days by slit lamp examination. There was positive modulation of biochemical parameters in the organ culture study. The results indicated that tea act primarily by preserving the antioxidant defense system.

Antifungal activity

Ethanol (50%) extract of the entire plant, in broth culture at a concentration of 1 mg/mL, was inactive on *Aspergillus fumigatus* and *Trichophyton mentagrophytes*. Hot water extract of the leaf on agar plate at a concentration of 1.0% was active on *Alternaria tenuis*, *Pythium aphanidermatum*, and *Rhizopus stolonifer*. Saponin fraction of the leaf on agar plate was active on *Microsporum audonini*, minimum inhibitory concentration (MIC) 10 mg/mL; *Epidermophyton floccosum* and *Trichophyton mentagrophytes*, MICs 25 μg/ mL.

Antihypercholesterolemic activity

Tea supplemented with vitamin E, administered to male Syrian hamsters, reduced plasma low-density lipoprotein (LDL) cholesterol concentrations, LDL oxidation, and early atherosclerosis compared to the consumption of tea alone by the hamsters. The antioxidant action of vitamin E is through the incorporation of vitamin E into the LDL molecule. The hamsters were fed a semi- purified hypercholesterolemic diet containing 12% coconut oil, 3% sunflower oil, and 0.2% cholesterol (control), control and 0.625% tea, control and 1.25% tea or control and 0.044% tocopherol acetate for 10 weeks. The hamsters fed the vitamin E diet compared to the different concentrations of tea significantly lower plasma LDL cholesterol concentrations, –18% ($p < 0.007$), –17% ($p < 0.02$), and –24% ($p < 0.0001$), respectively. Aortic fatty streak areas were reduced in the vitamin E diet group compared to the control, –36% ($p < 0.04$) and low tea –45% ($p < 0.01$) diets. Lag phase of conjugated diene production was greater in the vitamin E diet compared to the control, low tea, and high tea diets, 41% ($p < 0.0004$), 40% ($p < 0.0004$), and 39% ($p < 0.0008$), respectively. Rate of conjugated diene production was reduced in the vitamin E diet compared to the control, low tea, and high tea diets, –63% ($p < 0.002$), -57% ($p < 0.005$), and –59% ($p < 0.02$), respectively. Infusion of black tea leaves was taken by 31 men (ages 47 ± 14) and 34 females (ages 35 ± 13) in a 4-week study. Six mugs of tea were taken daily vs placebo (water, caffeine, milk, and sugar) and blood lipids, bowel habit, and blood pressure measured during a run-in period and at the end weeks 2, 3, and 4 of the test period.

Compliance was established by adding a known amount of *p*-aminobenzoic acid to selected tea bags and then measure it excretion in the urine. Mean serum cholesterol values during run-in, placebo and on tea drinking were 5.67 ± 1.05, 5.76 ± 1.11, and 5.69 ± 1.09 mmol/L ($p = 0.16$). There were also no significant changes in diet, LDL-cholesterol, high-density lipoprotein (HDL) cholesterol, triacylglycerols, and blood pressure in the tea intervention period compared with placebo. Stool consistency was softened with tea compared with the placebo, and no other differences were observed in bowel habit. The results were unchanged within 15 "non-compliers" whose *p*-aminobenzoic acid excretion indicated that fewer than six tea bags had been used, were excluded from the analysis, and when differenced between run-in and tea periods were considered separately for those who were given tea first or second.

Anti-inflammatory effect

Epigallocatechin-3-gallate was shown to mimic its anti- inflammatory effects in modulating the IL-I β-induced activation of mitogen activated protein kinase in human chondrocytes. It inhibited the IL-I β-induced phosphorylation of c-Jun N-terminal kinase (JNK) isoforms, accumulation of phosphoc-Jun and DNA-binding activity of AP-1 in osteoarthritis chondrocytes, IL-I β but not epigallocatechin-3-gallate, and induced the expression of JNK p46 without modulating the expression of JNK p54 in osteoarthritis chondrocytes. In immune complex kinase assays, epigallocatechin-3-gallate completely blocked the substrate phosphorylating activity of JNK but not p38-mitogen activated protein kinase (MAPK). Epigallocatechin-3-gallate had no inhibitory effect on the activation of extracellular signal-regulated kinase p44/p42 (ERKp44/p42) or p38-MAPK in chondrocytes. Epigallocatechin-3-gallate did not alter the total nonphosphorylated levels of either p38- MAPK or ERKp44/p42 in osteoarthritis chondrocytes. Epigallocatechin-3-gallate administered to primary human osteoarthritis chondrocytes at a concentration of 100 μM in cell Culture, inhibited the IL-I β-induced production of nitric oxide by interfering with the activation of nuclear factor (NF)κB. Tea, in culture with bovine nasal and meta-carpophalangeal cartilage and human nondiseased osteoarthritis and rheumatoid cartilage with and without reagents known to accelerate cartilage matrix breakdown, produced chondroprotective effect that may be beneficial for the arthritis patient by reducing inflammation and the slowing of cartilage breakdown. Individual catechins were added to the cultures and the amount of released proteoglycan and type II collagen were measured by metachromatic assay and inhibition enzyme-linked immunosorbent assay (ELISA), respectively. Possible nonspecific or toxic effects of the catechins were assessed by lactate output and proteoglycan synthesis. Catechins, particularly those containing a gallate ester, were effective at micromolar concentrations at inhibiting proteoglycan and type II collagen breakdown.

Antimutagenic activity

The anticarcinogenic activity of tea phenols has been demonstrated in rats and mice, transplantable tumors, carcinogen-induced tumors in digestive organs, mammary glands, hepatocarcinomas, lung cancers, skin tumors, leukemia, tumor promotion, and metastasis. The mechanisms of this effect indicated that the inhibition of tumors maybe the result of both extracellular and intracellular mechanisms indicting the modulation of metabolism, blocking or suppression, modulation of DNA replication and repair effects, promotion, inhibition of invasion and Metastasis, and induction of novel mechanisms. Green and black teas, administered orally to human adults, were effective. Between 60 and 180 minutes after the teas were administered, the antimutagenic active compounds were recovered from the jejunal compartment by means of dialysis. The dialysate appeared to inhibit the mutagenicity of the food mutagen 2-amino-3,8-dimethylimidazo[4,5-f]quinoxaline on *Salmonella typhimurium*. The maximum inhibition was measured at 2 hours after administration and was comparable for black and green teas. The maximum inhibition observed with black tea was reduced by 22, 42, and 78% in the presence of whole milk, semi-skimmed milk, and skimmed milk, respectively. Whole milk and skimmed milk abolished the antimutagenic activity of green tea by more than 90% and semi- skimmed milk by more than 60%.

When a homogenized breakfast was taken with black tea, the antimutagenic activity was eliminated. When tea and mutagen 2-amino-3,8-dimethylimidazo[4,5-f]quinoxaline were added to the system, 2-amino-3,8-dimethylimidazo[4,5-f]quinoxaline mutagenicity was efficiently inhibited, with green tea showing a slightly stronger antimutagenic activity than black tea. The addition of milk had only a small inhibiting effect on the antimuta-genicity. The antimutagenic activity corresponded with reduction in antioxidant capacity and with a decrease of concentration of catechin, epigallocatechin gallate, and epigallocatechin. Chinese white tea, tested on rat liver S9 in assay for methoxyresorufin *O*-demethylase, inhibited methoxyresorufin *O*-demethylase activity and attenuated the mutagenic activity of 3 - methylimidazo [4,5-f] quinoline (IQ) in absence of S9. Nine of the major constituents found in green and white teas were mixed to produce artificial teas according to their relative levels in white and green teas.

The complete tea exhibited higher antimutagenic potency compared with the corresponding artificial tea. Green and black tea polyphenols, applied to the surfaces of ground beef before cooking, inhibited the formation of the mutagens in a dose-related fashion. Green or black tea polyphenols sharply decreased the mutagenicity of a number of aryl- and heterocyclic amines, of aflatoxin B_1, benzo[a]pyrene, 1, 2-dibromoethane, and more selectively of 2-nitropropane, all involving an induced rat liver S9 fraction. Good inhibition was found with two nitrosamines that required a hamster S9 fraction for biochemical activation. No effect was found with 1-nitropyrene and with the direct-acting (no S9) 2-chloro-4-methylthiobutanoic acid. Hot water extract on the leaf was evaluated in cell cultures on various systems vs decaffeinated and caffeinated teas. On mouse mammary gland vs decaffeinated and caffeinated teas, ICs_{50} were 10 mg/mL and 10 μg/mL on CA-A427, IC_{50} 27 mg/mL and 31 μg/mL, and on epithelial cells, IC_{50} 0.01 ng/mL and 0.3 ng/mL. Hot water extract of the leaf, on agar plate at a concentration of 1 mg/plate, was active on Salmonella typhimurium TA98 vs 2-amino-3-methylimidazo [4,5-f]quinoline-induced mutagenesis and produced weak activity vs benzo[a]pyrene-induced mutagenesis. Infusion of the leaf, on agar plate at a concentration of 0.7 mg/plate, was active on *Salmonella typhimurium* TA98 and TA100 vs 2-amino-3-methylimidazo [4,5-f]quinoline-; 3-amino-1,4-dimethyl-5H-pyrid[4,3-b]indole(Trp-1); aflatoxin B1-; 2-amino-6-methyl-dipyrido[1,2-A:3,2-d] imidazole-, and benzo[a]pyrene-induced carcinogenesis. Infusion of the leaf, on agar plate at a concentration of 50 mg/plate, was active on *Salmonella typhimurium* TA98 vs 2-amino-3-methylimidazo[4,5-f]quinoline-; 2-amino-3,4-dimethyl-imidazo[4,5-f]quinoline-;2-amino-3,8-dimethylimidazo[4,5 - f]quinoxaline-; 2-amino-1-methyl-6-phenylimidazo [4,5-b]-pyridine-;2-amino-3,7,8-trimethylimidazo[4,5-f]quinoxaline-; 2-amino-3,4,7,8-tetramethyl-3H-imidazo-[4,5-f]quinoxaline-inoxaline-; 3-amino-1,4- dimethyl-5 H-pyrid[4,3-b] indole (Trp-P-I)- and 3-amino-1-methyl-5H-pyrido [4,3-b] indole-induced mutagenesis. Metabolic activation was required for positive results.

Anti-neoplastic effect

Green tea, administered orally at a dose of 6 g per day in six doses to 42 patients who were asymptomatic and had manifested, progressive prostate specific antigen elevation with hormone therapy, produced limited antineoplastic activity. Continued use of lute inizing hormone-releasing hormone agonist was permitted. However, patients were ineligible if they had received other treatments for their disease in the preceding 4 weeks or if they had received a long-acting antiandrogen therapy in the preceding 6 weeks.

The patients were monitored monthly for response and toxicity. Tumor response, defined as a decline of 50% or greater in the baseline prostate-specific antigen (PSA) value, occurred in a single patient, or 2% of The cohort (95% confidence interval [CI], 1–14%). This one response was not sustained beyond 2 months. At the end of the first month, the median change in the PSA value from baseline for the cohort increased by 43%. Infusion of the leaf, administered in the drinking of female mice at a concentration of 1.25%, was active vs UV radiation-induced papillomas and tumors[CS172]. Leaves in the drinking water of female mice at a dose of 0.6% reduced lung tumor multiplicity and volume in 4-(methyl-nitrosamine)-1-(3-pyridyl)-1-butanone (NNK) treated mice.

Antioxidative effect

Tea, administered orally to rats, decreased the thiobarbituric acid reactive substances (TBARS) contents in urine and lowered the esterified and total cholesterol contents in plasma as compared with a control group. TBARS contents in liver, plasma, and cholesterol levels in the liver were not affected. The lower plasma cholesterol concentration could not be explained by increased fecal excretion of cholesterol or bile acids. On the other hand, a relationship between decreased plasma cholesterol and significantly higher acetate concentrations in the cecum, colon, and portal blood of rats was assumed, Copper absorption was significantly increased while iron absorption was not affected. Epigallocatechin gallate, tea polyphenols, and tea extract were added to human plasma and lipid peroxidation induced by the water-soluble radical generator 2,2'-azobis (2-amidinopropane) dihydrochloride. Following a lag phase, lipid peroxidation was initiated and it occurred at a rate that was lower in a dose that was lowered in a dose-dependent manner by the polyphenols. Similarly, epigallocatechin gallate and the extract added to plasma strongly inhibited 2,2′-azobis(2-amidinopropane) dihydrochloride-induced lipid peroxidation.

The lag phase preceding detectable lipid peroxidation was the result of the antioxidant activity of endogenous ascorbate, which was more effective at inhibiting lipid peroxidation than the tea polyphenols and was not spared by these compounds. When eight volunteers consumed the equivalent of six cups of tea, the resistance of their plasma to lipid peroxidation did not increase over a period of 3 hours. Black tea leaves, administered to human red blood cells, was effective against damage by oxidative stress induced by inducers such as phenylhydrazine, Cu^{2+}-ascorbic acid, and xanthine/xanthine oxidase systems. Lipid peroxidation of pure erythrocyte membrane and of whole red blood cell was completely prevented by black tea extract. Similarly, the tea provided total protection against degradation of membrane proteins. Membrane fluidity studies as monitored by the fluorescent probe 1,6-diphenyl-hexa-1,3,5-triene showed considerable disorganization of its architecture that could be restored back to normal on addition of black tea or free catechins.

The tea extract in comparison to free catechin seemed to be a better protecting agent against various types of oxidative stress. Ethanol/water (7:3) extract of green tea, tested on 2,2-azino-di-3-ethylbenzthiazoline sulphonate, produced antioxidant activity compared with that of ascorbic acid (10 mmol/L). The Nonpolyphenolic fraction of residual green tea (after hot water extraction) produced a significant suppression against hydroperoxide generation from oxidized linoleic acid in a dose-dependent manner. Using silica gel TLC plate, chlorophylls a and b, pheophytins a and b, β-carotene, and lutein were isolated. All of these constituents exhibited significant antioxidant activites, the ranks of suppressive activity against hydroperoxide generation were chlorophyll a > lutein > pheophytin a > chlorophyll b > b-carotene > pheophytin b.

Antiproliferative activity

Green tea fractions, tested on human stomach cancer (MK-1) cells, indicated six active flavan-3-ols, epicatechin, epigallocatechin, epigallocatechin gallate, gallocatechin, epicatechin gallate, and gallocatechin gallate. Among the six active flavan-3-ols, epigallocatechin gallate and gallocatechin gallate produced the highest activity. Epigallocatechin, gallocatechin, and epicatechin gallate followed next, and the activity of epicatechin was lowest. This suggests that the presence of the three adjacent hydroxyl groups (pyrogallol or galloyl group) in the molecule would be a key factor for enhancing the activity.

Antiviral activity

Epigallocatechin-3-gallate, administered to Hep2 cells in culture, produced a therapeutic index of 22 and an IC_{50} of 25 μM. The agent was the most effective when added to the cells during the transition from the early to the late phase of viral infection suggesting that the polyphenol inhibits one or more late steps in virus infection. Ethanol (50%) extract of the entire plant, in broth culture at a concentration of 50 μg/mL, was inactive on Raniket and Vaccinia viruses. Hot water extract of the leaf in cell culture was active on Coxsackie A9, B1, B2, B3, B4, and B6 viruses, Echo type 9 virus, herpes simplex virus, poliovirus III, vaccinia virus, and REO type 1 virus.

Anti-yeast activity

Ethanol (50%) extract of the entire plant, in broth culture at a concentration of 1 mg/mL, was inactive on *Candida albicans*, *Cryptococcus neoformans*, and *Sporotrichum schenckii*. Ethanol extract of the leaf on agar plate produced MIC 9.3 mg/mL on *Candida albicans*.

Cytochrome P50 expression

Fresh leaves of green, black, and decaffeinated black tea enhanced lauric acid hydroxylation. The decaffeinated black tea produced no significant effect. Green tea and black tea but not decaffeinated black tea, stimulated the *O*-dealkylations of methoxy-, ethoxy-, and pentoxy-resorufin indicating upregulation of cytochrome P50 (CYP) 1A and CYP2B. Immunoblot analysis revealed that green and black tea, but not decaffeinated black tea, elevated the hepatic CYP1A2 apoprotein levels. Hepatic microsomes from green and black tea-treated rats, but not those from the decaffeinated black tea-treated rats, were more effective than controls in converting IQ into mutagenic species in the Ames test.

Dental enamel erosion

Herbal tea and conventional black tea, tested on teeth, resulted in erosion of dental enamel. After exposure to tea, sequential profilometric tracings of the specimens were taken, superimposed, and the degree of enamel loss calculated as the area of disparity between the tracings before and after exposure. Tooth surface loss resulted from herbal tea (mean 0.05 mm^2) was significantly greater than that which resulted from exposure to conventional black tea (0.01 mm^2), and water (0.00 mm^2). Tannin, catechin, caffeine, and tocopherol, tested in vitro on tooth enamel, demonstrated that these components possess the property of increasing the acid resistance of tooth enamel. The effects increased dramatically when the components were used in combination with fluoride. A mixture of tannic acid and fluoride showed the highest inhibitory effect (98%) on calcium release to an acid solution. Tannin in combination with fluoride inhibited the formation of artificial enamel lesions in comparison with acidulated phosphate fluoride (APF) as determined by electron probe microanalysis, polarized-light microscopy, and Vickers microhardness measurement.

DNA effect

Green tea extract, in cell culture at a dose of 10 mg/L corresponding to 15 mmol/L EGCg for 24 hours, did not protect Jurkat cells against H_2O_2-induced DNA damage. The DNA damage, evaluated by the Comet assay, was dose-dependent. However, it reached plateau at 75 mmol/L of H_2O_2 without any protective effect exerted by the extract. The DNA repair process, completed within 2 hours, was unaffected by supplementation.

Fluoride retention

Tea, used as a mouth rinse, demonstrated strong avidity of enamel for tea and salivary pellicle components. Thirty-four percent of the fluoride was retained in the oral cavity. Differences in retention at the tooth surface in the presence and absence of an acquired pellicle were not statistically significant at incisor or molar sites. Fluoride from tea showed strong binding to enamel particles, which was only partially dissociated by solutions of ionic strength considerably greater than that of saliva.

Gastrointestinal effect

Green tea, administered to rats fasted for 3 days, reverted to normal the mucosal and villous atrophy induced by fasting. Black tea ingestion had no effect. Ingestion of black tea, green tea, and vitamin E before fasting protected the intestinal mucosa against atrophy. Characterization of melanin extracted from tea leaves proved similarity of the original compound to standard melanin. The Langmuir adsorption isotherms for gadolinium (Gd) binding were obtained using melanin. Melanin–Gd preparation demonstrated low acute toxicity. LD_{50} for the preparation was in a range of 1.25–1.50 g/kg in mice.

Magnetic resonance imaging (MRI) properties of melanin itself and melanin-Gd complexes have been estimated. Gadolinium-free melanin fractions possess slighter relaxivity compared with its complexes. The relaxivity of lower molecular weight fraction was 2 times higher than relaxivity of Gd(DTPA) standard. Postcontrast images demonstrated that oral administration of melanin complexes in concentration of 0.1 m*M* provides essential enhancement to longitudinal relaxation times (T[1])-weighted spin echo image. The required contrast and delineation of the stomach wall demonstrated uniform enhancement of MRI with proposed melanin complex.

Hypocholesterolemic effect

Green tea, in human HepG2 cell culture, increased both LDL receptor-binding activity and protein. The ethyl acetate extract, containing 70% (w/w) catechins, also increased LDL receptor-binding activity, protein, and mRNA, indicating that the effect was at the receptor level of gene transcription and that the catechins were the active constituents. The mechanism by which green tea upregulated the LDL receptor was investigated. Green tea decreased the cell cholesterol concentration (–30%) and increased the conversion of the sterol-regulated element binding protein (SREBP-1) from the inactive precursor form to the active transcription-factor form. Consistent with this, the mRNA of 3-hydroxy-3-methylglutaryl coenzyme-A reductase, the rate limiting enzyme in cholesterol synthesis, was also increased by green tea.

Immunomodulatory effect

To determine the effects of tea on transplant-related immune function in vitro lymphocyte proliferation tests using phytohemagglutinin, mixed lymphocytes culture assay, IL-2, and IL-10 production from mixed lymphocyte proliferation were performed. Tea had immunosuppressive effects and decreased alloresponsiveness in the culture. The immuno-suppressive effect of tea was mediated through a decrease in IL-2 production. Tea, assayed in cell culture, enhanced neopterin production in unstimulated peripheral mononuclear cells, whereas an effective reduction of neopterin formation in cells stimulated with concanavalin A, phytohemagglutinin or interferon (IFN)-γ was observed. Theaflavins potently suppressed IL-2 secretion, IL-2 gene expression, and the activation of NF-κB in murine spleens enriched for CD4(+) T-cells. Theaflavins also inhibited the induction of IFN-γ mRNA. However, the expression of the T(H2) cytokines IL-4 and IL-5, which lack functional NF-κB sites within their promoters was unexpectedly suppressed by theaflavins as well.

Insulin-enhancing effect

Tea, as normally consumed, was shown to increase insulin activity more than 15-fold in vitro in an epididymal fat cell assay. The majority of the insulin-potentiating activity for green and oolong teas was owing to epigallocatechin gallate. For black tea, the activity was present in addition to epigallocatechin gallate, tannins, theaflavins, and other undefined compounds. Several known compounds found in tea were shown to enhance insulin with the greatest activity due to epigallocatechin gallate followed by epicatechin gallate, tannins, and theaflavins. Caffeine, catechin, and epicatechin displayed insignificant insulin-enhancing activities. Addition of lemon to the tea did not affect the insulin-potentiating activity. Addition of 5 g of 2% milk per cup decreased the insulin-potentiating activity one-third, and addition of 50 g of milk per cup decreased the insulin-potentiating activity approx 90%. Non-dairy creamers and soymilk also decreased the insulin-potentiating activity.

Iron absorption

Tea, administered by gastric intubation to rats, did not affect iron absorption when tea was consumed for 3 days but when delivered in tea the absorption was decreased. Rats maintained on a commercial diet were fasted overnight with free access to water and then gavaged with 1 mL of ^{59}Fe labeled FeCl3 (0.1 m*M* or 1 m*M*) and lactulose (0.5 *M*) in water or black tea. Iron absorption was estimated from Fe retention. Intestinal permeability was evaluated by lactulose excretion in the urine. Iron absorption was lower with given with tea at both iron concentrations but tea did not affect lactulose excretion.

Lipid peroxidation activity

Solubilized green tea, administered orally to rats for 5 weeks, reduced lipid peroxidation products. The treatment produced increased activity of glutathione (GSH) peroxidase and GSH reductase, increased content of reduced GSH, a marked decrease in lipid hydroperoxides and malondialdehyde in the liver, an increase in the concentration of vitamin A by about 40%. A minor change in the measured parameters was observed in the blood serum. GSH content increased slightly, whereas the index of the total antioxidant status increased significantly. In contrast, the lipid peroxidation products, particularly malondialdehyde, was significantly diminished. In the central nervous tissue, the activity of superoxide dismutase and glutathione peroxidase decreased, whereas the activity of GSH reductase and catalase increased after drinking green tea. Moreover, the level of lipid hydroperoxides, 4-hydroksynonenal, and malondialdehyde decreased significantly[CS036].

Neuromuscular-blocking action

Thearubigin fraction of black tea was investigated for neuro-muscular-blocking action of botulinum neurotoxin types A, B, and E in the mouse phrenic nerve-diaphragm preparations. On binding, A (1.5 n*M*), B (6 n*M*), and E (5 n*M*) abolished indirect twitches within 50, 90, and 90 minutes, respectively. Thearubigin fraction mixed with each toxin protected against the neuromuscular-blocking action of botulinum neurotoxin types A, B, and E by binding with the toxins.

Oral submucousal fibrosis effect

Tea, administered orally to 39 patients with oral submucous fibrosis, indicated that the treatment was effective for patients with abnormal hemorheology. The patients were divided into control and experimental groups. The control group included 22 oral submucous fibrosis patients who were treated by oral administration of vitamins A and D, vitamin B complex, and vitamin E. The experimental group included 17 patients who were treated with vitamins and tea pigment after their examination of hemorheology. The results showed that 7 of 12 patients in the experimental group with abnormal hemorheology had average 7.9 mm improvement on the open degree (58.3%), and the open degree of the other five patients whose hemorheology was normal only increased 2 mm (20%). The therapeutical results of the experimental group (58.3%) were significantly better than that of the control group (13.6%) ($p < 0.005$).

P-glycoprotein activity

Green tea polyphenols (30 μg/mL) inhibited the photo-labeling of P-gp by 75% and increased the accumulation of rhodamine-123 threefold in a multidrug-resistant cell line CH(R)C5, indicating that the polyphenols interact with P-gp and inhibit its transport activity. The modulation of P-gp transport by polyphenols was a reversible process.

Photoprotection effect

Tea extracts, administered topically, produced a dose- dependent inhibition of the erythema response evoked by UV radiation. The (–)- epigallocatechin-3-gallate and (–)-epicatechin-3 -gallate polyphenolic fractions were most efficient at inhibiting erythema, whereas (–)-epigallocatechin and (–)-epicatechin had little effect. On histological examination, skin treated with the extracts reduced the number of sunburn cells and protected epidermal Langerhans cells from UV damage. The extract also reduced damage that formed after UV radiation. Green tea polyphenols, applied topically to the human skin, prevented UVB-induced cyclobutane pyrimidine dimers, which are considered to be mediators of UVB-induced immune suppression and skin cancer induction. The treatment, prior to exposure to UVB, protected against UVB-induced local as well as systemic immune suppression in laboratory animals. Additionally, treatment of mouse skin inhibited UVB-induced infiltration of CD11b cells. CD11b is a cell-surface marker for activated macrophages and neutrophils, which are associated with induction of UVB-induced suppression of contact hypersensitivity responses. The treatment also resulted in reduction of the UVB-induced immunoregulatory cytokine IL-10 in skin as well as in draining lymph nodes, and an elevated amount of IL-12 in draining lymph nodes.

Protease inhibition

Epigallocatechin-3-gallate, in cell culture at a concentration of 100 μM, reduced virus yield by 2 orders of magnitude producing an IC_{50} of 25 μM and a therapeutic index of 22 in Hep2 cells. The agent was the most effective when added to the cells during the transition from the early to the late phase of viral infection, suggesting that it inhibited one or more late steps in virus infection. One of these steps appears to be virus assembly, because the titer of infectious virus and the production of physical particles were much more affected than the synthesis of virus proteins. Another step might be the maturation cleavages carried out by adenain. When tested on adenain, epigallocatechin-3-gallate produced an IC_{50} of 109 μM.

Radical scavenging activity

Green tea, evaluated using the 1,1-diphenyl-2-picrylhydrazyl radical, indicated that the galloyl moiety showed more potent activity. The contribution of the pyrogallol moiety in the B-ring to the scavenging activity seemed to be less than that of the galloyl moiety.

Tetanus toxin protection

Thearubigin fraction of black tea was investigated for neuromuscular-blocking action on tetanus toxin in the mouse phrenic nerve-diaphragm preparations and on binding of this toxin to the synaptosomal membrane preparations of rat cerebral cortices. Tetanus toxin (4 μg/mL) abolished indirect twitches in the mouse phrenic nerve–diaphragm preparations within 150 minutes. Thearubigin fraction mixed with tetanus toxin blocked the inhibitory effect of the toxin.

Toxicity

Green tea, administered orally at a dose of 6 g per day in six doses to 42 patients who were asymptomatic and had manifested, progressive prostate specific antigen elevation with hormone therapy, produced grade 1 or 2 toxicity in 69% of the patients and included nausea, emesis, insomia, fatigue, diarrhea, abdominal pain, and confusion. However, six episodes of grade 3 toxicity and one episode of grade 4 toxicity also occurred, with the latter manifesting as severe confusion.

Toxicity assessment

Ethanol (50%) extract of the entire plant, administered intraperitoneally to mice produced lethal dose $(LD)_{50}$ 316 mg/kg. Ethanol (95%) extract of the leaf, administered by gastric intubation to mice, produced LD_{50} 10 g/kg. Intraperitoneal administration produced CD_{90} 0.7 g/kg.

Cocos nucifera

Cocos nucifera is an unbranched monoecious plant of the *Palmae* family. It grows to 30 m tall, with a crown of 25–35 paripinnate leaves, producing 12–16 new leaves per year. There is a central bud, which if cut off, leads to the death of tree. The trunk is straight or gently curved, with marked foliar scars, 30–50 cm in diameter, rises from a thickened base, and increases in height at a decreasing rate with age. The leaves are horizontal or somewhat hanging, 4–8 m in length and divided. Segments of leaves are numerous, linear-lanceolate, 0.5–1 m long and tapering. In the axil of each leaf is a spathe enclosing a long, stout, straw, or an orange-colored spadix. The spadix is composed of up to

40 branches, each bearing up to 300 small, fragrant, male flowers, and a few female, 2 cm long, globose flowers. The male and female flowers are produced separately in the leaf axils, usually on a long stalk. Approximately one-third of the female flowers develop into four to eight ripe fruits in 12–13 months, per inflorescence. The fruit is ovoid, three-angled drupe, up to 30 cm long, usually with thick, fibrous mesocarp (husk) and a hard, green-brown endocarp (shell) enclosing one seed. The seeds consist of 10 to 20 mm-thick white, fleshy endosperm (meat), covered by thin brown testa, surrounding a cavity party filled with a watery, sweet fluid (coconut water or milk). The latter is found mainly in immature fruits.

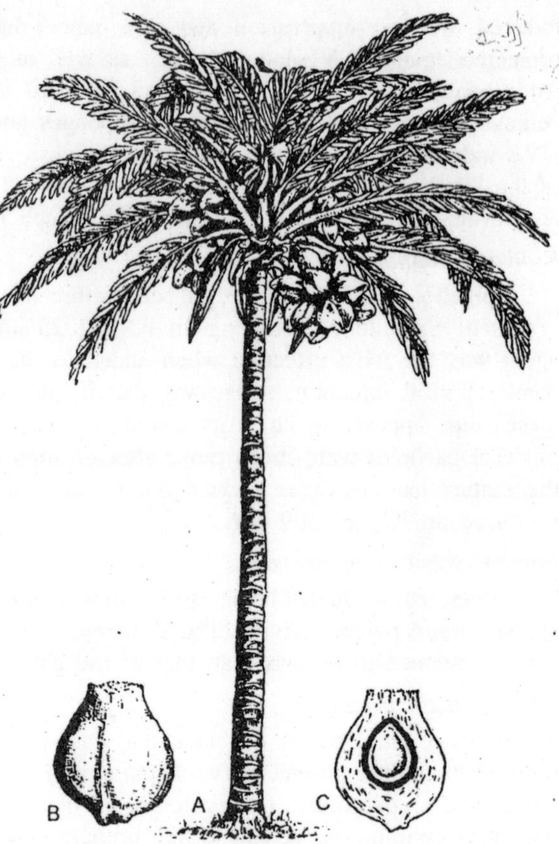

Fig. 17.11. Cocos nucifera. A–Plant a fruiting stage; B–Fruit (entire); C–Fruit (L.S.).

Origin and distribution

Evidence has been found that the place of origin is "submerged land to the north west of New Guinea." The major coconut areas lie between 20°N and 20°S of the equator. Although it is found beyond this region, 27° N and 27° S, cultivation has not been successful and the palm does not fruit. Many varieties are found in Melanesian region. It is most widely cultivated in the tropics: India, Ceylon, Malaysia, Indonesia, Philippines, South Sea Islands in the Pacific, East Africa, and Central and South Americas, up to 800 m above sea level, on humus-rich and porous soil or pure sand in coastal regions.

Traditional uses

Admiralty islands. The young root or leaves of the coconut plant are chewed for diarrhea.

Cook islands. Water extract of grated endosperm and *Citrus aurantium* juice is used to soak affected part in fractures and sprains. Endosperm is taken orally for asthenia. Oil, mixed with crushed *Phyllanthus virgatus*, is rubbed around the ear for ear infections. Extract of different dried parts of the palm are taken orally for filariasis. A water solution of the crushed dried bark or husk and grated bark of *Hibiscus tiliaceus* is used externally to soak fractures and sprains. Crushed aerial root tips of *Ficus prolixa* are fried with coconut cream made of fresh endosperm, and the resulting oil is taken orally as a laxative in treating serious diseases.

Fiji. Oil is used externally to prevent hair loss. The oil is warmed with crushed onion and garlic and applied aurally for earache. Water of the unripe fruit is taken orally for kidney problems.

Ghana. Coconut milk is taken orally for diarrhea.

Guatemala. Hot water extract of the dried fruit is taken orally as a febrifuge and sudorific and for renal inflammation and scrofula. Hot water extract of the dried fruit is applied externally on wounds, ulcers, bruises, sores, skin infections, mucosa, dermatitis, inflammations, abscesses, and furuncles.

Haiti. Decoction of the dried pericarp is taken orally for amenorrhea. Fresh essential oil is applied externally on burns.

India. Infusion of the inflorescence is taken orally every morning for 3 days, coinciding with the menstrual cycle for leukorrhea and problems associated with the menstrual cycle. A dose of 50 g daily of a mixture of *Cocos nucifera* fruit and *Ficus-benghalensis* latex is taken for 3 months to increase sexual potency in men. Fruit is taken orally as a remedy for tapeworms.

Indonesia. Coconut oil is applied externally to treat wounds and injuries by the ethnic group of Ngada. Shell is used as incense. Hot water extract of the root is taken orally for fever, bloody diarrhea, and dysentery. Milk is taken orally by adults for poisoning. Fruit milk is taken orally by females as a contraceptive. Fruit juice is believed to diminish libido or fertility. Seed oil with lemon juice and various tree roots is taken orally as an abortifacient. Fruit ointment is applied externally for swollen legs. Fresh flowers, chewed with *Borassus flbellifer*, are used for gonorrhea.

Jamaica. Hot water extract of the dried shell is taken orally for diabetes. Hot water extract of the root, with seven other plants, wine, and rum, is used as a tonic. Extract of different parts are taken orally for diabetes.

Marquesas islands. Fruit juice is mixed with *Cordia subcordata* and other plants and used for general menstrual disorders.

Mexico. A plaster made of fresh milk mixed with egg white is applied externally to prevent miscarriage.

Mozambique. Fruit is eaten by males as an aphrodisiac and used for relief of tumors.

Papua New Guinea. The fresh root of a young coconut is dug out and washed, then chewed and swallowed to relieve stomachache. Fruit milk of *Cocos nucifera* is taken orally together with leaves of *Cleroden* sp., *Pouzolzia microhylla*, or *Macaranga tanarius* by pregnant women as an abortifacient agent.

Peru. Hot water extract of the fresh fruit is taken orally for blennorrhagia and asthma and as a diuretic, tenifuge, and galactagogue.

Thailand. Hot water extract of the fresh fruit juice is taken orally as a cardiotonic and neurotonic.

Tonga. Infusion of fresh kernel of coconut and Euodia hortensis are taken orally to treat retention of blood clots in the uterus after childbirth (locally called "toka-ala"). A mixture of *Cocos nucifera*, *Glochidion concolor*, *Vigna marina*, *Morinda citrifolia*, *Euodia hortensis*, and *Premna taitensis* with lemon juice is taken orally by pregnant women to treat severe bleeding during early pregnancy. Infusion of fresh kernel, taken twice daily with "tongan oil" prepared from *Aleurites moluccana* is used for dysuria caused by "kahi," a locally described syndrome affecting the gastrointestinal and genitourinary systems.

Trinidad. Hot water extract of the root is taken orally for amenorrhea.

Vanuatu. Hot water extract of the fruit, drunk in large quantities when very hot, is said to induce abortion. Juice of the crushed root mixed with water is drank after delivery to restore strengh.

West Indies. Hot water extract of the root is taken orally for amenorrhea. Hot water extract of the mesocarp is taken orally by females for dysmenorrhea, amenorrhea, and menorrhagia.

Medicinal uses

Acquired immunodeficiency syndrome activity

Coconut oil and "monolaurin"—a coconut oil byproduct—were administered to 12 women and 3 men who were in the early stage of human immunodeficiency virus infection. Ten patients took different doses of monolaurin, and five patients took coconut oil. It was believed that the treatment would lead to higher CD4 counts and a lower viral load. The trial was abandoned because it received only lukewarm approval from the government.

Allergenic activity

Dried fruit juice, administered intraperitoneally to guinea pigs at a dose of 10 mL/animal, was active. Dried fruit juice, administered intravenously to guinea pigs at a dose of 5 mL/animal, was active[CN036]. A patient with coconut anaphylaxis was confirmed by skin prick test. In vitro serum specific immunoglobulin E (IgE) was present. Two patients with allergy manifested by life-threatening systemic reaction after consumption of coconut were investigated. Sera IgE from both patients indicated reduced coconut allergens with molecular weight of 35 and 36.5 kDa. IgE from 1 patient also bound a 55-kDa antigen. Preabsorption of sera with nut extracts suppressed IgE binding to coconut proteins. Preabsorption of sera with coconut produced a disappearance of IgE binding to protein bands at 35 and 36 kDa on a reduced immunoblot of walnut protein extract in one patient and suppression of IgE binding to a protein at 36 kDa in another patient. Three cases of individuals allergic to cocamide diethanolamide were investigated. In two of the cases, multiple other cutaneous allergies were present. In both instances, cocamide diethanolamide was present in several personal care products used by the patients. In the third case, occupational exposure was suspected.

Coconut diethanolamide, administered to six patients with occupational contact dermatitis caused by coconut diethanolamide, produced sensitization from a barrier cream in two patients, hand-washing liquid in three, and one had been exposed to a hand-washing liquid and to a metalworking fluid containing coconut diethanolamide. Leave-on products (hand-protection foams) produced sensitization more rapidly (2–3 months) than rinse-off products (5–7 years). There was no contact allergy to another coconut-oil-derived sensitizer (cocamidopropyl betaine). Coconut diethanolamide, administered to a dentist, produced an occupational allergic contact dermatitis for hand-washing liquids. Pollen extract, administered to 24 patients with allergy, asthma, and rhinitis produced positive skin prick test in all cases, and 19 of them were phadezym radioallergosorbent test-positive. Bronchial provocation test was positive in seven out of eight patients, and no late response or nonspecific reactions were observed. An 8-month-old baby fed from birth with maternal milk was investigated. The first milk induced a severe gastrointestinal disorder, which disappeared when second milk was used. The third milk caused a relapse.

The allergen was coconut, which was physicochemically modified in the second milk. It was confirmed by positive reintroduction test, positive skin test, and positive specific IgE test. Pollen extract immunotherapy was studied in 96 allergic patients for 6–12 months. The clinical status measured by the symptom-medication scores demonstrated that the patients had significant clinical improvement after pollen extract immunotherapy. Serological study indicated a significant reduction of specific IgE and elevation of specific IgG in posttherapeutic patients' sera. There was no correlation between symptom-mediation scores and changes in specific serum IgE or IgG levels. Proteins from fresh coconut and commercial extracts of coconut, administered to a patient with coconut anaphylaxis, produced a positive skin prick test. In vitro serum-specific IgE was present for coconut, hazelnut, Brazil nut, and cashew. Immunoblots demonstrated IgE binding to 35- and 50-kDa protein bands in the coconut and hazelnut extracts. Inhibition assays using coconut demonstrated complete inhibition of hazelnut specific IgE, but inhibition assays using hazelnut showed only partial inhibition of coconut-specific IgE. A total of 100 patients (59 females and 41 males, aged 10–59 years, mean age 27.9 years) with allergic rhinitis underwent a skin prick test with 30 aeroallergens.

Coconut produced 12% of positive results. Oil, administered to 3-lactoglobulin-treated brown Norway rats at a dose of 10% of diet supplemented with 0.5% curcumin for 3 weeks, lowered the circulatory release of rat chymase II in response to antigen. The triethanolamine (TEA) salt of the condensation product of coconut fatty acids with a complex of polypeptides and amino acids derived from collagen (TEA-Coco-hydrolyzed protein), administered to a 21-year-old woman, produced a severe dermatitis of the face after using a proprietary skin cleanser. Patch testing revealed delayed hypersensitivity to TEA-Coco-hydrolyzed protein but not to other ingredients of the cleanser and positive results with other condensates of fatty acids and protein hydrolysates.

Aminopeptidase activity influence

Oil, administered to mice testis using acrylamides as substrates, produced no difference in soluble glutamyl-aminopeptidase angiotensin among the groups tested. Soluble aspartyl-AP and soluble pyroglutamyl-AP progressively decreased with the degree of saturation of the fatty acids used in the diet. Membrane-bound glutamyl-AP progressively increased with the degree of saturation of the fatty acids used in the diet. For membrane-bound aspartyl-AP activity, mice that were fed diets containing fish oil showed significantly higher levels than those fed sunflower oil, olive oil, and lard, but not those fed coconut oil.

Antibacterial activity

Ethanol (50%) extracts of the leaf, on agar plate at concentrations above 25 μg/mL, were inactive on *Bacillus subtilis*, *Escherichia coli*, *Salmonella typhosa*, and *Staphylococcus aureus*. Tincture of the dried fruit (10 g plant material in 100 mL ethanol), on agar plate at a concentration of 30 μL/disc, was inactive on *Pseudomonas aeruginosa* and *Staphylococcus aureus* and produced weak activity on *Escherichia coli*. Water extract of the husk fiber and fractions from adsorption chromatography were active on *Staphylococcus aureus*. Hydrogenated oil, administered orally to Balb/c mice at a dose of 20% by weight for 4 wk and then infected with *Listeria monocytogenes* or treated with *N*-acetyl-L-cysteine (25 mg/mL intraperitoneally), produced no effect on survival. *N*-acetyl-L-cysteine reduced the recovery of *Listeria monocytogenes* from the spleen of the mice fed coconut oil diet. There was a reduction in lymphocyte proliferation. An important increase in the production of reactive oxygen species was found after 12 h of the incubation with *Listeria monocytogenes*. Hydrogenated oil, administered to *Listeria monocytogenes*-infected mice, produced a significant increase in peritoneal cells of coconut oil-fed mice and a reduction of bacterial recovery from the spleen. Oil, administered to mice injected with a nonlethal dose of *Escherichia coli* at a dose of 20% by weight for 5 weeks, produced a decrease of peak plasma tumor necrosis factor (TNF)-α, interleukin (IL)-1β, and IL-6 concentrations. Peak plasma IL-10 concentrations were higher in the coconut-fed group than in those fed the other diets, coconut oil diminished production of proinflammatory cytokines in vivo.

Anticarcinogenic effect

Coconut cake, administered to rat with 1,2-dimethylhydrazine-induced colon cancer at a dose of 25% of diet for 30 weeks, produced a significant decrease of the incidence and number of tumors, and β-glucuronidase and mucinase activities. Hydrogenated oil, administered to Wistar female rats at doses of 8% and 24%, with or without a 24 mg/day/rat phytosterol supplement, produced no significant influence. Colonic glands were found in area of lymphoid follicles in all the groups but were more frequently in rats on high-fat diet.

Antifungal activity

Ethanol (50%) extract of the leaf, on agar plate at a concentration of 25 μg/mL or more, was inactive on *Microsporum canis* and *Trichophyton mentagrophytes*. Oil, on agar plate at a concentration of 05 mL/plate, was active on *Absidia corymbifera*, *Aspergillus flavus*, *Aspergillus niger*, and *Penicillium nigricans*. Ethanol (95%) extract of the dried shell, on agar plate at a concentration of 100 μg/mL, was active on *Microsporum audouini*, *Microsporum canis*, *Microsporum gypseum*, *Trichophyton mentagrophytes*, *Trichophyton rubrum*, *Trichophyton tonsurans*, *Trichophyton violaceum*, and *Epidermophyton floccosum*. All fractions of the husk fiber, from adsorption chromatography, were inactive on *Candida albicans*, *Fonsecaea pedrosoi*, and *Cryptococcus neoformans*.

Antihypercholesterolemic activity

Oil was administered orally to male Wistar rats at doses of 12 or 24% of diet *ad libitum* for 4 weeks. Absorption of oleic acid in rats fed 24% oil was significantly greater than in controls during 0–8 hours but was not significantly different during 0–24 hours. There were no differences among groups in the distribution of cholesterol and oleic acid either in the lymph lipoproteins or in the lipid classes.

Oil was administered to 61 healthy males and 22 females aged 20–34 years, group I received a coconut–palm–coconut dietary sequence; group II, coconut–corn–coconut; group III, coconut oil during all three 5-week dietary periods. Compared with entry-level values, coconut oil raised the serum total cholesterol concentration greater than 10% in all three groups. The entry level of the ratio of low-density lipoprotein (LDL) to high-density lipoprotein (HDL) was not altered by coconut oil. Oil was administered to 6- month-old ovariectomized rats with or without taurine for 28 days. Body mass gain, food intake, liver weight, and plasma apoliprotein (apo) A-I, apo B, LDL, and very low-density lipoprotein (VLDL) concentrations were not affected by the diet. Taurine lowered the plasma total cholesterol and increased liver total lipid and triglyceride in rats that were fed corn oil but not in those fed coconut oil. Taurine increased the 3 -hydroxy-3-methylglutaryl coenzyme A (HMG-CoA) reductase messenger (m)RNA level in the liver of coconut-fed rats, but not in those fed corn oil. Structured lipids (10%) synthesized from oil triglycerides, coconut oil, and coconut oil–safflower oil blends (1:0.7 w/w) were administered to rats for 60 days. The structured lipids lowered serum and liver cholesterol levels. Most of the decrease observed in serum was found in LDL fraction. Oil, administered orally to male Wistar rats at a dose of 11% w/w for 6 months, produced a significant increase of serum total cholesterol (twofold), serum triglycerides (92.6%), LDL cholesterol (92.3%), and body weight gain (2.8-fold).

Antilipidemic activity

Triglycerides structured lipids from coconut oil, administered to rats at a dose of 10% of diet for 60 days, produced a 15% decrease in total cholesterol and a 23% decrease in LDL cholesterol levels in the serum compared to coconut oil-fed rats. Total and free cholesterol levels in the liver of structured lipid-fed rats were lowered by 31 and 36%, respectively. The triglycerides in the serum and liver were decreased by 14 and 30%, respectively.

Anti-nociceptive activity

Aqueous extract of the husk fiber, administered orally to mice at doses of 200 or 400 mg/kg, produced an inhibition of the acetic acid- induced writhing response.

Antioxidant activity

Aqueous extract of the husk fiber, in cell culture, was active vs 2,2-diphenyl-1 -picryl-hydrazyl-hydrate radicals. Juice, in cell culture, was active vs 1,1 -diphenyl-2-picrylhydrazyl, 2,2'-azino-*bis*(3-ethylbenz-thiazoline-6-sulfonic acid) and superoxide radicals but promoted the production of hydroxyl radicals and increased lipid peroxidation. The activity was most significant for fresh samples and diminished significantly when heated or treated with acid, alkali, or dialysis. Maturity of coconut drastically decreased the scavenging activity. Juice protected hemoglobin from nitrite-induced oxidation when added before the autocatalytic stage of the oxidation. Acid, alkali, or heat-treated or dialyzed juice showed a decreased ability in protecting hemoglobin from oxidation.

Antiparasitic activity

Polyphenolic-rich extract of the husk fiber, in cell culture at a concentration of 10 μg/mL, produced a reduction approx 44% of the association index between peritoneal mouse macrophages and *Leishmania amazonensis* promastigotes. It inhibited the growth of promastigote and amastigote developmental stages after 60 minutes. There was a concomitant increase of 182% in nitric oxide production by the infected macrophage in comparison to nontreated macrophages.

Antiproteinemic effect

Hydrogenated oil was administered orally to rats fed a protein- deficient diet at a dose of 200 g casein and 50 g coconut oil or 20 g casein and 50 g coconut oil for 28 days. The treatments produced a low concentration of protein and triacylglycerol (in serum VLDL, LDL–HDL 1 and 2–3), of cholesterol (in LDL–HDL1), and of phospholipids (in VLDL) in the protein-deficient groups. Relative amounts of linoleic and arachidonic acids in phospholipids of VLDL and HDL 2–3 were also lowered in the 20 g casein and 50 g coconut oil group. Coconut fat, administered to rats, produced an increase in plasma esterase-1 activity. Oil, administered to male Wistar rats at doses of 20% casein and 5% coconut oil or 2% casein and 5% coconut oil for 28 days, produced low concentration of protein, triacylglycerol, and VLDL in the plasma of 2% casein and 5% coconut oil group. Malondialdehyde content of the 2% casein and 5% coconut oil group was significantly higher than of control group. The lowest level of malondialdehyde was observed in the coconut oil group.

Anti-yeast activity

Tincture of the dried fruit, on agar plate at a concentration of 30 μL/disc, was inactive on *Candida albicans*. Extract of 10 g plant material in 100 mL ethanol was used. Ethanol (50%) extract of the leaf, at a concentration of 25 μg/mL or more, was inactive on *Candida albicans* and *Cryptococcus neoformans*. Seed oil, on agar plate at a concentration of 0.05 mL, was active on *Candida albicans*.

Apo B synthesis

Oil, administered to 1-month-old calves fed on a conventional milk replacer containing coconut oil, produced a twofold lower concentrations of total (^{35}S) proteins, (^{35}S) albumin, and (^{35}S) apo B in liver cells than in beef tallow-fed calves. The total amount of proteins secreted (including albumin) was similar in both groups. The amount of VLDL-(^{35}S) apo secreted was twofold lower in coconut oil-fed group. Oil, administered to rabbits at a dose of 14% of the diet for 4 weeks, produced an increase in HDL-cholesterol (C) level from 170 to 250% over chow-fed control, with peak differences occurring at 1 week. Plasma apo A-I levels were also increased from 160 to 180%. After 4 weeks, there was no difference in plasma VLDL-C or LDL-C levels in the both groups. Hepatic level of apo A-I mRNA was increased in the coconut-fed groups. Treatment of cultured rabbit liver cells and sera with various saturated fatty acids did not alter apo A-I mRNA levels as observed in vivo.

Atherosclerotic influence

Oil was administered orally to rabbits fed a semipurified, cholesterol-free atherogenic diet at a dose of 14% fat: coconut oil (CNO), corn oil (CO), palm kernel oil (PO), and cocoa butter (CB). Serum cholesterol levels (mg/dL) at 9 months were CO, 64; PO, 436; CB, 220; and CNO, 474. HDL cholesterol (%) was CO, 37; PO, 8.6; CB, 25; and CNO, 7. average artherosclerosis (arch + thoracic/ 2) was CO, 0.15; PO, 1.28; CB, 0.53; and CNO, 1.60. Oil, administered to British Halflop rabbits at a dose of 3% of the diet, produced an increase of cholesterol, triacylglycerol, apo B, apo C-III, and apo E as compared to chow-fed rabbits.

The apo A level did not differ from the chow-fed rabbits. There was a decrease in the low fractional catabolic rate of LDL-C. Oil, administered with cholesterol (30 g/kg) to male golden Syrian hamsters at a dose of 150 g/kg of diet, developed lipid-rich lesions in the ascending aorta and aortic arch after 4 weeks. The lesions continued to progress throughout the next 8 weeks. Removal of cholesterol from the diet halted this progression. Oil, administered without supplemental cholesterol in the same dose for 16 weeks, doubled the size of lesions in the ascending aorta and decreased linearly the lesion size in the aortic arch.

Blood pressure effect

Fruit juice, administered intravenously by infusion to dogs at a dose of 3 mL/minute for 100 minutes, was active. Initial effect was a decrease in blood pressure. Oil, administered to male weanling rats at a dose of 10% of diet for 5 weeks, produced significantly higher blood pressure than other groups. Systolic blood pressure was found related to the dietary intakes of saturated and unsaturated fatty acids. Prenatal exposure of the rats to a maternal low-protein diet abolished the hypertensive effect of the coconut oil diet.

Butyryl cholinesterase activity

Oil was administered to rats at different doses with or without clofibrate for 15 days. The hypolipidemic action of clofibrate was not influenced by the amount of fat. Clofibrate did not affect lower cholesterol concentration in rats fed the low fat diet, but it counteracted the rise in liver cholesterol seen in rats fed the high-fat diet. The high-fat diet produced slightly higher levels of butyryl cholinesterase in the small intestine but markedly raised intestinal esterase-1 activity.

Carcinogenic activity

Coconut oil acid diethanolamine condensate in ethanol was administered externally to 10 male and 10 female F344/N rats at doses of 25, 50, 100, 200, or 400 mg/kg body weight five times per week for 14 weeks. All of the rats survived the study. Final mean body weights and body weight gains of the 200 and 400 mg/kg males and females were significantly less than those of the controls. Clinical findings included irritation of the skin at the site of application in the 100, 200, and 400 mg/kg males and females. Cholesterol concentrations were significantly decreased in 200 and 400 mg/kg males. Histopathological lesions of the skin at the site of application included epidermal hyperplasia, sebaceous gland hyperplasia, chronic active inflammation, parakeratosis, and ulcer.

The incidences and severities of skin lesions generally increased with increasing dose in males and females. The incidences of renal tube regeneration in the 100, 200, and 400 mg/kg females were significantly greater than the vehicle control incidence, and the severities in the 200 and 400 mg/kg females were increased. Coconut oil acid diethanolamine condensate in ethanol was administered externally to 10 male and 10 female B6C3F1 mice at doses of the 50, 100, 200, 400, or 800 mg/kg body weight five times per week for 14 weeks. All mice survived until the end of the study. Final mean body weights and body weight gains of dosed males and females were similar to those of the vehicle controls. The only treatment-related clinical finding was irritation of the skin at the site of application in males and females administered the 800 mg/kg dose. Weights of the liver and kidney of 800 mg/kg males and females, the liver of the 400 mg/kg females, and the lung of the 800 mg/kg females were significantly increased compared to the controls. Epididymal spermatozoal concentration was significantly increased in the 800-mg/kg males. Histopathological lesions of the skin at the site of application included epidermal hyperplasia, sebaceous gland hyperplasia, chronic active inflammation, parakeratosis, and ulcer.

The incidences and severities of these skin lesions generally increased with increasing dose in males and females. Coconut oil acid diethanolamine condensate in ethanol was administered externally to 50 male and 50 female F344/N rats at doses of 50 or 100 mg/kg body weight five times a week for 104 weeks. The survival rates of treated male and female rats were similar to those of the vehicle controls. The mean body weights of dosed males and females were similar to those of the vehicle controls throughout most of the study. The only chemical-related clinical finding was irritation of the skin at the site of application in the 100-mg/kg females. There were marginal increases in the incidences of renal tubule adenoma or carcinoma (combined) in the 50-mg/kg females. The severity of nephropathy increased with increasing dose in the female rats. Nonneoplastic lesions of the skin at the site of application included epidermal hyperplasia, sebaceous gland hyperplasia, parakeratosis, and hyperkeratosis, and the incidences and severities of these lesions increased with increasing dose. The incidence of chronic active inflammation, epithelial hyperplasia, and epithelial ulcer of the forestomach increased with dose in female rats and the increases were significant in the 100-mg/kg group. Coconut oil acid diethanolamine condensate in ethanol was administered externally to 50 male and 50 female B6C3F1 mice at doses of 100 or 200 mg/kg body weight five times a week for 104 to 105 weeks. Survival of the mice was generally similar to that of the controls. Mean body weights of 100-mg/kg females from week 93 and 200-mg/kg females from week 77 were less than in the controls. The only clinical finding attributed to treatment was irritation of the skin at the site of application in males administered 200 mg/kg. The incidences of hepatic neoplasms (hepatocellular adenoma, hepatocellular carcinoma, and hepatoblastoma) were significantly increased in both sexes. Most of the incidences exceeded the historical control ranges. The incidences of eosinophilic foci in dosed groups of male mice were increased relative to that in controls. The incidences of renal tubule adenoma and renal tubule adenoma or carcinoma (combined) were significantly increased in the 200-mg/kg males. Several nonneoplastic lesions of the skin at the site of application were considered treatment related. Incidence of epidermal hyperplasia, sebaceous gland hyperplasia, and hyperkeratosis were greater in all dosed groups than in the controls. The incidence of ulcer in 200-mg/kg males and inflammation and parakeratosis in 200-mg/ kg females were greater than in the controls. The incidence of thyroid gland follicular cell hyperplasia in all of the dosed groups was significantly greater than those in the control groups.

Cardiovascular effect

Coconut and coconut oil, administered to 32 coronary heart disease patients in 16 age- and sex-matched healthy controls with no difference in the fat, saturated fat, and cholesterol consumption, produced no effect. Hydrogenated oil, administered to young male Wistar rats, at a dose of 10% of diet for 10 weeks, produced an increase in the risk of ventricular arrhythmias under conditions of both ischemia and reperfusion. The incidence of ventricular fibrillation was 67% in the oil fed group. The time until the first occurrence of extrasystole, the incidence of ventricular tachycardia, and the incidence of reperfusion-induced ventricular fibrillation were influenced in a similar manner between groups. The fatty acid composition of myocardial tissue, the ratio of *n*-3 to *n*-6 fatty acids, and the double-bond index were significantly affected by the various diets. Oil was administered by gastric intubation to male Sprague–Dawley rats at a dose of 86:14 w/w coconut oil/safflower oil for 10 days, containing either 0.8 mg Zn/kg or 111 mg Zn/kg. Zinc-deficient rats that were fed coconut oil had higher concentrations of triglycerides and total fatty acids in the heart than the control rats. The concentrations of phospholipids and total cholesterol were not different between zinc-deficient and control rats. Concentrations of lauric acid, myristic acid, palmitic acid, palmitoleic acid, and oleic acid were 65 to 192% higher in the hearts of zinc-deficient rats fed coconut diet than in the control rats. The level of arachidonic acid in phospholipids, which may represent desaturation activity, was not different in the zinc-deficient rats and control rats. Oil was administered orally to rats fed a copper-deficient diet at doses of 10 g/100 g coconut oil or 10 g/100 g coconut oil with 1 g/100 g cholesterol. Rats fed the diet with coconut and cholesterol had left ventricular chamber volumes that were twofold larger than those of rats fed diet with coconut oil only.

Copper deficiency reduced left ventricular chamber volume only in rats fed coconut oil and cholesterol. The results indicated that preload and contractility in the hearts of coconut oil-fed rats were greater than cardiac response to cholesterol addition to the coconut oil diet. Hearts in copper-deficient rats fed coconut oil and cholesterol exhibited eccentric hypertrophy and ventricular dysfunction. Oil, administered orally to rats for 4 weeks, produced a significant decrease in 5'-nucleotidase, phosphodiesterase I and *p*-nitrophenylphosphatase activity of cardiac sarcolemma. Sarcolemma from coconut-fed rats contained a significantly lower concentration of total polyunsaturated fatty acids (PUFAs) and a higher concentration of total monounsaturated fatty acids than that from safflower-fed rats. The fatty acid composition of the phosphatidylcholine exhibited the largest alterations because of coconut oil feeding. No dietary effect was observed in the sarcolemma content of cholesterol and phospholipids.

Cholestatic liver disease

Medium-chain fat from the oil, administered to bile duct-ligated rats, resulted in a decrease of consumption of the fat source compared to control rats; however, carbohydrate and protein intakes were not affected. Body weight gain was significantly greater in coconut-fed rats than in rats fed long-chain fat (Crisco vegetable shortening). Mortality was 44% in bile duct-ligated animals fed the long-chain fat and 0% in those fed medium-chain fat.

Cholesterol metabolism

Hydrogenated oil, administered orally to hamsters at a dose of 20% of diet for 4 weeks, induced hypercholesterolemia. Oil feeding had no effect on cholesterol synthesis but markedly inhibited cholesterol esterification in both the liver and the intestine. The diet-induced hypercholesterolemia was strongly correlated with an increase in acyl-CoA/cholesterol acyltransferase activity. The hypercholesterolemia increased aortic uptake of cholesterol and hence acyl-CoA/cholesterol acyltransferase activity. Coconut fat, administered orally to rabbits with partial ileal bypass, produced a significant increase of serum total cholesterol and phospholipids concentrations. The effect on serum lipids of the type of fat was similar in control and partial ileal bypass rabbits.

Coconut—a main source of energy for two Polynesian groups, Tokelauans and Pukapukans—was investigated. Tokelauans obtained a much higher percentage of energy from coconut than the Pukapukans, 63% compared with 34%, so their intake of saturated fat is higher. The serum cholesterol levels are 35–40 mg higher in Tokelauans than in Pukapukans. Analysis of a variety of food samples and human fat biopsies showed a high lauric (12:0) and myristic (14:0) acids content. Vascular disease is uncommon in both populations, and there is no evidence of the high saturated fat intake having a harmful effect in these populations. Oil, administered orally to growing male Sprague–Dawley rats fed a diet containing unoxidized or oxidized cholesterol (5 g/kg) with coconut or salmon oil (100 g/kg) for 5 weeks, produced an effect independent of the dietary fat. Hydrogenated coconut oil was administered to F(1)B Golden Syrian hamsters at a dose of 20 g/100 g for 10 weeks.

The hamsters were ranked according to their plasma VLDL and LDL cholesterol as a low or medium group. Low-coconut oil group had significantly higher aortic total and esterified cholesterol concentrations than the low-cholesterol-fed group. Hamsters in the low-cholesterolfed group had significantly higher aortic TNF-α concentrations than hamsters in the low-coconut oil group. Hamsters in the med-coconut oil group had significantly higher aortic IL-1-β concentrations than hamsters in the med-cholesterol group. Hamsters in both cholesterol fed groups had significantly lower plasma total cholesterol concentrations than hamsters in the low-coconut oil group.

Cholesterolemic effect

Oil, administered to phospholipids transfer protein knockout (PLTP0)-deficient mice, produced an increase of phospholipids and free cholesterol in the VLDL-LDL region of PLTP0 mice. Accumulation of phospholipids and free cholesterol was dramatically increased in PLTP0/HL0 mice compared to PLTP0 mice. Turnover studies indicated that coconut oil was associated with delayed catabolism of phospholipids and phospholipids/free cholesterol-rich particles. Incubation of these particles with hepatocytes of coconut-fed mice produced a reduced removal of phospholipids and free cholesterol by scavenger receptor BI, even though scavenger receptor BI protein expression levels were unchanged.

Coagglutination activity

Oil was administered to females at doses of a high-saturated fatty acids diet (HSAFA diet; 38.4% of energy from fat, polyunsaturated/saturated [P/S] fatty acid ratio 0.14) or low-saturated fatty acids diet (LSAFA; 19.7% of energy from fat, P/S ratio 0.17). The postprandial plasma concentration of tissue plasminogen activator (t-PA) antigen was decreased in the HSAFA-fed group. Plasma t-PA antigen was correlated with plasminogen activator inhibitor type 1 (PAI-1) activity when the participants consumed the HSAFA and LSAFA diet, although the diets did not affect the PAI-1 levels. There were no significant differences in postprandial variations in t-PA activity, factor VII coagulant activity, or fibrinogen levels as a result of the diets. Serum-fasting Lp(a) levels were lower in the HSAFA group and were lower in the LSAFA group. Serum Lp(a) concentrations did not differ when the women consumed the HSAFA and LSAFA diets.

Cytotoxic activity

Oil, in cell culture at a concentration of 300 μg/mL, was active on Ca-colon-HT29. Coir fiber, administered intratracheally to guinea pigs, resolved the granulomas. Coir fiber and ash, in cell culture, produced a hemolytic activity and macrophage cytotoxicity more marked with ash compared with the fiber alone. Extract of the husk fiber, in cell culture at a concentration of 10 μg/mL, inhibited the growth of promastigote and amastigote developmental stages of *Leishmania amazonensis* after 60 minutes. Extract of the fiber husk (rich in catechins), in erythroleukemia cell line (K562) and normal human peripheral blood lymphocytes activated by phytohemagglutinin or phorbol ester, produced a dose-dependent effect.

For phytohemagglutinin, this effect was irreversible, being already established on the first hours of culture. Oil, administered to C57B16 mice at a dose of 21% fat by weight, produced a significant decrease in macrophage-mediated death of P815 cells by nitric oxide and did not alter the death of L929 cell by macrophages. Liposaccharide-stimulated TNF-α production by macrophages decreased with increasing unsaturated fatty acid content of the diet: fish oil < safflower oil < olive oil < coconut oil < low-fat diet.

Desensitization effect

Saline extract of the dried pollen, administered subcutaneously to 96 allergic adults at variable doses, produced a clinical improvement and decreased IgE levels.

Dietary macronutrient distribution influence

Oil, administered to diet-induced overweight rats fed an energy-restricted diet with 60% of coconut oil, produced no difference between control and fat-fed group in weight loss and serum parameters. The coconut-fed group produced a greater reduction in the subcutaneous fat depot and of total body fat. Hepatic glycogen and glycogenic amino acid were altered in coconut-fed rats.

Diuretic activity

Decoction of the dried fruit, administered nasogastrically to rats at a dose 1 g/kg, was active. Fruit juice, administered intravenously by infusion to dogs at a dose of 3 mL/minute for 100 minutes, produced weak activity. Ethanol extract of the leaf, administered intraperitoneally to saline-loaded male rats at a dose of 0.185 mg/kg, was active. Urine was collected for 4 hours after treatment.

Erythrocytic effect

Hydrogenated coconut oil, administered orally to healthy rats for 10 weeks, produced a significant effect on five of the six classes of erythrocytes identified. The proportion of cells in each class was dependent on the diet. There was no significant effect of diet on erythrocyte filterability index and no statistical correlation between erythrocyte filterability index and morphology.

Exocrine pancreatic secretion

Oil, administered to piglets at a dose of 10 g/100 g of diet, did not affect the output of carboxylester hydrolase. Protein, chymotrypsin, carboxypeptidase A, elastase, and amylase outputs were not different among the dietary treatment groups. The outputs of trypsin and colipase were higher in the coconut-fed group. Oil, administered to three barrows at a dose of 15 g fat/100 g diet, produced a significant increase of chymotrypsin secretion.

Fatty acid composition influence

Oil was administered orally to mice bearing the L1210 murine leukemia cells at a dose of 16% of diet. A microsome-rich fraction prepared from the L1210 cells produced more monoenoic fatty acids (37% vs 12%) compared to mice fed the sunflower oil. Oil, administered to chicken at concentrations of 10 and 20% of diet, produced changes in fatty acid composition of free fatty acid and triglyceride fractions of chick plasma parallel to that of the experimental diet. Plasma phospholipids incorporated low levels of 12:0 and 14:0 acids, whereas 18:0, the main saturated fatty acid of this fraction, increased after coconut oil feeding.

The percentage of 18:2 acid significantly increased after coconut oil feeding. Oil, administered to rats at a dose of 15% of diet for 4 weeks, produced an increase of total cholesterol in the liver and the decrease of total liver phospholipids. Coconut/soy oil, administered by infusion into the duodenum of rats, produced the proportion of capric and lauric acids in the lymphatic triacylglycerol, reflecting the fatty acid composition in the diet. Results indicated that more than 50% of the capric and lauric acids could have been absorbed from the intestine as sn-monoacylglycerols. Hydrogenated coconut oil was administered to rats at a dose of 7% of the diet (essential fatty acids deficient in both *n*-6 and *n*-3) for 28 weeks (1 week gestation, 3 weeks lactation, and 24 weeks thereafter). The fatty acid compositional changes indicative of an essential fatty acid deficiency, such as the decreases in the levels of 18:2 *n*-6 along with an accumulation of 20:3 *n*-9 were observed in all the salivary glands. In the submandibular glands, the proportions of 16:1, 18:1 *n*-9 and 18:1 *n*-7 were higher in hydrogenated coconut oil-fed group than in the other groups. Some differences in the fatty acid composition of the three glands were found.

Fatty acid metabolism

Oil was administered to preruminant Holstein Friesian male calves fed a conventional milk diet containing coconut oil for 19 days. Fatty acid oxidation was determined by measuring the production of CO_2 (total oxidation) and acid-soluble products (partial oxidation). Production of CO_2 was 1.7–3.6-fold lower and acid soluble products tend to be lower in liver slices of coconut oil-fed than beef-tallow-fed calves. Fatty acid esterification as neutral lipids was 2.6- to 3.1-fold higher in liver slices of coconut oil-fed group. The increase in neutral lipid production did not stimulate VLDL secretion by the hepatocytes, leading to a triacylglycerol accumulation in the cytosol of the calves fed coconut oil. Oil, administered to preruminant calves fed a milk replacer containing coconut oil for 19 days, produced no significant difference in weight of the total body and tissue between the treated groups. Plasma glucose and insulin concentrations were lower in the coconut oil-fed group. Feeding on the coconut oil diet induced an 18-fold increase in the hepatic concentration of triacylglycerol.

The perixomal oxidation rate of oleate was 1.5-fold higher in the hearts of calves fed coconut oil. The cytochrome C oxidase/citrate synthase activity ratio was lower in the liver of the coconut oil-fed animals. Oil, administered as a ratio 7:1 w/w coconut oil/safflower oil by gastric intubation to zinc-deficient rats, reduced δ-desaturase activity in liver microsomes of rats fed coconut oil. Zinc-deficient rats on the coconut oil diet had unchanged δ-6-desaturase activity with linoleic acid as substrate and lowered activity with α-linolenic acid as substrate.

Genotoxic activity

Coconut oil acid diethanolamine condensate with or without S9 activation enzyme, in cell culture, produced no effect on *Salmonella typhimurium*. The treatment did not produce an increase in mutant L5178Y mouse lymphoma cell colonies, and no increased in the frequencies of sister chromatid exchanges or chromosomal aberrations in Chinese hamster ovary cells. In a peripheral blood micronucleus test in male and female mice from the 14-week test, positive results were obtained.

Genotype and diet effect

Coconut oil was administered to female Zucker rats throughout mating and lactation. Homozygous lean male and female rats, obese male, and lean heterozygous female rats were bred. Additional male rats were maintained on the same diet as their mothers until 11–12 days of age. Obese sucking rats had higher body weights than lean pups. Inguinal fat pad weights and pad-to-body weight ratios followed the pattern of obese greater than lean (FA/fa genes) pups that were greater than lean (FA/FA) pups. A similar relationship was found for adipose tissue lipogenic enzyme activities. At 11–12 weeks of age, measurements followed the general pattern of obese rats having greater value than lean rats (i.e., FA/fa = FA/FA). Coconut oil-fed fa/fa rats had lower hepatic lipogenic enzyme activities and lower fat cell numbers than safflower-fed fa/fa rats. High-fat diet did not result in a heterozygous effect in young adult lean male rats. Hydrogenated coconut oil, corn oil, or menhaden oil were administered to diabetes-prone BHE/ cdb and normal Sprague–Dawley rats. Both fat source and strain affected the temperature dependence of succinate-supported respiration. The transition temperature was greater in BHE/cdb rats than in the Sprague–Dawley rats. The efficiency of adenosine triphosphatase synthesis as reflected by the adenosine diphosphatase/O ratio was decreased in the BHE/cdb rats compared to Sprague–Dawley rats.

Glucose metabolism

Hydrogenated oil, administered to prediabetic weanling BHE rats fed a 6% fat and 64% sucrose diet, produced an increase of the fractional irreversible glucose turnover rates, fractional glucose carbon recycling, hepatic fatty acid synthesis rates, adipose fatty acid synthesis rate, lower muscle glycogen, and lower rates of incorporation of glucose into muscle glycogen than corn oil-fed rats. The diet had no effect on glucose mass and space, hepatic glycogen, or blood glucose levels. Oil, administered to male Wistar rats at a dose of 25% by weight for 26 days, produced a significant increase in serum total cholesterol, LDLs, liver cholesterol, and liver weight. There was a decrease in serum HDLs, triacylglycerol levels, and abdominal fat weight; an increase in 3-hydroxy-3- methylglutaryl-CoA reductase activity in the liver; reduction in plasma lecithin-cholesterol acyltransferase activity; lower level of serum insulin; and liver glycogen in the coconut oil-fed rats. Glucose use was altered because lower glucose-6-phosphatase and increased glucokinase activities in the liver of coconut oil-fed rats were found. Coconut palm wine was administered to rats at a dose of 24.5 mL/kg body weight/d for 15 days before conception and throughout gestation. On the 19th day of gestation, hypoglycemia was observed in both wine- and ethanol-treated groups. Synthesis of glycogen was elevated on exposure to ethanol/wine, but its degradation was enhanced only in ethanol-exposed rats. Key enzymes of the citric acid cycle and gluconeogenesis were inhibited on administration in both groups. The activities of glycolytic enzymes were increased. Hydrogenated oil (6%), administered to BHE rats at a dose of 5% of diet, produced no influence on glucose. Hepatocytes isolated from rats fed coconut oil had a significantly lower affinity for insulin than menhaden oil-treated rats.

Glycemic index

The glycemic index of different commonly consumed products supplemented with increasing levels of coconut flour was determined in 10 normal and 10 diabetic subjects. The test food with 200–250 g coconut flour/kg had significantly low, gastrointestinal (GI) (< 60); with 150 g coconut flour/kg had GI ranging from 61.3 to 71.4. A very strong negative correlation (r −0.85, $p < 0.005$) was observed between the GI and dietary fiber content of food. Oil, administered to lean Zucker rats at a dose of 5% of diet (87% saturated fatty acids) for 2 weeks, produced no differences in food intake, body weight, tissue level of glucagons-like peptide-1, plasma insulin, and glucagons levels in coconut oil- and olive oil-fed groups.

Hair damage prevention

Coconut oil application has a strong effect on hair as compared to sunflower and mineral oils. Among the three oils investigated, coconut oil was the only one that reduced the protein loss remarkably for both damaged and undamaged hair when used as a prewash and postwash grooming product.

Hemostatic effect

Coconut water, in citrated plasma of eight healthy volunteers, was observed. Replacement of up to 50% of diluted plasma by water did not influence initiation of coagulatión. Replacing 50% of citrated plasma by coconut water reduced maximum amplitude of thrombelastography recording dose by 39%.

Hepatic activity

Hydrogenated oil, administered orally to male weanling rats at a dose of 10% of diet for 9 weeks, produced no significant alteration of hepatic 5-, 6-, and 9- desaturase activity. Addition of oil to the diet, simultaneously with lowering of the carbohydrate level, diminished the stimulatory effect of dietary sucrose vs glucose on 9-desaturase activity.

Hepatic mitochondrial effect

Oil, administered to chicken at a dose of 20% of the diet, produced a clear damage to the hepatic mitochondria accompanied by an accumulation of glycogen and lipid droplets in the hepatocyte cytoplasm. Pharmaceutical coconut oil induced a high percentage of cellular death when administered for 14 days. Fatty acid profiles in liver and hepatic mitochondria changed during 24 hours after pharmaceutical and cooking oils supplementation to the diet. The accumulation of shorter chain fatty acids (12:0) and (14:0) was higher after pharmaceutical than after cooking oil diet feeding. Mitochondrial ratios of saturated/unsaturated and saturated fatty acids (SUFAs)/PUFAs rapidly changed in parallel to these ratios in both diets. Most of the mitochondrial parameters measured recuperate to the control values when diets were supplied for 5–14 days. The maintenance of these ratios after 14 days pharmacological oil diet feeding was significantly higher than those in control.

Hyperalphalipoproteinemic activity

Oil, administered orally to rabbits fed commercial chow or chow plus 14% w/w coconut oil, resulted in double increase the plasma levels of HDL cholesterol, phospholipids, and protein for up to 4 months without affecting HDL lipid and apoprotein composition. After 3 months also increased VLDL (107%) and LDL cholesterol (40%) levels, but the absolute increases in each of these lipoprotein fractions was less than half of that of HDL. Isotope kinetic studies of 125I-HDL protein indicated a double rate of production of HDL and no change in the efficiency of removal of HDL from plasma.

Hypercholesterolemic activity

Seed oil, administered by gastric intubation to dogs, was active. Seed oil, administered orally to adults, was active. Oil, administered orally to rats at a dose of 79 g/day for 3 weeks, produced a significant increase of the final plasma cholesterol in groups that consumed yeast with coconut oil (91 mg/dL), in comparison to group consuming soybean protein with coconut oil (36 mg/dL). Coconut fat, administered to hyporesponsive and hyperresponsive inbred strains of rabbits with high or low response of plasma cholesterol to dietary SUFAs vs PUFAs, produced no influence on the efficiency of cholesterol absorption. Fat, administered orally to young normolipidemic males at a dose of 30% of the diet with a polyunsaturated/saturated fat ratio of 4 or 0.25 for 8 weeks, produced a significant increase of total plasma cholesterol level. Oil, administered to Mongolian gerbils, produced a hypercholesterolemia associated with elevations in VLDL, LDL, and HDL.

The type of dietary fat did not influence lipoprotein composition and size. Fresh and thermally oxidized oil, administered to rats at a dose of 20% of diet, produced an increase of total cholesterol, LDL and VLDL cholesterol, and triacylglycerol and phospholipids levels and a decrease in HDL cholesterol. Oil, administered to 25 women at doses of 38.4% of energy from fat (HSAFA; PUFA/SUFA P/S ratio = 0.14) or 19.7% energy from fat (LSAFA; P/S ratio 0.17) for 3-week periods, produced no difference in serum total cholesterol, LDL cholesterol, and apo B concentrations between the diet periods. HDL cholesterol and apo A-I were 15% and 11%, respectively, higher during HSAFA diet period than during LSAFA diet period. The LDL/HDL-C and apo B/apo A-I ratios were higher during LSAFA diet period.

Hyperlipidemic activity

Palm wine was administered orally to female albino rats at a dose of 24.5 mL/kg body weight/day for 15 days before conception and during pregnancy. On days 13 and 19 of gestation, liver function and hyperlipidemia were seen in the fetuses. Hyperlipidemia was caused by increased biosynthesis since the incorporation of ^{14}C acetate into lipids and activity of HMG-CoA reductase and lipogenic enzymes were elevated. Oil, administered to miniature pigs fed a pig chow supplemented with 17.1% of coconut oil for 30 d, produced a significant increase of cholesterol, triglyceride, HDL cholesterol and subfractions, LDL cholesterol and subfractions, and lipoprotein lipase activity in both genders. For cholesterol, triglyceride, HDL cholesterol (HDL-C and HDL[2]-C), LDL cholesterol (LDL-C, LDL[1 and 2]-C), and hepatic lipase, the female response to the diet was exaggerated compared to the male response.

Hyperthermic effect

Coconut oil, administered orally to rats with human recombinant TNF-α at a dose of 190 g/kg for 12 weeks, produced an antihypothermic effect and changes in serum albumin and Cu content 8 hours after treatment and in muscle and liver protein after 24 hours. The results indicated that changes in ecosanoid metabolism may be involved in the modulatory effect of the coconut oil-enriched diet.

Hypertriglyceridemic activity

Coconut oil, administered orally to rats at a dose of 14%:0.5% oil/cholesterol diet, produced an increase of lipids and apo B in the VLDL and intermediate-density lipoprotein fractions. The particle diameters of lipoproteins were similar in coconut oil- and olive oil- fed groups. The rates of triglyceride hydrolysis of both groups' VLDL by postheparin lipoprotein lipase in vitro were the same. The average fractional removal of apo B did not differ between diet groups. Oil, administered to rabbits at a dose of 14%: 0.5% coconut oil/cholesterol of diet, produced an increase of plasma triglycerides 15 times higher than basal level. Postprandial triglyceride responses after the first high-fat/ cholesterol meal were more prolonged in coconut-fed rabbits than in olive-fed group. Postprandial triglyceride responses after chronic coconut oil/cholesterol feeding were significantly greater compared to the olive oil-fed group. One coconut oil/cholesterol meal was associated with a 40% increase of postheparin plasma lipoprotein lipase activity and changed little in chronically fed coconut oil/cholesterol group.

Hypocholesterolemic activity

Kernel protein, administered orally to rats on a coconut oil diet, lowered the levels of cholesterol, phospholipids, and triglycerides in the serum and most tissues when compared to casein-fed animals. The increase of hepatic degradation of cholesterol to bile acids and hepatic cholesterol biosynthesis and the decrease of esterification of free cholesterol were noted. In the intestine, cholesterogenesis was decreased. The kernel proteins also decreased lipogenesis in the liver and intestine.

Hypoglycemic activity

Ethanol extract of the leaf, administered orally to rats at a dose of 250 mg/kg, produced less than a 30% drop in blood sugar level. Fruit juice, administered intravenously by infusion to dogs at a dose of 3 mL/min for 100 min, was active. Hot water extract of the dried shell, administered by gastric intubation to dogs at a dose of 200 mL/animal (20 g of air-dried plant material), produced weak activity. The neutral detergent fiber from kernel, administered orally to rats at doses of 5%, 15%, and 30% of diet, resulted in significant decrease in the level of blood glucose and serum insulin, with increasing in the intake of fiber. The increase of fecal excretion of Cu, Cr, Mn, Mg, Zn, and Ca was present. Neutral detergent fiber from coconut kernel, administered to rats at doses of 5, 15, and 30% of diet, produced an increase of fecal excretion of Cu, Cr, Mn, Mg, Zn, and Ca.

Hypolipidemic activity

Protein, administered orally to hypercholesterolemic rats, reduced total, LDL, and VLDL cholesterol; triglycerides; and phospholipids levels in the serum and increased the level of serum HDL cholesterol. The concentration of total cholesterol, triglycerides, and phospholipids in the tissues was lower than in the control group. There was increased activity of superoxide desmutase and catalase. An increase of hepatic cholesterogenesis, conversion of cholesterol to bile acids and fecal excretion of bile acids, and excretion of urinary nitrate and an decrease of malonaldehyde level in the heart were observed. The neutral detergent fiber of kernel digested with cellulase and hemicellulase was administered orally to rats. Hemicellulose-rich fiber showed decreased concentration of total cholesterol and LDL and VLDL cholesterol and increased HDL cholesterol. Cellulose-rich fiber showed no significant alteration. There was increased HMG-CoA reductase activity and increased incorporation of labeled acetate into free cholesterol. Rats fed hemicellulose-rich fiber produced lower concentration of triglycerides and phospholipids and a lower release of lipoproteins into circulation. There were an increased concentration of hepatic bile acids and increased excretion of fecal sterols and bile acids.

Ileal oleic acid uptake

Hydrogenated oil, administered to rats at a dose of 5 g/100 g of diet, produced saturable kinetics in ileal brush border membrane vesicles: $V_{max} = 0.23 \pm 03$ μmol/mg protein/5 minutes and $K_m = 196 \pm 50.3$ nmol for controls, and $V_{max} = 04 \pm 01$ μmol/mg protein/5 minutes and $K_m = 206 \pm 85.3$ nmol for coconut oil-fed group.

Immune function

Coconut oil, administered to rats fed a fat-rich diet (corn oil) or a diet poor in linoleate (coconut oil) at high and low concentrations, completely abolished the responses to *Escherichia coli* endotoxin:

Intestinal brush border membrane

Oil, administered orally to rats at a dose of 10% for 5 weeks, produced an increase in level of saturated fatty acids in the brush border membrane from coconut oil-fed animals. Membrane fluidity was as follows: coconut oil less than commercial pellet diet less than corn oil less than fish oil. The membrane hexose content was high in the coconut-fed rats. Hexamines were elevated in coconut- treated rat brush borders. The activities of alkaline phosphatase, sucrase, and lactase were increased.

Intestinal esterase activity

Oil was administered to rats at different doses with or without clofibrate for 15 days. The hypolipidemic action of clofibrate was not influenced by the amount of fat. Clofibrate did not affect lower cholesterol concentration in rats fed the low-fat diet, but it counteracted the rise in liver cholesterol seen in rats fed the high-fat diet. The high-fat diet produced slightly higher levels of butyryl cholinesterase in the small intestine but markedly raised intestinal esterase-1 activity.

Intestinal neoplasia

Oil was administered to 8-week-old male Fischer rats divided into two groups of 60 each (sedentary and exposed to moderate exercise), at a dose of 21% of diet for 38 weeks. The exercising and sedentary rats fed coconut oil were significantly heavier than rats fed corn oil. In the rats fed coconut oil diet, nine carcinomas were recorded in the sedentary groups and five in the exercised rats, which developed significantly fewer neoplasms than corn oil-fed group.

Intestinal transport

Coconut water in different stages of maturation, administered to rats, produced a jejunal water absorption (17 ± 0.45 μL/minutes/cm), sodium excretion (–1694 ± 296 μEq/minutes/cm), and glucose absorption (5212.70 ± 2098.47 μg%/minutes/cm) in all the stages studied.

Intravenous hydration

The use of coconut water as a short-term intravenous hydration fluid for Solomon Island residents was investigated. Fresh young coconut water, administered to eight healthy male volunteers in three doses in separate trials representing 50, 40, and 30% of the 120% fluid loss at 30 and 60 minutes of the 2-hour rehydration period. The percent of body weight loss than was regained (used as index of percent rehydration) was 75 ± 5%. The rehydration index, which provided an indication of how much of what was actually ingested and used for body weight restoration, was 1.56 ± 0.14. There was no difference at any time in serum Na^+ and Cl^-, serum osmolality, and net fluid balance among the trials. Coconut water was significantly sweeter, caused less nausea and more fullness and no stomach upset, and was easier to consume in a larger amount compared to carbohydrate-electrolyte beverage and plain water. Water, administered to children with diarrhea, was inactive. The results indicated that coconut water composition, sodium and glucose concentrations, and osmolality values vary during maturation of the fruit. In no instance did the coconut water contain sodium and glucose concentrations of value as an oral rehydration solution.

Iron bioavailability

Oil, administered to suckling rats dosed with ^{59}Fe-labeled diet, produced a higher percentage of ^{59}Fe in the blood than those fed other fat sources. Administration to weanling rats produced a significantly higher percentage of ^{59}Fe retention than rats fed a formula-blend fat diet.

Jejunal oleic acid uptake

Hydrogenated oil, administered to rats at a dose of 5 g/100 g of diet, produced saturable kinetics in jejunal brush border membrane vesicles: V_{max} = 0.15 ± 01 μmol/mg protein/5 minutes, and K_m = 136 ± 29.1 nmol for controls, and V_{max} = 03 ± 01 μmol/mg protein/5 minutes and K_m = 124.5 ± 72.6 nmol for the coconut oil-fed group.

Lauric acid incorporation

Lauric acid (50%) from the oil, administered to rats for 6 weeks, produced no significant difference between the experimental distribution of triacylglycerol types and the random distribution, calculated from the total fatty acid composition.

Lipid metabolism

Oil, administered orally to female C57BL/6 mice weaned at 21 d of age at a dose of 15% w/w for 6 weeks, increased the total lipids, triglycerides, LDL and VLDL cholesterol, and thiobarbituric acid-reactive substances (TBARS) and reduced glutathione concentrations, without changes in phospholipids or total cholesterol concentrations compared to controls. The concentrations of total cholesterol, free and esterified cholesterol, triglycerides, and TBARS were increased in the macrophages of coconut-fed mice, whereas the content of total phospholipids did not change. The phospholipids composition showed an increase of phosphatidylcholine and a decrease of phosphatidyl-ethanolamine. Incorporation of [^{3}H]-cholesterol into the macrophages and into the cholesterol ester fraction was increased. The coconut oil diet did not affect [^{3}H]-AA uptake, induced an increase in [^{3}H]-AA release, and enhanced AA mobilization induced by lipopolysaccharide. Oil, administered to 28 persons with moderately elevated cholesterol level, decreased total cholesterol and LDL cholesterol (6.4 ± 0.8 and 4.2 ± 0.7 mmol/L), respectively, compared to butter diet (6.8 ± 0.9 and 4.5 ± 0.8 mmol/L). Apos A-1 and B were significantly higher on coconut oil and on butter than on safflower oil. In the group as a whole, HDL did not differ significantly in the three diets, whereas levels in women fed coconut oil were significantly higher than in the safflower oil group. Triacylglycerol level was lower in coconut oil group, but results were significant statistically only in women.

Lipid peroxide formation stimulation

Seed oil, administered to rats at a dose of 15% of diet for 6 weeks, was inactive on rat liver microsomes. Malondialdehyde concentration was unchanged among animals given different oils. Vitamin E level decreased among those fed soybean oil.

Lipogenetic effect

Kernel protein, administered orally to rats on a coconut oil diet, decreased lipogenesis in the liver and intestine. The kernel proteins also lowered the levels of cholesterol, phospholipids, and triglycerides in the serum and most tissues when compared to casein-fed animals. There was an increase in hepatic degradation of cholesterol to bile acids and hepatic cholesterol biosynthesis and a decrease in esterification of free cholesterol. In the intestine, cholesterogenesis was decreased.

Lipoprotein composition

Oil, administered to newborn chicken at a dose of 20% for 2 weeks, increased cholesterol concentration in all the lipoprotein fractions, whereas 10% coconut oil only increased cholesterol in LDL and HDL, an increase that was significant after 1 week of treatment. Similar results were obtained for triacylglycerol concentration after 2 weeks of treatment. Changes in phospholipids and total protein levels were less profound. Coconut oil decreased LDL and fluidity. Oil, administered with or without 0.5% cholesterol to 36 young male Syrian hamsters for 6 weeks, produced higher plasma total triglyceride and total cholesterol in coconut oil without cholesterol supplementation-fed group than in the fish oil-fed group. With cholesterol supplementation, there was no significant difference in plasma total triglyceride level among the three dietary groups. The hepatic cholesteryl ester content was higher, and there was lower liver microsomal acyl-CoA/cholesterol acyltransferase activity in the cholesterol-supplemented coconut oil group compared to other groups. There was no significant difference in the excretion of fecal neutral and acidic sterols among the three dietary groups.

Lipoprotein lipase activity

Oil, administered to preruminant calves, produced no effect on palmitate oxidation rate by whole homogenates and induced higher palmitate oxidation by intermyofibrillar mitochondria. Carnitine palmitoyltransferase I activity did not significantly differ between the groups. Heart and longissimus thoracis muscle of calves fed coconut oil had higher lipoprotein lipase activity but produced no differences in fatty acid-binding protein content or activity of oxidative enzymes.

Liver function effect

Palm wine was administered orally to female albino rats at a dose of 24.5 mL/kg body weight/day) for 15 days before conception and during pregnancy. On days 13 and 19 of gestation, liver function and hyperlipidemia were seen in the fetuses. Altered liver function was evidenced by the increased activity of alcohol dehydrogenase, aldehyde dehydrogenase, glutamic oxaloacetic transaminase (GOT) (aspartate amino transferase), and glutamic pyruvic transaminase (GPT) (alanine amino transferase).

Myocardial infarction

Coconut oil, administered orally to rabbits with myocardial infarction induced by isoproterenol, produced a higher level of phospholipids in the heart and aorta. The concentrations of cholesterol and triglycerides were lower in the safflower oil fed group.

Nasal absorption

Sucrose ester of coconut fatty acid in aqueous ethanol solution (sucrose cocoate SL-40) administered intranasally to anesthetized male Sprague–Dawley rats at a dose of 0.5% sucrose cocoate with insulin, produced a rapid and significant increase in plasma insulin level with a concomitant decrease in blood glucose levels. Administration of a dose of 0.5% sucrose cocoate with calcitonin produced a rapid increase in plasma calcitonin levels and a concomitant decrease in plasma calcium levels.

Nephrotoxic activity

Fruit juice, administered by intravenous infusion to dogs at a dose of 3 mL/minute for 100 minutes, produced weak activity. Albuminuria was observed just before the end of infusion administration.

Neutrophil functions

Oil, administered to rats 21 days old at a dose of 15% final fat content of the diet for 6 weeks, produced a reduction in spontaneous and phorbol myristate acetate-stimulated H_2O_2 generation in glycogen-elicited peritoneal neutrophils relative to neutrophils from rats fed the control diet. The activity of superoxide desmutase, glutathione peroxidase, and catalase did not change in animals fed the fat-rich diets. The initial rate of O_2 generation in both resting neutrophils and phorbol myristate acetate-stimulated cells was significantly reduced when animals were fed coconut oil.

Ophthalmic absorption

Sucrose ester of coconut fatty acid in aqueous ethanol solution (sucrose cocoate SL-40), administered ophthalmically to anesthetized Sprague–Dawley male rats at a dose of 0.5% sucrose cocoate with insulin, produced an increase in plasma insulin level and a decrease in blood glucose levels.

Ornithine decarboxylase activity

Fixed oil (4.5%), *Clupeidae brevortia tyrannus* (4%), and *Zea mays* (1.5%); fixed oil (7.5%), *Clupeidae brevortia tyrannus* (1%), and *Zea mays* (1.5%); fixed oil (8.5%) and *Zea mays* (1.5%), administered orally to mice for 1 year, were active vs benzoyl peroxide-induced ornithine decarboxylase activity. Oil, administered to 30 ultraviolet (UV)-irradiated Sencar and SKH-1 mice at doses of 1/14% (A diet), 7.9/7.1% (B diet), and 15/0% (C diet) corn oil/coconut oil for 6 weeks, produced no increase in enzyme activity. The level of ornithine decarboxylase activity in the UV-irradiated mice fed diet A was significantly higher than in mice fed the B or C diet. In the SKH-1 mice, ornithine decarboxylase activity was increased by 3 weeks and was significantly higher in mice fed diet C than in mice fed diet A. There was no significant effect of dietary fat on UV-induced skin tumor incidence.

Oxidative DNA damages

Oil, administered to Fischer F344 rats at a dose of 19.8% coconut oil and 2% corn oil for 12–15 weeks, produced an excretion of 8-oxo-7,8dihydro-2'-deoxyguanosine (8-oxodG) in male group equal to 954 ± 367 pmol/kg/ 24 hours in the coconut oil fed group compared to 403 ± 150 pmol/kg/24 hours in the control. Calculated per whole animal, the excretion was 328 ± 128 pmol/24 hours in the coconut oil-fed rats and 137 ± 51 pmol/24 hours in the control.

Phospholipidemic effect

Oil, administered to phospholipids transfer protein knockout (PLTPO)-deficient mice, produced an increase of phospholipids and free cholesterol in the VLDL–LDL region of PLTPO mice. Accumulation of phospholipids and free cholesterol was dramatically increased in PLTPO/HLO mice compared to PLTPO mice. Turnover studies indicated that coconut oil was associated with delayed catabolism of phospholipids and phospholipids/free cholesterol-rich particles. Incubation of these particles with hepatocytes of coconut-fed mice produced a reduced removal of phospholipids and free cholesterol by SRBI, even though SRBI protein expression levels were unchanged.

Plasma fatty acids

Oil, administered to chicken at doses of 10% and 20% of the diet, produced an increase in the percentages of lauric and myristic acids in free fatty acid and triacylglycerol fractions in chick plasma, whereas these changes were less pronounced in phospholipids and cholesterol esters. The percentage of arachidonic acid was higher in plasma phospholipids than in the other fractions and was drastically decreased by coconut oil feeding. Linoleic acid, the main fatty acid of cholesterol esters, was increased. Oil, administered to 37 children 1 year of age in the form of full vegetable-fat milk (3.5 g fat/dL, 100% vegetable fat from palm, coconut, and soybean oils), produced higher amounts of plasma linoleic acid and a plasma α-tocopherol concentrations than in the other milks tested. Oil, administered to male Wistar rats at a dose of 40% of diet for 2 months, increased apo A-I concentration in plasma and did not change apo A-I mRNA level.

Oil, administered to 38 healthy children in a form of full vegetable-fat milk (3.5 g fat/dL, 100% vegetable fat from palm, coconut, and soybean oils), produced a significantly lower percentage of SUFAs in plasma triglycerides than in children fed standard-fat milk. Plasma PUFA levels were significantly higher than in children fed standard-fat milk. Oil, administered to 41 healthy adults, produced a decrease of plasma lathosterol concentration, the ratio plasma lathosterol/cholesterol, LDL cholesterol, and apo B. Plasma total cholesterol, HDL cholesterol, and apo A levels were not significantly different between butter and coconut diets. Oil, administered to male golden Syrian hamsters at a dose of 15% w/w for 4 weeks, produced the highest triglyceride levels of the diets studied. Oil, administered to male golden Syrian hamsters at a dose of 4 g/kg of diet (12:0 and 14:0) for 7 weeks, produced the highest plasma cholesterol concentration compared to rapeseed and sunflower seed oil diets. Biliary lipids, lithogenic index, and bile acid profile of the gallbladder bile did not differ significantly among the six diets.

Platelets aggregation stimulation

Fruit juice, administered intravenously by infusion to dogs at a dose of 5 mL/min, was active. Total infusion was 300 mL. Oil, administered orally to six New Zealand white rabbits fed a commercial diet supplemented with 60 g/kg of coconut oil low in all PUFA for 60 days, produced a platelets aggregation induced by both thrombin and collagen significantly lower with either fish or linseed oil (*n*-3 PUFA), than with corn oil (*n*-6 PUFA) or the low PUFA coconut oil.

Prostaglandin outflow

Oil was administered to weanling male rats fed *ad libitum* a semisynthetic diet supplemented with 10% by weight of primrose oil, replaced partly or completely (25, 50, 75, or 100%) by hydrogenated coconut oil for 8 weeks. The release of prostanoids from the mesenteric vasculature was significantly reduced in the animals on the diet with the oil replaced by coconut oil.

Protective effect of vitamin A

Vitamin A, 240,000 IU, predissolved in 11.7 g of coconut oil and bolused directly into the rumen of mature wethers along with 4 g of chromic oxide or predissolved in 11.7, 23.4, or 35 g of coconut oil, produced significantly higher recoveries of vitamin A when dissolved in coconut oil (55.6%) compared to safflower oil (35 5%). Recoveries in abomasal digesta increased linearly with the amount of carrier coconut oil.

Semen cryopreservation

Coconut water extender, administered with glycerol to the semen of six adult dogs at concentrations of 4, 6, and 8%, produced satisfactory effect. There was no difference among groups in motility and vigor. A smaller percentage of total and secondary abnormalities were observed using 6% glycerol.

Sensitization (skin)

Fruit juice, administered subcutaneously to guinea pigs at a dose of 02 mg/animal, was active on skin. Edema occurred at the site of injection and recovered within 200 minutes. Fruit juice, administered subcutaneously to adults at a dose of 02 mg/person, was active on skin. Inflammation occurred at the site of injection and recovered within 90 minutes. Aqueous extract of the husk fiber, administered externally to rabbits, produced no significant dermic or ocular irritation.

Sickness behavior

Hydrogenated oil, administered to Swiss Webster mice at a dose of 17% w/w for 6 weeks, produced the bioactivity of plasma TNF-α equal to 32.6 $\pm$ 3.6 ng/mL in mice fed coconut oil diet compared to mice fed fish oil (98.2 $\pm$ 5.1 ng/mL).

Spasmogenic activity

Ethanol (95%) extract of the fresh leaf and stem, administered to guinea pigs at a dose of 0.5 mL/L, was active on ileum. Water extract of the fresh leaf and stem, administered intraperitoneally to guinea pigs at a dose of 0.5 mL/L, was active on ileum.

Subcellular membrane-bound enzymes activity

Oil, administered to male CFY weanling rats at a dose of 20% for 16 weeks, produced an increase of synaptosomal acetylcholinesterase activity in the coconut oil-fed group. The Mg^{2+}-adenosine triphosphate (ATPase) activity was similar among all groups in all the brain regions.

Toxicity assessment

Ethanol extract of the leaf, administered intraperitoneally to mice, was active, LD_{50} 0.75 g/kg. Ethanol extract of the fresh leaf and stem, administered intraperitoneally to mice at the minimum toxic dose of 1 mL/animal, was active. Water extract of the fresh leaf and stem, administered intraperitoneally to mice at the minimum toxic dose of 1 mL/animal, was active. Aqueous extract of the husk fiber, administered orally to mice, was active, LD_{50} 2.30 g/kg.

Tricarboxylate carrier influence

Oil, administered to rats at a dose of 15% of the diet for 3 weeks, produced a differential mitochondrial fatty acid composition and no appreciable change in phospholipids composition and cholesterol level. Compared with coconut oil-fed rats, the mitochondrial tricarboxylate carrier activity was markedly decreased in liver mitochondria from fish oil-fed rats. No difference in the Arrhenius plot between the two groups was observed.

Tumor prevention

The effect of kernel fiber on metabolic activity of intestinal and fecal β-glucuronidase activity during 1,2-dimethylhydrazine (DMH)-induced colon carcinogenesis was studied. Inclusion of fiber supported lower specific activity and less fecal output of β-glucuronidase than did the fiber-free diet. Kernel, administered to animals treated with DMH, resulted in higher average weight. A decrease of cholesterol and increase of phospholipids and cholesterol/phospholipids ratio in most of tissues was found. HMG-CoA reductase activity was decreased in most of the tissues of the kernel and DMH, kernel and chili, and kernel, chili, and DMH groups. Histopathological studies showed that kernel-fed animals had fewer papillae, less infiltration into the submucosa, and fewer changes in the cytoplasm with decreased mitotic figures. Oil, administered to rats for 4–8 weeks, produced a small but statistically insignificant reduction in TNF production. After 8 weeks, coconut oil suppressed production of the cytokine. Coconut oil produced no modulatory effect on the interleukin production. Oil, administered orally at a dose of 20% of diet to virgin female Balb/c mice treated with 7,12-dimethylbenz[a]anthracene (DMBA), produced no effect on body weight, feed intake, or survival to 44 weeks of age and 36 weeks after the six DMBA doses. Mammary tumor incidence was the same in the coconut oil or menhaden oil but significantly higher in the corn oil group. Oil was administered to female Wistar rats before mating and throughout pregnancy and gestation, and the male offspring were supplemented from weaning until 90 days of age. They were inoculated subcutaneously with Walker 256 tumor cells. Supplementation of the diet with coconut oil did not change cancer cachexia, except for a small decrease in serum triacylglycerol concentration.

Tumor-promoting effect

Fixed oil (4.5%) with 4% *Clupeidae brevortia tyrannus* and 1.5% *Zea mays*; 7.5% fixed oil, 1% *Clupeidae brevortia tyrannus*, and 1.5% *Zea mays*; and 8.5% fixed and 1.5% *Zea mays*, administered to mice in the diet for 52 weeks, were active. Tumors were initiated with dimethylbenzanthracene and promoted with benzoyl peroxide for 52 weeks. Oil, administered orally to female Sencar mice at doses of 5, 10, 15, and 20%, with addition of 5% corn oil for 1 week after initiation with 7,12-dimethylbenzanthracene and 3 weeks before the start of promotion with 12-0-tetradecanoylphorbol- 13-acetate, produced no significant difference in latency or incidence of papillomas or carcinomas between the saturated fat diet groups. Oil, administered to 30 Sencar and SKH-1 mice at doses of 1:14% (A diet); 7.9%:7.1% (B diet) and 15:0% (C diet) corn oil/coconut oil for 3 weeks before UV irradiation, produced tumor incidence that reached a maximum of 60, 60, and 53% for diets A, B, and C, respectively, with an average one to two tumors per Sencar mouse. For the SKH-1 mice, the diet groups reached 100% incidence by 29 weeks, with approx 12 tumors per mouse. No significant effect of dietary fat was found for tumor latency, incidence, or yield in either strain. Oil (17%) with 3% of sunflower seed oil, administered to DMBA-treated female Sprague–Dawley rats in the diet, produced twice as many tumors as those fed 3% sunflower seed oil or 20% of either saturated fat alone. Tumor yields in the rats fed these mixed-fat diets were comparable to rats fed a 20% lard diet, which provided about the same amount of linoleic acid.

Uncoupling protein expression

Oil, administered to female Wistar rats fed *ad libitum* a high-fat diet with coconut oil for 7 weeks, promoted an increase in body fat content, body weight, and uncoupling protein levels. At the completion of experiment I, oil was administered to high-fat diet rats for 3 weeks. Adipose depots were strongly reduced in the rats fed the high fat diet enriched with coconut oil. Specific uncoupling protein was 3.4 times higher than in controls.

Vascular permeability increased

Fixed oil (4.5%), 4% *Clupeidae brevortia tyrannus*, and 1.5% *Zea mays*; 7.5% of fixed oil, 1% *Clupeidae brevortia tyrannus*, and 1.5% *Zea mays*; 8.5% fixed oil and 1.5% *Zea mays*, administered to mice in the diet for 52 weeks, was active vs vascular permeability induced by benzoyl peroxide.

Cannabis sativa

Cannabis sativa is an annual herb of the *Moraceae* family that grows to 5 m tall. It is usually erect; stems variable, with resinous pubescence, angular, sometimes hollow, especially above the first pairs of true leaves; basal leaves opposite, the upper leaves alternate, stipulate, long petiolate, palmate, with 3–11, rarely single, lanceolate, serrate, acuminate leaflets up to 10 cm long, 1.5 cm broad. Flowers are monoecious or dioecious, the male in axillary and terminal panicles, apetalous, with five yellowish petals and five poricidal stamens; the female flowers germinate in the axils and terminally, with one single-ovulate ovary. Fruit is brown, shining achene, variously marked or plain, tightly embraces the seed with its fleshy endosperm and curved embryo; late summer to early fall; year-round in tropics. Drug-producing selections grow better and produce more drugs in the tropics; oil- and fiber-producing plants thrive better in the temperate and subtropical areas. The form of the plant and the yield of fiber from it vary according to climate and particular variety. Varieties cultivated for their fibers have long stalks, branch very little, and yield only small quantities of seed. Oil seed varieties are small, mature early, and produce large quantities of seed. Varieties grown for the drugs are small, much branched with smaller dark-green leaves. Between these three main types of plants are numerous varieties that differ from the main one in height, extent of branching, and other characteristics.

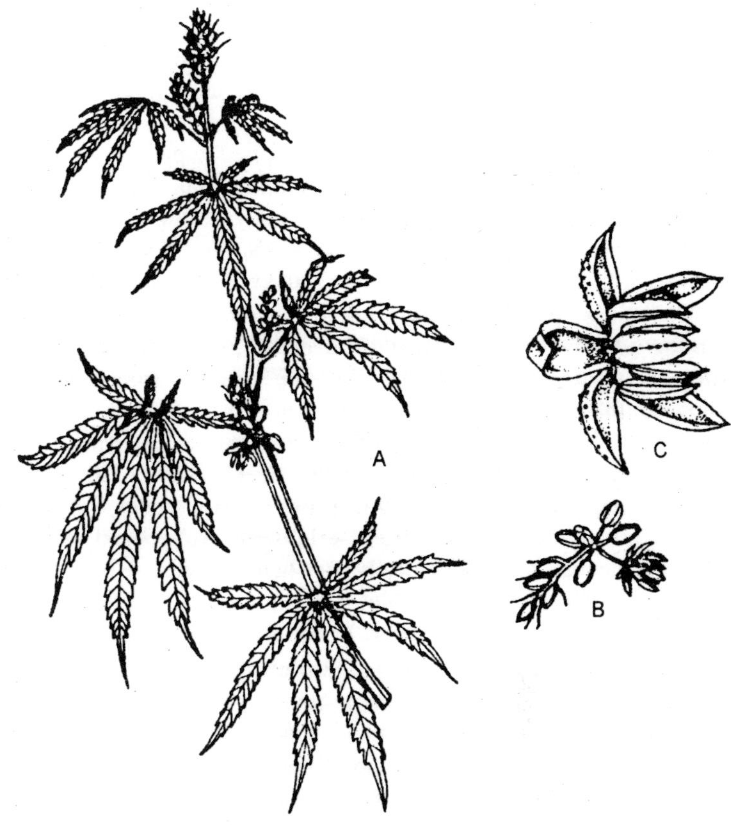

Fig. 17.12. Cannabis sativa. A–Male shoot; B and C–Flowers.

Origin and distribution

Native to Central Asia and long cultivated in Asia, Europe, and China. Now a widespread tropical, temperate, and subarctic cultivar. *Cannabis sativa* has been cultivated for more than 4500 years for different purposes, such as fiber, oil, or narcotics. The oldest use of hemp is for fiber, and later the seeds were used for culinary purposes. Plants yielding the drug were discovered in India, cultivated for medicinal purposes as early as 900 BC. In medieval times, it was brought to North Africa, where currently it is cultivated exclusively for hashish or kif.

Traditional uses

Afghanistan. Hot water extract of the resin is taken orally to induce abortion.

China. Hot water extract of the inflorescence is taken orally for wasting diseases, to clear the blood, to cool the temperature, to relieve fluxes, for rheumatism, to discharge pus, and to stupefy and produce hallucinations. The seed is taken orally as an emmenagogue. Decoction of the seed is taken orally as an anodyne, an emmenagogue, a febrifuge, for migraine, and for cancer. It is taken orally as a hallucinogen and externally for rheumatism.

Guatemala. The leaves are used externally to relieve muscular pains.

India. Hot water extract of the dried entire plant is taken orally as a narcotic and to relieve pain of dysmenorrhea. Hot water extract of the dried flower and leaf is taken orally for dyspepsia and gonorrhea and as a nerve stimulant. Hot water extract of the inflorescence of female plants is taken orally as an abortifacient. Hot water extract of the leaf is taken orally to relieve menstrual pain. For cuts, boils, and blisters, leaf paste is applied topically for 4 days. Hot water extract of the bark is taken orally for hydrocele and other inflammation. Extract of the leaves is used as an insect repellant. Hot water extract of the seed is taken orally as an emmenagogue. The powdered seed is taken orally as an aid in conception. One gram of seeds is powdered, then mixed with water, and given to women in the morning before breakfast for 7 days after menstruation.

The use of pepper and cane sugar is avoided. Paste of dried leaves is applied over the anus in the morning and evening for piles. The dried leaf juice is used externally on cuts and piles and taken orally as an anthelmintic. To eliminate cough, bronchitis, and other respiratory ailments, a half tablespoonful of powdered dried leaves is mixed with an equal amount of honey and taken orally three times daily. Seed oil is used externally for burns. The oil is extracted by roasting the seeds. Seeds are taken orally for diabetes, hysteria, and sleeplessness. The aerial parts are smoked to decrease nausea and vomiting induced by anticancer drugs. Hot water extract of the aerial parts is taken orally by males as an aphrodisiac. The dried aerial parts are smoked by women to increase their amorous prowess. The fresh leaves are taken orally for hemorrhoids. Hot water extract of the dried leaf and seed is taken orally for stomach troubles and indigestion. Fresh leaf juice is administered intraural to treat earache. The fruit is used externally for skin diseases. The unripe fruit is taken orally to induce sleep.

Iran. Fluidextract of the dried flowering top or the dried fruit is taken orally for abdominal pain associated with indigestion, for pain associated with cancer, for rheumatoid arthritis, for gastric cramps or neuralgia, for coughing, and as a hypnotic. Fluidextract of the dried fruit is taken orally for whooping cough, as a hypnotic, and a tranquilizer. The dried seed is taken orally as a diuretic. An infusion is taken orally as an analgesic in rheumatism or rheumatoid arthritis, a sedative, a diaphoretic, and for hysteric conditions, gout, epilepsy, and cholera. The seed oil is administered *per rectum* to reduce cramps associated with lead poisoning associated with constipation and vomiting. To reduce breast engorgement or reduce milk secretion, the seed oil is applied topically. In some cases, it would completely stop milk secretion. One to 2 g of seed oil is taken orally several times a day for urinary incontinency.

Jamaica. Hot water extract of the flower, leaf, and twig is taken orally as an antispasmodic and anodyne. Hot water extract of the resin is taken orally for diabetes.

Mexico. The aerial parts are smoked as a hallucinogen.

Morocco. The aerial parts are taken orally as a narcotic.

Nepal. Decoction of the leaf is taken orally by adults as an anthelmintic. The powdered leaf is mixed with cattle feed as a treatment for diarrhea. For headache, the dried leaves are ground with *Datura stramonium* leaves and *Picrorhiza schrophulariflora* stem and water then applied externally. The leaf juice is used externally as an antiseptic, as a hemostat on cuts and wounds, and to treat swelling of sprained joints. The seeds are crushed, mixed with curd, and taken orally for dysentery. Decoction of the seed is taken orally as an anthelmintic. To aid in parturition, 2 teaspoonfuls of powdered seeds are made into a paste with sesame oil (*Sesamum indicum* L.) and applied intravaginally during labor.

Pakistan. Hot water extract of the entire plant is taken orally as a parturifacient. Infusion of the leaf is taken orally for general weakness.

Saudi Arabia. The aerial parts, mixed with honey, sugar, and nutmeg, are taken orally as a psychotropic.

Senegal. The seed is taken orally as an emmenagogue.

South Africa. Hot water extract of the entire plant is taken orally for asthma[CS107]. Hot water extracts of the root and seed are taken orally to induce abortion, labor, and menstruation.

United States. Fluidextract of the inflorescence is taken orally as a narcotic, antispasmodic, analgesic, and aphrodisiac. Hot water extract of the flowering top is taken orally as a potent antispasmodic, anodyne, and narcotic. One teaspoon of plant material is steeped in 2 cups of boiling water, and 1 tablespoonful is taken two to four times a day. The dried aerial parts are smoked by both sexes as an aphrodisiac.

Vietnam. The seeds are taken orally as an emmenagogue.

West Indies. Hot water extract of the entire plant is taken orally as an antispasmodic.

Yugoslavia. Hot water extract of the seed is taken orally for diabetes.

Zimbabwe. Hot water extract of the aerial parts is taken orally as a treatment for malaria.

Medicinal values

Abortifacient activity

Alcohol extract of the dried leaf, administered intragastrically to pregnant rats at a dose of 125 mg/kg, produced teratogenic effects. Water extract of the dried leaf, administered intragastrically to pregnant rats at variable dosage levels on days 6–15 of pregnancy was active.

Acute cardiovascular fatalities

Six cases of possible acute cardiovascular death in young adults were reported where very recent cannabis ingestion was documented by the presence of Δ-9-tetrahydrocannabinol (Δ-9-THC) in postmortem blood samples. A broad toxicological blood analysis could not reveal other drugs.

Acute panic reaction (Koro)

Koro, an acute panic reaction related to the perception of penile retraction, was once considered limited to specific cultures. Over 70 American men responded by telephone to report negative reactions to cannabis. Three of them (Caucasians aged 22–26 years with considerable experience with cannabis) spontaneously mentioned experiencing symptoms of Koro after smoking cannabis. All three cases occurred after the participants had heard about cannabis-induced Koro and used the drug in a novel setting or atypical way. Two of the men had body dysmorphia, which may have contributed to symptoms. All three decreased their cannabis consumption after the Koro experience. Several factors may have interacted to create the symptoms. These include previous knowledge of cannabis-induced Koro, the use of cannabis in a way that might heighten a panic reaction, and poor body image.

Adverse effects

A causal role of acute cannabis intoxication in motor vehicle and other accidents has been shown by the presence of measurable levels of Δ-9-THC in the blood of drivers in the absence of alcohol or other drugs, by surveys of driving under the influence of cannabis, and by significantly higher accident culpability risk of drivers using cannabis. Evidence demonstrated that cannabis dependence, both behavioral and physical, occurred in about 7-10% of regular users, and that early onset of use—especially of weekly or daily use—is a strong predictor of future dependence. Cognitive impairments of various types are readily demonstrable during acute cannabis intoxication, but there is no suitable evidence yet available to permit a decision as to whether long-lasting or permanent functional losses can result from chronic heavy use in adults.

The gender effects on progression to treatment entry and on the frequency, severity, and related complications of the *Diagnostic and Statistical Manual of Mental Disorders*, 3rd edition revised drug and alcohol dependence among 271 substance-dependent patients (mean age: 32.6 years; 156 women) was studied. There was no gender difference among patients in the age at onset of regular use of any substance. Women experienced fewer years of regular use of opioids and cannabis and fewer years of regular alcohol drinking before entering treatment. Although the severity of drug and alcohol dependence did not differ by gender, women reported more severe psychiatric, medical, and employment complications. In a 3-day, double-blind, randomized, counterbalanced study, the behavioral, cognitive, and endocrine effects of 2.5 and 5 mg intravenous Δ-9-THC were characterized in 22 healthy individuals, who had been exposed to cannabis but had never been diagnosed with a cannabis abuse disorder. Prospective safety data at 1,3, and 6 months post-study was also analyzed. Δ-9-THC produced schizophrenia-like positive and negative symptoms, altered perception, increased anxiety and plasma cortisol, euphoria, disrupted immediate and delayed word recall, sparing recognition recall, impaired performance on tests of distractibility, verbal fluency, and working memory, but did not impair orientation.

This study examined the behavioral and neurochemical (cannabinoid *CB1* receptor gene expression) changes induced by spontaneous cannabinoid withdrawal in mice. Cessation of CP-55,940 treatment in tolerant mice induced a spontaneous time-dependent behavioral withdrawal syndrome consisting of marked increases (140%) in motor activity, number of rearings (170%), decreases in grooming (57%), wet-dog shakes (73%), and rubbing behaviors (74%) on day 1, progressively reaching values similar to vehicle-treated mice on day 3. This spontaneous cannabinoid withdrawal resulted in *CB1* gene expression up-regulation (20–30%) in caudate-putamen, ventromedial hypothalamic nucleus, central amygdaloid nucleus, and CA1, whereas in the CA3 field of hippocampus, a significant decrease (15–20%) was detected.

Alcohol interaction

The complementary DNA and genomic sequences encoding G protein-coupled cannabinoid receptors (CB1 and CB2) from several species were cloned. This has facilitated discoveries of endogenous ligands (endocannabinoids). Two fatty acid derivatives characterized to be arachidonylethanolamide and 2-arachidonylglycerol isolated from both nervous and peripheral tissues mimicked the pharmacological and behavioral effects of Δ-9-THC. The down-regulation of CB1 receptor function and its signal transduction by chronic alcohol was demonstrated. The observed down-regulation of CB1 receptor-binding and its signal transduction resulted from the persistent stimulation of receptors by the endogenous CB1 receptor agonists arachidonylethanolamide and 2-arachidonylglycerol, whose synthesis is increased by chronic alcohol treatment. The deletion of CB1 receptor has been shown to block voluntary alcohol intake in mice.

Allergenic effect

An "All India Coordinated Project on Aeroallergens and Human Health" was undertaken to discover the quantitative and qualitative prevalence of aerosols at 18 different centers in the country. Predominant airborne pollens were *Holoptelea*, *Poaceae*, *Asteraceae*, *Eucalyptus*, *Casuarina*, *Putanjiva*, *Cassia*, *Quercus*, *Cocos*, *Pinus*, *Cedrus*, *Ailanthus*, *Cheno/Amaranth*, *Cyperus*, *Argemone*, *Xanthium*, *Parthenium*, and others. Clinical and immunological evaluations revealed some allergenically important taxa. Allergenically important pollens were *Prosopis juliflora*, *Ricinus communis*, *Morus*, *Mallotus*, *Alnus*, *Querecus*, *Cedrus*, *Argemone*, *Amaranthus*, *Chenopodium*, *Holoptelea*, *Brassica*, *Cocos*, *Cannabis*, *Parthenium*, *Cassia*, and grasses. In the multitest routine skin-test battery, 78 of 127 patients tested (61%) were cannabis-test positive. Thirty of the 78 patients were randomly selected to determine if they had allergic rhinitis and/or asthma symptoms during the cannabis pollination period. By history, 22 (73%) claimed respiratory symptoms in July through September. All 22 of these subjects were also skin test-positive to weeds pollinating during the same period as cannabis (ragweed, pigweed, cocklebur, Russian thistle, marsh elder, or kochia).

Amnesic syndrome

A 26-year-old woman suffered disseminated intravascular coagulation (DIC) and a brief respiratory arrest following recreational use of 3,4-methylenedioxymethamphetamine (MDMA, or "ecstasy") together with amyl nitrate, lysergic acid (LSD), cannabis, and alcohol. She was left with residual cognitive and physical deficits, particularly severe anterograde memory disorder, mental slowness, severe ataxia, and dysarthria. Follow-up investigations have shown that these have persisted, although there has been some improvement in verbal recognition memory and in social functioning. Magnetic resonance imaging and quantified positron emission tomography investigations revealed severe cerebellar atrophy and hypometabolism accounting for the ataxia and dysarthria; thalamic, retrosplenial, and left medial temporal hypometabolism to which the anterograde amnesia can be attributed. There was some degree of frontotemporal–parietal hypometabolism, possibly accounting for the cognitive slowness. The putative relationship of these abnormalities to the direct and indirect effects of MDMA toxicity, hypoxia, and ischemia was considered.

Amyotrophic lateral sclerosis

One hundred thirty one respondents with amyotrophic lateral sclerosis—13 of whom reported using cannabis in the last 12 months—were examined. The results indicated that cannabis might be moderately effective at reducing symptoms of appetite loss, depression, pain, spasticity, and drooling. Cannabis was reported ineffective in reducing difficulties with speech and swallowing, and sexual dysfunction. The longest relief was reported for depression (approx 2–3 hours).

Analgesic activity

Ethanol (50%) extract of the entire plant, administered intra-peritoneally to mice at a dose of 250 mg/kg, was active vs tail pressure method. Flavonoid fraction of the leaf, administered intraperitoneally to mice, was active. The inflorescence, administered orally to male rats, produced weak activity vs paw pressure test, effective dose $(ED)_{50}$ 35.5 mg/kg and hot plate method, ED_{50} 53 mg/kg. Petroleum ether and ethanol (95%) extracts of the dried aerial parts, administered intragastrically to mice, was active vs phenylbenzoquinone-induced writhing, inhibitory concentration $(IC)_{50}$ 0.013 mg/kg and 0.045 mg/kg, respectively.

Analgesic effect

Ajulemic acid (AJA, CT-3, or IP-751), administered to healthy human adults and patients with chronic neuropathic pain, demonstrated a complete absence of psychotropic actions. It proved to be more effective than placebo in reducing this type of pain as measured by the visual analog scale. Signs of dependency were not observed after withdrawal at the end of the 1-week treatment period. Forty women undergoing elective abdominal hysterectomy were investigated in a randomized, double-blind, placebo-controlled, single-dose trial. Randomization took place when postoperative patient-controlled analgesia was discontinued on the second postoperative day. When patients requested further analgesia, they received a single, identical capsule of either 5 mg of oral Δ-9-THC (n = 20) or placebo (n = 20) in a double-blind fashion.

The primary outcome measure was summed pain intensity difference (SPID) at 6 hours after administration of the study medication derived from visual analog pain scores on movement and at rest. Secondary outcome measures were time-to-rescue medication and adverse effects of study medication. Mean (standard deviation [SD]) visual analog scale pain scores before medication in the placebo and Δ-9-THC groups were 6.3(2.6) and 6.4(1.3) cm on movement, and 3.2(1.9) and 3.3(0.9) at rest, respectively. There were no significant differences in mean (95% confidence interval [CI] of the difference) SPID at 6 hours between the groups (placebo 7.9, Δ-9-THC 4.3[−1.8 to 9] cm per hour on movement; placebo 8.8, Δ-9-THC 4.9[−0.2 to 8.1] cm per hour at rest) and time to rescue analgesia (placebo 217, Δ-9-THC 163[−22 to 130] minutes). Increased awareness of surroundings was reported more frequently in patients receiving Δ-9-THC (40 vs 5%, $p = 0.04$). There were no other significant differences with respect to adverse events.

THC, morphine, and a THC–morphine combination were administered to 12 healthy subjects using experimental pain models (heat, cold, pressure, and single and repeated transcutaneous electrical stimulation). THC (20 mg), morphine (30 mg), THC–morphine (20 mg THC + 30 mg morphine), or placebo were given orally as single dose. Reaction time, side effects (visual analog scales), and vital functions were monitored. For the pharmacokinetic profiling, blood samples were collected. THC did not significantly reduce pain. In the cold and heat tests, it even produced hyperalgesia, which was completely neutralized by THC–morphine. A slight additive analgesic effect was observed for THC–morphine in the electrical stimulation test. No analgesic effect resulted in the pressure and heat test, with neither THC nor THC–morphine.

Psychotropic and somatic side effects (sleepiness, euphoria, anxiety, confusion, nausea, dizziness, etc.) were common, but usually mild. Three cannabis-based extracts Δ-9-THC, cannabidiol [CBD], and a 1:1 mixture of them both) were given over a 12-week period in a randomized, double-blind, placebo-controlled, crossover trial. Extracts, which contained THC, proved most effective in symptom control. Regimens for the use of the sublingual spray emerged and a wide range of dosing requirements was observed. Side effects were common, reflecting a learning curve for both patient and study team. These were generally acceptable and little different to those seen when other psychoactive agents are used for chronic pain. Over a 6-week period 209 chronic noncancer pain patients were studied. Seventy-two (35%) subjects reported ever having used cannabis. Thirty-two (15%) subjects reported having used cannabis for pain relief (pain users), and 20 (10%) subjects were currently using cannabis for pain relief. Thirty-eight subjects denied using cannabis for pain relief (recreational users). Compared with nonusers, pain users were significantly younger ($p = 0.001$) and were more likely to be tobacco users ($p = 0.0001$). The largest group of patients using cannabis had pain caused by trauma and/or surgery (51%), and the site of pain was predominantly neck/upper body and myofascial (68 and 65%, respectively). The median duration of pain was similar in both pain users and recreational users (8 vs 7 years; $p = 0.7$). There was a wide range of amounts and frequency of cannabis use. Of the 32 subjects who used cannabis for pain, 17 (53%) used four puffs or less at each dosing interval, eight (25%) smoked a whole cannabis cigarette (joint), and four (12%) smoked more than one joint. Seven (22%) of these subjects used cannabis more than once daily, five (16%) used it daily, eight (25%) used it weekly, and nine (28%) used it rarely. Pain, sleep, and mood were most frequently reported as improving with cannabis use, and "high" and dry mouths were the most commonly reported side effects. Patients with chronic pain completed a questionnaire about the type of cannabis used, the mode of administration, the amount used and the frequency of use, and their perception of the effectiveness of cannabis on a set of pain-associated symptoms and side effects. Fifteen patients (10 males) were interviewed (median age, 49.5 years; range, 24–68 years). All patients smoked herbal cannabis for therapeutic reasons (median duration of use, 6 years; range, 2 weeks–37 years). Seven patients only smoked at night (median dose eight puffs, range two to eight puffs), and eight patients used cannabis mainly during the day (median dose of three puffs; range, two to eight puffs); the median frequency of use was four times per day (range, 1 to 16 times/day). Twelve patients reported improvement in pain and mood, whereas 11 reported improvement in sleep. Eight patients reported a "high;" six denied a "high." Tolerance to cannabis was not reported. THC was administered to six patients with chronic pain at doses 5–20 mg/day. A sufficient pain relief had been achieved in three patients. The other three suffered from intolerable side effects, such as nausea, dizziness, and sedation without a reduction of pain intensity. In these cases, the treatment was continued with other analgesics.

Ankylosing spondylitis

Ankylosing spondylitis is a systemic disorder occurring in genetically predisposed individuals. The disease course appears to be characterized by bouts of partial remission and flares. There were 214 patients questioned (169 men, 45 women; average disease duration, 25 years; age of disease onset, 22 years). The main symptoms of flare were pain (all groups), immobility (90%), fatigue (80%), and emotional symptoms, such as depression, withdrawal, and anger, (75%). All of patients experienced between one and five localized flares per year. Fifty-five percent of the groups contained patients ($n = 85$) who experienced a generalized flare. The main perceived triggers of flare were stress (80%) and "overdoing it" (50%). Patients reported that a flare might last anywhere from a few days to a few weeks and relief from flare were by analgesic injections (including opiates), relaxation, sleep, and cannabis. Three-quarters of the groups agreed that there was no long-term effect on the ankylosing sponylitis following a flare.

Anti-arthritic effect

Oral administration of AJA, a cannabinoid acid devoid of psychoactivity, reduced joint tissue damage in rats with adjuvant arthritis. Peripheral blood monocytes (PBM) and synovial fluid monocytes (SFM) were isolated from healthy subjects and patients with inflammatory arthritis, respectively, treated with AJA (0–30 m*M*) in vitro, and then stimulated with lipopolysaccharide. Cells were harvested for messenger RNA (mRNA), and supernatants were collected for cytokine assay. Addition of AJA to PBM and SFM in vitro reduced both steady-state levels of interleukin-1γ (IL-1γ) mRNA and secretion of IL-1γ in a concentration-dependent manner. Suppression was maximal (50.4%) at 10 m*M* AJA ($p < 0.05$ vs untreated controls, $n = 7$). AJA did not influence tumor necrosis factor-α (TNF-α) gene expression in or secretion from PBM.

Anticonvulsant activity

Ethanol (95%) extract of the entire plant, administered subcutaneously to male mice and rats at a dose of 2–4 mL/kg, was active vs metrazole and electroshock, respectively. A dose of 4 mL/kg was inactive vs strychnine convulsions in mice. The entire plant, smoked by 29 patients with epilepsy under the age of 30 years, was active. It must be noted that in some species, cannabinoids can precipitate epileptic seizures. Tincture of the resin, administered intraperitoneally to mice at a dose of 25 mg/kg, produced 80% protection vs pentyle-netetrazole convulsions.

Anti-emetic activity

In a qualitative study of self-care in pregnancy, birth, and lactation within a nonrandom sample of 27 women in British Columbia, Canada, 20 women (74%) experienced pregnancy- induced nausea. Ten of these women used antiemetic herbal remedies, which included ginger, peppermint, and cannabis. Only ginger has been subjected to clinical trials among pregnant women, although the three herbs were clinically effective against nausea and vomiting in other contexts, such as chemotherapy-induced nausea and post-operative nausea. CBD, a major non- psychoactive cannabinoid administered by oral infusion to rats with nausea elicited by lithium chloride, and with conditioned nausea elicited by a flavor paired with lithium chloride, was active[CS382]. Oral nabilone, oral dronabinol (THC), and intramuscular levonantradol were administered to 1366 patients. Cannabinoids were more effective antiemetics than prochlorperazine, metoclopramide, chlorpromazine, thiethylperazine, haloperidol, domperidone, or alizapride. Relative risk was 1.38 (95% CI 1.18–1.62), number-needed-to-treat (NNT) was 6 for complete control of nausea; relative risk was 1.28 (CI 1.08–1.51), NNT 8 for complete control of vomiting. Cannabinoids were not more effective in patients receiving very low or very high emetogenic chemotherapy. In crossover trials, patients preferred cannabinoids for future chemotherapy cycles: relative risk 2.39 (2.05–2.78), NNT 3. Some potentially beneficial side effects occurred more often with cannabinoids: "high" 10.6 (6.86–16.5), NNT 3; sedation or drowsiness 1.66 (1.46–1.89),

NNT 5; euphoria 12.5 (3–52.1), NNT 7. Harmful side effects also occurred more often with cannabinoids: dizziness 2.97 (2.31– 3.83), NNT 3; dysphoria or depression 8.06 (3.38–19.2), NNT 8; hallucinations 6.10 (2.41–15.4), NNT 17; paranoia 8.58 (6.38–11.5), NNT 20; and arterial hypotension 2.23 (1.75–2.83), NNT 7. Patients given cannabinoids were more likely to withdraw because of side effects (relative risk 4.67 [3.07–7.09]; NNT 11).

Antifungal activity

Ethanol (50%) extract of the dried leaf was active on *Rhizoctonia solani*, mycelial inhibition was 65.99%. Water extract of the fresh leaf on agar plate at a concentration of 1:1 was active on *Fusarium oxysporum*. The water extract also produced strong activity on *Ustilago maydis* and *Ustilago nuda*. Water extract of the fresh shoot on agar plate was inactive on *Helminthosporium turcicum*.

Antiglaucomic activity

Water extract of the dried entire plant, administered intravenously to Rhesus monkeys and rabbits at a dose of 0.01 μg/animal, was active. The intraocular pressure rose for 24 hours postinjection, then fell for 3 days. A dose of 25 μg/animal, administered intravenously to rabbits, was also active. The effect was not influenced by atropine, scopolamine, methysergide, haloperidol, chlorpromazine, spironolactone, yohimbine or dexamethasone. Partial inhibition was seen when galactose, glucose or mannose were administered intravenously, concurrently. Water extract of the dried leaf and stem, applied opthalmically to rabbits was active.

Antigonadotropin effect

Ethanol (80%) extract of the dried aerial parts, administered intra-gastrically to male langurs at a dose of 14 mg/kg daily for 90 days produced equivocal effect.

Anti-inflammatory activity

Petroleum ether and ethanol (95%) extracts of the dried aerial parts, applied externally on mice at a dose of 100 μg/ear, was active vs tissue plasminogen activator-induced erythema of the ear. CBD was administered orally to rats at doses of 5–40 mg/kg daily for 3 days after the onset of acute inflammation induced by intraplantar injection of 0.1 mL carrageenan (1% w/v in saline). CBD had a time- and dose-dependent antihyperalgesic effect after a single injection. Edema following carrageenan peaked at 3 hours and lasted 72 hours. A single dose of CBD reduced edema in a dose-dependent fashion and subsequent daily doses produced further time- and dose-related reductions. There were decreases in prostaglandin E2 (PGE2) plasma levels, tissue cyclo-oxygenase activity, production of oxygen-derived free radicals, and nitric oxide ([NO], nitrite/nitrate content) after three doses of CBD. The effect on NO seemed to depend on a lower expression of the endothelial isoform of NO synthase.

Antispermatogenic effect

Sixteen healthy chronic marijuana smokers were associated with a decline in sperm concentration and total sperm count during the fifth and sixth weeks after 4 weeks of high-dose smoking (8–20 cigarettes/day). The dried aerial part, taken by inhalation daily, decreases the quantity as well as quality of spermatozoa. Ethanol (80%) extract of the dried aerial parts, administered intragastrically to langurs at a dose of 14 mg/kg daily for 90 days, was equivocal. Ethanol (95%) extract of the dried aerial parts, administered intraperitoneally to mice at a dose of 2 mg/animal daily for 45 days, produced a complete arrest of spermatogenesis. The effect was reversible.

Antistress activity

The leaf smoke, in combination with hashish smoke, administered to rats housed in a wire cage inside a larger cage with a cat, was equivocal. The rats' brains were dissected and measured for protein and catecholamine levels.

Anti-tumor activity

Arachidonyl ethanolamide, in three cervical carcinoma (CxCa) cell lines at increasing doses with or without antagonists to receptors to arachidonyl ethanolamide, induced apoptosis of CxCa cell lines via aberrantly expressed vanilloid receptor-1. Arachidonyl ethanolamide-binding to the classical CB1 and CB2 cannabinoid receptors mediated a protective effect. A strong expression of the three forms of arachidonyl ethanolamide receptors was observed in ex vivo CxCa biopsies. Three cannabis constituents, CBD, Δ-8-THC, and cannabinol displayed anti-proliferative activity in several human cancer cell lines in vitro. They were oxidized to their respective paraquinones 2,4, and 6. Quinone 2 significantly reduced cancer growth of HT-29 cancer in nude mice. Δ-9-THC binds and activates membrane receptors of the 7-transmembrane domain, G protein-coupled superfamily. Several putative endocannabinoids have been identified, including anandamide (AEA), 2-arachidonyl glycerol, and noladin ether. Synthesis of numerous cannabinomimetics has expanded the repertoire of cannabinoid receptor ligands with the pharmacodynamic properties of agonists, antagonists, and inverse agonists. These ligands have proven to be powerful tools both for the molecular characterization of cannabinoid receptors and the delineation of their intrinsic signaling pathways. Much of the understanding of the signaling mechanisms activated by cannabinoids has been derived from studies of receptors expressed by tumor cells. Cannabinoids and their derivatives exerted palliative effects in cancer patients by preventing nausea, vomiting, and pain and by stimulating appetite. These compounds have been shown to inhibit the growth of tumor cells in culture and animal models by modulating key cell-signaling pathways. Cannabinoids are usually well tolerated, and do not produce the generalized toxic effects of conventional chemotherapies.

Anxiolytic activity

AEA, a primary endogenous ligand of the brain cannabinoid receptors, is released in selected regions of the brain and is deactivated through a two-step process consisting of transport into cells followed by intracellular hydrolysis. Pharmacological blockade of the enzyme fatty acid amide hydrolase (FAAH), which is responsible for intracellular AEA degradation, produced anxiolytic-like effects in rats without causing the wide spectrum of behavioral responses typical of direct-acting cannabinoid agonists. These findings suggest that AEA contributes to the regulation of emotion and anxiety, and that FAAH might be the target for a novel class of anxiolytic drugs.

Attention deficit hyperactivity disorder

Attention defict hyperactivity disorder has been considered a mental and behavioral disorder of childhood and adolescence. It is being increasingly recognized in adults, who may have psychiatric comorbidity with secondary depression, or a tendency to drug and alcohol abuse. A 32-year-old woman known for years as suffering from borderline personality disorder and drug dependence (including cannabis, LSD, and ecstasy) and alcohol abuse that did not respond to treatment was reported. Only when correctly diagnosed as attention defict hyperactivity disorder and appropriately treated with the psychotropic stimulant methylphenidate (Ritalin®), was there significant improvement. She succeeded academically, which had not been possible previously, her craving for drugs diminished, and a drug-free state was reached.

Auditory function

Eight male subjects (aged 22–30 years) who had previously used cannabis were investigated. They performed air conduction pure tone audiometry in both ears over 0.5–8 kHz. A simple test of frequency selectivity by detecting a 4-kHz tone under two masking noise conditions was also carried out in one ear. Three test sessions at weekly intervals were carried out, at the start of which they ingested a capsule containing either placebo, 7.5, or 15 mg of THC. These were administered in a randomized cross-over, double-blind manner. Auditory testing was carried out 2 hours after ingestion. Blood samples were also obtained at this time point and assayed for Δ-9-THC and 11-hydroxy-THC levels. No significant changes in threshold or frequency resolution were seen with the dosages employed in this study.

Behavioral effect

A four-page, self-completed questionnaire was designed to determine the drugs used (licit, illicit, and doping substances) along with beliefs about doping and the psychosociological factors associated with their consumption. The questionnaire was distributed to high school students enrolled in a school sports association in eastern France. The completed forms were received from 1459 athletes: 4% stated that they had used doping agents at least once in their life (their main source of supply being peers and health professionals). Thirty-four percent of the sample smoked some tobacco, 66% used alcohol, 19% used cannabis, 4% took ecstasy, 10% took tranquillizers, 9% used hypnotics, 4% used creatine, and 41% used vitamins against fatigue. Beliefs about doping did not differ among doping agent users and nonusers, except for the associated health risks, which were minimized by users. Users of doping agents stated that the quality of the relations that they maintained with their parents was sharply degraded, and they reported that they were susceptible to influence and difficult to live with. More often than nondoping-agent users, these adolescents were neither happy, nor healthy, although paradoxically, they seemed less anxious and were more self-confident. Maternal exposure to Δ-9- THC in rats resulted in alteration in the pattern of ontogeny of spontaneous locomotor and exploratory behavior in the offspring. Adult animals exposed during gestational and lactational periods exhibited persistent alterations in the behavioral response to novelty, social interactions, sexual orientation, and sexual behavior. They also showed a lack of habituation and reactivity to different illumination conditions. Adult offspring of both sexes also displayed a characteristic increase in spontaneous and water-induced grooming behavior. Some of the effects were dependent on the sex of the animals being studied, and the dose of cannabinoid administered to the mother during gestational and lactational periods. Maternal exposure to low doses of THC sensitized the adult offspring of both sexes to the reinforcing effects of morphine, as measured in a conditioned place preference paradigm.

β-Endorphin interaction

Δ-9-THC administered to rats produced large increases in extracellular levels of β-endorphin in the ventral tegmental area and lesser increases in the shell of the nucleus accumbens (Nac). In rats that had learned to discriminate injections of THC from injections of vehicle, the opioid agonist morphine did not produce THC-like discriminative effects, but markedly increased discrimination of THC. The opioid antagonist naloxone reduced the discriminative effects of THC. Bilateral microinjections of β-endorphin directly into the ventral tegmental area, but not into the shell of the Nac, markedly increased the discriminative effects of ineffective threshold doses of THC, but had no effect when given alone. The increase was blocked by naloxone.

Binocular depth inversion reduction

A study to assess whether the binocular depth inversion illusion (BDII) could detect subtle cognitive impairment owing to regular cannabis use was conducted. Ten regular cannabis users and 10 healthy controls from the same community sources, matched for age, sex, and premorbid intelligence quotient (IQ) were evaluated. The subjects were also compared on measures of executive functioning, memory, and personality. Regular cannabis users were found to have significantly higher BDII scores for inverted images. This was not to the result of a problem in the primary processing of visual information, as there was no significant difference between the groups for depth perception of normal images. There was no relationship between BDII scores for inverted images and time since the last dose, suggesting that the measured impairment of BDII more closely reflected chronic than acute effects of regular cannabis use. There were no significant differences between the groups for other neuropsychological measures of memory or executive function. A positive relationship was found between psychoticism as defined by the revised Eysenck Personality Questionnaire and cannabis, tobacco, and alcohol use. Cannabis users also used significantly larger amounts of alcohol. No relationship was found between BDII scores and drug use other than cannabis or psychoticism. Nabilone, a psychoactive synthetic 9-*trans*-ketocannabinoid, CBD, and a combined oral application of both substances on binocular depth inversion and behavioral states were investigated in nine healthy male volunteers. A significant impairment of binocular depth perception was found when nabilone was administered, but combined application with CBD revealed reduced effects on binocular depth inversion.

Birth-weight effect

A total of 32,483 cannabis-using women giving birth to live-born infants were investigated. The largest reduction in mean birth-weight for any cannabis use during pregnancy was 48 g (95% CI, 83–14 g), with considerable heterogeneity among the five studies. Mean birth-weight was increased by 62 g (95% CI, 8-g reduction – 132-g increase; p heterogeneity, 0.59) among infrequent users (≤ weekly), whereas cannabis use at least four times per week had a 131-g reduction in mean birth- weight (95% CI 52–209-g reduction; p heterogeneity, 0.25). From the five studies of low birth-weight, the pooled odds ratio for any use was 1.09 (95% CI 0.94–1.27; p heterogeneity, 0.19). In a cohort study consisted of a multiethnic population of 7470 pregnant women. Information on the use of drugs was obtained from personal interviews at entry to the study and assays of serum obtained during pregnancy. Pregnancy outcome data (low birth-weight [<2500 g], pre-term birth [<37 weeks gestation], and abruptio placentae) were obtained with a standardized study protocol. A total of 2.3% of the women used cocaine and 11% used cannabis during pregnancy. Cannabis use was not associated with low birth-weight (1.1, 0.9–1.5), pre-term delivery (adjusted odds ratio [OR] 1.1, CI 0.8–1.3), or abruptio placentae (1.3, 0.6–2.8).

Bladder dysfunction

Two whole-plant extracts of *Cannabis sativa* were administered to patients with advanced multiple sclerosis (MS) and refractory troublesome lower urinary tract symptoms. The patients took the extracts containing Δ-9-THC and CBD (2.5 mg of each per spray) for 8 weeks followed by THC-only (2.5 mg THC per spray) for a further eight weeks, and then into a long-term extension. Assessments included urinary frequency and volume charts, incontinence pad weights, cystometry, and visual analog scales for secondary troublesome symptoms. Twenty-one patients were recruited and data from 15 were evaluated. Urinary urgency, the number and volume of incontinence episodes, frequency, and nocturia all decreased significantly following treatment ($p < 0.05$, Wilcoxon's signed rank test). Daily total voided, catheterized and urinary incontinence pad weights also decreased significantly for both extracts. Patient self-assessment of pain, spasticity, and quality of sleep improved significantly ($p < 0.05$, Wilcoxon's signed rank test) with pain improvement continuing up to a median of 35 weeks. There were few troublesome side effects, suggesting that cannabis-based medicinal extracts are a safe and effective treatment for urinary and other problems in patients with advanced MS.

Blood pressure stress reactivity effect

Data from an ascorbic acid (AA) trial (Cetebe 3 g/day for 14 days, $n = 108$) were compared by substance use level regarding systolic blood pressure (SBP) stress reactivity to the anticipation and actual experience phases of a standardized psychological stressor (10 minutes of public speaking and arithmetic). Self-reported never users of cannabis, persons not currently smoking tobacco, and persons consuming three or more caffeine beverages daily all exhibited AA SBP stress reactivity protection to the actual stressor, but not during the anticipation phase. Self-reported ever cannabis users, current tobacco smokers, and persons consuming less than three caffeine beverages daily exhibited the AA SBP protection during the anticipation phase, but only the lower caffeine consumption group exhibited AA protection during both phases. Covariates (neuroticism, extraversion and depression scores, age, sex, body mass index) were not significant.

Blood-borne sexually transmitted infections

Substance use, including alcohol and illicit drugs, increases the risk for the acquisition and transmission of sexually transmitted infection (STI). The prevalence of blood-borne STI including human immuno-deficiency virus (HIV), human T-cell lymphotrophic virus type 1, hepatitis B virus, and syphilis in residents of a detoxification and rehabilitation unit in Jamaica were investigated. The demographic characteristics and the results of laboratory investigations for STI in 301 substance abusers presented during a 5-year period were reviewed. The laboratory results were compared with those of 131 blood donors. The substances used by participants were alcohol, cannabis, and cocaine. None of the clients was an intravenous drug user. Female substance abusers were at higher risk for STI.

The prevalence of STI in substance abusers did not differ significantly from that in blood donors (12% vs 10%). The prevalence of syphilis in substance abusers was significantly higher than that in blood donors (6% vs 3%, $p < 0.05$). The prevalence of syphilis was dramatically increased in female substance abusers and female blood donors (30%, $p < 0.001$ and 13%, $p < 0.05$, respectively). An excess of human T-cell lymphotrophic virus type 1 was also observed in female compared with male substance abusers. Unemployment was identified also as a risk factor for sexually transmitted disease in substance abusers.

Brain aging effect

The impact of duration of education, cannabis addiction and smoking on cognition and brain aging was studied in 211 healthy Egyptian volunteers with mean age of 46.4 ± 3.6 years (range, 20–76 years). The subjects were classified into two groups: Gr I (n = 174; mean age, 49.9 ± 3.8 years; range, 20–76 years), nonaddicts, smokers, and nonsmokers, educated and noneducated, and Gr II cannabis addicts (n = 37; mean age, 43.6 ± 2.6 years; range, 20–72 years) all smokers, educated and noneducated. Outcome measures included the Paced Auditory Serial Addition test for testing attention and the Trailmaking test A and Trailmaking test B (TMb) for testing psychomotor performance. Age correlated positively with score of TMb in the nonaddict group and in the addict group (Trailmaking test A and TMb). Years of education correlated negatively with scores of TMb in the nonaddict group (Gr I) but not the addict group (Gr II). Cannabis addicts (Gr II) had significantly poorer attention than nonaddict normal volunteers (Gr I). It was determined that impairment of psychomotor performance is age related whether in normal nonaddicts or in cannabis addicts. A decline in attention was detected in cannabis addicts and has been considered a feature of pathological aging.

Brain cannabinoid receptor

In humans, psychoactive cannabinoids produce euphoria, enhancement of sensory perception, tachycardia, antinociception, difficulties in concentration, and impairment of memory. The cognitive deficiencies persist after withdrawal. The toxicity of cannabis has been underestimated for a long time, since recent findings revealed that Δ-9-THC-induced cell death with shrinkage of neurons and DNA fragmentation in the hippocampus. The acute effects of cannabinoids, as well as the development of tolerance, are mediated by G protein-coupled cannabinoid receptors. The CB1 receptor and its splice variant, CB1A, are found predominantly in the brain with highest densities in the hippocampus, cerebellum, and striatum. The CB2 receptor is found predominantly in the spleen and in hemopoietic cells and has only 44% overall nucleotide sequence identity with the CB1 receptor. The existence of this receptor provided the molecular basis for the immunosuppressive actions of cannabis. The CB1 receptor mediates inhibition of adenylate cyclase, inhibition of N- and P/Q-type calcium channels, stimulation of potassium channels, and activation of mitogen-activated protein kinase. The CB2 receptor mediates inhibition of adenylate cyclase and activation of mitogen-activated protein kinase. The discovery of endogenous cannabinoid receptor ligands, AEA (*N*-arachidonyl-ethanolamine), and 2-arachidonylglycerol made the notion of a central cannabinoid neuromodulatory system plausible. AEA is released from neurons on depolarization through a mechanism that requires calcium-dependent cleavage from a phospholipid precursor in neuronal membranes.

The release of AEA is followed by rapid uptake into the plasma and hydrolysis by fatty-acid amidohydrolase. The psychoactive cannabinoids increase the activity of dopaminergic neurons in the ventral tegmental area–mesolimbic pathway. Because these dopaminergic circuits are known to play a pivotal role in mediating the reinforcing (rewarding) effects of the most drugs of abuse, the enhanced dopaminergic drive elicited by the cannabinoids is thought to underlie the reinforcing and abuse properties of cannabis. Thus, cannabinoids share a final common neuronal action with other major drugs of abuse such as morphine, ethanol, and nicotine in producing facilitation of the mesolimbic dopamine system.

Hippocampal slices from humans, guinea pigs, rats, and mice, and cerebellar, cerebro-cortical, and hypothalamic slices from guinea pigs were incubated with [^{3}H] noradrenaline and then superfused. Tritium overflow was evoked either electrically (0.3 or 1 Hz) or by introduction of Ca^{2+} ions (1.3 μM) into Ca^{2+}-free, K^+-rich medium (25 μM) containing 1 μM of tetrodotoxin. The cyclic adenosone monophosphate (cAMP) accumulation stimulated by 10 μM of forskolin was determined in guinea pig hippocampal membranes. The following drugs were used: the cannabinoid receptor-agonists (-)-*cis*-3-[2-hydroxy-4-(1,1- dimethylheptyl) phenyl]-*trans*-4-(3-hydroxypropyl)cyclo-hexanol (CP-55,940) and R(+) -[2,3 -dihydro-5-methyl-3 - [(morpholinyl) methyl]pyrrolo[1,2, 3-de]-1 ,4-benzoxazinyl]-(1-naphthalenyl)methanone (WIN 55,212-2 [WIN]), the inactive *S*(-)-enantiomer of the latter (WIN 55,212-3) and the CB1 receptor antagonist *N*-piperidino-5-(4-chlorophenyl)-1-(2,4-dichlorophenyl) -4-methyl-3-pyrazole-carboxamide (SR 141716). The electrically evoked tritium overflow from guinea pig hippocampal slices was reduced by WIN (peak inhibitory concentration 30%, 6.5) but not affected by WIN 55,212-3 up to 10 m*M*.

The concentration–response curve of WIN was shifted to the right by SR 141716 (0.032-μM) (apparent pA2 8.2), which by itself did not affect the evoked overflow. WIN (1 μM) also inhibited the Ca^{2+}-evoked tritium overflow in guinea pig hippocampal slices and the electrically evoked overflow in guinea pig cerebellar, cerebro-cortical, and hypothalamic slices, as well as in human hippocampal slices, but not in rat and mouse hippocampal slices. SR 141716 (0.32 μM) markedly attenuated the WIN-induced inhibition in guinea pig and human brain slices. SR 141716 (0.32 μM) by itself increased the electrically evoked tritium overflow in guinea pig hippocampal slices, but failed to do so in slices from the other brain regions of the guinea pig and in human hippocampal slices, but failed to do so in slices from the other brain regions of the guinea pig and in human hippocampal slices. The cAMP accumulation stimulated by forskolin was reduced by CP-55,940 and WIN.

The concentration-response curve of CP-55,940 was shifted to the right by SR 141716 (0.1 μM; apparent pA2 8.3), that by itself did not affect cAMP accumulation. In conclusion, cannabinoid receptors of the CB1 subtype occur in the human hippocampus, where they may contribute to the psychotropic effects of cannabis, and in the guinea pig hippocampus, cerebellum, cerebral cortex, and hypothalamus. The CB1 receptor in the guinea pig hippocampus is located presynaptically, was activated by endogenous cannabinoids, and may be negatively coupled to adenylyl cyclase. The acute administration of AEA or THC in rats increased the maximum binding capacity (B_{max}) of cannabinoid receptors in the cerebellum and, particularly, in the hippocampus. This effect was also observed after 5 days of a daily exposure to AEA or THC. The increase in the B_{max} after the acute treatment seemed to be caused by changes in the receptor affinity (high K_d). The increase after the chronic exposure may be attributed to an increase in the density of receptors. The [^{3}H]CP-55,940 binding to cannabinoid receptors in the striatum, the limbic forebrain, the mesencephalon, and the medial basal hypothalamus was not altered after the acute exposure to AEA or THC. The chronic exposure to THC significantly decreased the B_{max} of these receptors in the striatum and nonsignificantly in the mesencephalon. This effect was not elicited after the chronic exposure to AEA and was not accompanied by changes in the K_d.

Cannabinoid hyperemesis

Nineteen patients were identified with chronic cannabis abuse and a cyclical vomiting illness. Follow-up was provided with serial urine drug screen analysis and regular clinical consultation to chart the clinical course. Of the 19 patients, five refused consent and were lost to follow-up, and five were excluded based on cofounders. In all cases, chronic cannabis abuse predated the onset of the cyclical vomiting illness. Cessation of cannabis abuse led to cessation of the cyclical vomiting illness in seven cases. Three cases did not abstain and continued to have recurrent episodes of vomiting. Three cases rechallenged themselves after a period of abstinence and suffered a return to illness. Two of these cases abstained again and became, and remain, well. The third case did not and remains ill. A novel finding was that 9 of the 10 patients, including the previously published case, displayed an abnormal washing behavior during episodes of active illness.

Cannabinoid-induced fos expression

Cannabinoid CB1 receptor agonist CP-55,940 in Lewis and Wistar rats was investigated. A moderate (50 μg/kg) and a high (250 μg/kg) dose level were used. The 250-μg/kg dose caused locomotor suppression, hypothermia, and catalepsy in both strains, but with a significantly greater effect in Wistar rats. The 50-μg/kg dose provoked moderate hypothermia and locomotor suppression but in Wistar rats only. CP-55,940 caused significant Fos immunoreactivity in 24 out of 33 brain regions examined. The most dense expression was seen in the paraventricular nucleus of the hypothalamus, the islands of Callej a, the lateral septum (ventral), the central nucleus of the amygdala, the bed nucleus of the stria terminalis (lateral division), and the ventrolateral periaqueductal gray. Despite having a similar distribution of CP-55,940- induced Fos expression,

Lewis rats showed less overall Fos expression than Wistar rats in nearly every brain region counted. This held equally true for anxiety-related brain structures (e.g., central nucleus of the amygdala, periaqueductal gray, and the paraventricular nucleus of the hypothalamus) and reward-related sites (Nac and pedunculopontine tegmental nucleus). In a further experiment, Wistar rats and Lewis rats did not differ in the amount of Fos immunoreactivity produced by cocaine (15 mg/kg). These results indicate that Lewis rats are less sensitive to the behavioral, physiological and neural effects of cannabinoids.

Cannabis withdrawal effect

A 35-year-old male was cognitively assessed prior to cessation of 18 years of daily cannabis use and monitored for several weeks post- cessation. Brain event-related potential measures of selective attention reflecting a difficulty in filtering out complex irrelevant information showed no indication of improvement over 6 weeks of abstinence. When tested in the acutely intoxicated state prior to cessation of use, a dramatic normalization of the event-related potential signature was observed. A treatment program based on supportive–expressive psychotherapy was administered and depression, anxiety, and general psychological health were monitored over the course of withdrawal from cannabis.

Cannabis–amphetamine interaction

Cannabinoid–amphetamine interactions were studied as follows:

1. 30 minutes after acute injection of (-)-Δ-9-THC (0.1 or 6.4 mg/kg, intraperitoneally).

2. 30 minutes after the last injection of 14-daily treatment with (-)-Δ-9-THC (0.1 or 6.4 mg/kg).
3. 24 hours after the last injection of 14- daily treatment with (-)-Δ-9-THC (6.4 mg/kg).

Acute cannabinoid exposure antagonized the amphetamine-induced dose-dependent increase in locomotion, exploration, and the decrease in inactivity. Chronic treatment with (-)-Δ-9-THC resulted in tolerance to this antagonistic effect on locomotion and inactivity but not on exploration, and potentiated amphetamine-induced stereotypes. Lastly, 24 hours of withdrawal after 14 days of cannabinoid treatment resulted in sensitization to the effects of D-amphetamine on locomotion, exploration, and stereotypes.

Cannabis-induced coma

Two cases of cannabis-induced coma were reported following accidental ingestion of cannabis cookies. The possibility of cannabis ingestion should be considered in cases of unexplained coma in a previously healthy young child if signs of conjunctival hyperemia, pupillary dilatation, and tachycardia were present and other causes, such as central nervous system infection or trauma were unlikely.

Cannabis-related arteritis

A 19-year-old man who presented with plantar claudication associated with necrosis in a toe underwent diagnostic arteriography and surgery for popliteal artery entrapment type III was studied. Surgical clearance resolved the popliteal artery entrapment but left the clinical symptoms unchanged. Closer questioning disclosed a history of cannabis consumption and intravenous vasodilatory therapy was started. After the 21-day course of vasodilator agents, the pain disappeared and the toe necrosis regressed. The patient stopped taking cannabis and had no signs of recurrence. A 24-year-old woman who was a heavy cannabis smoker with progressive Raynauld's phenomenon and digital necrosis, was investigated. Systemic sclerosis and other connective tissue disorders, as well as arteriosclerosis and arterial emboli were excluded with appropriate laboratory examinations. Arteriography revealed multiple forearm, palmar and digital occlusions with corkscrew-shaped vessels. Based on the characteristic arteriography and clinical findings, the diagnosis of cannabis arteritis was retained. With careful necrectomy, conservative wound dressings and secondary prostacyclin therapy a complete healing of digital necrosis was observed.

There was no recurrence during the 6-month follow-up. Young men were presented with distal arteriopathy of the lower limbs in three cases, and of the left upper limb in the remaining patient. Symptoms occurred progressively, distal pulses had disappeared, and distal necrosis was constant. Three patients suffered from Raynauld's phenomenon, none of them presented with venous thrombosis. Radiological evaluation revealed distal abnormalities in all cases, and proximal arterial thrombosis in one case. The four patients were cannabis smokers for at least four years. With cannabis interruption and symptomatic treatment, lesions improved for three patients. For one of them, recurrence of arteriopathy occurred when he resumed smoking cannabis. For the fourth who never stopped cannabis, an amputation was necessary. Ten male moderate tobacco smokers and regular cannabis users with a median age of 23.7 years, developed subacute distal ischemia of the lower or upper limbs, leading to necrosis in the toes and/or fingers and sometimes to distal limb gangrene. Two of the patients also presented with venous thrombosis and three patients were suffering from a recent Raynauld's phenomenon. Biological test results did not show evidence of the classical vascular risk factors for thrombosis.

Arteriographic evaluation in all of the cases revealed distal abnormalities in the arteries of feet, legs, forearms, and hands resembling those of Buerger's disease. A collateral circulation sometimes with opacification of the vasa nervorum was noted. In some cases, arterial proximal atherosclerotic lesions and venous thrombosis were observed. Despite treatment with ilomedine and heparin in all cases, five amputations were necessary in four patients. The vasoconstrictor effect of cannabis on the vascular system has been known for a long time. It has been shown that Δ-8-THC and Δ-9-THC may induce peripheral vasoconstrictor activity. Cannabis arteritis resembles Buerger's disease, but patients were moderate tobacco smokers and regular cannabis users.

Cannabis-related flashback

A young man who offended a friend without any objective reason was reported. The report of the forensic psychiatrist demonstrated that the offense was committed under the influence of a cannabis flashback. The last time the offender had consumed cannabis was 2 weeks before the acts. A plasmatic detection was realized and showed a level of 6 ng/mL, 30 minutes after the beginning of the flashback.

Capgras syndrome

A report describes an apparently greater incidence of Capgras syndrome among the Maori population compared with the European population. Five cases of Capgras syndrome were identified in the eastern catchment area where 19% of the population identified as Maori, 75% as European, and 6% as other or nonspecified. All of the cases occurred in Maori patients. No cases were identified in the western catchment area where 12% of the population identified as Maori, 87% as European, and 1% as other or nonspecified. Four of five cases were females. Two cases had a history of cannabis use. Three cases had exhibited dangerous behavior towards family members.

Carcinogenic activity

The dried leaf, administered intraperitoneally to rats of both sexes at a dose of 7 mg/kg/week, was active. The animals were irradiated with y radiation between 40 and 50 days of age and observed for 78 weeks. There was a greater incidence of tumors in animals given marijuana extract and γ radiation than either marihuana or γ radiation alone.

Cardiorespiratory effect

Fifty stable patients (25 males, 25 females) with methadone maintenance treatment (MMT) programs were investigated. Forty-six MMT patients were current tobacco smokers, 19 were current cannabis users, and none were currently using opioids other than prescribed methadone. Abnormalities of respiratory function were defined as those results outside the 95% confidence interval of reference values for normal subjects adjusted for age, weight, height, and sex. Thirty-one (62%) MMT patients had reduced carbon monoxide transfer factor; 17 (34%) had elevated single breath alveolar volume, and 43 (86%) had a reduced carbon monoxide transfer factor–alveolar volume ratio. Six patients (12%) had reduced forced expiratory volume in 1 second (FEV1); one (2%) had reduced forced vital capacity (FVC); and nine (18%) had an obstructive ventilatory defect. Ten (20%) patients had arterial CO_2 pressure higher than 45 mmHg and 14 (28%) had alveolar to arterial oxygen gradient higher than 15 mmHg.

Chest X-ray, echo-cardiography, and electrocardiogram showed no significant abnormalities. The potent cannabinoid receptor agonists WIN55,212-2 (0.05, 0.5, or 5 pmol/50 nL) and HU-210 (0.5 pmol/50 nL) or the CB1 receptor antagonist/inverse agonist AM28 1 (1 pmol/100 nL) were microinjected into the rostral ventrolateral medulla oblongata (RVLM) of urethane-anesthetized, immobilized and mechanically ventilated male Sprague–Dawley rats ($n = 22$). Changes in splanchnic nerve activity, phrenic nerve activity, mean arterial pressure, and heart rate in response to cannabinoid administration were recorded.

The CB1 receptor gene was expressed throughout the ventrolateral medulla oblongata. Unilateral microinjection of WIN 55,212-2 into the RVLM evoked short-latency, dose-dependent increases in splanchnic nerve activity (0.5 pmol; 175 ± 8%, $n = 5$) and mean arterial pressure (0.5 pmol; 26 ± 3%, $n = 8$), and abolished phrenic nerve activity (0.5 pmol; duration of apnea: 5.4 ± 0.4 seconds, $n = 8$), with little change in heart rate ($p < 0.005$). HU-210, structurally related to Δ-9-THC, evoked similar effects when microinj ected into the RVLM ($n = 4$). Prior micro-injection of AM281 produced agonist-like effects, and significantly attenuated the response to subsequent injection of WIN (0.5 pmol, $n = 4$).

Cardiovascular effects

The leaf, smoked by adults of both sexes, at a dose of 600 mg/ person (1–1.5% THC), produced no adverse effects on blood pressure, electrocardiogram, and the heart. Cannabis and Δ-9-THC increase heart rate, slightly increase supine blood pressure, and on occasion produced marked orthostatic hypotension. Cardiovascular effects in animals are different, with bradycardia and hypotension the most typical responses. Cardiac output increases, and peripheral vascular resistance and maximum exercise performance decrease. Tolerance to most of the initial cardiovascular effects appears rapidly. With repeated exposure, supine blood pressure decreases slightly, orthostatic hypotension disappears, blood volume increases, heart rate slows, and circulatory responses to exercise and Valsalva maneuver are diminished, consistent with centrally mediated, reduced sympathetic, and enhanced parasympathetic activity. Receptor-mediated and probably nonneuronal sites of action account for cannabinoid effects. The endocannabinoid system appears important in the modulation of many vascular functions. Cannabis' cardiovascular effects are not associated with serious health problems for most young, healthy users, although occasional myocardial infarction, stroke, and other adverse cardiovascular events are reported.

CB1 cannabinoid receptor in human placenta

CB1 (G protein-coupled) receptor and FAAH expression in human term placenta were investigated by immunohistochemistry. CB1 receptor was found in all layers of the membrane, with particularly strong expression in the amniotic epithelium and reticular cells and cells of the maternal decidua layer. Moderate expression was observed in the chorionic cytotrophoblasts. The expression of FAAH was highest in the amniotic epithelial cells, chorionic cytotrophoblast, and maternal decidua layer. The results suggest that the human placenta is a likely target for cannabinoid action and metabolism. This is consistent with a placental site of action of endocannabinoids and cannabis being responsible, at least in part, for the poor outcomes associated with cannabis consumption and pathology in the endocannabinoid system during pregnancy.

Central nervous system depressant activity

Fluidextract of the aerial parts, administered intraperitoneally to rats at a dose of 25 mg/kg, was active. The fluidextract, administered orally to dogs, produced ataxia. The leaf, smoked by human adults, produced a decrease in psychomotor performance.

Central nervous system effect

Δ-9-THC activates the two G protein-coupled receptors CB1 and CB2. The endogenous ligands of these receptors were identified as lipid metabolites of arachidonic acid, named endocannabinoids. The two most studied endocannabinoids are AEA and 2-arachidonyl-glycerol. The CB1 receptor is massively expressed throughout the central nervous system, whereas CB2 expression seems restricted to immune cells. Following endocannabinoid binding, CB1 receptors modulate second messenger cascades (inhibition of adenylate cyclase, activation of mitogen-activated protein kinases and of focal-adhesion kinases), as well as ionic conductances (inhibition of voltage-dependent calcium channels, activation of several potassium channels). Endocannabinoids transiently silenced synapses by decreasing neurotransmitter release. They play major roles in various forms of synaptic plasticity because of their ability to behave as retrograde messengers and activate noncannabinoid receptors (such as vanilloid receptor type-1). Mice strain with a disrupted *CB1* gene (CB1 knockout mice) appeared healthy and fertile, but they had a significantly increased mortality rate. They also displayed reduced locomotor activity, increased ring catalepsy, and hypoalgesia in hotplate and formalin tests. Δ-9-THC-induced ring catalepsy, hypomobility, and hypothermia were completely absent in CB1 mutant mice. In contrast, Δ-9-THC-induced analgesia in the tail-flick test and other behavioral (licking of the abdomen) and physiological (diarrhea) responses after Δ-9-THC administration were found. Results indicate that most, but not all, central nervous system effects of Δ-9-THC are mediated by the CB1 receptor.

Central nervous system stimulant Activity

The resin, ingested by a 4-year-old girl, showed signs of stupor alternating with brief intervals of excitation and foolish laughing with atactic movements. Her temperature, blood pressure, pulse, hemoglobin, leukocytes, serum electrolytes, and serum urea were normal. Respiratory rate was 12 beats per minute. Blood sugar elevated. Recovery was complete within 24 hours with no treatment.

Cerebellar clock-altering effect

Twelve volunteers who smoked cannabis recreationally about once weekly, and 12 volunteers who smoked daily for a number of years performed a self-paced counting task during positron emission tomography imaging, before and after smoking cannabis and placebo cigarettes. Smoking cannabis increased regional cerebral blood flow in the ventral forebrain and cerebellar cortex in both groups, but resulted in significantly less frontal lobe activation in chronic users. Counting rate increased after smoking cannabis in both groups, as did a behavioral measure of self-paced tapping, and both increases correlated with regional cerebral blood flow in the cerebellum. Results indicate that smoking cannabis appears to accelerate a cerebellar clock-altering self- paced behaviors.

Clinical endocannabinoid deficiency

Clinical endocannabinoid deficiency, and the prospect that it could underlie the pathophysiology of migraine, fibromyalgia, irritable bowel syndrome, and other functional conditions alleviated by clinical cannabis were studied. Migraine has numerous relationships to endocannabinoid function. AEA potentiated 5 -hydroxytrayptamine (HT1A) and inhibited 5-HT2A receptors supporting therapeutic efficacy in acute and preventive migraine treatment. Cannabinoids also demonstrated dopamine-blocking and anti-inflammatory effects. AEA is tonically active in the periaqueductal gray matter, a migraine generator. THC modulated glutamatergic neurotransmission via *N*-methyl-D-aspartic acid-receptors. Fibromyalgia is now conceived as a central sensitization state with secondary hyperalgesia. Cannabinoids have similarly demonstrated the ability to block spinal, peripheral and gastrointestinal mechanisms that promote pain in headache, fibromyalgia, irritable bowel syndrome and related disorders.

Cognitive functioning

Cognitive performance was examined in 145 adolescents aged 13–16 years for whom prenatal exposure to cannabis and cigarettes had been ascertained. The subjects were from a low-risk, predominantly middle-class sample participating in an ongoing, longitudinal study. The assessment battery included tests of general intelligence, achievement, memory, and aspects of executive functioning. Consistent with results obtained at earlier ages, the strongest relationship between prenatal maternal cigarette smoking and cognitive variables was seen with overall intelligence and aspects of auditory functioning, whereas prenatal exposure to marijuana was negatively associated with tasks that required visual memory, analysis, and integration. A multisite, retrospective, cross-sectional, neuropsychological study was conducted among 102 near-daily cannabis users (51 long-term users: mean, 23.9 years of use; 51 shorter-term users: mean, 10.2 years of use), compared with 33 nonuser controls. Measures from nine standard neuropsycho-logical tests that assessed attention, memory, and executive functioning were administered prior to entry into a treatment program following a median 17-hour abstinence. Long-term cannabis users performed significantly less well than shorter-term users and controls on tests of memory and attention. On the Rey Auditory Verbal Learning Test, long-term users recalled significantly fewer words than either shorter-term users ($p = 0.001$) or controls ($p = 0.005$). There was no difference between shorter-term users and controls. Long-term users showed impaired learning ($p = 0.007$), retention ($p = 0.003$), and retrieval ($p = 0.002$) compared with controls. Both user groups performed poorly on a time estimation task ($p < 0.001$ vs controls). Performance measures often correlated significantly with the duration of cannabis use, being worse with increasing years of use, but were unrelated to withdrawal symptoms and persisted after controlling for recent cannabis use and other drug use. A patient with a history of traumatic brain injury along with current mood disorder and cannabis use was reported. The impact of cannabis use appeared to have a detrimental effect on his mood. Treatment of the mood disorder resulted in larger cognitive gains. Sixty healthy volunteers (a negative urine drug-screening test was prerequisite) were investigated. On the first day, baseline data were obtained from a physical examination and a psychological test battery for the investigation of visual and verbal memory and cognitive perceptual performance. On the second day, subjects received a regular cigarette or one containing 290 mg/kg body weight of THC. Physical and psychological assessments were performed immediately (15 minutes) after subjects smoked their cigarettes. Twenty-four hours later, physical and psychological examinations were repeated. Results suggest that perceptual motor speed and accuracy, two very important parameters of driving ability, seem to be impaired immediately after cannabis consumption. The analyses included 1318 participants under age 65 years who completed the Mini-Mental State Examination (MMSE) during three study waves in 1981, 1982, and 1993–1996. Individual MMSE score differences between waves two and three were calculated for each study participant. After 12 years, study participants' scores declined a mean of 1.20 points on the MMSE (standard deviation, 1.90), with 66% having scores that declined by at least one point. Significant numbers of scores declined by three points or more (15% of participants in the 18–29-year-old age group). There were no significant differences in cognitive decline between heavy users, light users, and nonusers of cannabis. There were also no male–female differences in cognitive decline in relation to cannabis use. From 250 individuals consuming cannabis regularly, 99 healthy, free of any other past or present drug abuse, or history of neuropsychiatric disease cannabis users were selected. After an interview, physical examination, analysis of routine laboratory parameters, plasma/urine analyses for drugs, and Minnesota Multiphasic Personality Inventory testing, users and respective controls were subjected to a computer-assisted attention test battery comprising visual scanning, alertness, divided attention, flexibility, and working memory. Of the potential predictors of test performance within the user group, including present age, age of onset of cannabis use, degree of acute intoxication (THC + THC–OH plasma levels), and cumulative toxicity (estimated total life dose), an early age of onset turned out to be the only predictor, predicting impaired reaction times exclusively in visual scanning. Early-onset users (onset before age 16; $n = 48$) showed a significant impairment in reaction times in this function, whereas late-onset users (onset after age 16; $n = 51$) did not differ from controls ($n = 49$). Male volunteers ($n = 5$) with histories of moderate alcohol and cannabis use were administered three doses of alcohol (0.25, 0.5, or 1 g/kg), three doses of cannabis (4.8, or 16 puffs of 3.55% Δ-9-THC), and placebo in random order under double blind conditions in seven separate sessions. Blood alcohol concentration (10–90 mg/dL) and THC levels (63–188 ng/mL) indicated that active drug was delivered to subjects dose dependently. Alcohol and cannabis produced dose-related changes in subjective measures of drug effect. Ratings of perceived impairment were identical for the high doses of alcohol and cannabis. Both drugs produced comparable impairment in digit–symbol substitution and word recall tests, but had no effect in time perception and reaction time tests. Alcohol, but not cannabis, slightly impaired performance in a number recognition test.

Comorbid dysthymia and substance disorder

A total of 642 patients were assessed. Thirty-nine had substance-related disorder and dysthymia (SRD-dysthymia) and 308 had SRD only. Data on past use were collected by a research associate using a questionnaire. The patients with SRD-dysthymia and SRD did not differ with regard to use of alcohol, tobacco, and benzodiazepines. The patients with SRD-dysthymia started caffeine use at an earlier age, had shorter "use careers" of cocaine, amphetamines, and opiates, and had fewer days of cocaine and cannabis use in the last year. They also had a lower rate of cannabis abuse/dependence. The results indicated that patients with dysthymia and SRD have exposure to most substances of abuse that was comparable to patients with SRD only. They selectively use certain substances less often than patients with SRD only. A course and severity of SRD among 642 patients with comorbid major depressive disorder (MDD) was analyzed by means of both retrospective and concurrent data. Data on course included lifetime use, age at first use, years of use, use in the last year, periods of abstinence, and current diagnosis. Data on severity included two measures of SRD-associated problems, substance abuse vs dependence, self-help activities, and number of substances being abused. SRD-MDD patients tended to manifest lower levels of cannabis, opiate, and cocaine use, and more SRD-only patients were abusing three or more substances. Men with SRD-MDD demonstrated longer mean durations of abstinence compared with men with SRD-only, whereas SRD-MDD women demonstrated shorter mean durations of abstinence, compared with women with SRD-only. MDD-SRD patients showed slightly less substance abuse, but SRD severity was comparable with SRD-only patients.

Covariation among risk behaviors

A sample of 913 sexually active high school students completed a self-administered questionnaire that required mainly "yes" or "no" answers to questions involving participation in a range of risk behaviors. Contraceptive nonuse was not significantly associated with use of cigarettes, alcohol, or inhalants; perpetration or being a victim of violence; exposure to risk of physical injury; and suicidality. For males only, there was a significant inverse association between contraceptive nonuse and use of cannabis in the previous month. This was not the case for lifetime cannabis use for either gender.

Cytochrome P450 and 2C6 expression

Hashish (cannabis) and heroin effect on the expression of cytochrome P450 2E1 (CYP 2E1) and cytochrome P450 2C6 (CYP 2C6) was measured after single (24 hours) and repeated-dose treatments (four consecutive days). The expression of CYP 2E1 was slightly induced after single-dose treatments and markedly induced after repeated-dose treatments of mice with hashish (10 mg/kg body weight). It is believed that *N*-nitrosamines are activated principally by CYP 2E1 and the activity of *N*-nitrosodimethylamine was found to be increased after single- and repeated-dose treatments of mice with hashish by 23 and 41%, respectively. Hashish treatments of mice increased the total hepatic content of CYP by 112 and 206%, respectively; aryl hydrocarbon hydroxylase activity by 110 and 165%, respectively; nicotinamide adenine dinucleotide phosphate–cytochrome c reductase activity by 21 and 98%, respectively, and glutathione level by 81 and 173%, respectively. The level of free radicals was potentially decreased after single- or repeated-dose treatments with either hashish or heroin.

Cytotoxic effect

THC, in leukemic cell lines (CEM, HEL-92, and HL60) and in peripheral blood mononuclear cells, 6 hours after exposure induced apoptosis, even at one times the IC_{50}. THC did not appear to act synergistically with cytotoxic agents, such as cisplatin. THC-induced cell death was preceded by significant changes in the expression of genes involved in the mitogen-activated protein kinase signal transduction pathways. Both apoptosis and gene expression changes were altered independent of p53 and the cannabinoid 1 and 2 receptors (CB1-R and CB2-R).

Depressant activity

Heavy cannabis use and depression are associated and evidence from longitudinal studies suggests that heavy cannabis use may increase depressive symptoms among some users. Participants (n = 1920) were reassessed as part of a follow-up study. The analysis focused on two cohorts: those who reported no depressive symptoms at baseline (n = 849) and those with no diagnosis of cannabis abuse at baseline (n = 1,837). Symptoms of depression, cannabis abuse, and other psychiatric disorders were assessed with the Diagnostic Interview Schedule.

In participants with no baseline depressive symptoms, those with a diagnosis of cannabis abuse at baseline were four times more likely than those with no cannabis abuse diagnosis to have depressive symptoms at the follow-up assessment, after adjusting for age, gender, antisocial symptoms, and other baseline covariates. These participants were more likely to have experienced suicidal ideation and anhedonia during the follow-up period. Among the participants who had no diagnosis of cannabis abuse at baseline, depressive symptoms at baseline failed to significantly predict cannabis abuse at the follow-up assessment.

The relationship between depressive symptoms and polydrug use (alcohol, cannabis, and cocaine) among blacks in a high-risk community was studied. A street sample (n = 570) from four high-risk communities was collected through personal interviews. Interviewers asked respondents about their drug use behavior during the past 30 days and their depressive symptoms during the past week. Odds ratios and logistic regressions, adjusted for age and sex, were used to assess the relationship between depressive symptoms and drug and polydrug use (drug use involving cocaine). Results showed that depressive symptoms are significantly associated with polydrug use. Depressive symptoms were not associated with alcohol use or with the combination of alcohol and cannabis use.

Diabetic ketoacidosis

One hundred fifty-eight young adults, aged 16–30 years, with type 1 diabetes, attending an urban diabetes clinic, were sent an anonymous confidential postal questionnaire to determine the prevalence of street drug use. Eighty-five completed responses were received. Twenty-nine percent of respondents admitted to using street drugs.

Of those, 68% habitually took street drugs more than once a month. Seventy-two percent of users were unaware of the adverse effects on diabetes. Results indicated that the street drug usage in young adults with type 1 diabetes is common and may contribute to poor glycemic control and serious complications of diabetes.

Digital necrosis

An 18-year-old woman, with a history of severe anorexia nervosa of 5 years' duration, who acknowledged regular use of tobacco and cannabis, was hospitalized for necrosis of the left index and thumb that had occurred shortly after left radial artery puncture for blood gas analysis. Acrocyanosis of the four limbs had been present since the onset of anorexia nervosa. Arteriography of the upper limbs showed major spasm of the left radial and cubital arteries and thromboses in the left inter-digital arteries of the left index and thumb. The distal portions of the arteries were then on the left and on the right. The necrotic lesions healed after intravenous administration of ilomedine and interruption of tobacco and cannabis. Acrocyanosis of the four limbs persisted.

Discriminative stimulus effect

Rhesus monkeys, trained to discriminate Δ-9-THC from vehicle in a two-lever drug discrimination procedure, were tested with a variety of psychoactive drugs, including cannabinoids or drugs from other classes. The results indicated that Δ-9-THC discrimination showed pharmacological specificity, in that none of the noncannabinoid drugs fully substituted for Δ-9-THC. The classical cannabinoids, Δ-9-THC and Δ-8-THC, and the novel cannabinoids, WIN and 1-butyl-2-methyl-3-(1-naphthoyl)indole, produced full dose-dependent substitution for Δ-9-THC in all monkeys. A heptyl indole derivative failed to substitute for Δ-9-THC, but it also did not displace [^{3}H] CP-55,940 from its binding site.

Dopamine metabolism

The effect of repeated administrations of THC or WIN, a synthetic cannabinoid receptor agonist, on dopamine turnover in the prefrontal cortex, striatum, and Nac in rats, was investigated. THC or WIN (twice daily for seven or 14 days) caused a persistent and selective reduction in medial prefrontal cortical dopamine turnover. No significant alterations of dopamine metabolism were observed in the Nac or striatum. These dopaminergic deficits in the prefrontal cortex were observed after a drug-free period of up to 14 days. The cognitive dysfunction produced by heavy, long-term cannabis use may be subserved, in part, by drug-induced alterations in frontal cortical dopamine turnover. Two weeks' administration of THC to rats, reduced dopamine transmission in the medial prefrontal cortex, whereas dopamine metabolism in striatal regions was unaffected.

Dopamine release

A 38-year-old drug-free schizophrenic patient took part in a single photon emission computerized tomographic study of the brain, and smoked cannabis secretively during a pause in the course of an imaging session. Cannabis had an immediate calming effect, followed by a worsening of psychotic symptoms a few hours later. A comparison of the two sets of images, obtained before and immediately after smoking cannabis, indicated a 20% decrease in the striatal dopamine D2 receptor-binding ratio, suggestive of increased synaptic dopaminergic activity.

Dopamine transmission modulation

The endogenous cannabinoid system is a new signaling system composed by the central (CB1) and the peripheral (CB2) receptors, and several lipid transmitters including AEA and 2-arachidonylglycerol. Cannabinoid CB1 receptors are present in dopamine projecting brain areas. In primates and certain rat strains it is also located in dopamine cells of the A8, A9, and A10 mesencephalic cell groups, as well as in hypothalamic dopaminergic neurons controlling prolactin secretion. CB1 receptors co-localize with dopamine D1/D2 receptors in dopamine projecting fields. Manipulation of dopaminergic transmission is able to alter the synthesis and release of AEA, as well as the expression of CB1 receptors. CB1 receptors can switch their transduction mechanism to oppose to the ongoing dopamine signaling. Acute blockade of CB1 receptor potentiates the facilitatory role of dopamine D2 receptor agonists on movement. CB1 stimulation results in sensitization to the motor effects of indirect dopaminergic agonists.

Dyskinetic activity

A 4-week dose escalation study was performed to assess the safety and tolerability of cannabis in six patients with Parkinson's disease (PD) with levodopa (L-DOPA)-induced dyskinesia. Then a randomized, placebo-controlled crossover study was performed, in which 19 patients with PD were randomized to receive oral cannabis extract followed by placebo or vice versa. Each treatment phase lasted for 4 weeks with an intervening 2-week washout phase. The primary outcome measure was a change in Unified Parkinson's Disease Rating Scale (UPDRS) (items 32 to 34) dyskinesia score. Secondary outcome measures included the Rush scale, Bain scale, tablet arm drawing task, and total UPDRS score following a levodopa challenge, as well as patient-completed measures of a dyskinesia activities of daily living scale, the PDQ-39, on–off diaries, and a range of category rating scales. Seventeen patients completed the study. Cannabis was well tolerated and had no pro- or antiparkinsonian action. There was no evidence for a treatment effect on L-DOPA-induced dyskinesia as assessed by the UPDRS, or any of the secondary outcome measures. An anonymous questionnaire sent to all patients attending the Prague Movement Disorder Center revealed that 25% of 339 respondents had taken cannabis and 45.9% of these described some form of benefit. 2,4,5-Trihydroxyphenethylamine (6-hydroxydopamine)-lesioned rats were treated with the enantiomers of the synthetic cannabinoid 7-hydroxy-Δ6-THC 1,1-dimethylheptyl. Treatment with its (-)- (3R, 4R) enantiomer (code name HU-210), a potent cannabinoid receptor type 1 agonist, reduced the rotations induced by L-DOPA/carbidopa or apomorphine by 34 and 44%, respectively. Treatment with the (+)-(3S, 4S) enantiomer (code name HU-211), an *N*-methyl-D-aspartate antagonist, and the psychotropically inactive cannabis constituent: CBD and its primary metabolite, 7-hydroxy-cannabinol, did not show any reduction of rotational behavior. The results indicate that activation of the CB1 stimulates the dopaminergic system ipsilaterally to the lesion, and may have implications in the treatment of PD.

Dystonic activity

The neural mechanisms underlying dystonia involve abnormalities within the basal ganglia—in particular, overactivity of the lateral globus pallidus. Cannabinoid receptors are located presynaptically on γ-aminobutyric acid receptor (GABA) terminals within the globus pallidus internus, where their activation reduces GABA reuptake. Cannabinoid receptor stimulation may thus reduce overactivity of the globus pallidus, and thereby reduce dystonia. A double-blind, randomized, placebo-controlled, crossover study using the synthetic cannabinoid receptor agonist nabilone in patients with generalized and segmental primary dystonia showed no significant reduction in dystonia following treatment with nabilone.

Endocrine effect

Animal models have demonstrated that cannabinoid administration acutely altered multiple hormonal systems, including the suppression of the gonadal steroids, growth hormone, prolactin, and thyroid hormone and the activation of the hypothalamic–pituitary–adrenal (HPA) axis. These effects were mediated by binding to the endogenous cannabinoid receptor in or near the hypothalamus. Despite these findings in animals, the effects in humans have been inconsistent, and discrepancies were likely owing in part to the development of tolerance. Intravenous administration of three cannabinoid agonists to nine castrated male calves under stress-free conditions provoked immediate increases of serum cortisol and respiration rate, and produced rapid hypoalgesia to cutaneous pain and thermal stimuli. AEA and methanandamide did not affect serum prolactin. Administration of WIN increased serum prolactin abruptly. None of the cannabinoid receptor agonists affected serum growth hormone.

Environmental stress and cannabinoids interaction

Anxiety and panic are the most common adverse effects of cannabis intoxication. Data suggest that cannabinoid CB1 receptor modulation of amygdalar activity contributes to these phenomena. Using Fos as a marker, it was tested the hypothesis that environmental stress and CB1 cannabinoid receptor activity interact in the regulation of amygdalar activation in male mice. Both 30 minutes of restraint and CB1 receptor agonist treatment (Δ-9-THC [2.5 mg/kg]) or CP-55,940 (0.3 mg/kg); by intraperitoneal injection) produced barely detectable increases in Fos expression within the central amygdala (CeA). The combination of restraint and CB1 agonist administration produced robust Fos induction within the CeA, indicating a synergistic interaction between environmental stress and CB1 receptor activation. An inhibitor of endocannabinoid transport, AM404 (10 mg/kg), produced an additive interaction with restraint within the CeA. In contrast, FAAH inhibitor-treated mice (URB597, 1 mg/kg) and FAAH (–/–) mice did not exhibit any differences in amygdalar activation in response to restraint compared with control mice. In the basolateral amygdala and medial amygdala, restraint stress produced a low level of Fos induction, which was unaffected by cannabinoid treatment. The CB1 receptor antagonist SR141 716 dose-dependently increased Fos expression in the BLA and CeA.

Epileptic effect

Δ-9-THC at a dose of 1 μM, significantly depressed evoked depolarizing postsynaptic potentials (PSPs) in rat olfactory cortex neurones. A standardized cannabis extract (SCE) and Δ-9-THC-free SCE significantly potentiated evoked PSPs (all results were fully reversed by the CB1 receptor antagonist

SR141716A, 1 μM). The potentiation by Δ-9-THC-free SCE was greater than that produced by SCE. On comparing the effects of Δ-9-THC-free SCE on evoked PSPs and artificial PSPs (aPSPs; evoked electrotonically following brief intracellular current injection), PSPs were enhanced, whereas aPSPs were unaffected, suggesting that the effect was not resulting from changes in background input resistance. Similar recordings made using CB1 receptor-deficient knockout mice and wild-type littermate controls revealed cannabinoid or extract-induced changes in membrane resistance, cell excitability and synaptic transmission in wild-type mice that were similar to those seen in rat neurones, but no effect on these properties were seen in CB1 receptor-deficient knockout mice cells.

Results indicated that the unknown extract constituent(s) effects over-rode the suppressive effects of Δ-9-THC on excitatory neurotransmitter release, which may explain some patients' preference for herbal cannabis rather than isolated Δ-9-THC (owing to attenuation of some of the central Δ-9-THC side effects) and possibly account for the rare incidence of seizures in some individuals taking cannabis recreationally. A SCE with pure Δ-9-THC, at matched concentrations of Δ-9-THC, and a Δ-9-THC-free extract (Δ-9-THC-free SCE) in in vitro rat brain slice model of epilepsy were examined. In the in vitro epilepsy model, in which sustained epileptiform seizures were induced by the muscarinic receptor agonist oxotremorine-M in immature rat piriform cortical brain slices, SCE was a more potent and again more rapidly-acting anticonvulsant than isolated Δ-9-THC. Δ-9-THC-free extract also exhibited anticonvulsant activity. CBD did not inhibit seizures, nor did it modulate the activity of Δ-9-THC in this model. These results demonstrated that not all of the therapeutic actions of cannabis herb might be a result of the Δ-9-THC content.

Estrogen receptors stimulating effect

THC, CBD, and desacetyllevonantradol, in estrogen-induced MCF-7 breast cancer cells at concentrations of no more than 10 μM, produced no effect. THC failed to antagonize the response to estradiol under conditions in which the antiestrogen LY156758 (keoxifene; raloxifene) was effective. The phytoestrogen formononetin behaved as an estrogen at high concentrations, and this response was antagonized by LY156758. THC, desacetyllevonantradol, or CBD did not stimulate transcription of an *EREtkCAT* reporter gene transiently transfected into MCF-7 cells.

Estrous cycle disruption effect

Ethanol (95%) extract of the dried aerial parts, administered intraperitoneally to gerbils at a dose of 2.5 mg/animal daily for 60 days, was active. Petroleum ether extract of the dried aerial, administered intraperitoneally to mice and rats at doses of 1 and 5 mg/animal, respectively, for 64 days, was active. Petroleum ether extract of the aerial parts, administered intraperitoneally to female rats, produced weak activity.

Petroleum ether extract of the entire plant, administered by gastric intubation to female mice at doses of 75 mg/kg and 150 mg/kg, was active. A dose of 3 mg/kg produced weak activity. Petroleum ether extract of the resin, administered intra-peritoneally to female rats at doses of 10 and 20 mg/kg, was active. Resin, administered orally to female rats at doses of 3, 15, and 75 mg/kg daily for 72 days, was active.

Familial mediterranean fever

A patient with familial Mediterranean fever was presented with chronic relapsing pain and inflammation of gastrointestinal origin. After determining a suitable analgesic dosage, a double-blind, placebo-controlled, crossover trial was conducted using 50 mg of Δ-9-THC daily in five doses in the active weeks and measuring effects on parameters of inflammation and pain. Although no anti-inflammatory effects of Δ-9-THC were detected during the trial, a highly significant reduction ($p < 0.001$) in additional analgesic requirements was achieved.

Food intake modulation

Cannabis sativa stimulates appetite, especially for sweet and palatable food. Cannabinoid action has proposed a central role of the cannabinoid system in obesity. Dronabinol, a commercially available form of a THC, has been used successfully for increasing appetite in patients with HIV wasting disease. Cannabinoid receptor antagonist may reduce obesity. To determine the prevalence of substance use in adolescents with eating disorders, the results of a data set of Ontario high school students were compared. One hundred and one female adolescents who met the *Diagnostic and Statistical Manual of Mental Disorders*, 4th edition's criteria for an eating disorder were followed up in a tertiary care pediatric treatment center. They were asked to participate in a cross-sectional study using a self-administered questionnaire assessing substance use and investigating reasons for use and nonuse; 95 agreed to participate and 77 completed the questionnaire (mean age, 15.2 years). The patients were divided into two groups: 63 with restrictive symptoms only, 17 with purging symptoms. The rates of drug use between subjects and their comparison groups were compared by Z-scores, with the level of significance set at 0.05. During the preceding year, restrictors used significantly less tobacco, alcohol, and cannabis than grade- and sex-matched comparison populations, and purgers used these substances at rates similar to those of comparison subjects. Other drugs seen frequently in the purgers included hallucinogens, tranquilizers, stimulants, LSD, phencyclidine, cocaine, and ecstasy. Both groups used caffeine and laxatives, but few used diet pills. Restrictors said they did not use substances because they were bad for their health, tasted unpleasant, were contrary to their beliefs, and were too expensive. Purgers generally used substances to relax, relieve anger, avoid eating, and "get away" from problems. Female adolescents with eating disorders who have restrictive symptoms use substances less frequently than the general adolescent population but do not abstain from their use. Those with purging symptoms use substances with a similar frequency to that found in the general adolescent population.

Gene expression effect

Cannabinoids can cross the placental barrier and be secreted in the maternal milk. Through this way, cannabinoids affect the ontogeny of various neurotransmitter systems leading to changes in different behavioral patterns. Dopamine and endogenous opioids are among the neurotransmitters that result more affected by perinatal cannabinoid exposure, which, when animals mature, produce changes in motor activity, drug-seeking behavior, nociception, and other processes. These disturbances are likely originated by the capability of cannabinoids to influence the expression of key genes for both neurotransmitters, in particular, the enzyme tyrosine hydroxylase and the opioid precursor proenkephalin. Cannabinoids seem to be able to influence the expression of genes encoding for neuroglia cell adhesion molecules, which supports a potential influence of cannabinoids on the processes of cell proliferation, neuronal migration or axonal elongation in which these proteins are involved. CB1 receptors, which represent the major targets for the action of cannabinoids, are abundantly expressed in certain brain regions, such as the subventricular areas, which have been involved in these processes during brain development. Cannabinoids might also be involved in the apoptotic death that occurs during brain development, possibly by influencing the expression of Bcl-2/Bax system. CB1 receptors are transiently expressed during brain development in different group of neurons which do not contain these receptors in the adult brain.

Glaucoma effect

Nine patients with glaucoma unresponsive to treatment were treated with orally administered Δ-9-THC capsules or inhaled cannabis in addition to their existing therapeutic regimen. An initial decrease in intraocular pressure was observed in all patients, and the investigator's therapeutic goal was met in four of the nine patients. The decreases in intraocular pressure were not sustained, and the patients elected to discontinue treatment within 1–9 months for various reasons.

Gliomatous effect

Gliomas, in particular glioblastoma multiform or grade IV astrocytoma, are the most frequent class of malignant primary brain tumors and one of the most aggressive forms of cancer. Cannabinoids and their derivatives slowed the growth of different types of tumors, including gliomas, in laboratory animals. Cannabinoids induced apoptosis of glioma cells in culture vía sustained ceramide accumulation, extracellular signal-regulated kinase activation and Akt inhibition. Cannabinoid treatment inhibited angiogenesis of gliomas in vivo. Cannabinoids killed glioma cells selectively and could protect nontransformed glial cells from death.

Gynecomastic effect

A retrospective analysis was carried out on 175 men over the age of 16 years who were presented with breast enlargement and/or "lumps" during a 7-year period to a single surgeon. The patients had complete biochemical assessment (liver function tests, γ-glutamyl transferase, prolactin, α-fetoprotein, and β-human chorionic gonadotropin), and mammography and/or ultrasound with fine-needle biopsy if indicated. Thirty-nine of the patients had bilateral true gynecomastia and 88 had unilateral gynecomastia (53% left). Carcinoma of the breast was diagnosed in eight, pseudo-gynecomastia in 18, 13 had physiological pubertal changes only, and 9 had other diagnoses. Adverse drug reactions were possibly implicated in the etiology of 47 patients, alcohol in seven patients, cannabis in one patient, testicular malignancy in four patients, and hepatocellular carcinoma in one patient. Five patients were found to have hyperprolactinemia. Twenty-four percent of patients were reassured without intervention; 18% failed to attend follow-up.

Hepatitis C risk factor

The study of a dually diagnosed population estimated the prevalence of hepatitis C virus (HCV) to be 29.7% or 16 times higher than that in the general population. A high correlation was found between the use of tobacco and HCV infection. This appears to be beyond the risk factor conveyed by intravenous drug use. Of the patients whose primary diagnoses were cocaine, opiate, amphetamine, or polysubstance dependence (drugs often used intravenously), 42% of the tobacco users were HCV-positive, whereas only 20% of the nontobacco using patients with similar primary diagnoses were HCV-positive. The association of tobacco use with HCV was found to be strong for females with alcohol, sedative/hypnotic, inhalant, or cannabis dependence, as none of the 17 nontobacco using female patients with these diagnoses were HCV-positive, whereas 14 of the 45 (31%) tobacco-using females with these diagnoses did test positive for HCV.

HIV involvement

The prevalence, predictors, and patterns of cannabis use—specifically medicinal cannabis use among patients with HIV—were examined. Any cannabis use in the year prior to interview and self- defined medicinal use were evaluated. A cross-sectional multicenter survey and retrospective chart review were conducted to evaluate overall drug utilization in HIV, including cannabis use. HIV-positive adults were identified through the HIV Ontario Observational Database; 104 consenting patients were interviewed. Forty-three percent of the patients reported cannabis use, whereas 29% reported medicinal use. Reasons for use were similar by gender although a significantly higher number of women used cannabis for pain management. The most commonly reported reason for medicinal cannabis use was appetite stimulation/weight gain. Male gender and history of intravenous drug use were predictive of any cannabis use. Age, gender, HIV clinical status, antiretroviral use, and history of intravenous drug use were not significant predictors of medicinal cannabis use. Despite the frequency of medicinal use, minimal changes in the pattern of cannabis use on HIV diagnosis were reported with 80% of current medicinal users also indicating recreational consumption. HIV patients (n = 252) were recruited via consecutive sampling in public health care clinics. Structured interviews assessed patterns of recent cannabis use, including its perceived benefit for symptom relief. Associations between cannabis use and demographic and clinical variables were examined using univariate and multivariate regression analyses. Overall prevalence of smoked cannabis in the previous month was 23%. Reported benefits included relief of anxiety and/or depression (57%), improved appetite (53%), increased pleasure (33%), and relief of pain (28%). Recent use of cannabis was positively associated with severe nausea (OR = 4, $p = 0.004$) and recent use of alcohol (OR = 7.5, $p < 0.001$) and negatively associated with being Latino (OR = 0.07, $p < 0.001$). No associations between cannabis use and pain symptoms were observed. No safety problems specific to HIV or protease inhibitors were found in a study in which volunteers stayed in a research hospital 24 hours a day and were randomly assigned to either smoke cannabis, take oral THC, or take an oral placebo. Cannabis and THC use was associated with weight gain.

Hyperglycemic activity

Ethanol (95%) extract of the leaf, administered intravenously to rats at a dose of 300 mg/kg, produced an increase of 40 mg percentage 2 hours postinjection and a corresponding decrease in liver glycogen. Ethanol (95%) extract of the dried leaf, administered by gastric intubation to rabbits, produced an increase followed by a gradual decrease in blood sugar levels. The dried leaves, smoked by human adults, produced elevated glucose levels in two out of four subjects and no impairment of insulin release or changes in growth hormone levels.

Hypoglycemic activity

Ethanol (95%) extract of the dried leaf, administered by gastric intubation to rabbits, produced an increase, followed by a gradual decrease, in blood sugar levels. Extract of the dried leaf, administered subcutaneously to rabbits at a dose of 0.5 mL/kg (approx 0.6 mg THC) for 9 weeks, further enhanced hypoglycemia induced by insulin. No hypoglycemic effect was seen in normal animals. Hot water extract of the resin, administered by gastric intubation to dogs at a dose of 20 g of air-dried resin/animal, produced weak activity. The dried leaf, smoked by adults at a dose of 2 g/person, was inactive.

Hypotensive activity

Ethanol (50%) extract of the entire plant, administered intravenously to dogs at a dose of 50 mg/kg, was active. Ethanol (95%) and water extracts of the dried aerial parts, administered intravenously to cats, were inactive. The ethanol extract stimulated respiration, and the water extract had no effect.

Ilicit drug in plasmapheresis donors

Seventy-five US plasma units from 10 different states in the United States and 75 German plasma units that had been analyzed principally for their protein composition were screened for drugs. Determinations were made, using automated immunoassays, of the presence of cannabis, cocaine, amphetamine, methamphetamine, MDMA, methyl enedioxy-ethylamphetamine (MDE), and opiates. Positive results were confirmed by gas chromatography–mass spectrometry. Eleven US plasma units were found to be positive for cocaine (14.6%), whereas all German samples were cocaine-negative ($p = 0.0007$). Fifteen US plasma units (20%) and one German unit (1,3%) were confirmed as positive for cannabis ($p = 0.0003$). Three out of 75 US plasma units were positive for both cannabis and cocaine. In none of the 150 samples were amphetamine, methamphetamine, MDMA, MDE, or opiates detected.

Immunomodulatory effect

The smoking of cannabis showed a significant local immuno-suppression of the bactericidal activity of human alveolar macrophages. In animal studies, cannabinoids were identified as potent modulators of cytokine production, causing a shift from T-helper-1 (Th1) to Th2 cytokines. In consequence, a compromised cellular immunity was observed in these animals, resulting in enhanced tumor growth and reduced immunity to viral infections. In vitro, immunosuppressive effects were shown in all immune cells, but only at high micro-molar cannabinoid concentrations not reached under normal clinical conditions. .

In conclusion, there was no evidence that cannabinoids induce a serious, relevant immunosuppression in humans, with the exception of cannabis smoking, which may affect local bronchoalveolar immunity. The immune function in 16 MS patients treated with oral cannabinoids was measured. A modest increase of tumor necrosis factor (TNF)-α in lipopolysaccharide-stimulated whole blood was found during cannabis plant-extract treatment ($p = 0.037$), with no change in other cytokines. In the subgroup of patients with high adverse event scores, an increase in plasma IL-12p40 was found ($p = 0.002$). The results indicate pro-inflammatory disease-modifying potential of cannabinoids in MS. THC and their metabolites inhibited production of IL-1 and γ-interferon, decreased a 33% of the lymphocytes activity and inhibited 66% of the lymphocytes adenylcyclase activity.

The consumption of cannabis decreased immunological competence of macrophages, and alternated their essential role of trophicity of the central nervous system. Inhibiting actions of cannabinoids on the cyclo-oxygenase, promoted production of arachidonic acid degradation products. This compound mimics the action of histamine, induced a raise of the vascular permeability and bronchospasm, and contributed at delayed reaction of anaphylaxia.

Infant mortality

For a period of 11 months, 2964 infants were enrolled and screened at birth for exposure to cocaine, opiate, or cannabinoid by meconium analysis. At birth, 44% of the infants tested positive for drugs, 30.5% positive for cocaine, 20.2% for opiate, and 11.4% for cannabinoids. Compared with the drug-negative group, a significantly higher percentage ($p < 0.05$) of the drug-positive infants had lower weight and smaller head circumference and length at birth and a higher percent of their mothers were single, multigravid, multiparous, and had little to no prenatal care. Within the first 2 years of life, 44 infants died: 26 were drug-negative (15.7 deaths per 1000 live births) and 18 were drug-positive (13.7 deaths per 1000 live births). The mortality rate among cocaine, opiate, or cannabinoid-positive infants were 17.7, 18.4, and 8.9 per 1000 live births, respectively. Among infants with birth-weight of 2500 g or less, infants who were positive for both cocaine and morphine had a higher mortality rate (OR = 5.9, CI = 1.4–24) than drug-negative infants. Eleven infants died from the sudden infant death syndrome (SIDS); 58% were positive for drugs, predominantly cocaine. The odds ratio for SIDS among drug-positive infants was 1.5 (CI = 0.46–5.01) and 1.9 (CI = 0.58–6.2) among cocaine-positive infants.

Infant neurobehavioral effect

The subjects and controls in this study were full- term infants of appropriate gestational age with no medical problems. At 1–2 days of age, 20 infants exposed to cocaine, alcohol, cannabis, and cigarettes, 17 infants exposed to alcohol and/or cannabis and cigarettes, and 20 drug-free infants were evaluated by using the Neonatal Intensive Care Unit Network Neurobehavioral Scale. Cocaine-exposed (CE) infants showed increased tone and motor activity, more jerky movements, startles, tremors, back arching, and signs of central nervous system and visual stress than unexposed infants. They also showed poorer visual and auditory following. There were no differences in how the examination was administered to CE and nonexposed infants. Reduced birth-weight and length were also observed in CE infants. Differences attributable to CE infants were related to muscle tone and motor performance, following during orientation, and signs of stress. CE infants were not more difficult to test, nor did they require an alteration in the examination. Both neurobehavioral patterns of excitability and lethargy were observed. The findings may have been a result of the synergistic effects of cocaine with alcohol and cannabis.

Inflammatory effect

A case of a 17-year-old male regular cannabis user who developed a large swollen uvula and partial upper airway obstruction after smoking cannabis was evaluated. Symptoms resolved with the administration of corticosteroids and antihistamines. A healthy 17-year-old man who inhaled cannabis prior to general anesthesia is described. In the recovery room, after an uneventful general anesthetic, acute uvular edema resulted in postoperative airway obstruction and admission to the hospital. The uvular edema was treated successfully with dexamethasone.

Information-processing effect

Information processes are thought to represent the basic building blocks of higher order cognitive processes. The inspection time task was used to investigate the effects of acute and subacute cannabis use on information processing in 22 heavy users compared with 22 nonusers. The findings indicated that users in the subacute state display significantly slowed information-processing speeds (longer inspection times) compared with controls. This deficit appeared to be normalized while users were in the acute state. These results may be explained as a withdrawal effect, but may also be owing to tolerance development because of long-term cannabis use.

Insecticidal activity

Leaf extract, administered to larvae of *Chironomus samoensis*, produced paralysis leading to death. The extract brought a drastic change in the morphology of sensilla trichoidea, the general body cuticle, and a significant reduction in the concentration of magnesium and iron, whereas manganese showed only slight average increase. Because the sensilla trichoidea has nerve connections, it was assumed that the toxic principle of the leaf extract has affected the central nervous system.

Intestinal motility activity

Rat intestinal epithelia mounted in an Ussing chamber attached with voltage/current clamp were used for measuring changes of the short-circuit current across the epithelia. The intestinal epithelia were activated with current raised by serosal administration of forskolin 5 μM. Ethanol extracts of cannabis augmented the current additively when each was added after forskolin. In subsequent experiments, ouabain, and bumetanide were added prior to ethanol extract of cannabis to determine their effect on Na^+ and Cl^- movement. The results suggested that the extract may affect the Cl^- movement more directly than Na^+ movement in the intestinal epithelial cells.

Intraocular pressure reduction

Polysaccharide fraction of the dried entire plant, administered intravenously to rabbits at a dose of 1 μg/animal was active. Water extract of the dried aerial parts, administered intravenously to rabbits at a dose of 250 μg/animal, was active. A dose of 5 μg/animal was inactive on Rhesus monkeys and active on rabbits. A dose of 10 mg/animal, administered *per rectum* to Rhesus monkeys and rabbits, was inactive.

IQ effect

Cannabis use for 70 individuals aged 17–20 years was determined through self-reporting and urinalysis. IQ scores were calculated by subtracting each person's IQ score at 9–12 years (before initiation of drug use) from his or her score at 17–20 years. The difference in IQ scores of current heavy users (at least five joints per week), current light users (less than five joints per week), former users (who had not smoked regularly for at least 3 months), and nonusers (who never smoked more than once per week and no smoking in the past 2 weeks) was compared. Current cannabis use was significantly correlated ($p < 0.05$) in a dose-related fashion with a decline in IQ over the ages studied. The comparison of the IQ difference scores showed an average decrease of 4.1 points in current heavy users ($p < 0.05$) compared with gains in IQ points for light current users (5.8), former users (3.5), and nonusers (2.6).

Lactate inhibition

The dried leaf, smoked by adults at a dose of 2 g/person, decreased blood lactic acid.

Leutinizing hormone-release inhibition

The dried aerial part, smoked by menopausal women at a dose of 1 g/person, was inactive. When administered to normal and castrated male rats, at a dose of 75 mg/kg, was active.

Lower limb occlusive arteriopathy

Seventy-three patients (60 males and 13 females less than 50 years of age) were divided into four groups: Buerger's disease (thromboangiitis obliterans [TAO]), atheromatous juvenile peripheral obstructive arterial diseases (POAD), autoimmune POAD, and arteriopathy of undetermined origin. The first symptoms occurred at 38 ± 8 years of age. Fourteen patients (20%) had TAO, 51 (70%) atheromatous POAD, 4 (5%) POAD with systemic or autoimmune disease, and 4 (5%) undetermined POAD. Age of onset was earlier in TAO (35 ± 8 vs 40 ± 8 years, $p = 0.046$), smoking was greater in the atheroma group (33 ± 16 vs 24 ± 14 pack/years, $p = 0.033$). Fifty-three patients with POAD had dyslipidemia and 26% had hypertension. Regular cannabis intake was more frequent in the TAO group (21% vs 8%). At the time of medical care,

Fontaine's stage was more frequently stage II in atheroma patients (57% vs 14%) and stage IV in TAO patients (86% vs 35%). TAO was diagnosed in 43% cannabis users and in 19% nonusers. Results indicated that the main etiology of juvenile POAD is atheroma, followed by TAO. Cannabis users accounted for at least 10% of these patients. They were characterized by lower tobacco intake, more distal lesions, more frequent involvement of the upper limbs. They presented more frequently as TAO. A case of a 30-year-old woman who smoked cannabis and developed intermittent claudication of the lower limbs was reported. Results indicated that cannabis could be involved not only in the pathogenesis of juvenile obstructive arteriopathy, but also in the development of atheromatous lesions.

Lung function

A group of over 900 young adults derived from a birth cohort of 1037 subjects were studied at age 18, 21, and 26 years. Cannabis and tobacco smoking were documented at each age using a standardized interview. Lung function, as measured by the FEV1–vital capacity (VC) ratio, was obtained by simple spirometry. A fixed effects regression model was used to analyze the data and to account for confounding factors. When the sample was stratified for cumulative use, there was evidence of a linear relationship between cannabis use and FEV1–VC ($p < 0.05$). In the absence of adjusting for other variables, increasing cannabis use over time was associated with a decline in FEV1–VC with time; the mean FEV1–VC among subjects using cannabis on 900 or more occasions was 7.2, 2.6 and 5% less than nonusers at ages 18, 21, and 26, respectively.

After controlling for potential confounding factors (age, tobacco smoking, and weight) the negative effect of cumulative cannabis use on mean FEV1–VC was only marginally significant ($p < 0.09$). Age ($p < 0.001$), cigarette smoking ($p < 0.05$), and weight ($p < 0.001$) were all significant predictors of FEV1–VC. Cannabis use and daily cigarette smoking acted additively to influence FEV1–VC. Results indicated that longitudinal observations over 8 years in young adults revealed a dose- dependent relationship between cumulative cannabis consumption and decline in FEV1–VC. When confounders were accounted for the effect was reduced and was only marginally significant, but given the limited time frame over which observations were made, the trend suggests that continued cannabis smoking has the potential to result in clinically important impairment of lung function.

Memory impairment

The effects of combined exposure to ethanol and Δ-9-THC in a memory task was investigated in rats. Ethanol, voluntarily ingested in alcohol-preferring rats, and THC, given by intraperitoneal injection, had a synergic action to impair object recognition when a 15-minute interval was adopted between the sample phase and the choice phase of the test. Ingestion of ethanol, or 2 or 5 mg/kg of THC were not able to modify object recognition in these experimental conditions. When voluntary ethanol ingestion was combined with administration of these doses of THC, object recognition was markedly impaired. THC impaired object recognition only at the dose of 10 mg/kg, when its administration was not combined with that of ethanol. The selective cannabinoid CB1 receptor antagonist SR 141716A (*N*-(piperidin-1-yl)-5-(4-chlorophenyl)-1(2,4-dichloro-phenyl)-4-methyl-1 H-pyrazole carboxamide HCl) at the dose of 1 mg/kg reversed the amnesic effect of 10 mg/kg of THC. This indicated that the effect is mediated by the receptor subtype. The synergism of ethanol and THC was not detected when an intertrial interval of 1 minute was adopted.

Memory improvement

Extract from fructus cannabis (EFC), administered intragastrically to mice with drug-induced dysmnesia at doses of 0.2, 0.4, and 0.8 g/kg, for 7 days, prolonged the latency and decreased the number of errors in the step-down test, and enhanced the spatial resolution of amnesic mice in water maze test. EFC at the dose of 0.2 g/kg overcame amnesia of three stages of memory process. EFC activated calcineurin activity at a concentration range of 0.01–100 g/L. The maximal value of EFC on calcineurin activity (35% ± 5 %) appeared at a concentration of 10 g/LCS320. EFC with activation of calcineurin, extracted from Chinese traditional medicine, was used to determine the effects on memory and immunity in mice. In the stepdown-type passive avoidance test, the plant extract (0.2 g/kg) significantly improved amnesia induced by drugs, and greatly enhanced the ability of cell-mediated type hypersensitivity and nonspecific immune responses in normal mice.

Mitochondrial Function Disruption

Δ-9-THC in the pulmonary transformed cell line A549 produced a rapid and extensive depletion of cellular energy stores. Adenosine 5'-triphosphatase levels declined dose dependently with an IC_{50} of 7.5 μg/mL of THC after 24 hours of exposure. Cell death was observed only at concentrations greater than 10 μg/mL. Studies using JC-1, a fluorescent probe for mitochondrial membrane potential, revealed diminished mitochondrial function at THC concentrations as low as 0.5 μg/mL. At concentrations of 2.5 and 10 μg/mL of THC, a decrease in mitochondrial membrane potential was observed 1 hour after THC exposure. Mitochondrial function remained diminished for at least 30 hours after THC exposure. Flow cytometry studies on cells exposed to particulate smoke extracts indicated that JC-1 red fluorescence was fivefold lower in cells exposed to cannabis smoke extract compared with tobacco smoke-exposed cells. Comparison with a variety of mitochondrial inhibitors demonstrated that THC produced effects similar to that of carbonyl cyanide *p*-trifluoromethoxyphenylhydrazone, suggesting uncoupling of electron transport. Loss of red JC-1 fluorescence by THC was suppressed by cyclosporin A, suggesting mediation by the mitochondrial permeability transition pore. This disruption of mitochondrial function was sustained for at least 24 hours after removal of THC by extensive washing.

Mitogenic effect

The resin was inactive on the human and rat white blood cells.

Molluscicidal activity

Ethanol (95%) and water extracts of the dried flowering tops, at a concentration of 1000 ppm, produced weak activity on *Biomphalaria straminea* and *Biomphalaria glabrata*. Water saturated with essential oil of the aerial parts, at a concentration of 1:2, produced weak activity on *Biomphalaria glabrata*.

Motor function

Nine cannabis smokers and 16 controls were studied to determine the attentional areas related to motor function, and primary and supplementary motor cortices. Echo planar images and high-resolution molecular resonance images were acquired. The challenge paradigm included left and right finger sequencing. Group differences in cerebral activation were examined for Brodmann areas (BA) 4, 6, 24, and 32 using region of interests analyses in statistical parametric mapping. Cannabis users, tested within 4–36 hours of discontinuation, exhibited significantly less activation than controls in BA 24 and 32 bilaterally during right- and left-sided sequencing and for BA 6 in all tasks except for left-sided sequencing in the left hemisphere. There were no statistically significant differences for BA 4. None of these regional activations correlated with urinary cannabis concentration and verbal IQ for smokers. The results suggested that recently abstinent chronic cannabis smokers produce reduced activation in motor cortical areas in response to finger sequencing compared with controls.

Multiple sclerosis

One hundred fifty-seven drug-naïve, first-episode schizophrenic patients were examined. A significantly elevated brain-derived neurotrophic factor (BDNF) serum concentrations in patients with chronic cannabis abuse ($n = 35$, $p < 0.001$) or multiple substance abuse ($n = 20$, $p < 0.001$) prior to disease onset were found. Drug-naive schizophrenic patients without cannabis consumption showed similar results to normal controls and cannabis controls without schizophrenia. Elevated BDNF serum levels were not related to schizophrenia and/or substance abuse itself but may reflect a cannabis-related idiosyncratic damage of the schizophrenic brain. Disease onset was 5.2 years earlier in the cannabis-consuming group ($p = 0.0111$). A cannabis-based medicinal extract (CBME) was administered to 160 patients with multiple sclerosis experiencing significant problems from at least one of the following: spasticity, spasms, bladder problems, tremor, or pain. The interventions were oromucosal sprays of matched placebo, or whole plant CBME containing equal amounts of Δ-9-THC and CBD at a dose of 2.5–120 mg of each daily, in divided doses. The primary outcome measure was a Visual Analogue Scale (VAS) score for each patient's most troublesome symptom. Additional measures included VAS scores of other symptoms, and measures of disability, cognition, mood, sleep and fatigue. Following CBME the primary symptom score reduced from mean 74.36 (11.1) to 48.89 (22.0) following CBME and from 74.31 (12.5) to 54.79 (26.3) following placebo. Spasticity VAS scores were significantly reduced by CBME (Sativex) in comparison with placebo ($p = 0.001$). There were no significant adverse effects on cognition or mood and intoxication was generally mild. A SCE with pure Δ-9-THC, at matched concentrations of Δ-9-THC, and a Δ-9-THC-free extract (Δ-9-THC-free SCE) in a mouse model of MS, were examined. Although SCE inhibited spasticity in the mouse model of MS to a comparable level, it caused a more rapid onset of muscle relaxation and a reduction in the time to maximum effect compared with Δ-9-THC alone. The Δ-9-THC-free extract or CBD caused no inhibition of spasticity. In an experimental allergic encephalomyelitis (EAE), an animal model of MS, it was demonstrated that the cannabinoid system is neuroprotective during EAE. Mice, deficient in the cannabinoid receptor CB1, tolerated inflammatory and excitotoxic insults poorly, and developed substantial neurodegeneration following immune attack in EAE. Exogenous CB1 agonists can provide significant neuroprotection from the consequences of inflammatory central nervous system disease in an experimental allergic uveitis model.

Mutagenic activity

Petroleum ether extract of the aerial parts, in the ration of *Drosophila* at concentrations of 0.5, 1, and 5% of the diet, was active. Petroleum ether extract of the dried leaf, administered by gastric intubation to male mice at a dose of 50 mg/kg, was active. Water and methanol extracts of the seed, on agar plate at a concentration of 100 mg/mL, were inactive on *Bacillus subtilis* H-17 (Rec+) and *Salmonella typhimurium* TA100 and TA98. Metabolic activation had no effect on the results.

Myocardial infarction

A young man who suffered a myocardial infarction after taking Viagra in combination with cannabis was investigated. Viagra is metabolized predominantly by the CYP450 3A4 hepatic microsomal isoenzyme. Cannabis is a known inhibitor of CYP450 3A4 isoenzyme. The effect of the Viagra was thus potentiated by the effect of cannabis.

Natural-killer cells effect

Leukemia susceptible BALB/c and resistant C57BL/6 mice were infected with Friend leukemia virus complex and its helper component Rowson-Parr virus. At different time points, their natural-killer cells were separated from spleens and treated with 0–10 μg/mL of THC, subsequently mixed with Yac-1 target cells for 4 and 18 hours. The natural-killer cell activity in both mouse strains infected by either virus complex or helper virus weakened on days 2–4 postinfection, normalized by day 8 and enhanced on days 11–14. Natural-killer cell activity on the effect of low concentration (1–2.5 μg/mL) of THC slightly increased in BALB/c, was unaffected in C57BL/6, especially in the 18 hour assays. In the combined effects of cannabis and retrovirus, damages by cannabis dominated over those of retroviruses. Inhibition or reactive enhancement of natural-killer cell activity on the effect of viruses were similar to those of infected but cannabis-free counterparts, but on the level of uninfected cells treated with cannabis. The effects of cannabis and retrovirus were additive resulting in anergy of natural-killer cells.

Neonatal abstinence syndrome

The relationship of maternal drug abuse to symptoms, the effectiveness of pharmacological agents in controlling symptoms, and the length of in-patient stay were investigated in infants with neonatal abstinence syndrome. Pharmacological treatment was oral morphine sulphate (0.2 mg four to six times hourly), phenobarbitone (3–7 mg/kg/day), or combination of the two were administered to infants with a serial Finnegan score greater than 8. The average maternal age was 24.6 years, (18–34 years). Drug use volunteered by the mothers was methadone alone in 6 cases, methadone and benzodiazepines in 14, methadone and heroin and benzodiazepines in 7, methadone and heroin in 10, heroin alone in 2, and other multiple drug use including oral morphine sulphate, dothiepin, and cannabis in 4. Average gestational age was 40.3 (35–42 weeks). The average birth-weight was 2.81 kg (1.89–3.91 kg). Time-to-onset of withdrawal symptoms was 2.8 (1–13) days. The duration of pharmacological treatment (oral morphine sulphate and/or phenobarbitone) was 21.8 (1–62) days. The total hospital stay for the 43 infants was 1011 days.

Neuroendocrine abnormalities

Prolactin response to D-fenfluramine was assessed in abstinent ecstasy (MDMA) users with concomitant use of cannabis only (13 males, 11 females) and in two control groups: healthy nonusers (13 females) and exclusive cannabis users. Prolactin response to D-fenfluramine was slightly blunted in female ecstasy users. Both male user samples exhibited a weak prolactin response to D-fenfluramine, but this was weaker in the group of cannabis users. Baseline prolactin and prolactin response to D-fenfluramine were associated with the extent of previous cannabis use. The results indicated that the endocrinological abnormalities of ecstasy users might be closely related to their coincident cannabis use.

Neurogenic symptoms alleviation

Whole-plant extracts of Δ-9-THC, CBD, 1:1 CBD: THC, or placebo were self-administered by sublingual spray to 24 patients with MS (n = 18), spinal cord injury (n = 4), brachial plexus damage

(n = 1), and limb amputation owing to neurofibromatosis (n = 1), at doses determined by titration against symptom relief or unwanted effects within the range of 2.5–120 mg/24 hours for 2 weeks. The patients recorded symptoms, well-being, and intoxication scores on a daily basis using visual analog scales. At the end of each two-week period an observer rated severity and frequency of symptoms on numerical rating scales, administered standard measures of disability (Barthel Index), mood, cognition, and recorded adverse events. Pain relief associated with both THC and CBD was significantly superior to placebo. Impaired bladder control, muscle spasms, and spasticity were improved by cannabis medicinal extract (CME) in some patients with these symptoms. Three patients had transient hypotension and intoxication with rapid initial dosing of THC-containing CME. The results indicated that cannabis could improve neurogenic symptoms unresponsive to standard treatments. Unwanted effects were predictable and generally well tolerated.

Neuropathic pain relief

Forty-eight patients with at least one avulsed root and baseline pain score of four or more on an 11-point ordinate scale participated in a randomized, double-blind, placebo-controlled, three-period crossover study. The patients had intractable symptoms regardless of current analgesic therapy. They entered a baseline period of 2 weeks, followed by three, 2-week treatment periods; during each period they received one of three oromucosal spray preparations. These were placebo and two whole plant extracts of *C. sativa* L.: GW-1000-02 (Sativex), containing Δ-9-THC: CBD in an approx 1:1 ratio and GW-2000-02, containing primarily THC. The primary outcome measure was the mean pain severity score during the last 7 days of treatment. Secondary outcome measures included pain related quality of life assessments. The primary outcome measure failed to fall by the two points defined in our hypothesis. Both this measure and measures of sleep showed statistically significant improvements. The study medications were well tolerated with the majority of adverse events, including intoxication type mild to moderate in severity and resolving spontaneous reactions.

Neuroprotective effect

The effect of cannabidiol on β-amyloid peptide-induced toxicity in cultured rat pheocromocytoma PC12 cells was investigated. Following exposure of cells to β-amyloid peptide (1 μg/mL), a marked reduction in cell survival was observed. This effect was associated with increased reactive oxygen species production and lipid peroxidation, and caspase 3 (a key enzyme in the apoptosis cell-signalling cascade) appearance, DNA fragmentation, and increased intracellular calcium. Treatment of the cells with CBD (10^{-7}–10^{-4} mol) prior to β-amyloid peptide exposure, significantly elevated cell survival, whereas it decreased reactive oxygen species production, lipid peroxidation, caspase 3 levels, DNA fragmentation, and intracellular calcium. CBD and other cannabinoids were examined as neuroprotectants in rat cortical neuron cultures exposed to toxic levels of glutamate. The psychotropic cannabinoid receptor agonist Δ-9-THC and cannabidiol, reduced *N*-methyl-D-aspartate, α-amino-3 -hydroxy-5 -methyl-4-isoxazole propionic acid and kainate receptor mediated neurotoxicities. Neuroprotection was not affected by cannabinoid receptor antagonist, indicating a (cannabinoid) receptor-independent mechanism of action. CBD demonstrated a reduction in hydroperoxide toxicity in neurons. In this trial of the abilities of various antioxidants to prevent glutamate toxicity, cannabidiol was superior to both α-tocopherol and ascorbate in protective capacity.

Neuropsychological effect

Cerebral blood flow was measured in 12 long-term cannabis users shortly after cessation of cannabis use (mean 1.6 days). The findings showed significantly lower mean hemispheric blood flow values and significantly lower frontal values in the cannabis subjects compared with normal controls. The results indicated that the functional level of the frontal lobes was affected by long-term cannabis use.

Neurotransmission inhibition

The BLA or the medial prefrontal cortex (PFC) stimulation in urethane-anesthetized rats induced generation of action potentials in the Nac neurons. This excitatory effect was strongly inhibited by the synthetic cannabinoid agonists WIN (0.062–0.25 mg/kg, iv [intravenously]) and HU-210 (0.125–0.25 mg/kg, iv), or Δ-9-THC (1 mg/kg, iv). D1 or D2 dopamine receptor antagonists (SCH23390 0.5–1 mg/kg, sulpiride 5–10 mg/kg, iv) or the opioid antagonist naloxone (1 mg/kg, iv) were not able to reverse the action of cannabinoids. The selective CB1 receptor antagonist/reverse agonist SR141716A (0.5 mg/kg, iv) fully suppressed the action of cannabinoid agonists, whereas *per se* had no significant effect.

Nicotine and D-9-THC interaction

Δ-9-THC administration to mice significantly decreased the incidence of several nicotine withdrawal signs precipitated by mecamylamine or naloxone, such as wet-dog-shakes, paw tremor, and scratches. In both experimental conditions, the global withdrawal score was significantly attenuated by Δ-9-THC administration. The effect of Δ-9-THC was not to the result possible adaptive changes induced by chronic nicotine on CB1 cannabinoid receptors. The density and functional activity of these receptors were not modified by chronic nicotine administration in the different brain structures investigated. The consequences of Δ-9-THC administration on *c-Fos* expression in several brain structures after chronic nicotine administration and withdrawal were examined. *c-Fos* was decreased in the caudate putamen and the dentate gyrus after mecamylamine precipitated nicotine withdrawal. Δ-9-THC administration did not modify *c-Fos* expression under these experimental conditions. Δ-9-THC also reversed conditioned place aversion associated to naloxone precipitated nicotine withdrawal. The results indicated that Δ-9-THC administration attenuated somatic signs of nicotine withdrawal and this effect was not associated with compensatory changes on CB1 cannabinoid receptors during chronic nicotine administration. Δ-9-THC also ameliorated the aversive motivational consequences of nicotine withdrawal.

Night vision improvement

In a double-blind study, graduated THC administration at doses of 0–20 mg (as Marinol) on measures of dark adaptometry and scotopic sensitivity was evaluated. Field studies of night vision were performed among Jamaican and Moroccan fishermen, and mountain dwellers with the LKC Technologies Scotopic Sensitivity Tester-1. Improvements in night vision measures were noted after THC or cannabis. The effect was dose-dependent and cannabinoid-mediated at the retinal level.

Nocturnal sleep effect

Eight healthy volunteers (four males, four females; aged 21–34 years) were taking placebo, 15 mg Δ-9-THC, 5 mg THC combined with 5 mg CBD, and 15 mg THC combined with 15 mg CBD. These were formulated in 50:50 ethanol to propylene glycol and administered using an oromucosal spray during a 30-minute period from 10 PM. Electroencephalogram was recorded during the sleep period (11 PM to 7 AM). Performance, sleep latency, and subjective assessments of sleepiness and mood were measured from 8:30 AM (10 hours after drug administration). There were no effects of 15 mg THC on nocturnal sleep. With the concomitant administration of the drugs (5 mg THC and 5 mg CBD to 15 mg THC and 15 mg CBD), there was a decrease in stage 3 sleep, and with the higher dose combination, wakefulness was increased. The next day, with a 15-mg THC dose, memory was impaired, sleep latency was reduced, and the subjects reported increased sleepiness and changes in mood. With the lower dose combination, reaction time was faster on the digit recall task, and with the higher dose combination, subjects reported increased sleepiness and changes in mood. Fifteen milligrams of THC appeared to be sedative, and 15 mg CBD appeared to have alerting properties as it increased waking activity during sleep and counteracted the residual sedative activity of the 15 mg THC.

Occipital stroke

A right occipital ischemic stroke occurred in a 37-year-old Albanese man with a previously uneventful medical history, 15 minutes after smoking a cigarette with approximately 250 mg of cannabis. Clinical manifestations of the stroke were left-sided hemiparesis, hemihypesthesia and blurred vision, which vanished spontaneously and almost completely after 3 days.

The patient has been smoking cannabis regularly from the age of 27, with a frequency of two to three cigarettes/cannabis per week during the 6 months that preceded his stroke. Except for cigarette smoking and slight dyslipidemia, classical risk factors for stroke/embolism were absent. The family history for cerebrovascular events, blood pressure, clotting tests, examinations for thrombophilia, vasculitis, extracranial and intracranial arteries, and cardiac investigations were normal or respectively negative; the stroke was attributed to the chronic cannabis consumption.

Oral cancer

A study of 116 patients aged 45 years and younger, diagnosed with squamous cell carcinoma of the mouth was conducted. Two hundred and seven controls who had never had cancer, matched for age, sex, and area of residence, were recruited. The self-completed questionnaire contained items about exposure to the following risk factors: tobacco products, cannabis, alcohol, and diet. Conditional logistic analyses were conducted adjusting for social class, ethnicity, tobacco, and alcohol habits. All tests for statistical significance were two-sided. The majority of oral cancer patients reported exposure to the major risk factors of tobacco and alcohol even at the younger age. The estimated risks associated with tobacco or alcohol were low among both males and females. Only smoking for 21 years or more produced significantly elevated odds ratios (OR = 2.1; 95% CI: 1.1–4). Exposure associated with other major risk factors did not produce significant risks in this sample. Long-term consumption of fresh fruits and vegetables in the diet appeared to be protective for both males and females.

Oral cytological effect

The effects of cannabis, methaqualone, or tobacco smoking on the epithelial cells in 16 patients were evaluated. The site samples included the buccal mucosa (left and right sides), the posterior dorsum of the tongue, and the anterior floor of the mouth. There was a significant prevalence of bacterial cells in the smears and a greater number of degenerate and atypical squamous cells in cannabis users compared with controls. Epithelial cells in smears taken from cannabis users and tobacco-smoking controls showed koilocytic changes.

Pancreatic effect

A 29-year-old man presented with acute pancreatitis after a period of heavy cannabis smoking. Other causes of the disease were ruled out. The pancreatitis resolved itself after the cannabis was stopped and this was confirmed by urinary cannabinoid metabolite monitoring in the community. There were no previous reports of acute pancreatitis associated with cannabis use in the general population. Drugs of all types are related to the etiology of pancreatitis in approximately 1.4–2% of cases.

Panic disorder

Sixty-six panic disorder patients were included in a study. All of whom met the DSM-IV diagnosis of panic disorder ($n = 45$) or panic disorder with agoraphobia ([PDA]; $n = 21$). Twenty-four patients experienced their first panic attack within 48 hours of cannabis use and then went on to develop panic disorder. All the patients were treated with paroxetine (gradually increased up to 40 mg/day). The two groups responded equally well to paroxetine treatment as measured at the 8 weeks and 12 months follow-up visits. There were no significant effects of age, sex, and duration of illness as covariates with response rates between the two groups. In addition, panic disorder or panic disorder with agoraphobia diagnosis did not affect the treatment response in either group. There were no significant differences in weight gain, sexual side effects, or relapse rates between patients according to gender or comorbid diagnosis.

Paroxysmal atrial fibrillation

A healthy young subject was observed for paroxysmal atrial fibrillation following cannabis intoxication. The abuse of this substance was the most possible and identifiable risk factor.

Place conditioning effect

THC was administered to female rats at doses of 1, 5, or 20 mg/kg) during gestation and lactation. Maternal exposure to low doses of THC (1 and 5 mg/kg), relevant for human consumption, produced an increased response to the reinforcing effects of a moderate dose of morphine (350 μg/kg), as measured in the place-preference conditioning paradigm (CPP) in the adult male offspring. These animals also displayed an enhanced exploratory behavior in the defensive withdrawal test. Only females born from mothers exposed to THC at a dose of 1 mg/kg exhibited a small increment in the place conditioning induced by morphine. The possible implication of the HPA was analyzed by monitoring plasma levels of adrenocorticotropic hormone (ACTH) and corticosterone in basal and moderate-stress conditions (after the end of the CPP test). Female offspring perinatally exposed to THC (1 or 5 mg/kg) displayed high basal levels of corticosterone and a blunted adrenal response to the HPA-activating effects of the CPP test. Male offspring born from mothers exposed to THC (1 or 5 mg/kg) displayed the opposite pattern: normal to low basal levels of corticosterone, and a sharp adrenal response to the CPP challenge. THC administration to rats at a low dose (1.5 mg/kg) resulted in failing to develop place conditioning, and developing a place aversion at a high dose (15 mg/kg). Administration of the cannabinoid antagonist SR141716A induced a CPP at both a low (0.5 mg/kg) and a high (5 mg/kg) dose.

Plant germination effect

Methyl chloride extract of the dried seed produced weak activity on *Amaranthus spinosus* (25.8%) inhibition. Methyl chloride extract of the dried leaves produced 17.5% inhibition of *Amaranthus spinosus*.

Plasma norepinephrine concentration

Forty-six newborn infants participated in a prospective study of the neonatal and long-term effects of prenatal cocaine exposure. Based on maternal self-report, maternal urine screening, and infant meconium analysis, 24 infants were classified as CE and 22 as unexposed. Between 24 and 72 hours postpartum, plasma samples for norepinephrine (NE), epinephrine, dopamine, and dihydroxyphenylalanine analysis were obtained. The Neonatal Behavioral Assessment Scale was administered at 1–3 days of age and at 2 weeks of age by examiners masked to the drug exposure status of the newborns. The CE newborns had increased plasma NE concentrations when compared with the unexposed infants (geometric mean, 923 pg/mL vs 667 pg/mL). There were no significant differences in plasma epinephrine, dopamine, or dihydroxyphenylalanine concentrations. Analysis for the effect of potential confounding variables revealed that maternal cannabis use was also associated with increased plasma NE, although birth-weight, gender, and maternal use of alcohol or cigarettes were not. Geometric mean plasma NE was 1164 pg/ mL in those infants with *in utero* exposure to both cocaine and cannabis compared to 812 pg/mL in those exposed to only cocaine and 667.0 pg/mL in those exposed to neither. Among the CE infants, plasma NE concentration correlated with an increased score for the depressed cluster ($r = 0.53$) and a decreased score for the orientation cluster ($r = -0.43$) of the Neonatal Behavioral Assessment Scale administered at 1–3 days of age. Adjusting for cannabis exposure had no effect on these relationships between plasma NE and the depressed and orientation clusters.

Pneumonic effect

A case–control study was conducted in 7001 individuals. Odds ratios were calculated by conditional logistic regression with substance use and social factors as cofounders. Pneumonia was not associated with kava use. Crude odds ratios = 1.26 (0.74–2.14, $p = 0.386$) increased after controlling for confounders (OR = 1.98, 0.63–6.23, $p = 0.237$) but was not significant. Adjusted odds ratios for pneumonia cases involving kava and alcohol users was 1.19 (0.39–3.62, $p = 0.756$). Crude odds ratios for associations between pneumonia and cannabis use (OR = 2.27, 1.18–4.37, $p = 0.014$) and alcohol use (OR = 1.95, 1.07–3.53, $p = 0.026$) were statistically significant and approached significance for petrol sniffing (OR = 1.98, 0.99–3.95, $p = 0.056$).

Postural syncope

Twenty-nine volunteers participated in a randomized, double-blind, placebo-controlled study. Cerebral blood velocity, pulse rate, blood pressure, skin perfusion on forehead and plasma Δ-9-THC levels were quantified during reclining and standing for 10 minutes before and after THC infusions and cannabis smoking. Both THC and cannabis induced postural dizziness, with 28% reporting severe symptoms. Intoxication and dizziness peaked immediately after drug. The severe dizziness group showed the most marked postural drop in cerebral blood velocity and blood pressure and showed a drop in pulse rate after an initial increase during standing. Postural dizziness was unrelated to plasma levels of THC and other indices.

Prenatal exposure

Data collected from the National Household Survey on Drug Abuse, a nationally representative sample survey of 22,303 non-institutionalized women aged 18–44 years, of whom 1249 were pregnant, were analyzed. During the 2-year study period, 6.4% of the non-pregnant women of childbearing age and 2.8% of the pregnant women reported that they used illicit drugs. Of the women who used drugs, the relative proportion of women who abstained from illicit drugs after recognition of pregnancy increased from 28% during the first trimester of pregnancy to 93% by the third trimester. However, because of postpregnancy relapse, the net pregnancy-related reduction in illicit drug use at postpartum was only 24%. Cannabis accounted for three-fourths of illicit drug use, and cocaine accounted for one-tenth of illicit drug use. Of those who used illicit drugs, over half of pregnant and two-thirds of non-pregnant women used cigarettes and alcohol.

Among the sociodemographic subgroups, pregnant and non-pregnant women who were young (18–30 years) or unmarried, and pregnant women with less than a high school education had the highest rates of illicit drug use. Over 12,000 women at 18–20 weeks of gestation were enrolled in an Avon Longitudinal Study of Pregnancy and Childhood. Five percent of the mothers reported smoking cannabis before and/or during pregnancy; they were younger, of lower parity, better educated, and more likely to use alcohol, cigarettes, coffee, tea, and hard drugs. Cannabis use during pregnancy was unrelated to risk of perinatal death or need for special care, but the babies of women who used cannabis at least once per week before and throughout pregnancy were 216 g lighter than those of nonusers, had significantly shorter birth lengths, and smaller head circumferences. After adjustment for confounding factors, the association between cannabis use and birth-weight failed to be statistically significant ($p = 0.056$) and was clearly nonlinear. The adjusted mean birth-weights for babies of women using cannabis at least once per week before and throughout pregnancy were 90 g lighter than the offspring of other women. No significant adjusted effects were seen for birth length and head circumference. In two hospitals, 12,885 pregnant women answered questionnaires regarding consumption of alcohol, tobacco, cannabis, and other drugs.

The prevalence of cannabis use was 0.8%. Women using cannabis, but no other illicit drugs were each retrospectively matched with four randomly chosen pregnant women in the same period and the same age group and with same parity. Eighty-four cannabis users were included. These women were socio-economically disadvantaged and had a higher prevalence of present and past use of alcohol, tobacco, and other drugs. No significant difference in pregnancy, delivery, or puerperal outcome was found. Children of women using cannabis were 150 g lighter, 1.2 cm shorter, and had 0.2 cm smaller head circumference than the control infants. A 27-year-old woman who smoked a joint (cannabis) and 20 cigarettes (tobacco) daily up to the time of a positive pregnancy test at 7 weeks and 4 days, was evaluated. On day 20 of pregnancy, she had a LSD minitrip. The patient had a spontaneous term delivery. The baby boy weight was between the 5th and the 50th percentile, length between the 50th and the 90th percentile, normal umbilical arterial and venous pH values, and Apgar scores of 7/9/10. There were no visible abnormalities, and behavior was normal. Eight hundred seven consecutive positive-pregnancy test urine samples were screened for a range of drugs, including cotinine as an indicator of maternal smoking habits. A positive test for cannabinoids was found in 117 (14.5%) of the samples. Smaller numbers of samples were positive for other drugs: opiates (11), benzodiazepines (4), cocaine (3), and one each for amphetamines and methadone.

Polydrug use was detected in nine individuals. Only two samples tested positive for ethanol. The proportion with a urine cotinine level indicative of active smoking was 34.3%. The outcome of the pregnancy was traced for 288 of the subjects. Cannabis use was associated with a lower gestational age at delivery ($p < 0.005$), an increased risk of prematurity ($p < 0.02$), and reduction in birth-weight ($p < 0.002$). Maternal smoking was associated with a reduction in infant birth-weight ($p < 0.05$). This was less pronounced than the effect of other substance misuse. A sample of low-income women attending a prenatal clinic was assessed. The majority of the women decreased their use of cannabis during pregnancy. The assessments of child behavior problems included the Child Behavior Checklist, Teacher's Report Form, and the Swanson, Noland, and Pelham checklist. Multiple and logistic regressions were employed to analyze the relations between cannabis use and behavior problems of the children at age 10, while controlling for the effects of other extraneous variables. Prenatal cannabis use was significantly related to increased hyperactivity, impulsivity, and inattention symptoms as measured by the Swanson, Noland, and Pelham, increased delinquency as measured by the Child Behavior Checklist, and increased delinquency and externalizing problems as measured by the Teacher's Report Form. The pathway between prenatal cannabis exposure and delinquency was mediated by the effects of cannabis exposure on inattention symptoms. Attention and impulsivity of prenatally substance-exposed 6-year-olds were assessed as part of a longitudinal study. Most of the women were light-to-moderate users of alcohol and cannabis who decreased their use after the first trimester of pregnancy. Tobacco was used by a majority of women and did not change during pregnancy.

The women, recruited from a prenatal clinic, were of low socioeconomic status. Attention and impulsivity were assessed using a Continuous Performance Task. Second and third trimester of tobacco exposure and first trimester of cocaine use predicted increased omission errors. Second trimester cannabis use predicted more commission errors and fewer omission errors. There were no significant effects of prenatal alcohol exposure. Lower Stanford-Binet Intelligence Scale composite scores, male gender, and an adult male in the household predicted more errors of commission. Lower Standford-Binet Intelligence Scale composite scores, younger child age, maternal work/school status, and higher maternal hostility scores predicted more omission errors. The neurophysiological effects of prenatal cannabis exposure on response inhibition were assessed in thirty-one participants aged 18–22. Ottawa Prenatal Prospective Study performed a blocked design Go/No-Go task while neural activity was imaged with functional magnetic resonance imaging.

The Ottawa Prenatal Prospective Study is a longitudinal study that provides a unique body of information collected from each participant over 20 years, including prenatal drug history, detailed cognitive/behavioral performance from infancy to young adulthood, and current and past drug usage. The functional magnetic resonance imaging results showed that with increased prenatal cannabis exposure, there was a significant increase in neural activity in bilateral PFC and right premotor cortex during response inhibition. There was also an attenuation of activity in left cerebellum with increased prenatal exposure to cannabis when challenging the response inhibition neural circuitry. Prenatally exposed offspring had significantly more commission errors than non-exposed participants, but all participants were able to perform the task with more than 85% accuracy. The findings were observed when controlling for present cannabis use and prenatal exposure to nicotine, alcohol, and caffeine, and suggest that prenatal cannabis exposure was related to changes in neural activity during response inhibition that last into young adulthood. The effects of prenatal cannabis and alcohol exposure on school achievement at 10 years of age were examined. Women were interviewed about their substance use at the end of each trimester of pregnancy, at 8 and 18 months, and at 3, 6, 10, 14, and 16 years.

The women were of lower socioeconomic status, high school-educated, and light-to-moderate users of cannabis and alcohol. At the 10-year follow-up, the effects of prenatal exposure to cannabis or alcohol on the academic performance of 606 children were assessed. Exposure to one or more cannabis joints per day during the first trimester predicted deficits in Wide Range Achievement Test- Revised reading and spelling scores and a lower rating on the teachers' evaluations of the children's performance. This relation was mediated by the effects of first-trimester cannabis exposure on the children's depression and anxiety symptoms. Second-trimester cannabis use was significantly associated with reading comprehension and under-achievement. Exposure to alcohol during the first and second trimesters of pregnancy predicted poorer teachers' ratings of overall school performance. Second-trimester binge drinking predicted lower reading scores.

There was no interaction between prenatal cannabis and alcohol exposure. Each was an independent predictor of academic performance. Pregnant rats were treated daily with Δ-9-THC from the fifth day of gestation up to the day before birth (GD21). Then rats were sacrificed and their pups removed for analysis of the neural adhesion molecule L1-mRNA levels in different brain structures. The levels of L1 transcripts were significantly increased in the fimbria, stria terminalis, stria medullaris, corpus callosum, and in gray-matter structures (septum nuclei and the habenula). It remained unchanged in most of the gray-matter structures analyzed (cerebral cortex, BAL nucleus, hippocampus, thalamic and hypothalamic nuclei, basal ganglia, and sub-ventricular zones) and also in a few white-matter structures (fornix and fasciculus retroflexus). The increase in L1-mRNA levels reached statistical significance only in Δ-9-THC-exposed males but not females, where only trends or no effects were detected.

The results supported evidence on a sexual dimorphism, with greater effects in male fetuses, for the action of cannabinoids in the developing brain. Fetal cannabis exposure has no consistent effect on outcome. Prenatal cocaine exposure has not been shown to have any detrimental effect on cognition, except as mediated through cocaine effects on head size. Although fetal cocaine exposure has been linked to numerous abnormalities in arousal, attention, and neurological and neurophysiological function, most such effects appear to be self-limited and restricted to early infancy and childhood. Opiate exposure elicits a well-described withdrawal syndrome affecting the central nervous, autonomic, and gastrointestinal systems, which is most severe among methadone-exposed infants. Executive functioning in cocaine/polydrug (cannabis, alcohol, and tobacco)-exposed infants was assessed in a single session, occurring between 9.5 and 12.5 months of age. In an A-not-B task, infants searched—after performance-adjusted delays—for an object hidden in a new location. The CE infants did not differ from non-CE controls recruited from the same at-risk population. Comparison of heavier-CE ($n = 9$) with the combined group of lighter-CE ($n = 10$) and non-CE ($n = 32$) infants revealed significant differences on A-not-B performance, as well as on global tests of mental and motor development.

Covariates investigated included socioeconomic status, marital status, race, maternal age, years of education, weeks of gestation, and birth-weight, as well as severity of prenatal cannabis, alcohol, and tobacco exposure. The relationship of heavier-CE status to motor development was mediated by length of gestation, and the relationship of heavier-CE status to mental development was confounded with maternal gestational use of cigarettes. The relationship of heavier-CE status to A-not-B performance remained significant after controlling for potentially confounded variables and mediators, but was not statistically significant after controlling for the variance associated with global mental development. Weight, height, and head circumference were examined in children from birth to early adolescence for whom prenatal exposure to cannabis and cigarettes had been ascertained. The subjects were from a low-risk, predominantly middle-class sample participating in an ongoing longitudinal study. The negative association between growth measures at birth and prenatal cigarette exposure was overcome, sooner in males than females, within the first few years, and by the age of 6 years, the children of heavy smokers were heavier than control subjects. Pre- and postnatal environmental tobacco smoke did not have a negative effect on the growth parameters; however, the choice of bottle-feeding or shorter duration of breastfeeding by women who smoked during pregnancy appeared to play an important positive role in the catch-up observed among the infants of smokers. Prenatal exposure to cannabis was not significantly related to any growth measures at birth, although a smaller head circumference observed at all ages reached statistical significance among the early adolescents born to heavy cannabis users.

Prolactin inhibition

The dried leaves, smoked by healthy female volunteers at a dose of 1 g/person, produced a decrease in plasma prolactin levels during the luteal phase of the menstrual cycle but not during the follicular phase. The results were significant at $p < 0.01$ level.

Propiospinal myoclonus

A 25-year-old woman with clusters of myoclonus induced by a single exposure to inhaled cannabis was evaluated. Investigations excluded a structural abnormality of the spine. Multichannel surface electromyogram with parallel frontal electroencephalogram recording confirmed the diagnosis of propriospinal myoclonus.

Psoriatic effect

Hot water extract of the dried seed, taken orally by 108 human adults with psoriasis at variable dosage level, was active. After 3–4 weeks of treatment, there was significant improvement. The extract was taken in combination with *Rehmannia glutinosa* (rhizome), *Salvia miltiorrhiza* (root), *Scrophularia ningpoensis* (root), *Isatis tinctoria* (branch and leaf), *Sophora subprostrata* (root), *Dictamnus dasycarpus* (rootbark), *Polygonum bistorta* (rhizome), and *Forsythia suspensa* (fruit).

Psychosocial morbidity association

Cannabis dependence is a prevalent comorbid substance use disorder among patients early in the course of a schizophrenia-spectrum disorder. Among 29 eligible patients, 18 participated in the study. First-episode patients with comorbid cannabis dependence ($n = 8$) reported significantly greater childhood physical and sexual abuse compared with those without comorbid cannabis dependence ($n = 10$). The result indicated the preliminary evidence of an association between childhood maltreatment and cannabis dependence among this especially vulnerable population. Childhood physical and sexual abuse may be a risk factor for the initiation of cannabis dependence and other substance use disorders in the early course of schizophrenia.

Psychotic effect

Thirty five hundred representatives 19 years of age were examined in a cohort study. The subjects completed a 40-item Community Assessment of Psychic Experiences, measuring subclinical positive (paranoia, hallucinations, grandiosity, first- rank symptoms) and negative psychosis dimensions, depression, and drug use. Use of cannabis was associated positively with both positive and negative dimensions of psychosis, independent of each other and of depression. An association between cannabis and depression disappeared after adjustment for the negative psychosis dimensions. First use of cannabis younger than age 16 years was associated with a much stronger effect than first use after age 15 years, independent of lifetime frequency of use. The association between cannabis and psychosis was not influenced by the distress associated with the experiences, indicating that self-medication may be an unlikely explanation for the entire association between cannabis and psychosis. Cross-sectional epidemiological studies indicated that individuals with psychosis use cannabis more often than other individuals in the general population. It has long been considered that this association was explained by the self-medication hypothesis, postulating that cannabis is used to self-medicate psychotic symptoms. This hypothesis has been recently challenged. Several prospective studies carried out in population-based samples, showed that cannabis exposure was associated with an increased risk of psychosis. A dose–response relationship was found between cannabis exposure and risk of psychosis, and this association was independent from potential confounding factors, such as exposure to other drugs and preexistence of psychotic symptoms. The brain mechanisms underlying the association have to be elucidated; they may implicate deregulation of cannabinoid and dopaminergic systems. Cannabis exposure may be a risk factor for psychotic disorders by interacting with a preexisting vulnerability for these disorders.

Refractory neuropathic pain

Seven patients (three women and four men) aged 60 ± 14 years suffering from chronic refractory neuropathic pain, received oral THC titrated to the maximum dose of 25 mg/day (mean dose: 15 ± 6 mg) during an average of 55.4 days (range: 13–128). Various components of pain (continuous, paroxysmal, and brush-induced allodynia) were assessed using visual analog scale scores. Health-related quality of life was evaluated using the Brief Pain Inventory, and the Hospital Anxiety and Depression scale was used to measure depression and anxiety. THC did not induce significant effect on the various pain, health-related quality of life and anxiety and depression scores. Numerous side effects (notably sedation and asthenia) were observed in five out of seven patients, requiring premature discontinuation of the drug in three patients.

Reproductive effect

Cannabis use during pregnancy in developed nations is estimated to be approx 10%. Recent evidence suggests that the endogenous cannabinoid system, now consisting of two receptors and multiple endocannabinoid ligands, may also play an important role in the maintenance and regulation of early pregnancy and fertility. Drugs of abuse, like alcohol, opiates, cocaine, and cannabis, are used by many young people for their presumed aphrodisiac properties. The opioids inhibit the hypothalamus–pituitary–gonads axis (HPG), and increase the prolactin levels, which interferes with the male and female sexual response. Cannabis, at high doses, could inhibit the HPG axis and reduce fertility. Cannabis initially increases libido and potency, but chronic use causes sexual inversion. Long-term use of cannabis has been found to cause physiological changes that can alter individual reproductive potential. The effects of cannabis depend on the dose and can include death from depression of the respiratory system. Cannabis is absorbed rapidly and eliminated very slowly. Δ-9-THC is highly liposoluble and fixes to the serum proteins, passing to the lungs and liver for metabolization and to the kidneys and liver for excretion. As with estrogens, there is an enterohepatic circuit for reabsorption and elimination. Ninety percent is eliminated in the feces, 65% within 48 hours. Because of the enterohepatic circuit and liposolubility, elimination requires 1 week for completion. The other important biotransformation of the active principle is hydroxylation. The hydroxylated derivatives are responsible for the psychoactivity of cannabis. Cannabis affects both neuroendocrine function and the germ cells. Studies on experimental animals have indicated that THC can cause a decline in the pituitary hormones, follicle stimulating hormone, luteinizing hormone, and prolactin, and in the steroids progesterone, estrogen, and androgens.

Human studies have shown that chronic users have decreased levels of serum testosterone. Because steroidogenesis can be restimulated with human chorionic gonadotropin, it appears that THC does not directly affect steroid production by the corpus luteum, but that its action is mediated by the hypothalamus. Because of its potent antigonadotropic action, THC is under study as an anovulatory agent. The same animal studies have shown that ovulation returns to normal 6 months after termination of use.

High rates of anovulation and luteal insufficiency have been observed in women smoking cannabis at least three times weekly. THC accumulates in the milk. Animal studies have shown that THC depresses the enzymes necessary for lactation and causes a diminution in the volume of the mammary glands. Significant amounts of the drug have been detected in both mothers' milk and the blood of newborns. Animal studies indicate that THC crosses the placenta, achieving concentrations in the fetus as high as those in the mother. Animal studies also demonstrated increasing frequency of abortions, intrauterine death, and declines in fetal weight. The effects were probably caused by an alteration in placental function. A human study likewise showed that cannabis use during pregnancy was significantly related to poor fetal development, low birth-weight, diminished size, and decreased cephalic circumference. Congenital malformations have been observed in experimental animals exposed to THC. Declines in sperm volume and count and abnormal sperm motility have been observed in chronic cannabis users. In vitro studies show that THC produces a marked degeneration of human sperm. Among sexually experienced girls, 39% (n = 123) reported using oral contraceptive pills(OCPs), 5.4% (n = 17) used Depo-Provera (medroxyprogesterone acetate) or Norplant (levonorgestrel), and 55.6% (n = 175) used no hormonal method. Logistic regression analysis revealed that the factors most significantly associated with the use of hormonal methods were older age (OR = 1.19; 95% CI, 1.07–1.33), not using a condom at last intercourse (OR = 0.55; CI, 0.34–0.90), and having had a well visit within 1 year (OR = 2.11; CI, 1.12–3.70). OCP users were less likely than Depo-Provera or Norplant users to have used alcohol ($p = 0.041$), cigarettes ($p = 0.002$), or cannabis ($p = 0.018$) in the past 30 days. OCP users were less likely than nonusers of hormonal methods to have smoked cigarettes ($p = 0.034$) or cannabis ($p = 0.052$). The school-based clinic had a greater proportion of subjects using long-acting progestins ($p < 0.001$).

Respiratory effect

Smoking a "joint" of cannabis resulted in exposure to significantly greater amounts of combusted material than with a tobacco cigarette. The histopathological effects of cannabis-smoke exposure included changes consistent with acute and chronic bronchitis. Cellular dysplasia has also been observed, suggesting that, like tobacco smoke, cannabis exposure has the potential to cause malignancy. Symptoms of cough and early morning sputum production are common (20–25%) even in young individuals who smoke cannabis alone. Almost all studies indicated that the effects of cannabis and tobacco smoking are addictive and independent. A small group of current male cannabis processors with a mean age of 43 years was studied. Questionnaire data, lung function, serial FEV1 and blood were collected from all workers. Seven workers (64%) complained of at least one respiratory symptom (one with byssinosis). The mean percentage predicted FEV1 was 91.5, FVC 97.7, peak expiratory flow 92.1, and forced expiratory flow between 25 and 75% of FVC 79.5. Serial FEV1 measurements in the two workers with work-related respiratory symptoms revealed a mean change in FEV1 on the first working day of –12.9%. This contrasted with +6.25% on the last working day. Respective values for the two workers without work-related symptoms were –1.4 and +3.2%. Nine hundred forty-three young adults from a birth cohort of 1037 were studied at age 21 years.

Standardized respiratory symptom questionnaires were administered. Spirometry and methacholine challenge tests were undertaken. Cannabis dependence was determined using DSM-III-R criteria.

Descriptive analyses and comparisons between cannabis-dependent, tobacco- smoking, and nonsmoking groups were undertaken. Adjusted odds ratios for respiratory symptoms, lung function, and airway hyperresponsiveness (PC20) were measured.

Ninety-one subjects (9.7%) were cannabis-dependent and 264 (28.1%) were current tobacco smokers. After controlling for tobacco use, respiratory symptoms associated with cannabis dependence included wheezing apart from colds, exercise-induced shortness of breath, nocturnal wakening with chest tightness, and early morning sputum production. These were increased by 61, 65, 72 (all $p < 0.05$), and 144% ($p < 0.01$) respectively, compared with non-tobacco smokers. The frequency of respiratory symptoms in cannabis-dependent subjects was similar to tobacco smokers of 1–10 cigarettes per day. The proportion of cannabis-dependent study members with an FEV1/FVC ratio of less than 80% was 36% compared with 20% for nonsmokers ($p = 0.04$). These outcomes occurred independently of coexisting bronchial asthma.

Reversal of cannabinoid addiction

Δ-9-THC was administered orally to mice at a dose of 10 mg/kg twice daily for 6 days to make them dependent on cannabinoids. Other groups of mice were administered orally with a Δ-9-THC and benzoflavone from *Passiflora incarnata* at doses of 10 or 20 mg/kg twice daily for 6 days. Mice receiving the Δ-9-THC and *Passiflora incarnata* extract developed significantly less dependence, worse locomotor activity, and less of typical withdrawal effects like paw tremors and headshakes, compared with mice receiving Δ-9-THC alone. Administration of SR-141716A, a selective cannabinoid-receptor antagonist (10 mg/kg, orally), to all groups on the seventh day resulted in an artificial withdrawal. Administration of 20 mg/kg of the *Passiflora incarnata* benzoflavone moiety to mice showing symptoms of withdrawal owing to administration of SR-141716A produced a marked attenuation of withdrawal effects.

Schizophrenic effect

The nerve growth factor (NGF) serum levels of 109 consecutive drug-naïve schizophrenic patients were measured and compared with those of healthy controls. The results were correlated with the long-term intake of cannabis and other drugs. Mean (± standard deviation) NGF serum levels of 61 control persons (33.1 ± 31 pg/mL) and 76 schizophrenics who did not consume illegal drugs (26.3 ± 19.5 pg/mL) did not differ significantly.

Schizophrenic patients with regular cannabis intake (> 0.5 g per day on average for at least 2 years) had significantly raised NGF serum levels of 412.9 ± 288.4 pg/mL ($n = 21$) compared with controls and schizophrenic patients not consuming cannabis ($p < 0.001$). In schizophrenic patients who abused not only cannabis, but also additional substances, NGF concentrations were as high as 2336.2 ± 1711.4 pg/mL ($n = 12$). On average, heavy cannabis consumers suffered their first episode of schizophrenia 3.5 years ($n = 21$) earlier than schizophrenic patients who abstained from cannabis. These results indicate that cannabis is a possible risk factor for the development of schizophrenia. This might be reflected in the raised NGF-serum concentrations when both schizophrenia and long-term cannabis abuse prevail.

Schizotypy correlation

Two hundred eleven healthy adults who used cannabis showed higher scores on schizotypy, borderline, and psychoticism scales than never- users. Multivariate analysis, covarying lie scale scores, age, and educational level indicated that high schizotypal traits best discriminated subjects who had used cannabis from never-users, whether or not they reported having used other recreational drugs. The results indicated that cannabis use was related to a personality dimension of psychosis-proneness in healthy people.

Sedative and stimulant effects

A double-blind, placebo-controlled study assessed subjective effects of smoking cannabis with either a long or short breath-holding duration. During eight test sessions, 55 male volunteers made repeated ratings of subjective "high," sedation, and stimulation, as well as rating their perceptions of motivation and performance on cognitive tests. The long, relative to the short, breath-holding duration increased "high" ratings after smoking cannabis, but not placebo. Cannabis smoking increased sedation and a perception of worsened test performance, and decreased motivation with respect to test performance. Paradoxical subjective effects were observed in those subjects reporting some stimulation, as well as sedation after smoking cannabis, particularly with the long breath-holding duration. Breath-holding duration did not produce any subjective effects that were independent of the drug treatment (i.e., occurred equally after smoking of cannabis and placebo).

Sexual receptivity

The effects of THC on sexual behavior in female rats and its influence on steroid hormone receptors and neurotransmitters in the facilitation of sexual receptivity was examined. Results revealed that the facilitatory effect of THC was inhibited by antagonists to both progesterone and dopamine D(1) receptors. To test further the idea that progesterone receptors (PR) and/or dopamine receptors (D[1]R) in the hypothalamus were required for THC-facilitated sexual behavior in rodents, antisense, and sense oligonucleotides to PR and D(1)R were administered intra-cerebroventricularly into the third cerebral ventricle of ovariectomized, estradiol benzoate-primed rats. Progesterone- and THC-facilitated sexual behavior was inhibited in animals treated with antisense oligonucleotides to PR or to D(1)R. Antagonists to cannabinoid receptor-1 subtype (CB1), but not to cannabinoid receptor-2 subtype (CB2) inhibited progesterone- and dopamine-facilitated sexual receptivity in female rats. Adult female and male rats that had been perinatally exposed to hashish extracts were investigated. Adult males perinatally exposed to hashish extracts exhibited marked changes in the behavioral patterns executed in the sociosexual approach behavior test; these changes did not exist in females.

Control males first visited the incentive male and took longer to visit the incentive female, whereas hashish-exposed males followed the opposite pattern. Hashish-exposed males spent more time in the vicinity of the incentive female, whereas they decreased their frequency of visits to, and the time spent in, the male incentive area. This behavior was observed during the first third of the test, but became normalized and even inverted during the last two-thirds. In the social interaction test, the normal reduction in the time spent in active social interaction following the exposure to a neophobic situation (high light levels) in controls did not occur in hashish-exposed males, although these exhibited a response in the dark-light emergence test similar to that of their corresponding controls. No changes were seen in spontaneous locomotor activity in both tests. These behavioral alterations observed in hashish-exposed males were paralleled by a significant decrease in L-3,4-dihydroxyphenylacetic acid contents in the limbic forebrain; this suggests a decreased activity of mesolimbic dopaminergic neurons. No effects were seen in females.

Smooth muscle relaxant activity

Ethanol (95%) and water extracts of the dried aerial parts, at a concentration of 1:1, produced weak activity on the rabbit duodenum. The ethanol extract was equivocal on the guinea pig ileum. Petroleum ether extract of the dried entire plant, administered intraperitoneally to rats at a dose of 0.89 mg/kg, was active vs corneo-palpebral reflex.

Spasticity treatment

Standardized plant extract was administered orally to 57 MS patients with poorly controlled spasticity, at a dose of 2.5 mg of THC and 0.9 mg of CBD. Patients in group A started with a drug escalation phase from 15 to a maximum of 30 mg of THC by 5 mg per day if well tolerated, being on active medication for 14 days before starting placebo. Patients in group B started with placebo for 7 days, crossed to the active period (14 days), and closed with a three-day placebo period (active drug-dose escalation and placebo sham escalation as in group A). Measures used included daily self-report of spasm frequency and symptoms, Ashworth Scale, Rivermead Mobility Index, 10-meter timed walk, nine-hole peg test, paced auditory serial addition test, and the digit span test.

There were no statistically significant differences associated with active treatment compared with placebo, but trends in favor of active treatment were seen for spasm frequency, mobility, and getting to sleep. In the 37 patients (per-protocol set) who received at least 90% of their prescribed dose, improvements in spasm frequency ($p = 0.013$) and mobility after excluding a patient who fell and stopped walking were seen ($p = 0.01$). Minor adverse events were slightly more frequent and severe during active treatment, and toxicity symptoms, which were generally mild, were more pronounced in the active phase. Six hundred thirty participants with stable MS and muscle spasticity were treated with oral cannabis extract ($n = 211$), Δ-9-THC ($n = 206$), or placebo ($n = 213$) for 15 weeks. Six hundred eleven of 630 patients were followed up for the primary end point.

No treatment effect of cannabinoids on the primary outcome ($p = 0.40$) was noted. The estimated difference in mean reduction in total Ashworth score for participants taking cannabis extract compared with placebo was 0.32 (95% CI, -1.04 to 1.67), and for those taking Δ-9-THC vs placebo it was 0.94 (-0.44 to 2.31). There was an evidence of a treatment effect on patient-reported spasticity and pain ($p = 0.003$), with improvement in spasticity reported in 61% ($n = 121$, 95% CI, 54.6–68.2), 60% ($n = 108$, 52.5–66.8), and 46% ($n = 91$, 39–52.9) of participants on cannabis extract, Δ-9-THC, and placebo, respectively.

Spatial working memory effect

Functional magnetic resonance imaging was used to examine brain activity in 12 long-term heavy cannabis users, 6–36 hours after last use, and in 10 control subjects while they performed a spatial working memory task. Regional brain activation was analyzed and compared using statistical parametric mapping techniques. Compared with controls, cannabis users exhibited increased activation of brain regions typically used for spatial working memory tasks (such as PFC and anterior cingulate). Users also recruited additional regions not typically used for spatial working memory (such as regions in the basal ganglia). The findings remained essentially unchanged when reanalyzed using the subjects ages as a covariate. Brain activation showed little or no significant correlation with subjects years of education, verbal IQ, lifetime episodes of cannabis use, or urinary cannabinoid levels at the time of scanning.

Spontaneous pneumomediastinum

Spontaneous pneumomediastinum is defined as pneumomediastinum in the absence of an underlying lung disease. It is the second most common cause of chest pain in young, healthy individuals (<30 years) necessitating hospital visits. Inhalational drug use (cocaine and cannabis) has been associated with a significant number of cases, although cases with no apparent etiological or incriminating factors are well-recognized. A case of an 18-year-old high school student with spontaneous pneumomediastinum was evaluated.

Sudden infant death syndrome

In a nationwide case–control study of 369 cases and 1558 controls, two-thirds of SIDS deaths occurred at night (between 10 PM and 7:30 AM). The odds ratio (95% CI) for prone sleep position was 3.86 (2.67–5.59) for deaths occurring at night, and 7.25 (4.52–11.63) for deaths occurring during the day; the difference was significant. The odds ratio for maternal smoking and SIDS deaths occurring at night was 2.28 (1.52–3.42), and for the day, 1.27 (0.79–2.03). If the mother was single, the odds ratio was 2.69 (1.29–3.99) for a nighttime death, and 1.25 (0.76–2.04) for a daytime death. Both interactions were significant. The interactions between time of death and bed sharing, not sleeping in a cot or bassinet, ethnicity, late timing of prenatal care, binge drinking, cannabis use, and illness in the baby were also significant. All were more strongly associated with SIDS occurring at night. In a nationwide case–control study, 393 cases and 1592 controls were analyzed. Adjusting for ethnicity and maternal tobacco use, the SIDS odds ratio for weekly maternal cannabis use since the infant's birth was 2.23 (95% CI = 1.39, 3.57) compared with nonusers, and the multivariate odds ratio was 1.55 (95% CI = 0.87, 2.75).

Suicidal effect

Standardized interview assessments were conducted with 2311 youths aged 8–15 years who used drugs before age 16. Approximately 15 years after recruitment, 1695 persons (mean age = 21 years) were reassessed. One hundred fifty-five of them made suicide attempts (SA) and 218 had onset of depression-related suicide ideation (SI). The relative risk, from survival analysis and logistic regression models, to study early use of tobacco, alcohol, cannabis, and inhalants, with covariate adjustments for age, sex, race/ethnicity, and other pertinent covariates were examined. Early-onset of cannabis use and inhalant use for females, but not for males, signaled a modest excess risk of SA (cannabis-associated RR = 1.9; $p = 0.04$; inhalant-associated RR = 2.2; $p = 0.05$). Early-onset of cannabis use by females (but not for males) signaled excess risk for SI (RR = 2.9; $p = 0.006$). Early-onset alcohol and tobacco use were not associated with later risk of SA or SI. Two hundred seventy-seven same-sex twin pairs (median age: 30 years) discordant for cannabis dependence and 311 pairs discordant for early-onset cannabis use (before age 17 years) were examined.

Individuals who were cannabis-dependent had odds of SI and SA that were 2.5–2.9 times higher than those of their noncannabis-dependent co-twin. Cannabis dependence was associated with elevated risks of major depressive disorder (MDD) in dizygotic, but not in monozygotic twins. Twins who initiated cannabis use before age 17 years of age had elevated rates of subsequent SA (OR, 3.5, 95% CI, 1.4–8.6) but not of MDD or SI. Early MDD and SI were significantly associated with subsequent risks of cannabis dependence in discordant dizygotic pairs, but not in discordant monozygotic pairs. The results indicated that the comorbidity between cannabis dependence and MDD likely arises through shared genetic and environmental vulnerabilities predisposing to both outcomes. In contrast, associations between cannabis dependence and suicidal behaviors cannot be entirely explained by common predisposing genetic and/or shared environmental predisposition.

Synergic cytotoxicity

THC, in A549 lung tumor cells culture at concentrations of less than 5 μg/mL, produced no cytotoxic effect. At higher levels it induced cell necrosis, with a lethal concentration $(LC)_{50}$of 16–18 μg/mL. Butylated hydroxyanisole ([BHA], a food additive)alone at concentrations of 10–200 μM, produced limited cell toxicity and significantly enhanced the necrotic death resulting from concurrent exposure to THC. In the presence of BHA at 200 μM, the LC_{50} for THC decreased to 10–12 μg/mL. Similar results were obtained with smoke extracts prepared from cannabis cigarettes, but not with extracts from tobacco or placebo cannabis cigarettes (containing no THC). Experiments were repeated in the presence of either diphenyleneiodonium or dicumarol as inhibitors of the redox cycling pathway. Neither of the compounds protected cells from the effects of combined THC and BHA, but rather enhanced necrotic cell death. Measurements of cellular ATP revealed that both THC and BHA reduced ATP levels in A549 cells, consistent with toxic effects on mitochondrial electron transport. The combination was synergistic in this respect, reducing ATP levels to less than 15% of the control. Exposure to cannabis smoke in conjunction with BHA may promote deleterious health effects in the lung.

Teratogenic activity

Resin, administered orally to pregnant rabbits at a dose of 1 mL/ kg, was active. Alcohol extract of the dried leaves, administered intragastrically to pregnant rats at a dose of 125 mg/kg from days 7 to 16 of gestation, was active. The fetuses showed several gross abnormalities, visceral anomalies, and skeletal malformations. Water extract of the dried leaf, administered intragastrically to pregnant rats at doses of 125, 200, 400, and 800 mg/kg, produced various types of malformations in the fetuses. Petroleum ether extract of the aerial parts, administered orally to rats and rabbits, was inactive.

Tourette syndrome

Tourette syndrome (TS) is a complex inherited disorder of unknown etiology, characterized by multiple motor and vocal tics. Involvement of the central cannabinoid (CB1) system was suggested because of therapeutic effects of cannabis consumption and Δ-9-THC-treatment in TS patients. The central cannabinoid receptor (CNR1) gene encoding the *CNR1* was considered as a candidate gene for TS and systematically screened by single-strand conformation polymorphism analysis and sequencing. Compared with the published *CNR1* sequence, three single-base substitutions were identified: 1326T→A, 1359G→A, 1419 + 1G→C. The change at position 1359 is a common polymor-phism (1359 G/A) without allelic association with TS. 1326T→A was present in only one TS patient and is a silent mutation, which does not change codon 442 (valine). 1419 + 1G→C affects the first nucleotide immediately following the coding sequence. It was first detected in three of 40 TS patients and none of 81 healthy controls. This statistically significant association with TS ($p = 0.034$) could not be confirmed in two subsequent cohorts of 56 TS patients (one heterozygous for 1419 + 1G→C) and 55 controls, and 64 patients and 66 controls (one heterozygous for 1419 + 1G→C), respectively. Transcript analysis of lymphocyte RNA from five 1419 + 1G→C carriers revealed no systematic influence on the expression level of the mutated allele.

In addition, segregation analysis of 1419 + 1G→C in affected families gave evidence that 1419 + 1G→C does not play a causal role in the etiology of TS. It was concluded that genetic variations of the *CNR1* gene are not a plausible explanation for the clinically observed relation between the cannabinoid system and TS. A single-dose, cross-over study in 12 patients, and a 6-week, randomized trial in 24 patients, demonstrated that Δ9-THC, the most psychoactive ingredient of cannabis, reduced tics in TS patients. No serious adverse effects occurred and no impairment on neuropsychological performance was observed. In the randomized, double-blind, placebo-controlled study, 24 patients with TS, according to DSM-III-R criteria, were treated over a 6-week period with up to 10 mg/day of THC. Tics were rated at six visits (visit 1, baseline; visits 2–4, during treatment period; visits 5–6, after withdrawal of medication) using the Tourette Syndrome Clinical Global Impressions scale (TS-CGI), the Shapiro Tourette-Syndrome Severity Scale (STSSS), the Yale Global Tic Severity Scale (YGTSS), the self-rated Tourette Syndrome Symptom List (TSSL), and a videotape-based rating scale. Seven patients dropped out of the study or had to be excluded, but only one because of side effects. Using the TS-CGI, STSSS, YGTSS, and video rating scale, there was a significant difference ($p < 0.05$) or a trend toward a significant difference ($p < 0.1$) between THC and placebo groups at visits 2, 3, and/or 4. Using the TSSL at 10 treatment days (between days 16 and 41) there was a significant difference ($p < 0.05$) between both groups.

Analysis of variance also demonstrated a significant difference ($p = 0.037$). No serious adverse effects occurred. In the randomized, double-blind, placebo-controlled study, the effect of a treatment with up to 10 mg Δ-9-THC over a 6-week period on neuropsychological performance in 24 patients suffering from TS was investigated. During medication and immediately, as well as 5–6 weeks after, withdrawal of Δ-9-THC treatment, no detrimental effect was seen on learning curve, interference, recall and recognition of word lists, immediate visual memory span, and divided attention. A trend towards a significant immediate verbal memory span improvement during and after treatment was found. A randomized double-blind placebo-controlled crossover single-dose trial of Δ-9-THC (5, 7.5, or 10 mg) in 12 adult TS patients was performed. Tic severity was assessed using the TSSL and examiner ratings (STSSS, YGTSS, TS-CGS).

Using the TSSL, patients also rated the severity of associated behavioral disorders. Clinical changes were correlated to maxi-mum plasma levels of THC and its metabolites 11-OH-THC and 11-nor-Δ-9-tetrahydrocannabinol-9-carboxylic acid. Using the TSSL, there was a significant improvement of tics ($p = 0.015$) and obsessive-compulsive behavior ($p = 0.041$) after treatment with Δ-9-THC compared with placebo. Examiner ratings demonstrated a significant difference for the subscore "complex motor tics" ($p = 0.015$) and a trend towards a significant improvement for the subscores "motor tics" ($p = 0.065$), "simple motor tics" ($p = 0.093$), and "vocal tics" ($p = 0.093$). No serious adverse reactions occurred. Five patients experienced mild, transient side effects. There was a significant correlation between tic improvement and maximum 11-OH-THC plasma concentration.

Toxic effect

Petroleum ether extract of the dried leaf, administered by gastric intubation to pregnant rats at a dose of 150 mg/kg, produced a reduction of food and water consumption and maternal weight gain. The weight of pups at birth was reduced by approx 10% of the litter size, and pup mortality at birth was not affected significantly. Water extract of the aerial parts, administered intravenously to male adults, was active. The resin, ingested by a 4-year-old girl, showed signs of stupor alternating with brief intervals of excitation and foolish laughing with atactic movements. Her temperature, blood pressure, pulse, hemoglobin, leukocytes, serum electrolytes, and serum urea were normal. Respiratory rate was 12 beats per minute. Blood sugar elevated. Recovery was complete within 24 hours with no treatment. Four patients suffered gastrointestinal disorders and psychological effects after eating salad prepared with hemp seed oil. The concentration of THC in the oil far exceeded the recommended tolerance dose. From January 1998 to January 2002, 213 incidences were recorded of dogs that developed clinical signs following oral exposure to cannabis, with 99% having neurological signs and 30% exhibiting gastrointestinal signs. The cannabis ingested ranged from 0.5 to 90 g. The lowest dose at which signs occurred was 84.7 mg/kg and the highest reported dose was 26.8 g/kg. Onset of signs ranged from 5 minutes to 96 hours, with most signs occurring within 1–3 hours after ingestion. The signs lasted from 30 minutes to 96 hours. Management consisted of decontamination, sedation (with diazepam as drug of choice), fluid therapy, thermo-regulation, and general supportive care. All followed animals made full recoveries. The suspension prepared from the benzene washing solution of cannabis seeds, administered intravenously to mice at a dose of 3 mg/kg, produced hypothermia, catalepsy, pentobarbital-induced sleep prolongation, and suppression of locomotor activity. These pharmacological activities of benzene washing solution of cannabis seeds were significantly higher than those of Δ-9-THC (3 mg/kg, iv).

Trauma injuries

An association between combat-related posttraumatic stress disorder (C-PTSD) and other mental disorders was studied in co-twin (male monozygotic twin pairs in the Vietnam Era Twin Registry). Logistic regression analyses demonstrated that combat exposure, adjusted for C-PTSD, was significantly associated with increased risk for alcohol and cannabis dependence and that C-PTSD mediated the association between combat exposure and both major depression and tobacco dependence. Sera from 111 patients with trauma injuries who presented during a 3-month period were screened for blood alcohol. Urine specimens were analyzed for metabolites of cannabis and cocaine. Sixty- two percent of patients were positive for at least one substance and 20% for two or more. Positivity rates were as follows: cannabis, 46%; alcohol, 32% (with 71% of these having blood alcohol levels >80 mg/ dL);

and cocaine (6%). Substance usage was most prevalent in the third decade of life. The patients who yielded a positive result were significantly younger than those negatives. There was no significant difference in age or substance usage between the victims of interpersonal violence or road traffic accidents. In the group designated "other accidents," patients were significantly older and had a lower incidence of substance usage than the other two groups. Cannabis was the most prevalent substance in all groups. Fifty and 55% of victims of road accidents and interpersonal violence, respectively, were positive for cannabis compared with 43 and 27% for alcohol, respectively. There was no significant difference in hospital stay or injury severity score between substance users and nonusers.

Trigeminovascular system effect

Arachidonylethanolamide is believed to be the endogenous ligand of the cannabinoid CB1 and CB2 receptors. Known behavioral effects of AEA are antinociception, catalepsy, hypothermia, and depression of motor activity, similar Δ-9-THC, the psychoactive constituent of cannabis. A role of the CB1 receptor in the trigeminovascular system, using intravital to study the effects of AEA against various vasodilator agents was examined. AEA inhibited dural blood vessel dilation brought about by electrical stimulation by 50%, calcitonin gene-related peptide (CGRP) by 30%, capsaicin by 45%, and NO by 40%. CGRP(8–37) attenuated NO-induced dilation by 50%. The AEA inhibition was reversed by the CB1 receptor antagonist AM251. AEA also reduced the blood pressure changes caused by CGRP injection, this effect was not reversed by AM251.

Tumor-promoting effect

A 28-year-old man who abused alcohol, nicotine, and cannabis for several years was investigated. He suffered simultaneously from a squamous cell carcinoma of the hypopharynx with bilateral cervical metastases, an adenocarcinoma of the transverse colon and a primary hepatocellular carcinoma. There were occurrences of three separate malignant tumors with different histologies in the aerodigestive tract, which could be related to a chronic abuse of cannabis.

Turning behavior

Cannabinoid agonists: WIN (1–100 ng/mouse), CP-55,940 (0.1– 50 ng/mouse), and AEA (0.5–50 ng/mouse), administered unilaterally into the mouse striatum, dose-dependently induced turning behavior. SR 141716A [*N*-(piperidin-1-yl)-5-(4-chlorophenyl)-1-(2,4-dichlorophenyl)-4-methyl-1H-pyrazole-3-carboxamide hydrochloride], the selective antagonist of CB1 receptor, antagonized the three cannabinoid receptor agonists-induced turning with similar effective $dose_{50}$ (0.13–0.15 mg/ kg, intraperitoneally). Spiroperidol (a D2 receptor blocker), (+)-SCH 23390 (a D1 receptor blocker), or prior 6-hydroxydopamine lesions of the striatum blocked WIN- and CP-55,940-induced turning, thus suggesting the involvement of DA transmission in cannabinoid-induced turning.

Uterine stimulant effect

Ethanol (50%) extract of the entire plant was inactive on the rat uterus. Ethanol (95%) and water extracts of the dried aerial parts, at a concentration of 1:1, produced strong activity on the non-pregnant rat uterus. Water extract of the flowering tops produced strong activity on the rat uterus.

Ventricular septal defect

A Birth Defect Case–Control Study was used to identify 122 isolated simple ventricular septal defect (VSD) cases and 3029 control infants. Exposure data on alcohol, cigarette, and illicit drug use were obtained through standardized interviews with mothers and fathers. Associations between lifestyle factors and VSD were calculated using maternal self-reports; associations were also calculated using paternal proxy reports of the mother's exposures. Maternal self-report of heavy alcohol consumption and paternal proxy report of the mother's moderate alcohol consumption were associated with isolated simple VSD. A twofold increase in risk of isolated simple VSD was identified for maternal self- and paternal proxy-reported cannabis use. Risk of isolated simple VSD increased with regular (≥3 days per week) cannabis use for both maternal self- and paternal proxy report, although the association was significant only for maternal self-report.

Visuospatial memory effect

Twenty-five college students who were heavy cannabis smokers (who had smoked a median of 29 of the last 30 days) were compared with 30 light smokers (1 day in the last 30 days). The subjects were tested after a supervised period of abstinence from cannabis and other drugs lasting at least 19 hours. Differences between the overall groups of heavy and light smokers did not reach statistical significance on the four subtests of attention administered. On examining data for the two sexes separately, marked and significant differences were found between heavy- and light-smoking women on the subtest examining visuospatial memory. On this test, subjects were required to examine a 6 × 6 "checkerboard" of squares in which certain squares were shaded. The shaded squares were then erased and the subject was required to indicate with the mouse which squares had formerly been shaded. Increasing numbers of shaded squares were presented at each trial. The heavy-smoking women remembered significantly fewer squares on this test, and they made significantly more errors than the light-smoking women. These differences persisted despite different methods of analysis and consideration for possible confounding variables.

Wilson's disease

A patient with generalized dystonia owing to Wilson's disease obtained mrked improvement in response to smoking cannabis.

Winiwarter-muerger disease

Two young men aged 18 and 20 years with juvenile endarteritis were evaluated. Both developed acute distal ischemia of the lower or upper limbs with arteriographic evidence suggestive of Winiwarter-Buerger disease. Both smoked regularly but not excessively, and both used cannabis regularly. In one case, the therapeutic response to with-drawal of cannabis was good. In the second, use of cannabis continued and arterial disease persisted. The main clinical and radiographical features in this condition are the same as in Winiwarter-Buerger disease.

INDEX

1

INTRODUCTION

Ancient civilisations, like modern society, had a keen interest in the health of man and other animals. Continuation of this interest over a period of time led to the discovery of a large number of therapeutic agents primarily from natural sources. In more recent times (about 50 years), with the involvement of a large number of pharmaceutical companies and many academic institutions, progress in the understanding of disease processes and mechanisms to control or eliminate the disease has accelerated. However, despite the advances and achievements of the last 50 years, the need to discover treatments for existing and evolving diseases has not decreased. This is primarily because of the inadequacies of current medicines. In many cases the treatment only leads to symptom relief and in various other cases the cure is associated with undesirable side-effects. In some cases (for example infectious diseases like tuberculosis, malaria and HIV), resistance/tolerance may develop to the existing treatments, thus making them ineffective against the infecting bacteria, parasite or virus. In addition, with the changing lifestyle and increasing life span, more and more pathological abnormalities that require entirely new treatments are being identified. For example, obesity and a number of cardiovascular diseases may have their origins in altered (more prosperous?) lifestyle habits, including environmental and psychosocial factors and diet. Changing social attitudes are also creating markets for the so called "lifestyle" drugs. Increasing knowledge about the underlying causes of diseases is enabling the discovery of more selective and less toxic drugs.

Progress in molecular biology (for example sequencing of human genome, proteomics, pharmacogenomics and protein engineering) is creating new avenues for the understanding of the precise disease mechanisms (biochemical pathways) and the discovery of new targets. Advances in this field are expected to lead to highly selective and efficacious medicines. Recombinant technologies are enabling the synthesis of larger biologically active proteins in sufficient quantities. Proteins and monoclonal antibodies are therefore becoming more important and common as therapeutic agents. Equally important is the progress being made in the fields of combinatorial chemistry, enabling the synthesis of millions of compounds, high-throughput screening technologies and other automation techniques facilitating more rapid drug discovery. In the longer run, a combination of all the new developments is likely to generate safer and more effective medicines, not only for the existing diseases but also for the diseases of the future which may become more important as a consequence of changes in lifestyle, and increasing age.

Malaria (caused in humans by single-celled *Plasmodium* protozoa parasites) can be considered an example of an "older" disease still in need of effective and cheaper treatments. Each year, 300–500 million people contract malaria and about 2–3 million die. A number of medicines, including chloroquine,

4-aminoquinolines, atovaquone, malarone, halofantrine, mefloquine, proguanil and artemisinin derivatives, are available. Three main types of vaccines, based on the three major phases of the parasite life cycle, are being developed: antisporozoite vaccines designed to prevent infection, anti-asexual blood-stage vaccines designed to reduce severe and complicated manifestations of the disease, and transmission blocking vaccines aimed at arresting the development of the parasite in the mosquito itself. Monoclonal antibodies against specific malarial antigens are being explored for diagnostic and potential therapeutic purposes. In addition, efforts are beginning to be made to shed light on the origin of the development of resistance in specific cases. Finally, with the availability of the malaria parasite genome map, researchers will be able to identify and validate good drug targets much more rapidly, leading to effective new therapies and vaccines.

Bone disorders like arthritis and osteoporosis are examples of diseases that are becoming increasingly important with the ageing population. Anti-inflammatory glucocorticoids like prednisolone and methylprednisolone, and immunosuppressants such as cyclosporin A and dexamethasone are used for the treatment. Although the treatment options have increased recently, most of these therapies, focus on addressing the symptoms rather than the underlying causes, of the disease. For example, cyclooxygenase (COX) 2 inhibitors like celecoxib and rofecoxib are being marketed as safer non-steroidal anti-inflammatory drugs (NSAIDs). Although the older NSAIDs are highly effective as analgesic, antipyretic and anti-inflammatory agents, long term ingestion causes gastric lesions. The discovery that the COX enzyme exists in two isoforms, with COX-2 being the primary isoform at sites of inflammation, led to a suggestion that inhibition of this isoform accounts for the therapeutic benefit of NSAIDs whereas inhibition of COX-1 results in adverse effects. The newer COX-2 selective agents appear to have a superior gastrointestinal safety profile. In addition to COX-2 inhibitors, inhibitors of matrix metalloproteinases (MMPs) are emerging for the treatment of many diseases, including arthritis. Enzymes that degrade the extracellular MMPs, are normally controlled by a set of tissue inhibitors that, if disrupted, will allow the enzymes to work unchecked, degrading the matrix and promoting not only arthritis but also tumour growth and metastasis. Another treatment option is inhibition of tumour necrosis factor (TNF)α, an inflammation promoting cytokine associated with multiple inflammatory events, including arthritis. Anti-TNFα therapies are already on the market. Finally, a variety of genes that code for antiarthritic proteins are under investigation, including interleukin (IL)-1Ra, IL-1sR, TNFsR, transforming growth factor β (TGFβ), IL-13, IL-10, and vIL-10, as are the vectors that will carry them to arthritic tissues.

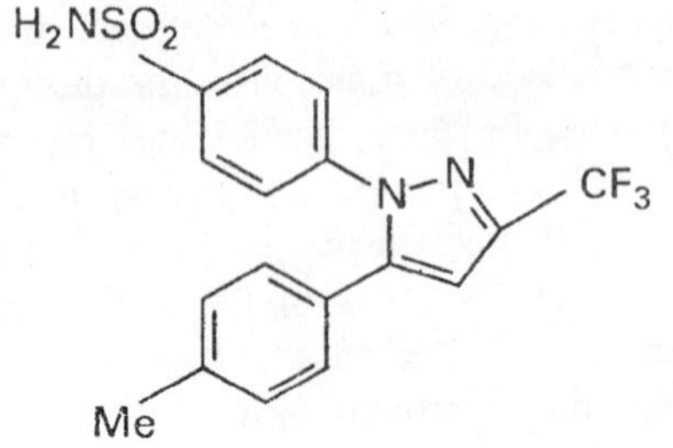

Celecoxib

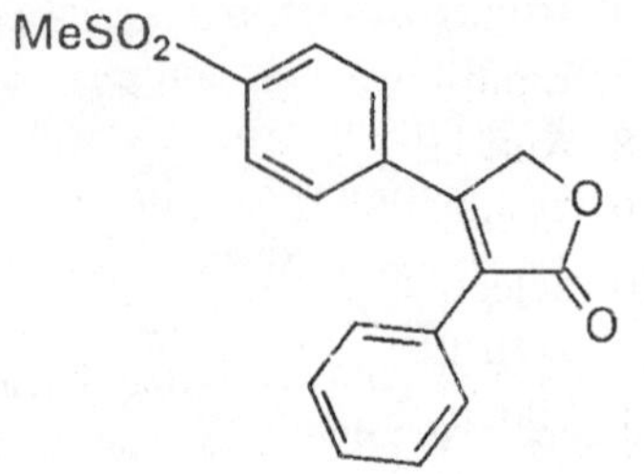

Rofecoxib

Recently, the process of drug discovery has been expanded to cover a range of molecular biology, biotechnology and medicinal chemistry (including combinatorial chemistry) techniques. The newer disciplines like genome analysis, proteomics, and bioinformatics are likely to lead to many new targets (receptors, enzymes, etc.) and therapeutically important proteins. Techniques like combinatorial chemistry and high-throughput screening are expected to identify hits/leads against various therapeutically important receptors and enzymes. Depending on the knowledge available on the receptor or the enzyme of interest, the hits/leads can then be modified in a random "*semi-rational*" or "*rational*" manner to generate the drug candidates. This chapter includes a short account of the historical aspects and a short introduction to some of the newer disciplines. The main theme/objective of the chapter is to give examples of receptor agonists and antagonists, enzyme inhibitors, including signal transduction inhibitors, and inhibitors of protein–protein interactions that have been discovered by random and semi-rational/rational approaches. This enables one to understand actual drug discovery procedures and the science that has led to many drugs currently on the market. Examples include:

1. COX inhibitors
2. Angiotensin converting enzyme (ACE) inhibitors, for example, antihypertensives such as captopril and lisinopril
3. Histamine H_1 receptor antagonists, for example antiallergy compounds such as fexofenadine
4. Histamine H_2 receptor antagonists – inhibitors of gastric acid secretion, such as cimetidine and ranitidine
5. Proton pump inhibitors – inhibitors of gastric acid secretion, such as omeprazole and esomeprazole
6. Activators of nuclear peroxisome proliferator activated receptor-γ, for example pioglitazone and troglitazone, used to treat type 2 diabetes
7. Lipid-lowering agents such as atorvastatin and cerivastatin
8. Anti-influenza treatments like zanamivir
9. Acetylcholinesterase inhibitors like donepezil for the treatment of Alzheimer's disease
10. Selective and competitive inhibitors of the cysteinyl leukotrienes (LTC_4, LTD_4 and LTE_4) such as zafirlukast and montelukast for the treatment of asthma
11. Sildenafil, an inhibitor of phosphodiesterase type 5 used to treat erectile dysfunction
12. Orlistat, an antiobesity compound
13. Atypical antipsychotic agents such as quetiapine and olanzapine for the treatment of schizophrenia.

It may be useful to mention at this stage that many of the highly successful drugs launched in the last 25 years were discovered in the pregenomic era and the real contribution of all the new technologies mentioned above remains to be proven. In some cases the drug was initially investigated for different indications. For example, sildenafil was being investigated in the clinic as an antianginal drug when its beneficial effects in improving erectile function were observed.

Historical Aspects

Early Discoveries

A number of early medicines, including morphine (analgesic) and quinine (antimalarial), were isolated from plants. Over the years the search for therapeutic agents has widened to isolate products from living agents such as bacteria, fungi, sea animals and even human beings. The important discoveries from this research not only include antibiotics such as penicillin but also many hormones and transmitters. Ivermectin (a drug used to treat tropical filariasis), lovastatin (HMG CoA reductase inhibitor), insulin, and cyclosporin A and FK 506 (immunosuppressants) are other examples of drugs originating from natural sources. Many of the biologically active peptides such as oxytocin, vasopressin, adrenocorticotropic hormone (ACTH), insulin, calcitonin, luteinising hormone releasing hormone (LHRH), growth hormone and erythropoietin are important examples of compounds isolated from humans and other animals that have led to medicines currently used in clinical practice. In addition, discoveries of many other agents like adrenaline, histamine and tryptamine and their receptors have led to extremely important medicines.

Many other early discoveries were primarily based on low-throughput random screening approaches. The mechanism of action was later rationalised when additional biochemical and pharmacological information became available. Examples of early drugs include sulfa drugs which led to the discoveries of several other classes of drugs. For example, the active metabolite of the sulfonamide prontosil inhibits the enzyme carbonic anhydrase, leading to an increase in natriuresis and the excretion of water. Sulfanilamide gave rise to better carbonic anhydrase inhibitors such as acetazolamide and later led to more effective diuretics such as hydrochlorothiazide and furosemide. Further chemistry in the field led to development of the sulfonylureas such as tolbutamide, used in the treatment of type 2 diabetes.

Impact of New Technology on Drug Discovery

Receptor Subtypes

Since the idea of a receptor as a selective binding site for chemotherapeutic agents was developed, huge progress has been made in the identification, characterisation and classification of receptors and receptor subtypes. In addition, knowledge has been gained about the downstream signalling pathways, most often involving transcription factors, that ultimately act on DNA and result in altered gene expression. Mapping the key signalling molecules in biochemical pathways and attempting to modulate their effects is resulting in new areas of drug discovery. The early assumption that a ligand acts at one receptor is no longer tenable and it is now well established that many endogenous ligands act at different receptor subtypes. The availability of more selective synthetic ligands, and cloning and amino acid sequencing technologies, has shown that different receptor subtypes exist for most of the receptors. The situation is further complicated by the existence of different receptor subtypes in different tissues in the same species, and by structural differences in receptor subtypes in different species of animals. Thus, the accumulated knowledge has not only provided many challenges for the drug discovery process but has also opened a way to many new drug discovery targets and much more selective treatments. From the point of view of drug discovery, ligands acting at the G-protein coupled receptors have resulted in the most successful drug candidates. Some of the examples illustrating how receptor research has led to more selective drugs and enhanced our understanding of the roles played by various receptor subtypes in disease processes are mentioned below. Early examples of different receptor subtypes that led to clinically useful drugs include α and β adrenoceptors and histamine H_1 and H_2 receptor subtypes. One of the more complicated and extensively studied area of receptor subtypes is the field of 5-hydroxytryptamine (5-HT; serotonin) receptors. The seven receptor subtypes, 5-HT_1 to 5-HT_7, have been characterised using selective ligands (agonists and antagonists); cloning and amino acid sequencing techniques have been used to define the molecular structures and intracellular transduction mechanisms. Several of the more selective compounds have reached the market for the treatment of various disorders of the nervous system (for example, antiemetics). Tryptamine 5-$HT_{1B/1D}$ receptor agonists like zolmitriptan, naratriptan and rizatriptan are marketed for the treatment of migraine.

Other more recent examples of new receptor subtypes include neurokinin, melanocortin and somatostatin receptor subtypes. Neurokinins (substance P, neurokinin A and neurokinin B) act at three receptor subtypes: NK_1, NK_2 and NK_3. Selective ligands are being explored for the treatment of pain, asthma, depression, etc. The natural melanocortic peptides are derived from the precursor peptide pro-opiomelanocortin (expressed in the pituitary) by proteolytic cleavage in three regions of the protein, generating ACTH, and α-, β- and γ-melanocyte stimulating hormone (MSH) peptides. Pro-opiomelanocortin also generates a number of other peptides including enkephalin and β-endorphin. Five melanocortin receptor subtypes (MC_1–MC_5) belonging to the G-protein coupled receptor family have been cloned (40–60% sequence identities), and selective ligands for the receptor subtypes have been synthesised. Early pharmacological studies have indicated that drugs selective for the MC_1 receptor may be useful for the treatment of inflammatory conditions, whereas compounds selective for the MC_4 receptor may be useful for controlling eating behaviour and body weight. These biological effects are very different to the involvement of MSH and ACTH in skin pigmentation and secretion of corticosteroids, respectively. Cloning studies have also identified five receptor subtypes of somatostatin (Ala-Gly-Cys-Lys-Asn-Phe-Phe-Trp-Lys-Thr-Phe-Thr-Ser-Cys, a cyclic peptide with a disulphide bridge), (hSSTR$_1$ selective) 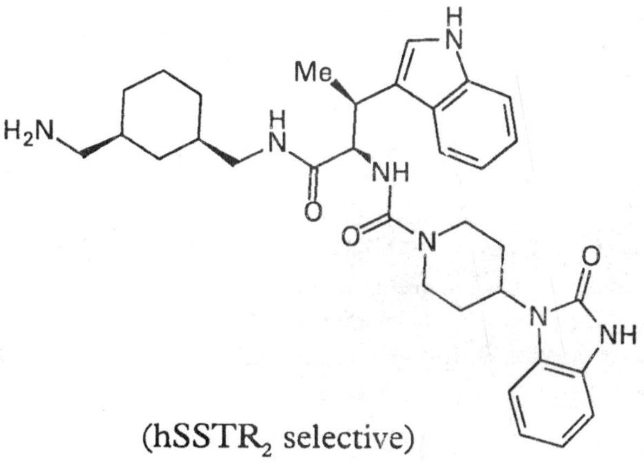 (hSSTR$_2$ selective)

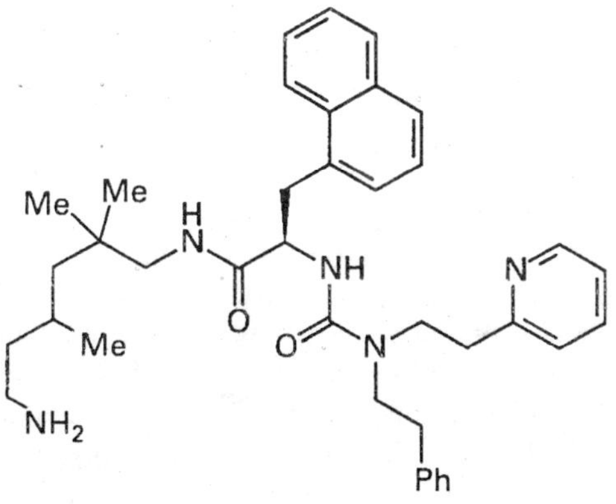

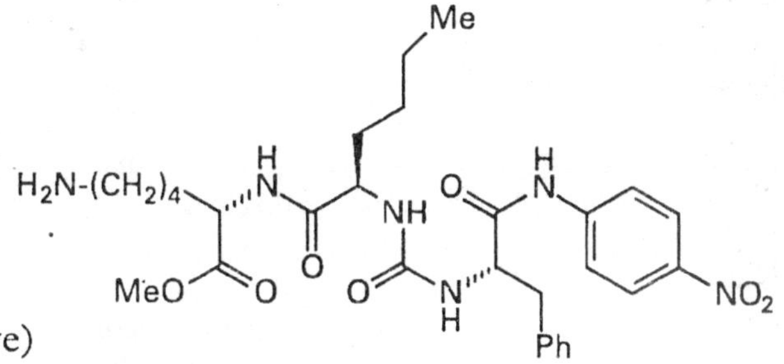

(hSSTR$_3$ selective)

a peptide discovered in 1971–72 and shown to be an inhibitor of growth hormone, insulin, glucagon and gastric acid secretion. Screening of heterocyclic β-turn mimetic libraries (based upon the Trp-Lys motif found in the turn region of somatostatin) against a panel of the five cloned human somatostatin receptors (hSSTR$_1$–hSSTR$_5$) led to the development of somatostatin receptor ligands that bind to the five receptor subtypes. Compound is relatively more selective for the hSSTR$_2$ receptor subtype and shows higher affinity against hSSTR$_3$ and hSSTR$_5$ subtypes. The turn mimetic is more potent at the hSSTR$_5$ receptor subtype. In another series of compounds, library screening followed by studies of structure–activity relationships (SAR) lead to the development of compounds selective for the hSST receptor subtypes. *In vitro* experiments using these selective compounds demonstrated the role of the hSST$_2$ receptor in inhibition of glucagon release from mouse pancreatic α cells and the hSST$_5$ receptor as a mediator of insulin secretion from pancreatic β cells. Both subtypes of receptor regulate release of growth hormone from the rat anterior pituitary gland. Some of the recent information has shown that the five receptor subtypes may fall into two classes or groups. One class (SRIF$_1$) appears to comprise SST$_2$, SST$_3$ and SST$_5$ and the other class (SRIF$_2$) consists of the other two recombinant receptor subtypes (SST$_1$ and SST$_4$).

More recently, attention has also been focused on orphan G-protein coupled receptors, a family of plasma membrane proteins involved in a broad array of signalling pathways. Novel orphan G-protein coupled receptors have continued to emerge through cloning activities as well as through bioinformatic analysis of sequence databases. Their ligands are unidentified and their physiological relevance remains to be defined. Methods are being developed to identify ligands acting at these receptors. One of these approaches identifies ligands by purification from biological fluids, cell supernatants or tissue extracts. The discoveries of endothelin (a vasoconstrictor peptide) and nociceptin (an orphan opioid-like receptor ligand) are examples of this type. Ligands can also be identified by screening the orphan receptor against a number of diverse chemical libraries. Once identified, the ligand is used to characterise physiological and pathological roles of the receptor, followed by the discovery of other agonist and antagonist analogues by medicinal chemistry approaches.

Currently the drug discovery process has progressed beyond the receptor stage and various steps that result from the interaction of the receptor with a specific ligand have been characterised. One of the more important processes, signal transduction, converts the external signals induced by hormones, growth factors, neurotransmitters and cytokines into specific internal cellular responses (for example, gene expression, cell division, or even cell suicide). The process involves a cascade of enzyme-mediated reactions inside the cell that typically includes phosphorylation and dephosphorylation of proteins (kinases and phosphatases) as mediators of downstream processes. Signal transduction inhibitors are currently being developed for the treatment of a number of diseases, including cancer and inflammation.

Genomics

Genetic factors influence virtually every human disorder (for example, Alzheimer's and Parkinson's diseases, diabetes, asthma and rheumatoid arthritis) by determining disease susceptibility or resistance and interactions with environmental factors. Gene transfer research ("*gene therapy*") holds promise for treating disorders through the transfer and expression of DNA in the cells of patients. Although some clinical trials have started, several important issues, including efficient delivery of the genetic material to the required sites, along with other chemical, biological, safety, toxicity and ethical issues, have not yet been fully resolved. From the point of view of drug discovery, mapping of the human genome is only the first step. It is likely that even when the human genomic sequencing has been fully completed and all genes have been identified, a substantial fraction of these, possibly up to 50%, will have complex biochemical or physiological functions. Therefore, only a proportion (about 20% of the genome) will be amenable to pharmacological exploitation. Another major problem is the involvement of many genes and environmental factors in various diseases. For example, with the exception of some diseases or traits resulting principally from specific and relatively rare mutations (for example, cystic fibrosis), most of the genetic disorders (for example, cardiovascular diseases, diabetes, rheumatoid arthritis and schizophrenia) develop as a result of a network of genes failing to perform correctly, some of which might have a major disease effect but many of which have a relatively minor effect. Complex diseases and traits result principally from genetic variation that is relatively common in the general population. Thus, completion of the human genome will not provide an immediate solution to the genetics of complex diseases. This can only be achieved by documenting the genetic variation of human genomes at the population level within and across ethnic groups and by characterising mutant genes. For further progress it is therefore essential to identify the function of each gene in the normal and disease situations and establish a link with the expressed protein (before and after post-translational modification) and its role in a disease pathway.

Since the complete genome of *Haemophilus influenzae* was published, sequencing of genomes from a wide range of organisms, from bacteria to man, has continued apace. Initial sequencing and analysis of the human genome has been published. Another more recent example is the genome sequence of *Escherichia coli* O157:H7, implicated in many outbreaks of haemorrhagic colitis. The functional characterisation of microbial genomics will have a significant impact on genomic medicine (new antimicrobial targets and vaccine candidates) and on environmental (waste management, recycling), food, and industrial biotechnology. In addition to the work on human and microbial genomes, progress is also being made on the sequencing of the mouse and rat genomes. Data from rodent species should speed the discovery of genes and regulatory regions in the human genome and make it easier to determine their functions. In addition, these sequences may have a significant impact on the disease models because these animal are most often used in the early discovery and preclinical testing of new drugs.

There are three main approaches to mapping the genetic variants involved in a disease: functional cloning, the candidate gene strategy and positional cloning. In functional cloning, identification of the underlying protein defect leads to localisation of the responsible gene (disease–function–gene–map). An example of functional cloning is the finding that individuals with sickle cell anaemia carry an amino acid substitution in the β chain of haemoglobin. Isolation of the mutant molecule led to the cloning of the gene encoding β globin.

In the candidate-gene approach, the most frequently used approach adopted to identify the predisposing or causal genes in the complex and multigenic and multifactorial diseases, genes with a known or proposed function with the potential to influence the disease phenotype are investigated for a direct role in a disease. In a small number of cases of type 2 diabetes, candidate-gene studies have identified mutations in, for example, the genes encoding insulin and the insulin receptor.

Marker genes not related to disease physiology and genome-wide screens are the starting points for mapping the genetic components of the disease. The aim is first to identify the genetic region within which a disease-predisposing gene lies and, once this is found, to localise the gene and determine its functional and biological role in the disease (disease–map–gene–function).

The introduction of functional genes for the restoration of normal function or the transfer of therapeutic genes to treat particular diseases such as cancer or viral infections is of growing interest. The hurdles to overcome in efficient gene therapy include successful transfer of the therapeutic genes, appropriate expression levels associated with sufficient duration of gene expression, and the specificity of gene transfer to achieve therapeutic effects in the patient. Viral vectors are still among the most efficient gene transfer vehicles. Because of the comparatively long history of characterisation of particular viruses and their genomes, their valuable characteristics for target cell infectivity, transgene capacity, and accessibility of established helper cell lines for the production of recombinant virus stocks to infect target cells, the most commonly used vectors are developed from retroviruses, lentiviruses, adenovirus, herpes simplex virus and adeno-associated virus. The advantages of retroviral vectors (stable integration into the host genome, generation of viral titres sufficient for efficient gene transfer, infectivity of the recombinant viral particles for a broad variety of target cell types, and the ability to carry foreign genes of reasonable size) are accompanied by several disadvantages, for example, instability of some retroviral vectors, possible insertional mutagenesis by random viral integration into host DNA, the requirement of cell division for integration of Moloney murine leukaemia virus-derived retroviral vectors, and targeting of retroviral infection and/or therapeutic gene expression. In addition to the viral transfection procedures, non-viral transfection procedures are also being developed. In a recent example, human monocyte-derived dendritic cells were transfected with genes encoding tumour-associated antigens. The transfection was achieved by dimerisation of a 35 amino acid cationic peptide (Lys-Lys-Lys-Lys-Lys-Lys-Gly-Gly-Phe-Leu-Gly-Phe-Trp-Arg-Gly-Glu-Asn-Gly-Arg-Lys-Thr-Arg-Ser-Ala-Tyr-Glu-Arg-Met-Cys-Asn-Ile-Leu-Lys-Gly-Lys) and then using a complex of this dimeric peptide with plasmid DNA expression constructs. Injection of transfected dendritic cells expressing a tumour-associated antigen protected mice from lethal challenge with tumour cells in a model of melanoma.

Identification of the genes that provide structural and regulatory functions in an organism are likely to be useful in obtaining genetically modified (transgenic) animals using gene knockout or knockin strategies. The transgenic animals are useful in the identification and validation of molecular drug targets, generation of animal models of disease for the testing of novel therapeutic strategies, and early recognition of toxicological effects.

Pharmacogenomics

Because different patients with the same disease symptoms may respond differently to the same drug, both in terms of therapeutic benefits and side-effects, understanding of the relationships between gene variation and the effect of such variation on drug responses within individuals is likely to lead to tailor made therapies for specific populations of patients. For example, a variety of antihypertensive drugs and drugs for congestive heart failure are now available, including calcium antagonists, ACE inhibitors, β-blockers, diuretics, α-blockers, centrally acting antihypertensives, and, more recently, angiotensin $(AT)_1$ receptor antagonists. Although all of these agents are effective in lowering blood pressure in most cases, there are significant differences between their therapeutic and side-effect profiles. A better knowledge of the mechanisms that influence the efficacy of the drugs in different individuals and understanding why some patients can tolerate the drug better than others may lead to more efficacious drugs with a better side-effect profile. The variation of the individual's response to such drugs may be caused by the heterogeneity of the mechanisms underlying hypertension, interindividual variation in the pharmacokinetics of the drug, or a combination of both.

The likely benefit of more efficacious tailormade drugs with fewer side-effects has led to the development of the science of pharmacogenomics, a name given to any drug-discovery platform that attempts to address the issues of efficacy and toxicity in individuals. The concept of individual variation at the molecular level is not new. Protein obtained from different individuals has been known to have different amino acid sequences. These protein isoforms originate either by genomic variation at the level of the actual gene sequence, or by variation in expression which results from changes in the promoter and control elements that regulate expression. Alleles differ from each other by structural features, such as single base-pair changes, or as the result of rearrangements or deletions of entire gene portions. Depending on the structure of regulatory sequences, some alleles may be expressed at very high levels, while others may be repressed. Similarly, depending on variation at the critical points in the assembly of genes, splicing variants may result from alternative arrangements of building blocks. Technologies that enable the monitoring of gene expression under different circumstances (based on high-throughput sequencing and screening approaches) are currently being developed and will enable systematic investigation of the patterns of gene expression between normal and disease states in a statistically meaningful way, along with the expression of the relevant proteins in different individuals. In addition, the potential of using single-nucleotide polymorphisms to correlate drug regimens and responses is also being investigated. The availability of precisely located single-nucleotide polymorphic sites spanning the genome holds promise for the association of particular genetic loci with disease states. This information, together with high-throughput gene-chip technologies, will offer new opportunities for molecular diagnostics and monitoring of disease predisposition in large sections of the population. It will also allow much earlier preventive treatment in many slowly evolving diseases.

Proteomics

The control mechanisms in health and disease are found at the protein level and, as mentioned above, genome sequencing does not provide sufficient information at the protein level. The tertiary structure and the type and extent of post-translational modifications (for example, glycosylation and phosphorylation) of a protein are critical to its function and cellular localisation but this information is not encoded in the protein's corresponding DNA. An additional complication between genes and proteins is the existence of alternative splice variants of messenger RNA which give rise to isomeric proteins that might contribute to regulatory processes in the cell. The processing of proteins may also be different in various tissues under different conditions. Some proteins may give rise to biologically active fragments and some may exert diverse functions in collaboration with other proteins. Therefore, the complete structure and function of an individual protein can not be determined by reference to its gene sequence alone. Thus, beyond genomics it is essential to compare the protein content of cells/tissues/organs in the normal and disease states and to generate the functional information on proteins required for various drug discovery processes. Proteomics is any protein-based approach that provides new information about proteins on a genome-wide scale, and addresses these difficulties by enabling the protein levels of cellular organisation to be screened and characterised. In a high-throughput manner, a large number of proteins from normal and disease samples (cells and tissue extracts) are separated on the basis of their charge and molecular weight by two-dimensional electrophoresis, and the amino acid sequences of proteins and their post-translational modifications are identified by mass spectrometry. The separated proteins are then stained and the maps of protein expression are digitally scanned into databases. These protein expression maps can be used to study cellular pathways and the perturbation of these pathways by disease and by drug action. Thus, an understanding of cellular pathways and protein changes resulting from the disease and from drug actions can not only lead to new drug targets but can also provide early markers for diseases and early indications of drug toxicity. It should be emphasised, however, that characterisation of a different protein in a disease state does not necessarily means that it plays a causal role or represents a potential therapeutic target. In many cases, the new protein may be a consequence of the disease rather than the cause. Further studies are required to check whether the activity of a candidate target eliminated by molecular/cellular techniques could reverse the disease phenotype. Moreover, even when a potential therapeutic target has been identified and a molecule capable of disrupting it has been obtained, we cannot assume that it will constitute an effective treatment for the disease under investigation. Alternative metabolic routes may provide cells with ways of circumventing blocked pathways.

The potential benefit of proteomics in predicting toxicity at an early stage may lead to accelerated drug discovery programmes. A comparison of the protein profiles of normal tissue with those of tissue treated with the known toxic agent might give an indication of the drug's toxic activity. Similarly, identification of a known toxic protein in drug-treated tissues may give an idea about the toxicity of the drug. As a first approach, an examination of liver and kidney, which are the major sites for metabolism and excretion of most drugs, before and after the drug administration may provide early indications about events that might result in toxicity. Proteomic analysis of the serum, where the majority of toxicity markers released from susceptible organs and tissues throughout the entire body collect, can be utilised to identify serum markers (and clusters thereof) as indicators of toxicity. The serum markers could subsequently be used to predict the response of each individual and allow tailoring of therapy whereby optimal efficacy is achieved whilst minimising adverse effects. Surrogate markers for drug efficacy could also be detected by this procedure and could be used to identify classes of patients who will respond favourably to a drug.

There is currently some debate about the ability of the techniques being used to detect all the proteins present in a given sample. It is possible that global proteome displays based on two-dimensional gel electrophoresis are largely limited to the more abundantly expressed and stable proteins. Thus, important classes of regulatory proteins involved in signal transduction and gene expression, for example, and other proteins of lower abundance remain undetected by current methodologies. Proteins of lower abundance are more likely to be detected by separating these from highly abundant proteins. The disadvantage of this strategy, however, is that it requires much larger amounts of protein, and many additional separations, and therefore may be impractical for studies of small cell populations or tissue samples. Efforts are underway to develop advanced proteomic technologies that do not rely on two-dimensional gel electrophoresis.

After the discovery of protein maps and characterisation of individual proteins, the most important aspect of proteomics is to define protein function. Although new proteins are likely to include receptors, ligands, enzymes, enzyme inhibitors, signalling molecules and pathways that may be therapeutic targets, precise functions of the individual proteins have to be identified. To discover and monitor the relevance of a protein to a disease-related process, it is important to find where, when and to what extent a protein is expressed. Many approaches are being used to discover protein function. Structural homology methods may be used to ascribe function to some proteins, since it is known that proteins of similar function often share structural homology (tertiary structure). Another approach to defining protein function is chemical proteomics, the identification of small molecules that interact with the proteins by screening new proteins against diverse chemical libraries using methods such as nuclear magnetic resonance (NMR) spectroscopy, microcalorimetry and microarrays. Another method for identifying ligand binding sites involves scanning the surface of a protein molecule for clefts. In many cases the largest cleft is the known primary binding site for small ligands. Further information about the ligand structures that can be accommodated in the binding site can be obtained by various computational programs like DOCK or HOOK.

Some of the proteins likely to have known enzyme activity or enzyme inhibition properties can be identified using screens for generic enzyme activities. Along with the structural and chemical library methods, several "*non-homology*" methods are being developed to identify protein functions. These are computational methods, and take advantage of the many properties shared among functionally related proteins, such as patterns of domain fusion, evolutionary co-inheritance, conservation of relative gene position, and correlated expression patterns. Protein function is defined by these methods in terms of context, that is, which cellular pathways or complexes the protein participates in, rather than by suggesting a specific biochemical activity. Large-scale functional analysis of new proteins can be accomplished by using peptide or protein arrays, ranging from synthetic peptide arrays to whole proteins expressed in living cells. Comprehensive sets of purified peptides and proteins permit high-throughput screening for discrete biochemical properties, whereas formats involving living cells facilitate large-scale genetic screening for novel biological activities. Protein arrays can be engineered to suit the aims of a particular experiment. Thus, an array might contain all the combinatorial variants of a bioactive peptide or specific variants of a single protein species (splice variants, domains or mutants), a family of protein orthologs from different species, a protein pathway, or even the entire protein complement of an organism.

Access to structural information on a proteome-wide scale is not only important for ascribing protein function but may also be useful in target validation and medicinal chemistry on hits/leads that require structural information for rational design processes. The most straightforward strategy for predicting structure is to search for sequence similarity to a protein with known three-dimensional structure. Additional information can be obtained by identifying known and novel folds in a protein. There are databases of structural motifs in proteins which contain data relevant to helices, β-turns, γ-turns, β-hairpins, ψ-loops, β-α-β motifs, β-sheets, β-strands and disulphide bridges extracted from proteins, which can be used for comparison. Novel folds can be identified by employing *ab initio* approaches used for prediction of protein structure. With the aim of extracting further information from protein sequences, sequence motif libraries have been developed. Advances in *x* ray crystallography, particularly the use of synchrotron radiation sources, and NMR spectroscopy also allow rapid determination of protein structures. Using protein crystals in which methionine residues are replaced by selenomethionine, and multiwavelength synchrotron experiments, electron-density maps for proteins can be generated in less than an hour instead of the weeks of experimental time required for a conventional structure determination by crystallography. Despite great improvements in *x* ray crystallography techniques, the rate-limiting step in structure determination remains the expression, purification and crystallisation of the target protein.

Many problems still remain to be solved before protein function can be confidently assigned by using the above techniques. For example, the idea of "one gene one protein one function" is not valid in many cases and increasing numbers of proteins are found to have two or more different functions.

The multiple functions of such moonlighting proteins can vary as a consequence of changes in cellular localisation, cell type, oligomeric state, or the cellular concentration of a ligand, substrate, cofactor or product. Multidrug transporter P-glycoprotein (a large 170 kD cell-surface molecule encoded by the human *MDR1* gene) is an example of a protein with multiple functions. It is well established that P-glycoprotein can efflux xenobiotics from cells and is one mechanism that tumour cells use to escape death induced by chemotherapeutic drugs. Recent observations have raised the possibility that P-glycoprotein and related transporter molecules may play a fundamental role in regulating cell differentiation, proliferation and survival. P-glycoprotein encoded by *MDR1* in humans and *Mdr1a* in mice can regulate an endogenous chloride channel. This activity of P-glycoprotein can be inhibited by phosphorylation by protein kinase C. MDR1 P-glycoprotein has also been proposed to play roles in phospholipid translocation and cholesterol esterification. Functional P-glycoprotein has also been suggested to play a role in regulating programmed cell death (apoptosis).

Bioinformatics and Data Mining Technologies

The availability of genomic data and the corresponding protein sequences from humans and other organisms, together with structure– function annotations, disease correlation and population variations, requires sophisticated data management systems (databases) for analytical purposes. Proteomics-oriented databases include data on the two-dimensional gel electrophoresis maps of proteins from a variety of healthy and disease tissues. Bioinformatic systems (computer-assisted data management and analysis) are used to gather and analyse this information in order to attach biological knowledge to genes, assign genes to biological pathways, compare the gene sets of different species, understand processes in healthy and disease states, and find new or better drugs. The currently available techniques have the capability to translate a given gene sequence into a protein structure, complete with predictions of secondary structure, and database comparisons. Progress is being made in devising systems that provide information on biological function derived from sequencing and functional analysis. In addition to the gene–function analysis studies, the need for data mining techniques (defined as "the non-trivial extraction of implicit, previously unknown, and potentially useful information from data") is becoming necessary in order to deal with the enormous amounts of information that the industry collects in individual databases (ranging, from, for example, databases of disease profiles and molecular pathways to sequences, chemical and biological screening data, including SAR, chemical structures of combinatorial libraries of compounds, individual and population clinical trial results and so on).

A large number of companies are developing data mining applications (software) which can identify cause–effect relationships between data sets and group together data points or sets based on different criteria. A time-delay data mining approach is used when a complete data set is not available immediately and in complete form, but is collected over time. The systems designed to handle such data look for patterns, which are confirmed or rejected as the data set increases and becomes more robust. This approach is geared towards analysis of long-term clinical trials and studies of multicomponent modes of action. It is also possible to overlay large and complex data sets that are similar to each other and compare them. This is particularly useful in all forms of clinical trial meta-analyses, where data collected at different sites over different time periods, and perhaps under similar but not always identical conditions, need to be compared. Here, the emphasis is on finding dissimilarities, not similarities. Predictive data mining programmes are available for making simulations, predictions and forecasts based on the data sets analysed.

Combinatorial Chemistry and High-throughput Screening

One of the earliest approaches to drug discovery was the random screening process. More recently, significant efforts were directed towards rational/semi-rational approaches. However, recent advances in high-throughput screening and synthesis techniques, coupled with large-scale data analysis and data management methods, have shifted the balance towards testing libraries of "diverse" chemical compounds in multiple screens (>20 000 compounds in a week) in the shortest possible time. This approach is expected to provide leads much more quickly for optimisation using combinatorial synthesis methods (targeted libraries) to generate drug candidates. Starting from the solid-phase peptide synthesis in the early sixties, which opened the way to chemical synthesis on solid supports, automated synthesis of diverse organic compounds has now become routine in many laboratories. Assays have been developed that make use of fluorescently labelled reagents (for example, receptors, ligands and enzyme substrates), allowing the rapid optical screening of large collections of compounds. Assays using microtitre plates (96–384 wells in each plate) have been designed to enable small quantities of compounds to be tested at a much reduced cost in terms of reagent use.

Combinatorial synthesis

Combinatorial chemistry is having a major impact in generating libraries containing large numbers of compounds in a relatively short period of time using solid phase-synthesis technologies. In addition, it is possible to buy readymade libraries built around specific molecular themes and consisting of many thousands of compounds, and to test these libraries in high-throughput screening systems using automated off-the-shelf instrumentation and reagents. The technique of combinatorial biocatalysis is also used to obtain diverse libraries. This approach takes advantage of natural catalysts (enzymes and whole cells), as well as the rapidly growing supply of recombinant and engineered enzymes, for the direct derivatisation of many different synthetic compounds and natural products. The types of reactions catalysed by enzymes and micro-organisms include reactions that can introduce functional groups (for example, carbon–carbon bond formation, hydroxylation, halogenation, cyclo additions, addition of amines), modify the existing functionalities (oxidation of alcohols to aldehydes and ketones, reduction of aldehydes or ketones to alcohols, oxidation of sulphides to sulphoxides, oxidation of amino groups to nitro groups, hydrolysis of nitriles to amides and carboxylic acids, replacements of amino groups by hydroxyl groups, lactonisation, isomerisation, epimerisation, dealkylation and methyl transfer) or addition onto functional groups (esterification, carbonate formation, carbamate formation, glycosylation, amidation and phosphorylation). Currently available technologies allow these biocatalysis reactions to be carried out in aqueous and non-aqueous solvents.

Techniques are available to screen individual compounds or mixtures in solution or still attached to the solid support. The main advantage of screening single compounds in solution (the technique most commonly used in the past) is that activity can be directly correlated with chemical structure. Screening mixtures of compounds has the advantage that fewer assays need to be performed and at the same time fewer synthetic steps are required to generate mixtures. However, it is not possible to synthesise mixtures that contain entirely different structures. Screening of mixtures can lead to false positives resulting from additive or cooperative effects of weakly active compounds. Thus, the most active mixture may not contain the most potent compound. An additional disadvantage of testing mixtures is that once an active mixture has been identified, the exact structure of the active compound, in most cases, can only be obtained by extensive deconvolution studies. There are some procedures like positional scanning approach which enable the active compound to be identified directly from screening. This method depends on the synthesis of a series of subset mixtures that contain a single building block (substituent) at one position and all the building blocks at the other positions. The structure of the most active compound is then assigned by selecting the building block from the most active subset at each position. The structure is confirmed by synthesis.

The most widely used solid phase method for the synthesis of libraries (originally used for peptides) has been termed the "*split-mix*", "divide, couple and recombine" and "one bead one compound" method. The resin beads display a linker to which building blocks are sequentially attached, to effectively grow molecules. As a first step, different batches of resin are reacted individually with a unique set of reagents (first set of building blocks); the resins are then combined and deprotected to liberate another reactive group. The resin is then divided into several components and each component is reacted individually by the second building block. This "divide, couple, recombine" strategy is continued until all the building blocks have been added. The resin batches are not combined after the final building blocks have been added. This strategy results in a resin library in which a single compound is attached to an individual bead. When a synthesis is complete, cleavage at the linker releases the molecule(s) from the bead(s). The screening of single beads, or the compounds derived from single beads, corresponds to screening of single compounds. Screening of these libraries can quickly identify the preferred last building block in the most active set. The subset library is then resynthesised by keeping this preferred final building block constant and screened to identify the penultimate preferred building block in each set. This deconvolution process, or iterative re-synthesis and screening, is repeated in order to define all the positions. The deconvolution process has to be repeated each time the library is tested in a new screen. Several different approaches have been investigated to avoid this inconvenient and time-consuming deconvolution method. One of these, using tagging/encoding strategies, involves the introduction of chemical tags at each stage of the "*split-mix*" synthesis either before the addition of each building block during the synthesis or before the subsequent mixing step. At the end of the synthesis any individual bead will possess a compound made up of a single combination of building blocks and an associated tag sequence with a specific tag corresponding to each specific building block. The identity of the compound on a single bead can be determined simply by analysing the tagging sequence. The original tagging methods, oligonucleotides (read by polymerase chain reaction (PCR) amplification and DNA sequencing) and peptides have now been replaced by using binary coding with chemical tags. This tagging strategy increases the number of steps in the synthesis of each library but allows more rapid identification of the active hits.

Library design

The design strategy may vary according to the information available on the target and the purpose of the library. For example, when the class of target is known (for example, an enzyme with a known mechanism of action and/or structural information or a known or similar receptor type/subtype), library design may be started from a known pharmacophore. For example, aspartyl proteinases like renin, HIV and cathepsin D proteases are inhibited by compounds containing a statine residue, a known transition-state analogue. Several libraries based on statine or a hydroxyethylamine core have been prepared and investigated against other aspartyl proteinases. The use of synthetic positional-scanning combinatorial libraries offers the ability to rapidly test and evaluate the extended substrate specificities of proteases. For example, a fluorogenic tetrapeptide positional-scanning library (containing a 7-amino-4-methylcoumarin-derivatised lysine) in which the P_1 amino acid was held constant as a lysine and the P_4-P_3-P_2 positions were positionally randomised was used to investigate extended substrate specificities of plasmin and thrombin, two of the enzymes involved in the blood coagulation cascade. The optimal P_4 to P_2 substrate specificity for plasmin was P_4-Lys/Nle/Val/Ile/Phe, P_3-Xaa, and P_2-Tyr/Phe/Trp. The optimal P_4 to P_2 extended substrate sequence determined for thrombin was P_4-Nle/Leu/Ile/Phe/Val, P_3-Xaa, and P_2-Pro. By three-dimensional structural modelling of the substrates into the active sites of plasmin and thrombin, it was possible to identify potential determinants of the defined substrate specificity. This method is amenable to the incorporation of diverse substituents at the P_1 position (all 20 proteinogenic and other non-proteinogenic amino acids) for exploring molecular recognition elements in various new uncharacterised proteolytic enzymes.

A similar approach can be adopted when a lead ligand has been identified by random screening. The structural template in the lead is modified to generate a targeted library. Many libraries have been synthesised around the so-called "*privileged structures*" which have shown activity against various targets. For example, compounds based on a benzodiazepine core have shown activity against a number of G-protein coupled receptors. However, when there is little information, or when entirely different structural leads are required, a larger diverse library is likely to be more suitable to increase the chance of success. The chemical diversity between the different members of the library is also very important to cover a wide chemical area and increase chances of success. In addition to some simple rules like incorporating acidic, basic, hydrophilic and hydrophobic groups of different sizes, a large number of computer-based methods are available for diversity analysis. Information is also available on the so-called "*drug-like molecules*" that tend to have certain properties. For example, log P, molecular weight, and the number of hydrogen bonding groups have been correlated with oral bioavailability. Analysis of a large number of compounds from the World Drug Index establishment resulted in the "rule of five" based on the assumption that compounds meeting these criteria have entered human clinical trials, and therefore must possess many of the desirable characteristics of drugs. A high percentage of compounds contained ≤ five hydrogen bond donors (expressed as the sum of OHs and NHs), ≤ 10 hydrogen bond acceptors, ≤ 500 relative molecular weight and log P of ≤ 5. Along with these measures, it is also desirable to exclude functional groups that tend to be undesirable because of chemical reactivity for example alkylating and acylating groups, and other unstable groups that lead to metabolism (solvolysis or hydrolysis).

The availability of complex large and diverse chemical libraries and ultra high-throughput screening technologies also provides an option whereby the biological pathways and proteins do not have to be fully characterised before starting the screening process. A number of preselected, incompletely characterised, disease-associated protein targets can be screened against many different libraries. Using the whole-cell systems and libraries containing membrane-permeable compounds, it is possible to identify compounds that perturb a cellular process or system, followed by identification of proteins required in cell function. From the perspective of drug discovery, this approach offers the means for the simultaneous identification of proteins that can serve as targets for therapeutic intervention ("*therapeutic target validation*") and small molecules that can modulate the functions of these therapeutic targets ("*chemical target validation*"). The overall process differs from the traditional methods of drug discovery in which biological methods are first used to select and characterise protein targets for therapeutic intervention, followed by chemical efforts to determine whether the protein target can be modulated by small molecules.

Structure-based Drug Design

The entire process of structure-based drug design requires identification and characterisation of a suitable protein target, determination of the structure of the target protein, the availability of an easy and reliable high-throughput screening assay, identification of a lead compound, development of computer-assisted methods for estimating the affinity of new compounds, and access to a synthetic route to produce the designed compounds. Progress has been made on many of these aspects. For example, expression systems are now available that allow the production of large amounts of naturally occurring proteins and modified proteins like isotope-labelled proteins required for NMR studies and proteins containing residues like selenomethionine (in place of methionine) that simplify determination of *x* ray structure. Advances in automation technologies have resulted in increased synthesis and screening capabilities. From the point of view of design, more important aspects of "*rational design*" strategy involve methods for using the information contained in the three-dimensional structure of a macromolecular target and of related ligand–target complexes, and predicting novel lead compounds. A variety of "docking" programmes now exist that can select from a large database of compounds a subset of molecules that usually includes some compounds that bind to the selected target protein. One such programme, DOCK, systematically attempts to fit each compound from a database into the binding site of the target structure, such that three or more of the atoms in the database molecule overlap with a set of predefined site points in the target binding site. The newer computational methods are aimed at using the information contained in the three-dimensional structure of the unligated target to design entirely new lead compounds *de novo*, as well as to construct large virtual combinatorial libraries of compounds that can be screened computationally (virtual screening) before going to the effort and expense of actually synthesising and testing them.

The *de novo* design of structure-based ligands involves fragment positioning methods, molecule growth methods, and fragment methods coupled to database searches. The fragment positioning methods determine energetically favourable binding site positions for various functional group types or chemical fragments. In the molecule growth methods, a seed atom (or fragment) is first placed in the binding site of the target structure. A ligand molecule is successively built by bonding another atom (or fragment) to it. Fragment positioning methods can also be coupled to database searching techniques either to extract from a database existing molecules that can be docked into the binding site with the desired fragments in their optimal positions or for *de novo* design.

Once a lead compound has been found by some means, an iterative process begins that involves solving the three-dimensional structure of the lead compound bound to the target, examining that structure, characterising the types of interactions the bound ligand makes, and using the computational methods to design improvements to the compound. A large number of examples that demonstrate the utility of this approach exist in the literature. Many inhibitors of enzymes, for example renin, HIV protease and thrombin, have been optimised using this approach.

Virtual screening

The virtual screening strategy involves construction or "synthesis" of molecules on the computer. The number of "synthesised" compounds is limited by synthesising focused libraries (for example, a hydroxamate library of MMP inhibitors) and concentrating on reactions that will work in high yield with reagents that are easily accessible, and incorporating "drug like" properties. Synthetic accessibility can be checked using programs such as computer-aided organic synthesis or computer-aided estimation of synthetic accessibility. As molecules are constructed, a variety of filters are applied to "weed out" compounds that do not meet certain criteria (for example, similarity and diversity analysis, presence of undesirable functional groups, molecular weight and lipophilicity). Once a virtual library has been created and the undesirable compounds removed, the next step is to generate three-dimensional conformations for each molecule. Since most molecules are quite flexible, a multiconformer docking approach is adopted. In this strategy, a set of conformations (typically 10–50) is generated and then each conformer is docked as a rigid molecule into the target enzyme or receptor, which is held fixed throughout. None of the docking approaches can take into account the important conformational changes that take place during the binding process of the ligand to its receptor. Before the three-dimensional conformational analysis, it is useful to get two-dimensional "shape" and "distance" information, to remove molecules that cannot possibly match the active site.

The factors taken into account for searching the virtual library include:

1. Knowledge about compounds that interact with the target, for example substrates, known classes of inhibitors, antagonists and agonists, SAR within various series, pharmacophores deduced from compound classes
2. Knowledge about receptor structure and receptor–ligand interactions, for example homology models, *x* ray and/or NMR structures, thermodynamics of ligand binding, effect of point mutations and dynamic motions of receptor and ligands

3. Knowledge about drugs in general, for example chemical structures and properties of known drugs, rules of conformational analysis and thermodynamics of receptor–ligand interactions.

In the early stages of the project when leads do not exist, computational methods can be used to select a diverse set of compounds from a large virtual library. If a compound shows activity, then other similar compounds from the library are synthesised and tested. If a lead already exists at the start of the programme, the size of the virtual library can be reduced by selecting a subset of compounds that are similar to the lead.

NMR, x ray and mass spectroscopic techniques

As a first step in structure-based design, the three-dimensional structure of the target macromolecule (protein or nucleic acid) is determined by *x* ray crystallography, NMR spectroscopy or homology modelling. Many examples of this type of research are well known in the literature. However, it should be emphasised that even after many cycles of the structure-based design process, when a compound that binds to the target with high affinity has been developed, it is still a long way from being a drug on the market. The compound may still fail in animal and clinical trials because of factors such as toxicity, bioavailability, poor pharmacokinetics (absorption, metabolism and half-life) and lack of efficacy.

In the lead generation phase, NMR methods are first used to detect weak binding of small molecule scaffolds to a target. The binding information is subsequently used to design much tighter binding inhibitors, or drug leads. SAR by NMR was the first NMR screening method disclosed in the literature. This is a fragment-based approach wherein a large library of small molecules is screened using two-dimensional ^{1}H or ^{15}N spectra of the target protein as a readout. From spectral changes one can identify the compounds that bind to the target. After deconvolution and identification of the active compound(s), a second screen of close analogues of the first "hit" is performed to optimise binding affinity to the first subsite. In order to identify small molecules that bind to another site on the target molecule, the screen is then repeated with the first site saturated. If small molecule fragments are identified that occupy several neighbouring subsites, one can then, based on the known structure, synthesise compounds that incorporate the small molecule fragments with various linking groups. If linked effectively, resulting compounds may have affinities for the target that are even stronger than the products of the binding constants of the individual unlinked fragments. As an example of the approach, several small fragments were discovered as ligands for the FK506 binding protein (K_i values 2–9500 μM). Linking these fragments led to more potent compounds like (K_i 49 nM).

The SHAPES strategy technique, like the above methods, relies on monitoring of ligand signals to determine which compounds in a mixture bind a drug target. The method uses standard one-dimensional line broadening and measurements of two-dimensional transferred nuclear Overhauser effect to detect binding of a limited (< 200) but diverse library of soluble low molecular weight scaffolds to a potential drug target. The scaffolds are derived largely from shapes or frameworks, most commonly found in known therapeutic agents, and as such represent approximations to "successful" regions of diversity space. This approach was used to identify p38 inhibitors. In the initial screen, the simple imidazole core did not appear to bind to p38. However, several tethered bicyclic compounds containing an imidazole (or close derivative) and an aryl moiety (pyridyl, phenyl or benzoic acid) exhibited weak binding (200 μM–2 mM). Since imidazole by itself did not bind, it was used as a core to fuse two of the tethered bicyclics or their derivatives, creating tricyclic molecules

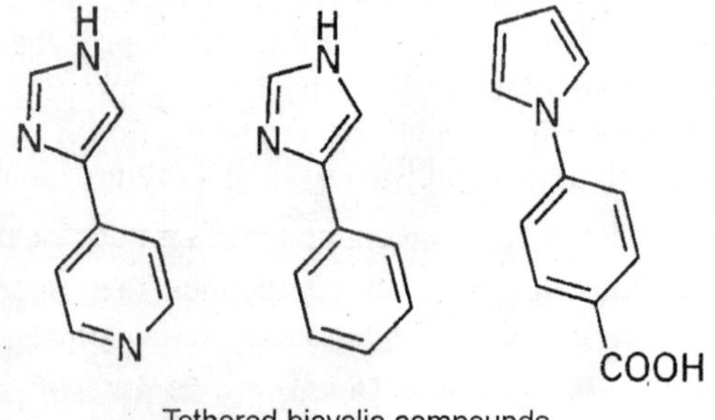

H N N H N N N N COOH

Tethered bicyclic compounds

with aryl derivatives as side chains and the imidazole as the binding core. Two such compounds showed improved binding. Further modifications resulted in more potent trisubstituted imidazoles like (K_i approximately 200 nM in a p38 enzyme assay).

Unlike in the past when *x* ray crystallography was used solely to study the structures of proteins and ligands, the technique is now being incorporated in all aspects of drug discovery, including lead identification, structural assessment, and optimisation. Crystallographic screening methods are being developed that enable experimental "*high-throughput*" sampling of up to thousands of compounds per day. One such technique, CrystaLEAD, has been used to sample large (≥ 10 000) compound libraries and detect ligands by monitoring changes in the electron density map relative to the unbound form. By careful design of the library, the technique leads to identification of the bound molecule from the primary data (electron density map) and eliminates the need for the deconvolution process. The electron density map yields a high-resolution picture of the ligand–protein complex and the resulting information on the ligand–target interactions can be used for structure-directed optimisation. As an example, the method was used for the discovery and optimisation of an orally active series of urokinase inhibitors for the treatment of cancer. The initially identified weaker 5-aminoindole and 2-aminoquinoline leads (K_i values 50–200 μM) were optimised. One of the 2-aminoquinoline inhibitors (K_i 0.37 μM) demonstrated oral bioavailability (38%). The 2-naphthamidine derivative did not show oral bioavailability.

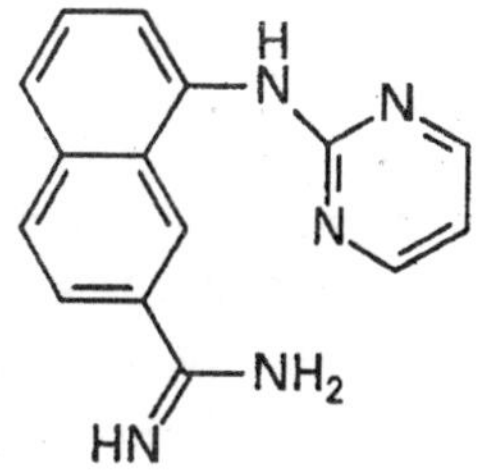

H
N
N
N
NH_2
HN
2-naphthamidine derivative

In addition to its application in drug discovery, crystallographic screening may also be applied in the structural genomics field, where crystal structures become available even in the absence of functional characterisation of the protein. In such cases, the ligands discovered could facilitate target validation, assay development, and the assignment of function.

Pharmacokinetics

The issues related to pharmacokinetics – drug absorption, distribution, metabolism, and excretion (ADME) – have always been important to the success of the drug discovery process. In many cases, not enough attention was paid to these factors in the early stages of the discovery process, leading to failures in the late stages of development. To avoid expensive late-stage failures and to cope with the high-throughput synthesis and screening technologies that result in many hits/leads, efforts are being directed to identify ADME problems at an early stage of the discovery process. It has become common practice to determine cytochrome P450 inhibition, blood levels after intravenous and oral administration, and identification of metabolites at an early stage. Some of this information may be useful in the lead optimisation process so that chemistry can be directed to overcome the problems. Bioavailability studies may be particularly important for evaluating the significance of the *in vivo* biological results, especially, if the results are negative or less convincing. Although ADME studies may be valuable in highlighting the shortcomings of the early hits/leads, these may sometimes result in inappropriate rejection of a lead. In many cases, the physicochemical and toxicological properties of the early hits/leads may be very different to those of the optimised drug candidates.

Examples of Drug Discovery

This section covers the discovery of many of the successful drugs on the market, together with some others which did not make it to the market for various reasons. Although medicinal chemistry along with structural (for example, *x* ray and NMR spectroscopy) and modelling studies has played a major part in all the cases, the starting leads and the final drugs were not always obtained by totally rational design processes. The structure–activity studies in the most relevant *in vitro* and *in vivo* models have played a significant role in converting the initial lead into the final drug that reached the market. Even today, because of the complexities of the drug discovery process, a totally rational approach leading to a marketed drug is not possible. In each of the examples discussed below, chosen to include different design strategies, an attempt has been made to highlight the origins of the starting leads and various rational/semi-rational discovery steps used in the optimisation process. Several interesting points emerge from the examples mentioned below. One of the more interesting and recent developments has been the discovery of non-peptide antagonists and agonists acting at the peptide receptors. Although non-peptide antagonists have been obtained in many cases (for example, ACTH, angiotensin, bradykinin, cholecystokinin, gastrin and LHRH), the agonists have only been obtained in a few cases (for example, angiotensin and bradykinin). These agonist/antagonist discoveries show how small chemical changes can convert an antagonist to an agonist and thus highlight the importance of the screening process.

Receptor Ligands (Agonists and Antagonists)

Early examples

In the past, a number of discoveries have been made in the absence of any knowledge about the receptors or ligands. One of the earliest examples of this kind is morphine which was used for many years as an analgesic (as a constituent of opium, extracted from the poppy plant, *Papaver somniferum*) without any knowledge about its mechanism of action. Only in the last 30 years have various opiate receptor subtypes (for example, μ-, δ-, κ- and σ-receptors) been identified. In addition, endogenous opiate-like peptides, for example enkephalins (Tyr-Gly-Gly-Phe-Met and Tyr-Gly-Gly-Phe-Leu) and endorphins, have been isolated and characterised. Many other opiate-like peptides have been isolated from different species, and enormous number of receptor-selective analogues (agonist and antagonist) have been synthesised in the hope of finding analgesic agents without the side-effects associated with morphine. However, no such compound has yet reached the market. Although there are some reports about peptides acting at the benzodiazepine receptor, the story of morphine and enkephalins is the only example so far where a non-peptide (morphine) acting at a peptide receptor was known before the peptide ligand (enkephalin) was isolated. In all the other examples (described below) the endogenous peptide ligand was isolated first from natural sources and the non-peptide ligands were obtained later by random screening or semi-rational approaches.

Another example of drug discovery without much knowledge of the receptor or the ligand is the discovery of benzodiazepines initially obtained by random (*in vivo*) screening of compounds for anxiolytic activity. The compounds were later found to act as modulators of γ-aminobutyric acid (GABA) at its receptor. Many years later, the discovery and characterisation of benzodiazepine receptors from brain tissue led to the development of *in vitro* receptor binding assays and drugs like diazepam. In a similar manner, histamine had been recognised as a chemical messenger and was shown to stimulate gastic acid secretion many years before the discovery of its receptors. Discovery of antihistamine compounds resulted in the classification of three receptor subtypes (H_1, H_2 and H_3). Histamine acting via H_1 receptors causes contraction in some smooth muscles (for example, in the gut, the uterus and the bronchi) and relaxation in other smooth muscles (for example, in some blood vessels), causing hypotension. Physiologically, histamine plays a role in regulating the secretion of gastric acid by stimulating the parietal cells to produce the acid. This effect is mediated by H_2 receptors. The role of the H_3 receptor is less well defined. Extensive work on antihistamine compounds has resulted in many successful drugs like fexofenadine, cimetidine and ranitidine.

In many cases, including the adrenergic receptors, the nature of the ligand/transmitter (dopamine R1 = R2 = H; epinephrine [adrenaline] R1 = OH, R2 = Me; norepinephrine [noradrenaline] R1 = OH, R2 = H) was known before starting the drug discovery programmes. The availability of many synthetic analogues led to receptor classification (α- and β-adrenergic receptors and other subtypes) and selective ligands. Many of these, for example salbutamol (a β_2-selective agonist used as a bronchodilator for the treatment of asthma), propranolol (a non-selective β-antagonist) and atenolol (a selective β_1-antagonist) both used in the treatment of angina and hypertension, have been successful drugs.

Selective oestrogen receptor modulators (oestrogen antagonists and aromatase inhibitors)

Another example of drug discovery in the absence of any significant knowledge about the receptors has been the discovery of selective oestrogen receptor modulators. Like the above examples, the structures of the ligands were known and were utilised, in some cases, for the discovery of drugs now on the market. The discovery of selective oestrogen receptor modulators (agonists and antagonists) highlights the impact of developing science in any area of drug discovery as new information emerges and new indications become obvious. In the case of oestrogens, over the years it has become clear that oestrogen is important not only in the growth, differentiation and function of tissues of the reproductive system but also plays an important role in maintaining bone density and protecting against osteoporosis. It also has beneficial effects in the cardiovascular (cardioprotective) and central nervous systems (protecting against Alzheimer's disease). In addition, the two isoforms of oestrogen receptor (ERα and ERβ) belonging to a family of nuclear hormone receptors that function as transcription factors on binding to their respective ligands have been identified. Thus tissue-selective oestrogen receptor modulators ranging from full agonist activity to pure antioestrogenic activity may be useful in the treatment and prevention of osteoporosis, treatment of breast cancer, and may reduce the risk of cardiovascular disease and Alzheimer's disease.

Tamoxifen, a non-steroidal anti-oestrogen, demonstrates antiproliferative effects in the breast and is widely used for the treatment of breast cancer. However, it does not show antioestrogenic properties in all tissues. For example, tamoxifen acts as an agonist on bone, liver and the endometrium. This mixed antagonist/agonist profile leads to many advantages in cancer patients. As an antagonist, tamoxifen prevents oestrogen-induced proliferation of breast ductal epithelium and breast cancer, and as an agonist in bone and liver it prevents bone loss in postmenopausal women and reduces cholesterol levels. However, the oestrogenic effects in the endometrium in postmenopausal women can result in an increased risk of endometrial cancer. Many other tamoxifen analogues, for example toremifene and droloxifene, show similar selectivity profiles. An orally active prodrug of the benzopyrene derivative (EM-652) showed a similar agonist/antagonist profile but with more antagonistic effects in the uterus. The activity of raloxifene is also similar to that of tamoxifen, except on the endometrium where it possesses less agonist activity. In comparison with the above mixed agonist/antagonist compounds, the steroidal anti-oestrogen Faslodex (ICI-182780) demonstrates a pure antioestrogenic profile in all tissues.

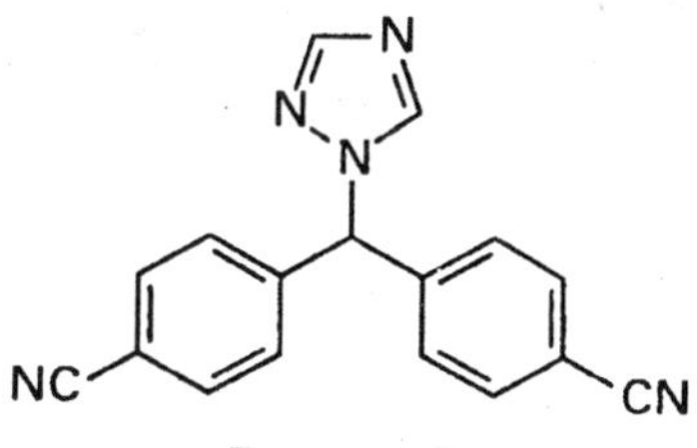

N N N NC CN

Letrozole

As an alternative to blocking the actions of oestrogen with compounds like tamoxifen, similar biological/clinical effects can be obtained by inhibiting aromatase, the enzyme that catalyses the final and rate-limiting step in oestrogen synthesis (conversion of androgens into oestrogens). Steroidal compounds such as formestane and exemestane, that are structurally related to the natural substrate of aromatase, and non-steroidal compounds such as for example anastrozole, letrozole, fadrozole and vorozole have been developed as aromatase inhibitors. Many of these are currently in use for the treatment of breast cancer.

LHRH agonists and antagonists

In more recent times, efforts have been directed towards finding receptor agonists and antagonists acting at the peptidergic receptors. In most of these cases (including LHRH), naturally occurring ligands were first isolated from various animal species, including humans, and crude receptor preparations were then used to screen for other agonist and antagonist ligands. Extensive structure–activity studies are carried out to identify the regions responsible for binding to the receptor and intrinsic activity. In general, SAR studies involve the synthesis of a large number of analogues by carrying out deletion studies (eliminating one or more amino acids from the chain), amino acid replacements with natural and unnatural amino acids, peptide bond replacements, and synthesis of conformationally restricting cyclic peptides. These studies are often followed by conformational studies using various spectroscopy and modelling techniques. Based on the results, further modifications are carried out in a semi-rational manner to obtain compounds with the desired properties.

LHRH [Pyr-His-Trp-Ser-Tyr-Gly-Leu-Arg-Pro-Gly-NH_2] is secreted from the hypothalamus and its action on the pituitary gland leads to the release of luteinising hormone and follicle stimulating hormone. Both of these hormones then act on the ovaries and testes and are responsible for the release of steroidal hormones. Early studies indicated that chronic administration of potent LHRH agonist analogues leads to tachyphylaxis or desensitisation of the pituitary receptors, leading ultimately to a suppression (not stimulation) of oestrogen and testosterone. This finding has led to the use of potent LHRH agonists in the treatment of hormone-dependent tumours. The LHRH antagonists are also expected to be useful for the treatment of these tumours but progress in the antagonist field has been relatively slow. Potent antagonists have been obtained by multiple amino acid substitutions in various positions of the LHRH molecule and a number of the best antagonists have between five and seven amino acid residues replaced by unnatural amino acids. These combinations of multiple substitutions were arrived at in a stepwise manner starting from the first antagonist, [des-His^2]-LHRH. Some antagonists like Abarelix [Ac-D-Nal(2)-D-Phe(p-Cl) -D-Pal(3) -Ser-MeTyr-D-Asn-Leu-Lys (å-isopropyl)-Pro-D-Ala-NH_2] and Ganirelix [Ac-D-Nal(2)-D-Phe (p-Cl)-D-Pal(3)-Ser-Tyr-D-hArg(Et_2)-Leu-hArg(Et_2)-Pro-D-Ala-NH_2] are currently in development for various indications, including as antitumour agents.

For the discovery of potent LHRH agonist and antagonist analogues, a large number of analogues were synthesised by incorporating amino acid changes in single and multiple positions. The most important SAR findings that led to these compounds were:

1. Replacement of the C-terminal glycinamide residue (-$NHCH_2CONH_2$) by a number of alkyl amide (-NH-R) or aza-amino acid amide residues (-NH-N(R)-$CONH_2$), which resulted in a 2–3-fold improvement in potency
2. Substitution of the glycine residue in position 6 by D amino acid residues [for example, D-Ala, D-Leu, D-Arg, D-Phe, D-Trp, D-Ser(Bu^t)], which led to a 2–100-fold improvement in potency
3. A combination of D amino acids in position 6 and an ethylamide or azaglycine amide.

The effects of multiple changes were not always additive. A combination of many of these changes led to the discovery of potent agonists which are currently on the market for the treatment of prostate cancer, breast cancer and some non-malignant conditions such as endometriosis and uterine fibroids. The marketed drugs include Zoladex {[D-Ser(Bu^t)^6, Azgly^{10}]-LHRH} Leuprolide {[D-Leu^6, des-Gly-NH_2^{10}]-LHRH(1-9)NHEt}, Nafarelin {D-Nal(2)^6]-LHRH}, Buserelin {[D-Ser(Bu^t)^6, des-Gly-NH_2^{10}]-LHRH(1-9)NHEt} and Triptorelin { [D-Trp^6]-LHRH}.

The potential of LHRH agonists in human medicine has been greatly enhanced by the development of convenient formulations for the delivery of these peptides. The most successful of these have been the biodegradable poly(d,l-lactide-co-glycolide) depot formulations which release the drug over a period of 1–3 months. A biodegradable poly(d,l-lactide-co-glycolide) sustained-release formulation of Zoladex can deliver 3.6–10.5 mg of the peptide over a period of 1–3 months. The formulation consists of a homogeneous dispersion of the drug (20% w/w) in a rod of the polymer and is administered by subcutaneous injection. Non-peptide antagonists of LHRH were discovered by directed or random screening approaches. A directed screening approach based on the Tyr-Gly-Leu-Arg region of LHRH followed by further medicinal chemistry on a weak lead gave a potent antagonist (T-98475). In binding assays (cloned human receptors and membrane fractions of monkey and rat pituitaries), was as potent as [D-Leu^6, Pro-NHEt] -LHRH. Oral administration of T-98475 (60 mg/kg) to castrated male cynomolgus monkeys resulted in >70% inhibition of plasma LH levels 8 hours after administration of the compound. Medicinal chemistry based on another series of weak non-peptide antagonist leads, discovered by screening the company collection for binding affinity to the rat gonadotrophin releasing hormone (GnRH) receptor, led to a potent compound that demonstrated an IC_{50} of 32 nM in the same binding assay.

Somatostatin agonists and antagonists

The cyclic peptide somatostatin [Ala-Gly-Cys-Lys-Asn-Phe-Phe-Trp-Lys-Thr-Phe-Thr-Ser-Cys, disulphide bridge between Cys^3 and Cys^{14}] and the 28 amino acid precursor containing 14 additional amino acid residues (Ser-Ala-Asn-Ser-Asn-Pro-Ala-Met-Ala-Pro-Arg-Glu-Arg-Lys) at the N-terminus were isolated from extracts of ovine and porcine hypothalamus, respectively. Both peptides are associated with a large number of biological activities, including inhibition of the secretion of growth hormone, insulin, glucagon and gastric acid. Thus, somatostatin may play an important role in many physiological and pharmacological systems. Five human receptor subtypes ($hSSTR_1$–$hSSTR_5$) for somatostatin have been characterised. A large number of analogues have been synthesised in the hope of finding drugs for various diseases. Examples of compounds which have reached the market include octreotide [sandostatin, D-Phe-cyclo(Cys-Phe-D-Trp-Lys-Thr-Cys)-Thr-ol], lanreotide [D-Nal-cyclo(Cys-Tyr-D-Trp-Lys-Val-Cys)-Thr-NH_2 and vapreotide (RC-160) [D-Phe-cyclo(Cys-Tyr-D-Trp-Lys-Val-Cys)-Trp-NH_2]. Daily and slow-release depot formulations of octreotide have been used for the treatment of growth-hormone secreting pituitary tumours, thyrotropin-secreting pituitary adenomas, pancreatic islet cell tumours and carcinoid tumours that express somatostatin receptors. A long-acting formulation of octreotide administered to acromegalic patients for 18 months (once every 4 weeks) suppressed growth hormone and insulin-like growth factor levels in all patients, and signs and symptoms of acromegaly improved during treatment. Reduction of the pituitary tumour was seen in all previously untreated patients.

Progress towards developing small cyclic peptides that are equipotent or more potent than somatostatin was made in several steps. Early SAR established that the Ala^1-Gly^2 residues and the disulphide bridge were not essential for biological activity. Amino acid substitution studies indicated that replacements of Lys^4 by Arg, Phe, Phe(F_5) or Phe(p-NH_2) residues, Asn^5 by Ala or D-Tyr, Phe^7 by Tyr, Trp^8 by D-Trp, D-Trp(5-F), D-Trp (6-F), D-Trp(5-Br), Phe^{11} by Phe(p-I) or Nal(2) and Cys^{14} by D-Cys gave compounds that were either equipotent or more potent than the parent peptide. Amino acid substitutions in other positions gave less potent analogues. For example, most of the analogues obtained by substituting the Phe^6 and Phe^7 residues, except by other aromatic amino acids like Phe (p-Cl), Phe(p-I) and Tyr, were less potent (<10%) than somatostatin. Deletion of the C-terminal carboxyl group or its replacement by an ethylamide group also resulted in compounds equipotent to somatostatin. An equally important finding, useful in designing smaller peptides, emerged by deleting various amino acid residues. Compounds lacking Lys^4 and Asn^5 were found to retain significant biological activity whereas the compounds lacking Phe^6, Trp^8, Lys^9, Thr^{10}, Phe^{11}, Thr^{12} were relatively poor agonists. The deletion and substitution studies led to much smaller peptides like cyclo(Aha-Phe-Phe-D-Trp-Lys-Thr-Phe), cyclo(Pro-Phe-D-Trp-Lys-Thr-Phe) and cyclo(Pro-Phe-D-Trp-Lys-Val-Phe). The most potent analogue, cyclo(MeAla-Tyr-D-Trp-Lys-Val-Phe) was 20–50-fold more potent than somatostatin in inhibiting growth hormone, 70 times more potent in inhibiting insulin and >80 times more potent in inhibiting glucagon. Other more potent cyclic peptides containing disulphide bridges, D-Phe-Cys-Phe-D-Trp-Lys-Thr-Cys-Thr(ol), D-Phe-Cys-Tyr-D-Trp-Lys-Val-Cys-Thr-NH_2, D-Phe-Cys-Tyr-D-Trp-Lys-Val-Cys-Trp-NH_2 and D-Phe-Cys-Tyr-D-Trp-Lys-Val-Cys-Thr-NH_2, were 8 0–200 times more potent than somatostatin. Since the discovery and availability of cloned multiple receptors, additional SAR studies have led to agonist and antagonist analogues that are selective for different receptors. For example, the cyclic peptide Cys-Lys-Phe-Phe-D-Trp-Phe(*p*-CH_2NH-CH$(CH_3)_2$-Thr-Phe-Thr-Ser-Cys with a disulphide bridge is a potent agonist at human $SSTR_1$ receptors and the N(α-Me)benzylglycine-containing analogue cyclo [(R)-βMeNphe-Phe-D-Trp-Lys-Thr-Phe] is an $hSSTR_2$-selective agonist. The $hSSTR_2$-agonist selectively inhibited the release of growth hormone in rats (equipotent to sandostatin) but had no effect on the inhibition of insulin at the same dose. Cyclo(Phe(N-aminoethyl)-Tyr-D-Trp-Lys-Val-Phe(N-carboxypropyl)-Thr-NH_2 (PTR 3046) a backbone-cyclic somatostatin analogue, and the lanthionine octapeptide displayed high selectivity for the $SSTR_5$ receptor.

In comparison with the agonist analogues, very few antagonists of somatostatin have been obtained by amino acid substitution. Two octapeptide derivatives, 4-NO_2-Phe-c(D-Cys-Tyr-D-Trp-Lys-Thr-Cys)-Tyr-NH_2 and Ac-4-NO_2-Phe-c(D-Cys-Tyr-D-Trp-Lys-Thr-Cys)-D-Tyr-NH_2 (inactive at the SST_1 and SST_4 receptor subtypes; high affinity for the $SSTR_2$ and $SSTR_5$ receptor subtypes) inhibited somatostatin-mediated inhibition of cAMP accumulation in a dose-dependent manner. The more potent antagonist, Ac-4-NO_2-Phe-c(D-Cys-Tyr-D-Trp-Lys-Thr-Cys)-D-Tyr-NH_2], displays a binding affinity to $SSTR_2$ comparable with that observed for the native hormone. H-Nal-c [D-Cys-Pal-D-Trp-Lys-Val-Cys]-Nal-NH_2 was also a more selective $hSSTR_2$ antagonist.

Angiotensin agonists and antagonists (peptides and non-peptides)

Angiotensin II and other members of the angiotensin family are produced by the processing of a protein called α_2-globulin or angiotensinogen, which is synthesised in the liver and found in the blood. The protein is first cleaved by the enzyme renin to generate a decapeptide called angiotensin I (Asp-Arg-Val-Tyr-Ile-His-Pro-Phe-His-Leu), which is further cleaved by ACE to produce the octapeptide angiotensin II [Asp^1-Arg-Val-Tyr-Ile-His-Pro-Phe^8], which is a potent vasoconstrictor. Angiotensin II acts at two receptor subtypes (AT_1 and AT_2). In the case of the agonist analogues, one of the most significant changes has been the replacement of the N-terminal Asp by Sar (N-methylglycine) to give [Sar^1]-angiotensin II, which in a number of *in vitro* tissue preparations was 1.5–2.5 times more potent than the natural ligand. AT_2-receptor selective analogues were obtained by modifications at the N-and C-termini of the peptide. The N-terminally modified compounds, [Me_2Gly^1]-, [Me_3Gly^1] - and [Me_3Ser^1] -angiotensin II, were > 1000-fold more potent at the AT_2 receptor. The analogue modified at positions 1 and 8, [Sar^1, Phe^8] -angiotensin II was 345-fold more potent than angiotensin II at the AT_2 receptor. Modifications of the C-terminal dipeptide (Pro^7-Phe^8) of [Sar^1, Val^5] angiotensin II with constrained aromatic (Tic) and hydrophobic (Oic) amino acids led to analogues with negligible affinity for the AT_1 receptor, but nanomolar affinity for the AT_2 receptor. The most potent and AT_2-selective analogue of the series was Sar-Arg-Val-Tyr-Val-His-Phe-Oic (IC_{50} values of 240 and 0·51 nM, at the AT_1 and AT_2 receptors, respectively).

A conformationally restricted analogue of angiotensin II, [$hCys^3$, $hCys^5$] - angiotensin II, was equipotent to angiotensin II in displacing [^{125}I]-angiotensin II from rat uterus membranes and in inducing contractions in the rabbit aortic rings (pD_2 8·48). Conformational analysis studies indicated that the cyclic peptide-like analogues {for example, c[$hCys^{3,5}$]-angiotensin II} may assume an inverse γ-turn conformation; thus, the amino acid residues 3–5 in angiotensin II were substituted with residues that induce different turns. Most of the analogues were either inactive or much less potent than angiotensin II. However, one of the analogues exhibited AT_1 receptor affinity (K_i 750 nM). A close analogue of containing a nine-membered ring in place of the central ten-membered ring was not active up to a concentration of 10 μM. This example illustrates one of the major difficulties in the synthesis of conformationally restricted analogues: even very small chemical changes lead to relatively large conformational changes and the resulting compounds are usually inactive. Such compounds do not provide much help in the design process. Antagonists of angiotensin II were initially obtained by eliminating the side chain from the C-terminal phenylalanine residue. Antagonists like [Gly^{8}] -angiotensin II, which competitively blocks the myotropic action of both angiotensin I and angiotensin II in *in vitro* test systems but did not antagonise the pressor response to angiotensin II in anaesthetised cats, were further modified in position 8 to give more potent antagonists, for example [Ile^{8}] -angiotensin II. A combination of positions 5 and 8 changes along with the N-terminal changes (Sar^{1}) discovered in the case of agonist series of compounds gave more potent antagonists like [Sar^{1}, Ala^{8}]-angiotensin II, [Sar^{1}, Ile^{8}] -angiotensin II (pA_2 9.48) and [Sar^{1}, Pen(SMe)^{5}, Ile^{8}]-angiotensin II. [Sar^{1}, Thr(Me)^{5}, Ile^{8}]-, [Sar^{1}, β-MePhe^{5}, Ile^{8}]- and [Sar^{1}, His^{5}, Ile^{8}]-angiotensin II were more potent than [Sar^{1}, Ile^{8}]-angiotensin II in the *in vivo* rat blood pressure test. In the cyclic series of antagonists many other cyclic compounds (except [Sar^{1}, hCys^{3}, hCys^{5}, Ile^{8}]-angiotensin II), for example [Cys^{1,5}, Ile^{8}] -, [D-Cys^{1}, Cys^{5}, Ile^{8}] -, [Sar^{1}, Cys^{5,8}]-, [Sar^{1}, Cys^{5}, D-Cys^{8}]- and [Sar^{1}, hCys^{5}, D-Cys^{8}]-angiotensin II, were much less potent.

Non-peptide antagonists of angiotensin II were obtained by random screening approaches. Despite all the progress achieved in discovering potent agonist and antagonist analogues and the information about ligand–receptor interactions derived from the above compounds, it was not possible to design non-peptidic molecules by this rational design procedure. The discovery from a random screening lead of DuP753 (losartan), which is selective for AT_1, opened the way to non-peptide antagonists. The SAR studies indicated that a considerable variation was allowed in the chemical structure of the antagonists. The synthetic medicinal chemistry approaches identified various replacements for the imidazole and the biphenyl tetrazole groups and highlighted chemical changes that led to AT_1- or AT_2-selective or mixed (AT_1 and AT_2) receptor antagonists. Compound (L-162,389) is an example of a mixed antagonist (AT_1 and AT_2 binding affinities of 2–4 nM). In a macrocyclic series of analogues, bound primarily to the AT_1 receptor (AT_1 and AT_2 receptor IC_{50} values 23 nM and 4000 nM, respectively) whereas a very similar analogue bound to both the receptors with similar affinity (IC_{50} 20–30 nM). Another interesting aspect of the non-peptide agonist/antagonist SAR studies has been the identification of both agonists and antagonists in the same series of compounds by minor structural

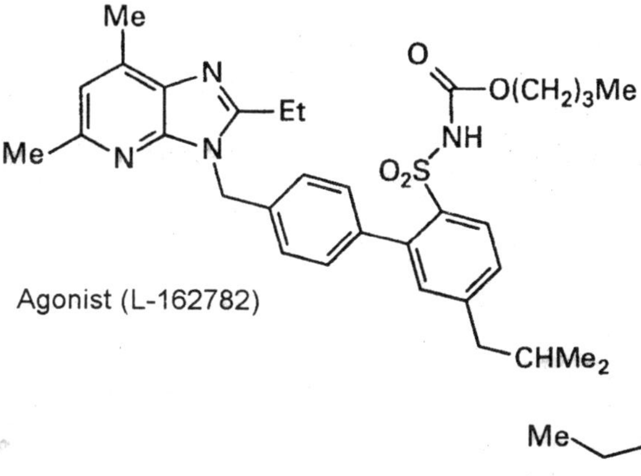

Agonist (L-162782)

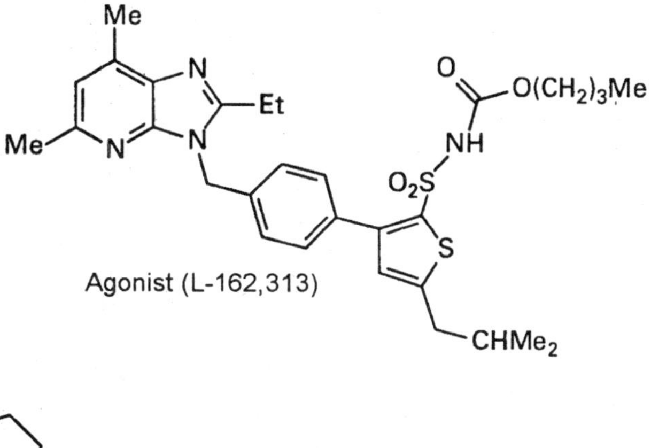

Agonist (L-162,313)

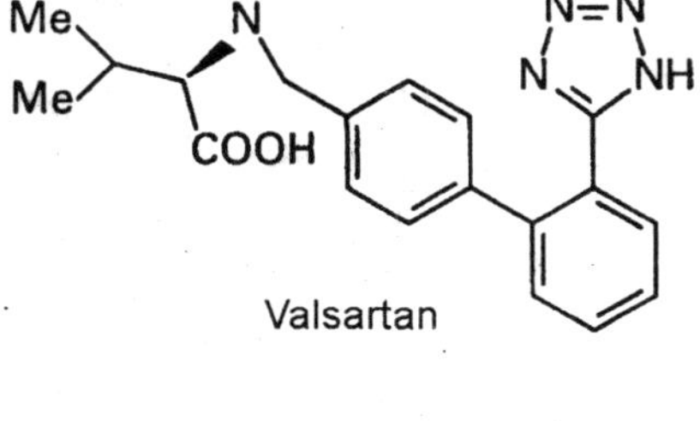

Valsartan

modifications. For example, compound (L-162782) is an agonist whereas a similar analogue that differs chemically by only a single methyl group (L-162,389) is an antagonist. Another close analogue (L-162,313) also displayed agonist activity. At present, it is not possible to predict changes that lead to agonist/antagonist analogues by any rational design approaches. Only by screening the compounds in appropriate tests can selective compounds with the desired biological profile be identified. A large amount of chemical effort in the angiotensin antagonist field has led to the discovery of many successful drugs like losartan, valsartan, candesartan, ibresartan and eprosartan for the treatment of high blood pressure and other cardiovascular complications.

Bombesin/neuromedin agonists and antagonists

Four subtypes of the bombesin receptor have been identified (gastrin-releasing peptide [GRP] receptor, neuromedin B receptor, the orphan receptor bombesin receptor subtype 3 and bombesin receptor subtype 4). The roles of individual receptor subtypes are under investigation and selective ligands for these receptor subtypes are being synthesised. Systematic SAR studies have provided many receptor antagonists. A semi-rational approach was used for the discovery of non-peptide antagonists of neuromedin B. The role of each amino acid side chain was defined by alanine scanning in bombesin(7-14)-octapeptide, Ac-Gln-Trp-Ala-Val-Gly-His-Leu-Met-NH_2 (minimum active fragment), and indicated that Trp^8, Val^{10} and Leu^{13} were most important for the binding affinity to the receptors. A search within the company's compound collection was then initiated for various templates containing Trp, Val/Leu types of side chains. This led to a moderately active lead. Changes at the C-terminus led to more potent (S) α-methyl-Trp derivative. Additional chemical modifications on resulted in a series of "balanced" neuromedin-B preferring (BB_1)/GRP preferring (BB_2) receptor ligands, as exemplified by PD 176252. Compound displays a BB_2 receptor affinity of 1 nM whilst retaining subnanomolar (0·17 nM) BB_1 receptor affinity and is a competitive antagonist at both receptor subtypes.

Bradykinin agonists and antagonists

Peptide SAR studies resulted in potent bradykinin B_2 receptor antagonists like HOE 140 D-Arg-Arg-Pro-Hyp-Gly-Thi-Ser-D-Tic-Oic-Arg. Replacement of some of the amino acids by substituted 1,3,8-triazaspiro[4,5]decan-4-one-3-acetic acids in the B_2 receptor antagonist D-Arg-Arg-Pro-Pro-Gly-Phe-Ser-D-Tic-Oic-Arg gave potent B_2 receptor antagonists like compound (NPC 18521, K_i 0·15 nM) which contains a phenethyl group at position 1 of the spirocyclic mimetic. Another example of a pseudopeptide analogue is compound NPC 18884, which contains three arginine residues. Given intraperitoneally or orally, compound inhibited bradykinin-induced leukocyte influx and exudation. The effects lasted for up to 4 hours and were selective for the bradykinin B_2 receptors. At similar doses compound had no significant effect against the inflammatory responses induced by des-Arg^9-bradykinin, histamine or substance P.

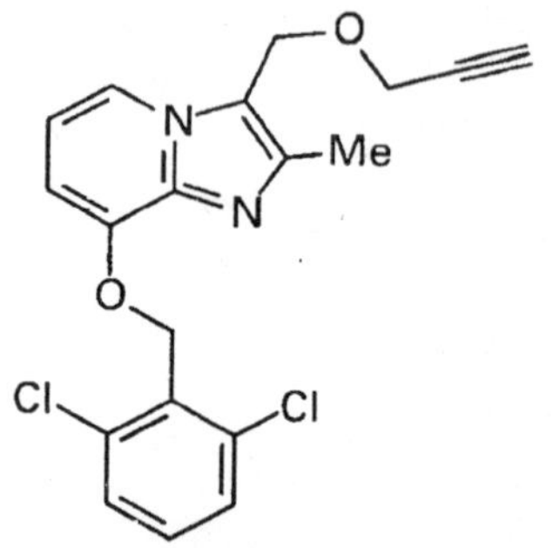

O N Me N O Cl Cl

Lead

Non-peptide B_2 receptor antagonists and agonists of bradykinin were obtained by random screening approaches. Chemical modifications on a random screening lead led to the non-peptide antagonist, which was active in a number of *in vitro* and *in vivo* test systems (for example, bradykinin-induced bronchoconstriction and carrageenin-induced paw oedema). The non-peptide agonist bound with high affinity to the B_2 receptor (IC_{50} 5·3 nM) but had no binding affinity for the B_1 receptor; at concentrations between 1 nM and 1 μM compound stimulated phosphatidylinositol hydrolysis in Chinese hamster ovary cells permanently expressing the human bradykinin B_2 receptor. The response was antagonised by the B_2 receptor selective antagonist Hoe 140. Intravenous administration of bradykinin or the agonist (both at 10 μg/kg) caused a fall in blood pressure. However, the duration of the hypotensive response was significantly longer than the response to bradykinin.

Cholecystokinin agonists and antagonists

Peptidomimetic agonist and antagonist analogues of cholecystokinin (CCK) were obtained from the C-terminal tetrapeptide of CCK/gastrin (Boc-Trp-Met-Asp-Phe-NH_2) and analogues like Boc-Trp-MeNle-Asp-Phe-NH_2 and by synthesising conformationally constrained analogues by replacing the Trp-Met/Trp-MeNle dipeptides. The diketopiperazine derivative and the constrained cyclic pseudopeptide CCK_B agonist [(*S*) at the α-carbon of the aminononane moiety (CCK_A/CCK_B = 147)] exhibited full CCK_B receptor agonist properties, and increased gastric acid secretion in anaesthetised rats.

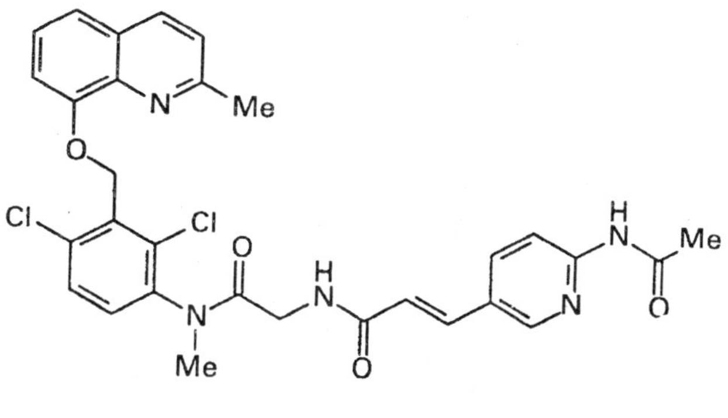

FR173657; antagonist

Non-peptide CCK agonists and antagonists based on a benzodiazepine skeleton were obtained by random screening and lead optimisation. 1,5-Benzodiazepine derivatives were shown to be agonists and antagonists of CCK_A and CCK_B. The substitution pattern at the anilinoacetamide nitrogen played an important role for the activity. While compounds with a hydrogen or methyl substituent were weak antagonists of CCK-8, the ethyl, propyl, *n*-butyl and cyanoethyl derivatives were agonists. Compound displayed 86% CCK-8 functional activity in the guinea-pig gallbladder assay at 30 μM (CCK-8 = 100% at 1 μM) and showed similar affinity for CCK_A and CCK_B receptors. When given orally to rats, the CCK_A agonist (GW5823) reduced food intake to 40% of that in vehicle-control treated animals. When administered orally, the CCK_B/! gastrin antagonist YF476 inhibited gastic acid secretion in a pentagastrin-induced acid secretion model and displayed a long duration of action (> 6 hours at a dose of 100 nmol/kg). In addition to the benzodiazepine derivatives, a number of other chemically distinct CCK antagonists have been prepared starting from the random screening leads. The nine-membered ring analogue was a potent CCK_B/gastrin antagonist (rat stomach pK_B 9·08, mouse cortex pIC_{50} 8·3). In comparison, the analogues containing six-, seven- and eight-membered rings were poor CCK_B/gastrin receptor antagonists.

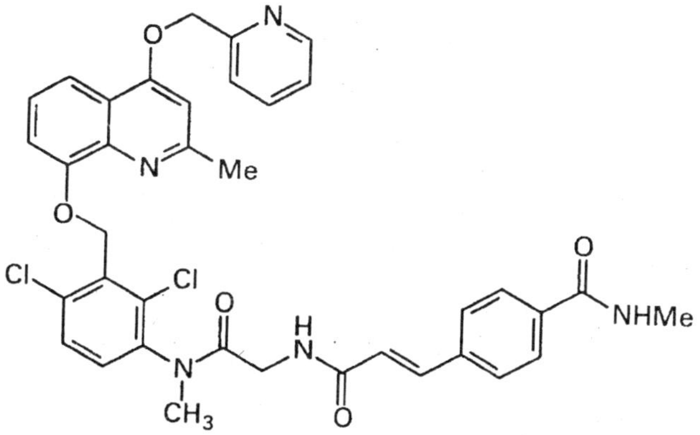

FR190997; agonist

Endothelin antagonists

Endothelin is one of the most potent vasoconstrictor peptides. Antagonists of this peptide are being sought for various cardiovascular disorders. Leads for antagonist design have originated from natural sources, rational design approaches and by random screening. ET_A and ET_B receptor selective antagonists were obtained from cyclic pentapeptides of microbial origin like the ET_A-selective peptide BQ 123 [c(D-Val-Leu-D-Trp-D-Asp-Pro)]. Linear tripeptide derivatives were subsequently developed as ET_A [BQ-485] or ET_B [BQ-788 and BQ-017] receptor selective or non-selective [BQ-928] antagonists. In the BQ-123 series, amino acid replacements converted the ET_A selective antagonist BQ-123 to ET_B selective and non-selective antagonists. For example, c(D-*t*-Leu-Leu-2-chloro-D-Trp-D-Asp-Pro) and c(D-Pen(Me)-Leu-2- bromo-D-Trp-D-Asp-Pro) were nearly equipotent at both the receptors whereas c(D-Pen(Me)-Leu-2-cyano-D-Trp-D-Asp-Pro) was much more potent at the ET_B receptor. In the *cis*-(2,6-dimethylpiperidino)carbonyl-Leu-D-Trp-D-Nle series of analogues, the 2-bromo-D-Trp, 2-chloro-D-Trp and 2-methyl-D-Trp analogues were potent antagonists at both receptors whereas the 2-cyano-D-Trp and 2-ethyl-D-Trp analogues were more potent at the ET_B receptor.

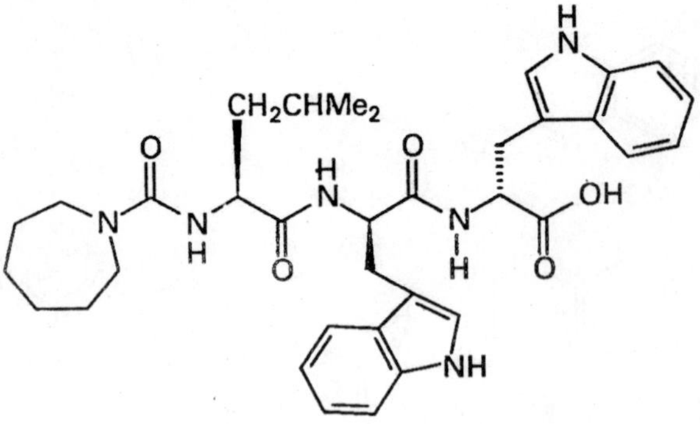

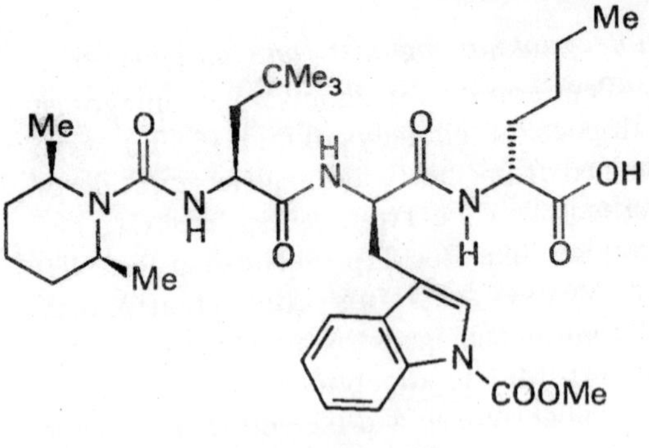

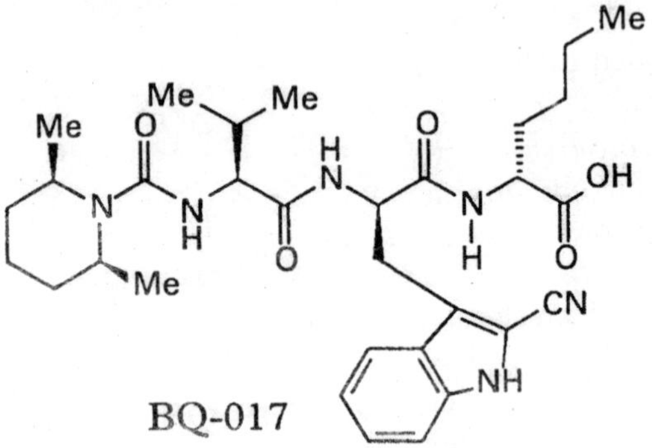

Antagonists were also discovered using a rational approach starting from the endothelin C-terminal dodecapeptide derivative, succinyl-Glu-Ala-Val-Tyr-Phe-Ala-His-Leu-Asp-Ile-Ile-Trp. Replacing each amino acid in turn with glycine indicated that Phe^{14}, $Ile^{19,20}$ and Trp^{21} were the most important residues. Based on this evidence, a series of compounds with an aromatic moiety attached through a spacer to the amino group of the Trp residue were synthesised. Further work around the initial weak antagonist lead, N-*trans*-2-phenylcyclopropanoyl-Trp, resulted in a 400-fold selective ET_B antagonist. Replacement of the biphenylalanine residue by 2-naphthylalanine, Met, Leu, Ile, Cha, Thr or ethylglycine gave antagonists that were 2–4-fold more potent at the ET_B receptor. The D-Phe-Val derivative displayed similar affinity for ET_A and ET_B receptors (K_i 1–2 nM).

Non-peptide antagonists of endothelin were discovered by random screening approaches. A comparison of compounds demonstrates that it is possible to obtain selective and non-selective compounds in the same series by chemical modifications. Carboxyindoline derivative was about 100-fold more selective antagonist for the ET_A receptor was a non-selective antagonist. Another series of ET_A-selective antagonists included a more selective (> 25000-fold) pyrrolidine carboxylic acid derivative, A-216546. A-216546 was orally available in rat, dog and monkey, and blocked the endothelin-1-induced presser response in the conscious rats. Replacement of the dialkylacetamide side chain in compound resulted in a complete reversal of receptor selectivity, preferring ET_B over ET_A. Compound (A-308165) demonstrated greater than 27000-fold selectivity favouring the ET_B receptor.

Enzyme Inhibitors

Converting Enzyme Inhibitors

Many biologically active peptides are obtained from their precursors by the actions of converting enzymes (zinc metallopeptidases). For example, ACE cleaves a dipeptide from the C-terminus of angiotensin I to generate the pressor peptide angiotensin II. In addition, some of the biologically active peptides (for example, bradykinin, atrial natriuretic peptide (ANP) and enkephalins) are degraded by the converting enzymes into inactive fragments. These enzymes are important in controlling many physiological and pathological processes. In the case of peptides that, in some pathological conditions, produce undesirable effects (for example, vasoconstriction in the case of angiotensin II and endothelin), it is beneficial to prevent the formation of such peptides from their precursors by inhibiting the enzymes involved in the process (for example, ACE and endothelin converting enzyme). On the other hand, in the case of peptides that produce therapeutically beneficial effects (for example, enkephalins and atrial natriuretic factor; ANF), inhibiting the enzymes that inactivate these peptides (for example, enkephalinase and atriopeptidase) is likely to increase the biological half-life of the peptide and thus extend the duration of action. From the point of view of drug discovery, ACE inhibitors, which prevent the formation of a pressor peptide angiotensin II, have been the most successful examples. From the point of view of medicinal chemistry, lessons learned from the ACE story have been very useful in the design of inhibitors of many other metalloproteinases like enkephalinase, atriopeptidase and MMPs.

ACE (peptidyl dipeptidase), known to catalyse the hydrolysis of dipeptides from the C-terminus of polypeptides, belongs to a family of zinc metalloproteinases, which require a zinc atom in the active site. In these enzymes a combination of three His, Glu, Asp or Cys residues creates a zinc binding site. The first major step in the discovery of ACE inhibitors was the isolation of bradykinin-potentiating peptides like $BPP5_a$ (Pyr-Lys-Trp-Ala-Pro) and SQ 20881 (Pyr-Trp-Pro-Arg-Pro-Gln-Ile-Pro-Pro) from the venoms of the Brazilian snake, *Bothrops jaraca* and the Japanese snake, *Agkistrodon halys blomhoffii*. SAR studies on these peptides indicated that a number of pentapeptide analogues of $BPP5_a$, for example Pyr-Lys-Phe-Ala-Pro, were equipotent to the parent peptide in inhibiting ACE. However, smaller di- or tri-peptides, for example Gly-Trp, Val-Trp, Ile-Trp, Phe-Ala-Pro and Lys-Trp-Ala-Pro, were less potent. Although SQ 20881 was studied extensively in the clinic, it could not be used as a drug because of a lack of oral activity. Progress towards the orally active ACE inhibitors was made after the discovery of D-benzylsuccinic acid as an inhibitor of another zinc metalloprotease, carboxypeptidase A. This led to the synthesis of proline derivatives by combining the features present in venom peptides and benzylsuccinic acid. One of the early compounds, succinylproline, was only a weak inhibitor of ACE (approximately 150-fold less potent than SQ 20881). Further modifications in this series led to 2-D-methylsuccinyl-proline and 2-D-methylglutaryl-proline (5- and 10-fold less potent, respectively, than SQ 20881). Replacement of the carboxyl group by a thiol group (a better zinc-ion ligand) resulted in potent ACE inhibitors like captopril (2-D-methyl-3-mercaptopropanoyl-proline), which produced dose-related inhibition of the pressor response to angiotensin I in normotensive male rats and produced marked antihypertensive effects in unanaesthetised Goldblatt two-kidney renal hypertensive rats. Captopril was the first ACE inhibitor to reach the market for the treatment of hypertension.

Since the discovery of captopril, a number of other analogues containing either a different chelating group or a proline replacement have been found to be potent inhibitors of ACE. Some of this work was based on a hypothetical model of the substrate (angiotensin I) binding at the active site of the enzyme. In the case of the ACE inhibitors containing a thiol function (for example, captopril), the thiol group interacts with the zinc ion and the methyl group binds at the S_1' subsite. The proline residue binds at the S_2' subsite and the C-terminal carboxyl group of the proline residue interacts with a positively charged group present in the enzyme. Over the years, medicinal chemistry approaches involving modifications of the chelating group and different groups binding in the S_1' and S_2' subsites have resulted in many potent inhibitors of ACE and many of these, including captopril, enalapril and lisinopril, have become highly successful drugs for the treatment of hypertension and other cardiovascular disorders. The design of phosphorus-containing ACE inhibitors, for example fosinopril, was based on the structure of phosphoramidon [N-α-L-rhamnopyranosyloxy-hydroxyphosphinyl)-Leu-Trp], an inhibitor of another zinc metalloproteinase (thermolysin) isolated from a culture filtrate of *Streptomyces tanashiensis*. In comparison with the effort required for the discovery of ACE inhibitors, progress in identifying potent inhibitors of the enkephalin-degrading dipeptidylcarboxypeptidase (enkephalinase) (used as analgesics) and ANF degrading enzyme (used as antihypertensive agents) was rapid because of the similarities between the enzymes. However, the similarities resulted in problems in achieving selectivity. The differences in the S_1' and S_2' subsites of metalloproteinases were exploited to achieve selectivity. The first potent inhibitor of enkephalinase (thiorphan) was about 30-fold more potent against enkephalinase (K_i approximately 4 nM) than against ACE. Another inhibitor, kelatorphan, was a potent inhibitor of enkephalinase and dipeptidylaminopeptidase and a weak inhibitor of aminopeptidase. Inhibitors like glycoprilat and their orally active prodrugs were potent inhibitors of ACE and enkephalinase; they prevented angiotensin I-induced pressor responses in rats and also increased urinary water and sodium excretion. Similarly, dual metalloproteinase inhibitors like CGS30440 (IC_{50} 19 and 2 nM against ACE and neutral endopeptidase, respectively) inhibited the angiotensin-1 pressor response, elevated the concentration of circulating ANP, and increased the excretion of urine, sodium and cGMP in rats injected with ANP. Candoxatrilat was an inhibitor of atriopeptidase.

It has been much more difficult to achieve complete selectivity in the case of inhibitors of MMPs (for example, collagenases, stromelysins and gelatinases), a family of zinc-containing proteinases involved in extracellular matrix remodelling and degradation. These enzymes have been implicated in diseases like rheumatoid arthritis, osteoarthritis, cancer and multiple sclerosis. The information generated in the case of converting enzyme inhibitors quickly led to inhibitors containing hydroxamate, thiol, N-carboxyalkyl and phosphorous groups for chelating the essential zinc metal and other peptidic and non-peptidic groups for binding to various binding pockets (S_1, S_1' -S_3') in the enzymes. The N-(X = NH) or C-carboxyalkyl (X = CH_2) series of inhibitors also inhibited several of the enzymes (MMP-1, -2 and -3). A proline derivative inhibited MMP-1, -2, -3, -7 and -13; a sulfonamide derivative inhibited MMP-1, -2, -3, -8 and -13, and a conformationally restricted inhibitor like compound (R = H, Ac, Boc or $PhSO_2$) inhibited MMP-1, -3, -8 and -9. Clinical trials on one of the broad-spectrum inhibitors, marimastat, for the treatment of pancreatic, lung, brain and stomach cancers failed to demonstrate efficacy in humans.

Aspartyl protease (renin and HIV protease) inhibitors

Aspartyl proteases are a family of enzymes which, in general, cleave peptide bonds between bulky hydrophobic amino acid residues. The cleavage of the peptide bond is mediated by a "*general acid-general base*" catalysis mechanism using the carboxyl groups of the aspartic acid residues at the active site. Enormous progress has been made in the discovery and optimisation of the pharmacokinetic properties of the inhibitors. Since the antihypertensive market is well served by a number of orally active agents like β-blockers, ACE inhibitors and angiotensin II antagonists, and the condition is chronic, requiring long-term treatment, it is essential to have orally active inhibitors for this indication. Many of the potent and selective renin inhibitors are now approaching the appropriate level of oral bioavailability after more than 25 years of research. In contrast, by using all the chemical information available in the case of renin inhibitors, it has been possible to discover potent orally bioavailable HIV protease inhibitors in a relatively short period of time, and many of these are already highly successful drugs.

Renin inhibitors

A number of chemical approaches have been used in the design of renin inhibitors. In the absence of the purified enzyme, most of the early search for inhibitors was carried out using crude renin preparations. The amino acid sequences of mouse, rat and human renin were obtained later on using either the traditional isolation and sequencing techniques or cDNA methodology. Various three-dimensional models of renin were constructed in the early stages, based on the *x* ray structures of other similar aspartyl proteases, for example endothia-pepsin and penicillopepsin. Later on, the *x* ray crystal structure of recombinant human renin was reported. The inhibitor design process has been based on some of these models.

Initial design of the inhibitors was based on a rational design strategy using the renin substrate as a starting point. Some of the early studies indicated that the octapeptide of horse angiotensinogen (His-Pro-Phe-His-Leu-Leu-Val-Tyr), cleaved slowly by renin between the two leucine residues, was a weak competitive inhibitor of renin. This led to the modifications in the P_1 and P_1' positions (Leu-Leu) of this peptide. The early work indicated that the two leucine residues could be replaced by other natural and unnatural amino acids (for example, Phe, D-Leu). Many of the resulting analogues, like His-Pro-Phe-His-Leu-D-Leu-Val-Tyr, His-Pro-Phe-His-Phe-Phe-Val-Tyr and Pro-His-Pro-Phe-His-Phe-Phe-Val-Tyr-Lys, although more potent than the original substrate-based compounds, were still weak inhibitors of renin. More potent inhibitors were obtained by replacing the peptide bond between the two leucine residues. Many of these peptides, for example Pro-His-Pro-Phe-His-Pheψ (CH_2NH)Phe-Val-Tyr-Lys, His-Pro-Phe-His-Leuψ (CH_2NH)Val-Ile-His and Pro-His-Pro-Phe-His-Leuψ(CH_2NH)Val-Ile-His-Lys (H-142), were potent and selective inhibitors of human renin. The two peptides containing a reduced Leu-Val peptide bond were 800–1000 times more potent inhibitors of human renin (IC_{50} 10–190 nM) than of dog renin (IC_{50} 10–150 mM) and H-12 did not inhibit cathepsin D up to a concentration of approximately 700 mM. One of the smaller peptides, Boc-Phe-His-Chaψ(CH_2NH)Val-NHCH$_2$CH(Me)-Et, approached the potency of H-142 in inhibiting human renin and lowered blood pressure in salt-depleted cynomolgus monkeys at a dose of 0·1–0·5 mg/kg. Unlike the reduced peptide bond [-ψ(CH_2NH)] analogues, replacement of the scissile peptide bond by -CH_2O-, -COCH_2-, -CH_2S- and -CH_2SO- did not lead to enhanced potency. The reduced peptide bond analogue, H-142, has been studied extensively in various animal and human models. At doses of 1 and 2·5 mg/kg/hr, H-142 produced a dose-related reduction in plasma renin activity and reduced the circulating levels of angiotensin I and II.

Another important step in the discovery of potent inhibitors of renin was the isolation of a naturally occurring aspartyl protease inhibitor pepstatin (Iva-Val-Val-Sta-Ala-Sta [Sta = (3S, 4S)-4-amino-3-hydroxy-6-methylheptanoic acid]), which was a relatively poor inhibitor of human renin but a potent inhibitor of pepsin. Incorporation of the statine residue in the angiotensinogen octapeptide resulted in potent inhibitors of renin. His-Pro-Phe-His-Sta-Val-Ile-His and Iva-His-Pro-Phe-His-Sta-Leu-Phe-NH_2 were equipotent to H-142 as inhibitors of human plasma and kidney renin. Another similar compound, Iva-His-Pro-Phe-His-Sta-Ile-Phe-NH_2, was a five-fold more potent inhibitor of human plasma and kidney renin than was H-142. However, the statine analogue was much less selective. In comparison with H-142, the statine analogue was about 300-fold more potent in inhibiting dog renin. The statine residue [-NH-CH(CH_2CHMe_2)-CH(OH)-CH_2CO-] in the above transition-state analogues was modified in various ways to assess the importance of the side chain isobutyl group, the hydroxyl group and the methylene group. In general, replacement of the isobutyl side chain (occupying the P_1 position) by cyclohexylmethyl or benzyl groups resulted in more potent compounds. The hydroxyl and the methylene groups were not essential for renin inhibition. Several compounds containing difluorostatine, for example difluorostatone, norstatine [(2R, 3S)-3-amino-2-hydroxy-5- methylhexanoic acid], cyclohexylnorstatine [(2R, 3S)-3-amino-4-cyclohexyl-2-hydroxybutyric acid], aminostatine (3,4-diamino-6-methylheptanoic acid) and α, α-difluoro-β-aminodeoxystatine, were potent inhibitors of human renin. Incorporation of the hydroxyethylene, dihydroxyethylene and other statine-like residues in place of the scissile peptide bond in substrate-based analogues, along with other amino acid or non-peptide changes at the N- and C-termini, led to more potent, selective and relatively small molecular weight inhibitors of renin. Examples of such compounds include Ro 42-5892, ICI 219623 and CGP38560. Ro 42-5892 was effective in lowering blood pressure in sodium-depleted marmosets and squirrel monkeys after oral administration (0·1 to 10 mg/kg.). ICI 219623 was effective in lowering blood pressure in anaesthetised sodium-depleted marmosets after intravenous (0·3–3·0 mg/kg) and oral (30 mg/kg) dosing. The indole-2-carbonyl derivative (JTP-3072) caused significant reduction in blood pressure in marmosets at an oral dose of 10 mg/kg for up to 3 hours. Compounds showed some oral absorption. Compound (IC_{50} 1.4 nM) displayed oral activity in a sodium-depleted normotensive cynomolgus monkey at a dose of 3 mg/kg.

In an attempt to design small molecular weight compounds, conformational analysis of the binding mode of CGP 38560 was carried out. This indicated that the S_1 and S_3 pockets constitute a large contiguous, hydrophobic binding site accommodating the P_1 cyclohexyl and the P_3 phenyl groups in close proximity to each other. This led to the synthesis of δ-amino hydroxyethylene dipeptide isosteres lacking the P_4–P_2 peptide backbone. Compound was a moderately potent inhibitor of human renin (IC_{50} 300 nM). Non-peptide inhibitors (R = $-OCH_2COOCH_3$, $-OCH_2CONH_2$ or $-OCH_2SO_2CH_3$) were 15–50- fold more potent inhibitors. Random screening approaches led to non-peptide inhibitors like the tetrahydroquinoline derivative (IC_{50} 0·7 nM [recombinant human renin] and 37 nM [human plasma renin]), which displayed long lasting (20 hour) blood pressure lowering effects after oral administration (1 and 3 mg/kg) to sodium-depleted conscious marmosets. The piperidine derivative also inhibited plasmepsin I and II from *Plasmodium falciparum*.

HIV protease inhibitors

In comparison with the discovery of renin inhibitors, the task of discovering inhibitors of HIV protease has been relatively easy. This is primarily because many of the approaches used successfully in the design of renin inhibitors were also applicable in the design of HIV protease inhibitors. In addition, samples of both HIV-1 and HIV-2 proteases (99 residue peptides), obtained by chemical synthesis and recombinant technology, were available in the early stages of the programme, along with the three-dimensional structure of the HIV-1 protease. Like renin, HIV protease was found to prefer a hydrophobic amino acid (Leu, Ile, Tyr, Phe) in the P_1 position of the substrate and was inhibited by pepstatin. However, unlike renin, incorporation of the statine residue in the P_1 position of the substrate, or the replacement of the scissile peptide bond in the substrate-like peptides with a -CH_2NH-group, did not lead to potent inhibitors. Potent inhibitors of the enzyme were obtained by replacing the scissile peptide bond with a hydroxymethylcarbonyl, hydroxyethylamine, hydroxyethylurea or a hydroxyethylene group. Many such compounds like saquinavir, indinavir, ritonavir, neflinavir and palinavir have reached the market or are in the late stages of clinical trials. In addition, various inhibitors of HIV protease were developed to overcome the problem of viral resistance by modifying the existing inhibitors like ritonavir and amprenavir. Computational studies using HIV-1 protease mutants ($Met^{46}Ile$, $Leu^{63}Pro$, $Val^{82}Thr$, $Ile^{84}Val$, $Met^{46}Ile/Leu^{63}Pro$, $Val^{82}Thr/Ile^{84}Val$ and $Met^{46}Ile/Leu^{63}Pro/Val^{82}Thr/Ile^{84}Val$) and known inhibitors of the enzyme (ABT-538 and VX-478) were used to design inhibitors with better binding affinity towards both mutant and wild-type proteases. ABT-378 inhibited wild-type and mutant HIV protease, blocked the replication of laboratory and clinical strains of HIV type 1, and maintained high potency against mutant HIV selected by ritonavir *in vivo*. Similarly, the allophenylnorstatine-containing dipeptide (JE-2147) (elimination half-life 94 minutes after intravenous administration; oral bioavailability 33–37% in non-fasting and fasting animals) was a potent inhibitor, active against a wide spectrum of HIV-1, HIV-2, SIV, and various clinical HIV-1 strains *in vitro*.

Many other non-peptide inhibitors of HIV protease (dihydropyrone, cyclic urea and sulfamide series of compounds) were obtained by modifications of random screening leads. Examples of these include a cyclic sulfone derivative and PNU-140690, which showed activity against a variety of laboratory strains of HIV-1, clinical isolates and other variants resistant to other protease inhibitors.

Thrombin Inhibitors (Serine Protease)

Thrombin inhibitors like D-Phe-Pro-Arg aldehyde have been known for a long time. However, the compounds lacked oral bioavailability. A semi-rational approach was adopted to modify P_1 to P_3 positions to improve the potency, selectivity and pharmacokinetic properties. Changes in individual positions were followed by multiple changes and synthesis of conformationally restricted analogues. Substitution of the C-terminal arginine aldehyde moiety (P_1 position) by *p*-amidinobenzylamine gave thrombin inhibitors comparable in potency with the transition-state aldehyde analogue but much less potent (130–400,000-fold) against trypsin, plasmin, tissue plasminogen activator and urokinase. Incorporation of a conformationally restricted analogue of arginine in the P_1 position, along with a six- or a seven-membered lactam sulphonamide moiety at P_3 to P_4 positions, gave inhibitors which showed much more selectivity against serine proteases like factor Xa and trypsin. Examples of other conformationally restricted thrombin inhibitors include compounds like (K_i 0·5 nM) which was approximately1 000-fold less potent against trypsin and inactive against plasmin, tissue plasminogen actiator, activated protein C, plasma kallikrein and chymotrypsin. Inhibitor containing conformationally restricting moieties in the P_3–P_2 region showed improved pharmacokinetics in the rat (61% oral bioavailability, elimination half-life 1 hour). A chemically similar inhibitor, inhibited thrombus formation when administered orally (30 mg/kg; bioavailability 55%; 4 hour duration of action) one hour before induction of stasis.

A number of P_3-position-modified thrombin inhibitors exhibited oral bioavailability in rats and dogs, and were efficacious in a rat $FeCl_3$-induced model of arterial thrombosis. Compounds and the corresponding analogues with an unprotected amino group at the N-terminus, showed selectivity (300–1500-fold selectivity for thrombin compared with trypsin) and oral bioavailability (40–76%) in rats or dogs. The arylsulfonylpropargylglycinamide derivative (K_i values 5, 19000, > 30000 nM, > 200000 and > 200000 nM against thrombin, factor Xa, trypsin, plasmin and tissue plasminogen actiator, respectively) also demonstrated oral activity at a dose of 30 mg/kg in rats. Compound containing a Phe(*p*-CH_2NH_2) residue in the P_1 position, was one of the more potent and selective inhibitors of thrombin (K_i values 6·6 and 14 200 nM against thrombin and trypsin respectively) and showed good oral bioavailability in rats (approximately 70%) but low oral bioavailability in dogs (10–15%). Some of the modified D-Phe-Pro-Arg aldehyde analogues like melagatran are undergoing clinical evaluation. Non-peptide inhibitors of thrombin (obtained by random screening procedures) include compounds based around benzothiophene and other ring systems and cyclic and linear oligocarbamate derivatives. The benzothiophene derivative showed antithrombotic efficacy in a rat model of thrombosis after infusion (ED50 2·3 mg/kg/h). The cyclic oligocarbamate tetramer inhibited thrombin with an apparent K_i of 31 nM.

Ras Protein Farnesyltransferase Inhibitors

Cysteine farnesylation of the ras oncogene product Ras is required for its transforming activity and is catalysed by the enzyme protein farnesyltransferase. The enzyme catalyses the transfer of a farnesyl group from farnesyl diphosphate to a cysteine residue of the protein substrate such as Ras. The enzyme recognises a tetrapeptide sequence (Cys-A-A-X, where A is an aliphatic amino acid and X is Met, Ser, Ala, Cys, or Gln) at the C-terminus of the protein. A closely related enzyme, geranylgeranyltransferase, recognises the Cys-A-A-X motif when X is either Leu or Phe, but transfers a geranylgeranyl group from geranylgeranyl diphosphate. Inhibition of farnesyltransferase represents a possible method for preventing association of Ras p21 to the cell membrane, thereby blocking its cell-transforming capabilities. Such inhibitors may have therapeutic potential as anticancer agents.

Semi-rational design approaches for the discovery of farnesyltransferase inhibitors were based on the tetrapeptide Cys-Val-Phe-Met. SAR studies, followed by the synthesis of conformationally restricted analogues, led to inhibitors, which was effective in prolonging the survival time in athymic mice implanted intraperitoneally with H-*ras*-transformed RAT-1 tumour cells. A non-thiol inhibitor (a methyl ester prodrug) showed activity in several *in vivo* tumour models. Examples of other conformationally restricted tetrapeptide analogues incorporating an N-alkyl amino acid residue include compound (HR-11). Further medicinal chemistry approaches on these modified peptides, including the synthesis of a library of secondary benzylic amines, led to orally active methionine derivatives like compound, which attenuated tumour growth in a nude mouse xenograft model of human pancreatic cancer. Compound showed 21–32% oral bioavailability in mice, rats, and dogs. The methyl ester prodrug suppressed the growth of human lung adenocarcinoma A-549 cells in nude mice by 30–90%, in a dose-dependent manner.

Random screening approaches also produced inhibitors of farnesyltransferase. SAR studies on the random screening lead Z-His-Tyr(OBn)-Ser(OBn)-Trp-D-Ala-NH_2 (PD083176) (IC_{50} 20 nM), including the replacement of the N-terminal Z group and the histidine and Trp residues, led to less potent peptides. However, substitution of the Tyr(OBn) and Ser(OBn) residues did not have much effect on the enzyme inhibitory activity. Based on the SAR and truncation studies, potent inhibitors of farnesyltransferase were obtained. The Z-His derivative inhibited isolated farnesyltransferase but was about 4000-fold less potent against geranylgeranyltransferase-1. Compound was also active in athymic mice implanted with H-ras-F cells. When administered intraperitoneally (150 mg/kg/day once daily) for 14 consecutive days after tumour implantation, the tumour growth was inhibited by approximately 90%.

Random screening approaches followed by medicinal chemistry also resulted in chemically distinct farnesyltransferase inhibitors. Compound was orally active in several human tumour xenograft models in the nude mouse, including tumours originating from colon, lung, pancreas, prostate, and urinary bladder. In the piperazine series of inhibitors, compound blocked tumour growth in mice implanted with H-*ras*-transformed cells (approximately 65% inhibition at 1.4 mg/kg/day). The benzodiazepine derivative inhibited anchorage-independent growth of H-*ras*-transformed Rat-1 cells (EC_{50} 160 nM).

Protein Kinase Inhibitors

The protein kinases are a family of proteins (serine/threonine kinases and tyrosine kinases) involved in signal transduction. Signal transduction via these proteins occurs through selective and reversible phosphorylation of the substrates by the transfer of γ-phosphate of ATP (or GTP) to the hydroxyl groups of serine, threonine and tyrosine residues. A large number of protein kinases (>150) have been identified from mammalian sources, and the human genome is expected to provide many more (>2000) in the future. These kinases play a key role in signal transduction pathways involved in many biological processes, such as control of cell growth, metabolism, differentiation and apoptosis. Along with approaches based on monoclonal antibodies, synthetic small molecule inhibitors of kinases are being actively developed for the treatment of various diseases.

A recent example of the antibody-based approach is the discovery of a monoclonal antibody against human epidermal growth factor receptor (HER2), a family of epidermal growth factor receptor tyrosine kinases, including the epidermal growth factor receptor. Many epithelial tumours, including breast cancer, express excess amounts of these proteins, particularly HER2. HER2 is a tyrosine kinase receptor with extracellular, transmembrane and intracellular domains. Initially, several monoclonal antibodies against the extracellular domain of the HER2 protein were found to inhibit the proliferation of human cancer cells that over-expressed HER2. The antigen binding region of one of the more effective antibodies was fused to the framework region of human IgG to generate a "humanised" monoclonal antibody. The antibody (trastuzumab) was investigated alone and in combination with chemotherapy in women with metastatic breast cancer that overexpressed HER2. Compared with chemotherapy alone, treatment with chemotherapy plus trastuzumab was associated with a significantly higher rate of overall positive response and a longer time to treatment failure. Treatment with trastuzumab was associated with some side-effects (chills, fever, infection and cardiac dysfunction).

Examples of compounds in various stages of clinical development include HER2 kinase inhibitors (ZD-1839, CP-358774 and PD-0183805], Bcr-Abl (CGP-57148) and vascular endothelial growth factor receptor kinase inhibitors (SU-5416). Although many of the starting leads were obtained by random screening approaches, further medicinal chemistry was aided by the availability of a number of crystal structures and other modelling approaches.

Protein–Protein Interaction Inhibitors

Many physiological and pathological processes are mediated by protein–protein interactions. The proteins involved in cell adhesion have been most widely studied. The interactions between the integrin family of heterodimeric cell surface receptors and their protein ligands are fundamental for maintaining cell function, for example by tethering cells at a particular location, facilitating cell migration, or providing survival signals to cells from their environment. Ligands recognised by integrins include extracellular matrix proteins (for example, collagen and fibronectin), plasma proteins like fibrinogen, and cell surface molecules like transmembrane proteins of the immunoglobulin family and cell-bound complement. A number of integrins and their ligands have been associated with many processes involved in cardiovascular diseases (for example, thrombosis involving platelet aggregation), inflammation, cancer (for example, metastasis) and bone disorders. The discovery of platelet aggregation inhibitors by blocking the interaction of platelet glycoprotein IIb/IIIa with its natural ligands (fibrinogen and von Willebrand factor) are examples of inhibitors of protein–protein interactions.

Novel inhibitors of glycoprotein IIb/IIIa and fibrinogen/von Willebrand interaction include injectable peptides (for example integrilin), orally active peptidomimetics that act as competitive inhibitors, and a monoclonal antibody c7E3 (abciximab), which irreversibly binds to GP IIb/IIIa. Administered intravenously, circulating abciximab has a plasma half-life of less than 10 minutes. However, the antibody binds tightly to platelets and provides receptor blockade for a period of up to 15 days.

The design of peptide and non-peptide inhibitors of platelet aggregation was based on the early observations that the integrins recognise peptide sequences like Arg-Gly-Asp present in the larger protein ligands like fibronectin and vitronectin. This led to the synthesis of a large number of analogues containing the Arg-Gly-Asp tripeptide or the chemical features of the tripeptide side chains (for example, the guanidino function and the carboxyl group). SAR studies indicated that a basic functional group that mimics the side chain of the arginine and a carboxylic acid group that mimics the Asp side chain are critical to the receptor binding and platelet aggregation activities of these compounds. In addition, a lipophilic group near the carboxylic acid function was found to enhance the potency of the antagonists. These findings led to the synthesis of more stable cyclic peptides like integrelin and many other compounds containing different non-peptide templates to hold the important functional groups in the proper spatial arrangements. All these approaches have resulted in potent injectable or orally active platelet-aggregation inhibitors. Examples of compounds that have reached the market include the antibody abciximab and the injectable peptide integrilin. Many of the orally active compounds like lamifiban, sibrafiban, xemilofiban, orbofiban and tirofiban have been studied extensively in the clinic. However, most of these failed in the late stages of development.

In addition to the well known examples of IIb/IIIa, antagonists of other integrins like $\alpha_v\beta_3$ (vitronectin receptor), $\alpha_v\beta_5$, $\alpha_v\beta_6$, $\alpha_4\beta_1$ and $\alpha_4\beta_7$ have been synthesised. The design of $\alpha_v\beta_3$ receptor antagonists was based on IIb/IIIa antagonists. Therefore some of the compounds, like isoxazoline-containing mimetic, were antagonists of both $\alpha_v\beta_3$ (IC_{50} 0·7 nM) and IIb/IIIa (IC_{50} 0·34 nM). Some other analogues, were more selective against the $\alpha_v\beta_3$ receptor. For example, the diaminopropionic acid derivative was > 500-fold more potent against $\alpha_v\beta_3$ integrin than against $\alpha_v\beta_5$, $\alpha_5\beta_1$ and GPIIb/IIIa integrins. Compound (SC56631) prevents osteoclast-mediated bone particle degradation. The imidazopyridine analogue was active in the $\alpha_v\beta_3$ binding assay (K_i 45 nM) and showed efficacy in an animal model of restenosis.

Further modifications in compounds such as led to non-peptide vitronectin receptor antagonists that had oral activity. For example, compound (K_i 3.5 nM for $\alpha_v\beta_3$ and 28000 nM for $\alpha IIb\beta_3$) showed between 4–14% oral bioavailability in the rat and dog. Another analogue, SB 265123 (K_i 4.1 nM for $\alpha_v\beta_3$, 1.3 nM for $\alpha_v\beta_5$, 18000 nM for $\alpha_5\beta_1$, and 9000 nM for $\alpha IIb\beta_3$), displayed 100% oral bioavailability in rats, and was active *in vivo* in the ovariectomised rat model of osteoporosis.

$\alpha_4\beta_1$ and $\alpha_5\beta_1$ Antagonists

Cyclic peptide inhibitors of VLA-4 and fibronectin/vascular cell adhesion molecule (VCAM)-1 interaction, for example c(Ile-Leu-Asp-Val-NH(CH_2)$_5$CO) were reported. Several of these inhibitors, for example c(Ile-Leu-Asp-Val-NH(CH_2)$_5$CO), c(Ile-Leu-Asp-Val-NH(CH_2)$_4$CO) and c(MePhe-Leu-Asp-Val-D-Arg-D-Arg), blocked VLA-4/VCAM-1 and VLA-4/fibronectin interactions in *in vitro* assays and inhibited oxazolone and ovalbumin-induced contact hypersensitivity responses in mice. The compounds did not affect cell adhesion mediated by two other integrins, VLA-5 ($\alpha_5\beta_1$) and LFA-1 ($\alpha_L\beta_2$). *p*-Aminophenylacetyl-Leu-Asp-Val derivatives containing various non-peptide residues at the N-terminus are reported to be inhibitors of integrin $\alpha_4\beta_1$. Compound (BIO-1211), showed activity in a model of antigen-induced bronchoconstriction and airway hyper-responsiveness in sheep. In various integrin adhesion assays, showed activity against $\alpha_4\beta_7$, $\alpha 1_5\beta_1$, $\alpha_5\beta_1$, $\alpha_6\beta_1$, $\alpha_L\beta_2$ and $\alpha IIb\beta_3$ integrins at much higher concentrations.

Drug discovery has been a continuously changing and evolving field of science over the years. More and more effective and safer treatments have been discovered. Although chemical and biological sciences have always played a major role in the discovery process, new scientific developments and technologies are altering the ways in which these sciences are applied to the discovery process. Advances in rapid DNA sequencing techniques have resulted in the sequencing of the human genome. Finding the disease-related genes, translating the gene sequences into biologically active proteins and evaluating their functions is likely to lead to new drug discovery targets based on new biochemical pathways. The genomic and proteomic studies may also lead to new therapeutic proteins and antibodies. Given the therapeutic success of the interferons, erythropoietin, granulocyte-macrophage colony-stimulating factor, herceptin (trastuzumab), rituximab, and many others, protein drugs are likely to make many additional therapeutic contributions.

Combinatorial library techniques and natural product libraries are providing large numbers of new compounds for screening. Automated high-throughput screening techniques are being developed continuously to test large numbers of available compounds in multiple screens. A combination of these two technologies, along with the discovery of new target proteins (receptors, enzymes, etc.), has the potential to generate leads for various drug discovery programmes. However, before the leads can be taken seriously, it is essential to validate the target appropriately. Otherwise, the optimised leads are likely to fail in the later stages of development. In many cases where some treatments exist along with some knowledge about the causes of the disease, the need for target validation and development of the relevant biological models is less stringent. The discovery of new medicines in these fields becomes a continuous process of identifying medicines that are more efficacious and convenient to administer in a larger number of patients, and display the best possible toxicity profile.

The availability of leads along with advances in multiple parallel solid-phase synthetic and purification techniques would enable the lead optimisation procedure to be carried out in a relatively short period of time. The design strategies for the lead optimisation are likely to be a combination of the types of approaches highlighted in the examples described above. SAR studies, along with structural and modelling studies using cloned proteins (receptors, enzymes, etc.), are likely to make the lead optimisation procedure somewhat more rational. The availability of cloned receptor subtypes and various members of the enzyme classes in the early stages of the programme can be used to build selectivity into the receptor ligands and enzyme inhibitors. Better understanding of the signalling processes will enable the cellular processes to be controlled in a more efficient manner.

2

Clinical Data Management System

This article is intended to be an overview of clinical data management systems and the processes they support. Data management systems are highly dependent on the size and complexity of the organization using them. Systems can range from a set of SAS data sets to a fully integrated, distributed set of applications using a relational database. The entire data management process may employ a variety of technical solutions.

Background

The information presented here is based on experience with processes and technology in a large international pharmaceutical company. Many of these concepts are employed in smaller pharmaceutical companies and contract research organizations (CROs) but on a lesser scale.

Re-engineering

The pharmaceutical industry is under constant pressure to bring drugs to market more quickly and less expensively, without compromising the quality of the products. The desire to achieve a profitable balance between these three objectives—speed, cost, and quality—results in perpetual "*re-engineering.*" The investment put into developing and implementing a solid database and streamlining data management tools and processes can contribute greatly to the success of this effort.

How Technology Is Driving Changes in Data Management

The introduction and proliferation of the Internet and web-based applications is having a profound impact on the conduct of clinical trials. The Internet provides us with the ability to communicate easily with CROs and investigators; and them with us, without compromising corporate security. Data sets can easily be placed on a secure web site for being reviewed and updated by a partner. Remote data entry will reach its full potential as a result of the introduction and acceptance of internet technology.

Study Setup

Standardization

To avoid redundancy, many parts of the study and setup processes can be standardized and reused. For example, as case report forms (CRFs) are developed for use across studies, the corresponding components of the study definition (questions, response values), the validation checks, reports, and extract data structures can be reused as well, especially within a drug project. This standardization allows for more efficient use of resources and systems, as well as realization of benefits in CRF design, study definition, validation, analysis, reporting, metrics, and training. Standards for data collection

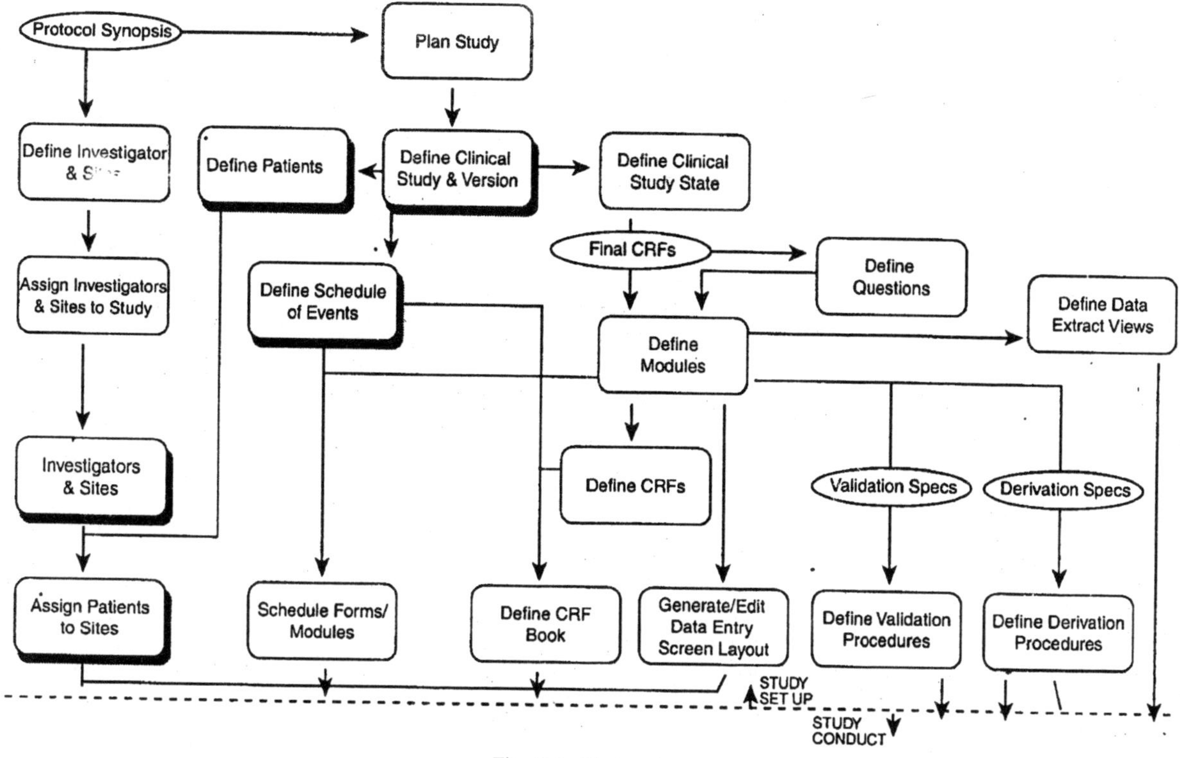

Fig. 2.1. Study setup.

and processing are also necessary to fulfill the reporting requirements for pooled analyses across a project (e.g., safety updates, integrated reports, summaries).

Protocol Development

The protocol must contain a clear statement of the objectives of the investigation (primary and secondary endpoints) and the methods of analysis to be used. The various sections may be written by the appropriate team members and assembled by the clinical representative who is the protocol author. Once the protocol is complete, the CRF is designed. The CRF is the principal document used to collect the study data and guide the study definition in the data management system.

In-House vs. Outsourcing to CROs

Once the project team completes a protocol synopsis, in-house resources should be evaluated. Consideration is given to the type of study required along with the study's priority within the project. The advantages of doing the data management in-house include:

1. All data for project resides on one database
2. Full control over study set-up
3. Re-use of tools already developed
4. Real-time access to data
5. Control over study costs.

If in-house resources are limited and the decision is made to outsource data management activities, the planning process begins by creating a detailed scope of work statement and issuing the request for proposal (RFP). Bids should be solicited from several CROs.

In choosing a CRO, consider the following:

1. Depth of experience in data management
2. Compatibility of computer systems
3. Qualified technical support for data transfer
4. SOPs and policies that meet GCP criteria
5. Interpersonal compatibility
6. Price

Previous sponsor experience with the CRO, the CRO's track record of delivering, and the CRO reputation within the industry are more important than price. When a CRO has been chosen, the contract should include a detailed definition of the scope of work required along with a clear understanding of when the data is considered clean and ready for analysis. A test run of data transfer from the CRO to the sponsor should be done early in the study to identify any problems in data formatting and transmission. The milestones and deliverables must be tracked closely during study conduct in order to ensure that appropriate progress payments are made. The importance of regular communication cannot be overemphasized. The early identification and resolution of technical or process problems is necessary for a smooth database closure and transfer of data. Transfer of data often contains more issues and surprises than anticipated.

The sponsor must take the time to gain a thorough understanding of the CRO's organization, work processes, and needs with respect to the project. In turn, the CRO must understand the sponsor's structure, organization of the project management team, and the rôle the CRO is expected to fill in the overall operational process of the clinical study. This building of mutual understanding takes time and effort but is crucial for project success. The project team requires reports to track the progress of the study including patient enrollment data, discrepancy counts, outstanding CRF pages, and terminated patients (including dropouts). If the CRO already has adequate tracking systems, the reports should be evaluated and adapted as needed. After study completion, a review of the CRO's performance and a written report of lessons learned will provide information for future planning of projects and outsourcing needs. There are several options for the transfer of CRO-processed data back to the sponsor. Most often, the final data are entered into the CRO's database to produce the final study reports with corresponding datasets. However, with the advances in the Internet and in distributed study conduct, it is possible, and generally desirable from the sponsor's viewpoint, for the CRO to enter data directly into the sponsor's database.

CRF Development

The CRF design process can begin either following or concurrent with the protocol development. Well-designed data collection forms are critical to achieve the objectives of the clinical trial. Consideration should be given to the content, format, and layout of the forms since all these factors contribute to the overall quality and accuracy of the data that will be collected, processed, and reported.

Many disciplines should participate in the CRF design stage. The core team will generally consist of representatives from statistics, data management, forms design, medical and clinical monitoring groups, with other specialists, consulting, as necessary. The primary objective of the team in this process is to optimize and balance the following requirements for the CRF:

1. To facilitate the investigational site in filling out the forms correctly
2. To allow for quick and accurate data entry
3. To ensure that data can be analyzed and that they represent the patient's experience for statistical and clinical reporting

4. To facilitate the pooling of data across a project for safety updates and integrated safety and efficacy reporting
5. Consistency within project or area (e.g., pharmacoeconomics, clinical pharmacology) to allow reuse of tools.

The forms should only collect data that are needed for reporting purposes and avoid collecting unnecessary or redundant data. The standardization of CRFs for use across multiple studies results in significant savings in the design, processing, reporting, and training resources required for a clinical study. Forms can be further broken down into modules (e.g., physical exam, vital signs, demography) or groups of questions. The use of these modules allows for greater flexibility when constructing the forms/pages while retaining the standard use of the question groups. A library of forms can be centrally gathered and maintained that includes "global" forms (those that can be used across projects—e.g., adverse events, demography), project or therapeutic standard forms (used across a project), and study specific forms. There are many applications and systems that can be used to design and generate the CRFs. These range from word processing and desktop publishing packages to customized systems that facilitate the maintenance and use of a library of modules/forms and enforce standards. The CRF may also be in an electronic format rather than on paper, as in the case of remote data entry systems.

Randomization

Randomization is the process by which patients are randomly assigned to a treatment group. It is used to reduce the possibility for investigators and study personnel to bias the results (consciously or unconsciously) in favor of one treatment over another in a study. Randomization also allows for maintaining the blinding of a study when the blind must be broken for an individual patient. In most trials, the randomization data will be kept blinded until data are considered clean and after exclusions are decided to avoid influencing the results of a study. At the end of the trial, it is a requirement to confirm the integrity of the blinding. There must be documentation or an audit trail of all blind breaks and of all data changes post unblinding. The statistician plays an important role in specifying appropriate parameters to be utilized in generating the randomization. The randomization specifications include treatments, centers, block size, study design, blinding requirements, and stratification factors. It is through the usage of stratification or grouping criteria that patient differences can be minimized between treatment groups. Randomization codes are used for packaging and labeling study medications. The systems that are used to generate labels for the treatment bottles may be independent of those that produce the randomization.

Study Definition

A study definition is used to identify to the system characteristics about the data fields stored within, criteria for acceptance of those data, as well as extract formats and file structures. These characteristics may include database variable name, data type (numeric, character, date/time), question name and label, short reference name (e.g., SAS variable name), format (e.g., ddmmyy), field length, acceptable response values (e.g., male/female), coding formats (e.g., 1 = yes, 2 = no), and validation information (e.g., validate against specific thesaurus). Data entry screen layout is also part of the study definition. The ease (or difficulty) of data entry must be balanced with the utility of the data extract file structure, both of which are greatly determined by this process. Therefore, good database design requires the close cooperation and compromise between data management and statistics to ensure quality and efficiency throughout the data processing, management, analysis, and reporting lifecycle.

Many database systems have a catalog of questions or other global library capabilities to facilitate the storage and retrieval of data definition objects. Using these objects as "*building blocks*," standard modules can be established and used across many studies.

This standardization saves considerable resources, not only in the study set-up process but also in training data entry personnel, coding validation checks, producing monitor reports, and for analysis/reporting. The continued usage of these standards can also allow for constant streamlining and improvement based on experience, with appropriate maintenance and controls. Related to the study definition process, most systems require a schedule of events to be defined to instruct the system when to expect certain forms for tracking purposes and to associate date/visit with the form.

Data Quality Specifications

A data quality plan is a tool to aid in the implementation of data quality. The plan should be developed as soon as the protocol is finalized. Data quality is a shared responsibility across all functions. For example, the monitor assures quality by source document verification (SDV), and the clinician reviews listings of individual patient profiles and study "*outliers.*" New data and corrections to data are usually processed nightly through a batch validation program in the clinical database. The batch validation program will identify new discrepancies that have appeared since the last execution of the validation. The program will also resolve any previously generated discrepancies that are no longer valid because either the data or the associated validation criteria have changed. Batch validation may also be run "on demand" if immediate validation of data is required. With the help of the study team, data management usually prepares the validation procedures document to identify specific variables that must be validated. Edit checks may be defined as part of the data structure and executed during data entry. Programmed checks are user-defined checks executed off-line during batch validation.

These programmed checks include

1. Standard checks developed for all standard CRF pages
2. Project specific checks used within each project
3. Study specific checks used for study specific pages of the CRF.

The completed validation checks should be run against test data to ensure they are written correctly. As the data is received and validated by these procedures, it is important to review the output and add or delete edit checks as appropriate.

Study Conduct

Receipt of Data

Technology is providing a number of options for the transmission of data from the investigator, CRO, or lab, back to the sponsor site. Imaging technology allows for the capture and efficient storage of all CRFs for use in data tracking and electronic submissions. Current and near future imaging technology will allow us to store an electronic copy of signed CRFs as well as easily archive all study-related documents. Images can be read using optical character recognition and bar coding techniques. These technologies, once perfected, will greatly reduce the manpower required to index and enter the data on CRFs into the data management systems. Imaging technology is currently being employed to route documents through the appropriate study conduct workflow.

There have been numerous advances in the area of remote data acquisition. Data can be collected at the site via an electronic CRF or a hand held electronic device. These data can then be transmitted back to the sponsoring company and batch loaded into the sponsor's clinical trial database. Remote data entry technology currently allows for the easy definition and distribution of the electronic CRFs to the investigator site. Some online cleaning can be performed as the data are entered before transmission to the sponsor site, where additional quality checks are applied and transmitted back to the investigator site. This iterative process allows for collection and generally faster cleaning of clinical data. Data can also be transmitted from the CRO, investigator, or lab via electronic data transfer. Laboratory data are most often transmitted this way due to the volume of the data. The data are then batch loaded into the sponsor's clinical trial database. Fax transmissions are often received from the investigator. The fax transmission can be printed out and then data entered, or the fax can go directly to a fax server or be passed through a scanner and an electronic image of the form/document can be created. This image can then be stored, or data entered either by optical character recognition, manual data entry, or a combination of the two. Many studies are still conducted by traditional paper-based methods. CRFs and documents are sent by post (often overnight) to the sponsor site where they are data entered and filed. Today's technology allows for the conduct at multiple sites, with the ability to pool data for interim analyses and integrated safety summaries. The size and complexity of a study should determine which technology should be employed. Most large pharmaceutical companies have a portfolio of study conduct technologies to employ.

Data Entry

In a paper-based data flow, as CRFs are received by the sponsor, the pages or forms can be "logged in" or identified to the system. A document number may be used to uniquely identify a page for further tracking within the database. This document identifier can be scanned from a barcode printed on a form, created using a document number generator, or manually entered. Once the form is recognized as received by the system, a data entry operator can start entry into the database. In the data definition process, screen layouts will have been defined to facilitate the accurate and speedy entry. Some validation or discrepancy checks can be designed to trigger at entry. For example, if a data entry operator attempts to violate the criteria defined to the system for a particular data field (e.g., entering character information into a numerically defined field), a discrepancy can be raised to alert the operator for acceptance or correction to the data. If the entry correctly reflects what is written on the CRF, the value can be accepted and a discrepancy noted for later follow up.

Many systems allow for the option to perform an independent second pass of data entry to ensure that data that is recorded on the CRF matches what is entered into the database. Second pass (double key) should be performed by a different data entry operator than the first pass. In the cases where the first pass and second pass do not match, the data entry operator is prompted and can accept either entry. An audit trail is kept by the system, and reports may be generated to document changes performed during the second-pass process. Data entry conventions are recommended to assist in the consistent handling of the data. These conventions should include guidelines and rules for dealing with expected (and unexpected) issues arising on the forms. Some examples include handling missing data, illegible text or data, investigator comments, acceptable abbreviations, etc.

Not all data are received by the sponsor site on CRFs or paper. For example, data may be entered remotely at the investigator site or generated as an output file from instrumentation and then electronically transferred to the sponsor site via the Web/Internet, other connections, or even diskettes. Alternatives to traditional data entry also include using optical character recognition (OCR) technology. This scanning technique used to populate the database may require the CRFs to be designed with special considerations as to the density of the forms, increased use of coded fields, and legibility of the completed forms.

Discrepancy Management

In addition to the discrepancies generated as a result of study definition (univariate discrepancies), discrepancies may also arise when a batch validation detects data inconsistencies (univariate and multivariate discrepancies). Discrepancies are also identified by a visual review of the data, e.g., monitoring lists, SDV review. Discrepancies may also be created by people responsible for data analysis (e.g., statisticians, pharmacoeconomists, clinical pharmacologists). All discrepancies and data fields requiring verification or clarification are tracked using the clinical database. Quality control for clinical data within data management includes computerized validation of data in the database and second-pass data entry. These activities are performed to ensure that data are complete, accurate, and compliant with the protocol. In addition to discrepancy reports, verification of randomly selected fields may be used to assess the data quality. Discrepancy reports are prepared for investigator review and correction. The sponsor translates the computer output into user-friendly reports. There is direct communication between the investigational site coordinator and the data manager for any error messages that may need clarification. Corrections are made by the site representative directly onto the CRF page and then faxed back to the sponsor. If fax technology is not used, a copy of the corrected CRF page is made and sent to the sponsor by mail or courier. Good clinical practice requires that all corrections must be dated and initialed by the site representative. Once the corrected copies are received, the data manager makes the change in the clinical database. An electronic audit trail is maintained in the clinical database of all data entered and changed. This audit trail tracks the date and time stamp and the identification of the person making the entry correction or change.

Ongoing Monitoring

A number of query tools may be used to track the quality and completeness of CRF and non-CRF data. Many of the tracking reports reside within the data management system, but tracking may also be done using simple ad hoc query tools such as Brio or even SAS. An example of on-going monitoring is the tracking of study enrollment by investigators. Inclusion and exclusion criteria are usually listed on the CRF. The investigator reviews the criteria and either admits or excludes the subject from continuing in the study. This may be reviewed and monitored manually by the monitor reviewing the subjects' medical records to confirm eligibility during source document verification or through reports/ listing of this particular patient data highlighting any irregularities.

Database Closure

At study completion, the data manager is responsible for assuring that the data are clean and then prepares to lock the study/close the database. The purpose of locking the study is to ensure that a full audit trail of any changes exists once the study/patients have been unblinded. Database closure marks the end of the study conduct phase and the beginning of the analysis and reporting phase. The standard definition of clean data is:

1. All outstanding data in-house
2. All outstanding discrepancies resolved
3. SDV completed
4. Clinical review of data complete
5. The allocation of preferred terms to CRF verbatim terms reviewed and complete
6. All non-CRF data revised and processed.

The data management system through a series of reports and internal checks provides the documentation and verification that data have been completely cleaned. When the criteria for clean data are met, a formal sign-off meeting is held for team members and ad hoc functional representatives. With the database closure form signed off, the data manager locks the database. Locking limits the ability to change values for specific privileged users. It also starts a new audit trail of any changes made after locking. The randomization codes may now be entered allowing the statistician to review the data in an unblinded fashion. Any pharmacokinetic data are also loaded at this time. Data management then freezes the database. No changes may be made to the existing database and no new data may be added.

Study Performance Metrics

Performance metrics are used by the study team to track and manage the study. The metrics will aid in the early identification and resolution of problems that may affect data quality and study timelines. For example, metrics involving patient enrollment, visits, forms flow, and discrepancies may be tracked using the clinical database.

Laboratory Data

It is common practice to employ outside laboratories to perform testing for safety and efficacy measures in clinical trials. Along with the results, these laboratories will also provide the units and normal ranges for the tests performed. Since the laboratories are typically utilized by many patients in a study or even across studies, it is practical for the units and ranges to be received and entered once in the system and then linked internally to the patient data to which they apply. This principle of centrally storing values that can be shared across the system is also desirable for maintaining the conversion factors used in deriving lab results into standardized units.

Thesaurus

Medical dictionaries are utilized extensively in clinical trials to assign common terminology to medical events such as adverse events reporting and clinical diagnoses, as well as to link medication trade names to their generic components. Thesaurus management systems facilitate both the ongoing maintenance of base dictionaries (e.g., COSTART, WHOART, MEDDRA) and the linkages to the reported and entered data.

Pharmacokinetic Data

In blinded studies, entering of pharmacokinetic (PK) data on an ongoing basis could jeopardize the blinding of the study. Consequently, the PK data are often entered into a separate database. The data is usually loaded into the data management system only after the study is closed and ready for analysis.

Analysis and Reporting

Extracting Data

A well-designed data management system typically will focus on the primary objective to facilitate the collection and cleaning of clinical data. Although it must also support analysis and reporting, it is not always possible to achieve an equal balance across all these requirements; therefore, data are usually analyzed outside of the clinical database. Data extraction is the process of selecting and copying data fields to an external file. Data extraction procedures generally produce files that are simply a reflection of the database. The data can then be manipulated and/or transposed to achieve an optimal structure for analysis and reporting requirements. Additional fields can be derived, response values standardized or decoded, and variables labeled more clearly. Data may be organized by type of data, such as adverse events, laboratory data, demography, physical exam, etc. Since many of these categories of data exist across clinical trials, standard file structures can be designed and implemented. This standardization allows for the reuse of validated software as well as facilitates the pooling of data across studies for use in project safety summaries and other data reporting across studies.

Derivations

The derivation of data points can be conducted in a number of different ways. Usually they are calculated either in the clinical trials database or as part of the creation of the analysis ready, value added data sets. It is advisable to store derivations for values that are not likely to change, and for which the derivation algorithm is commonly accepted in the clinical trials database. Derivations that are a result of a constantly changing database, or of a complex algorithm particular to a given study, should be conducted outside the clinical trials database and as part of the creation of the analysis ready, value added data sets.

Reporting Tools

Reporting and analysis is usually a continuous process throughout the life of a study. The "final report" is the culmination of the efforts involved in conducting a clinical trial. For ongoing reporting during the life of a study, there are a large number of reporting tools available on the market for the querying of clinical trials data. Each database has a number of tools that are appropriate for creating easy to mildly complex reports against the clinical trials database (i.e., Oracle has several reporting tools). There are also a number of user-friendly query tools that are designed to retrieve data from a number of different databases. Brio can generate query results that join multiple tables and give quite a bit of flexibility over report format and features such as sorting. More complex reports, such as a "missing and overdue forms report," are usually written in third generation language (3gl) such as C++, or taking the data outside the database and using external programming tools. For the final statistical listings and tables, SAS is the industry standard. Where reporting is concerned, the tool that best performs the job should be the one selected.

Electronic Submission of CRFs to Regulatory Agencies

Sponsors may be required to provide selected CRFs as part of the overall package submitted to the regulatory authorities. Recently, regulatory agencies have been encouraging the electronic submission of these CRFs. Given a comprehensive and well-indexed imaging system, it may be possible to subset the requested images and electronically transfer the file with relative ease. For the situations where these files must be manually compiled, a different process may be employed. As CRFs are identified for inclusion, a scanner can be used to produce .pdf files (via Adobe Acrobat Exchangez). An index is required to facilitate the retrieval of the forms, as desired. The collection of indexed images is then transferred onto CD-ROM for the electronic submission.

System Issues

Year 2000

The approach of 2000 A.D. had caused the technology industry to take an in-depth look at all of the automated solutions employed in the industry. Every place where a date was used in an application was examined. Two digit dates were particularly troublesome as we approached the new millennium. The validation effort consumed an enormous amount of resources, both in-house and at the software vendors.

Upgrades

Whether your clinical trials management system was developed in-house or purchased from a vendor, eventually you will have the opportunity to experience an upgrade. At some point you will probably need to upgrade the operating system on the PC or server, the version of the database that your application is built on, or the application software itself. Worst case is when you have to upgrade all of these at once. Ideally your application environment consists of a fully functional and separate test environment. It is in this area that you would test any upgrades. Testing should consist of executing documented test scripts with the goal of proving that existing functionality still works and any advertised new functionality also works. Ideally you would try to avoid upgrading multiple pieces of your environment at the same time, as in the worst case example above. Although multiple rounds of testing is resource intensive, it is much easier to determine the source of any problems and resolve them in a controlled environment. This is a point to be aware of when choosing clinical trial software: Will the vendor support multiple versions of an operating system and database? This will give you the time to test the worst case scenario in a two-phase approach.

Conversion vs. Migration vs. Upgrade

Over time software becomes obsolete, as does hardware. Upgrading to the latest version of the software or hardware is probably the easiest path. But when you find that you must move to a completely new hardware or application environment, there are several things to consider. Often software and hardware vendors can provide the service of migrating or converting your existing data from one system to another. One should carefully investigate what this process would entail. Conversion can be a painful and extremely resource intensive operation. You should realistically look at whether it is feasible to let ongoing trials complete in the legacy system or whether it is feasible to re-enter data into the new system for smaller studies. These strategies are often much more straightforward and less error prone than a conversion would be.

System Validation

Computer systems validation (CSV) is an ongoing process that involves the evaluation and documentation of all components of a system during its life cycle to ensure compliance with approved user requirements and quality standards. A system is defined not only by its hardware and software, but also by the processes surrounding its use. CSV is applicable to a system used to collect, process, capture, or manipulate data that may be included in a submission to a regulatory authority. Validation requires establishing documented evidence that a system meets its predefined specifications and quality attributes. Validation seeks to assure that a system has been developed, tested, and implemented in a controlled manner, performs and will continue to perform accurately and reliably, and is secure from unauthorized or accidental change. In addition to documenting the development and implementation of system components, validation includes documenting hardware and software change control, security management, and training.

Audit Trails and Change Control

It is important to be able to track the reason and source for any changes to data in your clinical trials database. Many applications have built in audit trail capabilities that track the date, time, and ID of the person entering or changing data through the application. Some applications will even prompt for a data change reason. Any changes or deletion of data should be done through the application whenever possible. Sometimes however, the volume of the data to be modified or complexity of the changes requires external intervention. If you plan to modify data in the clinical trials database from outside of the application, the process should be very carefully documented. As in any software development, the program or script that will be run to enter or update data should have a design document, that outlines the modules purpose and expected performance, as well as a set of fully executed test cases. It is common to keep all requests for manual data changes and data change scripts with their respective documents in one directory as backup for a data change log.

3

CLINICAL EVOLUTION OF DRUG

The process of developing a new drug, from the identification of a potential drug candidate to postmarketing surveillance, is extremely complex. The drug development process requires input from various members of a multidisciplinary team and the conduct of numerous studies. The time from drug discovery to marketing takes an average of 13 years. Once a chemical is identified as a new drug candidate, extensive preclinical analyses must be completed before the drug can be tested in humans. The pharmacology, toxicology, and preclinical pharmacokinetics must be characterized. The formulations of the drug product that were used in the preclinical studies may be different from the formulation of the final drug product, which may require that additional formulation work and pharmacokinetic analyses be performed. If the characteristics of the new drug candidate are acceptable for all of the preclinical assessments, it may then be tested in humans. The new drug candidate, at this point, enters the clinical research stage of drug development.

Clinical research represents a vital stage in the development process a stage that is no less daunting than the preclinical research stage. The data obtained from the first-time-in-human, Phase 1 pharmacokinetic studies, and initial safety evaluations in healthy volunteers can make or break the entire developmental program for a drug candidate. The sponsoring company, of course, hopes that the data collected in these initial studies will show minimal safety concerns over an adequate dose range. The pharmacokinetic data can then be used to help design future studies in which efficacy and long-term safety are assessed and additional pharmacokinetic and pharmacodynamic data are collected. Although the basic designs of the initial single and multiple dose-escalating studies are generally straight-forward (but the starting dose is often intensely debated), it is imperative that these studies and future studies be designed to address specific questions. The questions vary depending on numerous specific considerations, including the targeted disease characteristics (e.g., acute or chronic); desired safety, efficacy, and pharmacokinetic evaluations; and assessment of clinical pharmacology (e.g., dosage formulations or dose frequency).

Basic study procedures must also be considered. Thus, the design, conduct, data reporting and analysis, and production of the final study reports can be completed only through the coordinated efforts of a multidisciplinary drug development team. For every clinical study, input is required from multiple personnel with various areas of expertise. Members of a drug development team include physicians, scientists, pharmacists, project managers, statisticians, computer programers, study monitors, regulatory experts, and for some studies, a representative of the formulations group. While some team members may be able to perform multiple tasks, no one team member has the expertise or the time to do everything required to conduct a clinical study. In addition, some members may have overlapping abilities, but other members with particular expertise may be called upon. For example, pharmacokineticists are the experts in pharmacokinetics, but they may also be knowledgeable in pharmaceutics, biostatistics, and clinical care. However, scientists (PhDs) are trained primarily in basic research, while physicians (MDs) are trained in clinical medicine. Since a single drug development program is derived from both of these distinct disciplines, considerable overlap, cooperation, and coordination are necessary to take a drug successfully and efficiently from discovery to market.

Clinical drug development is generally divided into four phases: Phase 1 through Phase 4. For each study conducted within a particular phase, specific information is collected according to the requirements for individual drugs being developed. Collection of safety, efficacy, and pharmacokinetic data is the focus of most clinical trials. Although these topics appear to be distinct disciplines, they are intertwined and represent different ways of evaluating the intrinsic properties of a drug. While the safety, efficacy, and pharmacokinetics of a drug may be assessed in most studies, the team must establish the type and extent of information to be collected, which will vary based upon the specific objectives and designs of the studies. A critical function of the drug development team is the development of the study protocol. The study protocol must clearly describe the study design and methodology that will be used to achieve the study objectives. Input from non-medical and non-scientific members of the team, such as marketing and information technology experts, also is helpful in establishing development strategies and in designing and conducting of clinical studies. Finally, project planning efforts can synchronize team efforts, help contain the soaring costs of pharmaceutical research, and coordinate international development efforts.

The drug development team's primary goal is to gain approval to market the drug, which requires that a marketing application be submitted to a regulatory agency (e.g., a New Drug Application [NDA] is submitted to the Food and Drug Administration [FDA] in the United States and to the Health Products and Food Branch [HPFB] in Canada, while a Marketing Authorization Application [MAA] is submitted to European regulatory agencies). During the conduct of the studies and the compilation and analyses of the data, the team must consider and evaluate many issues, such as how to collect, categorize, and report adverse events. All of these decisions will affect the marketing application that is submitted and may ultimately define how the drug is to be administered. Many of the decisions to be made by the team, and particularly by the investigators, pose ethical dilemmas. Legislation has been enacted to protect human research subjects. Recently, the most pressing ethical dilemma facing the clinical research scientist concerned biotechnology and genetic engineering research. Frequent changes in the regulations and guidelines of various regulatory agencies, differences in interpretations of these rules, and special reporting mechanisms for adverse events represent only a few of the challenges facing a drug development team. Due to continuous advances in scientific information, understanding of disease processes, and gene therapy, change continues to be the rule in modern drug development. However, through the efficient application of sound scientific principles in an ethical manner and with a coordinated team effort, effective new therapies can continue to be developed and marketed.

Roles of the Drug Development Team Members

Physicians

The physician's contribution to drug development and the physician's role on a drug development team have changed over the last few decades. Before the 1960s, medical departments of pharmaceutical companies were primarily composed of physicians who were routinely involved in responding to drug information requests rather than developing new drugs. The Kefauver–Harris Amendment, enacted in 1962, required pharmaceutical companies to demonstrate before marketing that a drug was efficacious, which necessitated that physicians increase their presence on drug development teams. Along with the advent of additional governmental regulations, the increase in complexity of medical knowledge has mandated that physicians become an integral member of any drug development team. In fact, because of the different roles of the physician within an organization, companies may now have various departments (e.g., a clinical research department and a clinical safety department) within the medical department.

Although physicians are trained in patient care, physicians who are typically employed by pharmaceutical companies have more training in scientific methodology than those in the past. The physician on the team is the one qualified to follow the progress of each patient enrolled in a clinical trial and to interpret the results. Some physicians continue to spend time treating patients at a university hospital or a specific clinic where their specialty can be utilized and practiced, which allows these physicians to maintain sharp diagnostic skills. Also, some may perform basic research in academic settings to develop or maintain their knowledge and skills in basic research. However, much of today's clinical research is actually conducted by investigators who are not employed by the company sponsoring the development of the drug. The physician on the drug development team must help in the selection of appropriate investigators to conduct the clinical studies. Pharmaceutical physicians may rely on colleagues who are experts in their respective fields and who have appropriate patient populations and facilities for the targeted research project. The physician is also the expert who deals with emergency situations that may arise during the course of a clinical research project, such as an overdose or severe adverse experience (SAE) that might be experienced with the drug. Similarly, the physician assists investigators who are responsible for evaluating the severity of adverse experiences (AEs) and determining the causal relationship of the AEs to the drug under development.

The physician's involvement in clinical research does not end with the completion of the clinical study. Medical reports, clinical study reports, and sections of NDAs must be written. Interactions with regulatory agencies that require the physician's input may occur frequently. Physicians in clinical research may also be called upon to promote new drugs in a scientific environment by organizing symposia and workshops and by reviewing journal advertisements and promotional material for medical validity and accuracy. The role of the physician in a clinical drug development program has expanded and has been refined in the last 40 years. Physicians increasingly contribute clinical and scientific expertise and administrative skills. Many physicians on drug development teams today spend most of their time designing and implementing studies and interpreting and reporting data rather than being in direct contact with patients. An experienced clinician is an important member of any drug development team.

Scientists

While a drug development team may have only one primary physician, it may have multiple scientists. Pharmacokineticists, pharmacologists, toxicologists, and pharmaceutical scientists are all involved in the clinical development of drugs. The contributions of scientists to a drug development project are derived from their experience in both scientific methodology and basic research.

Although physicians are trained in patient care, scientists are trained in problem-solving skills related to scientific research. To obtain a doctoral degree, a scientist must conduct research and write a dissertation that covers a topic of sufficient scope and depth. During this process, the scientist learns how to solve problems from different perspectives. The scientist also collects extensive data and performs data analyses, thereby gaining valuable insight into the considerations necessary to determine the feasibility of collecting data in a clinical trial. Also, some scientists, such as pharmacokineticists with a pharmacy background, may receive some clinical experience during their training as a scientist.

Scientists help design major portions of study protocols and clinical case report forms (CRFs). The study protocol is the overall plan that the study follows, and it must contain certain types of information, including the following: (1) background data on the targeted disease; (2) the empirical and structural formula of the drug being studied; (3) preliminary pharmacology and toxicology of the drug (specific study objectives and designs); (4) the methods and materials to be used in the study; (5) information regarding drug packaging, labeling, dosage forms, and decoding procedures; (6) overdose management; (7) patient discontinuation procedures; (8) explanation of informed consent and provisions regarding institutional review board approval; and (9) any relevant references and appendices. The CRFs are the forms on which individual patient data are recorded during a clinical trial. From these data, clinical and statistical analyses are performed. All the information that is stipulated in the study protocol must be collected on the CRFs. In conjunction with non-scientific personnel, scientists are responsible for ensuring that the CRFs will capture the appropriate information for each study subject according to the objectives, tests, and evaluations stipulated in the protocol. Careful attention must be given to the administration of special tests or collection of samples so that the timing of the assessments or sample collections do not conflict.

Experience in basic research enables the scientist to function as an important link between the basic research labs within the company and the drug development team. Departments specializing in drug metabolism, microbiology, pharmacology, and toxicology need feedback from early human safety and pharmacokinetic studies so they can continue to plan and conduct appropriate long-term animal studies. Thus, communication between the clinical scientist and the basic scientist is important throughout the progress of the drug development program. Because clinical research has become increasingly more scientific, experts in the methodology of science are necessary for a complete research program. The drug development team's scientists may account for much of the scientific expertise, but the roles of the research team overlap to form a scientifically sound, medically astute cohesive group. In addition to scientific expertise, use of the scientist's administrative talents, such as organizational skills and familiarity with personnel practices, enables effective drug development. Thus, scientists with these skills are often employed in management positions in many organizations.

Pharmacists

The pharmacist's role on the drug development team has greatly expanded the professional opportunities of individuals with backgrounds in pharmacy. Pharmacists can provide valuable therapeutic insight into medical research. Training of pharmacists as clinical scientists with both clinical skills and scientific research skills continues to be an emphasis at many pharmacy schools. Several programs have been devised for the education and development of the pharmacist as clinical scientist. Pharmacists have a broad knowledge in both clinical medicine and pharmaceutics, and therefore are able to bridge the gap between the clinic and the laboratory. Pharmacists' training focuses on drug therapies in disease states, whereas physicians' training focuses on the diagnosis of disease states. Studies regarding drug interaction, positive control, or drug comparison involve drugs that have been studied and marketed. Pharmacists can help in the design of such trials because of their knowledge of marketed drugs. Additional roles of pharmacists appear in the areas of drug information and education and training. Pharmacists have the appropriate expertise in drug therapy to answer inquiries from physicians (and other health professionals) concerning both marketed and investigational drug products. Similarly, the clinic/laboratory bridge that the pharmacist builds makes this team member especially well suited to educate and train new employees in drug development. By offering both general and special skills, the research pharmacist blends clinical medicine with pharmaceutical science and is well qualified as an educator and drug information specialist.

Non-Scientific Personnel

Drug development includes many tasks that may not require the specialized expertise of a physician or a scientist. Administrative skills, creativity, and excellent communication abilities, which are qualities not necessarily emphasized within traditional medical and scientific educational curricula, may be required for many of these tasks. The administrative skills necessary for drug development include incorporating seemingly disparate but vitally linked concepts into a single overall plan. Integration planning may mean organizing study files into a logical sequence or helping to assemble the various parts of an NDA. In the first example, files must be set up in a way that can facilitate internal quality assurance audits and FDA inspections. In the second example, knowledge of the FDA's regulations and good abstracting capabilities are required.

Creativity is a quality that cannot be developed through formal training. Creativity requires bold conjecture and it expresses itself in newer, better ways to accomplish the same goals. An example of creativity in clinical drug research might involve the development of a variable report that could support all of the different research documents that are generated by drug research teams. With such a variable report, common information need not be recreated each time another document is generated. Excellent communication skills may be the most important quality for individuals working in drug development, even for these with strong medical backgrounds. Clinical research requires extensive interactions with personnel within the organization and with outside vendors or clinical sites. The information flow must be both efficient and accurate. For example, marketing departments must communicate frequently with medical departments so that marketing studies, advertising, and package inserts can be planned and evaluated. Individuals who lack strong science backgrounds but who have excellent communication skills often act as liaisons in these situations.

One aspect of clinical research that requires extensive contribution by the drug development team personnel is study monitoring. Study monitors oversee the planning, initiation, conduct, and data processing of clinical studies. While monitoring studies, monitors must communicate frequently with investigators and help ensure the data are being collected properly, FDA regulations are being followed, and any administrative problems are resolved as quickly as possible. Although monitors traditionally have had a non-scientific background, many monitors today have training in the basic sciences, and some even have advanced degrees, which allows them to better understand the scientific aspects of the project. Effective study monitors have a wide range of talents. The many facets of a clinical research program afford individuals with varying types of training, education, and experience, the opportunity to contribute to the drug development process. Although some tasks clearly require the clinical or scientific expertise of a physician or a scientist, other tasks are better suited to those individuals with less specialized and more general capabilities.

Stages in Clinical Drug Development

Before clinical drug development can begin, many years of preclinical development occur, millions of dollars are spent, and countless decisions are made. Basic research teams consisting of chemists, pharmacologists, biologists, and biochemists first identify promising therapeutic categories and classes of compounds. One or more compounds are selected for secondary pharmacology evaluations and for both acute and subchronic toxicology testing in animal models. A compound that is pharmacologically active and safe in at least two non-human species may then be selected for study in humans. Before the drug can be tested in humans, an Investigational New Drug (IND) application, which contains supporting preclinical information and the proposed clinical study designs, must be filed with an appropriate regulatory agency.

Clinical drug development follows a sequential process. By convention, development of a new drug in humans is divided into four phases: preapproval segments (Phases 1 through 3) and a postapproval segment (Phase 4). The definitions of the three preapproval phases have relatively clear separations. However, the different phases refer to different types of studies rather than a specific time course of studies. For example, bioequivalence studies and drug–drug interaction studies are both Phase 1 studies, but they may be conducted after Phase 3 studies have been initiated. The generalized sequence of studies may be tailored to each new drug during development.

Phase 1

After the appropriate regulatory agency has approved a potential drug for testing in humans, Phase 1 of the clinical program begins. The primary goal of Phase 1 studies is to demonstrate safety in humans and to collect sufficient pharmacokinetic and pharmacological information to permit the determination of the dose strength and regimen for Phase 2 studies. Phase 1 studies are closely monitored, are typically conducted in healthy adult subjects, and are designed to meet the primary goal (i.e., to obtain information on the safety, pharmacokinetics, and pharmacologic effects of the drug). In addition, the metabolic profile, adverse events associated with increasing dosages, and evidence of efficacy may be obtained. Because most compounds are available for initial studies as an oral formulation, the initial pharmacokinetic profile usually includes information about absorption. Additional studies, such as drug–drug interactions, assessment of bioequivalence of various formulations, or other studies that involve normal subjects, are included in Phase 1.

Generally, the first study in humans is a rising, single-dose tolerance study. The initial dose may be based on animal pharmacology or toxicology data, such as 10% of the no-effect dose. Doses are increased gradually according to a predetermined scheme, often some modification of the Fibonacci dose escalation scheme, until an adverse event is observed that satisfies the predetermined criteria of a maximum tolerated dose (MTD). Although the primary objective is the determination of acute safety in humans, the studies are designed to collect meaningful pharmacokinetic information. Efficacy information or surrogate efficacy measurements also may be collected. However, because a multitude of clinical measurements and tests must be performed to assess safety, measurements of efficacy parameters must not compromise the collection of safety and pharmacokinetic data. Appropriate biological samples for pharmacokinetic assessment, typically blood and urine, should be collected at discrete time intervals based upon extrapolations from the pharmacokinetics of the drug in animals. Depending on the assay sensitivity, the half- life and other pharmacokinetic parameters in healthy volunteers should be able to be evaluated, particularly at the higher doses. The degree of exposure of the drug is an important factor in understanding the toxicologic results of the study. Pharmacokinetic linearity (dose linearity) or non-linearity will be an important factor in the design of future studies.

Once the initial dose has been determined, a placebo-controlled, double-blind, escalating single-dose study is initiated. Generally, healthy male volunteers are recruited, although patients sometimes are used (e.g., when testing a potential anticancer drug that may be too toxic to administer to healthy volunteers). These studies may include two or three cohorts, with six or eight subjects receiving the active drug and two subjects receiving placebo. The groups may receive alternating dose levels, which allow assessment of dose linearity, intrasubject variability of pharmacokinetics, and dose- response (i.e., adverse events) relationship within individual subjects. Participants in the first study are usually hospitalized or enrolled in a clinic so that clinical measurements can be performed under controlled conditions and any medical emergency can be handled in the most expeditious manner. This study is usually placebo-controlled and double-blinded so that the drug effects, such as drug-induced ataxia, can be distinguished from the non-drug effects, such as ataxia secondary to viral infection. The first study in humans is usually not considered successfully completed until an MTD has been reached. An MTD must be reached because the relationship between a clinical event (e.g., emesis) and a particular dose level observed under controlled conditions can provide information that will be extremely useful when designing future trials. Also, the dose range and route of administration should be established during Phase 1 studies.

A multiple-dose safety study typically is initiated once the first study in humans is completed. The primary goal of the second study is to define an MTD with multiple dosing before to initiating well-controlled efficacy testing. The study design of the multiple-dose safety study should simulate actual clinical conditions in as many ways as possible; however, scientific and statistical validity must be maintained. The inclusion of a placebo group is essential to allow the determination of drug-related versus non-drug-related events. The dosing schedule, which includes dosages, frequency, dose escalations, and dose tapering, should simulate the regimen to be followed in efficacy testing. Typically, dosing in the second study lasts for 2 weeks. The length of the study may be increased depending on the pharmacokinetics of the drug so that both drug and metabolite concentrations reach steady state. Also, if the drug is to be used to treat a chronic condition, a 4-week study duration may be appropriate. To obtain information for six dose levels with six subjects receiving active drug and two receiving placebo for each of two cohorts, a minimum enrollment of 24 subjects should be anticipated. Similar to the first study in humans, these subjects would be hospitalized for the duration of the study.

Also similar to the first study, pharmacokinetic data must be obtained. These data will be used to help determine dosage in future efficacy trials. The new pharmacokinetic information that can be gathered includes the following: (1) determination regarding whether the pharmacokinetic parameters obtained in the previous acute safety study accurately predicted the multiple dose pharmacokinetic behavior of the drug; (2) verification of pharmacokinetic linearity (i.e., dose proportionality of C_{max} and AUC) observed in the acute study; (3) determination regarding whether the drug is subject to autoinduction of clearance upon multidosing; and (4) determination of the existence and accumulation of metabolites that could not be detected in the previous single-dose study. A number of experimental approaches can be used to gather this information, and all require frequent collection of blood and urine samples. The challenge to the clinical pharmacokineticist is to design an appropriate blood sample collection schedule that will maximize the pharmacokinetic information, yet can be gathered without biasing the primary objective—determination of clinical safety parameters.

Phase 2

After the initial introduction of a new drug into humans, Phase 2 studies are conducted. The focus of these Phase 2 studies is on efficacy, while the pharmacokinetic information obtained in Phase 1 studies is used to optimize the dosage regimen. Phase 2 studies are not as closely monitored as Phase 1 studies and are conducted in patients. These studies are designed to obtain information on the efficacy and pharmacologic effects of the drug, in addition to the pharmacokinetics. Additional pharmacokinetic and pharmacologic information collected in Phase 2 studies may help to optimize the dose strength and regimen and may provide additional information on the drug's safety profile (e.g., determine potential drug-drug interactions). Efficacy trials should not to be initiated until the MTD has been defined. In addition, the availability of pharmacokinetic information in healthy volunteers is key to the design of successful efficacy trials. The clinical pharmacokineticist assists in the design and execution of these trials and analyzes the plasma drug concentration data upon completion of the efficacy studies.

During the planning stage of an efficacy trial, the focus is on the dosage regimen and its relationship to efficacy measurements. Plasma drug concentrations for various dosages can be simulated based upon the data collected in the first two studies in humans. The disease or physiological states of the test patients (e.g., organ dysfunction as a function of age), concurrent medications (e.g., enzyme inducers or inhibitors), and the safety data obtained earlier must be considered when choosing an optimal dosage regimen for the study. In addition, if the targeted site of the drug is in a tissue compartment, theoretical drug levels in this compartment can be simulated, which may help scientists determine the appropriate times for efficacy measurements.

On completion of the efficacy trial, a therapeutic window for plasma drug concentrations can be defined by reviewing the correlation between plasma drug concentrations and key safety and efficacy parameters. The goal is to improve efficacy and safety of the drug by individualizing the dosage based upon previous plasma drug concentration profiles in the same patient.

Phase 3

If the earlier clinical studies establish a drug's therapeutic, clinical pharmacologic, and toxicologic properties and if it is still considered to be a promising drug—Phase 3 clinical trials will be initiated. Phase 3 studies enroll many more patients and may be conducted both in a hospital or controlled setting and in general practice settings. The goals of Phase 3 studies are to confirm the therapeutic effect, establish dosage range and interval, and assess long-term safety and toxicity. Less common side effects and AEs that develop latently may be identified. In addition, studies targeted to evaluate and quantify specific effects of the drug, such as drowsiness or impaired coordination, are conducted during this phase. Phase 3 studies are also used to identify the most appropriate population or subpopulation for the study drug and to establish a place for the drug in its therapeutic class. A drug may be developed in a therapeutic class that already has effective alternatives, but the investigative compound may have a better safety profile than its established competitors. A Phase 3 clinical study can be designed to assess relative safety profiles.

Closer inspection of drug interactions is warranted in Phase 3 clinical trials. In many disease states, the use of polytherapy is quite common, and the risk of drug–drug interactions is high, both from pharmacokinetic and pharmacodynamic perspectives. The likelihood of drug interactions and semiquantitative estimates of magnitude may be predicted from in vitro data. The potential for interactions needs to be evaluated from two perspectives: the potential that the new drug may affect the pharmacokinetics of other drugs, and the potential that other drugs may affect the pharmacokinetics of the new drug. The former generally depends on the ability of the new drug to affect various enzyme and carrier-mediated clearance processes. Most notably, this concerns the cytochrome P450 (CYP) isoforms but could also involve conjugative enzymes and transporters, such as p-glycoprotein. Drugs may be an effective inhibitor without being a substrate of a CYP isoform, as is the case for quinidine's inhibition of CYP2D6.

The potential for significant drug–drug interactions caused by other drugs requires knowledge of the components of clearance for the new drug and the likelihood that known inhibitors will be coadministered. For drugs with multiple pathways and a broad therapeutic index, the need for formal interaction studies may be limited. Population pharmacokinetic analyses of data obtained from Phase 3 studies may be used to help discover and quantify drug interactions due to classes of drugs often associated with inhibition (e.g., macrolides, systemic antifungals, calcium channel antagonists, fluoxetine, paroxetine) or induction (e.g., anticonvulsants, rifampin). Most early clinical trials are conducted at university medical centers with physicians who specialize in a certain area of medicine. When study drugs are eventually marketed, however, general practitioners will be prescribing them as well. Therefore, it is important that family physicians are exposed to study drugs during this phase because they represent the segment of clinicians who will be writing most of the prescriptions. Similarly, to maximize the commercial return on drug development, a multi-indication strategy may be pursued (sometimes designated as Phase 5 if conducted postapproval). In addition, testing of the drug in foreign countries is appropriate during Phase 3; however, other countries may operate under different regulatory obligations than in the United States.

Phase 4

Whereas Phase 1, 2, and 3 studies are conducted prospectively using subjects or patients whose entrance into the study depends on strict inclusion and exclusion criteria, Phase 4 studies employ mainly observational, rather than exclusionary, study designs. Post-marketing surveillance and any additional studies requested by the regulatory agency as conditional approval of the NDA are conducted during Phase 4. Data collection in premarketing clinical trials is an extensive, scientific exercise. Detailed blood work, special laboratory tests, and careful physiologic monitoring are typical in these studies.

Postmarketing studies, however, are often targeted for much larger patient populations (5000–10,000 or more), which limits extensive data collection from each patient and emphasizes collection of safety information. These studies are complemented by reports of AEs from patients not enrolled in a study. The large numbers of patients in Phase 4 studies make it easier for researchers to determine rare AEs and can help identify patient populations that are at particular risk for certain AEs. For example, demographic trends toward side effects involving geographic locus, gender, or race may be determined from postmarketing surveillance data.

Protocol Considerations

The task of designing a clinical study cannot be undertaken until the study objective of that trial has been rigorously defined. The objective should explicitly state what is being investigated and vague language should be avoided. Once an unbiased and specific objective has been developed, scientists can build the study design around it and then develop and write the protocol. One of the main considerations when designing an investigational study concerns the type and number of comparative groups that will be involved. A control group of subjects may be evaluated in addition to the group taking the investigational drug. Sometimes more than one control group is used in a study. The control groups take either placebo or active medication and are compared with the group taking the investigational drug. This design is used to rule out the possibility of a placebo effect or to assess the efficacy and safety of the investigational drug relative to other drugs currently marketed.

Regulatory agencies frequently require the pivotal Phase 3 studies, which will be used to support an NDA, to be placebo-controlled studies. Placebo medication should be as similar as possible to the drug being investigated (e.g., same color, taste, and shape). No statistically significant difference in response between this group and the subjects taking the investigational drug is evidence against that drug having any real effectiveness. Similar to the placebo considerations, active medication taken by the control group also should be as similar as possible to the drug being investigated (e.g., same color, taste, and shape). If the formulations cannot be made with similar appearances (e.g., tablet, suspension, etc.), a placebo of each formulation could be made so subjects would take one active formulation and the placebo of the other formulation to maintain the blind. No statistically significant difference in response in this group relative to the subjects taking the investigational drug is evidence that active medication has no advantage therapeutically over the existing therapy. However, a higher incidence of AEs in the control group and an equal rate of efficacy relative to the subjects taking the investigational drug are evidence of the new drug's advantage over the existing therapy.

In addition to determining the types and number of control groups that should be included in a study, the drug development team must decide between a parallel and a crossover design. For example, in a placebo- controlled clinical trial, a parallel design is one in which each study group takes the same medication (i.e., either placebo or active drug) throughout the study. With a crossover design, each study group eventually receives both placebo and active drug (e.g., one group may take placebo for a 6-week period and then cross over to receive active drug for the following 6-week period).

An advantage of the crossover design is that it allows each group to be its own control, thereby allowing a demonstration of efficacy to occur during the treatment with the drug. A disadvantage of the crossover design is that residual effects from one treatment period may carry over into the other treatment period. Absolute determination of efficacy and safety of the different treatments is difficult and sometimes impossible. One way to avoid the problem of residual effects on crossover studies is to have washout periods between the different treatment phases. During the washout period, the patient is either given a placebo or no treatment for several days or weeks so that any possible metabolite or effect of the drug is "washed out" of the patient before the next treatment phase begins. An advantage of the parallel design is that it avoids the problems associated with possible residual effects of one treatment period influencing the other treatment period(s) because each treatment group is only exposed to one drug. Compared with a crossover study, more patients may be required for a parallel study so that statistical significance can be established between the study groups. In a parallel study, recruiting the required larger numbers of patients who fit the study criteria takes longer, but the duration of that study is usually shorter than the duration of a crossover study. Crossover designs span greater periods of time because each group must sequentially take an active and a control medication over a period that is long enough to allow a treatment effect to emerge. When washout periods are added, the time required to conduct these studies becomes longer still, and more study subjects may drop out. These difficulties are often outweighed by the fact that statistical significance can be achieved with fewer patients in crossover studies.

Once the study design has been chosen, there are many other issues to consider when developing and writing clinical protocols. Among the topics to be considered are criteria for patient eligibility, efficacy and safety parameters, timing of the events, packaging and dispensing of the clinical trial material, and the informed consent form. Also, to be determined is how the study will be blinded. For most well- controlled studies, subjects are assigned to the various groups by using a randomization process so that biased selection is eliminated, the overall collection of the subjects' variables is comparable in each group, and statistical power is guaranteed. In these double- blind studies, neither the subject nor the investigating scientists know to which group the subject has been assigned. Thus, extensive input from the drug development team is required when designing studies and writing protocols.

Drug Development Considerations

Most drugs are tested in humans to treat a specific disease entity or some adverse clinical condition. Because the pathogenesis of diseases and the exact mechanisms of action of drugs are often poorly understood, the process of evaluating a drug's efficacy can be complicated. Upon treatment, a patient's adverse clinical condition may improve; however, for many diseases this occurrence can only be evaluated indirectly by clinical assessments (e.g., via blood pressure measurements in the treatment of hypertension). However, a drug's characteristics can also be measured directly. For example, measurement of blood concentrations of the drug enabling calculation of pharmacokinetic parameters is a direct evaluation of the drug.

Similar to efficacy assessments, evaluation of the safety of a drug may also involve indirect measurements. One of the primary methods of obtaining safety information in a clinical trial is through a patient's reporting of AEs. Although the exact biochemical mechanisms responsible for many AEs cannot be evaluated directly, the indirect evaluation of the drug's adverse effect can be seen clinically. Because clinical assessments are indirect measures, AE reporting leads to several complex questions. The degree of drug- relatedness or causality, the effect of concomitant medication, the severity of the AE, the complications of the disease state, and the effects of other clinical conditions or diseases are usually difficult to determine, particularly early in the drug development program. Also, all reports of AEs in a clinical drug research program are recorded, tabulated, and cross- referenced to form a safety database, regardless of whether the AE is determined to be drug related. The information contained in this database is used to generate the package insert.

Although the clinical effect of a drug is perhaps the primary concern of drug development, an understanding of the drug's biochemical and physicochemical properties and mechanism of action is also desired. These direct measures are of equal concern in drug development as are the indirect evaluations of a drug's clinical effects. The primary tool used to study the intrinsic physicochemical properties of a drug is pharmacokinetics, which is a branch of biopharmaceutics. Pharmacokinetics describes the relationship between the processes of drug absorption, distribution, metabolism (biotransformation), and excretion (collectively abbreviated ADME) and the time course of therapeutic or adverse effects of drugs. Efficacy is determined by the drug concentration at the site of action, which generally is correlated with the drug concentration in the blood. The ultimate goal of pharmacokinetics is to characterize the sources of variability in the concentration time profile, which may be correlated with variability in efficacy and adverse events.

Pharmacokinetics can be used to guide dosage regimen selection and thereby optimize pharmacologic effects and minimize toxicologic effects when a drug is administered to an individual patient. Thus, although the basic pharmacokinetic properties of a drug are identified during the earliest stage of clinical drug development, the many factors affecting the pharmacokinetics in the patient population must be identified throughout the drug development process to enable proper dose selection for individuals. Thus, both indirect and direct measures are used to evaluate a drug.

Marketing Input

A successful pharmaceutical company has an appropriate blend of both research and marketing to enable a symbiotic, rather than antagonistic, relationship. Because an effective scientific and clinical research team often designs and executes experiments and clinical trials that involve costly overhead expenses, it is essential for marketing decisions to be geared toward company profitability being made allow the company profitable so these expenses can be met. Therefore, both medical and marketing input are necessary if a pharmaceutical company is to be successful.

By gathering data on all facets of the needs in the marketplace from clinicians and by maintaining a profile awareness of new products under development by competitors, marketing personnel are in an excellent position to advise their colleagues in the research arena who are responsible for the drug development program. Also, a marketing expert can help identify the problems other companies are having in selling their product and thereby avoid the same difficulties. For instance, sales problems may be related to ineffective advertising or faulty packaging; therefore, they do not concern clinical research. However, problems in sales can also be related to a drug's undesirable effects. An effective drug that does not lead to the AEs associated with an already approved drug would have a marketing advantage. Someone in marketing research may suggest conducting clinical studies that would evaluate the relative incidence of the AE with the hope that the data could be used to support effective advertising.

Thus, research and marketing are mutually benefical in a successful pharmaceutical company. Marketing groups help clinical research teams by supplying them with information about competing products, the needs of the marketplace, and suggestions for new formulations. Clinical research teams provide the data to support therapeutic and marketing claims and act as chief advisors to marketing personnel concerning drug research studies and promotional claims.

Effective Global Planning

Because drugs are frequently marketed worldwide and the clinical development of drugs may involve studies that are conducted internationally effective global planning can present its own difficulties. Obviously, medical practice, regulatory guidelines, and the cultural environment may be different in various countries, but also the manner in which research is conceived can differ vastly between countries. Medical researchers in some countries may be more conservative than researchers in other countries, which could potentially lead to the underdosing of drugs. These differences in research approaches actually stem from differences in ethical standards. Another reason that international planning may be difficult in drug research concerns the way in which various countries view early clinical trials and drug safety. Some countries view volunteer subjects and patients differently from a regulatory perspective, making it easier to recruit and enroll subjects for Phase 1 studies than it is to recruit and enroll patients for Phase 2 or Phase 3 studies. In the United States, both patients and volunteers are viewed in the same way, and studies with patients and volunteers cannot be initiated until the FDA has authorized an IND. In addition to regulatory guidelines, the regulatory process is still another aspect of clinical drug development that can differ widely between countries. In England, sponsoring research firms do not interact very much with the British drug regulatory agency the Committee on Safety of Medicines. This lack of direct interaction stems from the desire to keep commercial influence away from the objective evaluation of a pharmaceutical company's study data. This lack of communication results in British companies treating government guidelines for conducting clinical research as a routine checklist rather than an aid in forming the most appropriate development strategy.

In the United States, federal guidelines (Code of Federal Regulations, CFR) have been established by the FDA to help sponsoring research firms conduct good, consistent clinical studies. However, some of the items in these guidelines may not be appropriate for all clinical studies, and some items that may be appropriate to include in a clinical study may not have been incorporated into the federal guidelines. These variations occur because each drug and disease state is unique, and complete guidelines cannot be established for all cases. For these reasons, several meetings are held between clinical research teams and the FDA before an NDA submission to ensure that all appropriate methodology and experimentation is being incorporated into the overall drug development project.

Beginning in the early 1990s, the FDA participated in a collaborative effort to harmonize the technical procedures for development and regulatory approval of human pharmaceuticals internationally. Forces that led the agency in this direction included increased trade, the multinational nature of the pharmaceutical industry, trade agreements such as the North American Free Trade Agreement and the General Agreement on Tariffs and Trade by the World Trade Organization, European activism, and pressures on the industry to control costs. These pressures included intense competition and health care reimbursement controls. This harmonization effort is the work of the International Conference on Harmonisation (ICH) of Technical Requirements for Registration of Pharmaceuticals for Human Use. ICH has focused on achieving harmonization of technical requirements in three major regions of the world: the United States, the European Union, and Japan. Some of the earliest ICH guidelines addressed the format and content of the Investigator's Brochure, stability testing, and genotoxicity testing. The FDA also works with the World Health Organization and other international organizations to set standards for health care products. Clinical drug research is a complicated, multidisciplinary task that may be conducted internationally. In fact, many pharmaceutical companies are multinational, with locations in several countries. Planning and coordination become even more complex for such global drug development programs. Despite the differences among countries in medical practice, regulation, and culture, international drug development and marketing are vital parts of many organizations. The successful multinational pharmaceutical company will plan its clinical research strategy according to any differences among nations before to implementing its international development plans.

Ethical Considerations

No topic in clinical drug development is more controversial and emotionally charged than the myriad ethical dilemmas that face physicians and scientists involved in clinical research. Given that clinical research has generally proved to have moral consequences through its direct and indirect influence on alleviating suffering, steps must be taken to ensure that abuses do not occur during the course of drug development. Therefore, guidelines for the protection of human subjects have been developed, proposed, and accepted worldwide. Because of the atrocities committed by Nazi medical researchers in the 1930s, the Nuremberg Code was written, and highlighted the importance of obtaining all research subjects' voluntary consent to their participation in clinical studies. The Declaration of Helsinki, which was published by the World Medical Association in 1964 and has been updated several times since, takes the informed consent issue one step further by giving only qualified medical scientists and physicians the right to conduct clinical research. However, similar concerns go back at least to the 1830s, when

Dr. William Beaumont developed a contract with a patient, and in the late 1800s, when a leprosy worker experimented on a patient without her consent.

Legislation that ensures the protection of human research subjects in the United States includes the 1979 publication of the Belmont Report on the Ethical Principles and Guidelines for the Protection of Human Subjects of Research. This report concerns the fine line between biomedical research and the routine practice of medicine and explores the criteria that determine the risk-benefit ratio in the consideration of conducting clinical research. It also addresses basic guidelines for the proper selection of human research subjects and further defines the elements of informed consent.

Other important legislation in the United States includes the FDA's Guidance for Institutional Review Boards (IRBs) for further guarantees of protection for human research subjects. IRBs are independent committees that review proposed clinical research projects before the commencement of the research. These committees decide whether the risk to research subjects outweighs the potential benefit of the research; they can suggest modifications in the research proposal or disapprove the project altogether. IRBs must consist of both men and women of varying professions. At least one member must have his or her primary concern in a non-scientific area (e.g., a lawyer or clergyperson), and at least one member must not be affiliated with the institution at which the research will be conducted. Closely related to the rights of human research subjects are the rights of routine patients involved in non-research medical matters. In 1973, the American Hospital Association published the Patient's Bill of Rights, which requires that the acting physician give his patients complete information concerning their diagnosis, treatment, and prognosis; that the patient be given respectful care; that the patient be given the opportunity to refuse treatment; and that the patient's records, condition, and medical care be treated confidentially.

Another ethical issue facing clinical research scientists concerns study design, in particular, the placebo-controlled clinical trial. The reason placebo-controlled clinical trials are conducted is quite compelling from a scientific standpoint: to ensure that the evidence supporting the efficacy of an experimental drug is actually due to the properties of the drug and not to the psychologic properties of the study subjects. In other words, if a placebo effect from the experimental drug occurs rather than a true therapeutic effect, then a comparison of the drug group with the placebo group will show statistically similar response rates. It is a way to help separate actual drug responses from placebo responses, especially in studies investigating psychiatric compounds, but also in other therapeutic areas with a clearer "*physiologic*" or "*biochemical*" basis.

One defense for conducting placebo-controlled clinical trials is that the subjects chosen for the placebo group are randomly chosen, so that no malicious withholding occurs. Also, many study protocols have provisions of study extension that guarantee subjects in placebo groups have the opportunity to take the drug as an extension of the study after they complete the original part, or they are offered the chance to receive alternative therapy. Study subjects may be given monetary compensation for their participation in studies, in addition to free, thorough physical exams, lab work, and physician visits.

Interestingly, experimental drugs have unknown side effects that can cause serious biochemical and physiologic problems, whereas placebo medication does not. This fact makes possible the contrary argument and objection, on purely ethical grounds, to giving study subjects experimental and hence unproven drugs. Of course, informed consent and careful monitoring by trained medical personnel help to alleviate the ethical problems associated with giving subjects an active, investigational drug. The most important aspect of all studies is that the patient be completely informed of all study procedures and agree to willingly participate in the study. The most recent pressing ethical dilemma facing the clinical research scientist surrounds the increasing amount of research that is being conducted in biotechnical and genetic engineering. Ethical issues will continue to play important parts in the medical and legal worlds. Whereas pure science is value-neutral, its application is always open to debate. Undesirable extremes are likely to exist at both ends of the spectrum.

Future Prospectives

To conduct a clinical study for the evaluation of a new drug, a vast array of personnel is required. Physicians are largely used because of their knowledge of clinical medicine and patient care, whereas scientists are used because of their knowledge of the methodology and the science. Pharmacists serve a bridging function due to their unique training in therapeutics and the pharmaceutical sciences. Non-scientific personnel are indispensable because of their ability to coordinate the many facets of a drug development project. The clinical evaluation of drugs involves many different levels of scrutiny before a drug product can be marketed. These levels include Phase 1 for safety testing, Phase 2 for evaluating efficacy and determining the correct therapeutic dose, Phase 3 for large-scale studies and determination of drug interactions, and Phase 4 for postmarketing surveillance. Phase 1 studies are typically conducted in healthy volunteers, and Phase 2 through 4 studies are conducted in patients. Study design plays a critical role in the clinical evaluation of drugs. A clinical study cannot be conducted without specifically outlined objectives and a definitive plan, which are vital components around which the study protocol is constructed. The use of placebo or active drug control groups in the study, and whether the design should be open, parallel, or crossover, must be determined. In most studies, patients are assigned to study groups randomly.

The developmental objectives facing the clinical research team include indirect evaluations of a drug's safety and efficacy, such as effects on vital signs or behavior, and direct evaluations of a drug's intrinsic properties, such as its pharmacokinetics and mode of action. Also, the marketing medical liaison is important if research is to support future sales plans and advertising is to reflect study results. Finally, effective global planning is necessary because drugs are more frequently developed and marketed worldwide, and therefore involve differing patient populations and different government regulations. ICH guidelines have helped to standardize regulations worldwide. The ethical dilemmas facing clinical research scientists affect much of the legislation that currently regulates the conduct of clinical trials. The goal of drug development research is to develop effective pharmacotherapy for mankind's ailments, and regulatory agencies have enacted legislation to prevent unethical research. Although traditional medicines continue to be discovered and developed, the fields of biotechnology and gene therapy continue to advance. In addition, new methods to collect and evaluate clinical data on a real-time basis will help to speed the development process.

4

Clinical Perspectives

The eventual clinical implications of the large efforts in pharmacogenomic research throughout the world described in other chapters may be profound and widespread, but the actual utility of pharmacogenetic knowledge in clinical practice to date remains limited and largely untested. Changes in clinical practice represented by changes in dose or in the drug administered that result in real changes in health outcomes would be important measures of progress toward the "*personalized medicine*" or "*precision prescriptions*" so frequently predicted. Such outcomes might include the avoidance of a specific toxicity or the achievement of a specific therapeutic effect, but, as with all measures of success in medicine, must also include real clinical outcomes. It seems inevitable that significant improvements will continue to be made in the proportion of patients that are treated well, as is heralded by the recent reports of the effectiveness of a generally *ineffective* drug, gefitinib (Iressa) in lung cancer in patients who carry sensitizing mutations of the tyrosin kinase domain of the epidermal growth factor receptor (EGFR). We would not be surprised at this progress, if we recognized that such improvements are actually part of a continuum of improvement in the quality and individualization of patient care.

Individualization of therapy to an individual patient is not a new concept in medicine, but one central to its practice since the beginning. The writings of Hippocrates, Garrod, Jenner, and Osler all emphasize the centrality of treating the patient as an individual. There are multiple recent successes in targeting therapy to individual patients, supported by outcomes data and in wide clinical use already. To take the field of breast cancer as an example, such advances would include the evolution from the simple individualization of dose of chemotherapy by weight and body surface area to the use of estrogen and progesterone receptor status to target endocrine therapy by specific estrogen receptor modulators or aromatase inhibitors, to the use of the Gail index to identify patients most worth of preventive treatment, and to the use of BRCA1 mutations and HER2 status to target trastuzumab (Herceptin) therapy. We should not delude ourselves either by thinking that pharmacogenetic testing will usher in a new revolution in therapy or that the need for it represents an insult to our collective ability to individualize treatments in the past. "*Personalized medicine*" is nothing new. We have been doing it all along. That said we have to admit that we have been doing it when we had time and when it was possible in busy clinical practice environments and that the pressures to adopt a "*one dose fits all*" approach are real. Quality has always mattered in health care, but now the quality of our performance as effective prescribers is being measured by hospitals, by health care systems and by government agencies.

Pharmacogenomics should be seen as a stimulus to quality prescribing, a salve to the impersonalization of mass health care, and an invitation to advance the quality of our care beyond what is possible when we have time to do it and less medication to choose from. It should be designed as a "*tool for quality improvement*" along with the legions of administrators monitoring the number of new and return patients we see, the multiple digital assistants marketed to us, and the digitizing of our medical records. A large number of potential pharmacogenetic tests have been proposed, and so it is necessary to have some simple means of separating, which tests are likely to be most valuable.

In guiding drug therapy, pharmacogenetic tests should help to prevent serious adverse reactions, reduce hospitalizations and mortality, and should thereby reduce health care costs, but also avoid the prescribing of drugs to patients who are likely not to respond. In fact, preventing ineffective treatment possibly is as effective in reducing costs of health care as adjusting doses to minimize adverse effects and improve efficacy. While tests that are robust, reliable and cheap to perform will inevitably have an edge over those that are not, it is also important that a test provides added value above what is currently available. If we can measure LDL-cholesterol as a metric to follow statin efficacy, or if the physician of a patient with hypertension can tell at the next weekly visit whether a diuretic or an *angiotensin converting enzyme* (ACE) inhibitor is working, it makes less sense to develop a pharmacogenetic test to predict the effects of statins and anti-hypertensive drugs, than to search for one that predicts the response to an antidepressant or cancer treatment, where our current predictive powers are more limited. However, we constantly learn and better understand the reasons for variability in drug response. For instance, the somewhat smaller reduction in total cholesterol and LDL cholesterol in some patients treated with pravastatin recently was explained by a common variant of the HMG-CoA reductase gene.

We should not be naïve to the fact that our scientific forbearers have developed numerous useful predictors of treatment response. To return to the example of breast cancer treatment: no pharmacogenetic test is likely to have value unless it can improve on the currently widely used and useful predictive clinical parameters: the number of lymph nodes, grade of tumor, etc. An excellent example of a rigorous approach has been provided by the group at the Netherlands Cancer Institute, who showed that a customized tumor gene expression array was a more powerful predictor of the outcome of disease in young patients with breast cancer than standard systems based on clinical and histologic criteria. Last, but NOT least, a pharmacogenetic test, as any other diagnostic procedure, must be economically viable for companies that make test kits and for laboratories that do the testing. With these criteria in mind we have reviewed the approximately 45 pharmacogenetic situations or genes that have been associated with drug response in more than one clinical study. Monogenic traits were considered in regard to their possible clinical impact or the potential that they may consistently affect the choice and/or dose of a drug treatment. Of the seven genes and situations, the role of CYP2D6 in the use of neuroleptics and antidepressants is discussed in other chapters, and the testing for the presence of HER2 in breast cancer or for variants of HCV is well established.

N-Acetyltransferase (NAT2) and Isoniazid

One of the first pharmacogenetic traits to be recognized more than 50 years ago was the slow acetylation of the antituberculosis drug isoniazid now known as the polymorphism of N-acetyltransferase 2 (NAT2) and inherited as an autosomal recessive trait. Isoniazid is the treatment of choice for latent tuberculosis infection and is included in most first-line therapy regimens in combination with rifampicin, ethambutol and pyrazinamide. However, acute or chronic hepatitis frequently develops in patients receiving these drugs, with an incidence of 1–36%, depending on different regimens and how one defines hepatic injury, from transient elevations of liver function tests to serious injury or even death. Of the various drugs used in the combination therapy, isoniazid appears to be the main drug to induce hepatotoxicity. Additional risk factors are alcohol consumption, advanced age and pre-existing chronic liver disease. In numerous studies, slow acetylators treated with isoniazid and rifampicin had a higher risk of hepatotoxicity than rapid acetylators and among patients with hepatotoxicity, slow acetylators had significantly higher serum aminotransferase levels. Additional genetic risk factors were a homozygous "wild-type" genotype for CYP2E1 (CYP2E1 c1/c1) conferring high activity to this enzyme. In other studies, the acetylator genotype was a good predictor of isoniazid plasma levels and isoniazid-induced hepatotoxicity. These data suggest that genotype-derived dosage regimens, e.g., 400, 300, and 200 mg per day for slow (homozygous for two defective alleles), intermediate (heterozygous) or rapid (homozygous for two active alleles) acetylators, should be considered in future prospective studies.

The resurgence of tuberculosis in many countries as a serious threat because of a growing prevalence of drug resistance and its association with high risk patients such as HIV-seropositive individuals, convicts, homeless, or drug users has reemphasized the role of genetic risk factors for the hepatotoxicity associated with antituberculous regimens. The incidence of NAT2 slow acetylators can vary from 5% to 95%, depending on the geographic/ethnic origin of the population studied. In addition to isoniazid, the NAT2 polymorphism affects the pharmacokinetics of a wide variety of arylamine and hydrazine drugs and chemical carcinogens. They include sulfonamides such as salazosulfapyridine, the anti arrhythmic procainamide and the anticancer drug amonafide, for all of which dose adjustments according to the acetylator genotype or phenotype have been recommended, but are not part of common practice.

CYP2C9 AND WARFARIN

Warfarin is a commonly used anticoagulant that requires careful clinical management to balance the potentially lethal risks of over-anticoagulation and bleeding with the equally daunting risks of under anticoagulation and clotting. It is a legitimate target for a pharmacogenetic test because the surrogate for clinical effect, the international normalized ratio (INR) of the prothrombin time takes several days to reach its steady state, and improvements in both adverse outcomes and efficacy would be obtained if a pharmacogenetic test could more accurately predict dose. The CYP2C9 is known to be the primary catalyst of the human metabolism of the S-enantiomer of warfarin, and the scientific association is sufficiently strong that warfarin was the substrate chosen for the crystallization of a human cytochrome

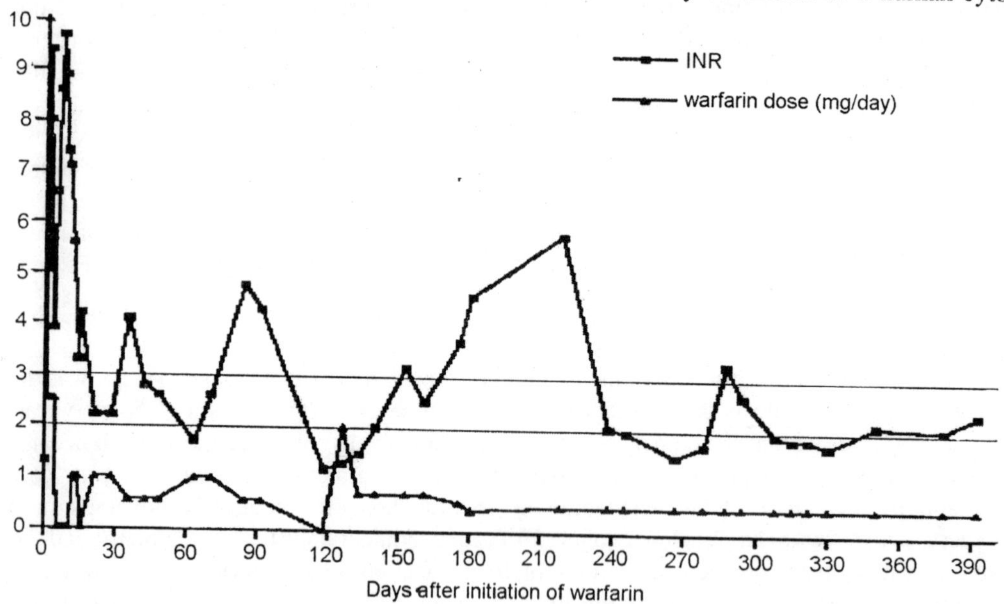

*Fig. 4.1. The INR values and warfarin doses of a patient with CYP2C9*3 allele variant requiring over 1 year to maintain a therapeutic INR.*

CYP2C9 with its bound substrate. Multiple retrospective studies from investigators all over the world have shown that variant alleles of the CYP2C9 gene encoding the *2 [Arg144Cys] and *3 [Ile359Leu] alleles increase the anticoagulant effect of warfarin and decrease the mean daily dose required to maintain the INR of the prothrombin time within the target therapeutic range. It is clear that the cost of caring for such a patient would likely outweigh the cost of a pharmacogenetic test. This anecdotal observation is supported by other case reports, and by a number of trials.

The more persuasive of these are studies that take into account the other clinically available predictive factors, including specifically Vitamin K intake. Aithal et al., the first group to report a clinical association between CYP2C9 genotype and warfarin dose went on to study the contribution of CYP2C9 genotype, age, body size, and vitamin K and lipid status to warfarin dose requirements. The multiple linear regression models for warfarin dose indicated significant contributions from age ($r = 0.41$, $p < 0.001$), genotype ($r = 0.24$, $p < 0.005$), and age and genotype together ($r = 0.45$, $p < 0.005$). The CYP2C9 genotype had a significant effect on S-warfarin clearance ($r = 0.34$, $p < 0.0001$) but none on R-warfarin clearance. In addition, Khan et al. studied the influence of dietary Vitamin K on dosage requirements and showed that, while dietary vitamin K had no effect, CYP2C9 genotype ($p = 2\%$) and age ($p < 1\%$) significantly contributed to inter-patient variability in warfarin dose requirements.

While data have been available for some time in relation to maintenance dose, the effect of CYP2C9 polymorphisms on dose requirements during the induction phase, when the danger of bleeding complications likely is greatest, has also been studied: patients with 2C9*2 or 2C9*3 variant alleles more frequently had INR values above the upper limit of the target range (3.0) (65% for 2C9*2/- and 66% for 2C9*3/- Vs. 33% for 2Cp*1/1; p = 0.006 and .012, respectively). In elderly patients, a genetic influence on response to warfarin does exist as in younger patients. In work carried out by Siguret et al. The CYP2C9 genotype was performed in 126 patients, with a mean age 87 ± 6 years. The mean daily dose of warfarin was 3.0 ± 1.4 mg, with 3.1 mg in patients with the wild type *1/*1 genotype ($n = 80$), 2.7 mg in *1/*2 heterozygotes ($n = 20$), 2.9 mg in *1/*3 heterozygotes ($n = 18$), 1.2 mg in *2/*2 homozygotes ($n = 2$), 2.3 mg in compound heterozygotes *2/*3 ($n = 6$).

Most importantly, the aggregated data prompted Higashi et al. to design a trial to test whether CYP2C9 genotyping could predict outcomes of patients on warfarin therapy. In this retrospective cohort study, 200 patients receiving long-term warfarin therapy for various indications underwent CYP2C9 genotyping and were evaluated by outcome measures, including anticoagulation status, measured by time to therapeutic INRs, rate of above-range INRs, and time to stable warfarin dosing or to serious or life-threatening bleeding events. They found that the mean maintenance dose varied significantly among the six-genotype groups (*1/*1 [$n = 127$], *1/*2 [$n = 28$], *1/*3 [$n = 18$], *2/*2 [$n = 4$], *2/*3 [$n = 3$], and *3/*3 [$n = 5$]) (by the Kruskall–Wallis test, $\chi^2 = 37.348$; $p < 0.001$). Compared with patients with the wild-type genotype, patients with at least one variant allele had an increased risk of above-range INRs of 1.40 (95% CI, 1.03–1.90). The variant group also required more time to achieve stable dosing (HR, 0.65; 95% CI, 0.45–0.94), with a median difference of 95 days ($p = 0.004$). In addition, patients with a variant genotype had a significantly increased risk of a serious or life-threatening bleeding event (HR, 2.39; 95% CI, 1.18–4.86).

More prospective studies are needed to test the feasibility and cost effectiveness of using algorithms based on these parameters for adjusting initial warfarin dose to meet individual needs, but the data at present make a strong case for the use of CYP2C9 genotyping testing prior to warfarin treatment, especially in the elderly. The main alternatives to warfarin, the coumarin derivatives acenocoumerol and phenoprocoumon, are widely or exclusively used instead of warfarin in certain European countries. Again the S-enantiomers of these closely related chemicals are substrates of CYP2C9. The presence of even one copy of CYP2C9*3 profoundly decreases the metabolic clearance of S-acenocoumarol. S-acenocoumarol, which normally is clinically inactive will now exert the main anticoagulant activity. The CYP2C9*3 allele therefore is related to low-dose requirements of racemic acenocoumerol, a higher frequency of over anticoagulation and an unstable anticoagulant response. Phenoprocoumon not significantly affected in its kinetics by the CYP2C9 polymorphism and appears to be a clinically useful alternative to warfarin in patients carrying CYP2C9*2 and *3 alleles.

Thiopurine S-Methyltransferase and Mercaptopurin

The therapy of cancer almost always involves multiple drugs with considerable toxicity. Pharmacogenomic approaches to cancer therapy have already briefly been discussed at the beginning of this chapter in regard to breast cancer. In general, these strategies include variations in germline DNA (e.g., genetic polymorphisms), acquired somatic mutations in tumor cells (e.g., sensitizing mutations in the tyrosine kinase domain of the EGFR gene that is the target of genitifib) or variations in RNA expression. Perhaps one of the best studied examples for the application of pharmacogenomic strategies to prevent adverse drug reactions is the polymorphism of the thiopurine S-methyltransferase (TPMT) gene, which has been extensively reviewed. The TPMT catalyses the S-methylation of thiopurine drugs such as mercaptopurine and its prodrug azathioprine. These drugs are successfully used to treat *acute lymphoblastic leukemia* (ALL) of childhood. Moreover, gastroenterologists prescribe thiopurine drugs as second-line (off-label) therapy for Crohn's disease and ulcerative colitis. Because methylation by TPMT is the pre-dominant pathway for inactivation of thiopurines, patients with TPMT deficiency accumulate active thioguanine nucleotides and this can lead to severe and life-threatening hematological toxicity. The TPMT activity in erythrocytes is trimodally distributed among Europeans, European-Americans, and African-Americans, which corresponds well to the genotypes or the respective presence of 2, 1, or 0 functional TPMT alleles.

In fact, the concordance rate between TPMT genotype and phenotype is >98%. Twenty mutant alleles of TPMT have been associated with low TPMT activity and three of these variants (TPMT*2, TPMT*3A, and TPMT*3C) account for approximately ~95% of low TPMT activity phenotypes. Approximately 1 in 150–300 individuals is homozygous for inactive TPMT alleles, approximately 10% of patients are heterozygous and have intermediate activity and ~90% are normal or high methylators in a Northern European Caucasian population. Interestingly, a subpopulation of ultrarapid TPMT metabolizers also was identified in these population studies. Because of the genotype–phenotype concordance and the severe toxicity associated with high concentrations of thioguanine nucleotides, several cancer centers routinely genotype patients for TPMT mutant alleles and use genotype-derived algorithms for dosing. Intermediate metabolizers receive ~65% and poor metabolizers 5–10% of standard doses of mercaptopurine. Dose reductions in patients with variant TPMT alleles lead to similar or superior survival compared to patients with wild-type alleles. Expectedly, there is considerable variability in the frequency of TPMT alleles in populations of different ethnic origins.

Despite the obvious robustness and cost-effectiveness of TPMT genotyping, additional factors and "*resistance of physicians to change*" so far have limited genotyping to specialized cancer centers. The arguments that full TPMT activity does not preclude possible myelotoxicity with multi-drug regimens and that partial TPMT activity does not always mandate reduced doses appear not very convincing. The information from genotyping obviously is only one type of information to be used in making decisions on drug and dosage regimens in following a patient with ALL, but it has an important function of telling the physician which patients have to be monitored more closely. Of major concern is a report of an increased incidence of secondary brain tumors after radiotherapy in children with decreased TPMT activity phenotypes and/or high concentrations of thioguanine nucleotides in blood cells. The implications for therapeutic decisions regarding prophylactic radiotherapy in ALL therefore must be further investigated.

UDP-Glucuronosyltransferase (UGT) 1A1 and Irinotecan

Results from several recently published trials suggest that patients who are homozygous for a UGT gene variant known as UGT1A1*28 (the "7/7" genotype) are at greater risk for irinotecan-induced severe diarrhea or neutropenia. Irinotecan is a camptothecin analog and inhibits topoisomerase I as an antineoplastic principle. It is used to treat several solid tumors. The disposition of irinotecan is quite complex and involves numerous metabolic enzymes and transport proteins. The SN-38 is the active metabolite of irinotecan and is eliminated via UGT1A1 conversion to SN-38G, an inactive glucuronide cleared via biliary excretion.

Reduced activity of UGT1A1 is linked to an approximately fourfold increased risk of severe toxicity, including dose-limiting diarrhea and neutropenia. Significant correlations between patients carrying one or two copies of the UGT1A1*28 allele and reduced UGT1A1 expression and reduced SW38 glucuronidation have been well documented. More than 50 mutations in UGT1A1 have been reported by Tukey and Strassburg, 2002 many of which are found in patients with Gilbert's syndrome, a form of mild non-hemolytic unconjugated hyperbilirubinemia. The most common mutant gene is UGT1A1*28, it contains seven dinucleotide repeats in the TATA box of the promoter [A$(TA)_7$TAA] instead of the normally six repeats, which leads to approximately 70% reduction of transcriptional activity. Many rare mutations also lead to Gilbert's syndrome, and individuals with this syndrome are pre-disposed to SN-38 initiated toxicity. Although, as always, a number of additional factors influence the toxicity of SN-38 in the intestine and bone narrow, assessment of the presence of the UGT1A1*28 allele in patients prior to irinotecan treatment will allow to start with lower dose or change to alternative therapies.

CYP2D6 and Codeine

It involves a large number of drugs, including many antidepressants and neuroleptics, antiarrhythmics, and many others commonly used drugs. In fact, recent recommendation for adjusting the doses for a number of antidepressant and neuroleptic drugs in the four genotypes/phenotypes poor metabolizers, extensive metabolizers, intermediate metabolizers, and ultrarapid metabolizers have been proposed. Prospective studies are planned to evaluate these recommendations, as genotyping tests for the multiple mutations of CYP2D6 are available. Here we discuss the striking differences in the responses to opioids that are associated with the CYP2D6 polymorphism. Dextromethorphan, codeine, hydrocodone, oxycodone, ethylmorphine, and dihydrocodeine all are dealkylated by polymorphic CYP2D6. The polymorphic O-demethylation of codeine is of clinical importance when this drug is given as an analgesic. About 5% of codeine is O-demethylated to morphine, and this pathway is deficient in poor metabolizers. Poor metabolizers therefore experience little analgesic benefit from treatment with codeine. Similarly, respiratory, psychomotor, and pupillary effects of codeine are decreased in poor metabolizers compared with extensive metabolizers.

Codeine is frequenctly recommended as a drug of first choice for treatment of chronic severe pain. Physicians must appreciate that no analgesic effect is to be expected in the 5–10% of Caucasians who are of the poor metaboliser phenotype, or who are extensive metabolizers receiving concomitant treatment with a potent inhibitor of CYP2D6. No morphine or morphine metabolites were detected in plasma when codeine was coadministered with quinidine. Although codeine may seem on the surface a poor candidate for a pharmacogenetic test, since the patient knows whether the medicine has worked or not, in fact there are many situations where analgesia is imperfect and even in situations where a patient can tell that codeine is having no analgesic benefit, his or her physician may not be aware, and self-reporting about pain is a notoriously variable and subjective phenomenon. It follows that the test may be valuable as a means of indicating which patients should not receive codeine as an analgesic, and who would most likely benefit.

Therapeutic Lessons

Pharmacogenetics has provided a number of therapeutic lessons that make us understand clinical drug response and it has influenced the drug development process. Among the therapeutic lessions are that most drug effects vary considerably from person to person and that all drug effects are influenced by genes. But it has also been realized that the most drug responses and toxicities are influenced by many genes interacting with environmental and behavioral factors. Genetic polymorphisms of single genes, including mutations in coding sequences, gene duplications, gene deletions, and regulatory mutations affect numerous drug-metabolizing enzymes. Several cytochrome-P450 enzymes, *N*-acetyltransferases 2 (NAT2), TPMT, and a UDP-glucuronosyltransferases (UDP-GT) are the examples discussed here. Individuals who possess these polymorphisms are at risk of experiencing more adverse drug reactions or inefficacy of drugs at usual doses.

Genetic polymorphisms of drug targets and drug transporters also are increasingly recognized (receptors, ion channels, and growth factors) as causing variation in drug responses, but they have not been studied enough in regard to their clinical importance that would advocate genotype-based dose adjustments. Several targets of cancer therapy, for example, the epidermal-growth-factor receptor, respond to treatment only in subgroups of patients who carry sensitizing mutations of these targets. Finally, the frequency of variation of drug effects, whether multifactorial, or genetic, varies considerably in populations of different ethnic origins.

Future Perspectives

One of the major challenges in the future is the interpretation of multigenic and multifactorial influences on drug responses. Indeed, as already mentioned, most drug effects and treatment outcomes, or the individual risk for drug inefficacy or toxicity are due to complex interactions between genes and the environment. Environmental variables include nutritional factors, concomitantly administered drugs, disease, and many other factors including lifestyle influences such as smoking and alcohol consumption. These factors act in concert with several individual genes that code for pharmacokinetic and pharmacodynamic determinants of drug effects such as receptors, ion channels, drug-metabolizing enzymes, and drug-transporters. The challenge will be to define polygenic determinants of drug effects and to use a combination of genotyping and phenotyping tests to assess environmental influences.

The increasing use of the term pharmacogenomics reflects the evolution of pharmacogenetics into the study of the entire spectrum of genes that determine drug response, including the assessment of the diversity of the human genome sequence and its clinical consequences. Rapid sequencing and genotyping of SNPs will have a major role in associating sequence variations with heritable clinical phenotypes of drug or xenobiotic response. The SNPs occur approximately once every 300–3000 bp if one compares the genomes of two unrelated individuals and represent 90–95% of all variant DNA sites. Any two individuals thus differ at approximately 3 to 10 million base pairs.

How can we use this information to predict drug responses particularly with the view that in a few years technologies will be available to sequence an entire human genome in a few hours and at a reasonable prize? Once a large number of SNPs and their frequencies in different populations are known, they can be used to correlate an individual's genetic "*fingerprint*" with the probable individual drug response.

It has been proposed that high density maps of SNPs or the so-called haplotype blocks in the human genome might allow the use of these SNPs as markers of xenobiotic responses even if the target remains unknown, providing a "*drug–response profile*" that is associated with contributions from multiple genes to a response phenotype. A recent "*proof of concept*" was provided by Xu et al. 2004 for tranilast-induced hyperbilirubinemia. Whole genome screening for regions of linkage disequilibrium associated with this adverse effect was used to identify three SNPs of UGT1A1 gene to be responsible for this drug-induced adverse reaction. In practice, and because of the complexities of defining disease phenotypes and clinical outcomes, the validity of this concept is limited.

Genomic technologies also include methods to study the expression of large groups of genes and indeed the entire complement of products (mRNAs) of a genome. Most drug actions produce changes in gene expression in individual cells or organs. This provides a new perspective for the way in which drugs interact with the organism and also provides a measure of the drug's biological effects.

For instance, numerous drugs induce their own metabolism and the metabolism of other drugs by interacting with nuclear receptors such as arylhydrocarbon receptor (AhR), peroxisome proliferator activated receptor (PPAR), pregnane × receptor (P × R), and constitutive androstane receptor (CAR). These receptors act as "*xenosensors*" and transcription factors that activate a response that includes increased biotransformation of drugs. The phenomenon of induction has major clinical consequences such as altered kinetics, drug–drug interaction or changes in hormone and carcinogen metabolism. Genomics is providing the technology to better analyze these complex multifactorial situations and to obtain individual genotypic and gene expression information to assess the relative contributions of environmental and genetic factors to variations in drug response.

Clinical Potential of Pharmacogenetics

Why is pharmacogenetics so rarely applied in clinical practice, in spite of well-established genetic polymorphisms and available genotyping methods? Numerous reasons for the slow acceptance of pharmacogenetic principles have been brought forward. The lack of large prospective studies to evaluate the impact of genetic variation on drug therapy is one reason for the slow acceptance of these principles. On the other hand, pharmacogenetic information is only reluctantly included in product information or drug data sheets alerting the physician to dosing problems.

A recent search for pharmacogenetic information in the prescribing information available to physicians provided the following bleak results. Seventy-six drug package inserts (PIs) from the Physician's Desk Reference (PDR) contained pharmacogenomic data. The gene usually was either a drug-metabolizing enzyme or the information was related to the variability in viral genomes as predictors of response to antiviral therapy or drug resistance. Information to guide treatment decisions was found in only 25 PIs, representing 22 drugs. Of these four were ranked in the top 200 prescribed drugs (celexocib, fluoxetine, pantoprazole, and divalproex sodium). Advice for treatment decisions based on specific genetic conditions were found in four PIs, namely that prolastin (α1-proteinase inhibitor) is not indicated in patients with certain α1-antitrypsin deficiency phenotypes, trastuzumab indicated only in patients with overexpression of the HER2 protein, tretinoin, and imatinib are to be given only in patients with either a specific subtype of acute myelogenous leukemia or Philadelphia chromosome-positive chronic myeloid leukemia, respectively.

Surprisingly, information on increased risk for potentially life- threatening adverse effects or treatment failures with conditional recommendations for genetic evaluation were found for only four drugs, namely recombinant factor X, somatotropin, divalproex sodium, and valproic acid. Only for one drug, thioridazine, did the PI contain a contraindication for a genetic subgroup, namely CYP2D6 poor metabolizers, which may develop QTc (prolonged heart-rate-corrected QT interval) interval prolongation in the electrocardiogram and develop ventricular arrhythmia.

Clearly, PIs at present do not contain useful information for gene-guided dose adjustments or therapeutic decisions. In particular, there are no explicit recommendations for drug dosing in TPMT deficient patients in the PIs for mercaptopurine or azathioprine or in the PI for warfarin for patients with low activity alleles of CYP2C9. Similarly, the PI for irinotecan does not contain information on the risk of patients with UGT1A1 deficiency. A major effort is underway at the Food and Drug

Administration to correct these obvious deficiencies in alerting physicians to potential problems, and this has included the first approval of a pharmacogenetic test: an oligonucleotide microarray test for CYP2D6 and CYP2C19 genotypes in December of 2004. In the future, not performing a pharmacogenetic test may have legal consequences.

Pharmacogenomics offers the potential to provide better health care through improved rational prescribing. We believe that is gradual acceptance in clinical practice will contribute to the education of health care professionals as prescribers. In addition, we must recognize an increasingly important source of pressure to improve pharmacotherapy: increasingly educated patients will come to expect the application of genomics and other technologies to drug selection and dosage when possible. The personalized medicine that many view as a new goal is actually what physicians always intended, and is becoming what patients, and the regulatory bodies that protect them, expect.

5

Molecular Diagnostics

Pharmacogenomics is a rapidly evolving area driven by the new genetic information and new molecular technologies arising from the mapping and sequencing of the human genome. The field of pharmacogenomics has a parallel with the more traditional area of molecular diagnostics, in which molecular techniques are used for identification of a disease mutation in a particular patient population with a genetic disorder. Both fields have been impacted greatly by new genetic information and technologies, and have certain similar challenges to overcome. This chapter will focus on describing technologies and general issues in molecular diagnostics, and similarities to pharmacogenomic molecular applications.

Molecular diagnostics is an integration of molecular genetic knowledge and technology and conventional laboratory medicine for patient diagnostics. Due to the cost of performing testing, molecular diagnosis has historically been restricted to testing of a limited number of individuals at high risk, typically people who are suspected of being affected or carriers of a particular monogenic inherited disorder. This scenario is beginning to change as diagnostics expands into higher-volume testing of larger patient groups and at-risk populations. For example, widespread population carrier screening for cystic fibrosis carriers using molecular diagnostic methods has recently been implemented in the United States, with the goal of identifying carrier couples prior to the birth of an affected child. The increased volume of testing produced by these new applications has required the development of higher-throughput and lower cost molecular diagnostic assays to detect nucleotide changes. Large-scale molecular diagnostic applications parallel molecular pharmacogenomic testing requirements for high throughput and cost-effective molecular diagnostic tests suitable for screening a large number of individuals for multiple genetic changes. An important issue in a discussion of typical molecular diagnostics and pharmacogenomics is the difference in the interpretation of testing for mutations in a single gene disorder vs. testing for mutations in one or more genes involved in multifactorial disorders.

The majority of current molecular diagnostic assays are used to test for mutations in monogenic disorders. For example, cystic fibrosis is a relatively common single gene disorder caused by mutations in the cystic fibrosis transmembrane conductance regulator (CFTR) gene. Many diagnostic laboratories routinely test for 25–30 of the most common CFTR mutations, which account for the majority of cystic fibrosis mutations in most populations. The finding of a mutation is diagnostic in that a prediction of disease can be made on the basis of finding two mutations in the CFTR gene carried by an individual. In contrast, multifactorial diseases such as hypertension and obesity are more complex as disease onset is likely to be dependent on changes in several genetic regions, each with a different influence on disease progression, plus environmental factors. Individuals with a family history of hypertension may carry mutations in several genetic regions that lead to an increased susceptibility for hypertension. However, due to environmental differences only a portion of the individuals who carry these mutations will develop hypertension. The interpretation of molecular testing in multifactorial diseases is complex, as it requires interpretation of the results of testing several genetic regions and involves gene–environment interactions that are difficult to predict. Many individual drug responses are likely to be multifactorial traits, and these same issues will complicate prediction of drug response outcome based on molecular testing results.

Types of Genetic Variations

Genetic diseases can be divided into two main groups based on whether they are caused by relatively few common mutations or by many unique mutations. Tay-Sachs disease, a fatal neurodegenerative disorder caused by a deficiency of hexosaminidase A, is common in the Ashkenazi Jewish population. Three hexosaminidase mutations account for ~96% of the disease in the Ashkenazi Jewish population. In contrast most patients with Fabry disease, a metabolic disorder caused by deficiency of the enzyme galactosidase A, have unique mutations in the galactosidase A gene. This distinction is significant, as the detection of a small number of known mutations in a gene requires quite different technologies than the analysis of a complete gene to search for unknown mutations. Other types of genetic variation known to cause genetic disorders include deletions and duplications that can range in size from a single base to large regions encompassing whole exons or entire genes.

Deletions and duplications are of particular significance in molecular diagnosis, as they require special assays for detection, such as quantitative PCR to determine gene copy number. Genetic mutations can also alter function at levels other than the DNA coding sequence, such as mutations at conserved splice site sequences, which alter RNA splicing. The methods of detection of these different types of genetic changes vary depending on the type of mutation to be detected. Methods of mutation detection include specific assays designed to identify a certain nucleotide change at a particular base pair in a sequence, or the use of direct sequencing to detect many unique mutations. Direct sequencing may be preceded by the scanning methods to highlight particular exons of a gene that may contain a mutation. If a genetic disease is caused by a few recurrent mutations that account for the majority of disease, it is often more appropriate to test for these few mutations by a specific assay rather than by sequencing. In contrast, diseases caused by a large number of mutations in a single gene are more appropriately tested by direct sequencing methods. Therefore, it is critical that a molecular diagnostic test be appropriately matched to the types of mutations to be detected for a particular gene.

Methods to Detect Known Mutations

There is a vast array of techniques that are currently being used to look for mutations for clinical molecular diagnostic use. The following overview of methods describes some of the most common techniques to detect recurrent mutations used in many diagnostic laboratories.

PCR-Restriction Enzyme Assays

Certain genetic changes alter a restriction enzyme recognition site, either by creating a new site or destroying an existing site. In these cases, a molecular diagnostic assay can be designed in which a region containing the potential mutation site is amplified via PCR and digested with the appropriate restriction enzyme to determine if the restriction digest pattern is altered due to the presence of the mutation. In some cases, designing a PCR primer containing a mismatch that anneals near a mutation site can artificially produce a restriction enzyme site. When combined with the mutant genetic sequence, the mismatched PCR primer sequence and the mutation alters a restriction enzyme site and so produces altered restriction enzyme patterns. Quality control for this type of assay requires that appropriate positive and negative control samples must be present in each assay in order to confirm that the enzyme is properly active. An example of a PCR-restriction enzyme assay to detect variation for a pharmacogenomic application is the original detection of mutations in the gene for the cytochrome isozyme P250D6 (CYP2D6), which cause the *"poor metabolizer"* of debrisoquine phenotype. Since this paper was published, many assays using different methods have been designed to detect mutant alleles in the P250D6 gene, highlighting the complexity in choosing a method for molecular analysis of mutations in a particular gene. The main advantage for molecular diagnostics using a PCR-restriction enzyme assay is that it is simple to develop and perform, likely accounting for its continued use in many diagnostic laboratories. The major disadvantage is that the assay is time consuming, as each mutation must be individually analyzed. Although this assay is effective for testing a small number of samples in specific cases, it is not suited for testing samples for multiple mutations or for screening large numbers of samples.

Allele-Specific Oligonucleotide Assay

The basis of the *allele-specific oligonucleotide* (ASO) assay is that DNA duplexes which contain a mismatch are destabilized and have a lower melting temperature than correctly paired duplexes. To test for mutations using ASO, two probes, one containing the normal sequence and one containing the mutant sequence, are produced and hybridized to the patient's DNA. For each normal and mutant probe, conditions can be found where the probe will hybridize to only its perfectly matched duplex. If the patient sample contains only normal sequence, only the normal probe will hybridize. In a heterozygous sample, both the mutant and normal probes will hybridize, and in a homozygous mutant sample only the mutant probe will hybridize. An advantage of the ASO method is that it can be used to simultaneously test samples for several different mutations by the use of multiple probes bound to a solid matrix.

In practice, the success of this method relies on precisely establishing conditions for optimal oligonucleotide hybridization in order to ensure specific probe hybridization, and so multiplex ASO assays can be difficult to develop. Molecular diagnostic kits for use in genetic disorders based on ASO methods are available. There have been improvements to the ASO assay, specifically by development of a multiplex allele-specific diagnostic assay (MASDA) in which the ASO technique is adapted to a solid support and multiple regions are probed simultaneously. This has been achieved by altering probe hybridization conditions, so that hybridization of multiple probes at a single temperature is feasible. Using these improvements, it has been possible to analyze >500 samples simultaneously for >100 known mutations in multiple genes.

Allele-Specific Amplification Assay

The *allele-specific amplification assay* (ASA) assay is based on the fact that Taq polymerase will not initiate amplification from a primer that has a mismatch at the 3' ends. Two primers are designed so that the 3' base of the primer corresponds to the site of the genetic mutation to be tested, with either the normal or the mutant sequence at the 3' base positions. An unknown sample can then be tested for the presence of the mutation by using both the normal and the mutant primers in PCR with a common reverse primer. If the sample contains only normal sequence, a PCR product will only be produced when the normal primer is used, and similarly when the sample contains mutant sequence a product will only result from use of the mutant primer. Like the PCR-restriction enzyme method discussed, the ASA approach has also been applied to the detection of mutations in the CYP2D6 gene.

In the original ASA protocols, the mutant and normal PCR primers were separated into two reactions, so that lack of amplification could occur in one PCR reaction depending on the sequence present in a test sample. This is not ideal for a diagnostic test due to the possible misinterpretation of a false negative result, and the ASA protocol is usually modified to be a multiplex reaction that includes a positive internal control in each PCR reaction. For example, an ASA assay has been developed, which detects 12 common CFTR mutations simultaneously. However in this assay, two reactions must still be run in parallel for every sample to be analyzed, since the mutant and normal products produced are the same size and so must be physically separated in order to be distinguished.

The ASA can be improved by the use of fluorescent-dye labeled primers, which avoids the need for two separate reactions by using flourochromes to distinguish normal and mutant sequences. We have developed molecular diagnostic ASA assays to detect mutations causing Tay-Sachs and Canavan disease using fluorescent-dye labeled PCR primers. The mutant and normal primers are labeled with different color dyes, so that the PCR products resulting from either the normal or the mutant allele-specific primer will be a different dye color, allowing discrimination of normal and mutant sequence. The use of fluorescent dyes thus simplifies the assay, and allows one sample to be tested for multiple mutations in a single reaction. The advantage of the ASA method is that multiplex reactions to detect several mutations simultaneously can be developed. Multiplex reactions reduce the labor and costs and so are ideal for detection of a larger number of mutations. The main disadvantage of the ASA method is that achieving specific product amplification can be problematic.

Oligonucleotide Ligation Assay

The *oligonucleotide ligation assay* (OLA) is similar to allele-specific amplification in that specific interrogation of a mutation site is achieved by two oligonucleotides that contain the normal or mutant base at the 3' end of the primer. However, in the OLA assay, the normal or mutant primer anneals directly downstream and adjacent to a common primer. The two primers are directly adjacent to one another, and thermostable ligase is able to join the annealed primers. In the case of a normal DNA sequence, only the normal and common primers will anneal and so be ligated, while a mutant DNA sequence will produce ligation of only the mutant and common primers. This method has also been applied to the detection of CYP2D6 alleles.

A recent improvement in the OLA assay is the use of sequence-coded separation (SCS), in which non-nucleic mobility altering compounds are attached to the specific primers. The mobility altering compounds are designed so that the products from each primer are a different size, and so will allow discrimination between primer pairs for different mutations. This technology is used in a diagnostic assay for cystic fibrosis in which 32 mutations in the CFTR gene can be detected simultaneously. This novel method of size separation may expand the utility of the OLA assay, as it will allow multiplex assays for a large number of mutations. The main advantage of the OLA technique is the ability to multiplex several mutations; while the disadvantage is that without SCS the assay is of somewhat limited application. Many diagnostic laboratories currently use the commercially available OLA assay for mutations causing cystic fibrosis.

Primer Extension/Minisequencing Assay

The primer extension assay is similar to the dideoxy method commonly used in sequence analysis. In the primer extension assay, a region containing the mutation to be assayed is amplified in a first PCR reaction. A specific primer, which is designed to anneal directly upstream of the base which is the site of a known mutation, is then used in a second reaction. Radioactively labeled dideoxy nucleotides corresponding to either the normal or the mutant base at the potential mutation site are added in separate tubes. During the reaction, the labeled nucleotide added to the 3' end of the primer will depend on the sequence at the potential mutation site. If the normal sequence is present at the potential mutation site, only the reaction containing the normal labeled dideoxy nucleotide will produce a labeled primer. Conversely, if the mutant sequence is present at the mutation site, only the reaction containing the mutant nucleotide will produce a labeled primer. Individuals who are heterozygous for the mutation will produce labeled primers in both dideoxy tubes, due to the presence of both sequences at the potential mutation site. Primer extension assays are very sensitive for mutation detection and may be advantageous for large-scale testing with some modifications to the basic protocol. Primer extension assays have been designed to use fluorescent dye labeled nucleotides to eliminate the need for radioactivity and may also be adaptable to use on solid supports. For molecular diagnostics purposes, there are also commercially available kits and protocols for diagnostic applications.

Technical Advances in Molecular Diagnostic Techniques

In recent years, there have been major technical advances in genetic analysis methods due primarily to use of new technologies developed for genomic applications. This is leading to an increased emphasis on faster, more efficient methods of detecting genetic mutations facilitated by the use of novel methods and equipment, with increased automation to reduce labor intensive steps in genetic analysis. Major technological advances will be essential as routine molecular diagnosis of genetic disorders adjusts to increasing volumes and large-scale population screening. Most current molecular diagnostics assays are not highly automated, and are generally labor-intensive and expensive. For large-scale molecular diagnostic testing, more automation with reduced personnel involvement is essential in order to reduce the cost of testing. Other requirements of large-scale testing will be improved software programs capable of dealing with large amount of data.

Capillary Electrophoresis

A significant advance in common molecular diagnostic applications is capillary electrophoresis, in which traditional slab electrophoresis gels are replaced by capillaries. The electrophoresis of samples is carried out in a thin capillary tube filled with a matrix, and the movement of DNA molecules through the tube is detected and recorded. Capillary electrophoresis is amenable to automation as samples can be automatically loaded from reaction plates. Capillary electrophoresis can be readily applied to many genetic tests that traditionally would be analyzed on a slab gel, including methods for recurrent mutation detection, fragment analysis and direct sequencing. Capillary electrophoresis with equipment containing 96–384 capillaries has greatly reduced the labor required for certain molecular diagnostics tests, particularly direct sequencing for mutation detection.

DNA Chip Technology

The DNA chips are high-density arrays, in which many nucleic acid sequences are anchored on glass supports similar in size to microscope slides. The DNA chips can be designed in certain formats depending on the application of the chip. The current applications of DNA chip technology of relevance to diagnostics include use in determining sequence of an unknown fragment by hybridization, detection of SNPs or gene expression profiling in various tissues. The major benefit of the use of DNA chips for these applications is that information on thousands of genetic regions can be obtained from a single chip experiment. For example, chips that are used to determine expression profiles from various genes can analyze thousands of RNA fragments on a single chip. This has been used for cancer applications, in which gene expression profiles from tumor tissues are compared to normal tissues to determine, which genes are differentially regulated in the cancer tissues. Currently, DNA chips for use in gene expression studies work well. However, sequencing and SNP chips are still not accurate enough for routine use in identifying genetic changes in a clinical molecular diagnostic laboratory. In addition, there are ethical considerations regarding provision of molecular diagnostic testing of a large number of genes or mutations on DNA chip, which need to be addressed.

Denaturing High Pressure Liquid Chromatography Analysis

New applications for Denaturing High Pressure Liquid Chromatography (HPLC) may also have important future applications for testing for genetic variation. The HPLC has been adapted to DNA fragment analysis for separation of fragments under partially denaturing conditions. Fragments to be analyzed for the presence of a mutation are amplified by PCR and then run on a denaturing HPLC column. The DNA heteroduplexes containing a mismatched base due to the presence of a mutation have a different mobility through the HPLC column from normal matched homoduplexes, due to the altered melting temperature of the heteroduplex. The mobility difference between the normal and the mutant sample allows for screening of fragments for genetic changes.

The main application of DHPLC technology for diagnostics is likely to be its use as a screening tool for genetic variation prior to sequencing, which is similar in principle to traditional methods of scanning such as single-strand conformational polymorphism (SSCP) and denaturing gradient gel electrophoresis (DGGE) assays. However, DHPLC also has the potential to be a method to screen samples for previously known mutations. The advantages of DHPLC are its automated nature, the simplicity of preparing fragments for analysis and the short run times required for fragment analysis.

MALDI-TOF Mass Spectrometry

Mass spectrometry is also being applied to genetic analysis by the use of matrix-assisted laser desorption/ionization time-of-flight (MALDI-TOF) mass spectrometry. The principle of this application is that sequence differences can be determined by analyzing the inherent mass differences of the four-nucleotide bases. For molecular diagnostic applications, the most obvious application of MALDI-TOF is the use of modified primer-extension assays, in which the base extended is at the nucleotide site of a known sequence change. MALDI-TOF is promising for high throughput applications, as more than one genetic region or mutation can be simultaneously analyzed and the assays. An example of the use of MALDI-TOF in diagnostics is in detection of mutations in CFTR causing cystic fibrosis.

Real-Time PCR

Additional developments in PCR technologies are also impacting on molecular diagnostics. One of the most important has been the development of PCR machines that have the capability of detecting product formation during the PCR reaction, known as real-time PCR. Assays can be designed in which the binding of a sequence-specific probe to its homologous PCR product results in an increase in fluorescence during the PCR reaction, allowing for real-time detection of the PCR product. This has been achieved using various probe designs that maintain a fluorescent reporter dye in close proximity to a quencher dye. Upon hybridization to its specific sequence the quencher is separated from the reporter thus generating a fluorescent signal from the reporter dye. This technology has been applied to detection of mutations causing genetic disease as well as for pharmacogenomic research. The advantage of real-time PCR techniques is that they do not require any post-PCR analysis such as gel electrophoresis, since the amplification and detection of the specific product are completed within the PCR reaction.

Robotics

A common objective of all of the new technologies discussed is to reduce the labor and expense required for large-scale testing. High-throughput detection machines require high sample input rates, which are not feasible without the use of robotics. Robotics will be required to automate the isolation of DNA, to prepare reactions for PCR, and to load detection machines after PCR. For example, the labor associated with manually preparing DNA samples for analysis on a 384-sample capillary electrophoresis machine would negate the benefit of using the advanced equipment. Robotics instruments are now available that can perform various functions, including nucleic acid extraction and preparation of PCR reactions. Robotics is likely to become more flexible in future, with robots specifically designed to interact with specialized equipment for specific applications. An important aspect of increased robotic use will be the development of software programs able to perform data analysis on the high volume of data generated. The increasing use of robotics will allow genetic diagnostic laboratories to increase the number of tests it is able to perform, without continually increasing laboratory staff, due to the ability to perform more tasks in less time. The methods listed above are some of the major areas of interest in the development of biotechnology-based molecular diagnostic procedures. Some private companies are currently offering genetic testing based on new biotechnology-based large-scale molecular diagnostic methods. An overview of some companies involved in developing diagnostic strategies for large-scale genetic testing for pharmacogenomics is provided in Persidis. The need to develop high-throughput, sensitive and cost-effective molecular testing for genetic variation remains a significant challenge in molecular diagnostics, which is shared with pharmacogenomic applications.

Since many individuals will require testing, and many genetic changes may need to be tested, the diagnostic methods will need to be robust, cost-effective and specific. Some of the new advances in genetic analysis, such as real-time PCR and MALDI-TOF, hold promise for meeting these demands. In addition, as the throughput of molecular diagnostic testing improves, testing is likely to still be limited by uncertain significance of new sequence changes detected. This is also an issue in common with pharmacogenetics, as the application of routine pharmacogenomics still requires a more thorough understanding of the genetic causes underlying drug response variations. The genetic variations may be simple changes, or they may be complex alterations that are also influenced by environmental factors. Significant research on the effect of genetic variation on enzyme activity and the resultant effect on drug response will be required. New technologies for DNA analysis and mutation detection, and improved understanding of the interpretation of mutations, will make it possible to meet the demands of both future molecular diagnostic and pharmacogenomic applications.

6

CLINICAL PHARMACOLOGY OVERVIEW

Clinical pharmacology is the branch of pharmacology that focuses on the study of drugs in humans. A comprehensive understanding of the principles of clinical pharmacology facilitates the clinician prescribing optimal therapy to an individual patient. Over the last 30 yr the clinical pharmacology of many drugs has been elucidated with advances in sophisticated, accurate, and precise analytical tools to determine plasma drug and/or metabolite concentrations in biological fluids. This has permitted a better understanding of the relationship between the pharmacokinetics (derived from the Greek *pharmakon* [drug] and *kinisis* [movement] and meaning drug concentration over time) and the pharmacodynamics (derived from the Greek *pharmakon* and *dynameostis* [power], meaning drug action or power) for many drugs. Oncology has, only somewhat belatedly, generated adequate data on these pharmacological properties of many widely used cytotoxic drugs. This is to some extent unfortunate, because cytotoxic drug therapy demands close attention to pharmacological principles as the therapeutic index of many anticancer agents is narrow, that is, $TD_{50}/ED_{50} \leq 2$. To achieve the primary therapeutic endpoint (tumor

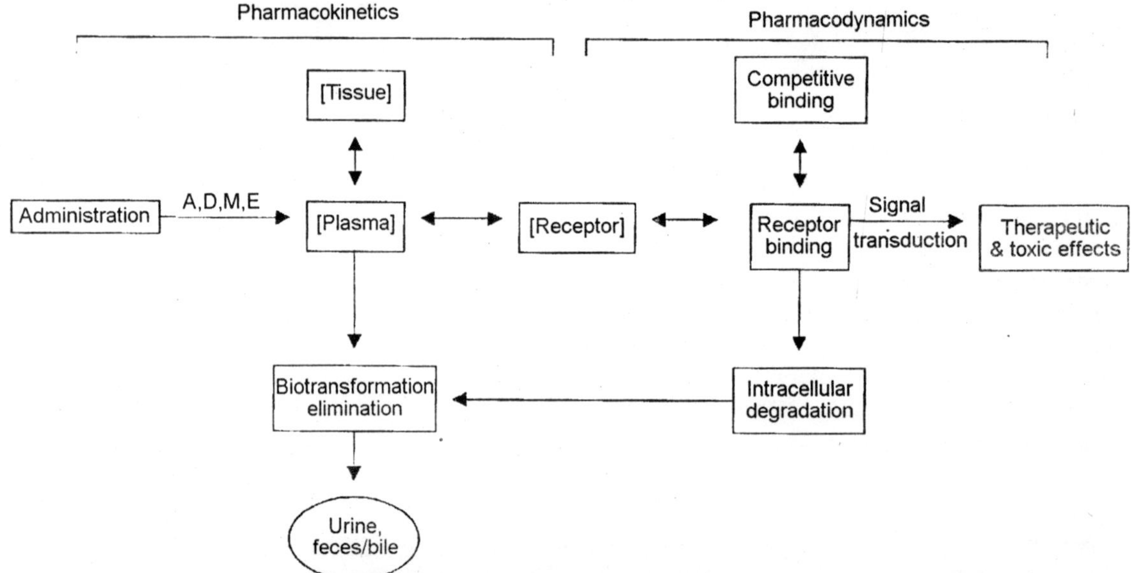

Fig. 6.1. Schematic representation of the physiologic processes determining drug disposition in the human body and the relationship of pharmacokinetics and pharmacodynamics to these processes.

cell death leading to tumor shrinkage), the limits of tolerable drug toxicity to normal tissues are often encroached. Importantly, adverse events, both anticipated and unexpected, must be integrated into therapeutic decisions to optimize patient outcome; thus ongoing assessment and reassessment of the cytotoxic drug effects on tumor and normal tissues are required. Drug–drug, drug–herb/food and drug–comorbid disease interactions, if not considered and anticipated, can have dire consequences for cancer patients. Furthermore, the rapidly increasing numbers of genetic polymorphisms in proteins involved either in the primary mechanism of a drug action and/or the processes that determine drug pharmacokinetics (absorption, distribution, metabolism, and excretion) further increase the complexity of optimal drug prescribing. This chapter focuses on the principles of clinical pharmacology applied to cytotoxic chemotherapy, and forms a basis as to why these principles assist the oncologist in optimizing the efficacy/toxicity ratio for cancer chemotherapeutic agents in individual patients.

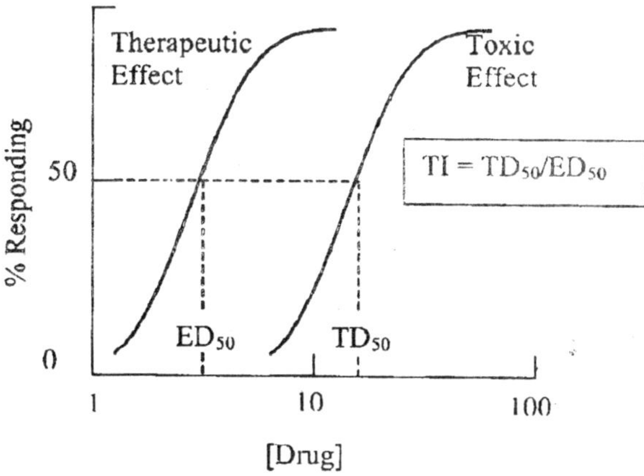

Fig. 6.2. Therapeutic index (TI): the ratio of the TD_{50} to the ED_{50} is an indicator of a drug's selectivity for producing the desired therapeutic effect in relation to its toxic effects.

Mechanisms of Drug Action (Pharmacodynamics)

The study of the effects of drugs on biologic and physiologic processes is termed pharmacodynamics. Most drug effects result from interactions with specific macromolecules or *targets* that induce a biochemical or physiologic change. The target of the drug may be an enzyme found in the plasma or sited intracellularly; a cell-membrane-located protein; an ion channel protein or a structural protein; or DNA, RNA, or other macromolecules (e.g., microtubules). The site of action of many drugs is a *receptor* which normally binds an endogenous regulatory ligand (e.g., hormones, growth factors, neurotransmitters); the receptor function is modified on drug binding. Drugs that bind to receptors and mimic the endogenous ligand are termed *agonists* (e.g., recombinant human erythropoietin [rhEPO], granulocyte colony stimulating factor [G-CSF], opioids). When a drug binds to a receptor and blocks the effects of the endogenous ligand, the drug is termed an *antagonist* (e.g., flutamide, an androgen receptor antagonist; ondansetron, a 5-hydroxytryptamine type 3 [5-HT3] antagonist, trastuzumab [Herceptin] monoclonal antibody against HER-2 /neu). Certain agents have both agonist and antagonist properties at receptors and are termed partial agonists (e.g., tamoxifen-mixed estrogen receptor agonist/antagonist, nalbuphine-mixed $\mu/\kappa/\delta$ opiate receptor agonist/antagonist). Many established and novel anticancer agents inhibit the function of endogenous enzymes by binding directly to an enzyme and are thus termed *enzyme inhibitors* (e.g., dihydrofolate reductase inhibitors—methotrexate; topisomerase I inhibitors, such as members of the camptothecin family; epidermal growth factor receptor [EGFR]-associated tyrosine kinase I inhibitors—OSI-774 [Tarceva] and ZD 1839 [Iressa]; and the farnesyl transferase inhibitor trifarnib).

Drug Action

The binding of a drug to its target is often highly specific and dictated by the three- dimensional structure of both the ligand and target as well as electrostatic, dipole–dipole, ionic, van der Waals, hydrophobic, and hydrogen bond forces. The greater the net sum of these forces, the higher the binding affinity of the drug to its target. Occasionally, a drug will form irreversible covalent bonds with its target, for example, alkylation of the 7-nitrogen and 6-oxygen atom in the guanine ring by ifosforamide

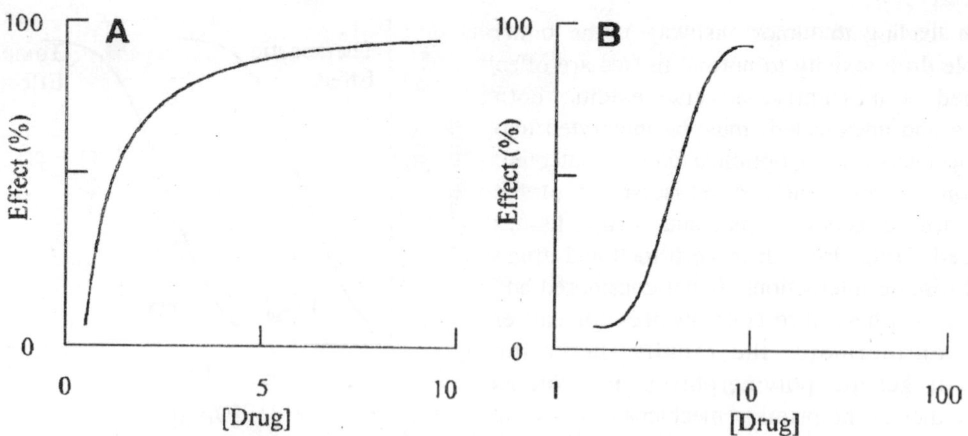

Fig. 6.3. Dose-response curves plotted (A) arithmetically and (B) semilogarithmically.

mustard, the active metabolite of the ifosfamide. The pharmacologic effects of any drug most often occur in a graded, effect site concentration-dependent manner. In many cases the plasma drug concentration is linearly related to the dose of the drug administered; the graphical representation of drug effect is thus often referred to as a *dose–response curve*. Agonist drugs produce a graded dose response up to a maximum value (E_{max}), above which increasing the drug concentration no longer produces a significant increase in effect. Antagonists produce no response and partial agonists have a reduced effect and reduced maximal effect–response. Each drug has a specific shape to its dose (concentration)–response curve at its target site. In clinical therapy its importance underpins the need for dose titration of a drug to optimize the desired response.

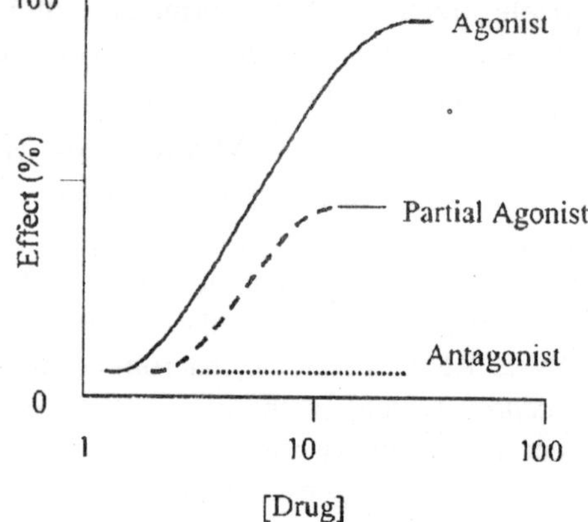

Fig. 6.4. Semilogarithmic plot of percent maximal effect vs drug concentration for an agonist, partial agonist, and antagonist.

Receptor Pharmacology and Function

Molecular cloning techniques, along with advanced biochemical methods, have greatly enhanced our ability to discover and characterize physiological receptors, signal transduction pathways, and effector proteins. Receptors for endogenous ligands are classified into four "*superfamilies*" with distinct functional properties. Three families are localized to the cell membrane: ligand gated ion channel receptors (e.g., glutamate, nicotinic acetylcholine, and γ-aminobutyric acid receptors); G-protein coupled receptors (e.g., opiate receptors), and receptors with enzymatic activity (e.g., EGFR and platelet derived growth factor receptor [PDGFr]). A fourth family of receptors is located within the cell and is known as nuclear transcription factor receptors (e.g., steroid hormone receptors, retinoic acid [RA] receptors, and retinoid X receptors [RXR]). Agonist binding to any one of these receptors, regardless of family, activates a signal transduction pathway, for example, activation of a specific enzyme or cascade of enzymes, release of a second messenger(s), or transcription of a particular gene, and it is this intracellular physiologic change that mediates the effect of a ligand stimulating the receptor.

Agonists

Agonists (e.g. morphine, bromocriptine, lutenizing hormone-releasing hormone agonist, [leuprolide]) produce an effect by interacting with and activating specific receptors for endogenous ligands. The particular signal transduction pathway linked to a receptor determines the process of receptor activation. Drugs that bind directly to and inhibit the activity of enzymes or proteins are not considered agonists because they do not first interact with an endogenous receptor. A useful parameter to compare drugs with equal maximal effect is EC_{50}, the concentration of drug at which a 50% maximal response is observed. Agonist properties can be quantified in terms of potency and magnitude of effect. Potency depends on four factors: receptor density, efficiency of receptor signal transduction, drug affinity for the receptor, and the degree of signal transduction induced by the drug binding to the receptor (*efficacy*). The latter two are properties of the drug itself and can be quantitated by plotting the percentage maximal effect vs log drug concentration for two comparison drugs, which will give relative potency or relative efficacy.

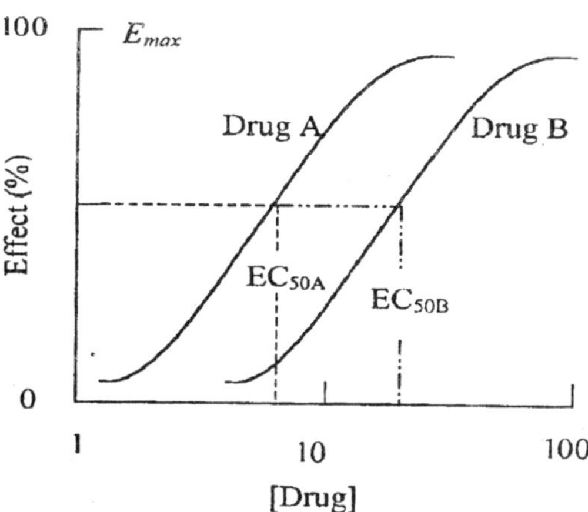

Fig. 6.5. Relative potency: semilogarithmic plot of percent maximal effect vs drug concentration for two drug (A and B) with equal maximum pharmacologic effect (E_{max}).

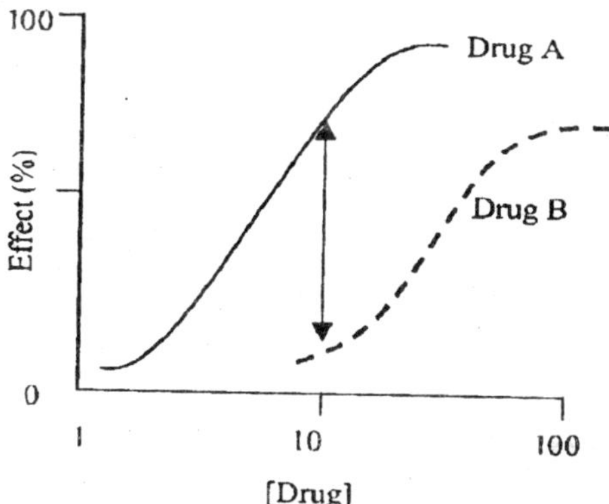

Fig. 6.6. Relative efficacy: semilogarithmic plot of percent maximal effect vs drug concentration for two drugs (A and B) with differing maximal effects.

Competitive antagonists

Competitive antagonists (e.g., trastuzumab, alemtuzumab, rituximab) bind the same endogenous receptors as agonists, but they fail to induce a response (i.e., there is no receptor-mediated downstream signal transduction). Agonists in the presence of competitive antagonists simultaneously compete for the same receptors. The drug concentration in the effect compartment and receptor affinity determine the degree of receptor occupancy of each agent at any given moment in time. The effects of a competitive antagonist can be overcome by increasing the concentration of the agonist. Noncompetitive antagonists, on the other hand, in effect decrease the number of "*effective*" receptors and attenuate the maximal response to an agonist. The effects of a noncompetitive antagonist cannot be overcome by increasing the agonist concentration.

Enzyme inhibition

Similar concepts can be applied to drugs that are enzyme inhibitors (e.g., methotrexate, camptothecins, EGFR tyrosine kinase inhibitors). Thus the drug and the endogenous substrate compete for the same binding site on the enzyme. When the drug is bound, the enzyme can no longer bind substrate and the rate of the enzymatic reaction is reduced. One of the most successful molecularly targeted agents that possesses such a mechanism is imatinib mesylate (STI571/Gleeve), which inhibits ATP binding to the tyrosine kinases activity of the protooncogene *KIT*, PDGFr, and BCR–ABL, inhibiting protein phosphorylation and signaling. Alternatively, some drugs (e.g., chloradenosine as its anabolite chlorodeoxy ATP and the non-nucleoside reverse transcriptase inhibitors [NNRTI] of HIV-

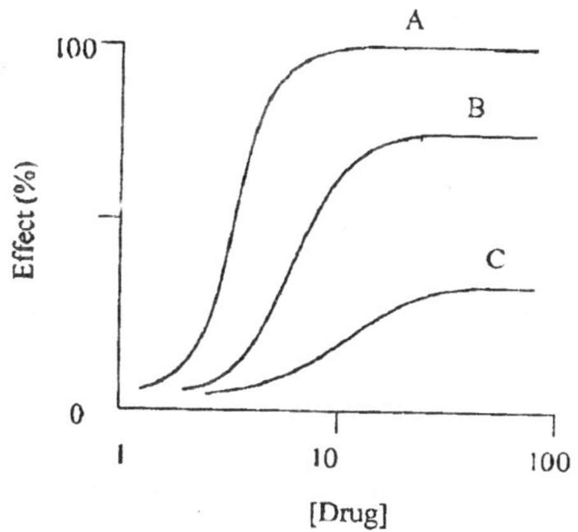

Fig. 6.7. Noncompetitive antagonism.

1, nevirapine, and efavirenz) bind to enzymes at sites other than the endogenous substrate-binding site and induce a conformational change in the enzyme structure. This structural change modifies the three-dimensional shape of the endogenous substrate binding site so that the endogenous substrate is no longer recognized and is unable to bind. These drugs are termed allosteric or noncompetitive enzyme inhibitors.

Partial agonists

Partial agonists (e.g., tamoxifen [a partial agonist at the estrogen receptor], bryostatin [a partial agonist of protein kinase C], certain opioids [nalbuphine, buprenorphine]) stimulate endogenous receptors, but to a lesser degree than full agonists because of their intrinsically low efficacy. When an agonist is administered in the presence of a partial agonist, the maximal effect of the agonist is diminished because some receptors are occupied by the less effective partial agonist, which implies that partial agonists are also partial antagonists. The partial agonist properties of a drug can be overcome by increasing the concentration of the pure agonist.

Non-Receptor-Mediated Drug Action

Some drugs exert their effects based solely on the physical or chemical nature of the drug. In cancer therapy, examples of drugs that work via this mechanism are purine analogs (e.g., 6-mercaptopurine and thioguanine) and certain pyrimidine analogs (e.g., fludaribine), which do not target specific endogenous receptors. They are incorporated into nucleic acids causing the impairment of DNA or RNA synthesis. This mechanism has been termed "*counterfeit incorporation.*"

Pharmacodynamic Models

Pharmacodynamic models quantify the pharmacologic effect of a drug as it relates to the concentration of drug at its site of action (effect compartment concentration). These models are dependent on the assumptions of receptor *occupancy theory*. This theory states that the intensity of the drug effect is proportional to the number of receptors bound by drug and that the maximum effect occurs when all receptors are occupied by the drug. The assumptions of the receptor occupancy theory are as follows: (1) drug--receptor association/dissociation is rapid and at equilibrium, (2) each receptor binds only one drug molecule at a time, (3) drug-receptor binding is reversible. The clinically most pertinent pharmacodynamic model is the E_{max} model, which is based on the hyperbolic relationship between pharmacologic effect and drug concentration. The effect (*E*) can be quantitated by the following equation:

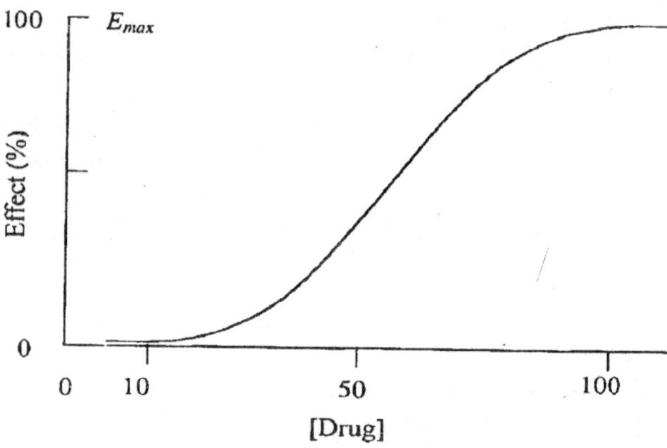

Fig. 6.8. Sigmoid E_{max} pharmacodynamic model.

$$E = (E_{max} \times C)/(EC_{50} + C)$$

where E_{max} is the maximal effect, C is the plasma drug concentration, and EC_{50} is the concentration of drug at which 50% maximal response is observed. If a receptor can bind more than one drug molecule simultaneously (e.g., oxygen binding to hemoglobin), then the sigmoid E_{max} model is used and the equation for effect becomes:

$$E = (E_{max} \times C^{\gamma}) / (EC_{50}^{\gamma} + C^{\gamma})$$

where γ is the "*Hill coefficient*" and relates to the number of drug binding sites per receptor; it determines the slope of the curvilinear relationship.

PHARMACOKINETICS

The study of the time course of drug absorption, distribution, metabolism, and elimination by the human body is termed *pharmacokinetics*. An adequate understanding of the basic principles of pharmacokinetics combined with the specific pharmacokinetic parameters for an individual drug enable the prescriber to choose the most appropriate route of administration, dose, and dosing frequency to obtain an optimal pharmacologic response while minimizing toxicity.

Absorption

Most drugs must enter the systemic circulation to reach specific sites of action (usually intracellular targets for cancer drugs), which are often distant from the site of administration. Drug absorption is a highly variable process dependent on the physicochemical properties of the drug such as molecular size and shape, lipid solubility, degree of ionization, and protein and tissue binding characteristics. Passive diffusion is by far the most important process by which drugs move across cell membranes. The thickness of the cell membrane and the presence or absence of drug efflux pumps (e.g., ATP binding cassette [ABC] transporters, e.g., ABCB1—also known as MDR-1 and P-glycoprotein) also determine the rate and extent of drug absorption. Oral (enteral) drug administration is the most common route of drug delivery because it is convenient, safe, and economical. The majority of cancer drugs, however, are either poorly absorbed from the gastrointestinal tract or undergo significant metabolism or excretion by the gastrointestinal mucosa and/or liver prior to entering the systemic circulation. This process is known as the *first-pass effect*. Drugs with a high first pass effect have low *bioavailability* (F), a term used to describe the fractional extent to which a dose of drug reaches the systemic circulation.

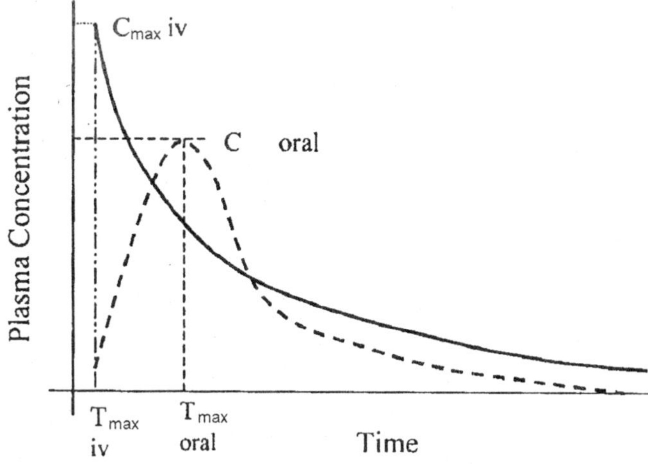

Fig. 6.9. Plasma drug concentration time curves following intravenous (solid line) and oral (dashed line) administration.

Examples of drugs with low oral bioavailability include morphine, many cytotoxics (e.g., paclitaxel, docetaxel, daunorubicin), and monoclonal antibodies (which are proteins and therefore degraded by acid in the stomach). Intravenous administration of drugs used in cancer chemotherapy circumvents the factors related to absorption and the first-pass effect, and by definition provides 100% bioavailability. Other routes of drug administration (e.g., subcutaneous, intramuscular, intra-arterial, intrathecal, and topical) are important in cancer therapeutics.

Distribution

Once a drug enters the systemic circulation, it begins to equilibrate (distribute) throughout the body. Many factors contribute to drug distribution including cardiac output, regional blood flow and blood flow within a tumor, pH of the local environment, presence of drug efflux pumps (especially ABCB1 [MDR-1/P-glycoprotein] and other ABC transporters that are present in many tumors), and the physicochemical properties of the drug, especially its lipid solubility. Binding to plasma proteins (mainly albumin for acidic drugs and α_1 acid glycoprotein for basic drugs) can limit the degree of drug distribution because only unbound (free) drug can passively diffuse through cell membranes. Some drugs accumulate in certain tissues preferentially, usually because they are highly lipophilic or secondary to tissue-specific binding (e.g., paclitaxel to beta-tubulin). Many chemotherapeutic agents have to enter tumor cells to produce a cytotoxic effect. Distribution into tumor cells can be facilitated by transport proteins (carriers) and may be energy dependent (i.e., active transport). Active transport moves drugs against electrochemical and concentration gradients, which can significantly increase drug concentration in tumor cells. Examples of drugs that are actively transported into cells in addition to their transmembrane flux by passive diffusion include fludarabine, gemcitabine, and methotrexate.

Metabolism (Biotransformation)

Many drugs undergo enzymatic modification (metabolism), which most commonly reduces their pharmacological activity and enhances the body's ability to excrete the drug. In some instances, the metabolite is more pharmacologically active than the parent drug (e.g., conversion of ifosfamide to ifosforamide mustard; CPT-11 to SN-38) or an active metabolite may be cleared more slowly than the parent compound (e.g., CPT-11 metabolite SN 38, morphine metabolite, morphine-6-glucuronide). Drug metabolism can be categorized into two phases: phase 1 reactions, which involve metabolic modifications of the drug (often oxidation, reduction, or hydrolysis), and phase 2 reactions, which are synthetic conjugation reactions involving the covalent linkage of a highly polar molecule (glucuronic acid, sulfate, amino acid, glutathione, acetate) to the drug or its metabolite. The products of phase 2 reactions have increased water solubility and are readily excreted in the urine (or bile). The primary site of drug metabolism (both phase 1 and phase 2 reactions) is the liver, although the gastrointestinal tract, kidney, and lungs play important roles for some drugs. Within the liver, the cytochrome P450 (CYP450) monooxygenase system accounts for the vast majority of phase 1 drug metabolism. There are more than 50 known functionally active cytochrome P450's in humans, with only eight isoforms accounting for more than 90% of all drug metabolism. CYP 3A4 and CYP 3A5 (nearly identical isoforms and also expressed in the intestinal epithelium) metabolize approx 50% of all drugs; CYP 2D6 (20% of drugs) and CYP2C9/19 account for the metabolism of another 20–25% of drugs; all the other active isoforms (CYP1A1/2, CYP2B6, CYP2A6, CYP2E1) accounting for the remaining CYP450 metabolic activity. Many drugs are substrates for (and thus metabolized by) more than a single member of the CYP450 enzyme family, having differing affinities for binding to the different CYP450s. Drugs can be both substrates for the CYP450 enzymes and inducers or inhibitors of these enzymes.

Concurrent use of drugs that interfere with the metabolism of another drug may result in significant toxicity or therapeutic failure. The recent identification of multiple genetic polymorphisms for many of the CYP450 enzymes has in part allowed us further insight into the interindividual variability in drug metabolism. The best example of this is the four different CYP2D6 phenotypes; which yield poor, intermediate, extensive, and ultrarapid metabolism of drugs that are substrates for this enzyme.

Phase 2 conjugation reactions also take place in the liver, the most important of which is glucuronidation. This involves the addition of a glucuronide group to the drug by uridine diphosphate glucuronosyltransferase (UGT). More than 15 isoforms of UGTs have been identified, and as with the CYP450 system, functional polymorphisms have been identified (UGT1A1 catalyzes the glucuronidation of SN-38 to SN-38 glucuronide). The same holds true for *N*-acetyltransferase (NAT) and accounts for the "slow and fast acetylator" phenotypes, which affects the metabolism of amonafide to *N*-acetylamonafide (NAT2) and its toxicity profile (fast acetylators experience greater myelosuppression). Intracellular metabolism is another important mechanism of drug biotransformation. Many antimetabolite drugs are dependent on intracellular anabolism/metabolism to yield pharmacologically active entities (e.g., 5-fluorouracil, gemcitabine, 6-mercaptopurine).

Excretion (Elimination)

Drugs can be eliminated from the body either in an unchanged form or as metabolites. Lipid-soluble drugs generally are metabolized to more polar compounds to facilitate their elimination from the body via the kidney. The kidneys are primarily responsible for the excretion of drugs and their metabolites while biliary excretion plays an important role for certain drugs (e.g., taxanes, SN-38 glucuronide). Elimination of drugs via the urine is dependent on three processes: glomerular filtration, active tubular secretion, and passive tubular reabsorption. The glomerular filtration rate is reduced in the elderly and many disease states and is dependent on cardiac output and intravascular volume. Drug molecules that are not protein bound ("free drug") can be filtered. Other physicochemical properties of drugs and metabolites that facilitate renal excretion include small molecular size (mol wt < 500 Da) and being unionized at physiological pH, which depends on the pK_a of the compound.

Pharmacokinetic Parameters

A simple plot of plasma drug concentration vs time offers the prescriber useful pharmacokinetic data. C_{max} is defined as the maximal plasma concentration following a specific dose and t_{max} is the time at which C_{max} is observed. The area under the plasma drug concentration vs time curve (AUC) is a useful measure of the body's total drug exposure.

Volume of distribution

The concept of volume of distribution can be demonstrated by the theoretical administration of a drug as a rapid intravenous bolus injection with sampling and measurement of plasma concentrations at specified time intervals. The resultant log plasma drug concentration vs time graph for a drug that rapidly distributes and equilibrates throughout the body (i.e., the one-compartment, well-stirred model with first-order elimination) will appear similar to the plot representing drug A. Extrapolation of the line back to time zero gives a theoretical plasma drug concentration (C_0) that would have occurred if drug equilibration were instantaneous. This theoretical concentration results from the dilution of a known amount of drug (usually milligrams) into an unknown volume of the human body, which is known as the *apparent volume of distribution* or V_d. Dividing the dose (D) by C_0 gives the value for V_d (usually expressed in liters): $V_d = D/C_0$. Factors affecting the volume of distribution include the physicochemical properties of the drug and many patient-dependent factors such as body size, fat composition, water content, and plasma protein concentration. The V_d is often referred to as the "apparent" volume of distribution because it does not represent a true physiologic single space or compartment within the human body, but rather a theoretical composite value for all the compartments to which the drug distributes. The one-compartment model is a convenient mathematical representation of drug distribution and elimination for many, but not all drugs. More complex models are required for drugs that have protracted distribution times (e.g., paclitaxel, daunorubicin). In the two-compartment model represented for drug B (e.g., docetaxel), the body is divided into two theoretical spaces, a smaller central compartment (blood volume plus the extracellular space of highly perfused tissues; heart, lung, liver, kidneys) and a larger peripheral compartment, which represents all other tissues. A semilogarithmic plot of plasma drug B concentration vs time reveals a biphasic decline in plasma drug concentration over time. The first phase, known as the alpha phase, represents redistribution of drug B out of the

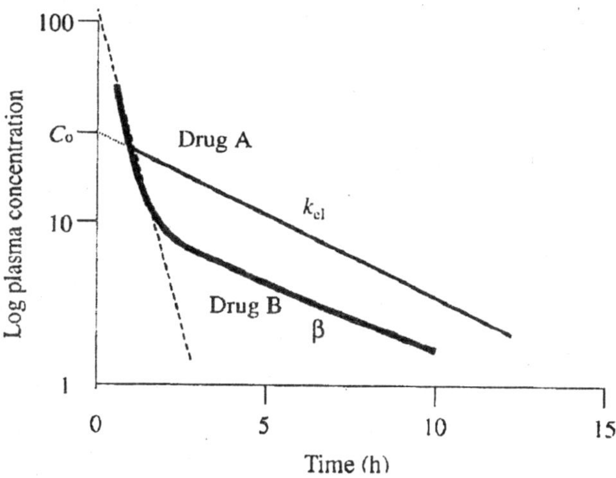

Fig. 6.10. Plasma drug concentration time curves following intravenous (solid line) and oral (dashed line) administration.

central (sampling) compartment and into the peripheral tissues. The beta phase, also known as the terminal elimination phase, occurs after drug B has equilibrated between the two compartments and primarily represents drug elimination. Three-compartment models are necessary to describe some drugs (e.g., paclitaxel, many anthracyclines) that have two distribution phases preceding the terminal elimination phase. The volume of distribution for drugs following a multicompartment model is conceptually the same as for one-compartment modeling, but calculated in a slightly different way.

Clearance

Clearance represents the rate at which a drug is eliminated from the body and is expressed in terms of volume per unit time for first-order elimination. The volume term represents the theoretical volume of blood (or more often plasma) totally cleared of drug during a given time interval, which remains constant and independent of plasma drug concentration. The amount or mass of drug removed from the body per unit time, however, is constantly changing (depending on plasma drug concentration) during first-order elimination and is therefore not a convenient means to express clearance. When clearance mechanisms are saturated (i.e., operating at full capacity), zero-order elimination kinetics is followed and a constant mass (milligrams) of drug is cleared from the body per unit time regardless of the plasma drug concentration.

Most drug pharmacokinetics fit a one-compartment, first-order elimination kinetics model with an elimination rate constant (k_e) equal to the slope of the line for the log plasma drug concentration vs time plot. The total body clearance, Cl_T (which is a summation of all clearance mechanisms; renal, hepatic, and other) of a drug is directly proportional to k_e and V_d: $Cl_T = k_e \times V_d$. Another useful equation to calculate Cl_T for first order elimination is:

$$Cl_T = F \times \text{dose/AUC}$$

where F is the bioavailability and AUC is the area under the log plasma drug concentration time curve.

Elimination half-life ($t_{1/2}$)

The amount of time it takes for the plasma drug concentration to decline by 50% is defined as the half-life ($t_{1/2}$). Half-life is also related to the ke: $t_{1/2} = 0.693/k_e$. Substitution of Cl_T/V_d for k_e yields the equation: $t_{1/2} = 0.693 \times V_d/Cl_T$.

$$t_{1/2} = 0.693 \times V_d/Cl_T$$

Thus, $t_{1/2}$ changes as a function of both Vd and Cl_T (under steady-state conditions). The half-life of a drug is useful in determining the dosing interval for many drugs that are dosed to a steady state and the time required to reach steady-state plasma concentrations (i.e., four half-lives to reach 94% of steady state) as well as being useful for estimating the time for a specific percentage of administered drug to be removed from the body (i.e., on cessation of drug therapy, the plasma drug concentration will decrease by 50% for each $t_{1/2}$ time interval).

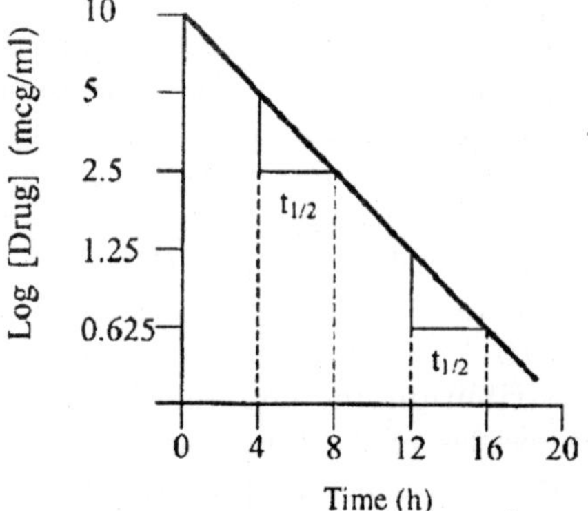

Fig. 6.11. Half-life: log plasma drug concentration vs time plot for a drug following first-order elimination kinetics and a half-life of 4 h.

Noncompartmental modeling

Noncompartmental modeling uses statistical moment theory to derive the same pharmacokinetic parameters and provides the additional parameters of AUMC or area under the first-moment curve (analogous to AUC) and the mean residence time (MRT). The primary advantage of noncompartmental modeling is the requirement for fewer model specific assumptions.

Nonlinear "dose-dependent" pharmacokinetics

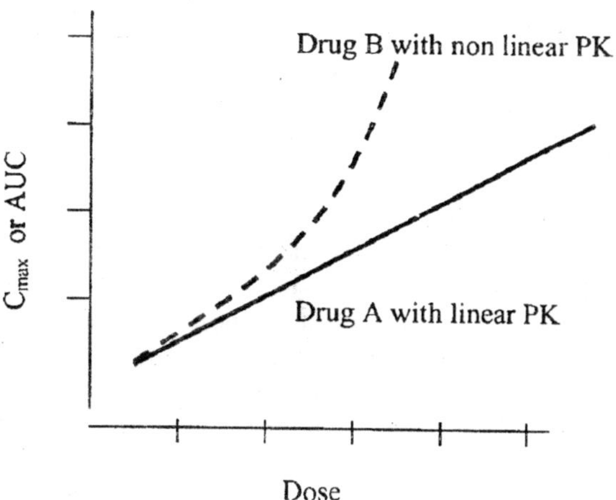

Fig. 6.12. Drug A has linear pharmacokinetics with dose proportional increases in C_{max} and AUC.

Clearance, for most drugs, remains constant (proportional to plasma drug concentration) over the therapeutic dose range and as a result, first-order kinetics are obeyed. Occasionally, clearance mechanisms become overwhelmed (i.e., saturated) and there is no longer an exponential decline in plasma drug concentration over time (i.e., zero-order kinetics are followed). Under such circumstances in which clearance mechanisms are saturated (e.g., enzyme saturation, Michaelis–Menton kinetics apply), small increases in dose can dramatically increase plasma drug concentration or AUC. In such cases (e.g. paclitaxel at doses > 135 mg/m^2 administered over 3 h), the pharmacokinetics are considered "*dose dependent*" or "*capacity-limited.*" This is also termed Michaelis–Menton pharmacokinetics as the nonlinear relationship of concentration and dose can be fitted to the classical enzyme kinetic model. The processes of drug absorption (e.g., oral methotrexate, melphalan), distribution, and excretion can also become saturated, which in turn leads to a drug exhibiting nonlinear pharmacokinetics.

Population Pharmacokinetics

Pharmacokinetic parameters can vary widely from one patient to the next, which may lead to significant toxicity in some patients and therapeutic failure in others. Population pharmacokinetic modeling of pharmacokinetic data from many different patients can help quantify some of this variability. This can be especially useful when the target population for the drug is heterogeneous or when the therapeutic window is narrow (i.e., effective plasma drug concentrations approach toxic concentrations). These models can simultaneously quantitate the effects of identifiable patient demographic variables (e.g., age, sex, weight, etc.), pathophysiological variables (e.g., renal or liver function, congestive heart failure, etc.), and therapeutic variables such as concomitant drug therapy on drug disposition. Another advantage is that the residual variability (the variability not accounted for by the other specified covariates) is quantitated, which includes intraindividual variability, model misspecification, and measurement error.

Pharmacokinetic-Pharmacodynamic Relationship

Pharmacokinetic modeling describes the change of plasma drug concentration over time and pharmacodynamic modeling relates drug concentration to pharmacologic effect (without regard to time). Pharmacokinetic–pharmacodynamic (PK–PD) modeling relates pharmacologic effect to the change of plasma drug concentration over time. The goal is to predict not only the magnitude but also the duration of pharmacologic effect based on the pharmacokinetic parameters of a particular drug. PK–PD models are predicated on the assumption that the concentration of drug in the plasma (accessible compartment) is proportional to the drug concentration at the receptor site (effect compartment). There are some drugs for which there is no correlation between plasma concentration and pharmacologic effect; however, toxicity may be correlated to plasma concentration in some cases (e.g., methotrexate). Such models have perhaps been best used in oncology to predict drug toxicity rather than antitumor effect.

Interpatient Variability

The pharmacokinetic parameters and the pharmacologic response from a specific dose of a drug may vary widely from patient to patient. There are multiple reasons for the observed interpatient variability in drug response that involves both pharmacokinetic and pharmacodynamic processes. These include organ dysfunction, disease state, concurrent medications, receptor and metabolic enzyme phenotype, age, sex, and other demographic characteristics. Drug bioavailability may vary from patient to patient secondary to increased or decreased expression or activity of intestinal enzymes that metabolize drugs or varying expression of drug efflux pumps (i.e., ABCB1-MDR-1 or P-glycoprotein). ABCB1 (P-glycoprotein) also pumps drugs out of cells, thus lowering the intracellular drug concentration, its overexpression in tumor cells is a well-documented mechanism of tumor cell resistance. One of the primary causes of pharmacokinetic variability is interpatient differences in the rate of drug clearance. In the case of drugs (or drugs with active metabolites) that are primarily cleared by the kidney, decreased renal function will dictate the need for dose reduction to avoid excessive toxicity (e.g., methotrexate). Drugs that undergo extensive hepatic biotransformation and/or biliary excretion may require dose modification in patients with severely compromised hepatic function (e.g., taxanes, anthracyclines, vinca alkaloids). Genetic polymorphisms in the CYP450 enzyme and other phase 2 enzyme systems (e.g., *N*-acetylation transferase-2, glutathione-*S*-transferase, and uridine diphosphate glucuronosyltransferase) will also contribute to differences in an individual's ability to metabolize anti-cancer drugs. Another major reason for altered CYP450 activity is the use of concurrent medications that either inhibit or induce one or more isoforms, which may result in significant changes in the rate of drug clearance.

Variability in the volume of distribution of a drug can also account for some of the observed interpatient variability. Age is particularly important for volume of distribution because infants have approx 70–80% total body water compared to 60% for adults. Elderly patients have relatively more adipose tissue and less water content as well as decreased muscle mass. Disease-related alterations in plasma protein concentrations in cancer patients can affect the volume of distribution of drugs that are highly protein bound (e.g., α_1-acid glycoprotein which binds docetaxel and UCN-01) influencing free drug concentrations and drug clearance. Pharmacodynamic variability is produced not only by differences between patients in the concentration of drug at the effect site as a result of pharmacokinetic variation but also by receptor/target polymorphisms. Examples of these polymorphisms include cases in which a receptor is more or less responsive to a certain drug concentration, as is the case for opioid receptors, or where paclitaxel resistance is linked to variants in the β-tubulin.

7

PROMISE OF PERSONALIZED MEDICINE

The concept of individualized drug therapy has been a central focus in clinical pharmacology and medicine for many decades. In practice, there are two key elements concerning customized therapies: choice of the dosing regimen and/or the drug itself. Both of these factors contribute to personalized medicine. Despite its apparent simplicity, individualization of treatment is a daunting challenge due to molecular heterogeneity in human diseases and marked patient-to-patient and between-population differences in drug effects as well as therapeutic dose requirements.

Therapeutics as a science relies on the degree of predictability of drug effects and the mechanisms governing their predictability. A clear understanding of the factors that influence dose–response and time-course of drug action allows rational choice of drugs and their dosages. There are also degrees of personalized medicine. The resolution of customization may vary, on the one hand, from drugs that are targeted for a very small group of individuals, to those that are intended for use in most members of the population without regard to individual characteristics of the patients. The latter group is also known as blockbuster drugs and represents majority of the medications that are currently in clinical use. Thus, the notion of personalized medicine reflects a fundamental conceptual departure from the traditional lore of pharmacotherapy that asserts the use of pharmaceuticals uniformly in broad patient populations, rather than smaller subpopulations wherein drugs may exhibit enhanced efficacy and optimal safety.

Interest in personalized medicine and rational choice of therapies can be traced back to the first formal comparative trial in the 18th century. James Lind, a naval surgeon, demonstrated in 1747 that citrus juice, and not the other leading remedies recommended by physicians of the day, cured scurvy. At the turn of the 20th century the British physician, Archibald Garrod wrote presciently on the topic of chemical individuality. More recently in the second half of the 20th century, the impetus for customized pharmacotherapy was fueled by adverse drug reactions (ADRs). The early reports of aplastic anemia in patients exposed to chloramphenicol, followed by the thalidomide disaster in 1961 led to recognition of at risk populations, or conditions (e.g., renal failure) and drug–drug interactions that may predispose to drug toxicity. These developments and the ensuing scientific scrutiny culminated in the publication, for the first time, of formal principles pertaining to individualization of drug treatment based on disease, genetic, or environmental chemical influences.

Why is there a strong emphasis on personalized medicine now? Interindividual variability in drug effects and the lack of reliable predictors of this variability are increasingly recognized as important barriers to science-based therapeutics. Moreover, the public health consequences of uncertainty in drug efficacy and safety have been increasingly documented by recent pharmacovigilance studies. A number of policy initiatives, particularly those on ADRs, further added to the momentum for personalized therapies in health care. Notably, present genetics-based efforts to individualize drug therapy have a more *mechanistic* focus in contrast to the previous empirical initiatives on personalized medicine using less precise demographic and descriptive clinical characteristics of the patients or the attendant disease. Hence, a common thread that runs through current pharmacogenomic strategies aimed at personalized medicine is the intent to relate the descriptive results of pharmaceutical interventions or patient characteristics to molecular and mechanistic underpinnings of drug response that, by extension, may allow more precise and rational predictions on clinical outcomes.

The advances made by completion of the Human Genome Project (HGP) 4 years ago and the high throughput genomic technologies that spun off from this effort now make it entirely feasible to apply this vast knowledge-base in the clinical practice and diagnosis of human diseases as well as drug efficacy and safety in each individual patient. The HGP presents unique research opportunities to identify novel drug targets for common complex diseases. This offers the promise in the near future for improvements not only in drug safety but also therapeutic efficacy by selective prescriptions in subpopulations identified by genetic testing of drug targets. The individualization of drug therapy is thus evolving from traditional dose titration methods to more radical approaches concerning prescription decisions and the choice of drugs based on individuals' genetic make-up. These changes, understandably, are attracting much attention from all stakeholders including patients, physicians, academic investigators, pharmaceutical industry, insurers and experts in regulatory science. Collectively, these recent developments have placed the study of human genetics and personalized medicine firmly on the social policy agenda, raising a vast amount of public interest as well as close scrutiny of its promises and actual impact on patient care.

Pharmacogenomics is a term introduced in late 1990s and is broadly defined as the study of variability in drug safety and efficacy using information from the entire genome of a patient. Variations in both gene sequence and expression are of interest to pharmacogenomic inquiries. By contrast, the term pharmacogenetics has been established since 1950s and refers to investigations on specific candidate genes in relation to individual differences in drug effects. Candidate genes in pharmacogenetic studies are selected based on a priori observations of disease susceptibility, drug absorption, metabolism, transport, and excretion as well as drug targets, as opposed to the genome-wide hypothesis-free approach in pharmacogenomics. Despite these differences, there is also interdependency between the two disciplines. Once the genes or genetic markers relevant to mechanism of drug action or safety are identified through the genome-wide pharmacogenomics search, each individual gene requires further clinical validation by focused and hypothesis-driven pharmacogenetic approaches before they can be routinely applied at point of care in the clinic. We herein chose to use the term pharmacogenomics but many of the ensuing discussion and concepts will also be applicable to pharmacogenetics.

The aim of the present chapter is to introduce the reader to (i) broad pharmacological, genetic and societal drivers as well as the promise of personalized medicine, (ii) specific pharmacogenomic strategies to individualize drug therapy early in drug discovery, clinical development and during routine therapy at point of care in the clinic, and (iii) conceptual and practical barriers to pharmacogenomic-guided personalized medicine and the broader ethical issues associated with customized therapies.

Drivers and Promise of Personalized Medicine

Rationale for Customized Drug Therapy: Variability and the Present State of Drug Safety and Efficacy in the Clinic

Most current medications and the recommended dosing regimens come with a significant risk of drug toxicity or treatment-failure in the clinic. Drug-related morbidity and mortality were estimated to cost up to $137 billion annually in the United States. A recent meta-analysis of prospective studies in the United States suggests that serious and fatal ADRs occur in 6.7% and 0.32% of hospitalized patients, respectively. This translates into more than two million serious ADRs and an annual death rate of 106,000 patients in the United States alone. These estimates rank ADRs as the fourth leading cause of death, ahead of accidents, diabetes and pneumonia. Subsequent extended analysis of pharmaco-epidemiology data in 32 non-U.S. studies from industrialized countries support the contention that fatal ADRs are a significant public health problem in many countries around the world. It is noteworthy that the serious ADRs noted above were observed during treatment with usual doses of drugs that had already been introduced for clinical use and despite the exclusion of cases due to intentional or accidental overdose, human errors in drug administration or non-compliance, drug abuse, and therapeutic failures. Similarly, an independent study of 2227 ADRs in hospitalized patients showed that about 50% had no readily discernible or preventable cause. Nearly 16% of the 1232 pharmaceutical products listed in the Physicians' Desk Reference in the U.S. were deemed to carry a significant ADR risk to warrant a "*black box*" warning on the drug label.

Table 7.1. Response rates of patients to major drug classes in selected therapeutic areas

Therapeutic area	*Efficacy rate (%)*
Alzheimer's	30
Analgesics (Cox-2)	80
Asthma	60
Cardiac arrhythmias	60
Depression (SSRI)	62
Diabetes	57
HIV	47
Incontinence	40
Migraine (acute)	52
Migraine (prophylaxis)	50
Oncology	25
Osteoporosis	48
Rheumatoid arthritis	50
Schizophrenia	60

The societal and global burden of ADRs can be compounded further by consideration of drug morbidity and mortality in ambulatory settings and nursing homes as well as non-industrialized countries. Collectively, these epidemiological observations suggest that more fundamental and previously unaccounted reasons, possibly genetic in nature, may underlie a significant portion of such unpreventable and apparently idiosyncratic ADRs in the clinic. Consistent with this hypothesis, a detailed analysis of 27 drugs frequently cited in ADR studies found that 59% are metabolized by one or more enzyme with a variant allele associated with deficient metabolism. By contrast, only 7–22% of drugs selected at random were influenced by a genetically polymorphic metabolic pathway. Although drug safety has traditionally received much research and media attention, drug efficacy is an equally important and yet, often overlooked dimension of pharmacotherapy. In comparison to ADRs, the public health consequences and economic costs of therapeutic-failure associated with drugs have not been well investigated. A recent review of published data on the efficacy of major drugs used in several important diseases is instructive in this regard. Spear et al. concluded that the response rates vary markedly across various therapeutic areas with 80% of patients responding to Cox-2 inhibitors while the response rate was as low as 25% in cancer chemotherapy and 30% in Alzheimer's disease. Overall, it appears that only about 50% of patients respond to drugs in major therapeutic classes (or conversely, 50% of patients, on average, do not respond to pharmacotherapy).

While drugs are often life-saving in some patients, the existing armamentarium of drugs, taken together, are only moderately effective in the general population and carry significant liabilities in the form of serious and fatal ADRs. The traditional notion of blockbuster drugs overlooks this interindividual variability in drug efficacy and safety despite its adverse public health consequences and economic burden on society at large. In fact, one may argue, in light of the pharmacovigilance data noted above, that there are really very few robust examples of blockbuster drugs in the clinic. The term "*blockbuster drug*" has more economic underpinnings and relates to the commercial promise of a medication. Unfortunately, this term is often misused in a scientific context to refer to a broad array of drugs that are assumed to work in most members of the population with optimal safety whereas, in essence, it indicates the pharmaceutical products that are developed and marketed with the general population in mind. The predicaments associated with safety and efficacy of the existing medications clearly call for more focused science-based therapeutics and rational approaches to selection of drugs and their dosing regimens to customize pharmacotherapy based on, for example, individual patient genetic make-up. Understanding the mechanisms and cause-effect relationships for apparently unpreventable and idiosyncratic ADRs and treatment-failures is crucial for early identification and prevention of such drug related problems in the 21st century healthcare.

Rationale for Genetics: Can it Explain and Predict Variability in Drug Efficacy and Safety?

A prerequisite implicit assumption for any pharmacogenomic study is that the targeted pharmacological trait (or phenotype) is subject to appreciable genetic control. To this end, it is important to recognize that drug effects are usually elicited against the background of disease phenomena. Many of the human diseases display genetic components with varying degrees. Further, some of the biological pathways underlying diseases may serve as targets for drug interventions or alternatively, hold the potential to modify, or counteract the direct pharmacological effects of drugs via homeostatic mechanisms. Thus, genetic regulation of diseases or physiological pathways may indirectly influence variability in drug effects.

More direct evidence for the role of heredity in pharmacology can be observed in pharmacokinetic processes. The origins of pharmacogenomics date to the 1950s when monogenic variations in drug metabolism were the primary focus of research interest. Early on, a number of seminal twin studies in healthy volunteers under uniform basal environmental conditions demonstrated a markedly higher reproducibility of pharmacokinetic indices in monozygotic twins (nearly 100% identity in the genome) compared to dizygotic twins who share, on average, only 50% of their genome. These observations provided the first unequivocal evidence that heredity plays a prominent role in drug metabolism, despite the multitude of other environmental and clinical factors that may potentially influence variability in drug exposure. Subsequently, the debrisoquine/sparteine (CYP2D6) polymorphism was first identified by Smith in London, England and Eichelbaum in Bonn, Germany. Since then, numerous genetic polymorphisms have been firmly documented and functionally characterized in various drug metabolizing enzymes and drug transporters. Most experts in the field of pharmacogenomics now agree that hereditary factors play an important role in drug disposition.

Although the focus of studies on the clinical relevance of genetic variations in pharmacokinetic pathways has been mostly on drug safety, there is both theoretical basis and empirical evidence to suggest that drug efficacy can also be influenced. In this regard, an early anecdotal observation made by Smith during the discovery of debrisoquine polymorphism can be instructive. In a pharmacokinetic study of debrisoquine in 1970s, a subtherapeutic dose resulted in unexpected and profound decrease in blood pressure of a subject, who, in fact, was one of the study investigators. Implicit in this historical account is that the side effect (hypotension) experienced by Smith himself is essentially an extension of the primary intended pharmacological effect of the antihypertensive drug debrisoquine. Such ADRs typified by an augmentation of the primary "*therapeutic*" effect of a drug are classified as Type A drug reactions. Type A reactions are common, dose- or concentration-dependent and also include ADRs due to overdose as well as drug–drug interactions. Thus, drug efficacy and toxicity are usually observed on a successive concentration gradient. This means that any genetic or environmental factor that can influence drug concentrations may also explain individual variations in both efficacy and safety. Dramatic differences in cure rates of helicobacter pylori infection and peptic ulcer with omeprazole (a CYP2C19 substrate) and amoxacillin among patients with different CYP2C19 genotypes further attest to the relevance of pharmacogenomic variability in drug metabolism with respect to drug efficacy.

Genetic variations in receptors, ion channels and other types of drug targets constitute a more recent but growing body of evidence in favor of heredity and its role in drug efficacy and safety. Already, there are accumulating data, for example, documenting the clinical significance of variations in genes encoding arachidonate 5-lipoxygenase (ALOX5) and β_2-adrenoreceptor for response to ALOX5 inhibitors and β_2-agonists, respectively, in asthma; serotonin receptors in response to atypical antipsychotic clozapine; and dopamine D3 receptor gene (DRD3) for predisposition to the movement disorder, tardive dyskinesia, induced by typical antipsychotic drugs. We note that the commonly occurring and unpreventable ADRs may be attributable in part to genetic variations in drug targets and/or presently unknown genetic differences in drug disposition, for instance, in phase II drug metabolizing enzymes and drug transporters.

Genes rarely act in isolation and hence, genetic contributions to pharmacological variability are subject to influences by gene–environment interactions as well as epistatic interactions among various genetic loci. Indeed, the most likely scenario is that the underlying basis of genetically determined variability in treatment response and common ADRs is polygenic. It is therefore often difficult to estimate the *composite genetic component* in pharmacological traits. This information is essential before decisions on further molecular pharmacogenomic work can be justified. Typically, heritability estimates are obtained using the twin method. Although twin studies are indeed very useful to establish the baseline heritability figures for common complex diseases, they may have limited applicability in pharmacological responses to drugs and other xenobiotics. Some of these limitations include difficulties in recruitment of twins, obtaining clinical outcome data in both twins (since the twin pairs may not suffer from the same disease at the same time) as well as the financial cost of twin investigations. To circumvent the difficulties associated with dissection of genetic components with the twin approach, a repeated-drug-administration (RDA) method has been earlier proposed wherein between- and within-subject variances in drug efficacy or safety are compared. A relatively larger between-subject variance as measured by the RDA analysis points to significance of hereditary factors in pharmacological variability. Recent applications of the RDA method demonstrate that genetics also plays a paramount role in pharmacological traits hitherto not subjected to pharmacogenomic analysis such as renal drug disposition.

Recognition of Molecular Heterogeneity in Human Diseases: The Need for New Drug Targets

The completion of the HGP 4 years ago provided the reference framework for the sequence of some 30,000–40,000 protein-coding genes in the human genome. At that time, a high-density map of the human genome consisting of 1.42 million single-nucleotide polymorphisms (SNPs) (now >3.7 million) have also been made available. These advances witnessed in parallel the development of high-throughput genomic technologies and the related infrastructure; this was favorably reflected in marked decreases in genotyping costs over the past several years. On the other hand, some of the alternative viewpoints consider the HGP more of an engineering triumph with the development of tools and technologies for genetic research. For translation of the human genome sequence to biology, clinical medicine and science-based therapeutics, a second additional layer of complexity, namely, interindividual and population-to-population variability in the genome will need to be addressed. The latter issue has recently culminated in the launch of the International HapMap project to identify the SNPs and their patterns (haplotypes) on individual chromosomes in various human populations from Africa, Asia and Europe. In the present post-genomic era, the ultimate goal is to utilize the haplotype map of the human genome as a foundation for future genetic association studies of human diseases as well as drug efficacy and safety. A further important consideration is that genetic variants underlying variability in drug effects are unlikely to be limited to the coding elements of genes. Variants in regulatory regions are most likely to be implicated and it is quite feasible that non-coding, intronic elements, which influence gene transcription, have an important role as well. These considerations greatly broaden the scope of genetic influences that will need to be considered.

Why do we need to know the genetic basis of human diseases? And how does this information contribute to rational therapeutics? A recent biochemical classification of drug targets found that the largest group was comprised of receptors (45%) followed primarily by enzymes (28%), hormones and related factors (11%), ion channels (5%), and nuclear receptors (2%). Overall, current drug targets across all therapeutic areas amount to only about 500 molecular targets. Considering the diversity of human diseases, there is no doubt that novel drug targets will be essential to develop drugs with improved efficacy. To this end, identification of the molecular genetic basis of diseases may have three fundamental contributions. First, knowledge of the genes will eventually help discern the identity of the corresponding proteins leading to disease and its clinical manifestations. In some cases, these proteins can serve as direct targets for therapeutic interventions by conventional small molecule drugs (<500 Da molecular weight). On the other hand, it is also reasonable to expect that not all disease-causing genes or their protein products will be druggable.

A second alternative therapeutic strategy in such cases may involve targeting other components of the biological pathway(s) containing the genes associated with disease. Third, in the absence of molecular genetic corollaries of disease, it is noteworthy that entry points for most therapeutic interventions have thus far been at the protein level. The knowledge of a specific disease- causing gene or mutation may allow interventions further upstream in the biological cascade at the level of gene expression before the corresponding proteins of pathophysiological significance are actually synthesized. For example, libraries of small inhibitory RNA (siRNA) molecules are now being investigated in the pharmaceutical and biotechnology industries as potential therapeutic agents to silence the genes whose expression may predispose to disease.

A glance at recent advances in human genetics can be instructive to gain a balanced context on the drivers of pharmacogenomics in the near future. In rare monogenic diseases, a clear pattern of Mendelian inheritance can be discerned wherein human genetic variation in one or both copies of a single gene will predictably lead to clinical manifestations of the attendant disease. Through positional cloning approaches, more than 1400 genes for some 1200 Mendelian traits have been identified by the year 2003. The majority of the mutations associated with monogenic diseases are in-frame amino-acid substitutions and nonsense codons (59%), deletions (22%) and insertions/duplications (7%) while only about 1% of the mutations linked to Mendelian traits were in regulatory regions of human genes. The remarkable success of the positional cloning strategy in monogenic diseases has not been uniformly reproducible upon application to multi- factorial complex human diseases such as diabetes, schizophrenia and non-familial, sporadic forms of common cancers. A hallmark of complex diseases is that a multitude of genetic loci as well as the environment and life-style importantly contribute to disease risk. The

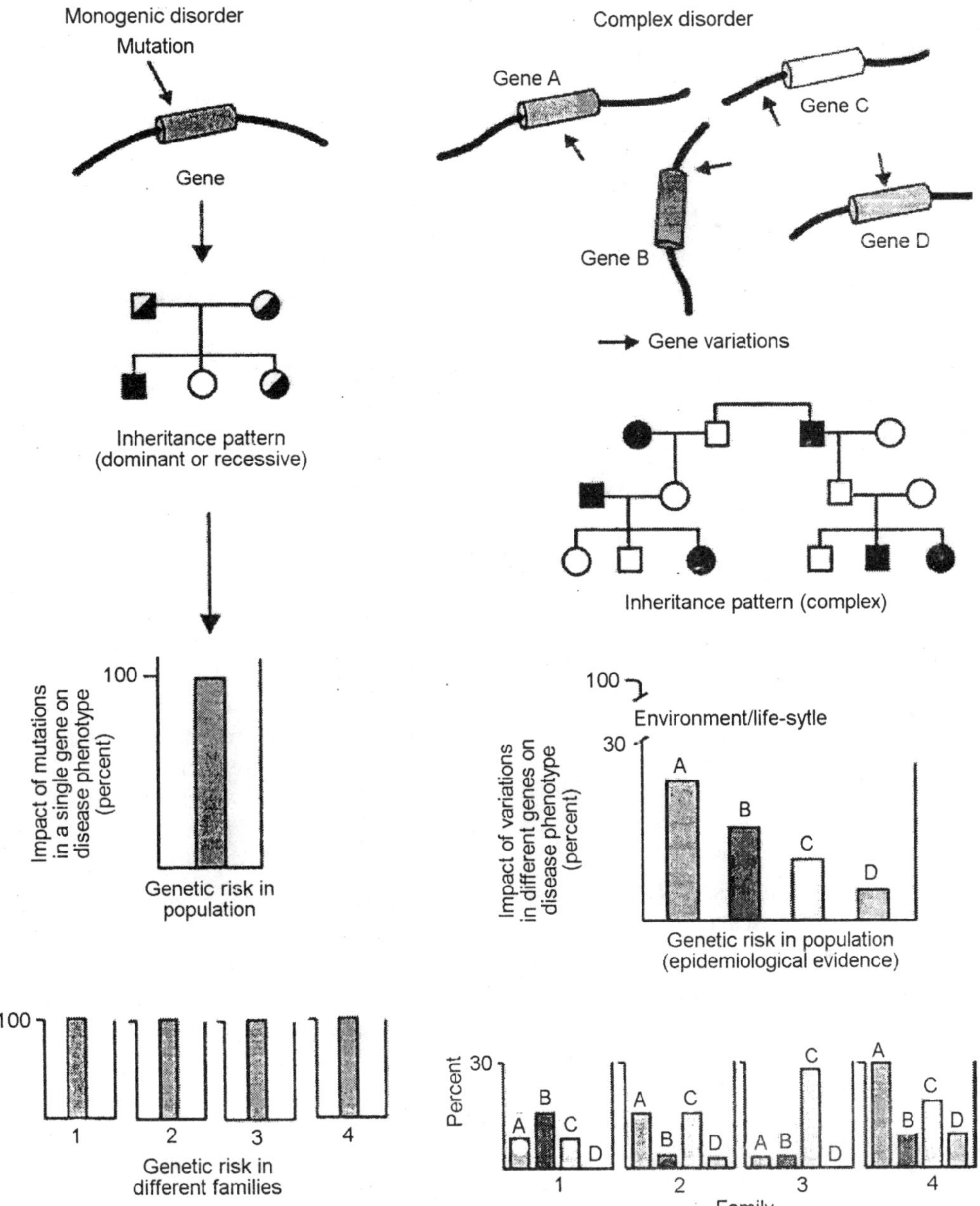

Fig. 7.1. Inheritance of monogenic and complex disorders.

multiplicity of contributory factors and their interactions result in non-Mendelian transmission of disease phenotypes in pedigrees. Further, genetic variations in regulatory regions of the genome that affect gene expression and translationally silent mutations are also likely to play a significant role in predisposition to multifactorial diseases. Hence, current nosologies based on clinical chemistry and symptoms reflect vastly divergent underlying molecular mechanisms leading to the final and ostensibly similar clinical syndromes among patients. This means that effective treatment of patient subpopulations typified by distinct molecular etiologies may require differential therapies with drugs that target a unique complement of biological targets. In the near future, we will therefore likely witness the emergence of genetic tests to assist and complement diagnosis of diseases with clinical nosology. To this end, a synergy between tests for genes associated with disease and drug effects can also be expected. For instance, the APOE4 allele of the APOE gene is associated with predisposition and a lower age of onset for sporadic or late onset familial forms of Alzheimer's disease as well as poor response to acetylcholinesterase enzyme inhibitor tacrine.

Shift in Emphasis on Health Care Policy Toward Disease Prevention

The dictum in the traditional folklore of medicine has been the treatment and alleviation of acute symptoms of disease. Aforementioned advances in our understanding of the risk factors and molecular basis of human diseases are now paving the way to develop medicines that can prevent or slow the progression of disease phenomena. Schizophrenia and some of the neurodegenerative diseases such as Alzheimer's or Parkinson's disease are being investigated in reference to neurodevelopmental theories to develop drugs that can halt the (patho)physiological processes leading to eventual clinical symptoms. The rise of statins and other lipid lowering drugs to prevent long-term cardiovascular morbidity and mortality is another example of preventative pharmacotherapies. It is thus noteworthy that the interest in personalized medicine does not happen in a vacuum and should be viewed within the larger framework of recent changes in health and therapeutic policies over the past decade.

Poised at the threshold of this upcoming and fundamental change in emphasis from treatment to prophylaxis in healthcare policy, pharmacogenomics will likely be shaped in the near future by particular attributes of the pharmacological interventions aimed at disease prevention. For instance, there will be an increasing demand to predict the long-term outcome and benefit-to-risk ratio of preventative therapies. Equally important, adherence to drug treatment by patients will need assurance beyond traditional physician visits and consultations, especially considering that such "future" patients will need to take drugs in the absence of acute symptoms and in the face of a probable disease risk in the far-too-distant future. It is in this very context that predictive pharmacogenomic tests will be essential for patients, physicians and insurers to make informed and rational decisions to subscribe to pharmacogenomically guided and customized therapies that may be offered at premium prices by drug manufacturers.

Asymmetry Between Genetics of Human Diseases and Pharmacological Phenotypes: An Impetus for Pharmacogenomic Research

The fundamental focus of human genetics is to establish the causal links between genes and phenotypes. Since its first introduction in late 1990s, the allure of pharmacogenomics has drawn a considerable number of human geneticists who have previously dealt with complex diseases. This importantly benefited and complemented the classical pharmacological approaches to questions of variability in drug effects. At the same time, a tendency has arisen to view pharmacological responses akin to disease phenotypes. There are however several fundamental differences unique to the field of pharmacology and the attendant phenotypes that may offer a relative advantage in application of genetic methodologies. It has long been known that most chronic human diseases initiate and progress over a considerable period of time before clinical findings become apparent. Thus, human genetics is essentially an observational science wherein molecular genetic markers are correlated with a disease process that is not experimentally controlled or reproducible for obvious ethical and practical reasons. A related corollary is that the scope of gene–environment interactions is often incalculable or difficult to estimate with adequate certainty.

For all the parallels between the disease traits and pharmacological phenotypes, the very difference between the observational nature of study designs in disease genetics and the ability to experimentally produce drug response phenotypes in a setting carefully controlled for environmental factors is perhaps one of the most salient tenets of pharmacology that may offer a marked opportunity to control for gene–environment interactions in pharmacogenomic investigations. For instance, it is feasible to quantify the baseline phenotypes prior to drug administration in humans, which can subsequently be subtracted from drug-induced phenotypes in biological systems. In theory, this can considerably facilitate correlative studies on human genetic variation and pharmacological phenotypes. By contrast, such experimental approaches are not applicable to the study of common multifactorial human diseases. This favorable asymmetry between disease genetics and pharmacogenomics is increasingly being recognized by scientists and clinicians with diverse backgrounds thereby coalescing interest in pharmacogenomics in various medical specialties in academia and the pharmaceutical industry.

Advances in Regulatory Science and Medicolegal Considerations

The transition from a new research idea to actual application in the clinic and drug development is a slow and arduous process. A recent search of the 2000 entries in the Physicians' Desk Reference (year 2003 electronic version) identified only 51 labels containing pharmacogenomic information. Moreover, presentations of the pharmacogenomic data in the labels were generally not in a form that could be readily applied in clinical practice. Although it is difficult to estimate the number of drug labels that should appropriately contain data on host genetic make-up for rational dose titration or choice of medications, the latter example suggests that pharmacogenomic information is likely underrepresented in current drug labels. This is an important issue of relevance for adoption of pharmacogenomics in the clinic because it is not clear whether and to what extent research findings available as off-label scientific publications can be applied in routine medical practice with busy schedules. Still, drug labels do not always reflect the best available evidence. Recent announcement of a guidance document in March 2005 by the U.S. Food and Drug Administration (FDA) to encourage regulatory pharmacogenomics data submission by drug developers is a welcome development in this regard. Advances in regulatory science over the past three decades have been instructive on the critical role of regulatory guidance in widespread implementation of new technologies on practices in the pharmaceutical industry and clinical medicine.

A case in point is the history of development of population pharmacokinetic approaches to explain variability in drug exposure. Despite the theoretical foundations established since the 1970s and the availability of statistical software capable of conducting such advanced pharmacokinetic analyses, the routine use of population pharmacokinetics in clinical drug development has been considerably facilitated in part through recent guidelines developed by regulatory agencies. The present heightened public awareness on societal ramifications of the HGP and the attendant genomic technologies is increasingly prompting governments and policy makers to provide further guidance on pharmacogenomics. Moreover, regulatory consideration may soon be given to drugs already in the clinic. This should further encourage drug manufacturers to adopt pharmacogenomics, with the realization that regulatory review will be applicable at all phases of a medication's life-cycle, both prior and subsequent to introduction for human use. Seen in this light, it is conceivable that developments on the regulatory policy front will importantly shape and drive the application of pharmacogenomics technology in the very near future.

As information on the molecular basis of human diseases and individual variability in drug effects continues to accumulate, a threshold may soon be crossed beyond which the standard of care will include predictive pharmacogenomic testing. Advances in accessibility of pharmacogenomic technologies may thus challenge the traditional questions of ethics and litigation standards. In fact, the clinical significance of genetic variability in certain drug metabolizing enzymes such as thiopurine methyl transferase are already (TPMT) well-established, e.g., in relation to life-threatening toxicity associated with thiopurine anticancer drugs. In such cases where research findings increasingly impact patient care, demands by insurers and government payers as well as legal liability and litigation by patients who suffer from drug toxicity or treatment-failure may set a strong precedent for pharmacogenomic testing by physicians and the pharmaceutical industry. Looking further, it is tempting to suggest that physicians who attend focused continuing medical education courses on pharmacogenomics may presumably be subject to reduced premiums for malpractice insurance in the future. Such complex medicolegal dynamics between patients, insurers, healthcare providers, and drug manufacturers may eventually catalyze the adoption of pharmacogenomics as part of science-based therapeutics.

A recently released survey of American consumers (n = 748) and physicians (n = 400) suggests that nearly 50% of consumers would be agreeable to undergo genetic testing to determine which medication would be most appropriate for them and that they would be willing to pay more for an individually tailored prescription. About 80% of physicians and consumers, on the other hand, expressed views that genetically guided personalized medicine would have a favorable impact on the U.S. healthcare system. It will be of interest to also characterize consumer and physician attitudes in other countries to determine the global patterns of acceptance of pharmacogenomics and the potential barriers to its implementation.

Strategies for Application of Pharmacogenomics to Customize Therapy

Drug Discovery and Preclinical Development

Drug discovery has long relied on serendipitous observations. For drugs introduced in the 1950s and onward, the mode of drug action has been typically discovered after some period of use in the clinic. Over the past two decades, routine application of high-throughput screening (HTS) methods together with combinatorial chemistry and a rich array of chemical libraries significantly accelerated the entry of therapeutic candidates with clearly defined molecular targets to early phase clinical evaluation. Despite these advances, out of 1035 new drug applications approved in the 12-year period from 1989 to 2000 in the United States, a sizable fraction (54%) were differentiated from existing drugs primarily on the basis of dosage form, route of administration, or as a combination product with another active ingredient. Moreover, direct-to-consumer promotions of pharmaceutical products occasionally rely on claims of higher therapeutic "*potency*." An improvement in potency means that the same drug effect can be elicited at a lower drug concentration. This may favorably influence drug selectivity and safety in certain cases.

The excessive emphasis on discovery of more potent compounds overlooks another basic currency of pharmacology: efficacy—the maximal effect that can be produced by a drug. This predicament is best exemplified by the moderate efficacy of current drugs in the clinic. Efficacy is reflected in the asymptotic plateau of concentration–effect curves; it is determined by both the chemical structure of the drug and the biological attributes of the targeted receptor–effector systems. No matter how many structurally diverse hit and lead compounds are synthesized in early discovery, large volumes of compound libraries will not make up for the limited diversity in drug targets (only some 500 at present) thereby markedly constraining the upper limits of therapeutic drug effects in patients. For improvements in drug efficacy, advances made by combinatorial chemistry and HTS need to be complemented by the discovery of novel drug targets, or better characterization of the subtypes of existing targets. Genome-wide association studies of drug response or common human diseases may provide clues for discovery of novel drug targets as well as entry points for the development of first-in-class compounds with unique pharmacological mode(s) of action. In efforts for customized therapies, it is clear that the identification of pharmacogenomic biomarkers should start very early, preferably in drug discovery and phase 2A/2B clinical studies for proof-of-concept.

In the present post-genomic period, another favorable influence of the HGP in drug discovery will likely be seen in preclinical studies of global gene expression before and after drug treatment in animal species. Shared patterns of gene expression among drugs within the same therapeutic class or alternatively, drugs that produce a similar form of toxicity may pave the way to map the attendant biological networks essential for drug efficacy and safety. Further, identification of genes related to common human diseases may contribute towards better preclinical models of drug efficacy, an area that needs much improvement for rational scaling of data obtained in animals to humans.

In the ideal case, the existing HTS processes in drug discovery may soon be tailored to accommodate the specific subtypes of novel or existing drug targets. This can then provide insights on optimal therapeutic candidates prior to clinical trials and create niche subpopulations in whom drugs can be used with greater efficacy and optimal safety. Focused pharmacogenetic testing in the clinic will be essential before such customized drugs can be prescribed. A reverse and complementary approach is to choose the compounds that will bind with high affinity and functionally interact with all subtypes of a given novel drug target. This alternative strategy for drug discovery may alleviate the need for pharmacogenetic testing at point of care: the lead compounds are chosen or customized (instead of the patients), in this case, to accommodate all variants of a biological target. Conversely, these early individualization attempts in drug discovery may be constrained by limits of medicinal and combinatorial chemistry to synthesize compounds that will be versatile enough to bind and activate all drug target subtypes, while demonstrating an adequate safety, bioavailability and drug–drug interaction profile.

All these technical advances and promises of pharmacogenomic-guided drug discovery also come with attendant ethical and social policy challenges. For example, if drugs are discovered and developed only for the most common subtypes of drug targets, this may potentially create therapeutic orphan subpopulations—will there be financial or legislative mechanisms in place to ensure that these individual patients also benefit from novel and mechanism-oriented therapeutic interventions? When developed, genetically tailored medications will likely be available at premium prices. Who will take the responsibility for ethical promotion of such personalized drugs?

It is interesting to note that among 1393 new drugs developed between 1975 and 1999, only 1.1% (16 drugs) was for tropical and other diseases prevalent in developing countries. While one-third of the world population live on less than US$2/day, and occasionally without access to essential drugs, it is foreseeable that some may question how pharmacogenomics may contribute to discovery of drugs that will benefit the patients in the developing world. To this end, it is worthwhile to bear in mind that the genomes from numerous parasitic pathogens, bacteria and viruses have been sequenced and available for the research community. Hence, pharmacogenomics offers much hope for novel drug target discovery and development against infectious agents affecting world's populations. In addition, concepts and technologies developed in parallel to pharmacogenomics may be instrumental for identification of individuals who may be more sensitive or resistant to infectious organisms in developing countries. It is hoped that these promises offered by pharmacogenomics will materialize and will be put into practice with a global public health policy in mind. Finally, although pharmacogenomics will likely revolutionize how new drug candidates are tailored for individual patients, serendipity and keen scientific insights will still continue to play a role in the drug discovery process.

Early Phase Clinical Drug Development

Allometric scaling of preclinical data to humans is often limited by marked interspecies differences in drug disposition, drug targets as well as the inevitable biological contrasts between outbred human populations and the inbred laboratory animals with a homogenous genetic background. First-in-human studies and the subsequent phase 2A/2B proof-of-concept clinical trials of therapeutic candidates in early stages of drug development play a bridging role with drug discovery efforts before large scale and confirmatory phase three clinical studies can be rationalized. The principal aims of these early investigations in humans include estimation of pharmacokinetic variability, the optimal dose ranges and administration schedules, the risk for drug–drug interactions, and provision of evidence on proof-of-concept for drug efficacy (or the lack thereof) and mode of action. Typically, single and multiple ascending doses of a *new molecular entity* (NME) are administered to healthy volunteer subjects and carefully selected groups of patients with a relatively uniform and usually mild to moderate disease state. On the other hand, even though these studies collectively provide preliminary insights into presumed effects of NMEs in humans, the complete range of pharmacokinetic and pharmacodynamic variability within and among human populations is seldom available at the end of phase two drugs development. This predicament, along with the occasional disconnect between the efficacy of NMEs in animal models, and the clinic, have recently stimulated a surge for identification of early indicators or biomarkers of drug activity and mode of action.

Per definitions provided by the U.S. National Institutes of Health expert working group, a biological marker (biomarker) is "a characteristic that is objectively measured and evaluated as an indicator of normal biological processes, pathogenic processes, or pharmacological responses to a therapeutic intervention". A surrogate endpoint represents a special subset of biomarkers that is intended to substitute for a clinical endpoint; this implies a stronger correlation between the surrogate biomarker and clinical outcome (e.g., therapeutic benefit, lack of efficacy, and toxicity). Insofar as the pharmacogenomic biomarkers are concerned, there is growing interest in characterizing changes in the expression of genes that encode known drug targets or other biological elements downstream from the immediate drug target–effector systems. A particular advantage in this regard is that the effects of drug treatment on expression of key pathways related to drug response may precede changes in clinical outcomes; this may alleviate the need for long-term clinical studies and expedite the drug development time frames. Moreover, genomic methodologies typically have a higher throughput than the conventional phenotypic or clinical endpoint-based measures of drug efficacy and safety. This may in effect provide a broader picture of drug effects in various pathophysiological pathways and in some cases, lead to discovery of hitherto unexpected additional mode(s) of drug action and indications for future therapeutic applications. It should be mentioned that all these exploratory and research-oriented applications of pharmacogenomics in early stage development contribute essentially to better characterization of NMEs and their effects in humans. The small study sample sizes in early phase clinical trials, however, are not sufficient to characterize the diagnostic sensitivity and specificity of genetic tests. On the other hand, these early pharmacogenomic investigations, if judiciously analyzed and interpreted, can be invaluable for hypothesis-generation and the initial identification of genetic biomarkers that may later be utilized for customization of drug therapy.

Early stage clinical studies typically describe the pharmacokinetic variability associated with a NME but these estimates, in most cases, remain limited to the study samples. Broader views of pharmacokinetic variations within and among human populations can be obtained only if the mechanisms of variability in drug disposition are discerned. To this end, panel studies in patients representative of the population extremes (e.g., poor metabolizers vs. rapid or ultrarapid metabolizers) for a given drug disposition pathway may help to define the upper limit of contribution of individual CYP450 and Phase II drug metabolizing isozymes or drug transporters to pharmacokinetic variability in the general population. These panel investigations in genetically stratified samples may inform several critical drug development decisions including: (1) extent of variability in dosages required for an optimal response in the targeted population, (2) risk for competitive drug–drug interactions and the list of concomitant medications that may cause a pharmacokinetic interaction upon co-administration with the NME under clinical development, and (3) prioritizing pharmacokinetic studies in different populations.

Pharmacokinetic bridging-studies are usually conducted when regulatory drug approval is sought in various countries. These data provide guidance for registration of new drugs in different populations based on similarities or differences in drug exposure. Consider, e.g., that an NME is found to be metabolized by CYP2C19 in early phase clinical studies. Because CYP2C19 displays marked inter-ethnic differences in the frequency of poor metabolizers (3% in Caucasians and 20–24% in Asians), this would immediately point towards the need to conduct highly focused and comparative pharmacokinetic studies in Asia, North America, Europe, and possibly in other countries. Without knowledge of the precise mechanisms governing interindividual variability in drug exposure, such inter-ethnic differences in drug disposition remain undetected during drug development. If dose adjustments are not made based on genetic or phenotypic differences in CYP450 function early in clinical development, drugs may face the risk of withdrawal from human use after their introduction in the clinic.

A notable application of pharmacogenomics in early phase drug development, which extends beyond personalized medicine, is in proof-of-concept investigations. Phase 2A/2B trials enriched for patients with certain genetic subtypes of drug targets previously shown to confer an increased likelihood of response can facilitate decisions on whether and to what extent a NME is a viable therapeutic candidate. Conversely, an inadequate response to a NME in such enriched samples may serve as an early indication of possible therapeutic failure in the general patient population.

Late Stage Clinical Drug Development—Phase Three Registration Trials

Phase three clinical trials form the centerpiece for overall clinical drug development programs. These pivotal late stage clinical studies are typically conducted in large patient samples and play an important role in registration of therapeutic candidates and confirming their efficacy and safety. This is also the stage of drug development when genetic tests for customization of therapy should be validated with adequate attention to their diagnostic sensitivity and specificity. Any new information learned on subpopulations identified with pharmacogenomic tests at this phase of development can favorably influence the customization of drug labels. Despite investments and enthusiasm for discovery of novel drug targets and pharmacogenomic applications in early phase clinical trials, direct stratification of patients using genetic tests in advanced stages of drug development is still rare. To date, a great majority of the pharmacogenomic biomarker development efforts have taken place in studies that were primarily designed for other purposes: demonstration of drug efficacy and safety.

The highly structured and defined time frames of the latter clinical trials may pose serious limitations for flexibility to accommodate statistical analysis and interpretation of pharmacogenomic data. Also, the high degree of population variability that characterizes the samples recruited for large-scale drug trials adds a further level of complexity to the interpretation of pharmacogenetic data, because of potentially spurious results due. Additionally, the statistical power of the traditional efficacy or safety-oriented clinical investigations may not always be sufficient to identify and validate predictive genetic tests to tailor drug therapy; in cases where epistatic effects are sought (a very likely scenario) there is a high likelihood that most current studies will be vastly underpowered for pharmacogenomic analysis. To achieve personalized medicines in the clinic, commitment to prospective pharmacogenomic testing in phase three trials designed specifically for biomarker validation and development is essential.

Through identification of patient subpopulations that are more likely to display a therapeutic response, pharmacogenomics holds the potential to conduct highly focused clinical trials enriched with "responder" patients. It is anticipated that this may reduce the required sample size and the time to obtain regulatory approval for new drug candidates. If and when successful, pharmacogenomic-guided drug development will also require companion genetic tests to tailor drug dosages or the choice of medicines. It is therefore crucial to coordinate in parallel the timely development of pharmaceutical and diagnostic products.

With the anticipated discovery of genes underlying some of the common complex human diseases over the next decade, we may increasingly witness NMEs with new drug targets and mode of action. These drugs, lacking clinical precedence on the therapeutic value of the targeted novel biological pathways, also bring along a considerable degree of risk for unexpected treatment failure or drug toxicity in the clinic. If predictive pharmacogenomic tests are available, these projected risks and promises associated with such first-in-class drugs can meet with enthusiasm and acceptance by clinicians, patients and drug manufacturers. The recent introduction of Herceptin for the treatment of patients with breast cancer who over-express the HER2 oncogene is a notable example in this regard. These critical drug development decisions can be further influenced by impact of genetic testing on the pharmaceutical patent life-cycle, the commercial promise of therapeutic candidates and the health policies in place for reimbursement of customized medicines and the companion pharmacogenomic diagnostic tests. Adoption of pharmacogenomics in drug development can be anticipated particularly in cases where severe drug toxicity is experienced in a small fraction of patients while the same drug may display adequate or remarkable efficacy in the majority of the patient population. Such therapeutic candidates can be brought to the clinic by genetic testing and identification of patients at risk for severe drug toxicity.

Applications Toward Drugs in the Clinic

A pivotal aim of pharmacogenomics is to provide the clinician with genetic tests that can be applied at relatively low cost in order to predict efficacy and adverse effects. The preceding sections have placed considerable emphasis on the anticipated contribution of pharmacogenomics to the development of new drugs. However, there exists a similarly great need to develop predictive tests that can be applied to existing agents. Antidepressant drugs are a highly illustrative example. Currently several classes of agents are in widespread use—these include specific serotonin uptake blockers, drugs with a putative action on brain norepinephrine as well as serotonergic systems, monoamine oxidase inhibitors and the older tricyclic antidepressants which are widely accepted to be highly effective but impose a significant adverse effects burden. The overall efficacy of all these drug classes is remarkably uniform with approximately 60% of patients meeting response criteria short of full remission and 10–15% less actually remitting. Some of these drugs are true "*blockbusters*" if one considers their annual sales and market share.

It is entirely unclear whether patients who fail to respond to one class of drug will respond to another class and whether there are differences between different drug classes in their efficacy. Patients who do not respond are administered a sequential series of drugs with little information available to the clinician who wishes to make an informed decision based on rational considerations. When response or remission eventually does occur, it is quite possible that this is due to natural termination of the depressive episode, which is ultimately self-limiting in most but not all cases and not to the drug administered at the time. It is highly feasible that response/remission rates to the initial drug could be raised well beyond their current levels by the availability of genetic predictors of response. For this scenario to materialize prospective trials would need to be conducted and it is entirely unclear that the motivation exists for the pharmaceutical industry to support such studies when their targets are drugs that are no longer protected by patents. It is likely that intellectual property issues in this regard have not been sufficiently thought through and there may be possibilities that justify the investment but have not been considered.

Barriers

Cost Factor and Access to Genomic Technologies

Despite the general enthusiasm and belief that pharmacogenomics will benefit drug therapy, the eventual decision to use genetic testing in the clinic may bear in part on cost-effectiveness analyses. This is not an unrealistic assumption because many of the newer therapies customized by genetic tests are anticipated to be offered at premium prices to recover the research and development costs by the pharmaceutical manufacturers. In countries with a publicly funded health care and reimbursement system, cost-effectiveness analyses may particularly be a significant consideration. Similar economical evaluations have contributed in the past to acceptance of molecular genetic tests for the diagnosis of infectious pathogens such as *Chlamydia* and *Mycobacterium tuberculosis* as part of the microbiology services. Insofar as the monogenic variability in drug metabolism is concerned, for example, inpatients in a psychiatry unit who are at extremes for CYP2D6 expression (poor and ultrarapid metabolizers) were found to incur, on average, $4000–$6000 higher healthcare costs when treated with drugs eliminated by CYP2D6. By contrast, virtually no pharmacoeconomic data are available concerning the cost of multigenic variability in drug effects.

Veenstra et al. recently proposed five basic requirements that may enhance the cost-effectiveness of a pharmacogenomic test: (i) provision of evidence that severe clinical or economic consequences can be avoided through the use of pharmacogenomics, (ii) current methods of therapeutic drug monitoring are inadequate, (iii) an unequivocal association between genotype and clinical phenotype, (iv) availability of a rapid and relatively inexpensive genetic test, and (v) a relatively common genetic variant. It is foreseeable that the insurers and other third-party payers of pharmacogenomic tests as well as hospital formularies may soon demand pharmacoeconomic data concerning the value and clinical impact of predictive pharmacogenomic testing on hospitalization rates, quality of life and daily functioning of patients, well beyond the direct pharmacological effects of drugs in clinical trials.

It may be argued that the current trends to characterize an increasing number of genetic variants, including the enthusiasm for genome-wide pharmacogenomic association studies, may add to the cost of genetic testing for research purposes, or at point of care as a diagnostic tool. On the other hand, the unit cost of genotyping and other genomic technologies have decreased considerably over the past several years. Additionally, broader inquiries of the human genome recently uncovered regions or blocks characterized by high linkage disequilibrium (LD) interspersed with short segments of very low LD (recombination hotspots). Within the high LD regions, there is limited haplotype diversity and the strong correlation between genetic markers creates redundancy in the informational value of each marker. This led to the recognition that common haplotypes within each block can be discerned with only a fraction of the markers, or a minimal set of SNPs named as haplotype tagging SNPs (htSNPs), present in a haplotype block. These advances may be advantageous to reduce the cost of pharmacogenomic studies further, especially in genome-wide association studies or when highly polymorphic candidate genes are being investigated. By contrast, for diseases that may result from rare haplotypes or in studies of genomic regions with low LD, characterization of all genetic markers may still be necessary. Collectively, it is reasonable to anticipate in the near future that the bottleneck in clinical pharmacogenomic studies will shift towards the rate-limiting step of collection of accurate clinical phenotypic information and relational analyses and interpretations of genetic and clinical datasets.

Pharmacogenomic Testing at Point of Care: Technical Standards and Expectations for Diagnostic Applications

Technical barriers in pharmacogenomic research are increasingly being overcome by declining costs and increased throughput of genotyping (or gene expression) methodologies. To date, much emphasis in pharmacogenomics has been placed on SNPs and their characterization in clinical samples. For genetic testing at point of care to become a reality, a broader scope of human genetic variation will need to be captured, including small insertions/deletions, and nucleotide repeat polymorphisms in the genome. For instance, certain commonly occurring CYF2D6 alleles are typified by insertions/deletion polymorphisms while the slow drug glucuronidation associated with the Gilbert's syndrome is a consequence of dinucleotide (TA) repeat polymorphism in the promoter region of UGT1A1. Attention to rare genetic variants will also be necessary particularly in cases where the test results inform critical decisions on choice of drug prescriptions or dosages. It is noteworthy that the required sensitivity and specificity of molecular genetic assays, in a diagnostic context, are markedly higher than the technical standards acceptable for pharmacogenomic research or biomarker discovery applications.

From a clinical standpoint, if there is a very toxic drug that can be prescribed by means of pharmacogenetic testing and exclusion of at risk patients, the only barrier between a patient and severe toxicity will be the pharmacogenetic test itself. Hence, in cases where the diagnostic sensitivity of the genetic test is not robust, a number of ethical and legal issues will readily emerge. Clinicians who are accustomed to high-throughput of diagnostic tests in clinical chemistry will understandably demand a comparable ease of interpretation of the test results, economic affordability and turn around times within several days or ideally, by the end of each patient's visit. These required standards for diagnostic pharmacogenomic tests at point of care are still not within reach in many countries and genetic testing largely remains restricted to specialized research laboratories or tertiary care medical centers.

Pharmacogenomics and Accelerated Drug Approval: Concerns for Long-Term Drug Safety

A key promise of pharmacogenomics for the pharmaceutical industry is accelerated drug approval in genetically stratified subpopulations or based on genomic surrogate markers of drug activity and efficacy. To be eligible for the accelerated approval program, the FDA however requires that "the medication must treat serious illnesses and show significant benefit over existing therapy for serious or life threatening illness, or provide benefit for serious or life threatening illness for which no therapy exists." The mandate for the latter program was established by the Prescription Drug User Fee Act of 1992 and the FDA Modernization Act of 1997. The published literature over the past 5 years tends to adapt the view that pharmacogenomic biomarkers will markedly reduce the time and number of patients required for drug approval. This is indeed a reasonable expectation but some cautionary restraint is necessary to establish adequate post-approval pharmacovigilance procedures, particularly for drug safety. The standard drug approval process evaluates no more than 3000 patients and healthy volunteers combined; this sample size is able to confirm the primary therapeutic benefits and detect only the common ADRs of new drugs. Rare ADRs (e.g., <1%) are typically detected after introduction of a new medication for routine clinical use. In fact, serious ADRs may be discovered as long as 36 years after regulatory approval.

The concern for drug safety during the post-marketing phase is also supported by the observation that a significant number of drugs carry black box warnings on the label. With this in mind, it is plausible that pharmacogenomic-guided accelerated approval of drugs based on surrogate markers of efficacy in studies with smaller sample sizes may be fraught with safety issues following regulatory approval. In accordance with this, serious ADRs were reported for 79% of accelerated approval cancer or anti-HIV drugs compared with 25% of similar drugs that received standard approval between the years 1996 and 2002. Taken together, this underscores the need to conduct confirmatory studies of efficacy and systematic post-marketing long-term safety evaluations for drugs that are developed by pharmacogenomic guidance. Consistency in definitions and collection of the data on safety endpoints should be planned and envisioned early in the drug development programs. This will ensure that both pre-registration and post-marketing safety data can be pooled to evaluate the broader population-based risks associated with customized therapies.

Clinical Barriers and Attention to Social, Legal, and Ethical Aspects

Studies that yield information relevant to pharmacogenetics might appear easy to perform. Ostensibly, the researcher simply needs to recruit a sample of patients treated with a particular drug, obtain a DNA sample, rate the clinical effect of the drug, document adverse effects and then determine the relationship between genetic variants and the clinical phenotypes of interest. In practice, the situation is considerably more complex. In different populations the frequency of genetic variants can differ greatly, rendering stratification and population admixture major headaches in the interpretation of studies. Stratification and admixture may also exist within samples that are apparently homogeneous from the ethnic standpoint. These considerations require great care in the selection of study populations, the application of tests for admixture and the use of appropriate statistical procedures to account for population differences when samples from different populations are pooled. Studies that take interaction among genes (epistasis) into account, an important requirement when the genetic basis of a phenotype is polygenic, require large samples in order to have sufficient statistical power. Placebo effects are another important consideration. In the absence of a placebo control, apparent association of a gene with a positive therapeutic outcome could represent association with the placebo effect of the drug and not with a true drug effect, as might be the case for the highly studied association of response to antidepressant SSRI drugs with a polymorphism in the serotonin transporter. While the association has been supported by several studies the only study to include a placebo group found an association with response among patients receiving placebo as well as patients receiving the active drug.

Definition of the clinical phenotype that is to be correlated with genetic variation may pose a significant challenge. Potential phenotypes include response to a drug (defined as improvement of symptoms to a predetermined degree), *remission* (defined as complete disappearance of the target disorder for a predetermined minimum time period) and also intermediate phenotypes such as *onset of therapeutic effect* and the *speed of response* or *remission*. It is conceivable that different genes may be implicated in each of these phenotypes particularly when the underlying genetic architecture is polygenic; there may also be varying degrees of overlap. Differentiating and applying these phenotypic definitions can be relatively straightforward, as in the case of cancer therapies but may be complex, as in psychiatric disorders, dementias, and other illness states where the etiology and pathology of the disorders is not known and the mechanisms of action of the drugs used to treat them not well established. Phenotypes may be defined categorically as presence or absence of response/remission or adverse effects or evaluated as continuous variables, the latter approach being more appropriate for analyzing genetic effects as QTLs. Consistent definition of the phenotype is a critical prerequisite for ensuring that studies are comparable and for facilitating meta-analysis which is a critical tool in evaluating the overall significance of ostensibly inconsistent results obtained by smaller, possibly under-powered studies. Thus, definition of the phenotype is a pivotal issue in pharmacogenetics. It needs to be addressed prospectively in the design of studies in order that the required information be collected in the course of the study.

From the social, legal and ethical standpoints the acquisition and storage of DNA samples and genetic information are issues that greatly concern the public. There is no doubt that as with any confidential information regarding an individual, the potential for abuse of genetic information is considerable. The individual has the right to expect that privacy will be strictly maintained and that DNA and genetic information will be used only for the purpose that was intended and for which permission was given. On the other hand there is concern that the steps taken to safeguard the rights of individuals in regard to their DNA and genetic information may be excessive and may impede scientific inquiry and deny important potential benefits. This process has been termed "*genetic exceptionalization*" and it can be discerned in overly stringent rules and regulations that are applied only in the context of genetic research whereas, if justified, they should be applied to other situations as well. In many countries stringent conditions and safeguards that are applied to genetic research by internal review boards are not demanded of non-genetic projects that place the participant at the same or even greater risk.

Many of the ethical concerns raised by pharmacogenomics are shared by genetic research into disease predisposition. Others are specific. The Nuffield Council on Bioethics outlined and discussed some of the major issues. Their report identified four central areas of concern: The first is information.

Since pharmacogenetic tests yield genetic information about individuals this raises issues of consent and confidentiality. The second area identified is resource. Pharmacogenetics may lower the cost of developing and delivering medicines but may also drive it up because of the need to incorporate pharmacogenetic testing at all pivotal stages and to design studies in accordance. The third concern is equity. Pharmacogenetics may significantly improve medical treatment for some people, but it may also result in more people falling into categories for which effective drugs are not developed, because of inadequate financial incentives to develop a drug that may be effective for only a small population, or for a large but economically poor population.

The fourth general category identified by the Nuffield Council is control. Who should decide whether a patient takes a pharmacogenetic test? Should patients be entitled to a drug if they do not wish to take an associated test? In their report the Nuffield Council addresses a comprehensive series of specific questions that are subsumed by these general areas of concern. Among the issues addressed are informed consent, privacy and confidentiality, regulation of pharmacogenetic tests, re-instatement of withdrawn medicines based on pharmacogenetic information, allocation of resources, stratification and the development of new medicines, implications for racial groups, and pivotal aspects of the implementation of pharmacogenetics in clinical practice.

Future Perspectives

Medical therapeutics has long followed an empirical tradition based on average values of pharmacological effects in the population. Unfortunately, this approach does not lend itself to predictable and science-based therapeutics due to marked variations in drug effects among patients and populations. An alternative and preferred strategy to achieve optimal drug safety and efficacy is to elucidate the mechanisms underlying variability in therapeutic outcomes which can inform the rational choice of drugs and their dosages in individual patients or subpopulations.

Pharmacogenomics provides the necessary conceptual framework and technical infrastructure to identify the previously unaccounted host-specific genetic factors underlying common (or rare) medication side effects and therapeutic failure otherwise attributed to idiosyncratic reasons. In this regard, the initial methodological approach was comprised of hypothesis- driven candidate gene studies of drug disposition, safety, or mode of action. Over the past several years, genome-wide hypothesis-free clinical pharmacogenomic association studies and analysis of gene expression before and after drug treatment have been increasingly utilized for discovery of unprecedented biological pathways of relevance to pharmacology and human diseases. It is interesting to note that tangible examples of customized therapies with novel modes of action are still limited in the clinic. However, a lag period should normally be anticipated before any new technology or scientific paradigm bears fruits. New drug development usually takes 10–15 years and for therapeutic candidates with novel molecular targets identified through pharmacogenomic approaches, it would be reasonable to see the first examples in the clinic over the next 10-year period. By contrast, for drugs that are already available for clinical use, it should be feasible to develop genetically customized treatment guidelines within a relatively shorter time frame. It is difficult to verify the practical validity of this theoretical prediction since it is uncertain whether and to what extent the pharmaceutical industry will be willing to adopt pharmacogenomic testing for therapeutic agents in the clinic.

Although patents provide protection for market exclusivity of a given pharmaceutical product, pharmacogenomic diagnostic tests for the same compound can be developed by more than one investigator or institution thereby limiting the economic promise of a genetic test. Because most drug effects are subject to polygenic control, it is foreseeable that a multitude of genetic tests may eventually be developed in various populations by different private or academic not-for-profit interest groups. Although this is certainly an advantageous situation for patients and consumers of pharmacogenomic tests, it may potentially decrease the interest on the part of the pharmaceutical industry to pursue customized therapies once a drug is available for human use. It remains to be seen how, and under which conditions, research funding will be available for pharmacogenomic investigations involving drugs available in the clinic. As aptly stated by several investigators in the field, "the promise of pharmacogenomics is already here—the reality is getting closer."

Customization of drug therapy by pharmacogenomics is an arduous but worthwhile task that requires commitment of substantial research and economic resources before tangible results at point of care can be obtained. During this process, it is crucial to adopt a longer term vision, beyond the immediate goal of obtaining regulatory approval, to enhance the entire life cycle, and quality of a medicinal product: i.e., both prompt and timely introduction of new drugs to patients as well as their sustainable use in the clinic, without post-registration withdrawal or black box warnings, should be taken into account as part of the evaluations on the overall success of pharmacogenomic-guided drug development programs. There will be several additional and foreseeable challenges on the path to targeted therapies. Pharmacogenomic biomarkers will likely be population-specific; divergent sets of genes and epistatic interactions may influence drug effects in different populations. Another crucial consideration is the recognition that the role of genetics in pharmacology depends on the environment (temporal, geographic, or therapeutic) in which drugs are being administered. Thus, the genetic components in pharmacological variability are not physical constants; their magnitude can vary depending on the gene-environment interactions at the time of a pharmaceutical intervention. Drug effects that are apparently under strong genetic control in a certain therapeutic setting may be controlled entirely by environmental factors in another context. This means that environmental components of pharmacological variability, along with the attendant genetic factors, have to be identified in concert to develop unequivocal diagnostic genetic tests and customized therapies in the clinic. The broader philosophical questions surrounding gene patents, commercial genetic testing in the clinic and how best to bring capital, morality and knowledge into a productive, and ethical relationship still need to be resolved. Despite these challenges, the next 10 years will be an exciting and yet decisive period for pharmacogenomics. The gains will be achieved in small but significant increments and will favorably influence therapeutics as a science.

8

Clinical Pharmacokinetics

Clinical response to medication in an individual patient is the net result of the interaction of a number of complex processes. These processes can be categorized into two broad areas: those affecting pharmacokinetics or the relationship between the administered dose and the concentrations of the drug in the systemic circulation, and those affecting pharmacodynamics or the relationship between concentrations of the drug in the systemic circulation and the observed pharmacologic response. Absorption, distribution, metabolism, and excretion of a drug determine its pharmacokinetics. Drug–receptor interactions, concentrations of the drug at the receptor, and homeostatic compensatory mechanisms determine a drug's pharmacodynamics. Pharmacokinetics and pharmacodynamics are affected by a number of patient-specific factors including age, sex, ethnicity, genetics, disease processes, and prior and present drug exposure. This chapter focuses on the effects of advanced age on pharmacokinetics.

In clinical decision-making for the elderly patient it is important to recognize that the elderly may also experience an unexpected clinical response to a medication owing to the impact of factors other than their age, such as concurrent diseases and coadministered medications. Despite the fact that much less is known about pharmacodynamic changes in the elderly than changes in pharmacokinetics, the potential for altered pharmacodynamics must also be considered.

Definition of "Elderly"

"*Elderly*" has generally been defined as age 65 yr or older, although many other chronological definitions have been applied. Some researchers have enrolled patients as young as 50 yr old as "elderly" whereas others have studied only those patients in their 80s or older as "elderly." Although a chronological age is most often used to define elderly, it is important to recognize that the elderly are a heterogeneous group, with individuals aging at varying rates. Interindividual variation is much larger in the elderly than in the young. The aging process has been described as a condition of "*incipient disease*" with a variety of deteriorative changes taking place. When decline occurs more obviously in one organ system than another, a disease is diagnosed.

It is therefore difficult to distinguish between normal age-related changes and pathological states. Biological or physiological definitions of elderly have proved difficult to formulate, so chronological definitions of elderly remain the standard. The Food and Drug Administration's "Guideline for Industry Studies in Support of Special Populations: Geriatrics" arbitrarily defines the geriatric population as comprising patients aged 65 yr or older, although the inclusion of older patients is encouraged to the extent possible.

Elderly Patient

Although many older adults age successfully and lead healthy, productive lives well into their later years, the elderly as a group are more likely to suffer from chronic diseases and take more medications than their younger counterparts. The aging process itself is associated with changes in physiology that may alter drug pharmacokinetics and pharmacodynamics. When applying general knowledge of pharmacokinetic alterations in the elderly to the care of an individual patient in the clinical setting, it is necessary to consider the patient's overall condition, "*physiologic age*," disease states, and concurrent medications.

The elderly are especially vulnerable to adverse reactions to medications. The incidence of adverse drug reactions is two to three times that found in younger adults but may be underestimated because of lack of detection and underreporting. Many adverse reactions are preventable. Examples of preventable adverse effects include consequences of known drug–drug interactions or prescribing an inappropriate dosage for the elderly. The increased incidence of adverse reactions in the elderly results from altered pharmacokinetics, altered pharmacodynamics, increased opportunity for drug interactions, and inappropriate prescribing. While the changes in pharmacokinetics and pharmacodynamics are well recognized, age-related differences in dosing often are not noted in compendia such as the *Physician's Desk Reference* (*PDR*) that are used by prescribers. One recent study found many examples of evidence-based recommendations for dose alterations in the elderly that were reported in the literature but were not noted in the product labeling included in the *PDR*. This could explain, in part, the significant increase in adverse events in the elderly. Knowledge of basic pharmacokinetic differences in the elderly associated with age-related changes in physiology can be used to choose appropriate dosing regimens for the elderly and avoid preventable adverse drug reactions.

Pharmacokinetic Studies in the Elderly

Almost all of the information known about age-related changes in humans, including pharmacokinetics, has been obtained from cross-sectional studies. In these studies, the variable under investigation is measured in groups of subjects of different ages at a single point in time. Age differences are then inferred from a comparison of the mean values for each group or from a regression of the variable on age. The cross-sectional approach assumes that average differences between age groups reflect the change that occurs in an individual with the passage of time, which may or may not be valid.

When studying chronological changes in a particular variable, there are three primary time-related factors that must be considered: the effects of age, the effects of an environmental change or historical event at a specified period in time (period effects), and the effects of being part of the group or cohort of individuals born at a particular time (birth cohort). Cross-sectional studies often confound age effects with birth cohort effects. Findings in a group of individuals aged 65 today may differ from those in a group of 65-yr-olds studied 25 yr from now. These groups would be the same age but from different birth cohorts with different group experiences. Cross-sectional studies can also suffer from selective mortality effects, because the oldest study cohorts include only those individuals who survived to reach old age, and these individuals may be unique regarding the variable of interest.

Another approach to studying age-related changes is longitudinal studies. In these studies repeated measurements of a variable are made on the same individual at various points in time. This approach measures individual rates of aging for the specified variable, rather than differences between age groups as in cross-sectional studies. Although the results of longitudinal studies may be a more reliable approach to studying age-related changes, longitudinal studies tend to confound age effects with the effects of an environmental change or historical event at a specified period in time (period effects). These studies are also very difficult to conduct, taking many years to complete. For this reason, pharmacokinetic studies are virtually always cross-sectional in design.

Two general cross-sectional approaches are used to study pharmacokinetics in the elderly. The first is a formal pharmacokinetic study conducted either in healthy geriatric subjects or in elderly patient volunteers with the disease the drug is intended to treat. A relatively small group of subjects is studied using intensive blood sampling in each individual. In this approach, very healthy elderly people are selected for participation in an attempt to ensure that advanced age, and not disease, is the primary factor under investigation. Often these studies include only relatively young geriatric subjects that can meet the stringent inclusion criteria, limiting the generalizability of the results to the very old or frail patient. Results of these studies must be considered along with pharmacokinetic studies in other populations, such as patients with renal impairment, when making therapy decisions for individual patients.

The second cross-sectional approach is the pharmacokinetic screening or population pharmacokinetic study. These studies are typically conducted in conjunction with the main Phase III (or Phase II) clinical trials program. Under steady-state conditions, a small number of samples for drug level determinations are collected and analyzed. When appropriately designed, the influence of demographic and disease factors on pharmacokinetics can be examined in this type of study. Although the data analysis is more difficult, the advantage to this approach is that age and other factors, as well as their interactions, can be evaluated.

General Pharmacokinetic Changes Associated with Aging

Normal aging is associated with changes in human physiology, and many of these changes contribute to altered pharmacokinetics in the elderly. These changes are even more evident in frail or very old patients. Drug absorption and bioavailability, distribution, metabolism, and renal excretion may be altered in geriatric patients. If these changes are not considered when dosing elderly patients, preventable medication-related problems may result.

Absorption and Bioavailability

The bioavailability of a drug is defined as the fraction of drug reaching the systemic circulation after drug administration. Age-related changes in bioavailability depend on the route of drug administration, age-associated changes in the gastrointestinal tract and other organs of drug absorption, and age-associated changes in metabolism during the first pass through the liver or intestine. Despite changes in physiology with age, oral absorption and bioavailability of most drugs appear to remain unchanged in the elderly owing in part to the large functional reserve capacity of the gastrointestinal tract.

Gastric pH, gastrointestinal blood flow, active transport processes, and gastrointestinal motility have been reported to be altered in the elderly to a variable extent. Atrophic changes in the gastric mucosa may result in decreased acid secretion. The resulting increase in gastric pH could affect the ionization and solubility of some drugs. Decreased perfusion of the gastrointestinal tract and diminished active membrane transport processes could result in decreased rate or extent of drug absorption. These effects may be offset, however, by longer gastrointestinal transit times, with decreased gastrointestinal motility resulting in increased contact time for drug absorption. Most drug absorption in the gastrointestinal tract occurs by passive diffusion, and the majority of studies indicate that there are no clinically significant changes in the rate or extent of drug absorption from the gastrointestinal tract.

Intragastric metabolism and hepatic first-pass metabolism may be reduced in the elderly, resulting in increased drug bioavailability. Studies with levodopa, for example, have shown that the elderly experience a threefold increase in availability of levodopa related to a reduction in gastric wall content of dopa decarboxylase. Intestinal metabolism of verapamil, however, was well preserved in the elderly. Drugs that undergo a high rate of first-pass metabolism, such as propranolol, demonstrate increased bioavailability owing to decreased first-pass extraction.

Absorption and bioavailability for nonoral routes of administration (intramuscular, rectal, buccal, transdermal) and sustained release dosage forms have not been as well studied in the elderly. The rate of intramuscular absorption of antibiotics may be reduced in the elderly, but there are insufficient data to draw conclusions regarding the potential for age- related changes in drug absorption and bioavailability by these routes.

Distribution

Age-related changes in body composition and plasma protein binding may affect drug distribution in the elderly. The elderly tend to have decreased lean body mass, increased body fat, and decreased total body water. Interestingly, elderly individuals with high levels of physical activity are not different from those with low activity levels with respect to fat-free mass and fat mass. Lipid-soluble drugs may show an increased volume of distribution and water-soluble drugs may show a decreased volume of distribution in elderly patients related to these changes in body composition. For example, the elderly have an approx 20% lower volume of distribution for ethanol, which distributes in body water, than young individuals. Changes in body composition resulting in changes in volume of distribution may necessitate changes in loading doses of some drugs for the elderly.

Age-related changes in protein binding do not generally result in clinically significant changes in drug therapy for elderly patients. Generally, plasma protein binding of drugs remains unchanged or is decreased in the elderly. Serum albumin concentrations may be decreased in the elderly by 15–20%, but this is often related to renal dysfunction, hepatic disease, or frailty.

Hepatic Metabolism

Hepatic metabolism is one of the major routes of drug clearance in humans. The rate and extent of hepatic drug biotransformation depend on hepatic blood flow and hepatic enzyme content, affinity, and activity rate. Hepatic inactivation of drugs and environmental toxins occurs through phase I oxidative pathways (oxidation, deamination, or hydroxylation) or phase II conjugative pathways (acetylation, glucuronidation, or sulfation). Not all pathways of hepatic drug metabolism are equally efficient. Hepatic biotransformation results in a metabolite, which may be pharmacologically active or inactive, and may be eliminated from the body or further metabolized before elimination.

Interest in potential age-associated changes in drug metabolism is significant because of the need to reduce the risk of adverse drug reactions and drug interactions in the elderly. A number of age-related changes in physiology that may impact hepatic drug metabolism in elderly patients have been reported, but the effect of age on hepatic metabolism remains controversial. Much of the literature in this area has been conflicting. Early studies attributed observed changes in drug clearance in the elderly to changes in hepatic enzyme activity, and more recently to decreased liver size and hepatic blood flow. In vitro tests of enzyme have been inconsistent with results of in vivo studies. Despite these controversies, several generally accepted principles of the affect of aging on hepatic drug metabolism have emerged.

Hepatic blood flow has been shown to decline by approx 40% with age, in parallel with a decline in cardiac output. For drugs with a high hepatic extraction ratio, where clearance depends primarily on the rate of drug presentation to the liver through hepatic blood flow, aging is associated with decreased drug clearance. Phase I oxidative metabolism of some drugs appears to decline with aging, despite the fact that in vitro hepatic enzyme activity does not appear to be altered by age. Reduction in hepatic oxygen diffusion resulting from age-related changes in hepatocyte volume and surface membrane permeability and conformation is one proposed explanation for reduced oxidative drug metabolism observed with aging. Hepatic enzymes can be inhibited and induced by drugs and other compounds. Changes in hepatic enzyme induction with aging remain controversial. Phase II conjugative metabolic pathways appear to be unchanged with aging.

When prescribing for the elderly patient, age-related changes in drug metabolism should be considered. From a pharmacokinetic point of view, drugs that are metabolized exclusively by phase II conjugative mechanisms are preferred in the elderly. For oxidatively metabolized drugs with a high extraction ratio (high clearance drugs), dosages should generally be reduced owing to decreased hepatic blood flow. Dosages for drugs with a low extraction ratio (low clearance drugs) should be reduced as well. After initial dosing, doses can be adjusted based on patient response and tolerability. The potential for significant drug interactions, particularly resulting from hepatic enzyme inhibition in elderly patients on multiple medications, must be carefully considered.

Renal Excretion

Altered renal elimination of drugs is the most clinically important pharmacokinetic difference between elderly and young patients. Renal clearance depends, in part, on renal blood flow, which delivers drugs and metabolites to the kidneys for elimination. Elimination from the kidneys then occurs through glomerular filtration, tubular secretion, and tubular reabsorption. With aging, renal blood flow declines as cardiac output declines, resulting in decreased glomerular filtration rate as measured by creatinine clearance in the elderly. Although there is considerable interindividual variability, declining creatinine clearance with age (about 10% per decade after age 20) is consistently reported in the literature. Changes in the kidneys that occur with aging include a decrease in kidney weight, a thickening of the intrarenal vascular intima, sclerogenous changes of the glomeruli, and fibrosis and infiltration of chronic inflammatory cells in the stroma. Altered tubular function may also be present in advanced age.

The most important aspect of renal function to monitor clinically is the glomerular filtration rate (GFR). Most decisions about drug dosing for renally excreted drugs can be made based on the estimated GFR. Clinically, creatinine clearance is used to estimate GFR. Serum creatinine alone is not a good indicator of renal function in the elderly population because muscle mass, and therefore creatinine production, declines with age. A normal serum creatinine can result when both creatinine formation and elimination are reduced. Several algorithms have been proposed to estimate creatinine clearance. One frequently used method was developed by Cockcroft and Gault, where creatinine clearance (CL_{cr}) is calculated based on the patient's age, weight, and serum creatinine concentration:

$$CL_{cr} = \frac{(140 - \text{age in yr}) \times \text{weight (kg)}}{72 \times \text{serum creatine (mg / 100 mL)}} \qquad \ldots(1)$$

For women, the result is multiplied by 0.85. This formula is less accurate for estimates in the very high or low range and when renal function is changing rapidly. For frail elderly patients with chronic muscle atrophy, an alternative formula has been proposed that takes into account serum albumin levels as well.

For men:

$$CL_{cr} = \frac{\{[19 \times \text{serum albumin (g / dL)}] + 32\} \times \text{body weight (kg)}}{100 \times \text{serum creatine (mg / dL)}} \qquad \ldots(2)$$

For women:

$$CL_{cr} = \frac{\{[13 \times \text{serum albumin (g / dL)}] + 29\} \times \text{body weight (kg)}}{100 \times \text{serum creatine (mg / dL)}} \qquad \ldots(3)$$

This approach provides more accurate and less biased estimates of CL_{cr} than the Cockcroft and Gault method in elderly patients with renal insufficiency or serum albumin levels < 2.8 g/dL.

Effects of Age on the Pharmacokinetics of Chemotherapeutics

Old age is playing an increasing role in the treatment of cancer, as the prevalence of cancer in elderly patients is high and increasing: 60% of all cancers occur in patients aged 65 yr and above, and the elderly constitute a growing portion of the overall population, with 20% of the population expected to be > 65 yr by the year 2030.

This will lead to an increased use of anticancer agents by elderly patients. In addition to the physiological effects that aging may have on the pharmacokinetic characteristics of these agents, it has to be noted that the likelihood of polypharmacy due to noncancer, age-related chronic illnesses may lead to an increased incidence of drug–drug interactions. Quite a few of these interactions are pharmacokinetically based, for example, inhibition of hepatic metabolism (cytochrome P450-dependent, CYP) by concurrent medications.

Examples

Previous articles have reviewed the primary literature describing the effects of aging on the pharmacokinetic properties of chemotherapeutic agents. Most of these clinical studies were small, cross-sectional trials and assess plasma concentrations of the drug of interest, and in some cases, their active metabolites. A large portion of these studies reports changes in systemic exposure (e.g., peak plasma concentration, area under the curve, and terminal half-life) rather than more meaningful pharmacokinetic parameters such as volume of distribution, specific organ clearances, and oral bioavailability, if appropriate. Therefore, as pointed out earlier, it is sometimes difficult to assess whether physiological aging, concurrent medications or other confounding covariates are responsible for the observed age differences in systemic exposure. In addition, it is sometimes very difficult to interpret the results mechanistically, that is, what pharmacokinetic process is affected by age-related changes.

Based on these general properties, individual drugs whose pharmacokinetics are known to be affected by age, the likely mechanism of that age effect, and the need for dose modification in the elderly. Note that f_e indicates the fraction of the total dose renally eliminated unchanged. The major reason for dose modification in the elderly is the age-related impairment in renal excretory function. Therefore, the dose modifications based on renal function for selected anticancer agents. Overall, it is apparent that age-related renal impairment is the major cause of dose modifications in the elderly, and the (estimated) creatinine clearance serves as a good predictor for a patient-individualized dosing regimen. Apparent age-related effects on hepatic metabolism/biliary excretion have been observed, but usually do not lead to dose adjustments. Age-related effects on absorption are rare since most agents are given intravenously, while age effects on drug distribution are difficult to observe and are unlikely to result in dose modifications. This overall conclusion may change in the future when cancer treatment will involve chemoprevention and disease modification, with the agents given orally and less likely to be renally eliminated. Furthermore, owing to polypharmacy the likelihood of clinically significant drug–drug interactions at the level of drug absorption, first-pass, and systemic metabolism will increase.

9

Clinical Practices

The Good Clinical Practice (GCP) regulations section in the Code of Federal Regulations (CFR) (21 CFR 312) outlines the respective responsibilities of the clinical investigator, the drug sponsor, and the clinical study monitor involved in investigational new product development. These obligations, along with each participant's moral and ethical responsibilities for the safety of subjects who participate in clinical studies, comprise the essence of GCPs. GCPs have long been the norm for the investigator, as written in the 1572 Form; however, the first proposed regulations pertaining to investigator, sponsor, and monitor were first circulated in 1977 and 1978. In 1987, 10 years later, GCPs were published as final regulations in the CFR. Today, investigators, sponsors, and monitors are obligated by law to follow these GCPs. To conduct clinical research that meets the requirements of the FDA for new product approval, it is essential to understand GCP regulations and their subsequent impact on the clinical development process of drugs, devices, and biologics.

The 1987, Investigational New Drug (IND), regulations specified within the current CFR identify (more clearly than in previously proposed GCP guidelines) the delegation of responsibilities in the conduct of clinical trials. Not only do investigators have a key responsibility in assessing patients' efficacy and safety response to new drugs, devices, or biologics, but the sponsor and monitor also have equal responsibility for the patients' safety and welfare. The key players who are obligated under GCP regulations are described below and will be referenced throughout this article:

Investigator. An investigator is the individual who conducts a clinical investigation (i.e., under whose immediate direction the drug is administered or dispensed to the subject). If an investigation involves many physicians at a particular institution, one physician is designated as the Prinicple Investigator (PI) and they are the responsible leader of the team of investigators. The subinvestigator is any other individual member of that team as identified by the PI. These individuals are usually licensed physicians or individuals working under a licensed physician.

Sponsor/Investigator. A sponsor/investigator is an individual who both initiates and conducts an investigation (i.e., under whose immediate direction the investigational drug is administered or dispensed). This category refers mostly to physician investigators who are conducting clinical research under an investigator IND.

Sponsor. A sponsor is an individual or organization that takes responsibility for and initiates a clinical investigation. This may be an individual, pharmaceutical company, governmental agency, academic institution, or a private or other organization.

Monitor. A monitor is the person selected by the sponsor who is qualified by training experience to facilitate and oversee the progress of the investigation.

Investigator Obligations

In 21 CFR 312.53, the regulations deal with the descriptive information provided on form FDA 1572, the Statement of Investigator form. Also included in 21 CFR 312.53 are the selection requirements for clinical investigators. Previously, to conduct studies designated as Phases 1 and 2, investigators were required to complete a Statement of Investigator form FDA 1572; investigators conducting studies designated as phase 3 or phase 4 completed a different Statement of Investigator form, which was known as form FDA 1573. As a result of the IND rewrite regulations, form FDA 1573 is no longer used for any clinical studies. At present, for Phases 1–4, only the Statement of Investigator form FDA 1572 is required. This document states the obligations of investigators conducting clinical research. In addition to the general information on the 1572, new information includes the following: the name and address of any clinical laboratory facility, the address of the Institutional Review Board (IRB) responsible for the review and approval of the protocol, the patient consent form, and the individual investigators participating in the study. This document also states that the sponsor is charged with the responsibility of selecting qualified investigators, who are defined as those who are capable of conducting the study by virtue of their training and experience. By using the phrase "training and experience," the FDA means that clinical investigators conducting a study of a particular disease should have enough experience in that clinical specialty to observe correctly the signs, symptoms, and progress of the disease being treated with a new investigational drug. For example, if a new drug is designed for an Obstetrics/ Gynecology practice, a pediatrician would not be expected to have the expertise to assess this drug, nor would a cardiologist have expertise in evaluating a gastrointestinal drug.

Investigators are defined as those who have signed and completed form FDA 1572 or sub- or coinvestigators listed on that form, who are considered to have the academic and experiential qualifications for participating in the clinical program.

The "fine print" on the reverse side of form FDA 1572 is a written agreement whereby the investigators assure the sponsor that they will conduct the study in accordance with the appropriate study plan (i.e., the protocol) and will observe the GCP tenets. Implicit in this agreement is the fact that the Investigator will have obtained signed Informed Consent (IC) forms from patients or subjects participating in the clinical research under their jurisdiction. Form 1572 also charges the investigator with the reporting of adverse experiences that occur during the investigation and provides assurance that the investigator has read and understood the investigator's brochure. In addition, he or she assures that all individuals participating in the supervision of any clinical study, under the direction of the investigator, are aware of their responsibilities. Once form 1572 has been signed by the investigator, he or she further assures compliance with the requirements of providing study materials, protocols, and other pertinent information to an authorized IRB for review. This information, along with a curriculum vitae, should be provided along with the assurance that the investigational plan set forth in the study protocol will be complied with.

To summarize, the primary responsibilities of investigators in clinical trials are the ethical and moral obligations to all the participating patients and subjects in the study. Investigators must provide a measure of safety for each participant in the study so that the patient is protected ethically and morally from any endangerment that might occur during a trial using an investigational drug. After the investigator's responsibilities are outlined and he or she has signed form FDA 1572, any additional information from the sponsor that might be necessary should be requested and any concerns regarding procedures should be raised. An investigator is responsible for. (1) ensuring that an investigation is conducted according to the signed investigator statement, the investigational plan, and applicable regulations; and (2) for protecting the rights, safety, and welfare of subjects participating in a clinical investigation on any unapproved product. Also, the investigators must maintain complete control and accountability of the experimental products under investigation. An investigator shall obtain the informed consent of each human subject to whom the drug is administered and shall administer the drug only to subjects under the investigator's supervision or under the supervision of a subinvestigator responsible to the investigator. The investigator shall not supply the investigational drug to any person not participating in the clinical program.

The investigators are required to maintain adequate records of the disposition of the experimental medications, including dates, quantity, and use by subjects. If the investigation is terminated, suspended, discontinued, or completed, the investigator shall account for and return the unused supplies to the sponsor, or otherwise provide written documentation for disposition of the unused supplies of the drug. An investigator is required to maintain accurate case histories designed to record all observations and other pertinent data on each individual treated with the investigational drug. (Usually, this is accomplished by completing case report forms and maintaining medical records).

All investigators shall retain records of all subjects enlisted in investigational trials for 2 years after a new drug application (NDA) is approved for the indication for which the drug is being investigated. If no application is to be filed or if the application is not approved for such indication, records must be maintained 2 years after the investigation is discontinued or the IND is closed and the FDA has notified the sponsor of the status of the application. The investigator shall furnish all reports to the sponsor of the drug. The sponsor is responsible for collecting and evaluating the results obtained. The sponsor also is required to submit annual reports to the FDA on the progress of the clinical investigations. Investigators shall promptly report to the sponsor any adverse effect that may reasonably be regarded as caused by, or probably caused by, the investigational drug. If the adverse effect is serious the investigator shall report the adverse effect immediately. An investigator shall provide the sponsor with an adequate report shortly after completion of the investigator's participation in the study.

Other Investigator Responsibilities

The investigator must assure that an IRB complies with the regulations established in the CFR and that the IRB is responsible for the initial and continuing review and approval of the proposed clinical study. The investigator must also assure that he or she will promptly report all changes in the research activity and all unanticipated problems involving risk to human subjects Adverse Reactions (ADRs) or others to the IRB. In addition, the investigator will not make any changes in the research protocol without IRB approval, except where necessary to eliminate apparent immediate hazards to human subjects.

An investigator will on request from any properly authorized officer or employee of the FDA, at reasonable times, permit such officer or employee to have access to, copy, and verify any records or reports made by the investigator. The investigator is not required to divulge subject names, unless the records of particular individuals require a more detailed study of the cases or unless there is reason to believe that the records do not represent actual case studies or do not represent actual results obtained.

Sponsor Obligations

The sponsor's primary responsibility is clearly delineated in 21 CFR 312.50 and ensures that clinical studies are conducted in compliance with FDA regulations. The sponsor is responsible for selecting qualified investigators and for providing them with the information they need to conduct an investigation in accordance with the published regulations. Usually, the sponsor accomplishes this task by supplying the potential investigator with an investigator's brochure and a protocol of the clinical investigation on the agent to be investigated. An investigator's brochure contains all information from non-clinical studies and reports and any previous human efficacy and safety study reports that reflect previous experiences of patients of the investigational agent. Of primary interest in the obligations is the option of a sponsor to transfer total or partial responsibility for the conduct of a clinical study to a Contract Research

Organization (CRO). During the last decade, CROs have played a significant role in new drug development. However, CROs who contract with sponsor companies are obligated under the same GCP regulations as defined in this chapter. A CRO may be the sponsor or the monitor with equal obligations as defined in 21 CFR 312. The current regulations noted in 21 CFR 312.52 are specific and require that any transfer, whether in total or in part, be described in writing and agreed to by both parties. The FDA states that any obligations not specifically described by the sponsor in the written transfer of responsibilities will be considered as not transferred to the CRO; the liability for these undefined responsibilities, therefore, remains with the sponsor. The FDA further requires the CRO (once any transfer of responsibilities has been made by the sponsor) to comply with all applicable regulations and notes that the CRO is subject to the same regulatory actions as a sponsor if a CRO does not satisfy FDA regulations in the fulfillment of its contracted duties. As a result of these regulations, it is possible for a CRO to act on behalf of a sponsor once this legal transfer of obligations has been completed. Although the CRO must assure complete compliance with the responsibilities assigned, it remains the sponsor's responsibility to ensure the quality and integrity of data generated under the supervision of a CRO. In this situation, the sponsor would be expected to act as a quality assurance auditor of the data, even though assignment for the conduct of a study has been delegated to the CRO. It is important to note the following: that any such transfer shall be described in writing; if not all obligations are transferred, the description of the specific obligations being assumed by the CRO must be clearly stated. Any obligation not covered by the written description shall be deemed not to have been transferred. The regulations also charge the sponsor with responsibility for the inventory and control of the drug. Only investigators participating in a clinical trial may receive and have access to investigational drug and materials.

Sponsor and Monitor Obligations

One of the most important responsibilities of the sponsor is to monitor the progress of every clinical investigation conducted under its direction (21 CFR 312.56). A monitor's obligations, under the auspices of the sponsor, are to ensure that the deficiencies created during the conduct of clinical investigations are corrected or justified by the investigator and that the investigator adheres to the investigational plan. The appointed monitors for any clinical investigation conducted under a sponsor's IND have an obligation to assure that an investigator is complying with the signed Form FDA 1572 and the general investigational plan and that the clinical protocol is being followed. If an investigator does not correct his or her errors and mistakes and no improvement is noted in the progress of the study, the monitor shall promptly secure compliance or discontinue shipment of the investigational new drug to the investigator and end the investigator's participation in the clinical program. In addition the monitors, while monitoring the progress of a clinical investigation, must evaluate the evidence relating to safety and effectiveness. At the same time, sponsors shall make such reports to the FDA regarding information relevant to the safety of the drug, as they are required to do under section 312.32 of the FDA regulations.

When a monitor reports an adverse effect to a sponsor during an investigational study, it is the sponsor's obligation to determine whether there is an unreasonable and significant risk to the subject or patient. At that time, the sponsor must determine if the investigational study is to be discontinued. Important among the procedures of reporting adverse effects is the sponsor's obligation to the FDA, the IRB, and to all investigators who, at any time, participate in clinical studies and who are prescribing the experimental drug. Subsequent to this, the sponsor should furnish the FDA with a full report of the sponsor's actions and shall determine whether or not to discontinue the investigation. If the decision to discontinue is made, based on the seriousness of the ADRs reported, the studies should be terminated as soon as possible and no later than 7 days after making the decision.

It is important to understand that the obligations of monitors include the responsibility for assuring that all records and data recorded on case report forms reflect valid data gathered by the investigator and that they coincide with corresponding medical and hospital records of the candidate participating in the investigational study. Detailed auditing and documentation assure the sponsor that the monitor is overseeing the clinical data collected by the investigator and that GCPs are being followed. One misconception of many monitors who audit clinical investigations is that their only task is to assure correct entry of data. In fact, it is of extreme importance among the monitor's obligations to note any adverse effects or any deviations in laboratory values that could signify a safety problem to investigational study subjects. This is especially true in large multiclinic studies, in which many centers are conducting investigational studies following the same protocol and many monitors are auditing data. If any abnormal reactions or laboratory deviations are noted from center to center, the monitors should compare observations and assess an accumulative percentage of occurrence of these deviations. At times, a sporadic, apparently minor deviation can turn out to be a significant deviation when calculated across all centers. If monitors are astute, they can often prevent recurrence of adverse events that might jeopardize the safety of the subjects participating in investigational drug studies.

Another responsibility of the monitor is to assure maintenance of accurate records showing the receipt, shipment, or other disposition of the investigational drug. These records are required to include, as appropriate, the name of the investigator to whom the drug is shipped, the date, the quantity, and the batch number of each shipment. The monitor/sponsor shall also assure the return of all unused supplies of the investigational drug from each investigator whose participation in the investigation is discontinued or terminated. The sponsor may authorize an alternative disposition of unused supplies of the investigational drug, provided this alternative disposition does not expose humans to risks. Although the overall responsibilities are assigned to sponsors, it is the monitors' underlying responsibility for drug accountability.

In turn, the investigators, during experimental research, are also responsible for record retention similar to that of the sponsor. They are required to maintain adequate records of the disposition of the drug, including dates, quantity, and use by the subjects or patients. The investigator is also obligated, if he or she is terminated, suspended, or discontinued or if he or she has completed a study, to return all unused supplies of the drug to the sponsor or otherwise provide documentation of how the unused supplies of the drug were disposed. (It is recommended always to return the unused study medication to the sponsor). An investigator is required to prepare and maintain adequate and accurate case histories (designed to record all observations and other data pertinent to the investigation) on each individual treated with the investigational drug. The monitor should assure that all the previous procedures are adhered to and reported in a timely fashion.

An often-neglected investigator responsibility is the requirement to submit periodic reports to the sponsor. An investigator should be prepared to provide the sponsor with progress reports. These should include an update of the ongoing investigational trial. Annual reports to the FDA on the progress of the clinical investigations are required to be submitted by the sponsor. These reports contain information based on the investigators' progress reports. Safety reports are another issue. An investigator should promptly report to the sponsor any adverse events that may reasonably be regarded as caused by or likely caused by the investigational drug. Alarming adverse events (i.e., severe adverse reactions that jeopardize a patient's safety in any way) must be reported immediately by the investigator to the sponsor. Lastly, when an investigator has completed or terminated an investigational study, a final report shall be provided to the sponsor. This comprehensive report should be submitted to the sponsor shortly after completion of an investigator's participation in the investigation. The report summarizes the final observations of the study and any adverse events that occurred during the course of the clinical investigation. Monitors should also be responsible for encouraging investigators to complete and submit all the reports listed above. Constant follow-up may be necessary by the monitor if these investigator responsibilities are to be fulfilled. In most cases, the clinical monitor usually will provide the investigator with these reports.

Legal repercussions can occur from any neglect of the obligations by investigators, sponsors, or monitors. The CFR stipulates in 21 CFR 312.58 that the FDA can inspect the sponsor's records or reports on request from any properly authorized officer or employee of the FDA. These inspections normally occur at reasonable times and permit the FDA to have access to copy and verify any records and reports relating to a clinical investigation conducted under an IND. On written request by the FDA, the sponsor may be asked to submit the records, reports, or copies of them to the FDA. Under these regulations, the sponsor is also obligated to discontinue shipments of the drug to any investigator who has failed to maintain or make available records or reports of the investigation. Subsequently, an investigator may, on request from any properly authorized officer or employee of the FDA, at reasonable times, permit such an officer or employee to have access to or copy and verify any records or reports made by the investigator. The investigator is not required to divulge subject or patient names unless the records of particular individuals require a more detailed study of the cases.

GCP Non-compliance

What are the consequences if an investigator has repeatedly or deliberately either failed to comply with these GCP requirements or has submitted false information in any report to the sponsor. Initially, the Center for Drug Evaluation and Research (CDER) or the Center for Biologics Evaluation and Research (CBER) will furnish the investigator with written notice of the matter complained of and offer the investigator an opportunity to explain the matter in writing or at the option of the investigator, grant an informal conference. If the explanation offered by the investigator is not accepted by the CDER or the CBER, the investigator will then be given an opportunity for a regulatory hearing. At this hearing, the issue of whether the investigator is entitled to receive investigational drugs will be addressed. After evaluating all available information, including any explanation presented by the investigator, the FDA commissioner determines whether the investigator has repeatedly or deliberately failed to comply with the GCP requirements or has deliberately or repeatedly submitted false information to the sponsor in any required report.

The commissioner will then notify the investigator and the sponsor of any investigation in which the investigator has been named as a participant that the investigator is not entitled to receive investigational drugs. The investigation can not be terminated without reasonable cause as set forth by the commissioner and committee. Sponsor can also suspend shipment of drugs to the investigator for non-compliance to the protocol. If there is reasonable cause for this action, the investigator becomes subject to further investigation for each IND and each approved application submitted to the FDA containing data reported by this investigator. Therefore, every investigational study conducted by this investigator will be examined to determine whether the investigator has submitted unreliable data. Other investigations that are conducted under the same protocol will be temporarily put on hold. Conversely, the commissioner may determine, after eliminating the unreliable data by the investigator, that the remaining data justify continuing other of the same investigations at other sites.

However, if a danger to the public health exists, the commissioner will terminate the IND immediately; the sponsor will be notified and will have an opportunity for a regulatory hearing before the FDA on the question of whether the IND should be reinstated. If the commissioner determines that the data submitted are unreliable and that the data submitted by the investigator cannot be justified, the commissioner will proceed to withdraw approval of the drug product in accordance with the provisions of the Food and Drug Cosmetic Act (FD&C). As a result, an investigator who has been deemed to be ineligible to receive investigational drugs will be blacklisted and unable to participate in any experimental studies. The investigator may be reinstated when the commissioner determines that the investigator has presented adequate assurances that the investigator will use investigational drugs in compliance with FDA regulations. In conclusion, before an investigator accepts the responsibilities to conduct a clinical investigation with an IND drug, he or she must be aware of the legal obligations he or she has agreed to when form FDA 1572 is signed. Investigators must comply with the protocol and the rules, regulations, and guidelines of GCPs. Investigators must realize that they are subject to a federal offense and can jeopardize their reputation and, ultimately, their ability to conduct further clinical research. Investigators must know that the precise collection of data is mandatory in the conduct of clinical research. Research must be designed to assess the efficacy of the product and, above all, to assure that the safety of the patient remains the primary concern.

Sponsors' and monitors' responsibilities in complying with GCPs are also subject to serious repercussions under 21CFR 312.58. FDA inspectors are allowed to examine sponsors' files and the interventions of monitors' site visits to assure that GCP compliance was executed. Case report forms and clinical results are subjected to the same scrutiny that are applied to the investigators' responsibilities. If during an FDA inspection discrepancies are found in any form among the investigator, sponsor, and, when appropriate, the CRO (i.e., its documents), all three parties will be held responsible, and the IND will be placed on hold until the findings are resolved. Investigators', sponsors', and monitors' obligations must be fulfilled by complying with GCP rules and regulations. Sponsors' and monitors' consistent and persistent managing roles are vital in assuring that each person involved in conducting clinical studies meet his or her legal obligations. The success of any clinical program will depend on the cooperation, understanding, and compliance of this triad working together. With this agreement of responsibilities and a well-organized clinical plan, the results can only conclude valid data in support of a new drug application.

10

Laboratory Practices

The Good Laboratory Practice Guidelines (GLP) have been in existence for non-clinical safety studies since 1976. They have progressed through various transitional phases to become guidelines in some countries and regulatory/statutory instruments in others. The current document is the Organisation for Economic Co-operation and Development (OECD) Principles of GLP and is currently accepted as the industry standard. This was reviewed and published in January 1997 but must be used in conjunction with the appropriate Scientific Guidelines for the scientific side of the study, i.e., the OECD Toxicology Guidelines etc. This sets out to cover all non-clinical safety studies and gives guidance as to how these studies should be conducted in conjunction with the appropriate regulatory toxicology guidelines and, on that basis, when encompassed in the various Directives of the European Union (EU) or in other Memorandum of Understanding, allow data generated under this program to be mutually accepted by other OECD countries. One must not forget, however, the other equally important Guidelines and Regulations of other countries, such as those of the U.S. Food and Drug Administration (FDA) and the U.S. Environmental Protection Agency (EPA), and similar organizations in Japan. All have basically similar rules and, being members of the OECD, data generated to the OECD principles will generally be accepted in the United States and Japan. The EPA regulations used to be quite different and were applied to agrochemical and pesticide products. However, having been revised recently, they have been brought in line with the documents of other agencies.

The guidelines themselves, with the exception of those in countries where they are featured as regulations, are, as stated, guidelines to the conduct of the study and aim to cover compliance with the GLP principles but in no way do they dictate how the science will be performed. It must be remembered that compliance is monitored by adherence to GLP, whereas the regulatory authority and the receiving authority of the dossier when submitted for the application of a marketing permit or similar document review the science.

Objective of the Guidelines

The general objective of the guidelines originates in the very early 1970s, when one pharmaceutical company in particular and a contract research organization (CRO) generated data that, when submitted to the FDA, gave them cause for concern in the accuracy of the data presented and, in certain instances, the honesty of the submission. At that time, a full review of companies and institutions conducting non-clinical safety studies (toxicology) was undertaken by the FDA and although, in general, the industry was found to be credible, one company was found to be generating extremely poor-quality data, in many instances, in a fraudulent manner. This, therefore, caused the FDA to put together and implement the GLPs.

Over the next 10 years, many countries introduced similar good-practices guidelines. The EU in general produced its guidelines and eventually, despite the fact that the world was operating according to similar principles, a standard document was produced by the OECD in the early 1980s and became the industry standard. The reason this was of benefit to the whole industry was because this now precluded the fact that every submitting company would have to be inspected by each relevant monitoring authority and, when implemented into several directives and legal statutes within the OECD, this allowed data generated by one company to be accepted by several receiving authorities without further inspection.

The objective of the GLPs is to ensure that a standard approach is undertaken covering traceability and accountability and, while still allowing freedom for the scientists, to impose certain restrictions on the generation of data and the experimental work.

It must be remembered that GLP is merely common sense in a formal environment. The key phrases that are currently seen in a GLP environment include good documentation, good training, maintenance and calibration of all equipment, the archiving and storing of data in a formal and retrievable manner, and the use of high-quality, validated equipment and accredited test systems (animals).

This in general is merely good science, and the GLPs have further enhanced this by the addition of an independent Quality Assurance Unit (QAU) and a study director/principal investigator who jointly controls and oversees the project and involves the management in putting together adequate resources and assuming overall responsibility for the study. This can be seen as good science, with several slight enhancements. The details of these individual subjects are addressed later in this article.

Who Does It Affect?

Any company or institution performing non-clinical safety studies for the submission of data for a new chemical entity; a new biological, immunological, pesticide, veterinary or agrochemical product; or, for that matter, a similar product that will eventually appear in the marketplace and be consumed by the general public must adhere to GLP in the conduct of their non-clinical safety study experimentation. Within a company, every person from senior management to the junior technician is bound by these GLPs and must exhibit clear understanding and training in these practices.

To ensure that the practices are followed, a regulatory inspection takes place on a 2 year basis in most countries, and the objective of this is to review, as an independent group, how these good practices are being followed. Certification or a guarantee that the company is operating according to these standards is the benchmark standard. This is also addressed later in this article. As we move into the twenty-first century, it is quite apparent that the industry will shrink as mergers and acquisitions take place, and, with this, the emergence of the now familiar CRO will become ever more popular in the conduct of non-clinical safety studies. It is, therefore, very important that, in this area, the sponsor has the assurance that these facilities are operating not only to the highest standard of science but also in compliance with GLP and that, as a subcontractor, the data they generate will be equally accepted as if the data were generated by the company itself.

Why Have It?

In general terms, for companies conducting non- clinical safety studies, it is, a regulatory requirement, and without this certificate or certification of compliance, data will generally not be accepted by the receiving/regulatory authorities. However, one should not embark on the process of obtaining or working to GLP with this sole aim in mind. It should be used as an ongoing improving and quality standard for the laboratory.

In fact, it is the author's experience over the past 5 years, that many companies have gone far beyond the requirements of GLP compliance and that the overall concept of good scientific design and good science has been superseded by the desire merely to obtain compliance. It is quite often seen that an extremely poor quality scientific study has been conducted in complete compliance with GLP. It has been seen on several occasions in a laboratory, for example, where the refrigerator has been located far from its permitted limits; where the temperature has been diligently recorded, signed, and dated as required by GLP, but where no attempt has been made to either document the excursions outside the accepted range or to rectify the problem. The operative was merely under the impression that as long as temperature is recorded, this is GLP despite the damage that excursions outside the temperature range may have caused to any investigational product stored in the refrigerator.

Over the years, those scientists who have worked according to the principles of GLP now readily admit without any prompting that they are unsure how they conducted scientific studies before the advent of these good practices. The ability to reconstruct studies, to work to a standard format across several differing laboratories or countries, and to be able to prove beyond reasonable doubt that these were the values obtained and the results submitted. Certainly, data with a GLP compliance statement are being accepted more readily by the receiving authorities, which has led to fewer repeated studies. This, in turn, is helping to achieve the aim of all scientists in reducing the use of animals. From a company's point of view, working according to the principles of GLP shows that it has an attitude that is both ethical and moral to the production of scientific data with products that will eventually enter the human food chain or be of benefit to mankind.

How is It Enforced?

In the OECD countries, for at least 14 years, an Inspectorate has been set up, varying in inspector numbers from several hundred in the United States to one or two in countries not conducting a great deal of scientific non-clinical research. All countries, however, have a regulatory group that, in some instances, also acts as the receiving authority for the review of data, and reports to the GLP Monitoring Authority. This regulatory group visits on a 2-year basis or, in Germany, a 4 year basis, those companies that have claimed compliance and will then be on a rolling program of review.

Unlike its role in many areas of regulatory compliance, it is still the responsibility of the sponsoring company to claim compliance from the Monitoring Authority. This claim is made for a particular company, laboratory, and/or series of tests. From the date of compliance when a letter is written to the Monitoring Authority, data generated from then are assumed by that company to be in compliance with GLP. This claim in then verified in a visit from the regulatory inspector. The inspection may be performed by one or two persons for 1 to 5 days. At the end of the inspection, an exit meeting is held, and the company is usually given an indication of its performance. Noncompliance points are noted in writing and discussed, and a report is then prepared. In view of the findings, three levels of compliance can be obtained:

1. Sufficient deviations have been seen to question the integrity of the data and, therefore, a complete rejection of the claim of compliance is made, with a revisit necessary.
2. Minor points of compliance have been seen that can be handled in a specified period in which case, the laboratory is placed under the category, of pending compliance.
3. Very minor points of compliance have been seen, which, when addressed in writing by the management in a 1 month period with supportive paperwork, etc., lead to the company being given a Statement of Compliance, a Certificate of Compliance, or an indication that the laboratory is in compliance. It depends on the specific country whether a Certificate of Compliance is given. If a certificate is given, it generally states that on the particular day that the inspection took place, the laboratory was found to be in compliance with the OECD Principles of GLP. Also, the address of the facility is given as well as a listing of areas in which compliance has been confirmed. This could be stated as analytical support facilities, acute toxicology, mutagenicity, or similar designations.

Naturally, the benchmark standard is either the OECD Guidelines or similar standards in Japan or the United States. The Inspectorate carries out inspections against these documents. It could be said that often it is merely a review of the procedure and an opinion of compliance given by the inspector versus the interpretation of the individual conducting the experimental work. To try to overcome this criticism and to ensure that all inspectors work according to a standard format, over the past 4 years, the OECD has instituted a series of mutual joint visits (MJVs).

The process of an MJV is that a company is inspected by its local inspector and that the inspector is accompanied by inspectors from two other countries as observers. At the conclusion of the inspection, the company is given their findings by its local inspector and, outside that meeting, a review of the performance of the inspector with positive and negative points is given by the two observing inspectors. To ensure continuity, one of these three inspectors would then be on the next MJV.

In the past, Memorandums of Understanding (MoUs) have been instituted between certain major countries, such as Japan and the UK, the United States and Japan or Canada, etc. However, these have generally fallen into non-use for a variety of reasons, especially in Europe, where it is now, or has been for some time, not possible for a country to negotiate directly with another country. Brussels, however, being the center of the European Community, has to carry out that discussion with a proposed partner in another country. As such, at the time of producing this overview, very few MoUs are currently in force.

What is GLP?

As noted in the Overview, GLP is a series of guidelines that cover the conduct and data production for non-clinical safety studies. The OECD covers a series of activities and personnel. Responsibilities, training, quality assurance (QA), standard operating procedures (SOPs), study plans and study reports, data production and recording, equipment maintenance and calibration, computers and validation, test systems and test substances, and archiving are the primary areas covered by the GLPs. A very brief overview of each of these areas is given hereafter.

Responsibilities

The prime players in a GLP scenario would be the management, the sponsor, the study director, the principal investigator, and the QA. In a hierarchical structure, management would be totally responsible for the conduct of the work and for the assurance that resources have been made available and that an active role is played by these people in overseeing the conduct of scientific research.

The sponsor is the company that places a contract with a CRO or requests from within a company that work in another department be undertaken. The sponsor is the person who is supplying the money and the request for the work.

The study director is the prime player and is ultimately responsible for the production of the study plan, the conduct of the study, and the overseeing or production of the final report. Naturally, a large amount of delegation may take place; however, this must always be in writing, and the overall responsibility for the conduct of the study; the daily contact with the study staff; the prevention of recording of problems and the assurance that the study has been conducted in line with the study plan, the GLP, and the scientific guidelines solely belongs to this individual.

The Principal Investigator is the next in line of responsibility after the Study Director in a multisite study. For example, they could be the person seen in a field study situation where the crop-spraying, for example, may be undertaken at a place remote from the GLP designated site where the study director works. The principal investigator is therefore the person responsible initially for that portion of the work, although under the direct control of the study director. It may also be that, within a company, work is subcontracted to the Analytical Department, for example, for the analysis of formulated material. The person responsible for this particular aspect of the scientific work is the principal investigator, who is involved in the study plan and responsible to the study director. Another typical scenario is work conducted in a CRO under the control of the study director, where samples of plasma are taken for toxicokinetics, for example, and these samples analyzed by the sponsor. The sponsor's analyst, therefore, may well be designated the principal investigator.

Quality assurance

This is an independent group that does not become involved in the conduct of the study but merely reviews the data, experimental work, and documents produced to ensure compliance with the SOPs, the study plans, and GLP. Other activities such as training and assistance in interpreting GLPs, etc., may be the responsibility of the QAU.

Training and recording

It is the responsibility of the management to ensure that training takes place and the responsibility of the Study Director to assure that the individuals conducting the work are adequately trained and have adequate records. At a minimum, there must be a CV, a training record, and a very clear job description. Specifically, with regard to a study director, there must be explicit details of how the study director position can be met and the responsibilities of that individual in carrying out the relevant duties. There should be procedures detailing how the training will take place; recording of the training must be made on a regular basis, the records must be stored in archives and regularly updated, and a complete and historical review of the trainee's activities, previous training, and ability to conduct the work according to GLP must be documented.

Quality Assurance

This function, as has already been stated, is an independent review. The responsibilities here start with a review of the study plan and continue through the review of the study in the in-life phase, data audits, and the final study report audit. In addition to these, systems audits and process audits can be undertaken. The aim of QA is to assure the management that compliance with GLP is maintained throughout the entire study, that the data integrity is maintained, and that compliance with the SOPs and the study plan is adhered to by all experimental study staff. The study audit is a specific audit of the study in direct relation to the study plan. A systems audit, however, rather than proceeding in a vertical line, takes a horizontal line across all studies and would include such tasks as archiving, training, SOPs, general computer validation, animal house operation, and management activities. These are but a few areas that would constitute a systems audit but, hopefully, gives an idea of the type of activities across studies that would be audited.

Process audits, on the other hand, have specifically been addressed in the revised 1997 GLPs, and these are basically aimed at auditing short-term studies of a repetitive nature, generally undertaken by similar teams of people. Here, that the system is working and that parts of the process are reviewed over a quoted period in the QA SOP are assured. The aim is to ensure that all critical aspects of this process are reviewed through different studies over a period of time. This, then, does not necessitate QA review of all short-term studies on every occasion, nor does it require the review of such areas as analytical analysis on a batch-by-batch basis or the analysis of hematology or biochemistry samples each time these come up for analysis.

QA itself is required to produce SOPs that clearly detail operation, method of selection of critical phases, and studies and to report its results to the management.

After every audit, a report is produced that is then discussed with the study director and circulated to the management with the overall agreement from the study director relating to the audit findings and their explanation of the resolution.

Standard Operating Procedures (SOPs)

These generally have been likened to a complete documented history of the entire aspect of conducting non- safety studies. Any activity needs to be described in one of these documents. There may be a compilation of activities, or they may address single items such as the calibration and use of an electronic balançe. They must be produced by the individual most familiar with the task, agreed on by the management, and counter-signed by a person senior to the author.

Once produced, SOPs must be reviewed on a regular basis, (approximately every 2 years) and any changes to these procedures must be made in writing, with the agreement of all parties and circulated to each owner or user of the SOP. The SOP itself must be filed in the archive and additional copies produced. An SOP management system must be set up, whereby a responsible person knows the whereabouts of all SOPs and can retrieve and replace them with amended or superseded revesions and can make sure that they are reviewed regularly and disposed of when no longer required.

The SOP must appear immediately in the area adjacent to the workplace to be readily available to all persons. Frequently, SOPs are the basis of training, and most companies now have SOP-based training schemes. The content and receipt of the SOP should be acknowledged immediately on receipt and a training program set up whereby confirmation of the understanding and the ability to perform the duties stated in the SOP is documented in the appropriate training record.

SOPs should be adequately controlled to prevent unauthorized photocopying, which may lead to the possibilities of a superseded copy not being administered to the known recipients. Someone making an illegal photocopy would not be on the distribution list and, therefore, would not always receive updated versions, with the possibility that an outdated method could be used.

The requirement for archiving historical copies is one of the key attributes of GLP in that traceability can be seen as originating at the archive. The dates and historical record of the SOPs can prove irrevocably that a particular action was the method in use at the time.

SOPs can be paper-based or electronic. The trend toward electronic record-keeping is becoming more common in laboratories. The only requirement made by the inspectorate is that accurate, controlled copies are available on the electronic media and that prevention of copying or unauthorized changing are built into the SOP system.

Study Plans and Reports

Before any study can be undertaken satisfactorily, a study plan must be produced. The study plan is merely an indication of all of the activities that will take place, resources required, time frames, and objectives. The study plan can be likened to a road map that, when given to all the participants, will allow them to start at the beginning and to proceed through the various mazes to the final completion point indicated by the study report. The one golden rule in GLP is one study plan, one study director, and one report. The study report itself is a mirror image of all the headings in the study plan and serves to confirm that the objectives of the study have been met and that the results and discussions of the data presented give an indication of the outcome of the particular experimental work. Both the study plan and the report are audited by QA, and each study plan and report are generally determined by the company's format.

Data

Raw data, or source data, are generally considered the first records made, either electronically in computer-readable form, or records created the first time that the "pen hits the paper."

These should be original signed and dated recordings that may be on any type of media. Cases in which media such as heat-sensitive paper contain the result, should be photocopied in the event of deterioration over a time.

Electronic data can be regarded as the disk, CD-ROM, or similar media provided that this material, when reintroduced to the computer and the software, can generate the images stored on the disk or electronic media in a 100% readable form. There are many types of electronic media, machines, and source data or raw data within the toxicological environment. However, ironically, the most common storage media and the most common raw data are paper. Paper and its storage partner, microfilm, have been around for many years, and their stability and reproducibility are well known. Other electronic media, however, do not have the same capability of reproduction known over a long period, and, thus, most industries and companies prefer paper. In regard to the data they should be recorded promptly, legibly, and signed and dated, and any corrections should be made in a format to allow the original record to be seen, the change described and justified where applicable, and the change signed and dated by the individual making the revision. This procedure, whether on paper or via computer, should have the same standards. With use of the computer, an audit trail is necessary to identify the change and the person making it, along with the reason.

Equipment

As can be imagined, equipment in a toxicological study may be varied, simple, or complex. As such, it is difficult to describe each individual type of equipment in this limited space.

GLP requires that equipment be maintained, calibrated, and generally demonstrated as fit for use.

Equipment such as high-pressure liquid chromatography (HPLC) should have system-suitability checks, installation qualifications, and operational qualifications performed at a minimum.

Other equipment such as centrifuges and balances should be maintained and calibrated and, with regard to the latter, regular checks should be made with known, standardized, regularly calibrated weights. These should be placed on the balance with a frequency to guarantee that data from the machine are accurate. Even if the balance is an electronic calibrating balance, regular manual check weights should be applied.

Each piece of equipment should have a log book that gives a historical record of its use, breakdown, repair, and service. Generally, it is acceptable that these log books be placed by the equipment generating critical data to be presented in the final report.

All equipment should be clearly identified as to the time that it started producing raw data for experimental use and, when no longer required, the equipment should be removed from the laboratory or suitably labeled "not for GLP use."

The calibration and validation of equipment have been addressed extensively but, equipment that can be shown as "fit for use," within the GLP environment is generally acceptable to most regulatory inspectors.

Computers

Over the past few years, computers have played a very important role in many aspects of toxicology. The general trend in the industry and particularly from the Inspectorate is to ensure that they are fully validated.

Validation, however, means different things to different people. Some companies and their Information Technology Group (ITG) will dismantle the computer and its software components, reconfigure them, test them, and then reinstall them. Others will take a more realistic approach and work on the basis that the computer was brought in for a specific task and, is considered validated provided that task is completed with the aid of the computer in a reproducible and acceptable manner.

However, in the most simplistic form, validation could be covered by "evidence that the computer will perform the task for which it was purchased and, more importantly, continue to perform that task for the foreseeable future." In other words, as with other equipment, is the computer fit for purpose?

Several documents have been written from a regulatory standpoint, the most useful being Monograph 10 of the OECD Principles, Application of GLP to Computer Systems. Many books are available and vary in detail and content to cover everything that one would wish to know about computers, but were afraid to ask, down to the simple documentation giving the essentials for validation and providing a disk with the SOPs to comply with GLP!

The prime concern of the Inspectorate is that the user responsible for performing the validation and producing the report is in control of the equipment and can ensure and prove the integrity of the data when entered into the computer and regenerated in some other form.

It is generally accepted in the industry that acceptance testing is perfectly satisfactory for most computers and assures that the computer, when installed on company premises, will perform the function for which it was purchased. However, each computer must be viewed in the role it will play in the company and suitable testing must be conducted to ensure that the data and integrity are of the highest quality and that total control over output is maintained.

As with all equipment, computer maintenance and calibration records are of paramount importance. If in-house software programs are produced, they are tested and validated, and the source code is made available. One of the key elements required in the computer record-keeping is that of change control and password protection and training. One very important rule is that the electronic signatures rule, and it must be observed when data are signed off electronically. This FDA requirement became effective August 20th, 1997, and covers all data for which signatures are made electronically and requires that the FDA is officially notified.

Test Systems

This really is a slightly complex name for what is generally considered the animal subject. Test system, however, has been utilized because in many instances in toxicology, GLP now applies to such subjects as ground water, soil, insects such as earthworms and honey bees, and microorganisms such as daphnia and, therefore, the use of the word animal is not always applicable.

The main criteria are that the origin of the test system is known with its breeding history, where applicable, that these are purchased from well-known and, if possible, accredited suppliers, and that the quarantine period is observed to ensure that test systems are of high quality and fit for use.

Care, husbandry, intermediate sacrifice if the test system is found to be "in extremis," and humane sacrifice before necropsy are essentials for the test system. Separate housing among species and experimentation is critical, and all aspects of manipulation of the animal from clinical observations, dosing, and special tests such as electrocardiogram (ECG) need to be well documented and outlined in SOPs.

Animal husbandry itself, the animal room, and the animal room diary giving an indication of exactly what occurred in the room and to the animal are essential items of documentation. Unique identification is also of paramount importance with the animals, cages, and the location of the cages.

Full and documented history of heating and ventilation are required and, in barrier-maintained rooms, signed and dated records of positive to negative pressures are to be kept. These records should also reference any malfunction and its rectification. Furthermore, excursions outside the permitted range must be documented, and the effect on the study and data integrity must be identified and addressed by the study director in the final report.

Test Substance

In most instances, the test substance can be the new chemical entity (NCE) or an existing product; a comparator, pharmaceutical, veterinary, or agrochemical product; or even a device. Knowledge of the composition, characterization, stability, and other physiochemical properties is essential. Stability, however, may be determined as the short-term studies progress, with the proviso that the overall stability is known, along with full characterization, by the time long-term toxicity studies are carried out. Stability testing may well be carried out in parallel as long as the stability of the active ingredient and formulated product is known sufficiently to allow for control of the dosing to be done within the period of stability known at that time.

One of the key elements of test substance control is accountability. A record of the amount received for toxicity testing should be accurately recorded, and 100% accountability of that product throughout the life of the testing is an essential element of GLP.

Again, formulation of the product is required to be covered in detail, and, in many companies, the elements of GLP are the benchmark standards when dealing with test substance. Use of the test substance in the animal facility, the maintenance of homogenity of suspensions, the mixing of the product in feed, and the testing of the product are all essential. This is one particular area in which within the toxicology testing area, support functions such as analytical studies then come under GLP. These functions will be required to test formulations and feedstuffs, etc. to ensure that the correct amount of the active ingredient is present as determined by the study plan for the various dosing groups. This requires that a validated method be available before any work is carried out, with the ability to analyze samples of the formulated product or plasma samples for toxicokinetics as the study progresses.

It is required that a reserve or retention sample of the active ingredient is retained. This should be retained for as long as it affords reasonable testing and within the expiry period determined by the analytical facility. It is also required that a retention sample be retained for studies that are not considered to be short term. This is one particular area in which revision of the GLPs is sometime not well-thought through. Originally, it had been stated that reserve samples should be taken for studies exceeding 4 weeks. This was subsequently revised to specify "studies that are not considered to be short-term." The glossary in the GLPs defines a short-term study as "a study of short duration with repetitive processes." This, one must admit, does not give a lot of guidance!

Archives

Having addressed all the various aspects of the study, one can see that much documentation, tissues, slides, and wax blocks could well be accumulating. The requirement is to store this material for "a period of time." Again, very little guidance is given in the GLP, and one is referred to the national guidelines for the storage of data. However, it is of great importance that this material is maintained in good condition in a retrievable format for at least 15 years for or 2 years past the availability of "the product," whichever is longer.

Generally, companies themselves are maintaining that material for far longer, or for 2 years past the availability of the product.

All the material must be retained in a secure location for easy access, under the responsibility of a management-designated archivist and deputy. The security aspect of the archive should preclude damage from outside sources, fire, water, rodents, etc. The entire aspect of archiving is basically one of common sense, and guidance on how to archive these materials can be obtained from government agencies that store personnel records or from libraries.

How can compliance be Maintained within a Facility?

Compliance, having been granted after an inspection, should be monitored on a daily basis. However, it is the author's opinion that many companies standards of compliance relax after the initial certificate has been granted only to find that, 2 years later, for example, an enormous rush 1 month before an announced inspection is required to generate the appropriate documentation and to update the system.

It is suggested that QC reviews be carried out on a regular basis to ensure that points likely to detract from the overall compliance are reviewed regularly and that project meetings be held where QA is invited to give a precis of the regular points seen during audits so that these can be addressed and rationalized.

Training and retraining, along with an awareness of the requirement to comply with GLP, are of immense importance. New equipment, major SOP revisions, and transfer of technicians or scientists among departments are always good signs that additional training be carried out. It must be remembered that GLP is team work. It is no good considering that there are the scientists and technicians on the one hand and, QA on the other. There is also no point in considering that whatever happens and however little QC is carried out, QA will discover all the mistakes in the final report and review. Remember, it is not QA's problem; that department's role is to ensure that compliance has been maintained; QC and data-checking are the responsibilities of every member of the staff team.

Improvement targets should be set in line with quality-control manuals used in other accreditation systems. It is always a good point to review internally and on a regular basis: (1) problems that have been encountered in experimentation; (2) audit findings; (3) ways to improve work by looking at new systems and reviewing SOPs to ensure that these are current; and (4) and areas where improvements can be made.

An example can be taken from the accreditation systems, in which, in addition to QA audits, departments become involved in self-inspection. Each department can identify a QA representative whose daily responsibility is to review compliance issues, to look at the overall quality policy of the company, and to ensure that between QA audits, self-inspection is performed and that a departmental review is made of these findings with action points and a time plan identified.

The primary impetus for the maintenance of compliance, however, is the regular external inspection by the Inspectorate. In addition, it is now becoming frequent for independent consultants to be brought in to do pre-regulatory inspections. Whichever way one views the system, whether through consultation or by assigning a department to perform inspections in one area and to conduct audits in another, the regular review of compliance should be maintained.

When using CROs, the whole aspect of auditing takes on a different light. Here, subcontracting is usually performed because of internal pressures, shortage of space, or lack of in-house expertise. Dealing with CROs is no different than setting up an in-house GLP system. The CRO should be regarded as an extension of the facility in which the sponsor is conducting its own research.

Pitfalls and Benefits

In conclusion, it is worthwhile to address the pitfalls and benefits of operating according to the principles of GLP. A pitfall could be seen as a restriction on the scientist against performing free research. It could also be seen as an intrusion by an independent body looking at why problems occur and at the sorts of problems that occur and carrying out regular reviews with senior management about these problems. Costs will increase because of time pressures and the necessity of involving third-party reviews. The recording of data will now be subject to more QC, more required approvals, extra costs, and, generally, more data presented. Time must be taken to write and review SOPs. This in itself can be a very costly exercise; the author knows of one company that, having spent more than 6 months writing its SOPs, classed them as capital pieces of equipment and put a value of $5500 on that volume.

Other companies and personnel may encounter similar pitfalls. The list is not intended to be exhaustive but merely to indicate areas in which additional time, money, and resources will be allocated. However, on the positive side, benefits can be seen immediately.

In talking to many people who have operated under the GLP system for the past 20 years, it is generally heard that the system allows for a better standard of research, less repeated work, the ability to have full accountability and traceability of everything within the experimental phase, and the knowledge that all documentation produced at the end of the study is now safe and secure in the archive and can be readily accessed for regulatory review or inspection.

Fewer studies are being repeated, and, therefore, the immediate benefit is the lowering of subject usage. The fact that data, when generated with a certificate or a compliance statement, will now be accepted by all OECD member countries means that once the study is completed and the regulatory submission made, the time for acceptance several countries (if submissions are made in a multistate procedure) will be reduced dramatically. Finally, it is considered that the initial bureaucratic straitjacket of GLP when thrust on the international research community in 1976 has rapidly turned full circle and now is seen as the quality standard to which all companies in all countries want to aspire. From that point of view, all non-clinical safety studies, when conducted according to the principles of GLP and adequately addressing science as well as compliance, can achieve a very high success rate both in the outcome of the science and in the acceptance of data for a regulatory submission

11

MANUFACTURING PRACTICES

The Current Good Manufacturing Practice (cGMP) regulations for finished pharmaceuticals that have been promulgated by the U.S. Food and Drug Administration (FDA) have been a subject of active discussion since they were first published with the passage of the Kefauver–Harris Drug Amendments in 1962. GMPs were intended to establish minimum manufacturing and control practices for the pharmaceutical industry and focus on what needed to be done rather than how it should be done. Failure to comply with the current Good Manufacturing Practice regulations as set forth in the "Code of Federal Regulations," 21 CFR Parts 210 and 211, constitutes adulteration of a drug that is entered into interstate commerce and is therefore subject to regulatory action. These requirements apply to human and animal drugs. The regulations in Part 210 are introductory in nature; Part 211 contains the more detailed and descriptive regulations.

In the late 1970s, the FDA organized a task force to study the GMPs. Revised GMPs were published in September 1978, and became official in March 1979. At that time, the FDA also considered establishing more specific GMP regulations for products such as small-volume parenterals, medicinal gases and drug substances, to supplement the existing umbrella regulations.

Today, separate GMPs are in effect for biologics and foods but have not yet been promulgated for small-volume parenterals, medicinal gases or drug substances. In attempting to create regulations for specific products, the FDA concluded that it would be better to first issue guidances and guidelines rather than to revise regulations. Thus, what is put forth in 21 CFR Part 211 is supplemented with a number of guidances, guidelines and Compliance Policy Guides. There remain some differences, however, between guidances and guidelines from the Center for Biologics Evaluation and Research (CBER), the Center for Drug Evaluation and Research (CDER), and the Compliance Policy Guides, sometimes leaving a firm's cGMP status subject to the interpretation of a field investigator.

Based on the amount of time needed to promulgate a revision of the regulations, it is understandable that it is preferable to work with guidances, guidelines, and compliance policy guides. Current GMPs are supposed to be, as their title indicates, a description of the current manufacturing and control practices that are acceptable for a pharmaceutical company selling products in the United States. Although these cGMPs are not enforced in some foreign countries, an FDA inspection in a foreign country, based on current GMPs, can be the key to importing and marketing a product in the United States.

The FDA is required to inspect a firm every 2 years for compliance to cGMPs. With the advent of programs such as the new drug preapproval inspection program implemented in 1990, inspections may be more frequent and have expanded into areas not previously investigated regularly by the FDA, such as clinical manufacturing. An unsatisfactory inspection can delay approval of new products and lead to further regulatory action by the FDA, such as seizure and injunction, for existing products. The penalties can apply to the individual or both the firm and individuals.

The GMPs as set forth in 21 CFR Part 211 also have been applied to drug substances and clinical products. Guidelines and guidances have been issued to describe the FDA interpretation of 21 CFR Part 211 pertaining to drug substances and the production of investigational drugs and reinforce the agency's understanding that cGMPs are applicable. The FDA has reinforced the connection between registration of drugs and the manufacture of active pharmaceutical ingredients by the issuance of guides to industry. Recently, the FDA has issued for comment a draft guidance for "Good Manufacturing Practice for the Manufacturing, Processing, and Holding of an Active Pharmaceutical Ingredient." Finalization of these draft cGMP principles is being written into a guideline that is being coordinated through the International Conference on Harmonization of Technical Requirements for the Registration of Pharmaceuticals for Human Use (ICH) toward publication of a guidance for active pharmaceutical ingredients that will be standardized and followed by manufacturers in the United States, Europe, and Japan. As a sidenote, active pharmaceutical ingredients have also been called drug substances and bulk pharmaceutical chemicals. The "Status of Current Good Manufacturing Practice Regulations for Finished Pharmaceuticals" is as follows:

(a) The regulations set forth in this part and in parts 211 through 226 of this chapter contain the minimum current good manufacturing practice for methods to be used in, and the facilities or controls to be used for, the manufacture, processing, packing, or holding of a drug to assure that such drug meets the requirements of the act as to safety, and has the identity and strength and meets the quality and purity characteristics that it purports or is represented to possess.

(b) The failure to comply with any regulation set forth in this part and in parts 211 through 226 of this chapter in the manufacture, processing, packing, or holding of a drug shall render such drug to be adulterated under section 501(a)(2)(B) of the act and such drug, as well as the person who is responsible for the failure to comply, shall be subject to regulatory action.

The "Applicability of Current Good Manufacturing Practice Regulations for Finished Pharmaceuticals" is as follows:

(a) The regulations in this part and in parts 211 through 226 of this chapter as they may pertain to a drug and in parts 600 through 680 of this chapter as they may pertain to a biological product for human use, shall be considered to supplement, not supersede, each other, unless the regulations explicitly provide otherwise. In the event that it is impossible to comply with all applicable regulations in these parts, the regulations specifically applicable to the drug in question shall supersede the more general.

(b) If a person engages in only some operations subject to the regulations in this part and in parts 211 through 226 and parts 600 through 680 of this chapter, and not in others, that person need only comply with those regulations applicable to the operations in which he or she is engaged.

This article reviews Part 211, Current Good Manufacturing Practice for Finished Pharmaceuticals. Title 21, Parts 600 through 680 for biological products, supplement but do not supersede the regulations in this part, unless the regulations explicitly provide otherwise. The focus of Good Manufacturing Practice for all products is on a quality control unit that has the responsibility and authority to approve or reject all components, drug product containers, closures, in- process materials, finished product, and production and control documentation. "Quality Control Unit" refers to any person or organizational element designated by the firm to be responsible for the duties relating to quality control. Specific subparts of Part 211 are summarized and described later. This article is not intended to reproduce the complete GMPs, but certain parts are excerpted for emphasis.

Organization and Personnel

Responsibilities of Quality Control Unit

(a) There shall be a quality control unit that shall have the responsibility and authority to approve or reject all components, drug product containers, closures, in-process materials, packaging material, labeling, and drug products, and the authority to review production records to assure that no errors have occurred or, if errors have occurred, that they have been fully investigated. The quality control unit shall be responsible for approving or rejecting drug products manufactured, processed, packed, or held under contract by another company.

(b) Adequate laboratory facilities for the testing and approval (or rejection) of components, drug product containers, closures, packaging materials, in-process materials, and drug products shall be available to the quality control unit.

(c) The quality control unit shall have the responsibility for approving or rejecting all procedures or specifications impacting on the identity, strength, quality, and purity of the drug product.

(d) The responsibilities and procedures applicable to the quality control unit shall be in writing; such written procedures shall be followed.

The intent of this subpart is to ensure that there is a group within the organization that can review and judge the acceptability of procedures used to produce pharmaceutical products on an independent basis, as well as judging the products themselves, before they are entered into interstate commerce. The FDA has emphasized separation of the quality control unit from production (organizationally). In addition, the FDA considers the organizational level to which the quality control unit reports very important. From a legal perspective, the chief executive officer (CEO) or president of a firm is considered the most responsible official and thereby becomes the most liable. Therefore, he is subject to criminal prosecution should the organization be found to violate the Food, Drug and Cosmetic (FDC) Act. One of the most serious infractions is fraud, that is, the intent to mislead the FDA. Hence, it is incumbent on the CEO to have well-qualified personnel in the organization and an organizational structure that reinforces quality.

Personnel Qualifications

This section emphasizes the training of personnel both in cGMP and in their specific responsibilities with regard to manufacturing, processing, packing or holding of a drug product and functions to provide assurance that the drug product has the safety, identity, strength, quality, and purity that it purports or is represented to possess. This section also requires that there be a sufficient number of qualified personnel.

(a) Each person engaged in the manufacture, processing, packing, or holding of a drug product shall have education, training, and experience, or any combination thereof, to enable that person to perform the assigned functions. Training shall be in the particular operations that the employee performs and in current good manufacturing practice (including the current good manufacturing practice regulations in this chapter and written procedures required by these regulations) as they relate to the employee's functions. Training in current good manufacturing practice shall be conducted by qualified individuals on a continuing basis and with sufficient frequency to assure that employees remain familiar with cGMP requirements applicable to them.

(b) Each person responsible for supervising the manufacture, processing, packing, or holding of a drug product shall have the education, training, and experience, or any combination thereof, to perform assigned functions in such a manner as to provide assurance that the drug product has the safety, identity, strength, quality, and purity that it purports or is represented to possess.

(c) There shall be an adequate number of qualified personnel to perform and supervise the manufacture, processing, packing, or holding of each drug product.

This section makes it clear that the quality control unit is not the only group responsible for the quality of products and conformance with GMP. Because the quality of a product must be "built in," control (at the manufacturing level) of raw materials and process control are important.

Buildings and Facilities

This section requires that the buildings and facilities are adequate, provide specifically defined areas for certain operations and are designed to prevent mix-ups. Included are design and construction features; lighting; ventilation, air filtration, air heating and cooling; plumbing; sewage and refuse disposal; washing and toilet facilities; sanitation; and maintenance. Lighting, ventilation, air filtration, and air heating and cooling must be adequate. Again, the word adequate is used frequently. This is where an individual investigator's and firm's interpretations can differ. This section also requires written procedures associated with sanitation and that the facilities should be maintained in a good state of repair. Although it may seem obvious that maintenance should be performed regularly, it can happen that preventative maintenance programs compete with production requirements for attention; however, an in-depth preventative maintenance program should be in place.

Equipment

This section addresses equipment design, size, and location, as well as construction, cleaning and maintenance. Similar to the requirements for buildings and facilities, it is necessary to provide appropriate equipment for the manufacture of a product and ensure that the equipment material of construction is not reactive, additive, or absorptive. In the 1978 version of the GMPs, requirements for equipment cleaning and use logs, as well as written procedures for equipment cleaning and maintenance were added. These requirements aid in the investigation and solution of problems by identifying batches that may also be implicated in a particular problem.

Control of Components and Drug Product Containers and Closures

This section relates to the receipt, identification, storage, handling, sampling, testing, and approval or rejection of components and drug product containers and closures, and the requirements for written procedures for each. It also covers the use of approved materials, retesting of approved material, and prevention of use of rejected materials. Although the requirements of this section indicate that each lot be appropriately identified as to its status and that materials in different statuses be stored separately, the implementation of computerized warehouses has made it possible to eliminate status labels and physical separation of quarantined and approved materials. Rejected materials are usually handled separately. These practices are not to imply that a computerized system can be used without appropriate assurance of controls. The current GMP requirement that materials must be tested or examined for all specifications and released prior to use is in conflict with the philosophy of vendor certification, which is based on a consistent, reliable record of good quality. Only vendors with well-controlled processes and a good record of acceptable batches qualify for such a program. Thus, a material could be put into use based on the quality record of the supplier (vendor), even if testing is only for identification. This section also requires the use of oldest approved stock first, retesting of approved stock "as appropriate," and controls for drug product containers and closures. It prohibits use of rejected components and drug product containers and closures.

Production and Process Controls

This section focuses again on the need for written procedures and formal authorization by the quality control unit for any deviation from written procedures. Areas covered are addition of components;

calculation of yield; equipment identification; sampling and testing of in-process materials and drug products; time limitations on production; control of microbiological contamination; and reprocessing.

Many drug companies are using electronic means of verifying component names or item codes, receiving and control numbers, weights, or measures, and even the verification of component addition to a batch. There is a range of acceptability on the part of the FDA of electronic means of verification and batch documentation; however, the validation of such systems must be performed to accept electronic means of identification and verification.

The process controls required in this section should be based on process capabilities rather than conforming with a checklist based on the regulations. This would mean that tests not typically used for a particular dosage form may be appropriate, whereas other more commonly used tests may be without any value. This not only depends on the validation of the process but also equipment and process qualification. In addition, the need for microbiological controls can be greatly reduced by knowing whether a product supports microbial growth and whether the environment in the production area is maintained at a sufficiently low bioburden. Clearly, certain products require close attention to the production environment because of the ingredients and the end use.

Many firms use the so-called clean-zone concept, in which the restrictions on personnel entering a production area and the required protective clothing are based on the nature of a product—whether the product is prone to the growth of microbes or whether it is required to be sterile. Even for products not required to be sterile or that are not supportive of microbial growth, this concept controls the production environment through reduction of bioburden.

Reprocessing frequently receives considerable attention from the FDA. Over the years, reprocessing appears to have decreased, not only because of FDA pressures, but also because more products and processes are being validated and better controls are being exercised during production. At times, however, there is the need to reprocess, but it requires authorization of the quality control unit.

For a product covered by a New Drug Application (NDA) or Abbreviated New Drug Application (ANDA), provision for reprocessing must be included in the approved registration document. Although it is not always possible in the filing of an NDA or ANDA to foresee all reasons why a product may need to be reprocessed, a procedure for reprocessing can be evaluated and included in the registration document. If not included in the approved registration document, the regulations require submission of a supplemental application and prior approval in order to market a reprocessed batch.

To some people, batch or lot yield may seem to be more of a business concern rather than a regulatory or technical matter. However, GMPs require that yield tolerances be established and that yields outside of the tolerances be investigated. The need for an investigation is to determine that yields outside of normal limits can be an indication of problems during production that would not be evident with routine testing. A minor deviation may be relatively insignificant and could simply mean that the yield tolerances need to be reevaluated, a procedure that should be followed periodically.

It may seem that the identification of equipment in the processing record is also a superfluous burden. If several pieces of equipment have been shown to be used interchangeably, one might question the reason for this additional documentation; however, when a problem arises, it is necessary to know exactly which equipment was used. It may be possible to trace this back by reviewing equipment cleaning and use logs, but the investigation is simplified by having this information in the batch record. Recording variable batch information concerning the equipment, such as tablet compressing speeds, is also necessary.

Packaging and Labeling Controls

This subpart covers one of the aspects of pharmaceutical production that has received much attention because of recalls, including an increase in recalls related to labeling errors or product mix-ups associated with the packaging and labeling operation. Specific requirements identified in this section recently include the following.

Materials Examination and Usage Criteria

1. Use of gang-printed labeling for different drug products, or different strengths or net contents of the same drug product, is prohibited unless the labeling from gang-printed sheets is adequately differentiated by size, shape, or color.
2. If cut labeling is used, packaging, and labeling operations shall include one of the following special control procedures:
   (a) Dedication of labeling and packaging lines to each different strength of each different drug product;
   (b) Use of appropriate electronic or electromechanical equipment to conduct a 100% examination for correct labeling during or after completion of finishing operations; or
   (c) Use of visual inspection to conduct a 100% examination for correct labeling during or after completion of finishing operations for hand- applied labeling. Such examination shall be performed by one person and independently verified by a second person.
4. Printing devices on, or associated with, manufacturing lines used to imprint labeling upon the drug product unit label or case shall be monitored to assure that all imprinting conforms to the print specified in the batch production record.

Labeling Issuance

Procedures shall be utilized to reconcile the quantities of labeling issued, used and returned, and shall require evaluation of discrepancies found between the quantity of drug product finished and the quantity of labeling issued when such discrepancies are outside narrow preset limits based on historical operating data.

Packaging and Labeling Operations

Identification and handling of filled drug product containers that are set aside and held in unlabeled condition for future labeling operations to preclude mislabeling of individual containers, lots, or portions of lots. Identification need not be applied to each individual container but shall be sufficient to determine name, strength, quantity of contents, and lot or control number of each container.

These requirements reflect an increased use of electronic means to ensure correct labeling and tight controls on the practice of filling containers that will be labeled at a later date. A time-consuming operation required in the current GMPs is associated with the reconciliation of labels. The recalls and associated investigations demonstrate that unless 100% accountability can be achieved in the reconciliation process, there will not be an effective means of ensuring correct labeling. Section 211.132 was revised on February 2, 1989, to describe tamper-resistant packaging and labeling requirements for over-the-counter (OTC) human drug products. Compliance Policy Guide 7132a. 17 was issued in 1992 to describe the standardized tamper-resistant packaging requirements. This section also covers information concerning requests for packaging and labeling exemptions. It allows changes in packaging and labeling to comply with the requirements for OTC products subject to approved NDAs to be implemented prior to FDA approval as provided for in Section 314.70(c). Manufacturing changes to provide for sealed capsules require prior FDA approval under Section 314.70(b). Section 211.132 states that none of the requirements for "*special packaging*" (child-resistant packaging), as defined in Section 310.3[1] and required under the Poison Prevention Packaging Act of 1970, are affected. Subpart G also covers drug product inspection and expiration dating. The expiration date that is required in Section 211.137 relates to stability studies performed on the drug product described in 21 CFR 211.166. It requires that expiration dates be related to storage conditions stated on the product labeling.

Furthermore, the programs established are to use stability-indicating methods, under controlled conditions, in the marketed container–closure system and on an adequate number of batches to determine the appropriate expiration date. The FDA has issued guidelines on stability testing which outline in more detail the requirement to establish a stability program to determine and support the expiration date of a product. A new draft guidance for stability testing was published by the FDA in 1998, and discussions with comments to finalize this guidance are still continuing.

Holding and Distribution

This section covers warehousing and distribution and the procedures required for the quarantine of drug products before release by the quality control unit, storage of drug products under appropriate conditions, procedures to ensure use of the oldest approved stock first, and a system for documenting the distribution of each lot of drug product. This is another area where computerized systems are being used extensively. During inspections, the FDA review includes evaluation of the validation of any computerized systems and controls.

Laboratory Controls

This entire section refers to the requirements covering the testing of drug products and their components prior to release for distribution. It also covers stability testing and special testing, including testing for penicillin, if a reasonable possibility exists that a non- penicillin drug product has been exposed to cross- contamination with penicillin and laboratory animals. Additional information can be found in the Good Laboratory Practices, 21 CFR 58. Reserve samples arc required to be maintained for active ingredients and drug products. These specific requirements are elucidated in 211.170. The section on reserve samples also requires that a visual inspection of reserve samples of drug products be conducted at least once a year for evidence of deterioration. Fundamental to the testing requirements is the need for validated methods with established and documented accuracy, sensitivity, specificity, and reproducibility. It is also necessary to have meaningful sampling and testing plans that meet statistical quality control criteria. Judgments made with regard to sampling procedures should be based on the quality of the process control or the reliability of the vendor who supplies a raw material, drug substance, or packaging component.

Records and Reports

This section details the records and reports required to be maintained for pharmaceutical drug products, their components, and the equipment used in the processing of a drug product. Through these records, the entire history of a batch can be traced. The records cover equipment cleaning and use logs; component, container, closure, and labeling records; master production and control records and production record review; laboratory records; distribution records; and complaint files. Because this amount of recordkeeping can be voluminous, Section 211.180(d) allows for microfilm, microfiche, or other accurate reproductions of the original records for storage. Many firms are using the electronic generation of batch and analytical records. It is important to be able to retrieve all of the above records easily during an FDA inspection. Electronic methods must be supplemented with proper procedures to ensure that the records do not deteriorate over a period of time and can be retrieved when the computer systems used to generate the records have been revised or replaced.

This section also requires a master production and control record for each product, from which the batch production and control records are generated. These records must include complete instructions concerning the manufacture of a batch and precautions to be followed. Prior to the commercial distribution of a drug product into interstate commerce, all executed production and control records must be reviewed. If there is a discrepancy or a failure of any batch or any of its components to meet specifications, there must be an investigation and a written report of the findings. The investigation are to extend to other batches of the same or other drug products that may have been associated with the out of specification batch or discrepancy. Another part of this section covers complaint files, which are reviewed regularly during FDA inspections. In fact, a complaint file review may be the sole reason for an inspection if the FDA receives a complaint directly from a pharmacist, which may be a cause for concern. Sometimes the FDA will visit a firm to follow up on a complaint, even though the firm may not have been informed by the complainant. In the event that a complaint is received by a firm, it should be evaluated and a response sent to the complainant. It may be necessary also to conduct an investigation and prompt further action regarding the product or batch in the marketplace.

Returned and Salvaged Drug Products

This section requires that extensive records be maintained on returned drug products including ultimate disposition. Again, if the reason that a drug product is returned implicates other batches, an investigation is to be conducted in accordance with 211.192. Drug product salvaging is not allowed for drug products that have been subjected to improper storage conditions. If there is a question as to whether drug products have been subjected to such conditions, they may be salvaged only if there is evidence from laboratory tests that all applicable standards of identity, strength, quality, and purity have been met. In addition, evidence is required from the inspection of the premises that the drug products and associated packaging were not subjected to improper storage conditions as a result of a disaster or accident. Understandably, the value of the material to be salvaged is taken into consideration when such rigorous requirements exist for salvaging. Compliance with GMP requires that responsible employees in a firm be knowledgeable about the practices that other firms follow in order to comply. FDA investigators visit many firms and find a broad picture of current manufacturing and control practices. Thus, Current Good Manufacturing Practices are "state of the art," constantly changing. To be in regulatory compliance, a firm must review their procedures and systems regularly and revise them as necessary.

12

DRUG INTERACTIONS

The setting of chemotherapy for cancer is rife with potential for significant drug interactions and this topic has been the subject of several excellent reviews. Most patients receive multidrug combinations for their malignancy. Also, many of these patients are treated with intercurrent medication for co-morbidity or for cancer-related disorders (coagulopathy, infection, pain, seizures, etc.). The clinical significance of these potential drug interactions is also all the more relevant in cancer chemotherapy because the cytotoxic agents traditionally used do not have clear therapeutic windows. That is, the doses selected produce toxicity in a significant proportion of patients without necessarily providing benefit. Drug interactions causing an increased exposure of the patient to the cytotoxic agent may produce more severe side effects, whereas those causing a decreased exposure may jeopardize tumor control. Unfortunately, both the good and bad effects of chemotherapy are unpredictable, and the influence of drug interactions in either eventuality is almost impossible to detect in individual patients. These, however, may be borne out in large-scale studies, or when combined with pharmacokinetic data. Therefore, most drug interactions in cancer chemotherapy may go undetected unless some *a priori* knowledge alerts the clinician or oncology pharmacist to their likelihood.

When we think of drug-drug interactions, we usually think about classical interactions with the cytochrome P450 enzymes, as these have been well recognized and characterized over the last few decades. Certainly, this mechanism remains at the forefront of clinically significant drug-drug interactions. However, the pathways involved in the classical ADME of drug disposition (absorption, distribution, metabolism, and elimination) are all candidates for drug interactions. In particular, our understanding of transporters and their role in the systemic disposition of anticancer drugs has evolved exponentially over the last few years. They are now recognized as a major locus of drug-drug interaction. Also, the routes of metabolism of importance for the elimination of anticancer drugs are almost as diverse as their mechanisms of action, and some unexpected drug interactions have arisen as a result.

The aim of this chapter is to review some of the potential mechanisms of drug-drug interactions and to illustrate these with published data. The focus here is to examine the possible loci of drug interactions that should be considered in the setting of drug development rather than an exhaustive listing of all the known interactions. In addition, the possibility of exploiting drug-drug interactions to improve cancer chemotherapy is raised.

LOCI FOR DRUG INTERACTIONS: PROCESS BY PROCESS

As mentioned briefly in the previous section, any of the traditional processes implicated in drug pharmacokinetics (i.e., ADME) is a potential locus for drug-drug interactions.

Drug Absorption

Drug interactions can occur at the site of absorption by a multitude of mechanisms. Although oral chemotherapy has traditionally been limited in the past, many of the newer agents are being developed with the possibility of oral administration. Part of this challenge has arisen following demonstration that some of the newer "targeted" therapies are likely to require protracted exposure to ensure maximal benefit. Repeated intravenous administration in this context is impractical and there has been a push toward orally bioavailable drugs.

Gastric transit time and environment

For oral drugs, interactions leading to significant pharmacokinetic changes may arise as a result of changes in the gastric emptying time. Food is the most widely accepted factor for increasing gastric transit time, but a number of drug-related factors may have similarly important roles. Drugs may affect directly the rate of gastric emptying with most slowing this process, although some, such as metoclopramide, actually speed it up. Many cancer drugs produce transient nausea and vomiting. Nausea produces a slowing down of gastric emptying and may influence the rate and extent of absorption of oral chemotherapy. Many of the anticancer drugs given orally to date display wide variability in their absorption (e.g., mercaptopurine), which would possibly mask these subtle effects. Small-intestinal transit time is also likely to be an important factor). Certainly, the advent of rationally developed oral chemotherapy may, in the future, require specific consideration of these factors.

Drug interactions during absorption may also follow from alterations in the gastrointestinal environment. For example, the camptothecins are unstable at physiological pH and drugs affecting intragastric pH could be of concern for the administration of these agents by the oral route. This was the basis for a study of oral topotecan with and without ranitidine. Conversely, temozolomide is unstable at low pH and ranitidine was examined for an effect on drug absorption. In neither case was there any significant effect. In some cases, the instability of drugs at acidic pH has led to the direct incorporation of inhibitors of gastric acid production into oral bioavailability studies. Antacids may also be worthy of investigation from this point of view. Other nonspecific interactions that may modulate drug absorption can arise from the coadministration of binding drugs such as cholestyramine. Some parenteral formulations have surfactants to solubilize hydrophobic drugs in aqueous solutions. Although it is attractive to use intravenous formulations to investigate the oral route of administration of these drugs by simply administering these, the nonspecific effects of these agents may significantly modify the absorption of the compound of interest. In the case of paclitaxel, coadministration with its intravenous formulation surfactant, Cremophor EL, was shown to decrease greatly paclitaxel bioavailability whereas polysorbate 80 (Tween 80) had the opposite effect.

Drug metabolism

During their absorption from the gastrointestinal tract, drugs run the gauntlet of gut mucosal and hepatic drug metabolism, the so-called "first-pass effect." As reviewed else where in this book, a multitude of pathways are implicated in the metabolism of anticancer drugs. One of the first drug interactions observed in oncology was that which occurs between 6-mercaptopurine and allopurinol. An important metabolic pathway for the catabolism of 6-mercaptopurine is mediated by xanthine oxidase, which is inhibited by allopurinol. In the study by Zimm et al., administration of allopurinol increased peak concentrations and the area under the concentration–time curve (AUC) of 6-mercaptopurine by fivefold, but only when 6-mercapoturine was administered orally. Methotrexate is another, albeit weaker, known inhibitor of xanthine oxidase.

Inhibition of gut wall and hepatic metabolism may well be a requisite for appreciable absorption of some drugs from oral formulations. For example, the bioavailability of oral 5-fluorouracil (5-FU), which is of the order of 20–30 %, is limited by intestinal and hepatic dihydropyrimidine dehydrogenase (DPD), the major catabolic pathway for 5-FU. Novel oral formulations of fluoropyrimides often contain a DPD inhibitor to minimize this loss of drug to improve bioavailability. In the case of UFT, uracil is added in a 4:1 molar ratio as a competitive inhibitor of DPD with the 5-FU prodrug tegafur. With the DPD inhibitor ethyniluracil, the bioavailability of orally administered 5-FU approaches 100%. These are examples of how drug interactions can be exploited to improve the pharmacokinetic properties of important drugs. Another major class of drug metabolizing enzymes present in the mucosa and liver is the cytochrome P450 (CYP450) superfamily. In general, drug–drug interactions occurring at the CYP450 locus have been documented mostly in the context of parenterally administered cytotoxic drugs and these are discussed later.

Drug transport

There has been a revolution in the pharmacology of drug interactions following the demonstration that several of the ABC transporters, including P-glycoprotein, line the gastrointestinal lumen. Aside from the context of multidrug resistance, there has been the realization that these transporters, in facilitating basal to apical fluxes of drugs, are able to reduce greatly drug absorption following oral administration. This mechanism is now being extensively manipulated in the experimental setting to try and achieve oral chemotherapy of drugs previously considered too poorly absorbed. The taxanes are avid substrates of P-glycoprotein and particularly suitable for testing the concept of modulation of this transporter on drug bioavailability. Cyclosporin A and its nonimmunosuppressive analog PSC833 were some of the first blockers of P-glycoprotein to be tested for this modulation, demonstrating impressive improvements in paclitaxel bioavailability in mice. Results in clinical trials of 60 mg/m^2 of oral paclitaxel combined with 15 mg/kg of oral cyclosporin also showed large increases in oral bioavailability of paclitaxel. The bioavailability of the combination was approx 30%, which may, however, have been under-estimated because of the nonlinearity of paclitaxel kinetics. Nevertheless, targeting relevant concentrations (i.e., those achieved by intravenous administration) may prove difficult although possible. Other P-glycoprotein modulators (e.g., GF120918) are being investigated in this setting.

In the same vein, topotecan is a substrate of both P-glycoprotein and the half-transporter breast-cancer-related protein (BCRP) and both these transporters are expressed in the gut mucosa. The P-glycoprotein modulator GF120918 is also a potent modulator of BCRP and caused a further increase in topotecan bioavailability in the mouse as a result of blocking this second transporter.

Drug Distribution

Transporters

Aside from controlling the transfer of drugs across the gastrointestinal mucosa, the same transporters also control the distribution of drugs into other compartments (e.g., central nervous system, placenta). Inhibition or induction of transporters may therefore have an impact on the distribution of anticancer drugs. An effect of drug distribution would be detectable either from an effect on the volume of distribution of the drug or its pharmacokinetics in a specific compartment (e.g., central nervous system [CNS], cerebrospinal fluid [CSF], etc.). In a study of PSC833, Advani et al. examined the effects of this P-glycoprotein blocker (5 mg/kg po four times per day for 3 d) on a regimen of doxorubicin and paclitaxel. Importantly, this was a crossover study and, although the sequences were not randomized, this design enabled the effect of PSC833 to be observed in each individual. The presence of PSC833 led to a doubling of the terminal half-lives of both doxorubicin and paclitaxel. In the case of paclitaxel, the effect was due primarily to a trebling of the volume of distribution, indicating a substantial interaction with the distribution of this drug. In contrast, in the case of doxorubicin, the effect was attributable mostly to changes in total clearance. Specific compartments may well be targeted by such drug interactions. Indeed, there is the exciting possibility of improving drug distribution into the CNS by coadministration of blockers of P-glycoprotein and other transporters located at the blood–brain barrier. Importantly, however, an increase in CNS toxicity may be a down side to such strategies. Also, issues in relation to the concentrations required need clarification. There are conflicting data in animal models on the potential of cyclosporin A to modulate brain uptake of drugs and this may reflect subtle differences in the probe drugs and their schedules of administration. However, this is a clear area of concern for potential drug–drug interactions.

Protein binding

In theory, the competition by two drugs for a plasma binding protein can lead to an increase in the free concentration of the displaced drug. This, however, depends largely on the physicochemical and pharmacokinetic properties of the drug in question. In most cases, the displaced drug distributes rapidly into tissue compartments and/or is eliminated more rapidly with no net effect on free plasma concentrations. If the tissue compartment contains the tumor or organs of toxicity, then there may be a clinical effect of this displacement. These are, however, relatively rare but may need to be considered for drugs with very high plasma binding and small volumes of distribution. Cyclosporin A has been reported as being able to cause an increase in the unbound fraction of teniposide and increase the myelosuppressant effect of the latter. In such cases, however, it is difficult to discern whether the effect is exclusively pharmacokinetic. Methotrexate is a drug suspected of being the subject of many drug–drug interactions, some of which may possibly be mediated in part through protein-binding alterations. However, the data on this mechanism are relatively sparse, although a significant effect was shown with trimethoprim–sulfamethoxazole in pediatric leukemia patients with the free fraction of methotrexate rising from 37% to 52 % in the presence of the antibiotic. The significance of this modest change is not evident. Other compounds can produce similar effects and these include the salicylates, other nonsteroidal anitiinflammatory drugs (NSAIDs), sulfonamides, phenytoin, tetracycline, chloramphenicol, and *p*-aminobenzoic acid (PABA).

Direct interactions

Thiol protective agents (e.g., amifostine) provide nucleophiles able to react directly with platinum drugs. This could potentially alter the distribution and activity of these drugs. However, studies looking at possible pharmacokinetic interactions have so far not revealed clinically significant interactions with either cisplatin or carboplatin or other drugs for that matter.

Nonspecific effects

Several of the formulation vehicles are membrane-active compounds that may modify drug solubility and disposition. This was discussed briefly earlier in relation to the oral absorption of drugs. Similar effects may be relevant with regard to peripheral distribution of drugs. In fact some of these can be significant and the cause of apparent drug–drug interactions.

Drug Metabolism

Arguably, the most clinically significant drug–drug interactions in medical oncology are caused by interference at this locus. Several specific and nonspecific mechanisms are possible. Although it is beyond the scope of this chapter to explore all the possible enzymatic interactions, it is worth differentiating between some of the major mechanisms.

Competitive inhibition

Competitive inhibition is the dominant mechanism when two drugs compete for the same metabolic enzyme and a reduction of the metabolism of one occurs due to competitive displacement by the other.

Erythromycin and cyclosporin A, for example, are competitive inhibitors of cytochrome P450 3A. A feature of many substrate inhibitors of CYP3A, however, is their ability to form a reversible nitrosoalkane intermediate, which forms a tight complex with the CYP3A heme. Although reversible in theory, this complex is almost impossible to dissociate under physiological conditions. This is true for many of the compounds that undergo *N*-dealkylation reactions such as the macrolide antibiotics (erythromycin, troleandomycin, clarithromycin), some local anesthetics (e.g., lidocaine), diltiazem, fluoxetine, and tamoxifen. The complex typically requires significant preincubation with NADPH and enzyme to form and so may not be detected on a casual screen, in which preincubations with drug are the exception rather than the norm. As a result, the screen may detect only the immediate competitive component and greatly underestimate the possible interaction in vivo. Indeed, this form of complex may explain why some drug interactions with drugs such as erythromycin are much more extensive than predicted from inhibition constants estimated from competitive inhibition experiments. Long-term treatment with such drugs depletes the affected CYP until an equilibrium of CYP synthesis and deactivation occurs. The most potent inhibitors of CYP3A activity are the azole antifungals and some of the HIV protease inhibitors (ritonavir, indinavir, etc.). Although the latter may be problematic in the setting of HIV-related malignancy, interactions with azole antifungals are much more likely in the routine setting where they are sometimes used in antifungal prophylaxis. This may lead to severe, occasionally fatal interactions. The clearance of cyclophosphamide in children receiving fluconazole is reduced by almost 50% relative to controls, and in vitro experiments were in support of a role of decreased CYP metabolism in this interaction.

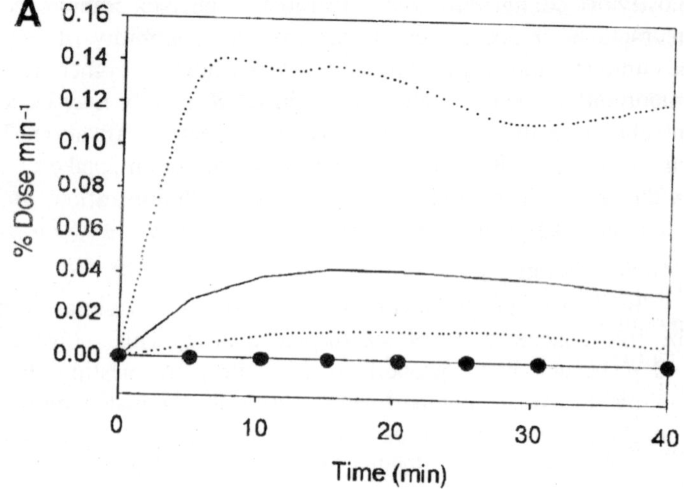

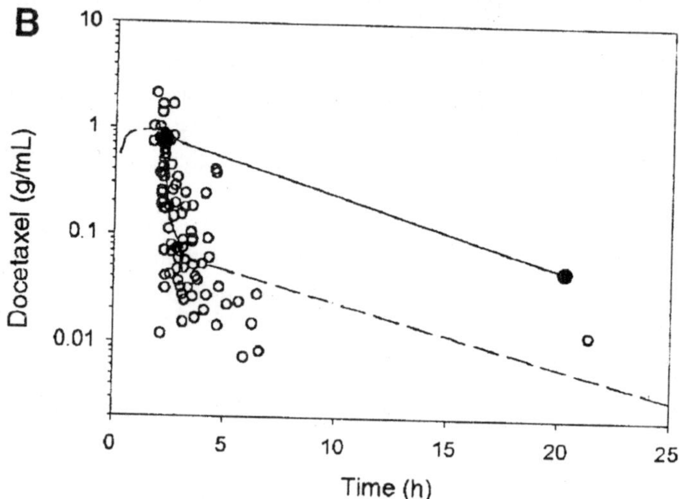

Fig. 12.1. A–The results of the [^{14}C]erythomycin breath test performed on 54 cancer patients prior to treatment with single-agent docetaxel. B–Sparse docetaxel plasma concentration data for the same individuals as in (A)

The azole antifungals are also inhibitors of CYP2C8, albeit at higher concentrations. Paclitaxel is metabolized more avidly by this isoform and an interaction with high-dose ketoconazole was thought possible on the basis of in vitro studies. However, acute administration of ketoconazole after paclitaxel or 200 mg orally 3 h prior to paclitaxel had no pharmacokinetic consequences. Whether this implies safety of paclitaxel with steady-state ketoconazole administration cannot necessarily be implied.

Other drugs metabolized by CYP3A include topotecan, irinotecan, paclitaxel, and docetaxel. With irinotecan, the importance of this pathway was recently made clear in a study of ketoconazole pretreatment. Administration of 200 mg of ketoconazole 1 h prior to and 23 h after the infusion of irinotecan did not impact on the clearance of irinotecan. However, it significantly shifted the metabolic profile away from CYP3A deactivation toward carboxylesterase-mediated activation. The apparent metabolic ratio for CYP3A was decreased approx 10-fold. Therefore, this interaction could provide a significant safety risk to patients receiving this combination.

Ketoconazole and the other azole antifungals are also inhibitors of P-glycoprotein (but possibly not substrates) and Kehrer et al. considered this as a potential factor in the drug interaction with irinotecan. Drug–drug interactions with azole antifungals may therefore be mediated at least partially through modulation of P-glycoprotein transport. For example, as mentioned previously, vinblastine does not readily penetrate into the CNS largely because of P-glycoprotein function, and mdr1a/1b knockout mice are at greater risk of neurotoxicity following administration of this agent. The clinical interaction between itraconazole and vincristine therefore may be due to modulation of CNS distribution of vincristine by P-glycoprotein. Fluconazole, in contrast, is a poor inhibitor of P-glycoprotein and given that doxorubicin is not appreciably metabolized by CYP450, a clinical interaction would not be predicted. This appears to be the case, at least in nonhuman primates.

Conversely, many of the investigated inhibitors of P-glycoprotein are inhibitors of CYP3A4, and this may contribute to drug–drug interactions. This includes some of the later generation inhibitors such as PSC833. The metabolism of thiotepa, which is at least partially mediated by CYP enzymes, has been shown to interfere with that of cyclophosphamide. Significant reductions in the *C*max and AUC of the active 4-hydroxycyclophosphamide metabolite were observed when thiotepa was administered 1 h prior to cyclophosphamide. Recently, it has been demonstrated that thiotepa is a potent, selective inhibitor of CYP 2B6, one of the key pathways in oxazaphosphorine metabolism. One of the issues with investigating drug–drug interactions involving the oxazaphosphorines is the fact that their metabolism is extremely complex, with some pathways responsible for both activation and deactivation reactions. Carmustine, which inhibits human aldehyde dehydrogenase 1, causes a reduction in the deactivation of the aldocyclophosphamide intermediate.

Suicide inhibition

Occasionally, the inhibiting drug is transformed into a highly reactive species by the action of the enzyme, and the two react to form a covalent complex. This type of inhibition is potentially more significant than competitive inhibition because the extent and duration of enzyme inactivation can both be extensive. In Japan, an interaction between an antiviral nucleoside, sorivudine, and 5-FU was suspected as being responsible for a series of 18 deaths. An investigation into the metabolism of sorivudine found that the drug was hydrolyzed into 5-(2-bromovinyl)uracil by intestinal bacteria. The latter is a potent suicide inhibitor of DPD, the major catabolic pathway of 5-FU. Blockage of DPD effectively transforms these patients to a DPD-deficient phenotype with possible lethal consequences. Ironically, 5-(2-bromovinyl)uracil was a well-recognized inhibitor of DPD and had previously been shown to be of benefit when combined with reduced doses of 5-FU in animal models. Indeed, tumoral overexpression of DPD is a recognized mechanism of resistance to fluoropyrimidines, and other suicide inhibitors of DPD have been developed clinically to reduce both the systemic and intratumoural metabolism of 5-FU.

Although suicide inhibition is an attractive mechanism to exploit in cancer chemotherapy (e.g., exemestane and aromatase), the situation with sorivudine exemplifies that drugs that produce suicide inhibition of key catabolic enzymes can have serious consequences unless they are administered for the specific purpose. Preclinical screening of compounds for their potential to inhibit DPD has become commonplace. Several 17α-ethinyl-substituted steroids such as gestodene and ethinylestradiol are suicide inhibitors of CYP3A and this would suggest potentially multiple drug–drug interactions. However, clinical studies looking for such effects with, for example, ethinylestradiol, have not been in support of a major effect under therapeutically relevant conditions.

Enzyme alkylation

Alkylating agents have the potential to interact with most cellular and extracellular macromolecules including enzymes and transporters. For example, the active product of cyclophosphamide, 4-hydroxyphosphoramide, and an eventual byproduct of its metabolism, acrolein, are able to react with cytochrome P450 enzymes. This can be blocked by the addition of thiol protective agents, suggesting a reaction with CYP sulfydryl groups. However, it is unclear what the clinical consequences of this are, if there are indeed any. Likewise, aquated platinum species can react with CYP enzymes leading to inactivation, but although these interactions can be demonstrated in vitro, pharmacokinetic interactions of this nature appear to be minor in vivo, as demonstrated with etoposide. Nevertheless, the demonstration that JM216, another recently developed platinum analog, also inhibits multiple CYP enzymes, indicates that some care should be taken with this class of drugs. Interaction of platinum compounds may extend to other enzyme systems, and, indeed, the clearance of 5-FU is reduced approx 25% by coadministration of oxaliplatin. The effect, however, does not appear to be mediated via an inhibition of DPD.

Reduced expression

Enzyme activity also relates to the expression of the protein and drugs able to modify the expression of the enzyme in question will also potentially lead to drug–drug interactions.

Cytotoxic drugs

Exposure of cells to cytotoxic agents may lead to differential expression of metabolic enzymes. In a rat model, Yoshisue et al. demonstrated that oral administration of 5-FU reduced the activity of several drug-metabolizing enzymes (phases I and II). The loss of activity was apparently mediated by a reduction of these proteins within the cells and displayed little specificity. The effect was more marked in enterocytes than hepatocytes, suggesting that interactions might be more pronounced for orally administered drugs. Certainly, some drug interactions involving fluoropyrimidines have been reported, but these have so far been limited to a handful of substrates, implying greater selectivity of this effect in human subjects. In particular, clinically significant interactions between fluoropyrimidines and substrates of CYP2C9 such as phenytoin and (*S*)warfarin have been reported.

In male rats, the mRNA expression of the sexually dimorphic CYP isoform 2C11 can be repressed by treatment with cisplatin whereas the expression of "female" cytochrome p450s is increased. Similar observations have been made by the same laboratory using cyclophosphamide. The mechanism and clinical relevance of these observations are both unclear and only serve to highlight the species differences that may cloud the investigation of drug–drug interactions in animal models.

Biological agents

Cytokines are able to down-regulate the expression of many cytochrome P450 enzymes, and this may explain the apparent link between inflammatory diseases and decreased metabolic drug clearance observed in several disease states including cancer. Exogenous cytokines can have the same effect and the administration of interferon-α to patients was associated with a significant 37% decrease in cyclophosphamide clearance. This was consistent with a reduction in metabolic activation, because the AUC of the activated metabolite 4-hydroxycyclophosphamide was correspondingly reduced by 45%. Similar data demonstrating a reduction in 5-FU clearance when administered with interferon-α have been reported, but this effect has varied between studies, possibly reflecting differences in schedules and doses.

Enzyme induction

Cytochrome P450s in general are inducible enzymes. In the case of CYP3A4, it is well recognized that glucocorticoids (dexamethasone), barbiturates, rifampicin, and several anticonvulsant agents (phenytoin, carbamazepine) are able to up-regulate enzyme activity transcriptionally. Indeed, drug interactions resulting from increased CYP3A-mediated metabolism following the administration of anticonvulsants and steroids are among the most commonly encountered and problematic drug–drug interactions in medical oncology. Among the CYP3A substrates that have been demonstrated as being affected are the *Vinca* alkaloids, cyclophosphamide, irinotecan, etoposide, and teniposide. In the study of Baker et al., the range of teniposide clearance in six children on anticonvulsants was 21–54 mL/min per m^2 (22 courses) as compared to 7–17 mL/min per m^2 in a control group matched for age and sex. The clearance of topotecan has also been shown to increase by approx 50% when phenytoin is coadministered with concomitant increases in the AUC of the CYP3A metabolite *N*-desmethyltopotecan. Steroids have been reported to induce the metabolism and/or clearance of other drugs, including paclitaxel. Many of these inducers also induce other CYP450 isoforms, including members of the CYP2C superfamily. The oxazaphosphorines ifosfamide and cyclophosphamide display autoinduction of metabolism with unregulated expression of several enzymes in vitro. However, this is a complex effect and its role in drug interactions is not well established. It is complicated by the fact that cyclophosphamide metabolites can also inactivate CYPs, as discussed previously.

A confounding factor for the interpretation of drug–drug interactions with drugs such as the anticonvulsants, steroids, and other CYP-inducing drugs (e.g., rifampin and phenobarbital) is that these compounds can coordinately up-regulate P-glycoprotein and other transporters. Hence, even drugs that are not extensively metabolized by the cytochrome P450 system may have altered pharmacokinetics, presumably through an effect on transporter- mediated excretion.

Excretion

Drug interactions leading to modified drug excretion generally relate to interference with transporter function. Specifically, drug transporters in the proximal tubule of the kidney and the bile canaliculi are most likely involved. A major problem is identifying the tissue and transporter most at play in any observed drug–drug interaction. For example, cyclosporin A is an inhibitor of not only CYP3A but also of the transporters MRP-2 and P-glycoprotein. In addition to the effects on drug distribution discussed previously, cyclosporin also modulates both the renal and nonrenal clearance of several drugs including etoposide.

Renal excretion

Many drugs undergo active tubular secretion in the kidney, and there is the potential for drug interactions at that locus. The interaction between methotrexate and probenecid is one of the best known examples. Several transporters of the *organic anion transporter* (OAT) family are present in the tubular epithelium of the kidney and their inhibition by probenecid, various antibiotics, and NSAIDs is the likely mechanism. These interactions are indeed now being determined at the molecular level, which was not possible until relatively recently. This type of interaction may be important for other antifolate analogues with significant tubular secretion, although there is a paucity of data on this subject. Alterations in tubular secretion may also be modified through less direct effects. For example, Beorlegui et al. reported an apparent interaction between omeprazole and methotrexate. They argued that inhibition of the tubular proton pump by omeprazole caused a reduction in methotrexate secretion because of the requirement for protons by the latter.

Biliary excretion

Biliary excretion is a major route of excretion of many anticancer drugs. As mentioned previously, several transporters are present at the canalicular membrane including P-glycoprotein, MRP1, MRP-2 (cMOAT), and MRP-3. The development and discovery of drugs that act on these transporters has recently enabled the elucidation and exploitation of drug interactions at this locus.

Inhibition of biliary excretion

There are no documented cases of drug interactions specifically involving biliary excretion of anticancer drugs. Mostly, the problem is that measurement of biliary excretion is not routinely possible. Therefore, some of the pharmacokinetic interactions that have been reported might be attributable to this locus, but confirmatory evidence is not available. Preclinical experiments using perfused rat liver preparations have shown that inhibitors of P-glycoprotein may reduce biliary excretion of compounds known to be excreted such as doxorubicin. Using a similar model, Smit et al. demonstrated the potential for interactions between *Vinca* alkaloids and doxorubicin.

Induction of biliary excretion

Transporters, as with metabolic enzymes, can be involved in drug–drug interactions as a result of induction of activity. It is increasingly recognized that the induction of transporters such as P-glycoprotein can be caused by agents that overlap substantially with those capable of inducing CYP3A. As a result, some interactions with anticonvulsants may actually be the results of up-regulation of important transporters. This is a possible mechanism for the interaction between methotrexate and anticonvulsants.

Predicting Interactions

The prediction and evaluation of significant drug–drug interactions has in many instances been a rather piecemeal process. However, significant inroads in our understanding of the loci of these interactions have been made in vitro through to in vivo and there are now instances of systematic screening for these interactions during drug development.

Historical Data

In assessing likely interactions for a new drug, it is enormously useful if the compound has metabolism and excretion similar to those of previously characterized analogs. In the absence of such information, the usual sequential processes of in vitro and preclinical studies need to be carried out. One of the major problems is the manner in which these experiments have been performed often varies significantly from study to study and the data often reported are in different formats. There is therefore a real need for consistent experimental design and reporting in such studies. In the absence of such a platform, however, other groups have assembled electronic databases, which at least should enable some qualitative predictions of potential drug–drug interactions. A drug–drug interaction locus identified in vitro will be relevant only if this pathway represents a major route of elimination for the candidate drug. This is one of the major issues that databases such as the one proposed by Bonnabry et al. are trying to address.

Predicted from In Vitro Experiments

The advantage of being able readily to obtain drug metabolism enzymes from recombinant sources (insect cells, human lymphoblastoid cells, yeast, bacteria) has greatly facilitated the task of establishing the important routes of metabolism likely to be encountered when administered to patients. Similarly, these systems can also be used to search for potential drug interactions. Rapid throughput systems have been developed that use specific fluorogenic substrates to facilitate the large-scale and thorough screening required. The much larger potential problem is that relating to drug transporters. Here, the best systems are likely to be panels of stably transfected cells expressing each known transporter, starting probably with P-glycoprotein, BCRP, and MRP-1 and MRP-2. Alternatively, cells mimicking the relevant in vivo system may be used to test simultaneously the effects of expression of transporters and metabolic enzymes. A specific problem with the in vitro testing of drug interactions with alkylating anticancer drugs relates to the fact that these have complex pharmacology featuring multiple, often unstable species. Comprehensive studies of metabolic interactions with such drugs are difficult to perform and to interpret.

In Silico

Ultimately, the structure–activity relationships for each enzyme/transporter may become sufficiently documented by the use of large databases to enable direct *in silico* predictions of the metabolic and transporter properties of new drugs. These in turn would enable extrapolation of likely in vivo disposition, pharmacogenetics, and possible drug interactions. As mentioned previously, predictions are complicated by the overlap between transporters and metabolism. The interaction of etoposide with cyclosporin reported by Bisogno et al. could, on the basis of other observations discussed above, be the result of interaction with metabolism, biliary and intestinal secretion, and protein binding. Likewise cimetidine, which is often used as a relatively nonselective CYP450 inhibitor, is also an inhibitor of OAT in the kidney. Hence the mechanism for the drug interaction reported between cimetidine and epirubicin is also difficult to identify. Ultimately, therefore, classical in vitro and in vivo approaches for the investigation of drug interactions are required.

Preclinical Studies

Animal models may enable certain drug–drug interactions to be examined in a more physiologically meaningful fashion. However, some major interspecies differences exist with respect to the metabolism and excretion of drugs. For example, rats are relatively deficient in the aldo–keto reductases that metabolize anthracyclines to their corresponding C-13 alcohols. The cytochrome P450 enzymes also often differ markedly between species, not only in terms of their substrate affinities and reaction products but also in their susceptibility to inducers and inhibitors. The regulation of CYP450 is also highly species dependent. For example, induction of CYP3A by rifampicin is pronounced in humans and rabbits but not in rats. Hence, investigations of drug interactions require the use of the most representative animal or in vitro system to ensure relevance.

Clinical Studies

Many of the clinical drug interactions reported have been detected on the basis on comparisons of relatively small patient groups. In most cases, data are compared to historical or case-matched groups. Even less reliable are isolated case reports that report suspected drug interactions on the basis of abnormal drug disposition. Because of the large interindividual differences in metabolism and disposition, many of these studies are underpowered and biased. Ideally, clinical studies should be performed using a randomized crossover design as is normally used in trials to support of registration of compounds. FDA guidelines are available for the design of such trials. However, in medical oncology, many of the drugs are inherently unsafe. Usually drug–drug interactions are investigated because they pose a threat either to the safety or the efficacy of a compound and it becomes ethically difficult to propose such trials in patients who cannot really afford either. One alternative is to incorporate extensive population pharmacokinetics as part of Phase II and III trials of anticancer drugs. This then enables the identification of patients with unusual pharmacokinetic data and the identification of possible interactions. One of the down sides of this approach is that studies may require a very large number of subjects (several hundred) unless the interacting drug is very commonly used in the intended setting (e.g., anticonvulsants in CNS malignancy).

The drug candidates most worthy of further study for possible interactions are obviously those that are likely to be coadministered and for which there is some support from *in silico*, in vitro, preclinical, or clinical data. Other factors to be considered include the doses of the agents, their dosing regimen (single or multiple doses), and the timing of the administration (A before B, A after B, or

A + B). The latter is particularly important when the drug interaction is modulated through alteration of gene expression. For example, a study on the effects of rifampicin on drug clearance would require several days of rifampicin treatment prior to administration of the test drug to ensure maximal induction of the relevant enzyme system.

When the Problem is Not the Drug

In some instances, apparently classical drug–drug interactions have subsequently been shown to have little to do with the drugs involved. Consideration of these alternate mechanisms should be part of the investigation of drug–drug interactions.

Vehicle Effects

Many drugs are not sufficiently soluble to be administered in purely aqueous solvents. Instead a formulation component is frequently a surfactant. These compounds should not be dismissed as inactive and inconsequential. For example, Cremophor EL has some membrane effects and has been investigated for its ability to reverse P-glycoprotein-mediated multidrug resistance. It also modulates differentially the toxicity of cisplatin to marrow and tumor cells. Cremophor EL has been shown to modulate the distribution and elimination of doxorubicin in both preclinical and clinical studies. In the study of Millward et al., 11 patients were randomized to receive either 50 mg/m^2 of doxorubicin alone or in combination with 30 mL/m^2 of Cremophor EL. They were then crossed over to the alternative regimen. Cremophor significantly reduced the clearance of doxorubicin by approx 20%. The metabolite doxorubicinol was present in higher concentrations after Cremophor EL administration, resulting in an almost doubling of its AUC. Cremophor EL is also the likely major component of the interaction between Taxol and anthracyclines. When Taxol is administered immediately prior to a doxorubicin infusion or as an infusion prior to bolus doxorubicin, the clearance of doxorubicin is reduced by 20–30% and concentrations of doxorubicinol are again greatly increased. The latter suggests a possible reduction in the biliary clearance of the metabolite or a redistribution phenomenon secondary to the membrane effects of the Cremophor EL. Indeed, even when paclitaxel is administered 24 h after doxorubicin, sudden rebound profiles of doxorubicinol are observed. The effects of Cremophor EL on the hepatic disposition of paclitaxel itself also appear to be due to nonspecific effects on distribution rather than direct effects on biliary excretion.

Polysorbate 80 (also known as Tween 80) is used in the current formulation of docetaxel and etoposide. The coadministration of polysorbate 80 by itself or in the etoposide formulation had up to a twofold effect on doxorubicin AUC, mainly through increased early tissue distribution. The effect of etoposide on methotrexate pharmacokinetics reported by Paal et al. may also be due to the nonspecific effects of the Tween 80 present in etoposide. Indeed, the rebound profile of plasma methotrexate that occurred a few hours following etopo side is qualitatively similar to the rebound of doxorubicinol concentrations when paclitaxel is administered in Cremophor EL.

Effects of Dose Form

Several drugs are now marketed in liposomal formulations (doxorubicin, daunorubicin, amphotericin B). Theoretically, drugs can self-load into preformed liposomes in the circulation, and this was first demonstrated in a mouse model. When combination therapy includes a liposomal agent, the fact that many anticancer drugs are amphiphilic compounds that can interact with membranes suggests that drug–liposome interactions could take place. By binding to liposomes, it is possible that the release of the encapsulated drug would be modified and this has indeed been demonstrated in vitro. In vivo, however, this appears less likely and the predominant effect appears to be the uptake of the free drug into the circulating liposomes. In the study of Waterhouse et al., mice administered idarubicin and liposomal vincristine had a 3.6-fold increase in circulating concentrations of idarubicin 15 min later.

Effects of Treatmeht Regimens

Apart from aspects of formulation composition, specific treatment regimens require additional procedures to ensure adequate safety. For example, fluid loading is usually undertaken prior to cisplatin or methotrexate to ensure adequate renal function. Therefore, administration of another drug also cleared by the kidneys with either cisplatin or methotrexate might possibly result in altered disposition relative to drug alone. Some data are in support of such an effect. For example, Hudes et al. reported an increase in the renal clearance of trimetrexate when administered with cisplatin. Paradoxically, the urinary recovery of pemitrexed was reduced and its total clearance increased when administered with cisplatin. It is expected that effects of volume loading on renal clearance would be most pronounced in patients with some degree of renal dysfunction. For example, Kaye et al. found greatly increased methotrexate clearance when coadministered with cisplatin and forced diuresis only in a patient with renal clearance < 60 mL/min.

Administration of premedication agents for nausea/vomiting and hypersensitivity reactions may also be implicated. For example, interaction studies of a drug regimen with or without cisplatin might reasonably introduce not only the cisplatin but also antiemetics in the regimen. Ondansetron, for example, has been suggested to cause a slight decrease in the clearance of cyclophosphamide in high-dose regimens as compared to historical controls. Other studies have also noticed similar modest effects on both cyclophosphamide and cisplatin elimination by ondansetron, again when compared to historical controls. Similarly, the requirement for steroid prophylaxis for hypersensitivity reactions with docetaxel has been suggested to be the mechanism behind the interaction between ifosfamide and docetaxel.

When the Cytotoxic Agent is Not the Victim

Because cytotoxic agents are potentially dangerous drugs we are actually more concerned about the effects of concomitant therapy on the cytotoxic drug rather than the reverse. However, many drugs that are used for the intercurrent treatment of the patient may also suffer from small therapeutic windows. As discussed above, there have been reports of perturbed coagulation parameters in patients on warfarin receiving capecitabine. Similarly, blood concentrations of phenytoin are increased under similar circumstances. The effect is unlikely to be mediated by an acute interaction, given that capecitabine does not inhibit the cytochrome involved in the metabolism of warfarin. However, as mentioned previously, it appears that oral fluoropyrimidines can affect the expression and activity of cytochrome P450s.

Can We Exploit Drug Interactions?

Oral Delivery of Drugs

Drug interactions, as shown in the relevant sections above can have both detrimental and beneficial effects in chemotherapy. In particular, the inhibition of gastrointestinal transporters and enzymes greatly improves the bioavailability of oral drugs and enables oral delivery of some drugs that could previously not be administered orally. Poor bioavailability is usually associated with highly variable systemic concentrations and an additional possible benefit could be a reduction in intra- and interpatient variability in pharmacokinetics, although this is unlikely to be reduced to less than that encountered with parenteral administration. An example of successful exploitation of this strategy is the development of orally administered fluoropyrimidines that incorporate an inhibitor of DPD.

Many transport and enzyme modulators are currently being investigated in the setting of oral chemotherapy, although analogues that are specifically not substrates for these pathways provide an alternative route of development. For example, several taxanes that are not P-glycoprotein substrates are currently being evaluated for oral chemotherapy.

Systemic Administration

As previously discussed for the DPD inhibitors, administration of an inhibitor may greatly reduce intratumoral metabolism that in some cases may act as a significant mechanism of resistance in vivo. The second possible advantage of the suicide inhibitors of DPD (e.g., ethinyluracil) is that when coadministered, the elimination of 5-FU is no longer mostly via DPD catabolism but by renal excretion. The latter pathway is inherently less variable and more predictable than DPD, thereby potentially facilitating the dose individualization of treatment, although this has not been exploited in Phase III trials of the combination. Other DPD inhibitors have been developed in combination with oral prodrugs of 5-FU. These combination products include S-1 and UFT. S-1 also contains potassium oxonate as an inhibitor of thymidine kinase, and this assists in reducing activation of the 5-FU in the gastrointestinal mucosa.

The reduction in fluoropyrimidine dose that is made possible with DPD inhibitors underscores another way in which drug interactions can be exploited. In the early years of cyclosporin A use, the interaction between diltiazem was characterized and exploited to enable substantial cost savings. However, interactions based on reversible mechanisms are very difficult to predict because of constantly varying profiles on the target and inhibitor drug. In oncology, because of the limited safety of many of these agents, introduction of an additional variable into the chemotherapy regimen may become counterproductive, and such strategies are used only in the experimental setting. Such interactions also need to be proven from the aspect of activity, and the substantial costs of the additional Phase III trials probably outweigh the savings. Ironically, cyclosporin has now been proposed as a modulator of several agents to improve their pharmacokinetic and pharmacodynamic properties.

FUTURE DIRECTIONS

From a drug development aspect, the most exciting proposition is that accumulated knowledge about current drugs and their metabolism will enable some *in silico* prediction of likely mechanism of clearance and the potential drug interactions that might arise. This could greatly assist the rational refinement of drug leads and reduce the expense of development. The possibility of using well-characterized drug–drug interactions to enable oral therapy may prove obvious potential advantages, but this has not yet been developed into the routine clinical setting. Finally, genomic advances are likely to advance greatly our understanding of drug–drug interactions, particularly as they relate to instances in which drug metabolism is induced. For example, cytochrome P450 3A expression is extremely sensitive to control from interactions of nuclear receptors with the RXR. Some of the nuclear factors involved (CAR, PXR, and PPAR) have recently been shown to be subject to functional polymorphic variation. The elucidation of genotype/phenotype associations may help ultimately enable prediction of drug–drug interactions in individual subjects.

13

INCRETIN MODULATORS

The stimulation of insulin secretion has been a therapeutic principle since the introduction of sulfonylureas in the 1950s, when tolbutamide and carbutamide were introduced. Second- and third-generation sulfonylureas like glibenclamide and glimeperide remain to be among the most commonly used antidiabetic agents, attesting to the fact that promoting β-cell secretory function is a feasible way of controlling plasma glucose in patients with type 2 diabetes. Nevertheless, sulfonylureas are far from ideal as antidiabetic agents, since their use is associated with weight gain and with the provocation of hypoglycemia. The latter is caused by the absence of a strict glucose dependency of the ability to promote insulin secretion, since sulfonylureas per se are able to close the ATP-dependent K^+ channel, even at rather low glucose concentrations.

The incretin concept was developed when it had become obvious that the oral ingestion of nutrients, especially carbohydrates (glucose, starch, etc.) releases insulinotropic hormones from the gut mucosa, which in turn augment the insulin secretory response induced by meal-related glycemic excursions. When the first incretin hormone to be described in detail, Glucose-dependent Insulinotropic Polypeptide (Gastric Inhibitory Polypeptide, GIP) was characterized, one of the remarkable properties was the strict glucose dependency of its insulinotropic actions, both in perfused rat pancreas and in human subjects in vivo. Werner Creutzfeldt, in his 1978 Claude–Bernard lecture to the European Association for the Study of Diabetes, made this characteristic of GIP a core component of the definition of incretin hormones in general. Obviously, with a peptide like GIP, it was impossible to provoke hypoglycemic episodes, even when it was administered at high doses. A natural compound that potently stimulates insulin secretion, however, without a risk of provoking hypoglycemia, attracted attention as a potential candidate parent compound for the development of antidiabetic drugs. Because GIP has lost most of its insulinotropic activity in patients with type 2 diabetes, it was not until the identification of glucagon-like peptide-1 (GLP-1) and the demonstration that GLP-1 had preserved insulinotropic (and additional) activities in patients with type 2 diabetes that the idea of using incretin hormones as the basis for novel antidiabetic drugs could be actively persued.

DEFINITION OF THE PROBLEM AND BASIC PATHOPHYSIOLOGY

Secretion and Action of Incretin Hormones in Physiology

Physiological roles of gastrointestinal peptide hormones

The ingestion of nutrients elicits the secretion of gastrointestinal hormones intimately involved in the regulation of gut and gallbladder motility, digestive juice secretion, and postprandial carbohydrate metabolism. In particular, incretin hormones stimulate insulin secretion from the endocrine pancreas.

Through the action of incretin hormones, enteral nutrition provides a more potent insulinotropic stimulus relative to an isoglycemic intravenous challenge. This phenomenon is named the "*incretin effect*".

GIP

The first incretin to be identified, GIP, was purified from porcine intestine extracts by virtue of its ability to inhibit gastric acid secretion (therefore, the original name was *gastric inhibitory polypeptide*). Soon, it was discovered that GIP displayed potent insulinotropic actions in animals and in human subjects. GIP was shown to be a 42 amino acid peptide hormone synthesized in duodenal and jejunal enteroendocrine K cells in the proximal small bowel (duodenum and jejunum).

GLP-1

Much later, the second incretin hormone, glucagon-like peptide-1 (GLP-1), was identified as a partial sequence of the cDNAs and genes encoding proglucagon. After posttranslational processing of proglucagon in gut endocrine L-cells, GLP-1 exists in two circulating equipotent molecular forms, GLP- 1 ("glycine-extended GLP-1") and GLP-1 amide ("amidated GLP-1"). The amidated form is more abundant in the circulation following meal ingestion in humans. Although the majority of GLP-1 is synthesized in the distal ileum and colon, plasma levels of GLP-1, like GIP, increase shortly after starting meals. This leaves two possibilities: Either there is an upper gut signal mediating GLP-1 release from more distal stores (i.e. the locations where GLP-1 is most abundant). Alternatively, GLP-1 is predominantly released from the sparse L-cells that are present in the upper gut. Quantitative considerations make it appear feasible that GLP-1 from gut segments coming into direct contact with chyme is the source of postprandial increments in GLP-1 concentrations.

Proteolytic degradation of incretin hormones by dipeptidyl peptidase-4

Plasma levels of total GLP-1 (including proteolytic degradation products) are low ("basal") in the fasted state (approximately 5 pmol/L) and increase rapidly following meal ingestion, reaching levels in plasma of 15–50 pmol/L. Only a minor proportion of circulating GLP-1 (approximately 10–20%) is intact, biologically active GLP-1. This is true after endogenous secretion as well as during exogenous administration, for example, during continuous intravenous infusion or after subcutaneous injection. The major reason is the rapid proteolytic degradation and inactivation by dipeptidyl peptidase-4 (DPP-4), an aminopeptidase recognizing peptides with a proline or alanine in the second aminoterminal position. It removes the first two aminoterminal amino acids, rendering the breakdown products (GLP-1 amide or GLP-1) biologically inactive or even weakly antagonistic. The circulating levels of intact GLP-1 and GIP are further kept low by rapid renal clearance. Whether additional proteases such as human neutral endopeptidase 24.11 are also essential determinants of GLP-1 inactivation remains under active investigation. Mice with targeted inactivation of the DPP-4 gene exhibit increased levels of plasma GIP and GLP-1, increased insulin secretion, and reduced glucose excursion following a glucose challenge.

GIP and GLP-1 receptors

GIP and GLP-1 exert their actions via engagement of structurally distinct G protein-coupled receptors. GIP receptors are predominantly expressed on islet β-cells, and to a lesser extent, in adipose tissue and in the central nervous system. In contrast, GLP-1 receptors are expressed in pancreatic endocrine β-cells and in several peripheral tissues including the central and peripheral nervous system, heart, kidney, lung, and the gastrointestinal tract. Activation of both incretin receptors on β-cells leads to rapid increases in levels of cyclic AMP and intracellular calcium, followed by insulin exocytosis, in a glucose-dependent manner. Incretin receptor signaling is associated with protein kinase A activation, induction of gene transcription, enhanced levels of (pro-)insulin biosynthesis, and the stimulation of β-cell proliferation. GLP-1 and GIP receptor activation protect β-cells against toxin-induced apoptosis (elicited by glucotoxicity – hyperglycemia, lipotoxicity – high concentrations of free fatty acids, streptozotocin, or hydrogen peroxide) and enhanced β-cell survival, findings observed in studies of both rodent and human islets.

Biological activity of GIP and GLP-1

The main functions of GIP are the glucose-dependent augmentation of insulin secretion during periods characterized by physiological hyperglycemia, the incretin function *sensu strictu*. Animal experiments suggest that GIP receptors on adipose tissue are essential for adipocyte triglyceride storage after meal ingestion: GIP receptor knock-out mice do not become obese when fed a high-fat diet.

GLP-1 does not only display glucose-dependent insulinotropic ("incretin") activity, but also inhibits glucagon secretion, decelerates gastric emptying and reduces food ingestion, and promotes enhanced glucose disposal via neural mechanisms involving receptors in the "*hepatoportal*" region. It is of interest that GLP-1 effects on glucagon secretion, like those on insulin secretory responses, are glucose-dependent, whereas counter-regulatory release of glucagon in response to hypoglycemia remains undisturbed even in the presence of pharmacological concentrations of GLP-1.

Effect of incretin receptor knock-out in mice

The physiological importance of endogenous GIP and GLP- 1 for glucose homeostasis can be examined using specific receptor antagonists or knock-out mice. Acute antagonism of either GIP or GLP-1 action lowers insulin secretion and increases plasma glucose following oral glucose ingestion in rodents. Similarly, mice with inactivating mutations in the GIP or GLP-1 receptors exhibit reduced glucose-stimulated insulin secretion and impaired glucose tolerance. GLP-1, but probably not GIP, is essential also for the control of fasting glucose concentrations, as acute antagonism or genetic disruption of GLP-1 action leads to increased levels of fasting glucose in rodents.

Effects of GLP-1 receptor antagonists in human subjects

The GLP-1 receptor antagonist exendin has been used to elucidate the role of endogenously secreted GLP-1 in human volunteers. Administration of exendin leads to a reduction in glucose-stimulated insulin secretion, diminished glucose clearance, and increased glucagon secretion. Indirect evidence suggests more rapid gastric emptying following disruption of GLP-1 action in humans as expected from the activity profile of GLP-1.

Activity of the Entero-Insular Axis and Incretin Hormones in Type 2-Diabetic Patients

Reduced incretin effect in patients with type 2 diabetes

In healthy human subjects oral glucose elicits a considerably higher insulin secretory response than does intravenous glucose (even if leading to the same glycemic increments). This incretin effect is substantially reduced or even completely lost in patients with type 2 diabetes. The reduction in the incretin effect probably is an acquired defect, since it is also found in patients with diabetes secondary to chronic pancreatitis, whereas chronic pancreatitis without diabetes is characterized by a normal incretin effect.

Secretion of incretin hormones in patients with type 2 diabetes

Cross-sectional analyses of larger cohorts suggest that there is a slight reduction in postprandial GLP-1 secretion following the ingestion of a mixed meal in patients with type 2 diabetes. Subjects with impaired glucose tolerance display intermediate results between healthy controls (normal response) and type 2-diabetic patients (reduced response). This is true for both total and intact GLP-1. However, the overall difference is small, and concerns the second and third hour after starting meal ingestion, whereas the characteristic differences in insulin secretory pattern are found in the early period after glucose or meal ingestion. Therefore, it cannot be considered likely that the slight reduction in postprandial GLP-1 secretion in patients with type 2 diabetes has any immediate impact on glycemic control. Along the same lines, any administration of GLP-1 receptor agonists should not be simply considered a replacement of an essential hormone (e.g. GLP-1) that is lacking in patients with type 2 diabetes.

GIP secretion in patients with type 2 diabetes has been reported as exaggerated, normal (on average), or reduced. In all cases, the differences were small in comparison with appropriate control subjects and are not likely to indicate any importance for the pathophysiology of the entero-insular axis in type 2 diabetes. Certainly, there is no complete lack in GIP in patients with type 2 diabetes.

Insulinotropic activity of GIP and GLP-1 in patients with type 2 diabetes

While the interaction of both GIP and GLP-1 with their respective receptors on healthy pancreatic endocrine β-cells leads to cAMP production and the augmentation of glucose-stimulated insulin release in a very similar manner, the insulinotropic activity of GIP is almost completely lost in patients with type 2 diabetes. This does not appear to indicate a lack of expression of GIP receptors on type 2-diabetic β-cells, since a bolus injection of GIP still elicits some insulin secretory response. However, prolonged infusion, even of highly pharmacological doses of GIP, is unable to meaningfully stimulate insulin secretion. This certainly is the fundamental defect underlying the reduced incretin effect in patients with type 2 diabetes.

On the other hand, a considerable proportion of the insulinotropic activity of GLP-1 as found in healthy subjects is preserved in patients with type 2 diabetes. Physiological concentrations of GLP-1 (as found after meal ingestion), however, have little if any effect on insulin secretion in patients with type 2 diabetes.

Upon a closer look, the insulinotropic activity of GLP-1 is also somewhat reduced in patients with type 2 diabetes compared with healthy control subjects. However, even a relatively low dose of GLP-1 can acutely restore the ability of β-cells to respond to increasing glucose concentrations with an insulin secretory response similar to healthy subjects. Nevertheless, the insulin response remains at approximately 20–25% relative to the effect in healthy subjects exposed to the same GLP-1 doses and concentrations. This partial preservation of insulin secretory effects is sufficient to make GLP-1 a potent insulinotropic agent in patients with type 2 diabetes.

Pharmacological doses of GLP-1 display the full spectrum of activities also in patients with type 2 diabetes. This includes effects on insulin and glucagon secretion, gastric emptying, appetite, and meal size. As a consequence, antidiabetic properties of pharmacological doses of GLP-1 have been examined in patients with type 2 diabetes.

Therapeutic Potential of Incretin Hormones

Owing to their pivotal role in the postprandial regulation of insulin secretion, both GIP and GLP-1 have been suggested as potential antidiabetic drug candidates. However, no significant reduction in glycemia could be achieved in studies with intravenous infusions of the GIP in hyperglycemic patients with type 2 diabetes. Indeed, while GIP exhibits potent insulinotropic properties in healthy subjects and probably mediates the major proportion of the incretin effect under physiological circumstances, its insulinotropic effect is markedly diminished in patients with type 2 diabetes. It is a current matter of debate whether this loss of incretin activity in type 2 diabetes is due to a specific defect, for example, in GIP signaling on pancreatic β-cells, or whether it goes along with a general decline in β-cell mass and function in such patients. In support of the latter hypothesis, the insuliotropic effect of GIP is not only reduced in patients with type 2 diabetes, but also in individuals with other forms of diabetes, such as MODY or type 1 diabetes. A number of GIP analogues exhibiting prolonged biological half-lives due to the chemical modifications, mostly at the N-terminal end of the peptide chain, have been proposed as potential drug candidates for the pharmacotherapy of type 2 diabetes, but as yet none of these compounds has been tested in patients with diabetes. Given the obvious inefficacy of native GIP in such patients, it is questionable whether GIP analogues will indeed exhibit a significant antihyperglycemic potential. Furthermore, unlike GLP-1, GIP even stimulates glucagon secretion, thereby potentially counteracting its insulinotropic effect.

Antidiabetic Actions of GLP-1

Short-term intravenous infusions of GLP-1 (approximately 1.2 pmol/kg/min, leading to pharmacological plasma concentrations of total GLP-1 of approximately 100 pmol/L, and intact biologically active GLP-1 of approximately 15 pmol/L) lower blood glucose in human subjects with type 2 diabetes through a transient glucose-dependent stimulation of insulin and suppression of glucagon secretion and gastric emptying. A 6-week subcutaneous infusion of GLP-1 in patients with type 2 diabetes achieving plasma levels of total GLP-1 of around 65 pmol/L was followed by a substantial improvement in insulin secretory capacity, insulin sensitivity, a reduction in HbA_{1c} by 1.2%, and weight loss. Although intravenous or subcutaneous GLP-1 infusions may be useful for the short-term control of hyperglycemia under a variety of clinical conditions, the long-term treatment of type 2 diabetes requires a more feasible approach for achieving sustained GLP-1 receptor activation. The proof-of-principle that GLP-1 can help lower, even normalize plasma glucose in a substantial number of patients with type 2 diabetes, has paved the way to explore the clinical efficacy of (i) peptides that act as GLP-1 receptor agonists, but have more suitable pharmacokinetic properties than are characteristic for the parent compound, GLP-1, and (ii) DPP-4 inhibitors (small molecules with substantial oral bioavailability).

THERAPEUTICAL APPROACH OF RELEVANT DRUGS, UNDERSTANDING AND PINPOINTING CLINICAL PHARMACOLOGY, CRITICAL EVALUATION OF DRUGS

GLP-1 Receptor Agonists

Exenatide (synthetic exendin-4)

Exenatide (synthetic exendin-4) was isolated from the salivary gland of the gila monster, a lizard found in the deserts of Arizona. Due to an ~50% amino acid homology with native human GLP-1, this peptide acts as a potent agonist at the mammalian GLP-1 receptor, but is not substrate to proteolytic cleavage by DPP-4. This leads to a circulating plasma half-life of 2–4 h, with exenatide levels being raised for ~6 h after a single subcutaneous injection.

The clinical effects of exenatide in the treatment of type 2 diabetes have been examined in phase 3 trials. In these studies, exenatide (5 or 10 μg s.c. twice daily) was added to an existing therapy with metformin, sulfonylureas, a combination of both, or thiazolidinediones. HbA_{1c}-reductions achieved after exenatide treatment over 30 weeks ranged from 0.8% to 1.0%, with HbA_{1c}-levels at baseline ranging between 8.2% and 8.6%. In addition, body weight was reduced by ~1-3 kg after 30 weeks (baseline weight: ~100 kg), and patients continuing in an open-label extension study for 80 weeks exhibited a total weight loss averaging ~4.5 kg. The latter effect is remarkable in that all other insulinotropic drugs (sulfonylureas and glinides) as well as insulin itself typically cause weight gain during long-term administration.

In an open-label comparison of exenatide with insulin glargine in diabetic patients suboptimally controlled with metformin and sulfonylurea, both treatment regimens led to a reduction in HbA_{1c} levels by ~1.1% after 26 weeks (baseline: 8.2%). However, while fasting glucose concentrations were reduced to a greater extent with insulin glargine, exenatide treatment elicited greater reductions in postprandial glycemia. The most striking differences between both treatment regimens were observed in body weight. Thus, patients treated with insulin glargine experienced a weight gain of 1.8 kg, whereas patients on exenatide lost on average 2.3 kg over the treatment period. Similar findings have been reported for the comparison of exenatide and premixed insulin aspart, both injected subcutaneously twice daily.

In April 2005, exenatide (trade name, Byetta) was approved by the FDA for the treatment of type 2 diabetic patients who have not achieved adequate glycemic control on maximally tolerated doses of metformin and/or a sulfonylurea. In Europe, exenatide was approved in November 2006.

Liraglutide

Liraglutide (NN221 1; Arg34, Lys26-[*N*-∈ (γ-Glu[*N*-α-hexadecanoyl])]-GLP-1) is a GLP-1 derivative developed by Novo Nordisk, which is currently undergoing phase 3 clinical trials. The plasma half-life of this compound has been extended to ~10–14 h through an amino acid substitution ($Arg_{34} \rightarrow Lys$) and the attachment of a glutamic acid and a 16-C-free fatty acid addition to Lys_{26}. The acyl moiety induces non-covalent binding to albumin with ~1–2% of Liraglutide circulating as the non-albumin bound, "free" peptide. These modified pharmacokinetic properties make the compound suitable for once-daily s.c. administration. In clinical studies in patients with type 2 diabetes, liraglutide reduced HbA_{1c} levels by up to 1.75%. Liraglutide induced a moderate weight loss during chronic administration, similar to the effects of native GLP-1 and exenatide.

Long-acting GLP-1 receptor agonists

As a single subcutaneous injection of exenatide does not produce effective glucose control for more than 6–8 h, there is considerable interest in the development of longer-acting GLP- 1 receptor agonists, which require less frequent parenteral administration. Exenatide LAR ("*long-acting release*") is a poly-lactide-glycolide microsphere suspension containing 3% exendin-4 peptide, which exhibits sustained dose-dependent glycemic control in diabetic fatty Zucker rats for up to 28 days following a single subcutaneous injection. Preliminary experience with exenatide LAR in 45 subjects with type 2 diabetes mellitus indicates a much greater reduction in fasting glucose concentrations and HbA_{1c} following once-weekly administrations of exenatide LAR for 15 weeks. However, long-term experience with exenatide LAR in larger numbers of patients has not yet been reported. Exenatide LAR is currently being examined in a Phase 3 trial head to head against twice-daily exenatide.

Additional strategies for development of long-acting GLP-1 receptor agonists include the use of chemical linkers to form covalent bonds between GLP-1 (CJC-1131) or exendin-4 (CJC-1134). Similarly, recombinant albumin-GLP-1 proteins (e.g., "albugon") have been developed, which mimic the full spectrum of GLP-1 actions in preclinical studies. Although these drugs are expected to exhibit a prolonged pharmacokinetic profile suitable for once-weekly dosing in diabetic patients, only limited clinical information is available about the efficacy and safety of these albumin-based drugs in human subjects.

DPP-4 Inhibitors

The therapeutic use of GLP-1 is primarily limited by its rapid in vivo degradation by the enzyme DPP-4. DPP-4 is a ubiquitous membrane-spanning cell-surface amino-peptidase widely expressed in many tissues including liver, lung, kidney, intestinal brush-border membranes, lymphocytes, and endothelial cells, which can also be found circulating in plasma. DPP-4 nonspecifically cleaves peptides displaying a proline or alanine residue in the second amino-terminal position, thereby making a number of gastrointestinal hormones, including GIP, GLP-1, GLP-2, PACAP, Neuropeptide Y, and Peptide YY substrates to DPP-4 degradation.

Endogenous GLP- 1 plasma levels typically increase by ~2–3-fold after meal ingestion and return to baseline values within ~3–6 h. Inhibiting DPP-4 activity extents the circulating half-life of the incretin hormone, thereby raising intact GLP-1 levels for up to 5 h after meal ingestion. While DPP-4 inhibitors primarily lower postprandial glycemic excursions, there is now evidence that basal concentrations of intact GLP-1 are also raised to some extent by DPP-4 inhibition, which may explain their (modest) effects on fasting glycemia. As a rule, DPP-4 inhibitors mimic many of the actions of native GLP- 1, such as the stimulation of insulin and inhibition of glucagon secretion. However, unlike

GLP-1 and its analogues, DPP-4 inhibitors do not typically influence body weight or gastric emptying. These discrepancies might be due to the nonspecific mode of action of the DPP-4 inhibitors, which also prevent the degradation of other peptides, especially GIP and NPY, which might exert opposite effects on gastric motility and the central nervous control of appetite. As an alternative explanation, it seems possible that the modest elevations in intact GLP-1 levels (approximately doubled) seen after DPP-4 inhibition are of insufficient magnitude to elicit significant effects on gastric emptying and food intake. A number of small molecule DPP-4 inhibitors suitable for oral administration are currently undergoing clinical trials. This article focuses on the two major compounds with available reports regarding phase 3 clinical trials.

Sitagliptin

The DPP-4 inhibitor sitagliptin has been developed by Merck Pharmaceuticals and was recently approved for the therapy of type 2 diabetes by the FDA under the name Januvia. The elimination half-life of sitagliptin is 12–14 h, thereby allowing for once-daily administration. In phase 3 trials enrolling drug-naïve patients with type 2 diabetes, sitagliptin led to HbA_{1c} reductions of 0.79% and 0.94% a dose of 100 and 200 mg, respectively (baseline: 8.0%). In diabetic patients inadequately controlled with metformin (baseline HbA_{1c}: 8.0%), HbA_{1c}-levels were reduced by 0.65% after 24 weeks of sitagliptin treatment. Likewise, patients pretreated with pioglitazone (baseline HbA_{1c}: 8.1%) exhibited a 0.7% HbA_{1c}-reduction after 24 weeks of sitaglitin treatment. Regarding the control of glycemia (HbA_{1c}), sitagliptin was equipotent to the sulfonylurea glipizide, when added to metformin pretreatment. Glipizide, however, caused significant weight gain. Similar to vildaglitin, sitagliptin does not have any systematic effect on body weight.

Vildagliptin

The DPP-4 inhibitor vildagliptin has been developed by Novartis Pharma and is currently awaiting approval. Vildagliptin has been studied at doses between 50 and 100 mg administered once or twice daily per os. In a study over 4 weeks, once-daily administration of 100 mg vildagliptin reduced fasting glucose by 0.70 mmol/L, and post-prandial glucose excursions by 1.45 mmol/L. This effect was accompanied by a significant reduction glucagon levels, whereas plasma insulin remained rather unchanged. However, similar insulin profiles at lower glucose concentrations indicate an improvement in glucose-stimulated insulin secretion. Consistent with this, indirect evidence from mathematical modeling studies suggested a significant improvement in β-cell function during vildagliptin treatment.

In metformin-treated patients with type 2 diabetes, the addition of vildagliptin led to a reduction of HbA_{1c} by ~0.8% (baseline: 7.7%), and this effect was maintained during an open-label extension for 52 weeks. Recent studies in patients with type 2 diabetes treated with the twice-daily administration of 50 mg vildagliptin also demonstrated a significant improvement in postprandial plasma triglyceride and apolipoprotein B-48-containing triglyceride-rich lipoprotein particle metabolism, suggesting that this compound might exert antiatherogenic effects beyond its glucose-lowering actions.

In a direct comparison, vildagliptin did not quite achieve noninferiority in comparison with metformin in terms of lowering HbA_{1c}-levels, but was associated with a lower frequency of GI-side effects. When compared with rosiglitazone, vildagliptin treatment elicited a similar reduction in HbA_{1c}-levels, but did not cause a similar increase in body weight.

Contrasting Properties of GLP-1 Receptor Agonists and DPP-4 Inhibitors

Twice-daily exenatide administered via subcutaneous injection is currently indicated for the treatment of patients with type 2 diabetes mellitus failing one or more oral agents, often as an alternative to institution of insulin therapy. In contrast, once-daily DPP-4 inhibitors may find use as first-line therapy or as add-on therapy to patients failing one or more oral agents. Although there does not appear to be a great difference in the HbA_{1c}-lowering capacity of GLP-1 receptor agonists versus DPP-4 inhibitors, the obvious difference between these classes of drugs is their effect on body weight. Weight loss is a common outcome of therapy with native GLP-1, exenatide, and liraglutide, whereas therapy with DPP-4 inhibitors is associated with prevention of weight gain. In contrast, gastrointestinal side effects, predominantly nausea, are frequently reported following treatment with injectable incretin mimetics, but have not been described with DPP-4 inhibition. These differences may be explained in part by the relatively modest stabilization of postprandial GLP-1 seen after DPP-4 inhibition versus the pharmacological increases in circulating levels of incretin mimetics exemplified by exenatide. Although nausea is a common side effect of exenatide therapy, many patients experience weight loss independent of nausea. Consistent with the above differences in circulating levels of GLP-1, incretin mimetics, but not DPP-4 inhibitors, profoundly decelerate gastric emptying.

Practical Outline in the Management

In this chapter, a suggestion will be developed on how incretin mimetics and DPP-4 inhibitors will fit into established treatment algorithms for glycemic control in patients with type 2 diabetes.

Choice of Patients

Incretin mimetics

Since incretin mimetics are injectable antidiabetic drugs, their use will most likely be considered, when oral antidiabetic agents in combinations do no longer assure glycemic control of the required quality. This is the moment, when - according to current guidelines - the start of insulin treatment would be considered according to most recommendations. However, such guidelines have, until now, not considered the availability of incretin mimetics or DPP-4 inhibitors. An attempt has been made to incorporate these novel antidiabetic treatment choices into a more complex algorithm.

Incretin mimetics (e.g. exenatide) would have some advantages over using insulin. In particular, they promote weight loss, whereas the initiation of insulin treatment must be expected to be associated with weight gain. This difference has been demonstrated in two head-to-head studies comparing twice-daily exenatide injections either with once-daily insulin *glargine* or twice-daily premixed insulin. It is, however, not known whether the resulting weight difference (approximately 5 kg) represents a significant health benefit in terms of cardiovascular risk or even outcome. Longer-term studies examining cardiovascular endpoints will be necessary to clarify this point. It can, however, be foreseen that for the obese type 2-diabetic patients, who has struggled to lose weight, an agent that will provide a good chance to lose rather than to gain body weight is an attractive choice. Along these lines, for patients in whom insulin therapy had been initiated recently, and in whom this has led to considerable weight gain, switching to incretin mimetics might be a reasonable alternative. However, studies examining the consequences of changing therapy from insulin to incretin mimetics in this particular situation are not yet available.

DPP-4 inhibitors

Given the fact that metformin is the established first-line drug for the anti-hyperglycemic treatment of obese type 2 diabetes, especially considering the reduction in the incidence of acute myocardial infarction and related mortality demonstrated in the UKPDS, the use of DPP-4 inhibitors may be considered, when metformin alone has failed to maintain adequate glycemic control, or is not likely to achieve treatment goals unless combined with additional agents. An early initiation of anti-hyperglycemic combination treatment is supported by the recent finding that metformin and sitagliptin achieved a higher likelihood of treatment success when given in combination to patients with type 2 diabetes not previously treated with oral agents. As a second oral antidiabetic agent, the use of DPP-4 inhibitors has to be weighed against the alternatives, sulfonylureas, glitazones, α-glucosidase inhibitors, and (basal, "bedtime") insulin. All other treatment choices (except acarbose or miglitol) will cause weight gain, whereas DPP-4 inhibitors generally can be considered weight-neutral. Sulfonylureas can provoke hypoglycemic episodes, and glitazones may precipitate fluid retention and congestive heart failure. Given the comparable antidiabetic potency of sitagliptin relative to the sulfonylurea glipizide and of vildagliptine in comparison with the thiazolidindione rosiglitazone, their weight-neutrality and unremarkable side-effect profile make DPP-4 inhibitors a serious contender for the second oral antidiabetic agent to be added to metformin treatment.

Given the fact that incretins (both GIP and GLP-1) are eliminated via the kidneys and that patients with impaired renal function have elevated circulating concentrations of GIP and GLP-1, treatment with usual doses of DPP-4 inhibitors might lead to further elevations in incretin plasma levels, potentially causing adverse events. Therefore, lower doses of DPP-4 inhibitors may be appropriate in such patients. Like in the case of renal functional impairment, not much is known on the use of DPP-4 inhibitors in patients with type 2 diabetes and associated diseases leading to severe organ failure (liver cirrhosis, heart failure, pulmonary disorders, etc.).

Initiation of Treatment

Incretin mimetics

Since starting exenatide injections may be associated with the provocation of nausea, it is better to start treatment at a lower dose (5 μg per injection, twice daily subcutaneously) and to increase the dose to 10 μg twice daily after 4 weeks. This has been shown to make the 10-μg dose more tolerable. Following this regimen has been associated with low withdrawal rates in studies using 10 μg twice daily. Initial studies using liraglutide had identified 0.75 mg once daily as a subcutaneous dose close to the maximum tolerated dose upon a single injection into treatment-naive subjects or patients. Later, a regimen starting at 0.5 mg once daily, and increasing the dose by 0.5 mg on a weekly basis, was used to extend the final dosage to 2 mg once daily for the majority of patients. Therefore, it appears advisable to start liraglutide at a low dose and titrate the daily dose up to the 2-mg range. The most recent trial has reported the use of 0.65, 1.25, and 1.9 mg once daily.

DPP-4 inhibitors

DPP-4 inhibitors can immediately be started at the target dose, since the initiation of treatment has not been associated with any untoward responses. Since studies examining effects of sitagliptin and vildagliptin at single (100 mg once daily orally) or divided doses (e.g., 50 mg twice daily orally) have not consistently resulted in different efficacy, once-daily dosing will probably be the standard.

Choice of Dose and Timing

Incretin mimetics

In studies examining the dose–response relationships for exenatide, 10 μg twice daily has uniformly been more effective than 5 μg twice daily. Therefore, for the majority of patients, exploiting the efficacy of 10 μg twice daily will be necessary to reach treatment targets. For those patients achieving their goals already at 5 μg twice daily, continuing at this dosage is an option.

Given the pharmacokinetics of exenatide injected subcutaneously into human subjects, a single injection is likely to be clinically effective over a period of 6–8 h. This can be inferred from the fact that the glycemic rise after breakfast and dinner is almost completely abolished when injecting exenatide before breakfast and dinner, whereas there remains a glucose excursion after lunch.

One consequence of the rather short duration of action of a single injection of exenatide is that timing the injection relative to meals is of some importance. Linnebjerg et al. demonstrated that exenatide should be injected within 60 min before starting meals. This appears plausible, since one important mode of action of exenatide is the deceleration of gastric emptying. Further, the question arises whether more frequent injections of exenatide (three or four per day) would provide even better glycemic control, including a more profound effect on fasting glucose concentrations and lunch-time glycemic control. One study had not found advantages of three over two injections. Rather than increasing the number of injections per day, the development has been in the direction of more extended-acting preparations of exenatide.

Preliminary results of using exenatide LAR indicate that doses of 0.8 and 2.0 mg per week (injected subcutaneously) are effective in reducing HbA_{1c} considerably. Interestingly, only the higher dose significantly reduced body weight, while the effect on HbA_{1c} after 15 weeks was relatively similar. This raises the question whether the dose–response relationship is different for glycemic control and for the reduction in body weight. If this were true, higher doses should be used, if weight reduction is among the treatment goals. Similarly, liraglutide reduced HbA_{1c} at doses of 0.65, 1.25, and 1.9 mg injected once daily subcutaneously, to a rather similar extent, while only the higher dose(s) significantly reduced body weight. Perhaps, the upper end of the dose–response relationship for weight reduction has not been characterized, and doses even higher than 2 mg daily would have more profound effects on body weight. Like with exenatide, the choice of the dose should consider whether or not weight loss is among the individual treatment goals.

DPP-4 inhibitors

Sitagliptin and vildagliptin exert their antidiabetic activity by inhibiting DPP-4 enzymatic activity. Since a single dose of 100 mg inhibits DPP-4 activity by >90% for most of a 24-h period, there is no obvious reason why higher doses should be more effective. As a consequence, a dose of 100 mg once daily will most likely be used rather uniformly, both for sitagliptin and vildagliptin, unless they are combined with other antidiabetic agents (like metformin), which are usually administered twice daily. Reduced doses may be necessary for patients with renal functional impairment.

Choice of Antidiabetic Agents to be Used in Combination

Incretin mimetics

Based on available clinical studies, a combining exenatide with metformin has the most obvious advantages: A substantial reduction in HbA1c is associated with the numerically largest weight loss (compared with combinations including sulfonylureas) and no increased risk of hypoglycemia (despite better glycemic control). Addition to thiazolidinediones is similarly possible. If exenatide is to be combined with sulfonylureas, the benefit of better glycemic control has to be weighed against the risk of hypoglycemia and less weight reduction. A combination of a short-acting incretin mimetic (to control postprandial rises in glycemia) and a long-acting insulin (to titrate fasting glucose into the target range) may theoretically appear to make sense, but no studies are available to report experience with this particular combination.

DPP-4 inhibitors

DPP-4 inhibitors can safely be combined with metformin and thiazolidinediones. A combination with sulfonylureas does not suggest particular advantages, since both agents, through different mechanisms, enhance insulin secretion. This combination would, most likely, not be as safe regarding hypoglycemic episodes. No studies are available regarding a potential combination with α-glucosidase inhibitors or insulin treatment.

Measures to Assure Metabolic Control (Self-Blood-Glucose Monitoring)

Although exenatide was approved by the FDA and introduced for use in the USA in 2005 (and other countries since) and sitagliptin has been approved in the USA and elsewhere in late 2006, no recommendations regarding metabolic control have been issued. The following suggestions, therefore, are based on the known properties of incretin mimetics and DPP-4 inhibitors.

Incretin mimetics

Since incretin mimetics will be used at fairly standardized doses (vide supra), and not based on individual titration (like in the case of insulin), and since incretin mimetics alone do not provoke hypoglycemic episodes, there will be a rather limited need for blood-glucose self-control in addition to regular determinations of HbA_{1c}. The frequency of glucose control will primarily depend on other antidiabetic agents used in combination and their potential to elicit hypoglycemia. Certainly, in comparison with any insulin regimen, the requirement for blood glucose-self control will be much smaller. This could affect the acceptability of such treatment regimens to patients and on the overall cost–benefit relationship.

DPP-4 inhibitors

DPP-4 inhibitors, in their most likely use, in combination with metformin, do not require additional measures of blood-glucose self-control, since they are administered at a standard dosage and do not provoke hypoglycemia. Thus, only occasional profiles to assess glycemic control are adequate.

Discontinuation of Treatment

With randomized clinical trials concerning incretin mimetics and DPP-4 inhibitors lasting up to 1 year, and open-label follow-up reported up to 2 years, it is obvious that these studies cannot provide an estimate of how long treatment with incretin mimetics and DPP-4 inhibitors can meaningfully control glycemia. It is, however, obvious that not all patients treated with such agents achieve their glycemic target, even within the time frame of the studies that have been reported. Therefore, preliminary thoughts on when incretin mimetics or DPP-4 inhibitors should be discontinued, and what the treatment alternatives would be, seem adequate, even in the absence of studies that would provide any firm guidance.

Incretin mimetics

Treatment with exenatide results in fairly stable fasting glucose and HbA_{1c} concentrations after approximately 3 months. If by then HbA_{1c} targets (e.g., $<7.0\%$) have not been met, intensification of treatment has to be considered. Since weight loss associated with the use of exenatide progresses at least up to a duration of 2 years, a secondary improvement of glycemic control appears possible with further weight reduction, although this is not clearly confirmed by serial HbA_{1c} measurements. Certainly, once weight becomes stable and HbA1c remains outside the target range, antidiabetic therapy needs to be intensified.

Adding more or other oral antidiabetic agents at this stage of type 2 diabetes does not seem to be helpful in achieving adequate glycemic control. Rather, insulin-based treatment regimens will most likely be needed. Since there is no reported experience with a combination of exenatide and insulin, this cannot be recommended. Established treatment regimens ranging from a combination of once-daily basal insulin and oral agents, twice-daily premixed insulin, or intensified regimens with multiple daily insulin injections should be initiated instead.

DPP-4 inhibitors

When a DPP-4 inhibitor added to metformin no longer adequately controls glycemia, the options for intensifying therapy include the start of basal insulin or an incretin mimetic. It is not known what continued treatment with DPP-4 inhibitors would add to a combination of metformin (continued) and basal insulin (newly initiated). In addition, there has been no published experience with a combination of a DPP-4 inhibitor and an incretin mimetic. Such studies are needed to justify a continuation of DPP-4 inhibitor treatment under these circumstances. Since there have been no head-to-head comparisons of the anti-hyperglycemic efficacy between DPP-4 inhibitors and incretin mimetics, one can only speculate whether switching from a DPP-4 to an incretin mimetic would improve glycemic control. Based on comparisons of the effects on fasting glucose and HbA_{1c} concentrations, one might assume that longer-acting incretin mimetics (exenatide LAR, liraglutide) would probably provide a better glycemic control than a DPP-4 inhibitor.

Side Effects of Treatment

Side Effects of Incretin Mimetics

Side effects of exenatide

As is typical for the administration of native GLP-1, a considerable proportion of patients receiving exenatide experience gastrointestinal side effects, such as nausea and more rarely vomiting or diarrhea. In the phase 3 trials with exenatide, the frequence of these adverse effects was reported to be as high as 48% during treatment with 10 μg of exenatide. However, it should be noted that, though frequent, these side effects were mostly mild to moderate in intensity and usually transient. Overall, the percentage of patients who discontinued exenatide treatment as a result of side effects was low. When considering all patients enrolled in the exenatide phase 3 trials, there also seemed to be an increase in the frequency of hypoglycemic events, but this was limited to the patients receiving additional treatment with sulfonylurea drugs. In contrast, the incidence of hypoglycemia was unchanged in patients treated with metformin.

Antibody formation has been reported in ~40–50% of patients receiving Exenatide treatment. However, these antibodies seemed to exhibit a weak binding affinity and have not been associated with severely impaired antidiabetic effectiveness of exenatide in the majority of treated subjects.

Side effects of liraglutide

In the published phase 2 trials with liraglutide, nausea, vomiting, and diarrhea were the most frequent adverse events reported, with the incidence of events being dose-related. Only a small proportion of patients (<5%) discontinued treatment due to these side effects. The frequency of hypoglycemia was not increased during liraglutide treatment. Side reactions of urticarial injection were reported in 1 out of 135 patients exposed to liraglutide in one trial and did not occur in the other published studies. No antibody formation has been reported after exposure to liraglutide.

Side Effects of DPP-4 Inhibitors (Sitagliptin and Vildagliptin)

A number of theoretical concerns have been expressed regarding potential adverse effects of DPP-4 inhibitors. In particular, the large number of physiological substrates of DPP-4 gave rise to speculations that inhibiting the action of this protease might interfere with numerous other hormonal axes, thereby potentially causing adverse reactions. Furthermore, since DPP-4 is also expressed on T-lymphocytes as CD26, it was speculated that chronic DPP-4 inhibition might alter immune functions. Against these theoretical considerations, the DPP-4 inhibitors have so far proven to be safe and well tolerated in clinical studies, and no characteristic pattern of adverse events has been observed. Thus, in patients with diabetes pretreated with metformin, the incidence of adverse effects during 12 weeks of treatment with sitagliptin was similar to the placebo group. Likewise, the frequency of side effects was not different from the placebo group in diabetic patients previously treated with a dietary regimen. With sitagliptin, the frequency of gastrointestinal side effects was slightly higher compared with placebo in one, but not all studies. Overall, the gastrointestinal side effects typically reported during the treatment with GLP-1 analogues do not represent a problem during DPP-4 inhibitor administration. Nevertheless, further long-term studies will be required to confirm the absence of a potential to cause clinically important adverse reactions before these drugs can unequivocally be accepted as safe, especially with regard to their potential effects on other hormonal axes and immune functions.

Key Issues in the Treatment Strategy

Based on presently available study results, the clinical benefit of using incretin mimetics is determined by their ability to control glycemia (i.e., lower HbA_{1c}), their inability to cause hypoglycemia unless combined with other antidiabetic agents that have the potential to initiate hypoglycemia, their weight effects (promotion of weight loss in the case of incretin mimetics, weight neutrality in the case of DPP-4 inhibitors), and their safety and tolerability, especially the absence of a potential to cause specific severe adverse events.

The novel classes of antidiabetic agents, incretin mimetics and DPP-4 inhibitors, may hold two additional promises: A reduction in cardiovascular complications typically associated with type 2 diabetes and the metabolic syndrome, and a positive influence on the natural history of type 2 diabetes, which with current treatment options is characterized by a steady loss of β-cell function, which in turn determines a rather short "*durability*" of successful glycemic control with any choice of antidiabetic agents.

Possible Effects of Incretin Mimetics and DPP-4 Inhibitors on β-Cell Mass

Both type 1 and type 2 diabetes are caused by a significant deficit in β-cell mass, caused by increased β-cell apoptosis. Strategies to inhibit β-cell apoptosis and/or increase the rate of β-cell replication may therefore allow for the prevention or even reversal of diabetes. A number of studies have suggested that GLP-1 might exhibit such properties. Thus, in β-cell lines (INS-1 cells), GLP-1 increased the rate of proliferation through induction of phosphatidylinositol 3-kinase, protein kinase C zeta, and activation of PDX1 gene expression. In rodent models of diabetes, GLP-1 led to an increase in β-cell replication, a stimulation of islet neogenesis, and an inhibition of β-cell apoptosis. An inhibition of β-cell apoptosis by GLP-1 was also noted in isolated human islets. These actions therefore raised hopes that GLP-1 analogues and DPP-4 inhibitors might halt or even reverse the progression of diabetes.

With exenatide, an increase in β-cell replication and neogenesis resulting in increased β-cell mass has been reported after partial pancreatectomy in rats, and a diminished recovery of β-cell mass after partial pancreatectomy was shown in GLP-1 receptor knock-out mice. Likewise, exendin-4 stimulated β-cell neogenesis in streptozotocin-induced diabetic rats as well as in Goto–Kakizaki diabetic rats. The effects of liraglutide on β-cell mass and turnover were studied as well. In db/db mice, liraglutide treatment significantly increased β-cell mass and proliferation resulting in improved diabetes control. In addition, liraglutide inhibited both cytokine- and free fatty acid-induced apoptosis in isolated rat islets.

Not only GLP-1 and its analogues, but also the DPP-4 inhibitors have been shown to exert beneficial effects on β-cell mass and turnover. Along these lines, Pospisilik and colleagues reported a significant increase in β-cell mass in strepozotocin-induced diabetic rats following 7 weeks of treatment with the DPP-4 inhibitor P32/98, and recently a significant increase in β-cell mass was reported after treatment with des-fluoro-sitagliptin in high-fat diet (HFD)/streptozotocin (STZ)-induced diabetic mice.

Taken together, these studies suggest that both incretin mimetics and DPP-4 inhibitors might indeed have a potential to induce β-cell regeneration in patients with diabetes during long-term treatment. It is, however, difficult to draw firm conclusions from these studies in rodents or in vitro for the situation in humans. In fact, the rates of β-cell turnover seem to be much lower in humans than in rodents, and the overall capacity for islet regeneration in humans appears to be limited. Furthermore, it is yet impossible to directly measure changes in β-cell mass or turnover, since the human pancreas are inaccessible for repeated biopsy sampling, and since the functional assessment of insulin secretion might only partly relate to the actual β-cell mass. Therefore, while current evidence strongly suggest that the GLP-1 analogues and DPP-4 inhibitors will indeed induce β-cell regeneration in patients with diabetes, this question will ultimately have to be answered in further long-term trials.

The recommendation of an extended and perhaps earlier use of incretin mimetics, for example, starting an injection therapy instead of using oral antidiabetic agents although oral agents would provide adequate glycemic control, would require the demonstration of unique benefits. In principle, the demonstration that exenatide and liraglutide, like GLP-1, can inhibit β-cell apoptosis and increase β-cell mass in isolated pancreatic islets and rodents, would provide a rationale to counteract the progressive loss of β-cell function (and presumably, β-cell mass) typical of type 2 diabetes. However, although some experiments with human islets or islet cell precursors have reported similar findings, only preliminary hints have been gained from clinical studies examining the long-term effect of incretin mimetics on parameters of "β-cell health."

Whether the reported decreases in the proportion of proinsulin (relative to insulin) can be used as makers of improvements in "functional β-cell mass," and whether these changes reflect specific actions of the treatment with incretin mimetics or mainly the removal of glucolipotoxicity as a consequence of improved metabolic control, remain to be demonstrated in long-term studies. Islet and β-cell turnover appear to be much slower in human subjects than in rodents. Certainly, the demonstration of profound improvements in β-cell mass and function, possibly associated with a longer durability of anti-hyperglycemic effects of incretin mimetics relative to other antidiabetic agents, would suggest their use at earlier stages of type 2 diabetes, perhaps even including prediabetes.

A similar reasoning seem to apply to DPP-4 inhibitors: In selected animal models, effects of using sitagliptin or vildagliptin on the rate of β-cell apoptosis and β-cell mass have been demonstrated. In one clinical study an improvement in meal-related β-cell function after a year of treatment has been reported. If substantial benefits in terms of "β-cell health" could be demonstrated, this could broaden the indications for the use of DPP-4 inhibitors.

Cardiac Effects of GLP-1: Consequences of the Treatment with Incretin Mimetics and DPP-4 Inhibitors

The GLP-1 receptor is expressed in the heart. In GLP-1 receptor knock-out mice structural and functional cardiac abnormalities are typical. In animals, exposure to GLP-1 reduces the size of myocardial necroses in the case of induced infarction. In a pilot study with patients treated for acute myocardial infarction, a 48-h infusion of GLP-1 improved left-ventricular function and a wall-motility index. In a dog model of dilated cardiomyopathy, GLP-1 increased glucose uptake and left-ventricular function. These findings, together with the cardiovascular benefit expected from significant weight loss, make it appear possible, that incretin mimetics and/or DPP-4 inhibitors may be agents with the potential to reduce the incidence of cardiovascular events in patients with type 2 diabetes, thus targeting one of the main clinical problems of this metabolic disease. Such potential benefits should be studied in randomized controlled trials of appropriate size and duration.

With incretin mimetics and DPP-4 inhibitors, two novel classes of antidiabetic agents have been developed and are in the course of being approved for the treatment of patients with type 2 diabetes, which will certainly broaden the armamentarium of anti-hyperglycemic therapy. This is valid based on their properties that have already been characterized in clinical trials. Some additional properties need to be explored in future studies, but hold the promise to make a substantial contribution to changing the course of type 2 diabetes, from the prevention of the transition between the prediabetic state to manifest diabetes, to improved and more durable metabolic control with less unwanted side effects and the prevention of diabetic complications.

GLP-1 is an intestinal incretin hormone that stimulates insulin ("incretin") and suppresses glucagon secretion, inhibits gastric emptying, and reduces appetite and food intake. In contrast to the other incretin hormone, GIP, GLP-1 remains active in patients with type 2 diabetes. GLP-1 itself, however, cannot be used for therapeutic purposes because of its rapid proteolytic degradation and inactivation (DPP-4) and renal elimination, leading to a $t_{1/2}$ of 1–2 min. Therapeutic use of the antidiabetic properties of incretins, especially GLP-1, can be made using degradation-resistant GLP-1 receptor agonists ("*incretin mimetics*"), or inhibitors of DPP-4 activity ("*incretin enhancers*").

Clinical studies with exenatide (two injections per day or long-acting release form administered once-weekly) and liraglutide (one injection per day) have proven the antidiabetic efficacy with reductions in fasting and postprandial glucose concentrations and HbA_{1c} (~1–2%), associated with weight loss (2–5 kg). Treatment with incretin mimetics is associated with mild nausea, which occurs early, mostly transiently, after initiation. Orally administered DPP-4 inhibitors (e.g., sitagliptin, vildagliptin) reduce HbA_{1c} by approximately 0.6–1.0%. DPP-4 inhibitors are weight-neutral. There are no specific safety of tolerability concerns emerging from clinical trials. Both incretin mimetics and DPP-4 inhibitors have the potential to increase β-cell mass as shown in animal studies. However, long-term clinical studies are required to ascertain specific benefits of using novel antidiabetic agents derived from the enteroinsular axis, in particular incretin hormones like GLP- 1, in the treatment of type 2 diabetes.

14

PHARMACOGENETICS

The use of drugs to treat cardiac arrhythmias is characterized by highly variable efficacy and serious toxicity. Both of these are difficult to predict in an individual patient. Studies of the mechanisms underlying this variability and unpredictability in drug action have been important platforms for defining the role of genetics in drug action and have also pointed to general mechanisms in the initiation and maintenance of abnormal cardiac rhythms. In practical terms, the past decade has seen a decline in the use of antiarrhythmic drugs, in part because of their unpredictable efficacy and toxicity. As well, "*non-pharmacologic*" techniques, including ablation of abnormal tissues underlying arrhythmias and implantable defibrillators, have matured and are increasingly used.

A common feature of most antiarrhythmic drugs is that they were developed without a clear understanding of the cellular and molecular mechanisms underlying cardiac arrhythmias. As a result, the molecular targets with which they interact to suppress (or occasionally exacerbate) arrhythmias and cause other forms of toxicity are only now being defined. Virtually all antiarrhythmic drugs target membrane proteins, including adrenergic receptors and ion channels, structures that generate ion-specific permeation pathways (pores) in response to changes in their environment; common examples of such changes include alterations in transmembrane voltage (generated by other ion channels) or the presence of ligands such as acetylcholine. Studies defining the genetics of variable antiarrhythmic drug responses have not only pointed to new disease mechanisms, but also to strategies for development of new drugs lacking serious adverse effects and targeting underlying disease processes that culminate in arrhythmias. This review will first summarize the impact of variants in genes determining drug disposition on the effects of therapies used in the treatment of arrhythmias. The role of genetics in determining variable pharmacodynamics will then be considered.

GENETICS OF ANTIARRHYTHMIC DRUG DISPOSITION

CYP3A

Therapeutic drug monitoring was developed to optimize treatment with drugs that have a narrow margin between dosage required to produce efficacy and those producing adverse effects. Examples of such drug classes to which this approach has been applied include antibiotics, anticonvulsants, and antiarrhythmics. Initial descriptions of variable drug disposition as a consequence of disease or of drug interactions generally did not include a clear understanding of the specific molecular mechanisms underlying such variability. Thus, for example, anticonvulsants were recognized 30 years ago to strikingly lower concentrations of quinidine and to reduce its therapeutic efficacy. In contemporary terms, this interaction reflects induction of CYP3A4 by anticonvulsant drugs, likely acting through orphan nuclear hormone receptors. While functionally important polymorphisms in the coding region of CPY3A4 have not been identified, there are such variants in CYP3A5, a closely related enzyme with overlapping substrate specificity and a prominent role in drug disposition in intestine. Given this view, variability in CYP3A expression becomes a logical candidate mechanism for modulating antiarrhythmic drug concentrations and hence effects; such variability could arise from polymorphisms in the promoter region of the CYP3A complex or in the genes encoding nuclear hormone receptors that mediate enzyme and transporter expression. Specific studies addressing these possibilities have not, however, been conducted.

CYP2D6

CYP2D6 is responsible for the biotransformation of a number of drugs used to control cardiac arrhythmias, notably some beta-adrenergic receptor antagonists (metoprolol, timolol, and carvedilol) as well as the sodium channel blocking antiarrhythmics encainide (no longer marketed), propafenone, and flecainide. The CYP2D6 poor metabolizers (PMs) making up 7% of Caucasian and African-American populations (and rare in Asian populations) display higher plasma concentrations and greater pharmacologic effects during treatment with CYP2D6 substrate beta-blockers. The molecular basis of variable CYP2D6 activity is discussed in detail elsewhere in this volume. The "*third-generation*" beta-blocker carvedilol is increasingly used in the treatment of heart failure and may be especially effective because of some vasodilator activity, possibly attributable to alpha-blockade. The extent of alpha- and beta-blockade by this drug does appear to be at least in part CYP2D6-mediated, although clinical trial data demonstrating that variable outcomes during carvedilol therapy in heart failure can be related to this polymorphism have not yet been developed.

Propafenone is another example of a drug that exerts multiple actions, and displays genetically determined variability in its clinical effects. In vitro, propafenone not only blocks sodium channels but also exerts beta- blocking activity. Initial reports of clinically significant adverse effects (such as bradycardia or bronchospasm) due to beta-blockade during propafenone therapy emphasized the unpredictable nature of this adverse effect. However, when CYP2D6 phenotype is considered, it becomes clear that PM subjects are at greater risk than extensive metabolizers (EMs) for clinically significant beta-blockade during treatment with the drug since they develop much higher concentrations of the parent drug than do EMs. It is also possible that consistent incorporation of beta-blockade into an antiarrhythmic molecule might improve its efficacy. Indeed, combining propafenone with low-dose quinidine (a CYP2D6 inhibitor) can result in phenocopying to the PM phenotype, and small trials have been undertaken to test the antiarrhythmic effects of the combination.

The antiarrhythmic drug encainide is biotransformed by CYP2D6 to a potent active metabolite, O-desmethyl encainide. Interestingly, this active metabolite, in turn, also undergoes CYP2D6-mediated biotransformation to a second active metabolite, 3-methoxy O-desmethyl encainide. Thus, variable CYP2D6 activity is a likely contributor to variable levels of the parent drug and its two active metabolites, and this may underlie some of the variability observed when the drug was used clinically. Flecainide, a compound with similar electrophysiologic properties, is bio-transformed to inactive metabolites by CYP2D6 and also undergoes renal excretion of parent drug. Thus, CYP2D6 phenotype has much less impact on flecainide plasma concentrations and effect, except in the rare patient with coexisting renal dysfunction.

CYP2C9

The anticoagulant warfarin is increasingly used to prevent thromboembolic complications in patients with atrial fibrillation. The drug is administered as racemate, and bio-inactivation of the active S-enantiomer is accomplished by CYP2C9. Relatively common variants in CYP2C9 that reduce its function have been described, and homozygotes for reduction of function alleles appear to be at increased risk for bleeding complications with the drug.

N-Acetyltransferase

Plasma concentration monitoring of procainamide and its metabolite, N-acetylprocainamide (NAPA), led to the recognition that acetylator status is the major determinant of the development of anti-nuclear antibodies and the drug-induced lupus syndrome during procainamide therapy. This finding, in turn, pointed to the metabolism of procainamide by non-acetyl transferase pathways as an important modulator of this form of drug toxicity and also formed the rational for considering NAPA as a potentially less toxic antiarrhythmic entity. NAPA was found to exert electrophysiologic activity in vitro and to suppress some arrhythmias in patients; importantly, the clinical studies also showed that NAPA was not back-converted to procainamide and did not cause antinuclear antibodies. However, NAPA was not an especially potent antiarrhythmic, and it commonly caused non-cardiovascular adverse effects such as nausea. Interestingly, while both procainamide and NAPA prolong cardiac repolarization (manifest on the surface ECG as QT, interval prolongation, thought at the time to correlate with antiarrhythmic activity), only the parent drug blocked cardiac sodium channels. Thus, the NAPA structure did provide a starting point for the development of a series of new and highly potent QT-prolonging anti- arrhythmic drugs that saw some enthusiasm for their use in the 1980s and 1990s.

Importantly, these clinical studies were executed at a time when the molecular basis of the slow and fast acetylator phenotypes were not well understood. We now know that there are two isoforms of the *N*-acetyltransferase enzyme arising from two different genes, NAT1 and NAT2. Constitutive expression of NAT1 accounts for basal enzyme function, and functionally important polymorphisms in NAT2, are thought to contribute to variability in overall enzymatic activity and thus to define the slow- and fast-acetylators phenotypes.

P-Glycoprotein

Digoxin is the prototypical substrate for transport by P-glycoprotein, the product of expression of the MDR1 gene. Elevation of serum digoxin concentration and increased risk of serious toxicity result from co-administration of drugs that inhibit P-glycoprotein; these include quinidine, amiodarone, verapamil, itraconazole, erythromycin, and cyclosporine. MDR1 DNA polymorphisms that are linked to variability in serum digoxin concentrations have been described, although whether the polymorphisms are causative or in linkage disequilibrium to regulatory sites in the gene is not yet fully established.

Antiarrhythmic Drug Pharmacodynamics

Even at equivalent plasma concentrations of parent drug (and relevant active metabolites) the effect of antiarrhythmic therapies still vary considerably among individuals. There are a number of mechanisms that may underlie such variability. One is variable uptake or efflux transporter function, responsible for delivery to and removal from key intercellular sites of action. Drug effects may be different in normal vs. diseased (e.g., scarred or hypertrophied) hearts. Finally, a substantial body of knowledge has been accumulating over the past decade attesting to a prominent role of genetic factors in modulating normal and abnormal cardiac electrophysiology and, in turn, their responses to drug exposure.

An extraordinarily important starting point for this work has been identification of specific genes whose expression results in key proteins determining cardiac electrogenesis. Ion channels, pore-forming structures that respond to ligands or changes in voltage to permit transmembrane movement of specific ions, are the most important class of these proteins. One very important approach to identifying ion channel and related genes has been the study of rare monogenic (familial) arrhythmia syndromes.

Most currently available antiarrhythmic drugs were developed at a time when molecular mechanisms underlying arrhythmias were not appreciated. As a consequence, these drugs interact with a very limited number of molecular targets: the cardiac sodium channel, beta-1 adrenergic receptors, L-type calcium channels, and one specific potassium current (termed I_{Kr}). The genes whose expression results in these currents or receptors are now well understood. Many other genes have been identified whose expression generates or modulates ion currents in heart or otherwise prominently modulates overall cardiac electrical behavior. Indeed, this work has generated a lengthy list of potential "new" antiarrhythmic drug targets: these include potassium currents (I_{Ks} and I_{Kur}), pacemaker current (I_f), novel calcium currents (I_{Ca-T}; the A1D isoform of I_{Ca-L}), and cardiac connexins C×43.

Study of the rare congenital arrhythmia syndromes has been important for ion channel biologists because it identifies genes whose expression plays a crucial role in normal cardiac electrophysiology. It has also been interesting to demonstrate that mutations in these genes may result not only in manifest congenital arrhythmia syndromes, but also subclinical phenotypes that can then be uncovered by drug administration. These are discussed next, followed by a consideration of how more common DNA polymorphisms, in these and other genes, might modulate drug responses.

Pharmacogenetics of QT Prolongation

One important implication of this increasingly complex view of the molecular basis of cardiac electrophysiology is that variations in many genes may modulate not only basal cardiac electrophysiology but also its response to drugs. One interesting and important example relates to the occasional development of marked prolongation of the QT interval on the surface electrocardiogram, a finding that is associated with a high risk of morphologically distinctive, potentially fatal, polymorphic ventricular tachycardia termed "*torsades de pointes.*" Torsades de pointes characteristically occurs in one of two clinical settings: in patients with a familial arrhythmia syndrome (the congenital Long QT Syndrome) and in patients exposed to drugs that have the potential to prolong the QT interval. The latter includes not only antiarrhythmic drugs, but a wide range of "*non-cardiovascular*" agents. Indeed, unexpected QT prolongation, torsades de pointes, and sudden death with the use of such drugs has been the single commonest reason for drug withdrawal in the United States over the past decade. Hence, evolving concepts with respect to the underlying molecular mechanisms of this distinctive arrhythmia syndrome have implications not only for management of patients with a relatively uncommon familial syndrome, but also have important implications for drug development in general.

The QT interval on the surface electrocardiogram represents the integrated behavior of a number of important ion currents active during the repolarization phase of a typical cardiac action potential. These include L-type calcium currents, a small contribution by sodium current, and several repolarizing potassium currents, notably the rapid component of the delayed rectifier (I_{Kr}), the slow component of the delayed rectifier (I_{Ks}), and the inward rectifier (I_{K1}). Studies of the congenital Long QT Syndrome in the mid-1990s identified mutations in the genes whose expression underlies I_{Kr}, I_{Ks}, and the cardiac sodium channel as the commonest causes of the syndrome. Importantly, cloning of the gene whose expression results in I_{Kr}, the Human Ether-a-go-go-Related Gene, or HERG (now known as KCNH2), was followed shortly thereafter by the recognition that virtually all drugs that prolong the QT interval do so by interacting with this particular ion channel protein. This work, then, provides an important link between a drug-induced syndrome and the congenital syndrome.

Another key observation made in the course of studying patients with the congenital syndrome was the identification of family members of pro-bands in whom mutations could be identified but the QT interval appeared normal. This "*incomplete penetrance*" then raises the question of whether some or all of patients developing "*idiosyncratic*" drug-induced QT prolongation and torsades de pointes represent individuals with a subclinical form of the congenital syndrome. Addressing this issue is not straight-forward, in part because several hundred mutations, in seven different genes, have now been identified in kindreds with this disease. Thus, unlike other common genetic diseases like cystic fibrosis or sickle cell anemia, there is a not a single predominant disease-associated mutation. As a result, any DNA variant identified in a patient with drug-associated torsades de pointes may be a disease-associated mutation, a predisposing polymorphism, or an irrelevant polymorphism, and distinguishing among these may be difficult. Nevertheless, case reports and one systematic survey of approximately 100 individuals with drug-induced torsades de pointes do support the concept of a genetic predisposition increasing susceptibility to this arrhythmia syndrome in approximately 10% of subjects. Some of these individuals do, indeed, have variants that alter channel function in vitro and that are absent in large numbers of ethnically matched controls; such patients can therefore be viewed as having the congenital syndrome, clinically inapparent in absence of drug challenge. In fact, in some instances, other family members may have manifest QT-interval prolongation in the absence of drugs, further confirming the diagnosis of the congenital syndrome. DNA polymorphisms may also predispose to drug-induced torsades de pointes, as discussed further below.

Clinical studies have identified a multitude of risk factors for drug-induced torsades de pointes, including female gender, congestive heart failure, left ventricular hypertrophy, hypokalemia, bradycardia, and subclinical ion channel dysfunction. A unifying framework to account for how these multiple factors may modulate risk is that of "*repolarization reserve*," which suggests that the normal expression and function of multiple gene products—with potentially redundant function—ordinarily acts to maintain a QT interval within the normal range. Subtle dysfunction of such gene products may be clinically inapparent and only be exposed by administration of a QT-prolonging drug. Thus, an individual harboring a subclinical loss of function mutation or polymorphism in the gene encoding I_{Ks} may not display any clinical phenotype at baseline, because of a robust I_{Kr}. Administration of an I_{Kr} blocker to such an individual might leave them with very little repolarizing current and hence would cause marked QT-interval prolongation. The concept of "*reduced repolarization reserve*," developed to provide a unified approach to thinking about torsades de pointes risk, can be readily adapted to many other biological systems; in general, highly variable clinical responses to drug challenge may reflect subtle dysfunction of genes whose products modulate a highly complex phenotype like the QT interval.

Altered Sodium Channel Function

Mutations that result in a "*gain of function*" in the cardiac sodium channel gene (SCN5A) cause the long QT Syndrome. By contrast, mutations in the same gene may result in loss of function and a different congenital syndrome, the "*Brugada syndrome*". Individuals with Brugada Syndrome have structurally normal hearts, a high risk of ventricular fibrillation, and a morphologically distinctive electrocardiogram. As in the Long QT Syndrome, mutation carriers who have a normal baseline electrocardiogram have been identified. In such cases, exposure to a sodium channel-blocking drug (e.g., flecainide or procainamide) is often used to unmask the Brugada Syndrome ECG phenotype. Indeed it was the observation that sodium channel block may unmask the ECG phenotype that led to consideration of SCN5A as a candidate in the Brugada Syndrome; in ~20% of pro-bands, mutations can be found in this gene. Occasional patients treated clinically with sodium channel-blocking drugs such as drugs such as flecainide, procainamide, or tricyclic depressants do develop the typical Brugada Syndrome ECG pattern; whether such individuals actually harbor subclinical Brugada Syndrome or are otherwise predisposed to sudden death during administration of these agents is a logical possibility.

From Rare Syndromes to Common Polymorphisms

Cases of subclinical congenital arrhythmia syndromes exposed by drug challenge are quite rare, but nevertheless constitute an important "*proof of concept*" of a genetic basis for variable drug responses. On the other hand, intensive study of monogenic arrhythmia syndrome disease genes, as well as other genes whose expression contributes to normal electrophysiology, has identified polymorphisms, some quite common, that may also modulate arrhythmia susceptibility. Population and association studies have identified such polymorphisms, with minor allele frequencies of 1.5–13% in control populations that appear to be over-represented among patients with drug-induced torsades de pointes. In such cases, in vitro studies have provided further support for the idea that the variant allele predisposes to the arrhythmia, especially in the presence of environmental triggers. The best-studied trigger for such arrhythmia susceptibility remains drug challenge, although other environmental stimuli, such as adrenergic activation or acute myocardial ischemia, could well play a role in other patients.

S1102Y in SCN5A is present in 13% of African Americans, but is absent or extremely rare in other ethnic groups. In vitro electrophysiologic studies showed that this variant does alter channel function, and clinical association studies suggest an overrepresentation of the Y allele in African-American subjects with a variety of arrhzythmia syndromes, including drug-induced arrhythmias, compared to African-American controls. Similarly, Q9E was initially identified as a mutation in KCNE2 (encoding a function-modulating potassium channel subunit). The proband was an elderly African-American woman who displayed torsades de pointes on exposure to an I_{Kr}-blocking antibiotic (clarithromycin), and further study revealed that Q9E does, in fact, alter I_{Kr} function in vitro. More recently, Q9E has been recognized as a relatively common polymorphism (5% minor allele frequency), again detected only in African-Americans. Other polymorphisms have been described that appear to modulate normal cardiac electrophysiology, although none have yet been linked convincingly to increased susceptibility to drug-induced arrhythmias. Thus, for example, K897T in HERG has been associated with longer QT intervals, particularly among women. H558R in SCN5A does not appear to alter baseline sodium channel function, but does modulate the clinical and in vitro phenotype of a disease-associated mutation in the same channel. A promoter polymorphism in the gene encoding the connexin C×40, whose normal function underlies cell–cell communication especially in atrium, appears to reduce gene expression. This polymorphism thus becomes a logical candidate gene for modulating the development of the very common arrhythmia atrial fibrillation and thus its response to drugs. Polymorphisms in the promoter region of cardiac sodium channel have been described that modulate expression of the channel in vitro; whether such polymorphisms underlie variable expression of the channel in patients and thus variable responses to challenges such as sodium channel-blocking drugs or acute myocardial ischemia is not yet known. Finally, recent clinical and mechanistic studies implicate activation of a number of key signaling pathways, such as the beta-adrenergic system, the renin-angiotensin-aldosterone system, oxidant stress, or inflammation, as potential arrhythmia triggers. Variants in these pathways then become new candidates for modulating arrhythmia susceptibility.

Currently available arrhythmic drugs were developed at a time when the molecular basis of cardiac arrhythmias was not understood. Thus, therapy has been largely empiric, efficacy has been unpredictable, and serious side effects have been common. Some of variability in clinical action of antiarrhythmic drugs can be attributed directly to variable drug disposition, through specific pathways whose activity is now well recognized to be modulated by common DNA polymorphisms. An in-depth understanding of the molecular basis or normal cardiac electrophysiology has come from a number of approaches, notably including the intensive study of families with rare monogenic arrhythmia syndromes. Variations in the complex physiologic signaling system that results in normal electrical activity now appears to be a proximate cause of most cardiac arrhythmias. DNA variants in genes encoding elements of this system may result in disease, or may more commonly modulate arrhythmia risk in the face of exogenous stressors, including drugs, in the susceptible patient. Further definition of these molecular mechanisms and the polymorphisms that underlie such susceptibility should lead to the development of drug therapies targeting underlying pathophysiologic mechanisms, and lacking common and serious adverse effects. As in many areas of pharmacogenetics, real advances require a partnership between clinical and basic investigators to precisely identify variable and important clinical phenotypes and then define mechanisms underlying that variability.

15

NEW ANTICANCER AGENTS

Development of new anticancer and cancer prevention agents presents significant challenges to clinical trialists. The correct design of all phases of clinical trials is essential to ensure as rapid and as successful a development as possible. One must have a plan that will give the new agent the best chance of matching its preclinical activity. Because there have been problems with this in the past, it is virtually certain that many promising new agents were dismissed as being inactive because of flaws in clinical trial design. This chapter provides information on multiple types of clinical trial designs that can and have been used for approval of new anticancer (and prevention) agents.

METHODS TO SELECT AGENTS THAT WILL BE ACTIVE IN THE CLINIC

Of course, if people knew for certain how to select agents that would definitely work in the clinic it is likely we would be much further along in our treatment of patients with cancer. However, there are some techniques that have been reported in the literature and that our drug development teams in San Antonio and in Tucson have used to increase the chances of bringing agents into clinical trials that will eventually be approved for clinical use. In the period of 1978–1983 our team just took the "next agent to come along" into the Phase I clinical trials. Unfortunately, only 3 of the 26 agents (12%) we took into Phase I trials during that time period were subsequently approved by the Food and Drug Administration (FDA). Clearly, we needed to do better than that.

In 1983, a significant publication by Staquet and colleagues reviewed the success of the various murine or human tumor cell lines that were being utilized as in vivo systems by the National Cancer Institute to evaluate all of the potential antineoplastic agents. In that study they noted that murine leukemias L1210 and P388, the murine B 16 melanoma, and the MX-1 mammary human tumor xenograft were the most predictive for antitumor activity in the clinic. These models were even more predictive if one used tumor regression or percent cure (≥ 45-d survivors) as an endpoint.

Models that were not predictive included the murine colon cancers Co26 and Co38, the CX-1 and LX-1, human tumor xenografts, and the Lewis lung model. When we utilized the Staquet suggested models to select agents for Phase I trials, the success rate for our program (as judged by the percent of new agents that were eventually approved by the FDA divided by all of the agents that we took into Phase I trials during that period) increased to 31%. In 1990 our team had the clinical impression that every time we took a new agent with a new mechanism of action into a Phase I clinical trial (e.g., tubulin inhibitors, such as docetaxel or paclitaxel, topoismerase I inhibitors such as topotecan or CPT11, or a chain terminator such as gemcitabine) it was very likely that the drug would eventually be approved. Using the additional parameter of a new mechanism of action, the success rate again appeared to improve.

The introduction of targeted monoclonal antibodies (MAbs) has also appeared to increase success rates. As is noted, by using the Staquet criteria plus the new mechanisms of action criteria, plus MAbs, it is estimated that nearly 67% of all new agents brought into Phase I trials will eventually demonstrate antitumor activity significant enough for approval by the FDA (provided that the appropriate pivotal trials are designed for the agent).

The point of MAbs is worth emphasizing. If one has a MAb specific to a particular cell surface antigen or receptor, it appears to be an excellent prognostic factor for activity and for approval. In summary, with some rather simplistic approaches, we believe some of the risk of development of new anticancer agents can be taken out of the process. In fact the likelihood of success can be very high.

Table 15.1. Example of new mechanism of action against specific targets: monoclonal antibodies against specific targets

Target	*Monoclonal antibody(s)*	*Clinical activity*
CD20	Rituximab (Rituxan)	Lymphoma
Her2/*neu*	Trastuzumab (Herceptin)	Breast, others
CD52	Alemtuzumab (CAMPATH)	CLL
CD20	Radiolabeled ibritumomab (Tiuxetan, Zevalin)	Lymphoma
EGFR	IMC-255; ABX-EGF	Colorectal
17-1A	Edrecolomab (Panorex)	Colorectal cancer
VEGF	Bevacizumab (Avastin)	Colorectal cancer renal cell, lung
Other	Many other	Other

General Aspects of Clinical Trial Design for Approval

It was stated above that agents with new mechanisms of action had a high probability of success—if the pivotal trials with the agent were designed correctly. To achieve that high probability of success some important aspects of clinical trial design include:

1. Try to select a clinical situation that closely mimics what was found in the preclinical data package. For example, if the new agent demonstrated only growth delays in an animal system, one should probably not design pivotal trials with response rate (e.g., tumor shrinkage) as a primary endpoint. Rather, one should utilize median survival or time to tumor progression (TTP) or time to treatment failure (TTF) as primary endpoints. The TTP or TTF endpoints are usually acceptable to regulatory agencies only if the trial is double-blinded. This is because clinicians caring for patients, and patients themselves, are most anxious to get off of a control arm and on to the new agent arm. This frequently will lead to a declaration that the control arm is not working so the patient can be crossed over to the new agent arm of the study. Thus, double-blinding is very helpful if it is at all possible. Another, more cumbersome method is to use an outside, independent, blinded review panel to assess tumor progression.
2. Make sure the sample size is large enough to give the new agent a real chance. For example, a sample size that allows one to detect only a 50% improvement in survival is too small of a sample size because that hurdle for any new agent is almost certainly too high (50% improvement). This is a setup for failure. Sample size must be large enough to give the new agent a chance e.g., a 25% improvement.
3. It is clear that if you are expecting an agent to be used to change the upfront treatment for patients with a specific type of tumor, two well controlled (and randomized) Phase III trials will need to

be performed. Normally two *well controlled* trials does not necessarily mean they have to be randomized trials. For example, well controlled could mean a well monitored study, or a study in which patients serve as their own controls. However, in the upfront situation, where the new agent is planned to change standard treatment, it is very likely that two *randomized* Phase III trials will be a necessity. There may be one exception to the two well controlled randomized Phase III trials requirement. It might be possible to obtain approval for the new agent to be used in an "upfront" situation if the level of significance for the primary endpoint of the Phase III trial is $p < 0.001$. As many experienced investigators can attest, a p value of that magnitude is indeed unusual in most Phase III trials.

4. It is frequently said that one must have an improvement in survival for a new agent to be approved. That is, of course, desirable. However, survival has not always been required. Table 3 details the new agents brought to the FDA Oncology Advisory Board for approval, the type of study(ies) that lead to approval, and the parameters used for that approval. As can be seen in that Table 3, there were 69 approvals and 16 disapprovals (note that some agents were brought multiple times for approval in different indications). As can be seen in that table there were 25 approvals based primarily on response, 16 on survival, 10 on TTP, and 18 based on other primary endpoints. There were 27 approvals based on Phase II trials and 42 approvals based on Phase III trials. One can also note that a variety of other endpoints have been used as primary parameters for approval (e.g., control of pleural effusion, reduction in dysplasia, etc.).

   It is this investigator's personal experience that regulatory agencies will entertain endpoints other than survival (see below) if that new endpoint is discussed prospectively with and in detail with the regulatory agencies. They, like us, like challenges.

5. As is noted above, the FDA and other world regulatory agencies have approved new agents based on response (as a surrogate for survival or for benefit for the patient). The landmark publication that really codified response rate as a surrogate was the article by O'Shaugnhessy and colleagues in which the general guidelines were put forth for approval based on Phase II results. There are many FDA observers who feel that response is no longer an approvable strategy, but it does document that it still can be a strategy for approval under the right circumstances, including:
   (a) a very high response rate or a substantial/complete response rate (where the responses are durable) which is something unexpected for a new agent. The best example of this is the high response rates noted with arsenic trioxide for patients with refractory acute promyelocytic leukemia.
   (b) a lower response rate but a low incidence of side effects. An excellent example of this is the Phase II experience with Herceptin for patients with refractory breast cancer (with response rates of 11% but with no significant side effects).

If you plan to use a Phase II strategy for approval, in general it is better to utilize a Phase II trial design with a reference arm. Otherwise there is a concern about patient selection (e.g., selection of long-term survivors regardless of treatment). Two possible strategies to give most reviewers confidence that it is indeed your new agent that is making a difference include trial designs such as:

(a) Patients with a refractory malignancy ↗ High dose of the new agent ↘ Lower dose of the new agent

Endpoints: response rate or time to tumor progression (if the arms are blinded).

(b) Patients with a refractory malignancy ↗ New agent ↘ Clinician's choice

Endpoint: response rate—as it is more difficult to blind the trial. (*Note*: this could be a 2:1 randomized of new agent vs clinician's choice.)

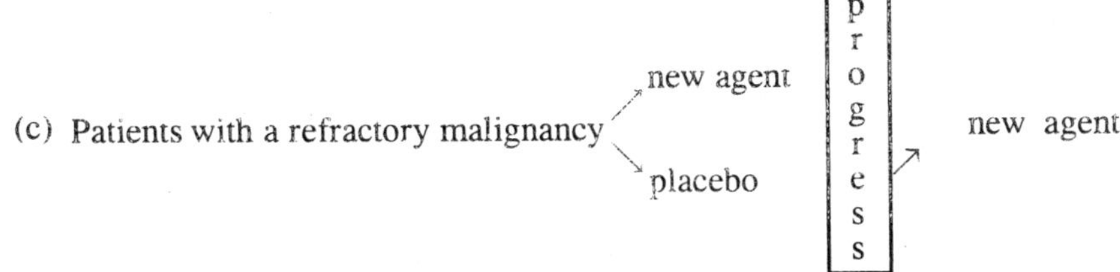

Endpoint: Time to tumor progression with a crossover allowed.

These types of randomized Phase II trials help (page 587) ensure everyone that there is no super-selection of your study population to select for patients who would have a favorable outcome irrespective of which treatment they were given.

Special Trial Designs, Particularly Suited for Cytostatic Agents

Patients as their Own Controls

This is a trial design that, until recently, was all but forgotten. There are at least two versions of this trial design. As can be seen, version 1, any patient who has a longer time on treatment on regimen B than on regimen A is considered a positive result (it is usually not an expected result for a patient to remain on treatment with a second- line regimen for a longer time than on a first-line regimen). This is certainly an inexact situation, as time on treatment is not the same as time to progression, but it is easier to measure when one does not have scans and X-ray films at regular intervals for the first regimen, as one usually has for the second regimen. Even though this is an inexact clinical trial situation, this trial design might offer some insight on whether or not the agent is having an effect on the natural history of the patient's disease. Based on past experience, if ≥30% of patients have a longer time on the new agent than on the regimen they received just prior to the new agent, that is a promising result that should be pursued.

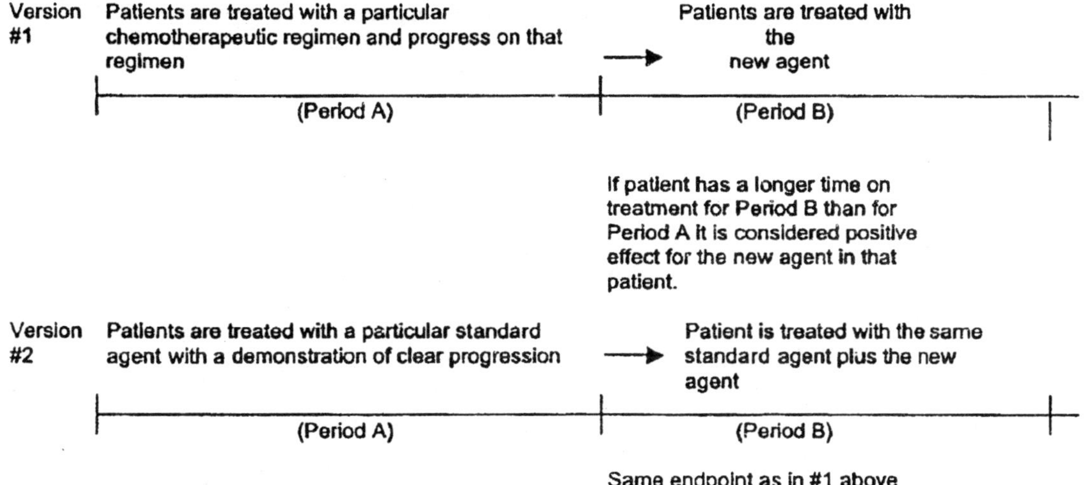

Fig. 15.1. Two versions of patients as their own control type of trial design.

To try version 2 of patients as their own controls one must have some preclinical information demonstrating that there is some synergy between the new cytostatic agent and the agent the patient is currently receiving. It is also critical in this design to make *very certain* that the patient is progressing on regimen A (best ascertained by an independent committee). It needs to be emphasized again that this type of trial is only an *exploratory trial*—but a trial that may again give hints of the agent changing the natural history of the disease. It is not a definitive trial design. This latter (version 2) design has already had a checkered start in that it was utilized for the design for the initial filing of the anti-epidermal growth factor receptor monoclonal antibody C225. The problem with that filing, however, was that it appears that there was unclear documentation as to whether or not the patient progressed on the initial regimen of CPT11 (period A) to which the C225 was added (during period B). That particular situation should not discourage the clinical investigator from trying version 2 of patients as their own controls *if* the new cytostatic agent demonstrates synergy with the standard cytotoxic agent (or other cytostatic agents for that matter).

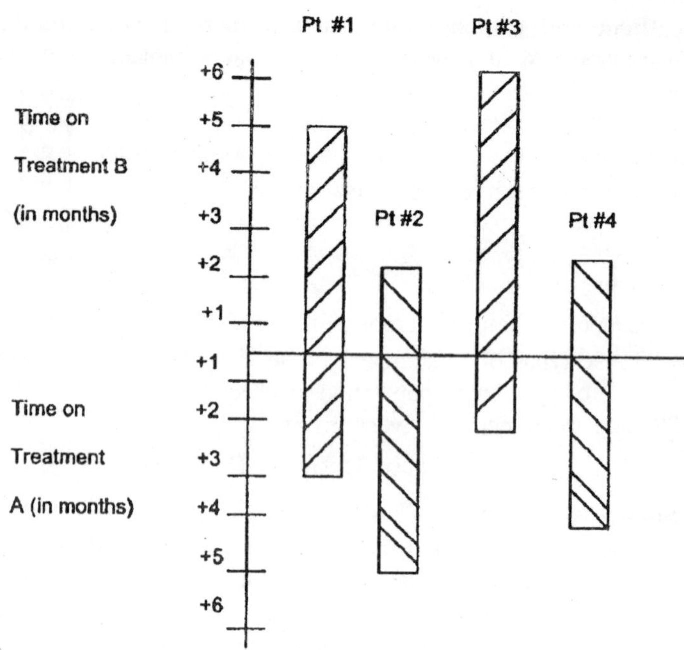

Fig. 15.2. Suggested manner for plotting time on treatment for period B vs time on treatment for period A.

Randomized Phase II Trial

This type of trial design was mentioned above. With some clever additional variations it can yield a great deal of information. As noted, the study was a three-arm study of chemotherapy vs chemotherapy plus a low dose of a MAb to VGEF vs chemotherapy plus a high dose of a MAb to VGEF. As can be seen, one of the endpoints for the study, in addition to toxicities, was the TTP. Once again, TTP can be a somewhat inexact endpoint and one that is not usually acceptable to a regulatory agency (except if the arms of the study are blinded—and this study was not). However, the above study design can provide information as to what sample sizes may be needed for an new drug application (NDA)-directed study. Such a study design can also provide information as to whether patients will participate in such a study, accrual rates, and so forth. Such a study design also yields valuable information on the safety of the various arms of the study.

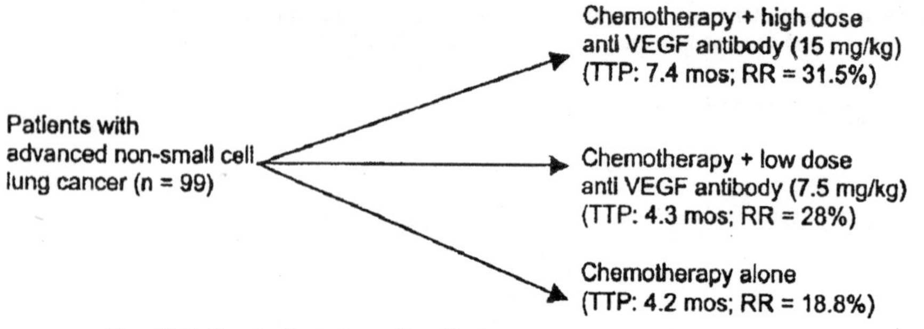

Fig. 15.3. Randomized phase II trail of a monoclonal antibody to VEGF.

An important option for the study is to continue with the study in a randomized fashion, selecting only one of the MAb-containing arms for comparison with the chemotherapy alone arm. This approach can save significant activation time for a new protocol (e.g., continue the randomized Phase II trial and power it up to be large enough for a Phase III trial rather than writing and activating a whole new Phase III trial). Another randomized Phase II trial that yielded very important information and which serves as an excellent model for solving drug development issues is a trial performed with the agent capecitabine (Xeloda). After results became available from the Phase I clinical trials with several different schedules of the agent, there was uncertainty as to just which schedule was the best. Therefore a randomized Phase II trial was conducted to determine which schedule (and dose) of capecitabine would be best to take into expanded Phase II and Phase III clinical trials. Patients were randomized to receive either: (a) 1331 mg/m^2/d continually; (b) 2510 mg/m^2/d intermittently, or (c) 1657 mg/m^2/d plus leucovorin 60 mg/d p.o. intermittently. The specific aims were to evaluate the safety and efficacy of each schedule. Cleverly, one of the efficacy endpoints utilized (in addition to response rate) was TTP. Utilizing TTP as a parameter of efficacy allowed a finer tuning because it allowed for a continuous assessment (in days) vs the dichotomous variable of response (response or no response). This clever randomized Phase II design showed that schedule "b" was the best schedule in terms of toxicities and efficacy. That schedule was then taken on into successful Phase II and Phase III trials, which led to the very rapid approval of capecitabine.

Randomized Discontinuation Trial Designs

This is a unique trial design for the development of cytostatic agents that has several very desirable features and yet seems as though it might be a very very difficult trial to complete. In reality, our team at the Arizona Cancer Center just participated in placing patients on a clinical trial utilizing this randomized discontinuation design and we have found excellent patient participation in the study. The design is particularly well suited for a new cytostatic agent that everyone wants to receive (just as the new agent endostatin was). All eligible patients initially received the new agent. Those who progress before 4 mo of treatment are completed are removed from the study. Those patients who do have a response or have stable disease for 4 mo are then randomized to continue the therapy or receive a placebo. The patients are carefully observed and if they have progressive disease (and are receiving placebo), they are placed back on the new agent. The endpoint for the study is the TTP for patients who continue on the therapy vs the TTP for patients who receive placebo.

The randomized discontinuation trial design has been used for testing new agents against the AIDS virus but it is just beginning to be used to evaluate new anticancer agents. Obviously when used in the situation with a new AIDs drug(s) one has viral titers to follow (vs computed axial tomography [CAT] scans and other imaging techniques for oncologists to follow a patient's tumor). The viral titers are more sensitive than our scans are. Also, some investigators question the ethics of randomizing patients who are responding to the new agent to continue, or discontinue that therapy. This problem can be addressed by randomizing only the patients with stable disease (and not the responders). Very carefully administered informed consent is obviously a necessity. One other potential problem with the randomized discontinuation design is that there is a theoretical problem in comparing the patients continued on

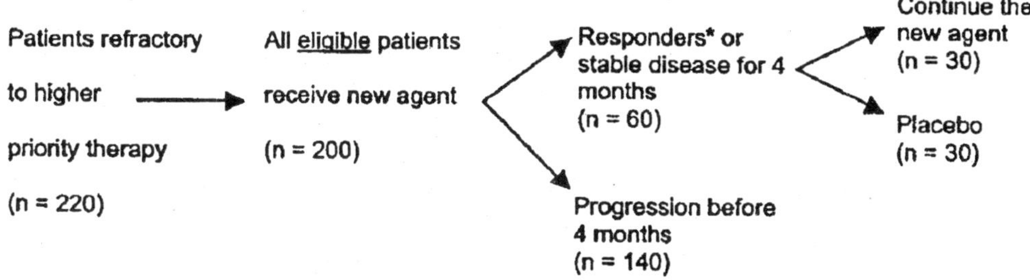

Fig. 15.4. Randomized discontinued design.

therapy vs those on placebo if there is a carryover effect of the agent (i.e., it could still be having an effect on the placebo group).

Regardless of its downsides, the randomized discontinuation trial design is one that should be considered for a new cytostatic agent. It does allow for a greater number of patients to have access to a potentially exciting new agent.

A Unique Endpoint for Approval

Clinical Benefit

In the early development of the chain terminator gemcitabine there were some patients with pancreatic cancer who demonstrated a decrease in their tumor-related pain and an increase in their appetite and weight. Gemcitabine had a new mechanism of action. It did not cause regression of pancreatic cancer growing in nude mice but rather it caused a slowing of growth of the pancreatic cancer xenografts growing in nude mice (MIA Pa Ca, PANC-1 and PAN C02). Therefore, it was likely that one would not see a complete or partial response in patients. In conversations with Dr. Bob Temple at the FDA and Dr. Gregory Burke our team was alerted to the fact that one endpoint they could accept in a trial was "fixing what bothers the patient." The term *clinical benefit* was derived from that conversation. Clinical benefit was not necessarily a quality of life parameter but it was an attempt to measure "fixing what bothers the patient." Because the three most common problems experienced by patients with pancreatic cancer included pain, weight loss, and a deterioration in performance status, Dr. John Anderson at Eli Lilly devised an algorithm to measure clinical benefit. This algorithm utilized pain performance status (measured by the Karnofsky scale because it had a broader range of 0–100 in increments of 10 rather than the ECOG or SWOG scales which have a range of only 0–5), and a direct measurement of weight (with clear cut definitions of what constituted weight gain or weight loss). The pivotal trial design for gemcitabine was as follows:

Patients with advanced, symptomatic pancreatic cancer → Weekly gemcitabine
→ Weekly 5 - FU

The primary endpoint for the study was an improvement in clinical benefit, with the secondary endpoints including response rate, median survival, and percentage of patients alive at 1 yr.

The study was positive for clinical benefit as well as for the other parameters. Gemcitabine was approved for use for treatment of patients with locally advanced or metastatic pancreatic cancer by the Oncology Drug Advisory Committee (ODAC) and by the FDA on the basis of this one study. In addition, there was a Phase II trial that was uncontrolled but demonstrated a similar survival (and response) to that found in the randomized phase III study. Gemcitabine was approved for treatment of patients with locally advanced or metastatic pancreatic cancer. Many observers who were present at the ODAC felt that gemcitabine would not have been approved if clinical benefit were the only parameter that was improved by gemcitabine. The other item of note is that gemcitabine was approved for frontline treatment of patients with advanced pancreatic cancer based on only one randomized trial. Observers at the ODAC felt that was because there were very few options for patients (and no prior controlled trials ever demonstrated an improvement in survival for any single agent) with advanced pancreatic cancer that gemcitabine was approved.

It is of note that no other attempts have been made to bring a new agent to the FDA using the clinical benefit parameter as the primary endpoint of the study. However, this investigator believes that with the proper algorithm it could be a solid primary endpoint for other pivotal trials with a new agent.

Special Challenges in Clinical Trial Designs for Approval

Analogs

Unfortunately in anticancer drug development we are still in the sulfonamide era—meaning that it is probably more productive to find agents with new mechanisms of action (for greater progress) than to work on analogs. However, there have been many commercial successes with analogs, largely based on less (or different) toxicities rather than on improved efficacy. The types of trials for approval for an analog program could be:

(a) Patients whose tumors are progressing on the parent compound (with very clear documentation of that progress) → Patient is treated with analog
Endpoint: Response rate

Endpoint: Response rate

Issues with this design include a very refractory patient population. However, if the analog has activity in that setting, it will certainly have a substantial chance for approval.

(b) Treat patients with the new analog who have a tumor type that is not responsive to the parent compound → Patient is treated with the analog
Endpoint: Response rate

Endpoint: Response rate

The issue here is that it is unlikely the analog will work in this situation. However, if it does work in this situation it also will have an excellent chance for eventual approval.

(c) Patient with a disease usually responsive to the parent compound ↗ New analog ↘ Parent compound

Endpoints: Survival, response rate, TTP toxicities

This is the best way to evaluate a new analog and the most likely way for an analog to be approved by regulatory agencies. Of course, superiority in one of the endpoints (not equivalence) is usually more convincing for approval.

Other Comments on Clinical Trials for Approval

Given the difficulty of treating patients with cancer, this author (as do many others in the field) believes that we should do everything we can to gain approval for new agents so patients have options. There are frequently numerous criticisms passing back and forth between investigators, regulators, educators, survivors, and others. At times their criticisms are valid—that perhaps we are asking for so much proof that an agent works (e.g., an improvement in survival) that it is discouraging to all involved and actually dampens any enthusiasm for development of new agents. It is this author's belief that the more these different constituencies communicate and work together (without assigning blame), the better chance we will have to develop innovative endpoints and trial designs for more rapid approval. Our job, together, is to obtain more options for clinical trial designs that allow development of new agents that work for our patients.

16

ANTIHYPERTENSIVE DRUGS

Recently, much attention has been focused on the interaction of small molecules with biological macromolecules. The search for selective enzyme inhibitors and receptor agonists or antagonists is one of the keys for target-oriented research in the pharmaceutical industry. Increased understanding of the mechanism of drug interaction on a molecular level has led to wide awareness of the importance of chirality as the key to the efficacy of many drug products. It is now known that in many cases only one enantiomer of a drug substance is required for efficacy and the other enantiomer is either inactive or exhibits considerably reduced activity. Pharmaceutical companies are aware that, where appropriate, new drugs for development should be homochiral to avoid the possibility of unnecessary side effects due to an undesirable enantiomer. In many cases where the switch from racemate drug substance to enantiomerically pure compound is feasible, there is the opportunity to extend the use of an industrial process. The physical characteristics of an enantiomer versus racemic compound may confer processing or formulation advantages.

Chiral drug intermediates can be prepared by different routes. One approach is to obtain them from naturally derived chiral synthons, produced mainly by fermentation processes. The chiral pool refers primarily to inexpensive, readily available, optically active natural products. A second approach is to carry out the resolution of racemic compounds. This approach can be achieved by preferential crystallization of enantiomers or diastereomers and by kinetic resolution of racemic compounds by chemical or biocatalytic methods. Finally, chiral synthons can also be prepared by asymmetric synthesis by either chemical or biocatalytic processes using microbial cells or enzymes derived therefrom. The advantages of microbial or enzyme-catalyzed reactions over chemical reactions are that they are stereoselective and can be carried out at ambient temperature and atmospheric pressure. The biocatalytic approach minimizes problems of isomerization, racemization, epimerization, and rearrangement that may occur during chemical processes. Biocatalytic processes are generally carried out in aqueous solution. These types of processes will avoid the use of environmentally harmful chemicals currently implemented in chemical processes and subsequent solvent waste disposal. Furthermore, microbial cells or enzymes derived therefrom can be immobilized and reused for many cycles. Recently, a number of review articles have been published on the use of enzymes in organic synthesis. This chapter provides some specific examples of preparation of chiral drug intermediates required for our antihypertensive agents.

VASOPEPTIDASE INHIBITOR

Enzymatic Synthesis of L-6-Hydroxynorleucine

L-6-Hydroxynorleucine is a chiral intermediate that is useful for the synthesis of a vasopeptidase inhibitor now in clinical trial and for the synthesis of C-7–substituted azepinones as potential intermediates

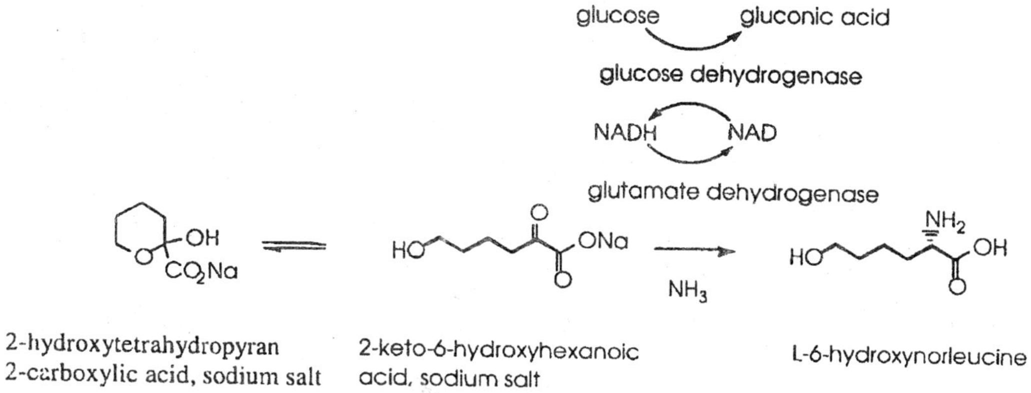

glucose → gluconic acid
glucose dehydrogenase
NADH ⇄ NAD
glutamate dehydrogenase

2-hydroxytetrahydropyran 2-carboxylic acid, sodium salt ⇌ 2-keto-6-hydroxyhexanoic acid, sodium salt → (NH_3) L-6-hydroxynorleucine

Fig. 16.1. Preparation of chiral synthon for vasopeptidase inhibitor.

for other antihypertensive metalloprotease inhibitors. It has also been used for the synthesis of siderophores, indospicines, and peptide hormone analogs. Previous synthetically useful methods for obtaining this intermediate have involved synthesis of the racemic compound followed by enzymatic resolution. D-Amino acid oxidase has been used to convert the D-amino acid to the ketoacid, leaving the L-enantiomer which was isolated by ion-exchange chromatography. In a second approach, racemic N-acetyl hydroxynorleucine has been treated with L-amino acid acylase to give the L-enantiomer. Both of these resolution methods give a maximum 50% yield and require separation of the desired product. Reductive amination of ketoacids using amino acid dehydrogenases has become a useful method for synthesis of natural and non-natural amino acids.

We have developed the synthesis and conversion of 2-keto-6-hydroxyhexanoic acid to L-6-hydroxynorleucine by a reductive amination process using beef liver glutamate dehydrogenase. 2-Keto-6-hydroxyhexanoic acid was converted completely to L-6-hydroxynorleucine by beef liver glutamate dehydrogenase. A nicotinamide adenine dinucleotide (NAD^+)-dependent formate dehydrogenase from *Candida boidinii* or glucose dehydrogenase from *Bacillus megaterium* was used for regeneration of reduced nicotinamide adenine dinucleotide (NADH) required for this reaction. The beef liver glutamate dehydrogenase was used for preparative reactions at 100 g/liter substrate concentration. 2-keto-6-hydroxyhexanoic acid, sodium salt, in equilibrium with 2-hydroxytetrahydropyran-2-carboxylic acid, sodium salt, is converted to L-6-hydroxynorleucine. The reaction requires ammonia and NADH. NAD^+ produced during the reaction was recycled to NADH by glucose dehydrogenase from *B. megaterium*. Reaction was completed in about 3 hr with reaction yields of 89–92%, and enantiomeric excess (e.e.) of >98% for L-6-hydroxynorleucine.

Chemical synthesis and isolation of 2-keto-6-hydroxyhexanoic acid required several steps. In a second, more convenient process, the ketoacid was prepared by treatment of racemic 6-hydroxynorleucine [produced by hydrolysis of 5-(4-hydroxybutyl)hydantoin] with D-amino acid oxidase and catalase. After the e.e. of the remaining L-6-hydroxynorleucine had risen to >99%, the reductive amination procedure was used to convert the mixture containing 2-keto-6-hydroxyhexanoic acid and L-6-hydroxynorleucine entirely to L-6-hydroxynorleucine with yields of 91–97% and e.e. of >98%. Sigma porcine kidney D-amino acid oxidase and beef liver catalase or *Trigonopsis variabilis* whole cells (source of oxidase and catalase) were used successfully for this transformation.

Enzymatic Synthesis of Allysine Ethylene Acetal

(*S*)-2-Amino-5-(1,3-dioxolan-2-yl)-pentanoic acid [allysine ethylene acetal] is one of three building blocks used for an alternative synthesis of omapatrilat, a vasopeptidase inhibitor. It has previously

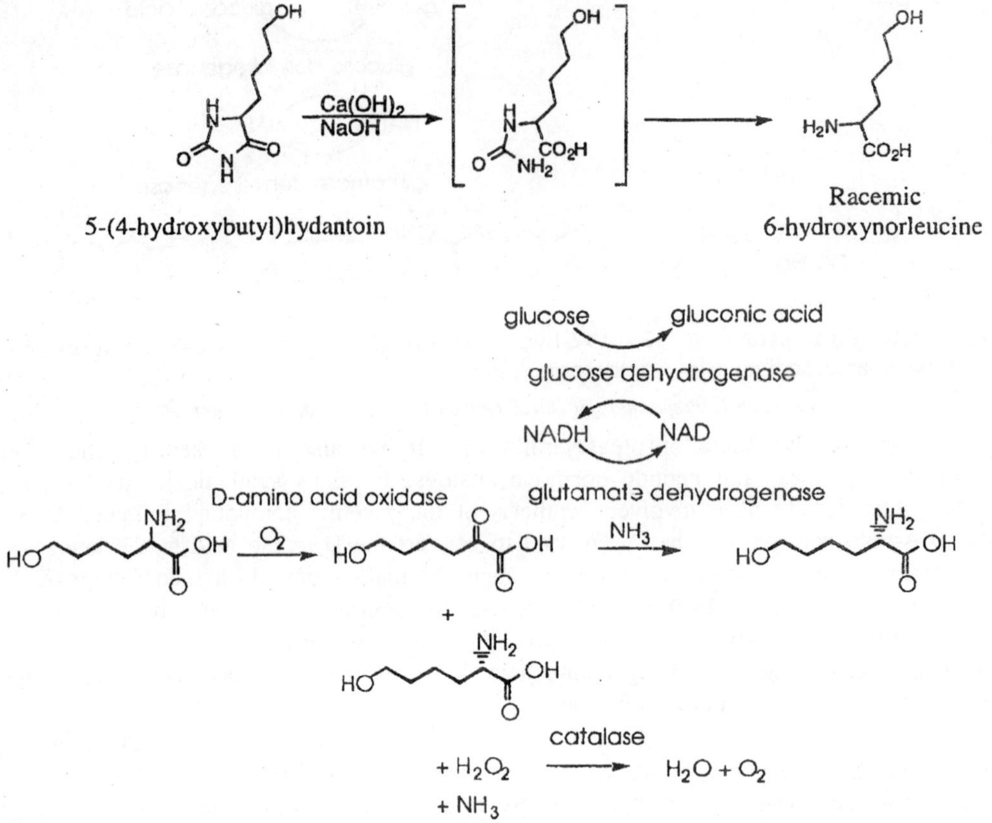

5-(4-hydroxybutyl)hydantoin

Racemic 6-hydroxynorleucine

Fig. 16.2. Chemical conversion of 5-(4-hydroxybutyl)hydantoin to racemic 6-hydroxynorleucine.

been prepared in an eight- step synthesis from 3,4-dihydro-2H-pyran. The reductive amination of ketoacid acetal to acetal amino acid was demonstrated using phenylalanine dehydrogenase from *Thermoactinomyces intermedius*. The reaction requires ammonia and NADH. NAD^+ produced during the reaction was recycled to NADH by the oxidation of formate to CO_2 using formate dehydrogenase from *C. boidinii*. An initial process was developed using heat-dried cells of*T. intermedius* ATCC 33205 as a source of phenylalanine dehydrogenase, and heat-dried cells of methanol-grown *C. boidinii* as a source of formate dehydrogenase.

An improved process was also developed using phenylalanine dehydrogenase from *T. intermedius* expressed in *Escherichia coli BL21 (DE3)* (pPDH155K) [SC16144] in combination with *C. boidinii* as a source of formate dehydrogenase. A third-generation process using methanol-grown *Pichia pastoris* as a source of endogenous formate dehydrogenase and *E. coli* SC16144 expressing *T. intermedius* phenylalanine dehydrogenase was also developed.

Glutamate, alanine, leucine, and phenylalanine dehydrogenases converted to the desired amino acid. Using an extract of *T. intermedius* ATCC 33205 as a source of phenylalanine dehydrogenase and formate dehydrogenase from *C. boidinii* for NADH regeneration, the reaction yield of 80% was obtained, and the process was developed using this enzyme combination. Heat-dried cells of*T. intermedius* and *C. boidinii* SC13822 grown on methanol were used for the reaction.

Phenylalanine dehydrogenase activities in cells recovered from fermentations. *T. intermedius* gave useful activity on a small scale (15 liters), but lysed soon after the end of the growth period, making

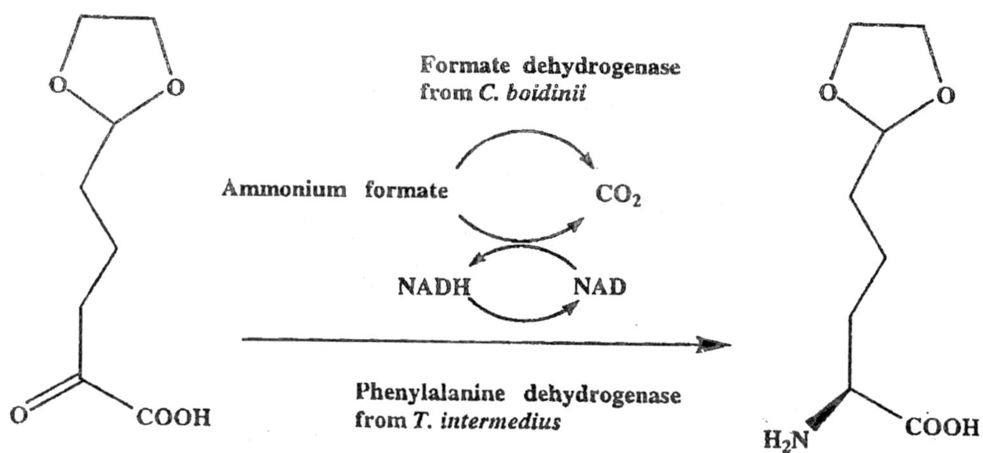

Fig. 16.3. Preparation of chiral synthon for vasopeptidase inhibitor.

recovery of activity difficult or impossible on a large scale (4000 liters). The problem was solved by cloning and expressing the *T. intermedius* phenylalanine dehydrogenase in *E. coli*, inducible by isopropyl thiogalactoside. Fermentation of *T. intermedius* yielded 184 units of phenylalanine dehydrogenase activity per liter of whole broth in 6 hr. At harvest, because the activity was unstable, the fermentor needed to be cooled rapidly. In contrast, the recombinant *E. coli* produced over 19,000 units per liter of whole broth in about 14 hr, and the activity was stable at harvest. *C. boidinii* grown on methanol was a useful source of formate dehydrogenase as described previously. In order to recover the cells on a large scale, 0.5% methanol was added to stabilize the cells.

P. pastoris grown on methanol was also a useful source of formate dehydrogenase. Expression of *T. intermedius* phenylalanine dehydrogenase in *P. pastoris*, inducible by methanol, allowed both enzymes to be obtained from a single fermentation. Formate dehydrogenase activity per gram of wet cells was 2.7-fold greater than for *C. boidinii*, and fermentor productivity was increased by 8.7-fold compared to *C. boidinii*. Fermentor productivity for phenylalanine dehydrogenase in *P. pastoris* was about 28% of the recombinant *E. coli* productivity.

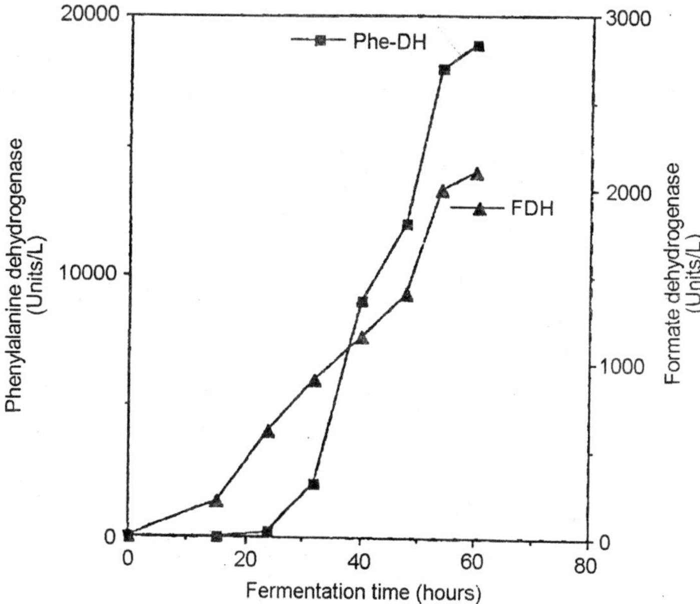

Fig. 16.4. Production of phenylalanine dehydrogenase and formate dehydrogenase in P. pastoris.

Formate dehydrogenase has been reported to have a pH optimum of 7.5–8.5. The pH optimum for the reductive amination of by an extract of *T. intermedius* was found to be about 8.7. Reductive amination reactions were carried out at pH 8.0. The time course for a representative batch showing conversion of ketoacid to amino acid using *E. coli/C. boidinii* heat-dried cells.

The procedure using heat-dried cells of *E. coli* containing cloned phenylalanine dehydrogenase and heat-dried *C. boidinii* was scaled up. A total of 197 kg of was produced in three 1600-liter batches using a 5% concentration of substrate with an average yield of 91 M% and e.e. of >98%.

Third-generation procedure, using dried recombinant *P. pastoris* expressing *T. intermedius* phenylalanine dehydrogenase inducible with methanol, and endogenous formate dehydrogenase induced when *P. pastoris* was grown in medium containing methanol, allowed both enzymes to be produced during a single fermentation. The two enzymes were conveniently produced in about the right ratio that was used for the reaction. The *Pichia* reaction procedure had the following modifications of the *E. coli*/*C. boidinii* procedure: concentration of substrate was increased to 100 g/liter, one-fourth the amount of NAD was used, and dithiothreitol was omitted. The procedure with *P. pastoris* was also scaled up to produce 15.5 kg of with 97 M% yield and e.e. >98% in a 180 liter batch using 10% ketoacid concentration.

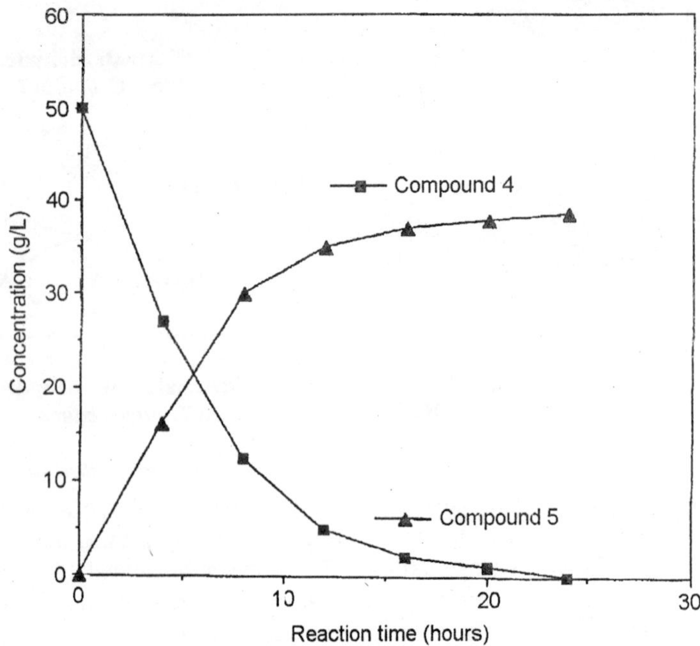

Fig. 16.5. Kinetics of enzymatic conversion of ketoacid acetal to amino acid acetal by phenylalanine dehydrogenase from recombinant E. coli and formate dehydrogenase from C. boidinii.

For reusability, formate dehydrogenase could be immobilized on Eupergit C and phenylalanine dehydrogenase on Eupergit C250L. The immobilized enzymes were tested for reusability in a jacketed reactor maintained at 40° C, and were used five times for the conversion without much loss of any activity and productivity. At the end of each reaction, the solution was drained from the reactor through a 80/400-mesh stainless steel sieve, which retained the immobilized enzymes, then the reactor was recharged with fresh substrate solution. After the fifth reuse, the reaction rate was decreased; however, the original reaction rate was restored in the seventh-reuse studies by addition of formate dehydrogenase.

β-3-Receptor Agonist

β-Adrenoceptors have been classified as β1 and β2. Increased heart rate is the primary consequence of β1-receptor stimulation, while bronchodilation and smooth muscle relaxation are mediated from β-2 receptor stimulation. Rat adipocyte lipolysis was initially thought to be a β-1-mediated process. However, recent results indicate that this type of lipolysis is neither β1 nor β2 receptor-mediated, but is due to "atypical" receptors, later called β3-adrenergic receptors. β3-Adrenergic receptors are found on the cell surface of both white and brown adipocytes and are responsible for lipolysis, thermogenesis, and relaxation of intestinal smooth muscle. Consequently, several research groups are engaged in developing selective β-3 agonists for the treatment of gastrointestinal disorders, type II diabetes, and obesity. Efficient biocatalytic syntheses of chiral intermediates required for the total chemical syntheses of β-3 receptor agonists have been reported by us.

The biocatalytic approaches include (1) the microbial reduction of 4-benzyloxy-3-methanesulfonylamino-2'-bromoacetophenone to the corresponding (*R*)-alcohol by *Sphingomonas paucimobilis*

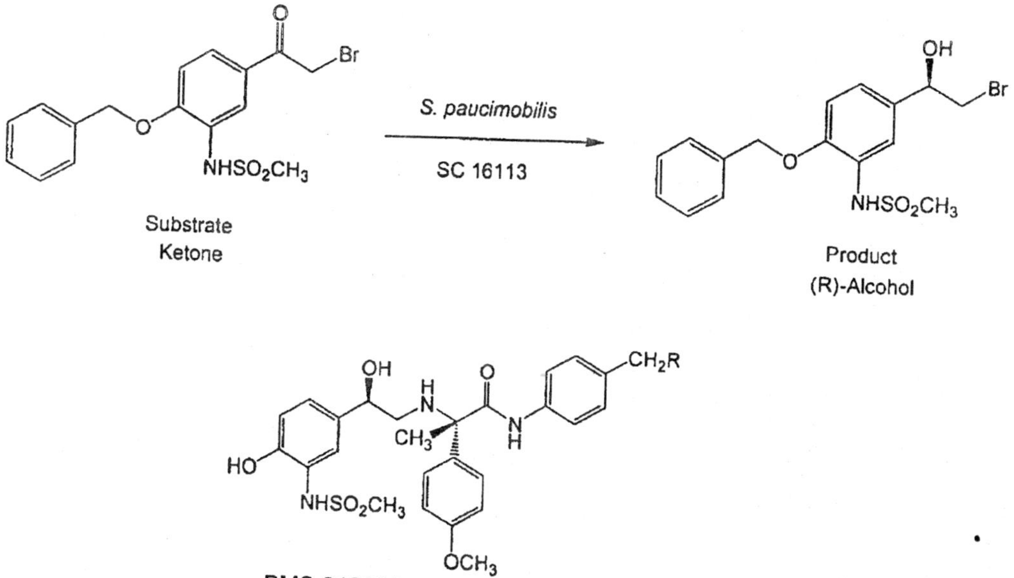

S. paucimobilis
SC 16113
Substrate
Ketone
Product
(R)-Alcohol

BMS-210620

Fig. 16.6. Preparation of chiral synthon for β-3-receptor agonist.

SC 16113; (2) the enzymatic resolution of racemic (α-methyl)phenylalanine amide and α-(4-methoxyphenyl) alanine amide by amidase from *Mycobacterium neoaurum* ATCC 25795 to prepare the corresponding (*S*)-amino acids, the asymmetric hydrolysis of methyl-(4-methoxyphenyl)-propanedioic acid, diethyl ester, to the corresponding (*S*)-monoester by pig liver esterase.

(A)
M. neoaurum
ATCC 25795
Substrate
Product
(B)
M. neoaurum
ATCC 25795
Substrate
Product
(C)
Pig Liver Esterase
Diester

S-(-)-Monoester

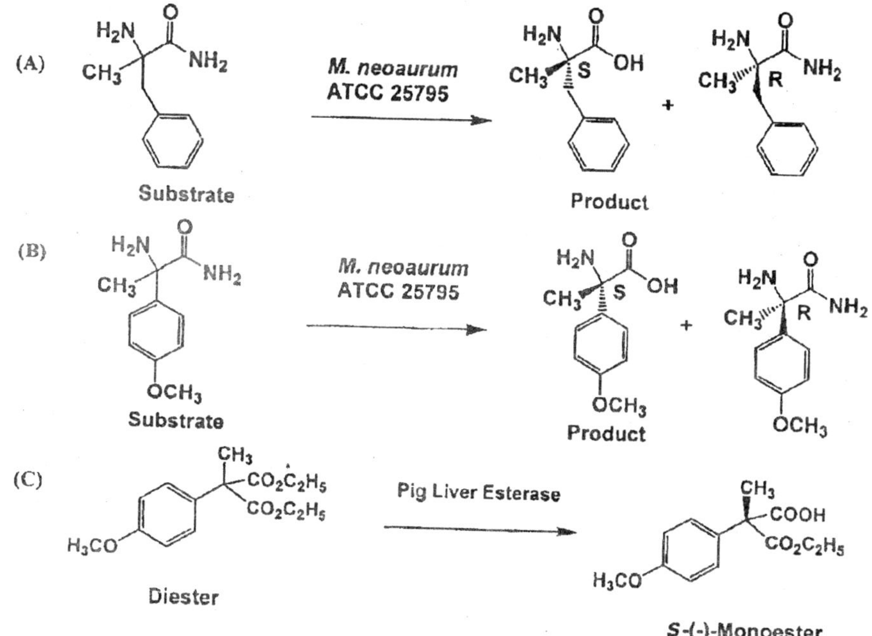

Fig. 16.7. Preparation of chiral synthon for β-3-receptor: (A) enzymatic resolution of racemic amino acid amide by amidase from M. neoaurum ATCC 25795; (B) enzymatic resolution of racemic amino acid amide by amidase from M. neoaurum ATCC 25795; (C) enzymatic asymmetric hydrolysis of diester to the corresponding (S)-monoester by pig liver esterase.

Microbial Reduction of 4-Benzyloxy-3-Methanesulfonylamino-2'-Bromoacetophenone

The microbial reduction of 4-benzyloxy-3-methanesulfonylamino-2'-bromoacetophenone to the corresponding (*R*)-alcohol was demonstrated by *S. paucimobilis* SC 16113. Among cultures evaluated, *Hansenula anamola* SC 13833, *H. anamola* SC 16142, *Rhodococcus rhodochrous* ATCC 14347, and *S. paucimobilis* SC 16113, gave desired alcohol in >96% e.e. and >15% reaction yield. *S. paucimobilis* SC 16113, in the initial screening, catalyzed the efficient conversion of ketone to the desired chiral alcohol in 58% reaction yield and >99.5% e.e.

The fermentation of *S. paucimobilis* SC 16113 culture was carried out in a 750-liter fermentor. From each fermentation batch, about 60 kg of wet cell paste was collected. Cells harvested from the fermentor were used to conduct the biotransformation in 1-, 10-, and 210-liter preparative batches under aerobic or anaerobic conditions. The cells were suspended in 80 mM potassium phosphate buffer (pH 6.0) to 20% (w/v, wet cells) concentration. Compound (1–2 g/liter) and glucose (25 g/liter) were added to the fermentor and the reduction reaction was carried out at 37°C. In some batches, at the end of the fermentation cycle, the cells were concentrated sevenfold by ceramic crossflow microfiltration using a 0.2-μm filter, diafiltered using 10 mM potassium phosphate buffer (pH 7.0), and used directly in the bioreduction process. In all batches of biotransformation, the reaction yield of >85% and the e.e. of >98% were obtained. The isolation of compound from the 210-liter preparative batch was carried out to obtain 100 g of product. The isolated gave 83% chemical purity and an e.e. of 99.5%.

In an alternative process, frozen cells of *S. paucimobilis* SC 16113 were used with resin adsorbed (XAD-16 resin) substrate at 5- and 10-g/liter substrate concentrations. In this process, an average reaction yield of 85% and an e.e. of >99% were obtained for product. At the end of the biotransformation, the reaction mixture was filtered on a 100-mesh (150-m) stainless steel screen, and the resin retained by the screen was washed with 2 liters of water. The product was then desorbed from the resin and crystallized in an overall 75 M% yield with 91% homogeneity and 99.8% e.e.

Enzymatic Resolution of Racemic (α-Methyl)phenylalanine Amides

The enzymatic resolution of racemic (α-methyl)phenylalanine amide and α-(4-methoxyphenyl)alanine amide to the corresponding (*S*)-amino acids, respectively, by an amidase from *M. neoaurum* ATCC 25795 has been developed. The chiral amino acids are intermediates for the syntheses of β-3-receptor agonists. The cells (10%, w/v, wet cells) of *M. neoaurum* ATCC 25795 were evaluated for biotransformation of compound. The reaction was completed in 75 min with a reaction yield of 48 M% (theoretical max. 50%) and an e.e. of 95% for the desired product. Freeze-dried cells of *M. neoaurum* ATCC 25795 were suspended in 100 mM potassium phosphate buffer (pH 7.0) at 1% concentration and cell suspensions were used for the biotransformation of compound. The reaction was completed in 60 min with a reaction yield of 49.5 M% (theoretical max. 50%) and an e.e. of 99% for the desired product. Biotransformation of compound was also carried out using a purified amidase. A reaction yield of 49 M% and an e.e. of 99.8% were obtained for desired product after 60 min of reaction time.

Freeze-dried cells of *M. neoaurum*ATCC 25795 and partially purified amidase were used for the biotransformation of compound. A reaction yield of 49 M% and an e.e. of 78% were obtained for the desired product using freeze-dried cells. The reaction was completed in 50 hr. Using partially purified amidase, a reaction yield of 49 M% and e.e. of 94% were obtained for desired product after a 70-hr reaction time.

Asymmetric Hydrolysis of Racemic Methyl-(4-Methoxyphenyl)-Propanedioic Acid, Diethyl Ester

The enzymatic asymmetric hydrolysis of methyl-(4-methoxyphenyl)-propanedioic acid, diethyl ester to the corresponding (*S*)-monoester by pig liver esterase (PLE) has been demonstrated. Chiral (*S*)-monoester is a key intermediate for the syntheses of β-3-receptor agonists.

Various organic solvents were tested for the PLE-catalyzed asymmetric hydrolysis of diester in a biphasic system. The results indicate that the reaction yields and e.e. of monoester were dependent on the solvent used in the asymmetric hydrolysis. Tetrahydrofuran (THF), methyl isobutyl ketone (MIBK), hexane, and dichloromethane inhibited PLE. Lower reaction yields (28–56 M%) and lower e.e. (59–72%) were obtained using *t*-butyl methyl ether, dimethylformamide (DMF), and dimethylsulfoxide (DMSO) as cosolvent. Higher e.e. (>91%) was obtained using methanol, ethanol, and toluene as cosolvent. Ethanol gave highest reaction yield (96.7%) and e.e. (96%) for monoester.

The effect of temperature and pH were evaluated for the PLE-catalyzed hydrolysis of diester in a biphasic system using ethanol as cosolvent. It was observed that the e.e. of desired monoester was increased with decreasing temperature from 25°C to 10°C. The optimum pH for asymmetric hydrolysis of diester in a biphasic system using ethanol as a cosolvent was 7.2 at 10°C. A semipreparative-scale asymmetric hydrolysis of diester was carried out in a biphasic system using 10% ethanol as cosolvent. Substrate (3 g) was used in a 300-ml reaction mixture. The reaction was carried out at 10°C, 125 rpm agitation, and at pH 7.2 for 11 hr. Reaction yield of 96 M% and an e.e. of 96.9% were obtained. From the reaction mixture, 2.6 g of monoester were isolated in 86.3 M% overall yield. The e.e. of isolated *S*-(–)-monoester was 96.9%.

Angiotensin Converting Enzyme (ACE) and Neutral Endopeptidase Inhibitors

Captopril is designated chemically as 1-[(2*S*)-3-mercapto-2-methylpropionyl]-L-proline. It is used as an antihypertensive agent through suppression of the renin–angiotensin–aldosterone system. Captopril and other compounds such as enalapril and lisinopril prevent the conversion of angiotensin I to angiotensin II by inhibition of ACE. The potency of captopril as an inhibitor of ACE depends critically on the configuration of the mercaptoalkanoyl moiety; the compound with the S-configuration is about

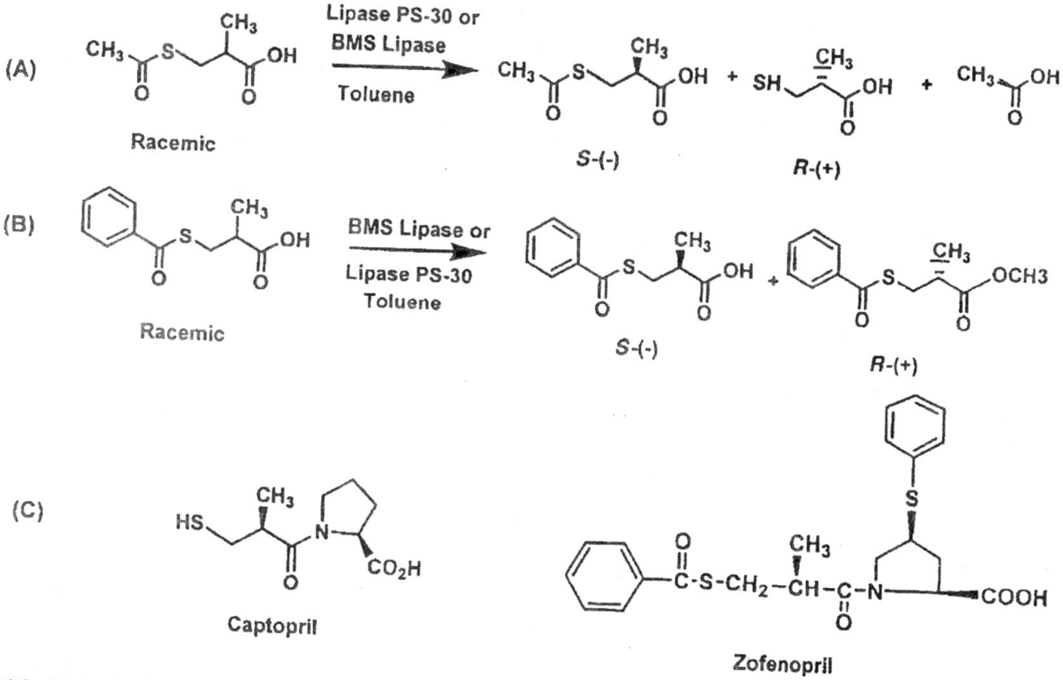

(A) Racemic → Lipase PS-30 or BMS Lipase, Toluene → S-(-) + R-(+)

(B) Racemic → BMS Lipase or Lipase PS-30, Toluene → S-(-) + R-(+)

(C) Captopril; Zofenopril

Fig. 16.8. (A) Synthesis of captopril side-chain S-(–): stereoselective enzymatic hydrolysis of racemic 3-acylthio-2-methylpropionoic acid. (B) Synthesis of zofenopril side-chain S-(–); stereoselective enzymatic esterification of racemic 3-behzylthio-2-methylpropionic acid. (C) Structures of captopril and zofenopril.

100 times more active than its corresponding *R*-enantiomer. The required 3-mercapto-(2*S*)-methylpropionic acid moiety has been prepared from microbially derived chiral 3-hydroxy-(2*R*)-methylpropionic acid, which is obtained by the hydroxylation of isobutyric acid.

The use of extracellular lipases of microbial origin to catalyze the stereo- selective hydrolysis of esters of 3-acylthio-2-methylpropionic acid in an aqueous system has been demonstrated to produce optically active 3-acylthio-2-methylpropionic acid. The synthesis of the chiral side chain of captopril by the lipase-catalyzed enantioselective hydrolysis of the thioester bond of racemic 3-acetylthio-2-methylpropionic acid to yield *S*-(–) has been demonstrated. Among various lipases evaluated, lipase from *Rhizopus oryzae* ATCC 24563 (heat-dried cells), BMS lipase (extracellular lipase derived from the fermentation of *Pseudomonas* sp. SC 13856), and lipase PS-30 from *Pseudomonas cepacia* in an organic solvent system (1,1,2-trichloro-1,2,2-trifluoroethane or toluene) catalyzed the hydrolysis of thioester bond of undesired enantiomer of racemic to yield desired *S*-(–), *R*-(+)-3-mercapto-2-methylpropionic acid and acetic acid. The reaction yield of >24% (theoretical max. 50%) and e.e. of >95% were obtained for *S*-(–) using each lipase in an independent experiment.

In an alternative approach to prepare the chiral side chain of captopril and zofenopril, the lipase-catalyzed stereoselective esterification of racemic 3-benzoylthio-2-methylpropionic acid in an organic solvent system was demonstrated to yield *R*-(+)-methyl ester and unreacted acid enriched in the desired *S*-(–)-enantiomer. Using lipase PS-30 with toluene as solvent and methanol as nucleophile, the desired *S*-(–) was obtained in 37% reaction yield (theoretical max. 50%) and 97% e.e. Substrate was used at 22-g/ liter concentration. The amount of water and the concentration of methanol supplied in the reaction mixture was very critical. Water was used at 0.1% concentration in the reaction mixture. More than 1% water led to the aggregation of enzyme in the organic solvent, with a decrease in the rate of reaction which was due to mass transfer limitation. The rate of esterification decreased as the methanol to substrate ratio was increased from 1:1 to 4:1. Higher methanol concentration probably inhibited the esterification reaction by stripping the essential water from the enzyme. Lower e.e. of product *S*-(–) was obtained at higher methanol concentration. Crude lipase PS-30 was immobilized on three different resins, XAD-7, XAD-2 and Accurel polypropylene (Accurel PP) in absorption efficiencies of about 68%, 71%, and 98.5%, respectively.

These immobilized lipases were evaluated for the ability to stereoselectively esterify racemic. Enzyme immobilized on Accurel PP catalyzed efficient esterification, giving 36– 45% reaction yield and 97.7% e.e. of *S*(–). The immobilized enzyme under identical conditions gave similar e.e. and yield of product in 23 additional reaction cycles without any loss of activity and productivity. *S*-(–) is a key chiral intermediate for the synthesis of captopril or zofenopril.

The *S*-(–)-α-[(acetylthio)methyl]phenylpropionic acid is a key chiral intermediate for the neutral endopeptidase inhibitor. We have demonstrated the lipase-catalyzed stereoselective hydrolysis of thioester bond of racemic α-[(acetylthio)methyl]phenylpropionic acid in organic solvent to yield *R*-(+)-α-[(mercapto)methyl]phenylpropionic acid and *S*-(–). Using lipase PS-30, the *S*-(–) was obtained in 40% reaction yield (theoretical max. 50%) and 98% e.e.

The *S*-(–)-2-cyclohexyl-1,3-propanediol monoacetate and the *S*-(–)-2-phenyl-1,3-propanediol monoacetate are key chiral intermediates for the chemoenzymatic synthesis of Monopril, a new antihypertensive drug which acts as an ACE inhibitor. The asymmetric hydrolysis of 2-cyclohexyl-1,3-propanediol diacetate and 2-phenyl-1,3-propanediol diacetate to the corresponding *S*-(–)-monoacetate and *S*-(–)-monoacetate by porcine pancreatic lipase (PPL) and *Chromobacterium viscosum* lipase have been demonstrated by Patel et al. In a biphasic system using 10% toluene, the reaction yield of >65% and e.e. of 99% were obtained for *S*-(–) using each enzyme. *S*-(–) was obtained in 90% reaction yield and 99.8% e.e. using *C. viscosum* lipase under similar conditions.

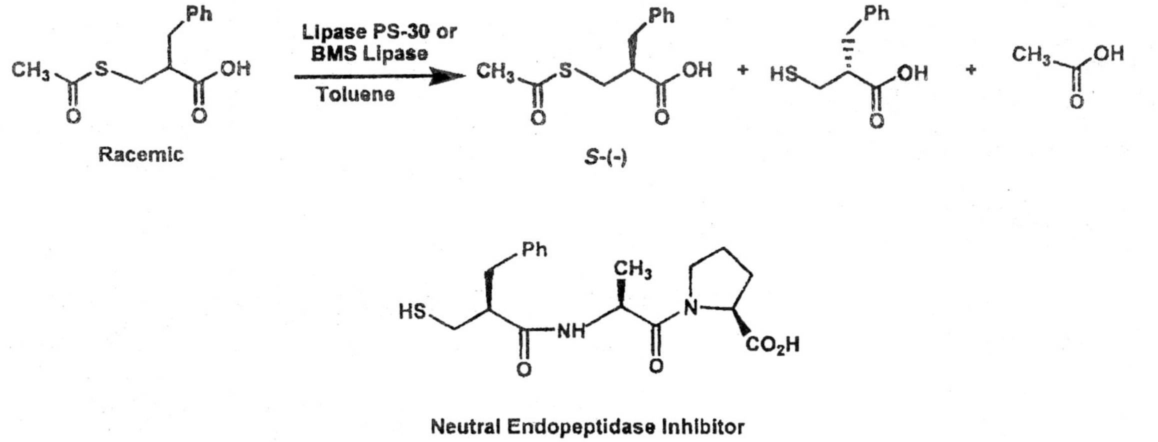

Racemic

Lipase PS-30 or BMS Lipase

Toluene

S-(-)

Neutral Endopeptidase Inhibitor

Fig. 16.9. Preparation of chiral synthon for neutral endopeptidase inhibitor: stereoselective enzymatic hydrolysis of racemic α-[(acetylthio)methyl]phenylpropionic acid.

Ceranopril is another ACE inhibitor which requires chiral intermediate 2-(*S*)-hydroxy-6-(carbobenzyloxyamino)-hexanoic acid. A biotransformation process was developed by Hanson et al. to prepare the 2-(*S*)-hydroxy-6-(carbobenzyloxyamino)-hexanoic acid. N-ε-carbobenzoxy(CBZ)-L-lysine was first converted to the corresponding keto acid by oxidative deamination using cells of *Providencia alcalifaciens* SC 9036 which contained L-amino acid oxidase and catalase. The keto acid was subsequently converted to 2-(*S*)-hydroxy-6-(carbobenzyloxyamino)-hexanoic acid using L-2-hydroxyisocaproate (HIC) dehydrogenase from *Lactobacillus confusus*. The NADH required for this reaction was regenerated using formate dehydrogenase from *C. boidinii*. The reaction yield of 95% with 98.5% e.e. was obtained in the overall process.

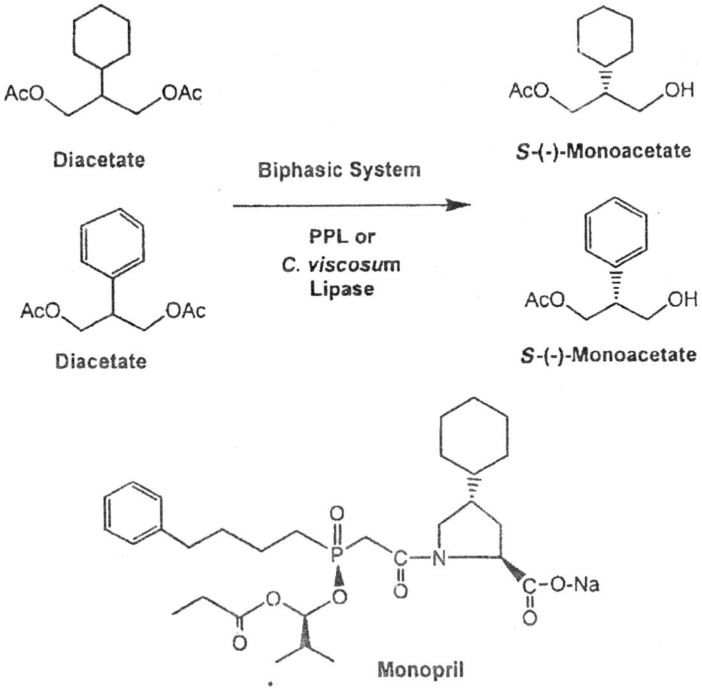

Diacetate

Biphasic System

PPL or *C. viscosum* Lipase

S-(-)-Monoacetate

Diacetate

S-(-)-Monoacetate

Monopril

Fig. 16.10. Preparation of chiral synthon for monopril: asymmetric enzymatic hydrolysis of 2-cyclohexyl- and 2-phenyl-1,3-propanediol diacetate and the corresponding S-(–)-monoacetates.

Thromboxane A2 Antagonists

Thromboxane A2 (TxA2) is an exceptionally potent pro-aggregatory and vasoconstrictor substance produced by the metabolism of arachidonic acid in blood platelets and other tissues. Together with potent anti-aggregatory and vasodilator compounds, TxA2 plays an important role in the maintenance of vascular homeostasis and contributes to the pathogenesis of a variety of vascular disorders. Approaches toward limiting the effect of TxA2 have focused on either inhibiting its synthesis or blocking its action at its receptor sites by means of an antagonist. The lactol or lactone are key chiral intermediates for the total synthesis of

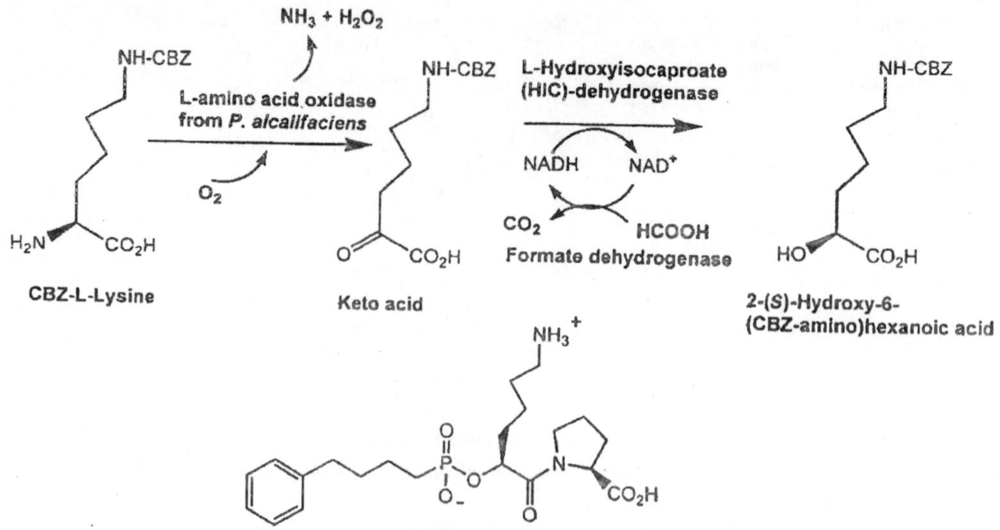

NH-CBZ
$NH_3 + H_2O_2$
L-amino acid oxidase from *P. alcalifaciens*
O_2
H_2N CO_2H
CBZ-L-Lysine
NH-CBZ
O CO_2H
Keto acid
L-Hydroxyisocaproate (HIC)-dehydrogenase
NADH NAD$^+$
CO_2 HCOOH
Formate dehydrogenase
NH-CBZ
HO CO_2H
2-(S)-Hydroxy-6-(CBZ-amino)hexanoic acid
NH_3^+
O P O O$^-$ N CO_2H O
Ceranopril

Fig. 16.11. Synthesis of chiral synthon for ceranopril: enzymatic conversion of CBZ-L-lysine to (S)-hydroxy-6-(carbobenzyloxyamino)-hexanoic acid.

compound, a new cardiovascular agent useful in the treatment of thrombolic disease. Horse liver alcohol dehydrogenase (HLADH) catalyzes the oxidoreduction of a variety of compounds. It has been demonstrated that HLADH catalyzes the stereospecific oxidation of only one of the enantiotopic hydroxyl groups of acyclic and monocyclic meso-diols. The authors demonstrated the oxidation of meso exo- and endo-7-oxabicyclo [2.2.1]heptane-2,3-dimethanol to the corresponding enantiomerically pure γ-lactones by HLADH. NAD and flavin adenine dinucleotide (FAD) at concentrations of 1 and 20 mmol, respectively, were required for the stereoselective oxidation of 12.7 mmol of substrate. Due to the high cost of enzyme and required cofactors, this process for preparing chiral lactones was economically not feasible for scale-up. Patel et al. described the stereoselective oxidation of (exo,exo)-7-oxabicyclo[2.2.1]heptane-2,3-dimethanol to the corresponding chiral lactol and lactone by cell suspension (10% w/v, wet cells) of *Nocardia globerula* ATCC 21505 or *Rhodococcus* sp. ATCC 15592. The reaction yield of 70 M% and e.e. of 96% were for chiral lactone after a 96-hr biotransformation process at 5-g/liter substrate concentration using cell suspensions of *N. globerula* ATCC 21505. An overall reaction yield of 46 M% (lactol and lactone combined) and e.e. of 96.7% and 98.4% were obtained for lactol and lactone, respectively, using cell suspensions of *Rhodococcus* sp. ATCC 15592. Substrate was used at 5-g/ liter concentration.

The asymmetric hydrolysis of (exo,exo)-7-oxabicyclo[2.2.1]heptane-2,3-dimethanol, diacetate ester to the corresponding chiral monoacetate ester has been demonstrated with lipases. Lipase PS-30 from *P. cepacia* was most effective in asymmetric hydrolysis to obtain the desired enantiomer of monoacetate ester. The reaction yield of 75 M% and e.e. of >99% were obtained when the reaction was conducted in a biphasic system with 10% toluene at 5 g/liter of the substrate. Lipase PS-30 was immobilized on Accurel PP and the immobilized enzyme was reused (5 cycles) without loss of enzyme activity, productivity, or e.e. of product. The reaction process was scaled up to 80 liters (400 g of substrate) and monoacetate ester was isolated in 80 M% yield with 99.3% e.e. The product was isolated in 99.5% chemical purity. The chiral monoacetate ester was oxidized to its corresponding aldehyde and subsequently hydrolyzed to give chiral lactol. The chiral lactol obtained by this enzymatic process was used in chemoenzymatic synthesis of thromboxane A2 antagonist.

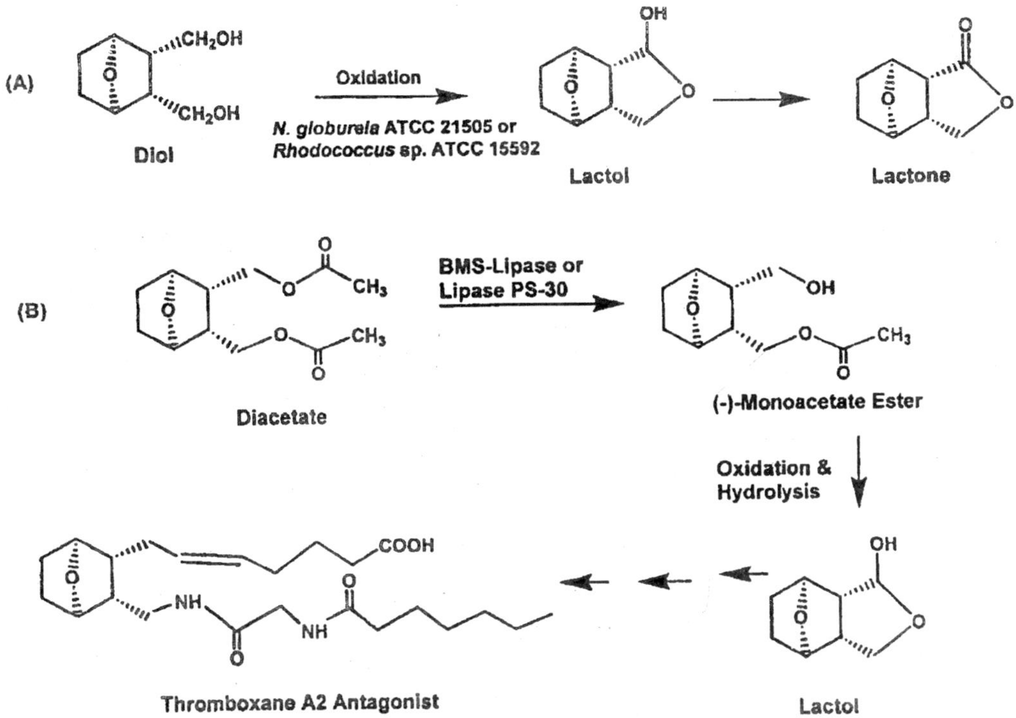

(A) Diol — Oxidation, *N. globurela* ATCC 21505 or *Rhodococcus* sp. ATCC 15592 → Lactol → Lactone

(B) Diacetate — BMS-Lipase or Lipase PS-30 → (-)-Monoacetate Ester — Oxidation & Hydrolysis → Lactol → Thromboxane A2 Antagonist

Fig. 16.12. Synthesis of chiral synthon for thromboxane A2 antagonist: (A) stereoselective microbial oxidation of (exo,exo)-7-oxabicyclo[2.2.1]hepatane-2,3-dimethanol to the corresponding lactol and lactone; (B) asymmetric enzymatic hydrolysis of (exo,exo)-7-oxabicyclo[2.2.1]heptane-2,3-dimethanol, diacetate to the corresponding S-(–)-monoacetate ester.

ANTICHOLESTEROL DRUGS

Chiral β-hydroxy esters are versatile synthons in organic synthesis, specifically in the preparation of natural products. Recently, we have described the reduction of the methyl ester of 4-chloro-3-oxobutanoic acid to the methyl ester of *S*-(–)-4-chloro-3-hydroxybutanoic acid by cell suspensions of *Geotrichum candidum* SC 5469. *S*(–) is a key chiral intermediate in the total chemical synthesis of a cholesterol antagonist (SQ 33600), which acts by inhibiting hydroxymethylglutaryl CoA (HMG CoA) reductase. In the biotransformation process, a reaction yield of 95% and e.e. of 96% were obtained for *S*-(–) by glucose, acetate-, or glycerol-grown cells (10% w/v) of *G. candidum* SC 5469. Substrate was used at 10-g/liter concentration. The e.e. of *S*-(–) was increased to 98% by heat treatment of cell suspensions (55°C for 30 min) prior to conducting the bioreduction.

Glucose-grown cells of *G. candidum* SC 5469 have also catalyzed the stereoselective reduction of ethyl-, isopropyl-, and tertiary-butyl esters of 4- chloro-3-oxobutanoic acid and methyl and ethyl esters of 4-bromo-3-oxobutanoic acid. A reaction yield of >85% and e.e. of >94% were obtained. NAD^+-dependent oxido-reductase responsible for the stereoselective reduction of â-keto esters of 4-chloro- and 4-bromo-3-oxobutanoic acid was purified 100-fold. The molecular weight of purified enzyme is 950,000. The purified oxido-reductase was immobilized on Eupergit C and used to catalyze the reduction. The cofactor NAD^+ required for the reduction reaction was regenerated by glucose dehydrogenase.

So far, most microorganisms and enzymes derived therefrom have been used in the reduction of a single keto group of β-keto or α-keto compounds. Recently, Patel et al. have demonstrated the stereoselective reduction of 3,5-dioxo-6-(benzyloxy)hexanoic acid, ethyl ester, to (3*S*,5*R*)-dihydroxy-6-(benzyloxy)hexanoic acid, ethyl ester. The compound is a key chiral intermediate required for the

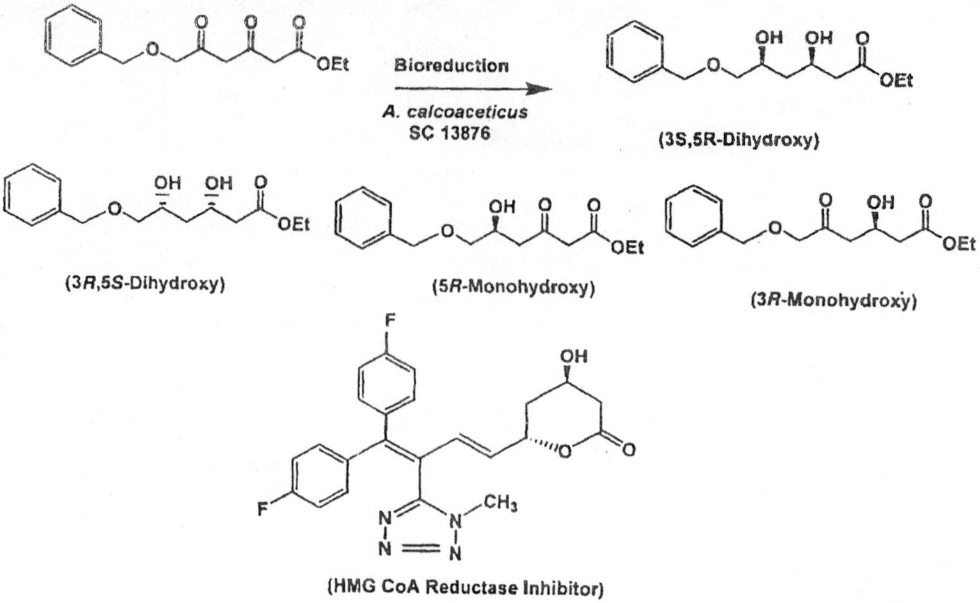

Bioreduction

A. calcoaceticus SC 13876

(3S,5R-Dihydroxy)

(3R,5S-Dihydroxy)

(5R-Monohydroxy)

(3R-Monohydroxy)

(HMG CoA Reductase Inhibitor)

Fig. 16.13. Synthesis of chiral synthon for anticholesterol drug R-(+): stereoselective microbial reduction of 3,5-dioxo-6-(benzyloxy)hexanoic acid, ethyl ester.

chemical synthesis of [4-[4α,6β(E)]]-6-[4,4-bis(4-fluorophenyl)-3-(1-methyl-1H-tetrazol-5-yl)-1,3-butadienyl]-tetrahydro-4-hydroxy-2H-pyran-2-one, compound *R*-(+), a new anticholesterol drug that acts by inhibition of HMG CoA reductase. Among various microbial cultures evaluated for the stereoselective reduction of diketone, cell suspensions of *Acinetobacter calcoaceticus* SC 13876 reduced. The reaction yield of 85% and e.e. of 97% were obtained using glycerol-grown cells. The substrate was used at 2 g/liter and cells were used at 20% (w/v, wet cells) concentration.

Cell extracts of *A. calcoaceticus* SC 13876 in the presence of NAD^+, glucose, and glucose dehydrogenase reduced to the corresponding monohydroxy compounds and [3-hydroxy-5-oxo-6-(benzyloxy)hexanoic acid ethyl ester and 5-hydroxy-3-oxo-6-(benzyloxy)hexanoic acid ethyl ester]. Both were further reduced to (3*S*,4*R*)-dihydroxy compound using the cell extracts. The reaction yield of 92% and the e.e. of 98% were obtained when the reaction was carried out in a 1-liter batch using cell extracts. The substrate was used at 10 g/liter. Product was isolated from the reaction mixture in 72% overall yield. The HPLC area percent purity of the isolated product was 99% and the e.e. was 98.5%. The reductase which converted was purified about 200-fold from cell extracts of *A. calcoaceticus* SC 13876. The purified enzyme gave a single protein band on SDS-PAGE corresponding to 33,000 Da.

Using an enzymatic resolution process, chiral alcohol *R*-(+) was also prepared by the lipase-catalyzed stereoselective acetylation of racemic in organic solvent. We evaluated various lipases, among which lipase PS-30 and BMS lipase (produced by fermentation of *Pseudomonas* strain SC 13856) efficiently catalyzed the acetylation of the undesired enantiomer of racemic to yield *S*-(−)-acetylated product and unreacted desired *R*-(+). A reaction yield of 49 M% (theoretical max. 50 M%) and e.e. of 98.5% were obtained for *R*-(+) when the reaction was conducted in toluene as solvent in the presence of isopropenyl acetate as acyl donor. Substrate was used at 4 g/ liter concentration. In methyl ethyl ketone at 50-g/liter substrate concentration, a reaction yield of 46 M% and e.e. of 96% were obtained for *R*-(+).

Lipase PS-30 was immobilized on Accurel PP and the immobilized enzyme was reused five times without any loss of activity or productivity in the resolution process to prepare *R*-(+). The enzymatic

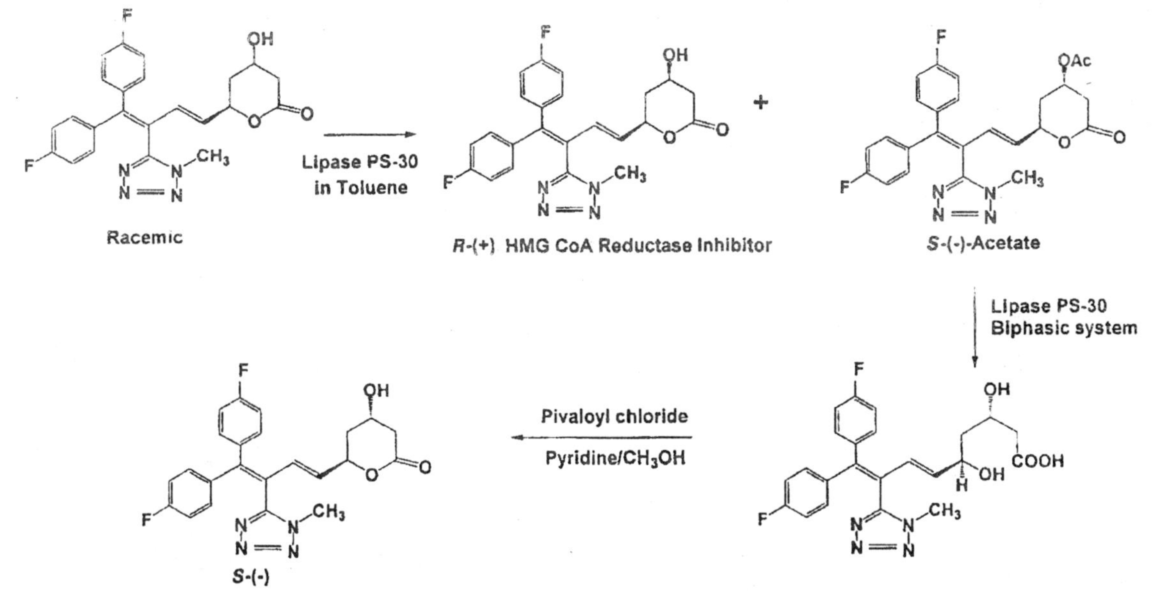

Fig. 16.14. Synthesis of chiral anticholesterol drug R-(+)-racemic: stereoselective enzymatic acetylation of racemic.

process was scaled up to a 640- liter preparative batch using immobilized lipase PS-30 at 4 g/liter racemic substrate in toluene as a solvent. From the reaction mixture, *R*-(+) was isolated in 35 M% overall yield with 98.5% e.e. and 99.5% chemical purity. The undesired *S*-(–)-acetate produced by this process was enzymatically hydrolyzed by lipase PS-30 in a biphasic system to prepare the corresponding *S*-(–)-alcohol. Thus both enantiomers of alcohol were produced by the enzymatic process.

Pravastatin and Mevastatin are anticholesterol drugs which act by competitively inhibiting HMG CoA reductase. Pravastatin sodium is produced by two fermentation steps. The first step is the production of compound ML-236B by *Penicillium citrinum*. The purified compound was converted to its sodium salt with sodium hydroxide and in the second step was hydroxylated to Pravastatin sodium by *Streptomyces carbophilus*. A cytochrome P-450–containing enzyme system has been demonstrated from *S. carbophilus* which catalyzed the hydroxylation reaction.

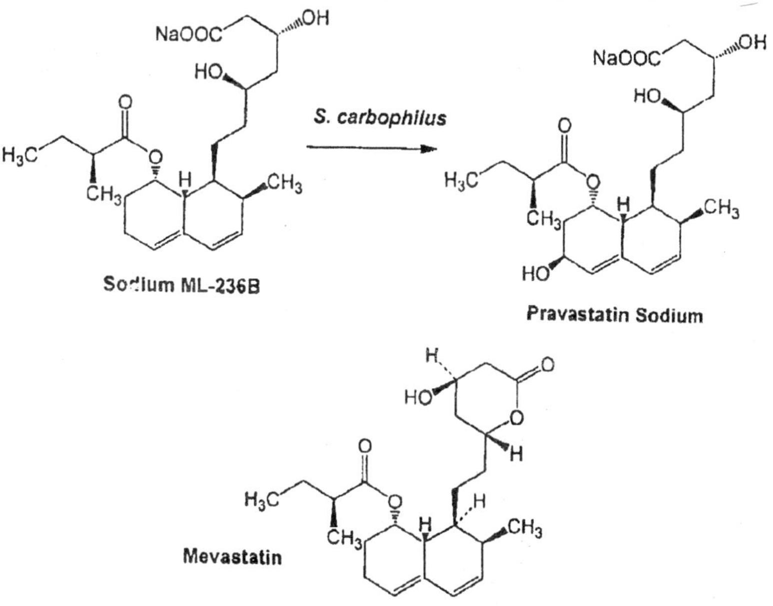

Fig. 16.15. Stereoselective microbial hydroxylation of ML-236B to Pravastain.

Squalene synthase is the first pathway-specific enzyme in the biosynthesis of cholesterol and catalyzes the head-to-head condensation of two molecules of farnesyl pyrophosphate (FPP) to form squalene. It has been implicated in the transformation of

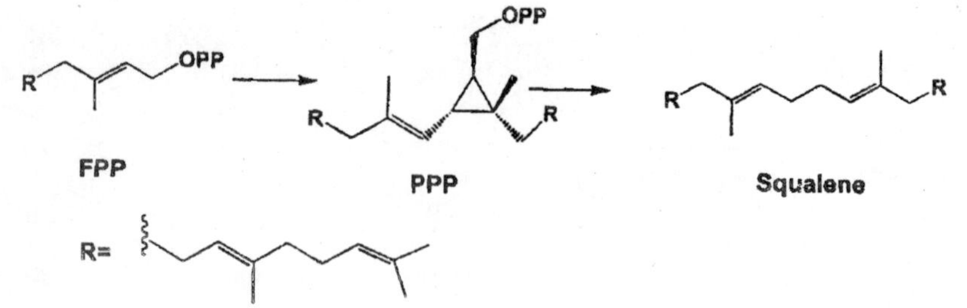

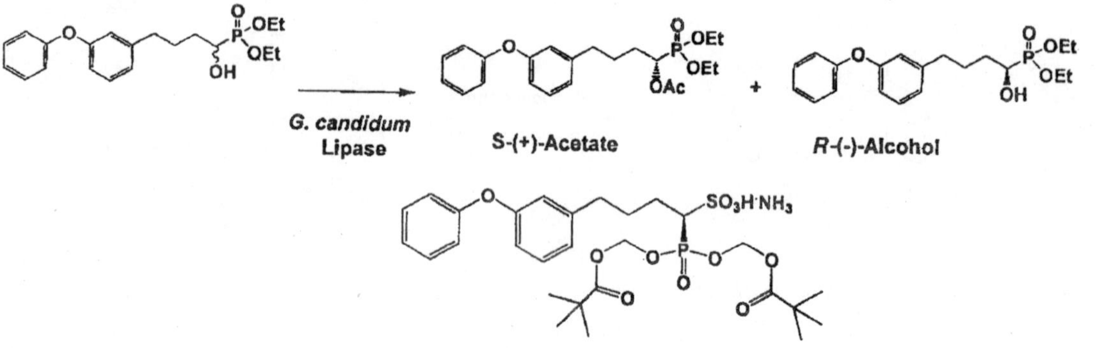

FPP PPP Squalene

R=

G. candidum Lipase S-(+)-Acetate R-(-)-Alcohol

BMS-188494

Fig. 16.16. Enzymatic synthesis of chiral synthon for BMS-188494, a squalene synthase inhibitor: stereoselective acetylation of racemic.

FPP into presqualene pyrophosphate (PPP). FPP analogs are a major class of inhibitors of squalene synthase. However, this class of compounds lacks specificity and are potential inhibitors of other FPP consuming transferases such as geranyl-geranyl pyrophosphate synthase. To increase enzyme specificity, analogs of PPP and other mechanism-based enzyme inhibitors have been synthesized. BMS-188494 is a potent squalene synthase inhibitor that is effective as an anticholesterol drug. (*S*)[1-(acetoxy)-4-(3-phenoxyphenyl)butyl]phosphonic acid, diethyl ester is a key chiral intermediate required for the total chemical synthesis of BMS-188494. The stereoselective acetylation of racemic [1-(hydroxy)-4-(3-phenoxyphenyl)butyl]phosphonic acid, diethyl ester, was carried out using *G. candidum* lipase in toluene as solvent and isopropenyl acetate as acyl donor. A reaction yield of 38% (theoretical max. 50%) and an e.e. of 95% were obtained for chiral.

Calcium Channel Blocking Agents

Dilthiazem, a benzothiazepinone calcium channel blocking agent that inhibits influx of extracellular calcium through L-type voltage-operated calcium channels, has been widely used clinically in the treatment of hypertension and angina. Since dilthiazem has a relatively short duration of action, recently an 8-chloro derivative has been introduced in the clinic as a more potent analog of dilthiazem. Lack of extended duration of action and little information on structure–activity relationships in this class of compounds led Floyd et al. and Das et al. to prepare isosteric 1-benzazepin-2-ones which resulted in the identification of a 6-trifluoromethyl-1-benzazepin-2-one derivative as a longer-lasting and more potent antihypertensive agent. A key chiral intermediate [(3*R*-*cis*)-1,3,4,5-tetrahydro-3-hydroxy-4-(4-methoxyphenyl)-6-(trifluoromethyl)-2H-1-benzazepin-2-one] was required for the total chemical synthesis of the new calcium channel blocking agent [(*cis*)-3-(acetoxy)-1-[2-(dimethylamino)ethyl]-1,3,4,5-tetrahydro-4-(4-methoxyphenyl)-6-(trifluoromethyl)-2H-1-benzazepin-2-one]. A stereoselective microbial process was developed for the reduction of 4,5-dihydro-4-(4-methoxyphenyl)-6-(trifluoromethyl)-1H-1

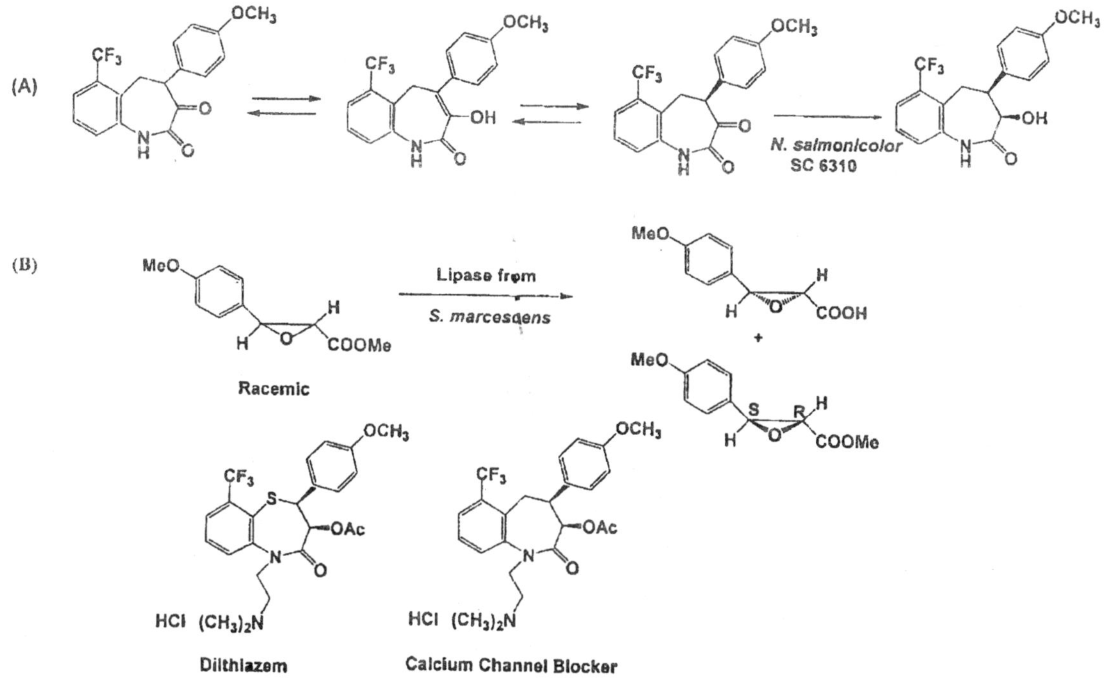

(A)

(B)

Fig. 16.17. Synthesis of chiral synthon for calcium channel blocker.

-benzazepin-2,3-dione to chiral. Compound exists predominantly in the achiral enol form, which is in rapid equilibrium with the two keto-form enantiomers. Reduction of could give rise to formation of four possible alcohol stereoisomers. Remarkably, conditions were found under which only the single alcohol isomer was obtained by microbial reduction. Among various cultures evaluated, microorganisms from the genera *Nocardia*, *Rhodococcus*, *Corynebacterium*, and *Arthrobacter* reduced compound to compound with 60–70% conversion yield at 1-g/liter substrate concentration. The most effective culture, *Nocardia salmonicolor* SC 6310, catalyzed the bioconversion in 96% reaction yield with 99.8% e.e. at 2-g/liter substrate concentration. Product was isolated and identified by NMR and MS. A preparative-scale fermentation process for growth of *N. salmonicolor* and a bioreduction process using cell suspensions of the organism were demonstrated.

A chiral intermediate (2*R*,3*S*)-3-(4-methoxyphenyl)glycidic acid methyl ester [(–)-MPGM] is required for the synthesis of dilthiazem. Matsumae et al. screened over 700 microorganisms and identified a lipase from *Serratia marcescens* which catalyzed the enantioselective hydrolysis of racemic MPGM in a biphasic system using toluene as organic phase. The reaction yield of 48% and the e.e. of 99.8% were obtained for (–)-MPGM.

Potassium Channel Openers

The study of potassium K-channel biochemistry, physiology, and medicinal chemistry has flourished, and numerous papers and reviews have been published in recent years. It has long been known that K-channels play a major role in neuronal excitability and a critical role in the basic electrical and mechanical functions of a wide variety of tissues, including smooth muscle, cardiac muscle, and glands. A new class of highly specific pharmacological compounds has been developed which either open or block K-channels. K-channel openers are powerful smooth muscle relaxants with in vivo antihypertensive and bronchodilator activities. Recently, the synthesis and antihypertensive activity of a series of novel K-

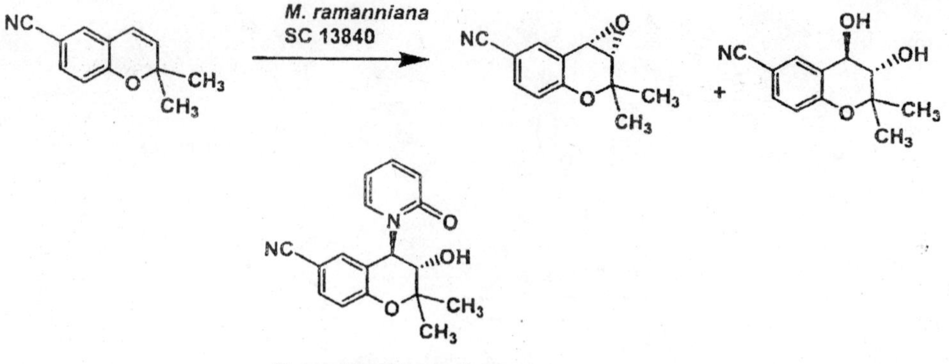

M. ramanniana
SC 13840

Potassium Channel Opener

Fig. 16.18. Oxygenation of 2,2-dimethyl-2H-1-benzopyran-6-carbonitrile to the corresponding chiral expoxide and (+)-trans-diol by M. ramanniana SC 13840.

channel openers based on monosubstituted *trans*-4-amino-3,4-dihydro-2,2-dimethyl-2H-l-benzopyran-3-ol have been demonstrated. Chiral epoxide and diol are potential intermediates for the synthesis of K-channel activators that are important as antihypertensive and bronchodilator agents. The stereoselective microbial oxygenation of 2,2-dimethyl-2H-1-benzopyran-6-carbonitrile to the corresponding chiral epoxide and chiral diol has been demonstrated. Among microbial cultures evaluated, the best culture, *Mortierella ramanniana* SC 13840, gave reaction yields of 67.5 M% and e.e. of 96% for the (+)-*trans*-diol. A single-stage process (fermentation/epoxidation) for the biotransformation was developed using *M. ramanniana* SC 13840. In a 25-liter fermentor, the (+)-*trans*-diol was obtained in the reaction yield of 60.7 M% and e.e. of 92.5%.

Using a 3-liter cell suspension (10% w/v, wet cells) of *M. ramanniana* SC 13840, the (+)-*trans*-diol was obtained in 76 M% yield with an e.e. of 96%. The reaction was carried out in a 5-liter Bioflo fermentor with 2-g/liter substrate and 1 0-g/liter glucose concentrations. Glucose was supplied to regenerate NADH required for this reaction. From the reaction mixture, (+)-*trans*-diol was isolated in 65 M% (4.6 g) overall yield. An enantiomeric excess of 97% and a chemical purity of 98% were obtained for the isolated (+)-*trans*-diol. In an enzymatic resolution approach, chiral (+)-*trans*-diol was prepared by the stereoselective acetylation of racemic diol with lipases from *Candida cylindraceae* and *P. cepacia*. Both enzymes catalyzed the acetylation of the undesired enantiomer of racemic diol to yield monoacetylated product and unreacted desired (+)-*trans*-diol. A reaction yield of 40% and an e.e. of >90% were obtained using each lipase.

Antiarrhythmic Agents

Larsen and Lish reported the biological activity of a series of phenethanolamine-bearing alkyl sulfonamido groups on the benzene ring. Within this series, some compounds possessed adrenergic and antiadrenergic actions. D-(+)-sotalol is a β-blocker that, unlike other β-blockers, has antiarrhythmic properties and has no other peripheral actions. The β-adrenergic blocking drugs such as propranolol and sotalol have been separated chemically into the dextrorotatory and levorotatory optical isomers, and it has been demonstrated that the activity of the levo isomer is 50 times that of the corresponding dextro isomer. Chiral alcohol is a key intermediate for the chemical synthesis of D-(+)-sotalol. The stereoselective microbial reduction of N-(4-(2-chloro-acetyl)phenyl)methanesulfonamide to the corresponding (+)-alcohol has been demonstrated. Among numbers of microorganisms screened for the transformation of ketone to (+)-alcohol, *Rhodo coccus* sp. ATCC 29675, *Rhodococcus rhodochrous* ATCC 21243, *N. salmonicolor* SC 6310, and *Hansenula polymorpha* ATCC 26012 gave the desired (+)-alcohol in >90% e.e. *H. polymorpha* ATCC 26012 catalyzed the efficient conversion of ketone to (+)-alcohol in 95% reaction yield and >99% e.e. Growth of *H. polymorpha* ATCC 26012 culture was carried out in a 380-liter fermentor and cells harvested from the fermentor were used to conduct transformation in a 3-liter preparative batch. Cell suspensions (20% wet cells in 1 liter of 10 mM potassium phosphate buffer, pH 7.0) were supplemented with 12 g of ketone and 225 g of glucose and the reduction reaction was carried out at 25°C, 200 rpm, and pH 7. Complete conversion of ketone to (+)-alcohol was obtained in a 20-hr reaction. Using preparative HPLC, 8.2 g of (+)-alcohol were isolated from the reaction mixture in overall 68% yield with >99% e.e.

The production of optically active chiral intermediates is a subject of increasing importance in the pharmaceutical industry. Increasing regulatory pressure by the Food and Drug Administration to market homochiral drugs has led to the use of alternative approaches, including biocatalysis for the synthesis of chiral compounds. Organic synthesis has been one of the most successful scientific disciplines and has enormous practical utility. One can ask the question, then, why biocatalysis? What does biocatalysis have to offer to synthetic organic chemists? Biocatalysis gives an added dimension and enormous opportunity to prepare industrially useful chiral compounds. The advantages of biocatalysis over chemical catalysis are that enzyme-catalyzed reactions are stereoselective and regioselective and can be carried out at ambient temperature and atmospheric pressure. In biocatalytic processes, microbial cells and enzymes can be immobilized and an immobilized biocatalyst can be reused for many cycles. In addition, enzymes can be overexpressed to make biocatalytic processes economically efficient. The use of different classes of enzymes in catalysis of different types of chemical reactions is essential to generate a variety of chiral compounds for chemoenzymatic synthesis of pharmaceutical products. This includes the use of hydrolytic enzymes such as lipases, esterases, proteases, dehalogenases, acylases, amidases, nitrilases, lyases, epoxide hydrolases, decarboxylases, and hydantoinases in resolution of racemic compounds and in asymmetric synthesis of optically active compounds. Oxidoreductases and aminotransferases have been used in synthesis of chiral alcohols, aminoalcohols, amino acids, and amines. Aldolases and decarboxylases have been effectively used in asymmetric synthesis by aldol condensation and acyloin condensation reactions. Oxygenases such as monooxygenases have been used in stereoselective and regioselective hydroxylation and epoxidation reactions and dioxygenases in the chemoenzymatic synthesis of chiral diols.

The idea of designing biocatalysts that act specifically in desired reactions of interest can change the face of synthesis. Tailored enzymes made by random and site-directed mutagenesis with modified activity and preparation of thermostable and pH stable enzymes can lead to the production of novel stereoselective biocatalysts. The use of enzymes inorganic solvents has led to hundreds of publications on enzyme-catalyzed asymmetric synthesis and resolution processes. Molecular recognition and selective catalysis are key chemical processes in life which are embodied in enzymes. In the course of the last decades, the progress in biochemistry, protein chemistry, molecular cloning, random and site-directed mutagenesis, and fermentation technology has opened up unlimited access to a variety of enzymes and microbial cultures as valuable tools in organic synthesis.

17

Pharmacology of Central Nervous System

The central nervous system (CNS) is responsible for controlling bodily functions as well as being the center for behavioral and intellectual abilities. Neurons within the CNS are organized into highly complex patterns that mediate information through synaptic interactions. CNS drugs often attempt to modify the activity of these neurons in order to treat specific disorders or to alter the general level of arousal of the CNS. This chapter presents a simplified introduction to the organization of the CNS and the general strategies that can be used with drugs to alter activity within the brain and spinal cord.

CNS Organization

The CNS can be grossly divided into the brain and spinal cord. The brain is subdivided according to anatomic or functional criteria. The following is a brief overview of the general organization of the brain and spinal cord, with some indication of where particular CNS drugs tend to exert their effects. This chapter is not intended to be an extensive review of neuroanatomy—a more elaborate discussion of CNS structure and function can be found in several excellent sources.

Cerebrum

The largest and most rostral aspect of the brain is the *cerebrum*. The cerebrum consists of bilateral hemispheres, with each hemisphere anatomically divided into several lobes (frontal, temporal, parietal, and occipital). The outer cerebrum, or cerebral cortex, is the highest order of conscious function and integration in the CNS. Specific cortical areas are responsible for sensory and motor functions as well as intellectual and cognitive abilities. Other cortical areas are involved in short-term memory and speech. The cortex also operates in a somewhat supervisory capacity regarding lower brain functioning and may influence the control of other activities such as the autonomic nervous system. With regard to CNS drugs, most therapeutic medications tend to affect cortical function indirectly by first altering the function of lower brain and spinal cord structures. An exception is the group of drugs used to treat epilepsy; these drugs are often targeted directly for hyperexcitable neurons in the cerebral cortex. In addition, drugs that attempt to enhance cognitive function in conditions such as Alzheimer disease (cholinergic stimulants) might also exert their primary effects in the cerebrum.

Basal Ganglia

A group of specific areas located deep within the cerebral hemispheres is collectively termed the *basal ganglia*. Components of the basal ganglia include the caudate nucleus, putamen, globus pallidus, lentiform nucleus, and substantia nigra. The basal ganglia are primarily involved in the control of motor activities; deficits in this area are significant in movement disorders such as Parkinson disease and Huntington chorea. Certain medications used to treat these movement disorders exert their effects by interacting with basal ganglia structures.

Diencephalon

The area of the brain enclosing the third ventricle is the *diencephalon*. This area consists of several important structures, including the thalamus and hypothalamus. The thalamus contains distinct nuclei that are crucial in the integration of certain types of sensations and their relay to other areas of the brain (such as the somatosensory cortex). The hypothalamus is involved in the control of diverse body functions including temperature control, appetite, water balance, and certain emotional reactions. The hypothalamus is also significant in its control over the function of hormonal release from the pituitary gland. Several CNS drugs affecting sensation and control of the body functions listed, manifest their effects by interacting with the thalamus and hypothalamus.

Mesencephalon and Brainstem

The *mesencephalon*, or *midbrain*, serves as a bridge between the higher areas of the brain (cerebrum and diencephalon) and the *brainstem*. The brainstem consists of the pons and the medulla oblongata. In addition to serving as a pathway between the higher brain and spinal cord, the midbrain and brainstem are the locations of centers responsible for controlling respiration and cardiovascular function (vasomotor center).

The reticular formation is also located in the midbrain and brainstem. The reticular formation is comprised of a collection of neurons that extend from the reticular substance of the upper spinal cord through the midbrain and the thalamus. The reticular formation monitors and controls consciousness and is also important in regulating the amount of arousal or alertness in the cerebral cortex. Consequently, CNS drugs that affect the arousal state of the individual tend to exert their effects on the reticular formation. Sedative-hypnotics and general anesthetics tend to decrease activity in the reticular formation, whereas certain CNS stimulants (caffeine, amphetamines) may increase arousal through a stimulatory effect on reticular formation neurons.

Cerebellum

The *cerebellum* lies posterior to the brainstem and is separated from it by the fourth ventricle. Anatomically it is divided into two hemispheres, each consisting of three lobes (anterior, posterior, and flocculonodular). The function of the cerebellum is to help plan and coordinate motor activity and to assume responsibility for comparing the actual movement with the intended motor pattern. The cerebellum interprets various sensory input and helps modulate motor output so that the actual movement closely resembles the intended motor program. The cerebellum is also concerned with the vestibular mechanisms responsible for maintaining balance and posture. Therapeutic medications are not usually targeted directly for the cerebellum, but incoordination and other movement disorders may result if a drug exerts a toxic side effect on the cerebellum.

Limbic System

So far, all of the structures described have been grouped primarily by their anatomic relationships with the brain. The *limbic system* is comprised of several structures that are dispersed throughout the brain but are often considered as a functional unit or system within the CNS. Major components of the limbic system include cortical structures (such as the amygdala, hippocampus, and cingulate gyrus), the hypothalamus, certain thalamic nuclei, mamillary bodies, septum pellucidum, and several other structures and tracts. These structures are involved in the control of emotional and behavioral activity. Certain aspects of motivation, aggression, sexual activity, and instinctive responses may be influenced by activity within the limbic system. CNS drugs affecting these aspects of behavior, including some antianxiety and antipsychotic medications, are believed to exert their beneficial effects primarily by altering activity in the limbic structures.

Spinal Cord

At the caudal end of the brainstem, the CNS continues distally as the *spinal cord*. The spinal cord is cylindrically shaped and consists of centrally located gray matter that is surrounded by white matter. The gray matter serves as an area for synaptic connections between various neurons. The white matter consists of the myelinated axons of neurons, which are grouped into tracts ascending or descending between the brain and specific levels of the cord. Certain CNS drugs exert some or all of their effects by modifying synaptic transmission in specific areas of gray matter, while other CNS drugs, such as narcotic analgesics, may exert an effect on synaptic transmission in the gray matter of the cord as well as on synapses in other areas of the brain. Some drugs may be specifically directed toward the white matter of the cord. Drugs such as local anesthetics can be used to block action potential propagation in the white matter so that ascending or descending information is interrupted (i.e., a spinal block).

Blood-Brain Barrier

The *blood-brain barrier* refers to the unique structure and function of CNS capillaries. Certain substances are not able to pass from the bloodstream into the CNS, despite the fact that these substances are able to pass from the systemic circulation into other peripheral tissues. This fact suggests the existence of some sort of unique structure and function of the CNS capillaries that prevents many substances from entering the brain and spinal cord—hence, the term *blood-brain barrier*. This barrier effect is caused primarily by the tight junctions that occur between capillary endothelial cells; in fact, CNS capillaries lack the gaps and fenestrations that are seen in peripheral capillaries. Also, nonneuronal cells in the CNS (e.g., astrocytes) and the capillary basement membrane seem to contribute to the relative impermeability of this barrier. Functionally, the blood-brain barrier acts as a selective filter and seems to protect the CNS by limiting the harmful substances that enter into the brain and spinal cord.

The blood-brain barrier obviously plays an important role in clinical pharmacotherapeutics. To exert their effects, drugs targeted for the CNS must be able to pass from the bloodstream into the brain and spinal cord. In general, nonpolar, lipid-soluble drugs are able to cross the blood-brain barrier by passive diffusion. Polar and lipophobic compounds are usually unable to enter the brain. Some exceptions occur because of the presence of carrier-mediated transport systems in the blood-brain barrier. Some substances (such as glucose) are transported via facilitated diffusion, while other compounds (including some drugs) may be able to enter the brain by active transport. However, the transport processes that carry drugs into the brain are limited to certain specific compounds, and the typical manner by which most drugs enter the brain is by passive lipid diffusion.

Several active transport systems also exist on the blood-brain barrier that are responsible for *removing* drugs and toxins from the brain. That is, certain drugs can enter the brain easily via diffusion or another process, but these drugs are then rapidly and efficiently transported out of the brain and back into the systemic circulation. This effect creates an obvious problem because these drugs will not reach therapeutic levels within the CNS, and won't be beneficial. Hence, the blood-brain barrier has many structural and functional characteristics that influence CNS drugs, and researchers continue to explore ways that these characteristics can be modified to ensure adequate drug delivery to the brain and spinal cord.

CNS Neurotransmitters

The majority of neural connections in the human brain and spinal cord are characterized as chemical synapses. The term *chemical synapse* indicates that a chemical neurotransmitter is used to propagate the nervous impulse across the gap that exists between two neurons. Several distinct chemicals have been identified as neurotransmitters within the brain and spinal cord. Groups of neurons within the CNS tend to use one of these neurotransmitters to produce either excitation or inhibition of the other neurons. Although each neurotransmitter can be generally described as either excitatory or inhibitory within the CNS, some transmitters may have different effects depending on the nature of the postsynaptic receptor involved. The interaction of the transmitter and the receptor dictates the effect on the postsynaptic neuron. The fact that several distinct neurotransmitters exist and that neurons using specific transmitters are organized functionally within the CNS has important pharmacologic implications. Certain drugs may alter the transmission in pathways using a specific neurotransmitter while having little or no effect on other transmitter pathways. This allows the drug to exert a rather specific effect on the CNS, so many disorders may be rectified without radically altering other CNS functions. Other drugs may have a much more general effect and may alter transmission in many CNS regions. To provide an indication of neurotransmitter function, the major categories of CNS neurotransmitters and their general locations and effects are discussed subsequently.

Acetylcholine

Acetylcholine is the neurotransmitter found in many areas of the brain as well as in the periphery (skeletal neuromuscular junction, some autonomic synapses). In the brain, acetylcholine is abundant in the cerebral cortex, and seems to play a critical role in cognition and memory. Neurons originating in the large pyramidal cells of the motor cortex and many neurons originating in the basal ganglia also secrete acetylcholine from their terminal axons. In general, acetylcholine synapses in the CNS are excitatory in nature.

Monoamines

Monoamines are a group of structurally similar CNS neurotransmitters that include the *catecholamines* (dopamine, norepinephrine) and 5-hydroxytryptamine (serotonin). *Dopamine* exerts different effects at various locations within the brain. Within the basal ganglia, dopamine is secreted by neurons that originate in the substantia nigra and project to the corpus striatum. As such, it is important in regulating motor control, and the loss of these dopaminergic neurons results in symptoms commonly associated with Parkinson disease. Dopamine also influences mood and emotions, primarily via its presence in the hypothalamus and other structures within the limbic system. Although its effects within the brain are very complex, dopamine generally inhibits the neurons onto which it is released.

Norepinephrine is secreted by neurons that originate in the locus caeruleus of the pons and projects throughout the reticular formation. Norepinephrine is generally regarded as an inhibitory transmitter within the CNS, but the overall effect following activity of norepinephrine synapses is often general excitation of the brain, probably because norepinephrine directly inhibits other neurons that produce inhibition. This phenomenon of *disinhibition* causes excitation by removing the influence of inhibitory neurons.

Serotonin (also known as 5-hydroxytryptamine) is released by cells originating in the midline of the pons and brainstem and is projected to many different areas, including the dorsal horns of the spinal cord and the hypothalamus. Serotonin is considered to be a strong inhibitor in most areas of the CNS and is believed to be important in mediating the inhibition of painful stimuli. It is also involved in controlling many aspects of mood and behavior, and problems with serotonergic activity have been implicated in several psychiatric disorders, including depression and anxiety.

Amino Acids

Several amino acids, such as glycine and gamma-aminobutyric acid (GABA), are important inhibitory transmitters in the brain and spinal cord. Glycine seems to be the inhibitory transmitter used by certain interneurons located throughout the spinal cord, and this amino acid also causes inhibition in certain areas of the brain. Likewise, GABA is found throughout the CNS, and is believed to be the primary neurotransmitter used to cause inhibition at presynaptic and postsynaptic neurons in the brain and spinal cord. Other amino acids such as aspartate and glutamate have been found in high concentrations throughout the brain and spinal cord; these substances cause excitation of CNS neurons. These excitatory amino acids have received a great deal of attention lately because they may also produce neurotoxic effects when released in large amounts during CNS injury and certain neurologic disorders (epilepsy, amyotrophic lateral sclerosis, and so forth).

Peptides

Many peptides have already been established as CNS neurotransmitters. One peptide that is important from a pharmacologic standpoint is substance P, which is an excitatory transmitter that is involved in spinal cord pathways transmitting pain impulses. Increased activity at substance P synapses in the cord serves to mediate the transmission of painful sensations, and certain drugs such as the opioid analgesics may decrease activity at these synapses. Other peptides that have important pharmacologic implications include three families of compounds: the endorphins, enkephalins, and dynorphins. These peptides, also known as the endogenous opioids, are excitatory transmitters in certain brain synapses that inhibit painful sensations. Hence, endogenous opioids in the brain are able to decrease the central perception of pain. Finally, peptides such as galanin, leptin, neuropeptide Y, vasoactive intestinal polypeptide (VIP), and pituitary adenylate cyclase–activating polypeptide (PACAP) have been identified in various areas of the CNS. These and other peptides may affect various CNS functions, either by acting directly as neurotransmitters or by acting as cotransmitters moderating the effects of other neurotransmitters.

Other Transmitters

In addition to the well-known substances, other chemicals are continually being identified as potential CNS neurotransmitters. Recent evidence has implicated substances such as adenosine and adenosine triphosphate (ATP) as transmitters or modulators of neural transmission in specific areas of the brain and in the autonomic nervous system. Many other chemicals that are traditionally associated with functions outside the CNS are being identified as possible CNS transmitters, including histamine, nitric oxide, and certain hormones (vasopressin, oxytocin). As the function of these chemicals and other new transmitters becomes clearer, the pharmacologic significance of drugs that affect these synapses will undoubtedly be considered.

CNS Drugs: General Mechanisms

The majority of CNS drugs work by modifying synaptic transmission in some way. Most drugs that attempt to rectify CNS-related disorders do so by either increasing or decreasing transmission at specific synapses. For instance, psychotic behavior has been associated with overactivity in central synapses that use dopamine as a neurotransmitter. Drug therapy in this situation consists of agents that decrease activity at central dopamine synapses. Conversely, Parkinson disease results from a decrease in activity at specific dopamine synapses. Antiparkinsonian drugs attempt to increase dopaminergic transmission at these synapses and bring synaptic activity back to normal levels. A drug that modifies synaptic transmission must somehow alter the quantity of the neurotransmitter that is released from the presynaptic terminal or affect the stimulation of postsynaptic receptors, or both. When considering a typical synapse, there are several distinct sites at which a drug may alter activity in the synapse. Specific ways a drug may modify synaptic transmission are presented here.

Presynaptic Action Potential

The arrival of an action potential at the presynaptic terminal initiates neurotransmitter release. Certain drugs, such as local anesthetics, block propagation along neural axons so that the action potential

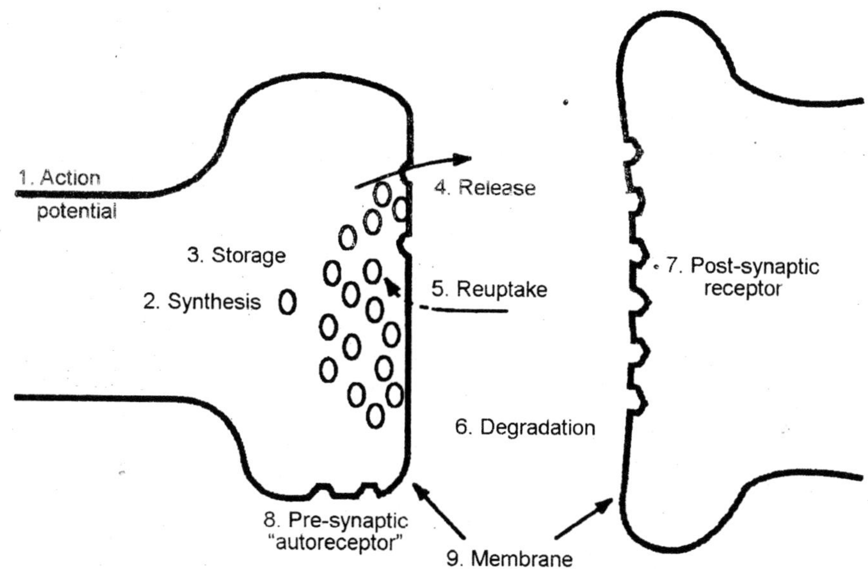

Fig. 17.1. Sites at which drugs can alter transmission at a CNS synapse.

fails to reach the presynaptic terminal, which effectively eliminates activity at that particular synapse. Also, the amount of depolarization or the height of the action potential arriving at the presynaptic terminal is directly related to the amount of transmitter released.

Any drug or endogenous chemical that limits the amount of depolarization occurring in the presynaptic terminal will inhibit the synapse because less neurotransmitter is released. In certain situations, this is referred to as *presynaptic inhibition*, because the site of this effect is at the presynaptic terminal. The endogenous neurotransmitter GABA is believed to exert some of its inhibitory effects via this mechanism.

Synthesis of Neurotransmitter

Drugs that block the synthesis of neurotransmitter will eventually deplete the presynaptic terminal and impair transmission. For example, metyrosine (Demser) inhibits an enzyme that is essential for catecholamine biosynthesis in the presynaptic terminal. Treatment with metyrosine results in decreased synthesis of transmitters such as dopamine and norepinephrine.

Storage of Neurotransmitter

A certain amount of chemical transmitter is stored in presynaptic vesicles. Drugs that impair this storage will decrease the ability of the synapse to continue to transmit information for extended periods. An example of this is the antihypertensive drug reserpine (Serpalan, Serpasil), which impairs the ability of adrenergic terminals to sequester and store norepinephrine in presynaptic vesicles.

Release

Certain drugs will increase synaptic activity by directly increasing the release of neurotransmitter from the presynaptic terminal. Amphetamines appear to exert their effects on the CNS primarily by increasing the presynaptic release of catecholamine neurotransmitters (e.g., norepinephrine). Conversely, other compounds may inhibit the synapse by directly decreasing the amount of transmitter released during each action potential. An example is botulinum toxin (Botox), which can be used as a skeletal muscle relaxant because of its ability to impair the release of acetylcholine from the skeletal neuromuscular junction.

Reuptake

After the neurotransmitter is released, some chemical synapses terminate activity primarily by transmitter reuptake. Reuptake involves the movement of the transmitter molecule back into the presynaptic terminal. A drug that impairs the reuptake of transmitter allows more of it to remain in the synaptic cleft and continue to exert an effect. Consequently, blocking reuptake actually increases activity at the synapse. For instance, tricyclic antidepressants impair the reuptake mechanism that pumps amine neurotransmitters back into the presynaptic terminal, which allows the transmitter to continue to exert its effect and prolong activity at the synapse.

Degradation

Some synapses rely primarily on the enzymatic breakdown of the released transmitter to terminate synaptic activity. Inhibition of the enzyme responsible for terminating the transmitter allows more of the active transmitter to remain in the synaptic cleft, thereby increasing activity at the synapse. An example is using a drug that inhibits the *cholinesterase* enzyme as a method of treating myasthenia gravis. In myasthenia gravis, there is a functional decrease in activity at the skeletal neuromuscular junction. Anticholinesterase drugs such as neostigmine (Prostigmin) and pyridostigmine (Mestinon) inhibit acetylcholine breakdown, allowing more of the released neurotransmitter to continue to exert an effect at the neuromuscular synapse.

Postsynaptic Receptor

Chemical antagonists can be used to block the postsynaptic receptor, thus decreasing synaptic transmission. The best-known example of this is the use of beta blockers. These agents are antagonists that are specific for the beta-adrenergic receptors on the myocardium, and they are frequently used to treat hypertension, cardiac arrhythmias, and angina pectoris. Other drugs may improve synaptic transmission by affecting the receptor directly so there is a tendency for increased neurotransmitter binding or improved receptor–effector coupling, or both. For instance, benzodiazepines (e.g., diazepam [Valium], chlordiazepoxide [Librium, others]) appear to enhance the postsynaptic effects of the inhibitory neurotransmitter GABA.

Presynaptic Autoreceptors

In addition to postsynaptic receptors, there are also receptors on the presynaptic terminal of some types of chemical synapses. These presynaptic receptors seem to serve as a method of negative feedback in controlling neurotransmitter release. During high levels of synaptic activity, the accumulation of neurotransmitter in the synaptic cleft may allow binding to the presynaptic receptors and limit further release of chemical transmitter. Certain drugs may also be able to attenuate synaptic activity through presynaptic autoreceptors. For instance, clonidine (Catapres), may exert some of its antihypertensive effects by binding to presynaptic receptors on sympathetic postganglionic neurons and impairing the release of norepinephrine onto the peripheral vasculature. The use of drugs that alter synaptic activity by binding to these autoreceptors is still somewhat new, however, and the full potential for this area of pharmacology remains to be determined.

Membrane Effects

Drugs may alter synaptic transmission by affecting membrane organization and fluidity. Membrane fluidity is basically the amount of flexibility or mobility of the lipid bilayer. Drugs that alter the fluidity of the presynaptic membrane could affect the way that presynaptic vesicles fuse with and release their neurotransmitter. Drug-induced changes in the postsynaptic membrane would affect the receptor environment and thereby alter receptor function. Membrane modification will result in either increased or decreased synaptic transmission, depending on the drug in question and the type and magnitude of membrane change. Alcohol (ethanol) and general anesthetics were originally thought to exert their effects by producing reversible changes in the fluidity and organization of the cell membranes of central neurons. Although this idea has been challenged somewhat, these drugs may still exert some of their effects via neuronal membranes. A CNS drug does not have to adhere specifically to only one of these methods of synaptic modification. Some drugs may affect the synapse in two or more ways. For example, the antihypertensive agent guanethidine (Ismelin) impairs both presynaptic storage and release of norepinephrine. Other drugs such as barbiturates may affect both the presynaptic terminal and the postsynaptic receptor in CNS synapses.

SEDATIVE-HYPNOTIC AND ANTIANXIETY AGENTS

Drugs that are classified as sedative-hypnotics are used both to relax the patient and to promote sleep. As the name "*sedative*" implies, these drugs exert a calming effect and serve to pacify the patient. At higher doses, the same drug can produce drowsiness and initiate a relatively normal state of sleep (hypnosis). At still higher doses, some sedative-hypnotics (especially barbiturates) will eventually bring on a state of general anesthesia. Because of their general central nervous system (CNS)-depressant effects, some sedative- hypnotic drugs are also used for other functions such as treating epilepsy or producing muscle relaxation. However, the sleep-enhancing effects will be of concern here.

By producing sedation, many drugs will also decrease the level of anxiety in a patient. Of course, these anxiolytic properties often cause a decrease in the level of alertness in the individual. However, certain agents are available that can reduce anxiety without an overt sedative effect.

Sedative-hypnotic and antianxiety drugs are among the most commonly used drugs worldwide. For example, it is estimated that insomnia affects between 10 to 15 percent of the general population, and that pharmacological management can be helpful in promoting normal sleep. Moreover, people who are ill, or who have recently been relocated to a new environment (hospital, nursing home), will often have difficulty sleeping and might need some form of sedative-hypnotic agent. Likewise, a person who sustains an injury or illness will certainly have some apprehension concerning his or her welfare. If necessary, this apprehension can be controlled to some extent by using antianxiety drugs during the course of rehabilitation. Consequently, many patients receiving physical therapy and occupational therapy take sedative-hypnotic and antianxiety agents to help promote sleep and decrease anxiety; rehabilitation specialists should understand the basic pharmacology of these agents.

SEDATIVE-HYPNOTIC AGENTS

Sedative-hypnotics fall into two general categories: benzodiazepines and nonbenzodiazepines. At present, benzodiazepines are typically used to promote normal sedation and sleep, especially in relatively acute or short-term situations. These agents will be addressed first, followed by a description of the nonbenzodiazepine hypnotics.

Benzodiazepines

Benzodiazepines are a family of compounds that share the same basic chemical structure and pharmacological effects. Although the more famous members of this family are associated with treating anxiety (e.g., diazepam), several benzodiazepines are indicated specifically to promote sleep. These agents exert hypnotic effects similar to those of nonbenzodiazepines—such as the barbiturates—but benzodiazepines are generally regarded as safer because there is less of a chance for lethal overdose. Benzodiazepines, however, are not without their drawbacks, and they can cause residual effects the day after they are administered; prolonged use can also cause tolerance and physical dependence.

Mechanism of benzodiazepine effects

The benzodiazepines exert their effects by increasing the inhibitory effects at CNS synapses that use the neurotransmitter gamma-aminobutyric acid (GABA). These inhibitory synapses are associated with a membrane protein complex containing three primary components: (1) a binding site for GABA, (2) a binding site for benzodiazepines, and (3) an ion channel that is specific for chloride ions. GABA typically exerts its inhibitory effects by binding to its receptor site on this complex and by initiating an increase in chloride conductance through the channel. Increased chloride conductance facilitates chloride entry into the neuron and results in hyperpolarization, or a decreased ability to raise the neuron to its firing threshold. By binding to their own respective site on the complex, benzodiazepines potentiate the effects of GABA and increase the inhibition at these synapses.

Consequently, the presence of the GABA-benzodiazepine–chloride ion channel complex accounts for the specific mechanism of action of this class of sedative-hypnotics. By increasing the inhibitory effects at GABAergic synapses located in the reticular formation, benzodiazepines can decrease the level of arousal in the individual. In other words, the general excitation level in the reticular activating system decreases, and relaxation and sleep are enhanced.

Research has also indicated that there are at least three primary types of GABA receptors, and these receptors are classified as GABA A, B, and C according to their structural and functional characteristics. $GABA_A$ and $GABA_C$ receptors, for example, cause inhibition by increasing chloride entry, whereas $GABA_B$ receptors may cause inhibition by increasing potassium *exit* (efflux) from CNS neurons. At the present time, it appears that benzodiazepines act primarily on the $GABA_A$ subtype and that the therapeutic effects of these drugs (sedation, hypnosis, decreased anxiety) are mediated through the $GABA_A$ receptor, which is found in the brain. Hence, clinically used benzodiazepines are basically $GABA_A$ receptor agonists.

Furthermore, the $GABA_A$ receptor is composed of several subunits (alpha, beta, gamma); it appears that individual subunits on this receptor mediate specific effects. Sedation, for example, seems to be mediated by the alpha 1 subunit, whereas other beneficial effects such as decreased anxiety might be mediated by the alpha 2 and alpha 3 subunits. Benzodiazepines seem to affect all of these subunits, hence their ability to produce sedative and antianxiety effects.

These drugs, however, might also exert certain side effects (tolerance, dependence) by affecting other subunits on the $GABA_A$ receptor. A drug that is selective for only the alpha 1 subunit might exert sedative effects without producing as many side effects. Some of the newer nonbenzodiazepine drugs such as zolpidem (Ambien) and zaleplon (Sonata) appear to be more specific for the alpha 1 subunit, and might therefore produce sedative effects with fewer side effects.

Because of these new advances, scientists continue to study the molecular biology of the $GABA_A$ receptor, and clarify how benzodiazepines affect these receptors. Likewise, differences between the principal GABA receptors (A, B, C) has encouraged the development of drugs that are more selective to GABA receptors located in certain areas of the CNS. The muscle relaxant baclofen (Lioresal), for example, may be somewhat more selective for $GABA_B$ receptors in the spinal cord than for other $GABA_A$ or $GABA_C$ receptors that are found in the brain. Future drug development will continue to exploit the differences between the GABA receptor subtypes so that drugs are more selective and can produce more specific beneficial effects with fewer side effects.

Finally, the discovery of a CNS receptor that is specific for benzodiazepines has led to some interesting speculation as to the possible existence of some type of endogenous sedative-like agent. The presence of a certain type of receptor to indicate that the body produces an appropriate agonist for that receptor makes sense. For instance, the discovery of opiate receptors initiated the search for endogenous opiate-like substances, which culminated in the discovery of the enkephalins. It has been surmised that certain endogenous steroids such as allopregnanolone (a metabolic byproduct of progesterone) can bind to the GABA receptors in the CNS and produce sedative-hypnotic effects. Continued research in this area may someday reveal the exact role of steroids and other endogenous substances, and the focus of pharmacologic treatment can then be directed toward stimulating the release of endogenous sedative-hypnotic agents

Nonbenzodiazepines

Barbiturates

The barbiturates are a group of CNS depressants that share a common chemical origin: barbituric acid. The potent sedative-hypnotic properties of these drugs have been recognized for some time, and their status as the premier medication used to promote sleep went unchallenged for many years. However, barbiturates are associated with a relatively small therapeutic index; approximately 10 times the therapeutic dose can often be fatal. These drugs are also very addictive, and their prolonged use is often a problem in terms of drug abuse. Consequently, the lack of safety of the barbiturates and their strong potential for addiction and abuse necessitated the development of alternative nonbarbiturate drugs such as the benzodiazepines.

Despite their extensive use in the past, the exact mechanism of the barbiturates remains somewhat unclear. When used in sedative-hypnotic doses, barbiturates may function in a similar fashion to the benzodiazepines in that they also potentiate the inhibitory effects of GABA. This idea suggests that barbiturates may affect the GABA-benzodiazepine–chloride ion channel complex described above. Indeed, considerable evidence exists that barbiturates bind directly to the $GABA_A$ receptor at a site that is different from the binding site for GABA or benzodiazepines. Barbiturates may, however, also exert effects that are not mediated through an effect on the GABA-benzodiazepine–chloride ion channel. At higher doses, for instance, barbiturates may also directly increase the release of inhibitory transmitters such as glycine, and increase the release of excitatory transmitters such as glutamate. Regardless of their exact mechanism, barbiturates are effective sedative-hypnotics because of their specificity for neurons in the midbrain portion of the reticular formation as well as some limbic system structures. At higher doses, barbiturates also depress neuronal excitability in other areas of the brain and spinal cord.

Newer, nonbenzodiazepine sedative-hypnotics

Several drugs including zolpidem (Ambien) and zaleplon (Sonata) were developed recently as sedative-hypnotics. These drugs are chemically different from the benzodiazepines, but still seem to affect the $GABA_A$ receptors in the brain. That is, these newer drugs bind to the $GABA_A$ receptor, which then causes GABA to bind more effectively, thus increasing chloride conductance and the level of inhibition in the neuron. Increased inhibition in certain areas of the brain results in less arousal and the promotion of sleep. These newer drugs appear to be as effective as the benzodiazepines in promoting sleep. The drugs also seem to have a lower risk of producing certain side effects and causing problems when discontinued. This difference might be explained by the fact that newer, nonbenzodiazepine drugs bind preferentially to the alpha 1 subunit of the $GABA_A$ receptor. As discussed earlier, stimulation of this particular subunit seems to mediate sedation without producing other side effects. Hence, drugs like zolpidem and zaleplon are gaining acceptance for the treatment of sleep disorders, and efforts continue to develop other nonbenzodiazepine drugs that selectively affect this receptor.

Other Nonbenzodiazepines

Several other nonbenzodiazepine compounds can be prescribed for their sedative-hypnotic properties. These compounds are chemically dissimilar from one another, but share the ability to promote relaxation and sleep via depressing the CNS. Cyclic ethers and alcohols (including ethanol) can be included in this category, but their use specifically as sedative-hypnotics is fairly limited at present. The recreational use of ethanol in alcoholic beverages is an important topic in terms of abuse and long-term effects. However, since this area is much too extensive to be addressed here, only their effects as sedative-hypnotics is considered.

Alcohol (ethanol) and other sedative-hypnotics— neither benzodiazepine nor barbiturate in nature— work through mechanisms that are poorly understood. In the past, it was thought that alcohols exerted their CNS-depressant effects directly on neuronal membrane composition and fluidity. These and other highly lipid-soluble substances could simply dissolve in the lipid bilayer and inhibit neuronal excitability by temporarily disrupting membrane structures in the presynaptic and postsynaptic regions of CNS neurons. Recent evidence, however, suggests that alcohol may act on protein receptors much in the same way as the benzodiazepines and barbiturates. That is, alcohol may exert most of its effects by activating $GABA_A$ receptors and increasing GABA-mediated inhibition in the CNS. In any event, alcohol and similar agents bring about a decrease in neuronal transmission, which causes fairly widespread CNS depression which accounts for the subsequent sedative effects of such compounds.

Pharmacokinetics

Benzodiazepine and nonbenzodiazepine sedative-hypnotics are usually highly lipid soluble. They are typically administered orally and are absorbed easily and completely from the gastrointestinal tract. Distribution is fairly uniform throughout the body, and these drugs reach the CNS readily because of their high degree of lipid solubility. Sedative-hypnotics are metabolized primarily by the oxidative enzymes of the drug-metabolizing system in liver cells. Termination of their activity is accomplished either by hepatic enzymes or by storage of these drugs in non-CNS tissues; that is, by sequestering the drugs in adipose and other peripheral tissues, their CNS-depressant effects are not exhibited. However, when the drugs slowly leak out of their peripheral storage sites, they can be redistributed to the brain and can cause low levels of sedation. This occurrence may help explain the "hangoverlike" feelings that are frequently reported the day after taking sedative-hypnotic drugs. Finally, excretion of these drugs takes place through the kidney after their metabolism in the liver. As with most drug biotransformations, metabolism of sedative-hypnotics is essential in creating a polar metabolite that is readily excreted by the kidney.

Problems and Adverse Effects

Residual Effects

The primary problem associated with sedative- hypnotic use is the residual effects that can occur the day after administration. Individuals who take a sedative-hypnotic to sleep at night sometimes complain of drowsiness and decreased motor performance the next day. These hangoverlike effects may be caused by the drug being redistributed to the CNS from peripheral storage sites or may simply occur because the drug has not been fully metabolized.

Anterograde amnesia is another problem sometimes associated with sedative-hypnotic use. The patient may have trouble recalling details of events that occurred for a certain period of time before the drug was taken. Although usually a minor problem, this can become serious if the drug-induced amnesia exacerbates an already existing memory problem, as might occur in some elderly patients.

These residual problems can be resolved somewhat by taking a smaller dose or by using a drug with a shorter half-life. Also, newer nonbenzodiazepine agents such as zolpidem and zaleplon appear to have milder effects, perhaps because of their relatively short half-life and the limited duration of action. These newer drugs have therefore been advocated in people who are prone to residual effects (e.g., older adults), and people who need to use these drugs for an extended period of time.

Tolerance and Physical Dependence

Another potential problem with long-term sedative- hypnotic drug use is that prolonged administration may cause tolerance and physical dependence. *Drug tolerance* is the need to take more of a drug to exert the same effect. *Dependence* is described as the onset of withdrawal symptoms if drug administration is ceased. Although these problems were originally thought to be limited to barbiturates, benzodiazepines and other sedative-hypnotics are now recognized as also causing tolerance and dependence when taken continually for several weeks.

The manner and severity of withdrawal symptoms varies according to the type of drug and the extent of physical dependence. Withdrawal after short-term benzodiazepine use may be associated with problems such as sleep disturbances (i.e., so-called rebound insomnia). As discussed earlier, withdrawal effects seem to be milder with the newer nonbenzodiazepine agents (zolpidem and zaleplon). Newer agents, however, are not devoid of these problems and care should be taken with prolonged use, especially in people with psychiatric disorders or a history of substance abuse.

Consequently, the long-term use of these drugs should be avoided, and other nonpharmacologic methods of reducing stress and promoting relaxation (e.g., mental imagery, biofeedback) should be instituted before tolerance and physical dependence. If the sedative-hypnotic drug has been used for an extended period, tapering off the dosage rather than abruptly stopping it has been recommended as a safer way to terminate administration.

Other Side Effects

Other *side effects* such as gastrointestinal discomfort (nausea and vomiting), dry mouth, sore throat, and muscular incoordination have been reported, but these occur fairly infrequently and vary according to the exact drug used. Cardiovascular and respiratory depression may also occur, but these problems are dose-related and are usually not significant, except in cases of overdose.

ANTIANXIETY DRUGS

Anxiety can be described as a fear or apprehension over a situation or event that an individual feels is threatening. These events can range from a change in employment or family life to somewhat irrational phobias concerning everyday occurrences. Anxiety disorders can also be classified in several clinical categories including generalized anxiety disorder, social anxiety disorder, panic disorder, obsessive-compulsive disorder, and posttraumatic stress syndrome. Antianxiety drugs can help decrease the tension and nervousness associated with many of these syndromes until the situation is resolved or until the individual is counseled effectively in other methods of dealing with his or her anxiety. Many drugs—including sedative-hypnotics—have the ability to decrease anxiety levels, but this is usually at the expense of an increase in sedation. Frequently, alleviating anxiety without producing excessive sedation is desirable so that the individual can function at home, on the job, and so on. Consequently, certain drugs are available that have significant anxiolytic properties at doses that produce minimal sedation. Benzodiazepine drugs and other nonbenzodiazepine strategies for dealing with anxiety are discussed here.

Benzodiazepines

As discussed previously, because of their relative safety, the benzodiazepines are typically the front-line drugs used to treat many forms of anxiety. In terms of anxiolytic properties, diazepam (Valium) is the prototypical antianxiety benzodiazepine. The extensive use of this drug in treating nervousness and apprehension has made the trade name of this compound virtually synonymous with a decrease in tension and anxiety. When prescribed in anxiolytic dosages, diazepam and certain other benzodiazepines will decrease anxiety without major sedative effects. Some sedation, however, may occur even at anxiolytic dosages; these drugs can be used as sedative-hypnotics simply by increasing the dosage.

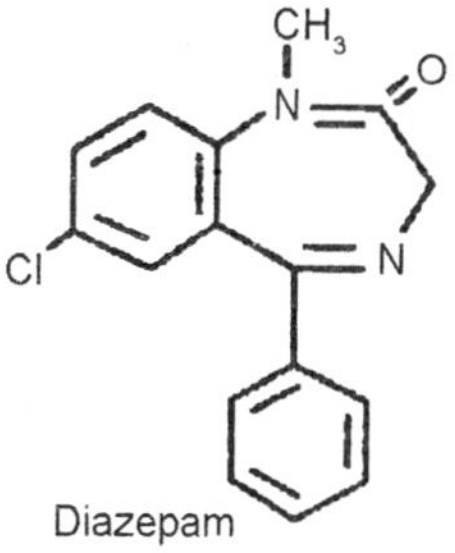

CH$_3$ N O Cl N

Diazepam

Fig. 17.2. Dizepam.

The mechanism of action of the benzodiazepines was discussed previously in this chapter. The antianxiety properties of these drugs involve a mechanism similar or identical to their sedative-hypnotic effects (i.e., potentiating GABAergic transmission). Benzodiazepines also seem to increase inhibition in the spinal cord, which produces some degree of skeletal muscle relaxation, which may contribute to their antianxiety effects by making the individual feel more relaxed.

Buspirone

Buspirone (BuSpar) is an antianxiety agent that was approved in 1986 for treating general anxiety disorder. This agent is not a benzodiazepine. It belongs instead to a drug class known as the azapirones. Therefore, buspirone does not act on the GABA receptor, but exerts its antianxiety effects by increasing the effects of 5-hydroxytryptamine (serotonin) in certain areas of the brain. Buspirone is basically a serotonin agonist that stimulates certain serotonin receptors, especially the 5-HT1A serotonin receptor subtype. This increase in serotonergic influence is beneficial in treating general anxiety disorder and possibly in panic disorder, obsessive-compulsive disorder, posttraumatic stress syndrome, and various other disorders that are influenced by CNS serotonin levels. More importantly, buspirone has a much better side-effect profile than traditional antianxiety drugs. Buspirone seems to produce less sedation and psychomotor impairment than benzodiazepine agents. There is a much smaller risk of developing tolerance and dependence to buspirone and the potential for abuse is much lower than with other anxiolytics. Buspirone has only moderate efficacy, however, and this drug may not take effect as quickly in patients with severe anxiety. Nonetheless, buspirone offers a safer alternative to traditional antianxiety drugs such as benzodiazepines, especially if patients need to receive treatment for an extended period of time. Development of additional azapirones and other drugs that influence serotonin activity may continue to provide better and safer antianxiety agents in the future.

Use of Antidepressants in Anxiety

Many patients with anxiety also have symptoms of depression. It therefore seems reasonable to include antidepressant drugs as part of the pharmacological regimen in these patients. Hence, patients with a combination of anxiety and depression often take a traditional antianxiety agent such as a benzodiazepine along with an antidepressant. Antidepressant drugs, however, might have direct anxiolytic effects. That is, certain antidepressants such as paroxetine (Paxil) or venlafaxine (Effexor) can help reduce anxiety independent of their effects on depression. These antidepressants have therefore been advocated as an alternative treatment for anxiety, especially for people who cannot tolerate the side effects of traditional anxiolytics, or who might be especially susceptible to the addictive properties of drugs like the benzodiazepines. Moreover, antidepressants such as paroxetine or venlafaxine are now considered effective as the primary treatment for several forms of anxiety, including generalized anxiety disorder, social phobia, and panic disorder. Antidepressants, either used alone or in combination with antianxiety drugs, have become an important component in the treatment of anxiety.

Other Antianxiety Drugs

The ideal antianxiety agent is nonaddictive, safe (i.e., relatively free from harmful side effects and potential for lethal overdose), and not associated with any sedative properties. Drugs such as meprobamate (Miltown) and barbiturates are not currently used to any great extent because they do not meet any of these criteria and are no more effective in reducing anxiety than benzodiazepines. As indicated earlier, buspirone and certain antidepressants currently offer an effective and somewhat safer method of treating anxiety, and the use of these agents has increased dramatically in recent years. Another option includes the beta-adrenergic antagonists (beta blockers) because these drugs can decrease situational anxiety without producing sedation. In particular, beta blockers such as propranolol (Inderal) have been used by musicians and other performing artists to decrease cardiac palpitations, muscle tremors, hyperventilation, and other manifestations of anxiety that tend to occur before an important performance. Beta blockers probably exert their antianxiety effects through their ability to decrease activity in the sympathetic nervous system, that is, through their sympatholytic effects. These drugs may exert both peripheral sympatholytic effects (e.g., blockade of myocardial beta-1 receptors) as well as decreasing central sympathetic tone. In any event, beta blockers may offer a suitable alternative to decrease the effects of nervousness without a concomitant decrease in levels of alertness or motivation. Again, these drugs have gained popularity with performing artists as a way to blunt the symptoms of performance anxiety without actually diminishing the anticipation and excitement that is requisite for a strong performance.

Problems and Adverse Effects

Most of the problems that occur with benzodiazepine anxiolytic drugs are similar to those mentioned regarding the use of these agents as sedative-hypnotics. Sedation is still the most common side effect of anxiolytic benzodiazepines, even though this effect is not as pronounced as with their sedative-hypnotic counterparts. Still, even short-term use of these drugs can produce psychomotor impairment, especially during activities that require people to remain especially alert, such as driving a car. Addiction and abuse are problems with chronic benzodiazepine use, and withdrawal from these drugs can be a serious problem. Also, anxiety can return to, or exceed, pretreatment levels when benzodiazepines are suddenly discontinued, a problem known as rebound anxiety. The fact that chronic benzodiazepine use can cause these problems reinforces the idea that these drugs are not curative and should be used only for limited periods of time as an adjunct to other nonpharmacologic procedures such as psychologic counseling. Problems and side effects associated with buspirone include dizziness, headache, nausea, and restlessness. Antidepressants such as paroxetine and venlafaxine also produce a number of side effects depending on the specific agent. Nonetheless, these newer, nonbenzodiazepine anxiolytics tend to produce less sedation, and their potential for addiction is lower compared to benzodiazepines. Hence, nonbenzodiazepine drugs might be an attractive alternative, especially in patients who are prone to sedation (e.g., older adults), patients with a history of substance abuse, or people who need chronic anxiolytic treatment.

Special Consideration of Sedative-Hypnotic and Antianxiety Agents in Rehabilitation

Although these drugs are not used to directly influence the rehabilitation of musculoskeletal or other somatic disorders, the prevalence of their use in patient populations is high. Any time a patient is hospitalized for treatment of a disorder, a substantial amount of apprehension and concern exists. The foreign environment of the institution as well as a change in the individual's daily routine can understandably result in sleep disturbances. Likewise, older adults often have trouble sleeping, and the use of sedative- hypnotic agents is common, especially in patients living in nursing homes or other facilities. Individuals who are involved in rehabilitation programs, both as inpatients and as outpatients, may also have a fairly high level of anxiety because of concern about their health and ability to resume normal functioning. Acute and chronic illnesses can create uncertainty about a patient's future family and job obligations as well as doubts about his or her self- image. The tension and anxiety produced may necessitate pharmacologic management.

The administration of sedative-hypnotic and antianxiety drugs has several direct implications for the rehabilitation session. Obviously the patient will be much calmer and more relaxed after taking an antianxiety drug, thus offering the potential benefit of gaining the patient's full cooperation during a physical or occupational therapy treatment. Anxiolytic benzodiazepines, for example, reach peak blood levels 2 to 4 hours after oral administration, so scheduling the rehabilitation session during that time may improve the patient's participation in treatment. Of course, this rationale will backfire if the drug produces significant hypnotic effects. Therapy sessions that require the patient to actively participate in activities such as gait training or therapeutic exercise will be essentially useless and even hazardous if the patient is extremely drowsy. Consequently, scheduling patients for certain types of rehabilitation within several hours after administration of sedative-hypnotics or sedative-like anxiolytics is counter-productive and should be avoided.

Finally, benzodiazepines and other drugs used to treat sleep disorders and anxiety are often associated with falls and subsequent trauma including hip fractures, especially in older adults. The risk of falls is greater in people who have a history of doing so or who have other problems that would predispose them to falling (vestibular disorders, impaired vision, and so forth). Therapists can identify such people and intervene to help prevent this through balance training, environmental modifications (removing cluttered furniture, throw rugs, and so forth), and similar activities. Therapists can help plan and implement nonpharmacological interventions to help decrease anxiety and improve sleep. Interventions such as regular physical activity, massage, and various relaxation techniques may be very helpful in reducing stress levels and promoting normal sleep. Therapists can therefore help substitute non-pharmacological methods for traditional sedative-hypnotic and antianxiety drugs, thus improving the patient's quality of life by avoiding drug-related side effects.

Sedative-hypnotic and antianxiety drugs play a prominent role in today's society. The normal pressures of daily life often result in tension and stress, which affects an individual's ability to relax or cope with stress. These problems are compounded when there is some type of illness or injury present. As would be expected, a number of patients seen in a rehabilitation setting are taking these drugs. Benzodiazepines have long been the premier agents used to treat sleep disorders and anxiety; they all share a common mechanism of action, and they potentiate the inhibitory effects of GABA in the CNS. With regard to their sedative-hypnotic effects, benzodiazepines such as flurazepam and triazolam are commonly used to promote sleep. Although these drugs are generally safer than their forerunners, they are not without their problems. Newer nonbenzodiazepine sedative-hypnotics such as zolpidem and zaleplon may also be effective in treating sleep disorders, and these newer agents may be somewhat safer than their benzodiazepine counterparts. Benzodiazepines such as diazepam (Valium) leave as are also used frequently to reduce anxiety, but the introduction of newer drugs such as buspirone and specific antidepressants (paroxetine, venlafaxine) have provided an effective but somewhat safer alternative for treating anxiety. Because of the potential for physical and psychologic dependence, sedative-hypnotic and antianxiety drugs should not be used indefinitely. These drugs should be prescribed judiciously as an adjunct to helping patients deal with the source of their problems.

18

Skeletal Muscle Relaxants

Skeletal muscle relaxants are used to treat conditions associated with hyperexcitable skeletal muscle—specifically, spasticity and muscle spasms. Although these two terms are often used interchangeably, spasticity and muscle spasms represent two distinct abnormalities. The use of relaxant drugs, however, is similar in each condition because the ultimate goal is to normalize muscle excitability without a profound decrease in muscle function. Considering the number of rehabilitation patients with muscle hyperexcitability that is associated with either spasm or spasticity, skeletal muscle relaxants represent an important class of drugs to the rehabilitation specialist.

Drugs discussed in this chapter are used to decrease muscle excitability and contraction via an effect at the spinal cord level, at the neuromuscular junction, or within the muscle cell itself. Some texts also classify neuromuscular junction blockers such as curare and succinylcholine as skeletal muscle relaxants. However, these drugs are more appropriately classified as skeletal muscle *paralytics* because they eliminate muscle contraction by blocking transmission at the myoneural synapse. This type of skeletal muscle paralysis is used primarily during general anesthesia. Skeletal muscle relaxants do not typically prevent muscle contraction; they only attempt to normalize muscle excitability to decrease pain and improve motor function.

Increased Muscle Tone: Spasticity Versus Muscle Spasms

Much confusion and consternation often arise from the erroneous use of the terms "spasticity" and "spasm." For the purpose of this text, these terms will be used to describe two different types of increased excitability, which result from different underlying pathologies. *Spasticity* occurs in many patients following an injury to the central nervous system (CNS), including cord-related problems (multiple sclerosis, spinal cord transection) and injuries to the brain (CVA, cerebral palsy, acquired brain injury). Although there is considerable controversy about the exact changes in motor control, most clinicians agree that spasticity is characterized primarily by an exaggerated muscle stretch reflex. This abnormal reflex activity is velocity-dependent, with a rapid lengthening of the muscle invoking a strong contraction in the stretched muscle.

The neurophysiologic mechanisms underlying spasticity are complex, but this phenomenon occurs when supraspinal inhibition or control is lost because of a lesion in the spinal cord or brain. Presumably, specific upper motor neuron lesions interrupt the cortical control of stretch reflex and alpha motor neuron excitability. Spasticity, therefore, is not in itself a disease but rather the motor sequela to pathologies such as cerebral vascular accident (CVA), cerebral palsy, multiple sclerosis (MS), and traumatic lesions to the brain and spinal cord (including quadriplegia and paraplegia).

Skeletal muscle *spasms* are used to describe the increased tension often seen in skeletal muscle after certain musculoskeletal injuries and inflammation (muscle strains, nerve root impingements, etc.) occur. This tension is involuntary, so the patient is unable to relax the muscle. Spasms differ from spasticity because spasms typically arise from an orthopedic injury to a musculoskeletal structure or peripheral nerve root rather than an injury to the CNS. Likewise, muscle spasms are often a continuous, tonic contraction of specific muscles rather than the velocity-dependent increase in stretch reflex activity commonly associated with spasticity. The exact reasons for muscle spasms are poorly understood. According to some authorities, muscle spasms occur because a vicious cycle is created when the initial injury causes muscular pain and spasm, which increases afferent nociceptive input to the spinal cord, further exciting the alpha motor neuron to cause more spasms, and so on. Other experts believe that muscle spasms occur because of a complex protective mechanism, whereby muscular contractions are intended to support an injured vertebral structure or peripheral joint. Regardless of the exact reason, tonic contraction of the affected muscle is often quite painful because of the buildup of pain-mediating metabolites (e.g., lactate). Consequently, various skeletal muscle relaxants attempt to decrease skeletal muscle excitation and contraction in cases of spasticity and spasm. Specific drugs and their mechanisms of action are discussed here.

Specific Agents Used to Produce Skeletal Muscle Relaxation

Skeletal muscle relaxants are categorized in this chapter according to their primary clinical application: agents used to decrease spasms and agents used to decrease spasticity. One agent, diazepam (Valium), is indicated for both conditions and will appear in both categories. Finally, the use of botulinum toxin (Botox) as an alternative strategy for reducing focal spasms or spasticity will be addressed.

Agents Used to Treat Muscle Spasms

Diazepam

The effects of diazepam (Valium) on the CNS and its use as an antianxiety drug are discussed in Chapter 6. Basically, diazepam and other benzodiazepines work by increasing the central inhibitory effects of gamma-aminobutyric acid (GABA); that is, diazepam binds to receptors located at GABAergic synapses and increases the GABA-induced inhibition at that synapse. Diazepam appears to work as a muscle relaxant through this mechanism, potentiating the inhibitory effect of GABA on alpha motor neuron activity in the spinal cord. The drug also exerts some supraspinal sedative effects; in fact, some of its muscle relaxant properties may derive from the drug's ability to produce a more generalized state of sedation.

Uses

Diazepam is one of the oldest medications for treating muscle spasms, and has been used extensively in treating spasms associated with musculoskeletal injuries such as acute low-back strains. Diazepam has also been used to control muscle spasms associated with tetanus toxin; the use of valium in this situation can be life-saving as well by inhibiting spasms of the larynx and other muscles.

Adverse effects

The primary side effect with diazepam is that dosages successful in relaxing skeletal muscle also produce sedation and a general reduction in psychomotor ability. However, this effect may not be a problem and may actually be advantageous for the patient recovering from an acute musculoskeletal injury. For example, a patient with an acute lumbosacral strain may benefit from the sedative properties because he or she will remain fairly inactive, thereby allowing better healing during the first few days after the injury. Continued use, however, may be problematic because of diazepam's sedative effects. The drug can also produce tolerance and physical dependence, and sudden withdrawal after prolonged use can cause seizures, anxiety, agitation, tachycardia, and even death. Likewise, an overdose with diazepam can result in coma or death as well. Hence, this drug might be beneficial for the short-term management of acute muscle spasms, but long-term use should be discouraged.

Polysynaptic Inhibitors

A variety of centrally acting compounds have been used in an attempt to enhance muscle relaxation and decrease muscle spasms. Some examples are carisoprodol (Soma, Vanadom), chlorphenesin carbamate (Maolate), chlorzoxazone (Paraflex, Parafon Forte, others), cyclobenzaprine (Flexeril), metaxalone (Skelaxin), methocarbamol (Carbacot, Robaxin, Skelex), and orphenadrine citrate (Antiflex, Norflex, others). The mechanism of action of these drugs is not well defined. Research in animals has suggested that these drugs may decrease polysynaptic reflex activity in the spinal cord, hence the term "*polysynaptic inhibitors.*" A polysynaptic reflex arc in the spinal cord is comprised of several small interneurons that link incoming (afferent) input into the dorsal horn with outgoing (efferent) outflow onto the alpha motor neuron. By inhibiting the neurons in the polysynaptic pathways, these drugs could decrease alpha motor neuron excitability and therefore cause relaxation of skeletal muscle.

It is not clear, however, exactly how these drugs inhibit neurons involved in the polysynaptic pathways. There is preliminary evidence that one of these compounds (cyclobenzaprine) might block serotonin receptors on spinal interneurons, thereby decreasing the excitatory influence of serotonin on alpha motor neuron activity. Although this effect has been attributed to cyclobenzaprine in animals (rats), the effect of this drug and other muscle relaxants in humans remains to be determined.

On the other hand, these compounds have a general depressant effect on the CNS; that is, they cause a global decrease in CNS excitability that results in generalized sedation. It therefore seems possible that some of their muscle relaxant effects are caused by their sedative powers rather than a selective effect on specific neuronal reflex pathways. This observation is not to say that they are ineffective, because clinical research has shown that these drugs can be superior to a placebo in producing subjective muscle relaxation. However, the specific ability of these drugs to relax skeletal muscle remains doubtful, and it is generally believed that their muscle relaxant properties are secondary to a nonspecific CNS sedation.

Uses

These drugs are typically used as adjuncts to rest and physical therapy for the short-term relief of muscle spasms associated with acute, painful musculoskeletal injuries. When used to treat spasms, these compounds are often given with a nonsteroidal anti-inflammatory agent (NSAIDs), or sometimes incorporated into the same tablet with an analgesic such as acetaminophen or aspirin. For instance, Norgesic is one of the brand names for orphenadrine combined with aspirin (and caffeine). Such combinations have been reported to be more effective than the individual components given separately.

Adverse effects

Because of their sedative properties, the primary side effects of these drugs are drowsiness and dizziness. A variety of additional adverse effects, including nausea, light-headedness, vertigo, ataxia, and headache, may occur depending on the patient and the specific drug administered. Cases of fatal overdose have also been documented for several of these drugs, including cyclobenzaprine and metaxolone. Long term or excessive use of these medications may also cause tolerance and physical dependence. In particular, carisoprodol should be used cautiously because this drug is metabolized in the body to form meprobamate, which is a controlled substance that has sedative/anxiolytic properties but is not used extensively because it has strong potential for abuse. Hence, use of carisoprodol represents a rather unique situation where the drug itself or its metabolic byproduct (meprobamate) can produce effects and side effects that lead to addiction and abuse, especially in people with a history of substance abuse. Likewise, discontinuing carisoprodol suddenly after long term use can lead to withdrawal symptoms such as anxiety, tremors, muscle twitching, and hallucinations. Consequently, polysynaptic inhibitors can help provide short-term relief for muscle spasms associated with certain musculoskeletal conditions, and they may work synergistically with physical therapy and other interventions during acute episodes of back pain, neck pain, and so forth. Nonetheless, they have some rather serious side effects and potential for abuse, and the long-term use of these drugs should be discouraged.

AGENTS USED TO TREAT SPASTICITY

The three agents traditionally used in the treatment of spasticity are baclofen, diazepam, and dantrolene sodium. Two newer agents, gabapentin and tizanidine, are also available for treating spasticity in various conditions. All of these agents are addressed below.

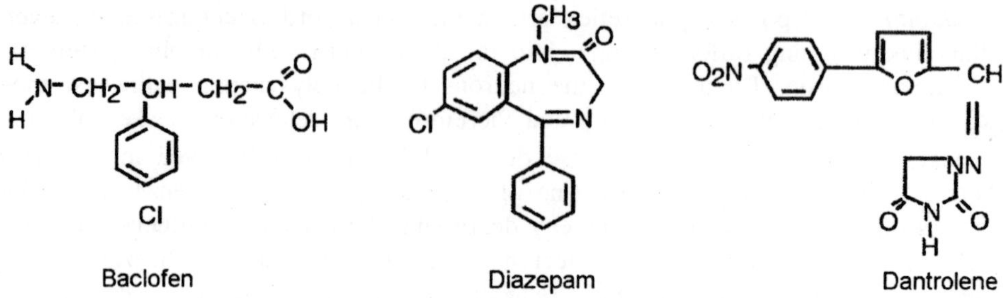

Fig. 18.1. Structure of three primary antispasticity drugs.

Baclofen

The chemical name of baclofen is beta (*p*-chlorophenyl)-GABA. As this name suggests, baclofen is a derivative of the central inhibitory neurotransmitter GABA. However, there appear to be some differences between baclofen and GABA. Baclofen seems to bind preferentially to certain GABA receptors, which have been classified as GABA$_b$ receptors (as opposed to GABA$_a$ receptors). Preferential binding to GABA$_b$ receptors enables baclofen to act as a GABA agonist, inhibiting transmission within the spinal cord at specific synapses. To put this in the context of its use as a muscle relaxant, baclofen appears to have an inhibitory effect on alpha motor neuron activity within the spinal cord. This inhibition apparently occurs via inhibiting excitatory neurons that synapse with the alpha motor neuron (presynaptic inhibition), as well as directly affecting the alpha motor neuron itself (postsynaptic inhibition). The result is decreased firing of the aipha motor neuron, with a subsequent relaxation of the skeletal muscle.

Uses

Baclofen is administered orally to treat spasticity associated with lesions of the spinal cord, including traumatic injuries resulting in paraplegia or quadriplegia and spinal cord demyelination resulting in MS. Baclofen is often the drug of choice in reducing the muscle spasticity associated with MS because it produces beneficial effects with a remarkable lack of adverse side effects when used in patients with MS. The drug also does not cause as much generalized muscle weakness as direct-acting relaxants such as dantrolene, which can be a major advantage of baclofen treatment in many patients with MS. Baclofen also appears to produce fewer side effects when used appropriately to reduce spasticity secondary to traumatic spinal cord lesions, thus providing a relatively safe and effective form of treatment. When administered systemically, baclofen is less effective in treating spasticity associated with supraspinal lesions (stroke, cerebral palsy), because these patients are more prone to the adverse side effects of this drug and beoause baclofen does not readily penetrate the blood-brain barrier.

Oral baclofen has also been used to reduce alcohol consumption in people who are chronic alcohol abusers. Apparently, relatively low doses of baclofen can reduce the cravings and desire for alcohol consumption via the effects of this drug on CNS GABA receptors. Future studies will help clarify the role of this drug in treating chronic alcoholism.

Adverse effects

When initiating baclofen therapy, the most common side effect is transient drowsiness, which usually disappears within a few days. When given to patients with spinal cord lesions, there are usually few other adverse effects. When given to patients who have had a CVA or to elderly individuals, there is sometimes a problem with confusion and hallucinations. Other side effects, occurring on an individual basis, include fatigue, nausea, dizziness, muscle weakness, and headache.

Abrupt discontinuation of baclofen may also cause withdrawal symptoms such as hyperthermia, hallucinations, and seizures. Increased seizure activity has also been reported following baclofen overdose, and in selected patient populations such as certain children with cerebral palsy and certain adults with multiple sclerosis.

Intrathecal Baclofen

Although baclofen is administered orally in most patients it can also be administered intrathecally in patients with severe, intractable spasticity. Intrathecal administration is the delivery of a drug directly into the subarachnoid space surrounding a specific level of the spinal cord. This places the drug very close to the spinal cord, thus allowing increased drug effectiveness with much smaller drug doses. Likewise, fewer systemic side effects occur because the drug tends to remain in the area of the cord rather than circulating in the bloodstream and causing adverse effects on other tissues.

When baclofen is administered intrathecally for the long-term treatment of spasticity, a small catheter is usually implanted surgically so that the open end of the catheter is located in the subarachnoid space and the other end is attached to some type of programmable pump. The pump is implanted subcutaneously in the abdominal wall and is adjusted to deliver the drug at a slow, continuous rate. The rate of infusion is adjusted over time to achieve the best clinical reduction in spasticity.

Intrathecal baclofen delivery using implantable pumps has been used in patients with spasticity of spinal origin (spinal cord injury, multiple sclerosis), and in patients with spasticity resulting from supraspinal (cerebral) injury, including cerebral palsy, CVA, and traumatic brain injury. Studies involving these patients have typically noted a substantial decrease in rigidity (as indicated by decreased Ashworth scores, decreased reflex activity, and so forth). Patient satisfaction is generally favorable, and caregivers for younger children report ease of care following implantation of intrathecal baclofen pumps. There is growing evidence that intrathecal baclofen can also reduce pain of central origin in people with spasticity; that is, continuous baclofen administration to the subarachnoid space may inhibit the neural circuitry that induces chronic pain in people with stroke and other CNS injuries.

Uses

Intrathecal baclofen can result in decreased spasticity and increased comfort in many people with severe spasticity. This intervention can also result in functional improvements, especially in cases where voluntary motor control was being masked by spasticity. Ambulatory patients with spasticity resulting from a CVA, for example, may be able to increase their walking speed and increase their functional mobility after intrathecal baclofen therapy.

These functional improvements, however, may not occur in all types of spasticity. Patients with severe spasticity of spinal origin, for example, may not experience improvements in mobility or decreased disability. If these patients do not have adequate voluntary motor function there is simply not enough residual motor ability to perform functional tasks after spasticity is reduced. Nonetheless, these patients may still benefit from intrathecal baclofen because of decreased rigidity and pain, which can result in improved self-care and the ability to perform daily living activities.

Adverse effects

Despite these benefits, intrathecal baclofen is associated with a number of potential complications. Primary among these is the possibility of a disruption in the delivery system; that is, a pump malfunction or a problem with the delivery catheter can occur. In particular, the catheter can become obstructed, or the tip of the catheter can become displaced so that baclofen is not delivered into the correct area of the subarachnoid space. Increased drug delivery due to a pump malfunction could cause overdose and lead to respiratory depression, decreased cardiac function, and coma. Conversely, abruptly stopping the drug due to pump failure, pump removal, or delivery catheter displacement/blockage may cause a withdrawal syndrome that includes fever, confusion, delirium, and seizures.

A second major concern is the possibility that tolerance could develop with long-term, continuous baclofen administration. Tolerance is the need for more of a drug to achieve its beneficial effects when used for prolonged periods. Several studies have reported that dosage must indeed be increased progressively when intrathecal baclofen systems are used for periods of several months to several years. Tolerance to intrathecal baclofen, however, can usually be dealt with by periodic adjustments in dosage, and tolerance does not usually develop to such an extent that intrathecal baclofen must be discontinued.

Hence, intrathecal baclofen offers a means of treating certain patients with severe spasticity who have not responded to more conventional means of treatment including oral baclofen. Additional research will help determine optimal ways that this intervention can be used to decrease spasticity. Further improvements in the technologic and mechanical aspects of intrathecal delivery, including better pumps and catheter systems, will also make this a safer and more practical method of treating these patients.

Dantrolene Sodium

The only muscle relaxant available that exerts its effect directly on the skeletal muscle cell is dantrolene sodium (Dantrium). This drug works by impairing the release of calcium from the sarcoplasmic reticulum within the muscle cell during excitation. In response to an action potential, the release of calcium from sarcoplasmic storage sites initiates myofilament cross-bridging and subsequent muscle contraction. By inhibiting this release, dantrolene attenuates muscle contraction and therefore enhances relaxation.

Uses

Dantrolene is often effective in treating severe spasticity, regardless of the underlying pathology. Patients with traumatic cord lesions, advanced MS, cerebral palsy, or CVAs will probably experience a reduction in spasticity with this drug. This drug is also invaluable in treating malignant hyperthermia, which is a potentially life-threatening reaction occurring in susceptible individuals following exposure to general anesthesia, muscle paralytics used during surgery, or certain antipsychotic medications (a condition also called neuroleptic malignant syndrome). In this situation, dantrolene inhibits skeletal muscle contraction throughout the body, thereby limiting the rise in body temperature generated by strong, repetitive skeletal muscle contractions. Dantrolene is not prescribed to treat muscle spasms caused by musculoskeletal injury.

Adverse effects

The most common side effect of dantrolene is generalized muscle weakness; this makes sense considering that dantrolene impairs sarcoplasmic calcium release in skeletal muscles throughout the body, not just in the hyperexcitable tissues. Thus, the use of dantrolene is sometimes counterproductive because the increased motor function that occurs when spasticity is reduced may be offset by generalized motor weakness. This drug may also cause severe hepatotoxicity, and cases of fatal hepatitis have been reported. The risk of toxic effects on the liver seems to be greater in women over 40 years of age, and in individuals receiving higher doses of this drug (over 300 mg). Other, less serious sid effects that sometimes occur during the first few days of therapy include drowsiness, dizziness, nausea, and diarrhea, but these problems are usually transient.

Diazepam

As indicated earlier, diazepam is effective in reducing spasticity as well as muscle spasms because this drug increases the inhibitory effects of GABA in the CNS.

Uses

Diazepam is used in patients with spasticity resulting from cord lesions and is sometimes effective in patients with cerebral palsy.

Adverse effects

Use of diazepam as an antispasticity agent is limited by the sedative effects of this medication; that is, patients with spasticity who do not want a decrease in mental alertness will not tolerate diazepam therapy very well. Extended use of the drug can cause tolerance and physical dependence, and use of diazepam for the long-term treatment of spasticity should be avoided whenever possible.

Gabapentin

Developed originally as an antiseizure drug, gabapentin (Neurontin) has also shown some promise in treating spasticity. This drug appears to cause inhibition in the spinal cord in a manner similar to GABA, but the exact mechanism of this drug remains to be determined. That is, gabapentin does not appear to bind to the same receptors as GABA, and this drug does not appear to directly increase the release or effects of endogenous GABA. Nonetheless, gabapentin may decrease spasticity by raising the overall level of inhibition in the spinal cord, thereby decreasing excitation of the alpha motor neuron with subsequent skeletal muscle relaxation. The exact way that this drug exerts its antispasticity effects, however, remains to be determined.

Uses

Gabapentin is effective in decreasing the spasticity associated with spinal cord injury 102 and multiple sclerosis. Additional research should clarify how this drug can be used alone or with other agents to provide optimal benefits in spasticity resulting from various spinal, and possibly cerebral, injuries.

Adverse effects

The primary side effects of this drug are sedation, fatigue, dizziness, and ataxia.

Tizanidine

Tizanidine (Zanaflex) is classified as an alpha-2 adrenergic agonist, meaning that this drug binds selectively to the alpha-2 receptors in the CNS and stimulates them. Alpha-2 receptors are found at various locations in the brain and spinal cord, including the presynaptic and postsynaptic membranes of spinal interneurons that control alpha motor neuron excitability. Stimulation of these alpha-2 receptors inhibits the firing of interneurons that relay information to the alpha motor neuron; that is, interneurons that comprise polysynaptic reflex arcs within the spinal cord. Tizanidine appears to bind to receptors on spinal interneurons, decrease the release of excitatory neurotransmitters from their presynaptic terminals (presynaptic inhibition), and decrease the excitability of the postsynaptic neuron (postsynaptic inhibition). Inhibition of spinal interneurons results in decreased excitatory input onto the alpha motor neuron, with a subsequent decrease in spasticity of the skeletal muscle supplied by that neuron.

Uses

Tizanidine has been used primarily to control spasticity resulting from spinal lesions (multiple sclerosis, spinal cord injury), and this drug may also be effective in treating spasticity in people with cerebral lesions (CVA, acquired brain injury). There is some concern, however, that tizanidine might slow neuronal recovery following brain injury, and some practitioners are therefore reluctant to use this drug during the acute phase of stroke or traumatic brain injury. Because it may inhibit pain pathways in the spinal cord, tizanidine has also been used to treat chronic headaches and other types of chronic pain (fibromyalgia, chronic regional pain syndromes, and so forth).

As an antispasticity drug, tizanidine appears to be as effective as orally administered baclofen or diazepam, but tizanidine generally has milder side effects and produces less generalized muscle weakness than these other agents. Tizanidine is also superior to other alpha-2 agonists such as clonidine (Catapres) because tizanidine does not cause as much hypotension and other cardiovascular side effects. Clonidine exerts antispasticity as well as antihypertensive effects because this drug stimulates alpha-2 receptors in the cord and brainstem, respectively. Use of clonidine in treating spasticity, however, is limited because of the cardiovascular side effects, and clonidine is used primarily for treating hypertension.

Adverse effects

The most common side effects associated with tizanidine include sedation, dizziness, and dry mouth. As indicated, however, tizanidine tends to have a more favorable side effect profile than other alpha-2 agonists, and this drug produces less generalized weakness than oral baclofen or diazepam. Tizanidine may therefore be a better alternative to these other agents in patients who need to reduce spasticity while maintaining adequate muscle strength for ambulation, transfers, and so forth.

Use of Botulinum Toxin as a Muscle Relaxant

Injection of botulinum toxin is a rather innovative way to control localized muscle hyperexcitability. Botulinum toxin is a purified version of the toxin that causes botulism. Systemic doses of this toxin can be extremely dangerous or fatal because botulinum toxin inhibits the release of acetylcholine from presynaptic terminals at the skeletal neuromuscular junction. Loss of presynaptic acetylcholine release results in paralysis of the muscle fiber supplied by that terminal. Systemic dissemination of botulinum toxin can therefore cause widespread paralysis, including loss of respiratory muscle function. Injection into specific muscles, however, can sequester the toxin within these muscles, thus producing localized effects that are beneficial in certain forms of muscle hyperexcitability.

Mechanism of Action

The cellular actions of botulinum toxin at the neuromuscular junction have recently been clarified. This toxin is attracted to glycoproteins located on the surface of the presynaptic terminal at the skeletal neuromuscular junction. Once attached to the membrane, the toxin enters the presynaptic terminal and inhibits proteins that are needed for acetylcholine release. Normally, certain proteins help fuse presynaptic vesicles with the inner surface of the presynaptic terminal, thereby allowing the vesicles to release acetylcholine via exocytosis. Botulinum toxin cleaves and destroys these fusion proteins, thus making it impossible for the neuron to release acetylcholine into the synaptic cleft. Local injection of botulinum toxin into specific muscles will therefore decrease muscle excitation by disrupting synaptic transmission at the neuromuscular junction. The affected muscle will invariably undergo some degree of paresis and subsequent relaxation because the toxin prevents the release of acetylcholine.

It has been suggested that botulinum toxin might have other effects on neuronal excitability. This toxin, for example, might also inhibit contraction of intrafusal muscle fibers that are located within skeletal muscle, and help control sensitivity of the stretch reflex. Inhibiting these intrafusal fibers would diminish activity in the afferent limb of the stretch reflex, thereby contributing to the antispasticity effects of this intervention. Through its direct action on muscle excitability, botulinum toxin may also have other neuro-physiological effects at the spinal cord level. That is, reducing spasticity might result in complex neurophysiologic changes at the spinal cord, ultimately resulting in more normal control of

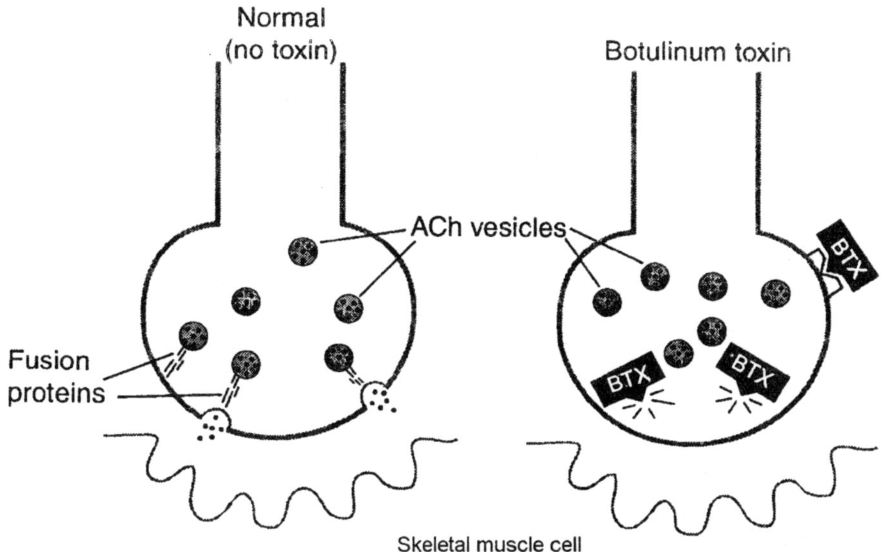

Fig. 18.2. Mechanism of action of botulinum toxin at the skeletal neuromuscular junction.

motor function in both the injected muscle and its antagonist. In other words, reduction of excessive afferent discharge from the spastic muscle might help reestablish a more reasonable level of excitation at the cord level, thus improving efferent discharge to the injected muscle and its antagonist. More research will be needed to help clarify how local administration of botulinum toxin can have direct effects on the injected muscle as well as reflex neurophysiological effects on the spinal cord.

Clinical Use of Botulinum Toxin

Seven strains (serotypes) of botulinum toxin have been identified, but only two types are currently available for clinical use: botulinum toxin types A and B. These types differ somewhat in their chemistry, duration of action, and so forth. The most commonly used therapeutic type is botulinum toxin type A; this agent is marketed commercially under trade names such as Botox and Dysport. Botulinum toxin type B (Myobloc) is also available, and can be useful in patients who develop immunity to the type A form of this toxin.

Botulinum toxin has been used for some time to control localized muscle dystonias, including conditions such as spasmodic torticollis, blepharospasm, laryngeal dystonia, strabismus, and several other types of focal dystonias. When used therapeutically, small amounts of this toxin are injected directly into the dystonic muscles, which begin to relax within a few days to 1 week. This technique appears to be fairly safe and effective in many patients, but relief may only be temporary. Symptoms often return within 3 months after each injection, necessitating additional treatments. Still, this technique represents a method for treating patients with severe, incapacitating conditions marked by focal dystonias and spasms.

More recently, there has been considerable interest in using botulinum toxin to reduce spasticity in specific muscles or muscle groups. This treatment has been used to treat spasticity resulting from various disorders including cerebral palsy, traumatic brain injury, CVA, and spinal cord injury. As with treatment of focal dystonias, the toxin is injected directly into selected muscles. If necessary, electromyography or ultrasonography can be used to identify specific muscles and guide the injection to the desired site within the muscle belly (e.g., the motor point of the muscle). There is also some evidence that electrical stimulation of the nerve supplying the muscle for the first few days following injection may help increase the efficacy of the toxin, presumably by enhancing its uptake by the presynaptic nerve terminals.

Botulinum toxin injection has been documented as a means to control severe spasticity in various clinical situations. This intervention, for example, can help remove spastic dominance in certain patients so that volitional motor function can be facilitated. For example, judicious administration of botulinum toxin can result in improved gait and other functional activities in selected patients with cerebral palsy, stroke, or traumatic brain injury. Even if voluntary motor function is not improved dramatically, reducing spasticity in severely affected muscles may produce other musculoskeletal benefits. For example, injection of botulinum toxin can reduce spasticity so that muscles can be stretched or casted more effectively, thus helping to prevent joint contractures and decreasing the need for surgical procedures such as heel-cord lengthening and adductor release.

These injections can likewise enable patients to wear and use orthotic devices more effectively. Injection into the triceps surae musculature can improve the fit and function of an ankle-foot orthosis by preventing excessive plantar flexor spasticity from "pistoning" the foot out of the orthosis. Injections into severely spastic muscles can also increase patient comfort and ability to perform ADL and hygiene activities. Consider, for example, the patient with severe upper extremity flexor spasticity following a CVA. Local injection of botulinum toxin into the affected muscles may enable the patient to extend his or her elbow, wrist, and fingers, thereby allowing better hand cleansing, ability to dress, decreased pain, and so forth.

Finally, local botulinum toxin administration has been advocated as a way to control muscle hyperexcitability in other clinical situations. There has, of course, been considerable interest in using this toxin for cosmetic reasons. Injection of botulinum toxin into specific facial muscles can paralyze these muscles, thereby reducing the appearance of wrinkles around the eyes, mouth, and so forth. Nonetheless, patients undergoing physical rehabilitation may also benefit from uses of this toxin. For example, patients with hyperactive (neurogenic) bladder following spinal cord injury can be treated by injecting botulinum toxin directly into the bladder detrussor muscle or external urethral sphincter. This intervention may help normalize bladder function and promote more effective voiding. Botulinum toxin has also been used to treat patients with chronic pain syndromes, including chronic headache, migraine, and various musculoskeletal disorders (back pain, whiplash injuries, and so forth). Clearly, this intervention has many potential benefits in many different clinical situations, and additional research will be needed to document how botulinum toxin can be used to reduce muscle hyperexcitability and improve function in various patient populations.

Limitations and Side Effects

Botulinum toxin does not cure spasticity and there are a number of limitations to its use. In particular, only a limited number of muscles can be injected during a given treatment because only a limited amount of botulinum toxin can be administered during each set of injections. For example, the total amount of botulinum toxin type A injected during each treatment session is typically between 200–300 units in adults, with proportionally smaller amounts used in children depending on his or her size and age. The typical dose of the type B form is 2500–5000 units. Exceeding these doses will cause an immune response whereby antibodies are synthesized against the toxin, making subsequent treatments ineffective because the patient's immune system will recognize and inactivate the toxin. The number of muscles that can be injected is therefore often limited to one or two muscle groups; for example, the elbow and wrist flexors in one upper extremity of an adult, or the bilateral triceps surae musculature of a child.

As indicated earlier, the relaxant effects of the toxin are likewise temporary, and these effects typically diminish within 2 to 3 months after injection. The effects apparently wear off because a new presynaptic terminal "sprouts" from the axon that contains the originally affected presynaptic terminal. This new terminal grows downward, reattaching to the skeletal muscle and creating a new motor end plate with a new source of acetylcholine. The effects of the previous injection are overcome when this new presynaptic terminal begins to function. Another injection will be needed to block the release from this new presynaptic terminal, thus allowing another 2 to 3 months of antispasticity effects. This fact raises the question of how many times the injection cycle can be repeated safely and effectively. At the present time, there is no clear limit to the number of times a muscle can be injected, providing, of course, that sufficient time has elapsed between each series of injections. Longitudinal studies will be needed to determine if there are any detrimental effects of long-term use of this intervention.

Consequently, botulinum toxin represents a strategy for dealing with spasticity that is especially problematic in specific muscles or groups of muscles. Despite the rather ominous prospect of injecting a potentially lethal toxin into skeletal muscles, this intervention has a remarkably small incidence of severe adverse effects when administered at therapeutic doses. Botulinum toxin can therefore be used as part of a comprehensive rehabilitation program to provide optimal benefits in certain patients with severe spasticity.

Pharmacokinetics

Most muscle relaxants are absorbed fairly easily from the gastrointestinal tract, and the oral route is the most frequent method of drug administration. In cases of severe spasms, certain drugs such as methocarbamol and orphenadrine can be injected intramuscularly or intravenously to permit a more rapid effect. Likewise, diazepam and dantrolene can be injected to treat spasticity if the situation warrants a faster onset. As discussed earlier, continuous intrathecal baclofen administration may be used in certain patients with severe spasticity, and local injection of botulinum toxin is a possible strategy for treating focal dystonias and spasticity. Metabolism of muscle relaxants is usually accomplished by hepatic microsomal enzymes; and the metabolite or intact drug is excreted through the kidneys.

Skeletal muscle relaxants are used to treat the muscle spasms that result from musculoskeletal injuries or spasticity that occurs following lesions in the CNS. Depending on the specific agent, these drugs reduce muscle excitability by acting on the spinal cord, at the neuromuscular junction, or directly within the skeletal muscle fiber. Diazepam and polysynaptic inhibitors are used in the treatment of muscle spasms, but their effectiveness as muscle relaxants may be because of their nonspecific sedative properties. Agents used to treat spasticity include baclofen, dantrolene, diazepam, gabapentin, and tizanidine. Each drug works by a somewhat different mechanism, and the selection of a specific antispasticity agent depends on the patient and the underlying CNS lesion (e.g., stroke, MS). Local injection of botulinum toxin can also be used to treat focal dystonias and spasticity, and this technique may help control spasms and spasticity in specific muscles or muscle groups. Physical therapists and other rehabilitation personnel will frequently work with patients taking these drugs for the treatment of either spasticity or spasms. Although there are some troublesome side effects, these drugs generally facilitate the rehabilitation program by directly providing benefits (muscle relaxation) that are congruent with the major rehabilitation goals.

19

METABOLIC ENGINEERING FOR CEPHALOSPORIN C

Improving product yield in an antibiotic fermentation relies on an understanding and exploitation of the basic biology of the producing microorganism. Traditionally, microbiologists and biochemical engineers optimize the productive phase of fermentations by manipulating the nutrition and environment of the producing microorganism. Genetic manipulation of the producing fungus or bacterium through natural selection or deliberate random mutation and screening for enhanced yield or favorable metabolite profile have been companions to fermentation optimization for decades. The success of these traditional techniques is typified by the two-orders-of-magnitude increase in the production of penicillin by *Penicillium chrysogenum* since the early 1950s.

Biochemical pathways leading from basic metabolic precursors to finished products are deduced through chemical structural analysis of the products and by-products coupled with biochemical and genetic investigation. Highly sensitive bioanalytical techniques allow biochemists to characterize many of the enzymes responsible for antibiotic production. Similar techniques also help to identify product precursor pools that can indicate rate-limiting steps in the production of an antibiotic. With the introduction of recombinant DNA techniques in the 1970s, the genes coding for the various enzymes responsible for the biochemical steps became targets for antibiotic yield improvement investigations.

The term *metabolic engineering* refers to the deliberate genetic manipulation of one or more steps in a biosynthetic pathway leading to a desired product. Such manipulations may include gene deletions to reduce or eliminate undesirable by-products, an increase in gene copy number to enhance conversion of rate- limiting precursor pools to end products, or the introduction of a non-natural gene resulting in a novel product. In this chapter we will discuss the metabolic engineering of the cephalosporin C (CPC) biosynthetic pathway for yield improvement and production of economically important intermediates for semisynthetic cephalosporin synthesis.

ENZYMES OF CEPHALOSPORIN C BIOSYNTHESIS

Cephalosporin C, characterized by β-lactam-dihydrothiazine fused ring, is produced via a multistep biosynthetic pathway by *Cephalosporium acremonium*. This pathway shares several steps with the pathway that diverges to penicillin produced commercially by *Penicillium chrysogenum* and again diverges and is extended by several steps to yield cephamycin C by *Streptomyces clavuligerus*. All of the enzymes in the CPC pathway have been purified and characterized, and the genes coding for each enzyme have been cloned using the so-called reverse genetics approach and by traditional genetic methodologies.

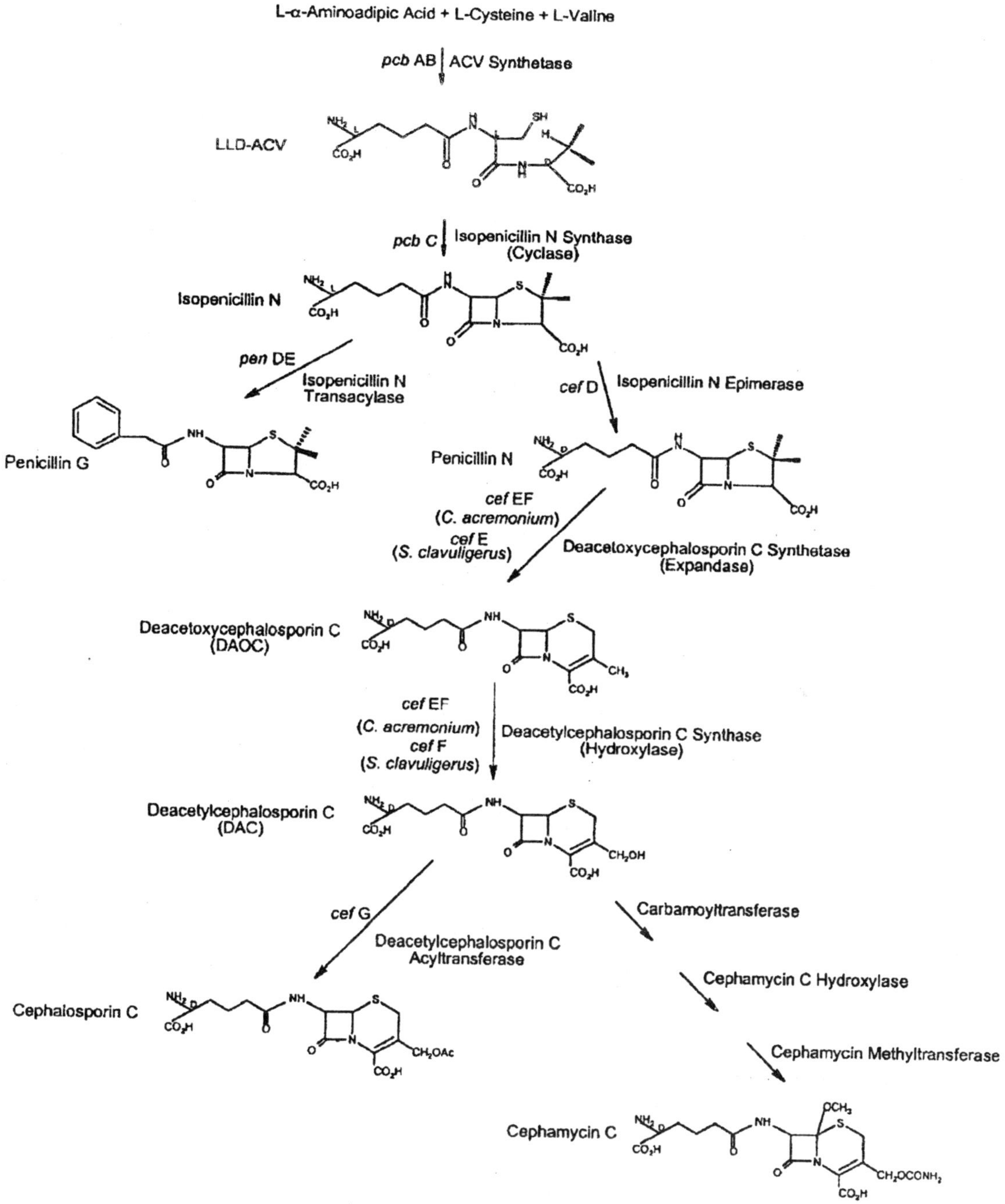

L-α-Aminoadipic Acid + L-Cysteine + L-Valine

pcb AB | ACV Synthetase

LLD-ACV

pcb C | Isopenicillin N Synthase (Cyclase)

Isopenicillin N

pen DE — Isopenicillin N Transacylase

cef D — Isopenicillin N Epimerase

Penicillin G

Penicillin N

cef EF (*C. acremonium*) *cef* E (*S. clavuligerus*) — Deacetoxycephalosporin C Synthetase (Expandase)

Deacetoxycephalosporin C (DAOC)

cef EF (*C. acremonium*) *cef* F (*S. clavuligerus*) — Deacetylcephalosporin C Synthase (Hydroxylase)

Deacetylcephalosporin C (DAC)

cef G — Deacetylcephalosporin C Acyltransferase

Carbamoyltransferase

Cephamycin C Hydroxylase

Cephamycin Methyltransferase

Cephalosporin C

Cephamycin C

Fig. 19.1. Biosynthetic pathway for cephalosporin C in C. acremonium, penicillin G in P. chrysogenum, and cephamycin C in S. clavuligerus.

Ingolia and Queener proposed the current nomenclature for the genes in this pathway. Genes common to both penicillin and cephalopsorin biosynthesis are named *pcb*, the genes unique to penicillin are designated *pen*, while those involved only in cephalosporin biosynthesis are named *cef*.

ACV Synthetase

In 1971 it was shown that incubating the dipeptide δ-(L-α-aminoadipyl)-L-cysteine (AC) with DL-[^{14}C]-valine and ATP in a particulate fraction from *C. acremonium* protoplast extracts yielded labeled δ-(L-α-aminoadipyl)-L-cysteinyl-D-valine (ACV), implying that AC was an intermediate in ACV biosynthesis. This notion was substantiated when Abraham identified AC from β-lactam-producing actinomycete. Later, soluble extracts of *C. acremonium* were shown to generate both AC and ACV from labeled amino acid precursors. These data led to the generally accepted conclusion that ACV synthesis was analogous to the two-enzyme process for glutathione biosynthesis.

Banko et al. speculated that the putative dual-enzyme process was instead catalyzed by a single, multifunctional enzyme. Their data clearly showed that in cell-free extracts of *C. acremonium* the rate of ACV synthesis was significantly greater when the precursor amino acids were provided than it was when AC and valine were used as substrates for the reaction. Jensen and her coworkers demonstrated a similar result using cell-free extracts of *S. clavuligerus*.

The issue was resolved when van Liempt et al. partially purified the enzyme responsible for the multifunctional synthesis of the ACV tripeptide from *Aspergillus nidulans*. The enzyme was later purified and characterized from *C. acremonium* and *S. clavuligerus* by Baldwin et al. The gene was cloned by reverse genetics from *A. nidulans* and by conventional methods from *P. chrysogenum* and *C. acremonium*. The name for the gene coding ACV synthetase, *pcb*AB, is reminiscent of the understanding of the biochemistry prior to 1987. To summarize, the enzyme activates the three component amino acids utilizing ATP, assembles the tripeptide, and epimerizes L-valine to D-valine prior to releasing the tripeptide.

Isopenicillin N Synthase (IPNS)

Isopenicillin N synthase (IPNS) or "*ACV cyclase*" catalyzes the oxidative cyclization of ACV by the removal of four hydrogens from the tripeptide with the consumption of one molecule of oxygen. The newly formed C—N and C—S bonds of the respective β-lactam and thiazolidine rings are putatively made in a stepwise manner while the intermediates are enzyme bound. IPNS from *C. acremonium* was purified and its N-terminal sequence reported in the early 1980s. Samson et al. utilized the sequence data to clone the IPNS gene *pcb*C. IPNS has been extensively characterized with respect to its enzymology, substrate specificity, and catalytic mechanism.

Isopenicillin N Epimerase (IPNE)

The generation of cephalosporin from penicillin is dependent on the epimerization of the L-α-aminoadipyl side chain of isopenicillin N to the D-α-aminoadipyl side chain of penicillin N, since penicillin N but not isopenicillin N is the substrate for ring expansion enzymes. This reaction is catalyzed by IPNE and is coded for by the *cef*D gene. While the activity of the IPNE from *C. acremonium* has been studied in cell-free extracts, it has not been purified to date. Jensen et al. described a partial purification and characterization of IPNE from *S. clavuligerus* and noted that it did not share cofactor requirements with other β-lactam biosynthetic enzymes. The enzyme was purified to homogeneity by Usui and Yu and was determined to be a racemase, converting isopenicillin N and/or penicillin N to an equimolar ratio of the two substrates/products, shifting to the direction of penicillin N by its further metabolism to DAOC. The gene was cloned by Kovacevic et al.

Ring Expansion/Hydroxylation Enzymes (DAOCS/ DACS)

The conversion of penicillin N to CPC is initiated by the oxidative ring expansion of penicillin N to deacetoxycephalosporin C (DAOC). Subsequent hydroxylation of the 3'-methyl carbon of DAOC generates deacetylcephalosporin C (DAC). Kohsaka and Demain described the enzymatic ring expansion activity from cell-free extracts of *C. acremonium*. Two reports of partial purification of the "*expandase*" enzyme by Kupka et al. and Scheidegger et al. and their respective co-workers suggested that ring expansion and hydroxylation activities were catalyzed by a single enzyme. They also described an inherent instability of the enzyme preventing sufficient purification to definitively determine the bifunctional nature of the enzyme. In contrast, ring expansion and hydroxylation activities from *S. clavuligerus* were clearly separable by anion-exchange chromatography. *S. clavuligerus* DAOC synthetase ("*expandase*") and DAC synthase ("*hydroxylase*") were subsequently purified to near homogeneity, biochemically characterized, and cloned and expressed in *E. coli*. Dotzlaf and Yeh devised a stabilizing cocktail that was modified as the purification progressed, allowing the purification of DAOC synthetase/ DAC synthase from *C. acremonium*to near-homogeneity. The highly purified protein retained its bifunctional nature, an observation also reported by Baldwin et al. in a nearly simultaneous publication. The bifunctionality of the DAOC synthetase/DAC synthase from *C. acremonium* was conclusively demonstrated by cloning and expressing its structural gene in *E. coli*. The gene coding for the two activities in *C. acremonium* is named *cef*EF, while the separate genes coding for ring expansion and hydroxylation activities in *S. clavuligerus* are named *cef*E and *cef*F, respectively.

DAC Acyltransferase (DAC-AT)

The final step in the biosynthesis of CPC is catalyzed by acetyl CoA: deacetylcephalosporin C *O*-acetyltransferase (DAC-AT). Fujisawa et al. showed that cell-free extracts of a CPC-producing strain readily converted DAC and acetyl-l-[^{14}C]-CoA to labeled CPC. They utilized this novel assay system to characterize several mutants that accumulated DAC and correctly proposed that DAC was an intermediate in the CPC pathway and was converted to CPC by DAC-AT.

Scheideggar et al. purified DAC-AT approximately 15-fold and estimated the molecular mass of the enzyme to be ~70 kDa. By incorporating 7-aminocephalosporanic acid (7-ACA) in the purification buffers, Matsuyama and his co-workers were able to stabilize DAC-AT, allowing a 1300-fold purification to apparent homogeneity. They estimated the mass to be ~55 kDa based on gel filtration and determined that the enzyme was a heterodimer composed of 14-kDa and 27-kDa subunits based on SDS-PAGE. The difference in mass as measured by the two methods was not discussed by the authors. In a related article, the cloning of the *cef*G gene and expression of DAC-AT activity in *Saccharomyces cerevisiae* using the reverse genetics approach based on the amino acid sequence of the purified protein was reported. In a third paper the disruption of *cef*G gene expression by insertional mutagenesis causing an accumulation of DAC and a lack of CPC production in the mutant *C. acremonium* strain was described.

Gutierrez et al. and Mathison et al cloned the *cef*G gene using traditional genetics by first searching for potential open reading frames (ORF) flanking the *pcb*C (IPNS) and *cef*EF (expandase/hydroxylase) genes. A likely ORF was located upstream of the *cef*EF gene by DNA sequence analysis. Both groups demonstrated that the cloned gene complemented DAC-AT deficient mutants of *C. acremonium* by restoring CPC production. Gutierrez and his co-workers cloned and expressed DAC-AT activity in *P. chrysogenum*, while Mathison and her co-workers reported similar results in *Aspergillus niger*.

Based on DNA sequencing, the mass of the *cef*G gene product was deduced to be 49,269 Da, which correlated well with the value reported by Matsuyama et al. Subsequently, Velasco et al. demonstrated the mass of immunoaffinity purified DAC-AT to be 49–52 kDa based on SDS-PAGE and gel filtration. However, unlike Matsuyama et al., DAC-AT purified from three different *C. acremonium* strains by Velasco et al. was monomeric.

Metabolic Engineering for CPC Yield Improvement

Isolation and structural elucidation of the active components from antibiotic- producing microorganisms begins the study of the biosynthetic pathway leading to the desired end product. The abundance of the various intermediate products of an antibiotic biosynthetic pathway can be accurately determined throughout the fermentation cycle by techniques such as high-performance liquid chromatography (HPLC). This and other analytical techniques allow identification of potential rate-limiting steps in the pathway. Three rate-limiting steps in the CPC pathway that are catalyzed by ACV synthetase, DAOC synthetase/DAC synthase, and DAC acetyltransferase are discussed below.

ACV Synthetase

Mounting evidence established the formation of ACV to be a rate-limiting step in CPC biosynthesis. Because ACV synthetase catalyzes the transitional step between primary and secondary metabolism in the β-lactam-producing microorganisms, it is likely to be a major regulatory site for β-lactam biosynthesis. Martin and Liras documented that increased ACV synthetase activity paralleled higher levels of cephalosporin or penicillin production in sequential strains. Zhang and Demain showed that ACV synthetase from various cell-free extracts of *C. acremonium* and *S. clavuligerus* possessed from 1% to 10% of the specific activity of isopenicillin N synthase, isopenicillin N epimerase, and deacetoxycephalosporin C synthetase. Finally, analysis of a mathematical model of CPC biosynthesis based on *in vitro* enzyme kinetic data led Malmberg and Hu to conclude that ACV synthesis is the major rate-limiting step in the pathway. At this writing, there are no reports of improved CPC yields in industrial strains by increasing the copy number of *pcb*AB. However, MacCabe et al. described the restoration of penicillin production in *A. nidulans* transformed with the *pcb*AB gene or the *pcb*AB plus *pcb*C genes together. They also claimed that certain transformants expressed a higher level of antimicrobial activity than the corresponding wild-type strain and suggested that extra copies of *pcb*AB might improve yields in the wild-type *A. nidulans*. In related work, Kennedy and Turner overexpressed ACV synthetase when the promoter for *pcb*AB in *A. nidulans* was replaced with the ethanol dehydrogenase promoter and reported up to a 30-fold increase in penicillin yields.

Isopenicillin N Synthetase and Epimerase

Isopenicillin N synthase and epimerase have not been implicated as rate-limiting enzymes for CPC biosynthesis. Although ACV was found in the mycelia of *P. chrysogenum* and *C. acremonium*, an excessive accumulation of ACV in fermentation broths has not been reported. Furthermore, pools of excreted penicillin were determined to be mostly penicillin N, not isopenicillin N, favoring the synthesis of the next intermediate, DAOC. In addition, *in vitro* kinetic data exclude both IPNS and IPNE as potential rate-limiting enzymes.

DAOC Synthetase/DAC Synthase

Metabolite analysis of ultrafiltered broth from a high-yielding CPC fermentation showed, in addition to CPC, the accumulation of penicillin, DAOC, and DAC. Further analysis of the accumulated penicillin indicated that >80% was penicillin N, the substrate for the DAOCS. Skatrud et al. described the elegant first use of metabolic engineering of an industrially important antibiotic producing strain when they successfully cloned an additional copy of the *cef*EF gene into *C. acremonium* strain 394-4 (a derivative of *C. acremonium* ATCC 11550). Their cloning efforts resulted in a twofold increase in the DAOCS activity in 150-liter pilot-scale fermentations. Doubling the DAOCS activity translated into a 16-fold reduction in level of penicillin N, a 6-fold decrease of accumulated DAOC, and a 15% increase in CPC yields. There was no effect on the level of DAC. These data predated and confirmed the mathematical model of CPC biosynthesis of Malmberg and Hu.

DAC Acyltransferase

As stated above, Skatrud et al. clearly showed that, while penicillin N accumulation was significantly reduced and CPC yields were substantially enhanced, the level of DAC was unchanged. The authors suggested that limitation in the carbon flow at the DAC-AT step could be causing the accumulation of DAC; however, they cautioned that DAC present at the end of the fermentation could be the result of degradation of CPC. Cephalosporin C degradation to DAC can result from either or both enzymatic hydrolysis by an extracellular acetylhydrolase and chemical hydrolysis due to a rapid rise in pH at the end of the fermentation. Skatrud and his co-workers suggested that cloning and expression of the *cef*G gene in a strain similar to 394-4 would be a practical way to address this question, but DAC-AT had not been purified or cloned at that time. By 1993, the means to address this issue were available. The enzyme had been purified, characterized, and cloned in several laboratories by both traditional and reverse genetics. Mathison et al. and later Gutierrez et al. successfully cloned and expressed the *cef*G gene in *C. acremonium*. Both groups showed enhanced conversion of DAC to CPC compared to untransformed strains. Mathison and her co-workers speculated that, since the DNA fragment used by Skatrud et al. to clone the *cef*EF gene unknowingly contained the *cef*G gene, the reduced penicillin N pool and improved CPC yields reported could have been the result of enhanced DAC-AT rather than enhanced DAOCS activity. They suggested that increased DAC-AT activity might reduce DAC levels to a point below a theoretical repression level for *cef*EF expression. This interesting hypothesis would not account for the lack of reduction in the DAC pool in the Skatrud strain. Velasco et al. showed that the *cef*G gene is poorly transcribed during both early- and late-phase growth in three low-producing *C. acremonium* strains compared to the *cef*EF gene. Gutierrez and his co-authors reported that introduction of extra copies of the *cef*G gene with its native promoter region only marginally improved reduction of the DAC pool with a corresponding increase in the CPC product. However, when the promoter was replaced with four different promoters, including the promoter for the *P. chrysogenum pcb*C gene (IPNS), high steady-state levels of DAC-AT expression and activity for each construct were found. The report by Gutierrez et al. implies that Skatrud et al. correctly interpreted their data. However, to paraphrase Mathison et al., it will be interesting to see if incorporating an altered promoter region will increase *cef*G expression and improve titers in industrial production strains of *C. acremonium*.

Metabolic Engineering for Production of 7-ADCA

The manufacture of several semisynthetic oral cephalosporin antibiotics involves the chemical ring expansion of penicillin V to 7-aminodeacetoxycephalosporanic acid (7-ADCA). This is a costly and potentially environmentally damaging process. Cloning of the *C. acremonium cef*EF gene (DAOCS/DACS) and the *S. clavuligerus cef*D (IPNE) and *cef*E gene (DAOCS) opened the possibility for biosynthetic/enzymatic processes for production of 7-ADCA.

DAOC Generation

Early *in vitro* data indicated that ring expansion of adipyl-6-APA or penicillin G was either nonexistent or barely detectable. Therefore, an alternative route to 7-ADCA through the enzymatic deacylation of DAOC requiring the fermentative production of DAOC at economically feasible levels was pursued. Elimination of DACS activity would allow *C. acremonium* to produce DAOC as its end product. Before it was known that DAOCS and DACS activities in *C. acremonium* were catalyzed by a single bifunctional enzyme, Queener et al. conducted mutagenesis and screening for mutants blocked in DACS activity. They effectively eliminated CPC production in some mutants, but DAOC production was only slightly enhanced. Attempts to eliminate DACS activity of the bifunctional DAOCS/DACS by *in vitro* mutagenesis of the cloned *cef*EF gene always resulted in a concomitant loss of DAOCS activity as well. It was later revealed through the use of inhibition kinetics that the two activities probably share a common active site. A simple disruption or deletion of the *cef*F gene in *S. clavuligerus* would result in the desired effect, since DAOCS of that organism produces only minimal amounts of DAC; however, to date this result has not been reported. A second approach involved expressing the *S clavuligerus cef*D and *cef*E genes in *P. chrysogenum*. Cantwell et al. transformed *P. chrysogenum* with a hybrid *cef*E gene containing the promoter sequence from *P. chrysogenum pcb*C gene and reported DAOCS specific activities from 4.3% to 10.3% relative to *S. clavuligerus*. Cantwell et al. later cloned the *S. clavuligerus cef*D gene into the *P. chrysogenum* strain that contained the *S. clavuligerus cef*E gene and demonstrated IPNE activity. This pioneering work was the first demonstration of cephalosporin production by fermentation of *P. chrysogenum*. The DAOC production was at the expense of penicillin V production but much less than the normal end product. The authors concluded that DAOC production would be greatly enhanced if isopenicillin N-to-penicillin V conversion could be prevented.

DAOG Generation

A second potential bio-synthetic/enzymatic route to 7-ADCA involves the enzymatic ring expansion of penicillin G or V *in vivo* followed by *in vitro* deacylation. Little or no *in vitro* ring expansion activity with these substrates was shown for either the bifunctional DAOCS/DACS or monofunctional DAOCS. It was proposed that, through site-directed mutagenesis, DAOCS could be "*enzyme engineered*" to convert penicillin G or V to DAOG or DAOV, which would then be enzymatically deacylated *in vitro* to yield 7-ADCA. Improved expression of native DAOCS in *P. chrysogenum* was the first goal in the proposed scheme. Queener et al. reconstructed the hybrid gene described by Cantwell et al. by inserting the *cef*E ORF between the *pcb*C promoter and terminator sequences. One *P. chrysogenum* isolate transformed with the new hybrid gene produced DAOCS specific activities 70-fold higher than the best transformant

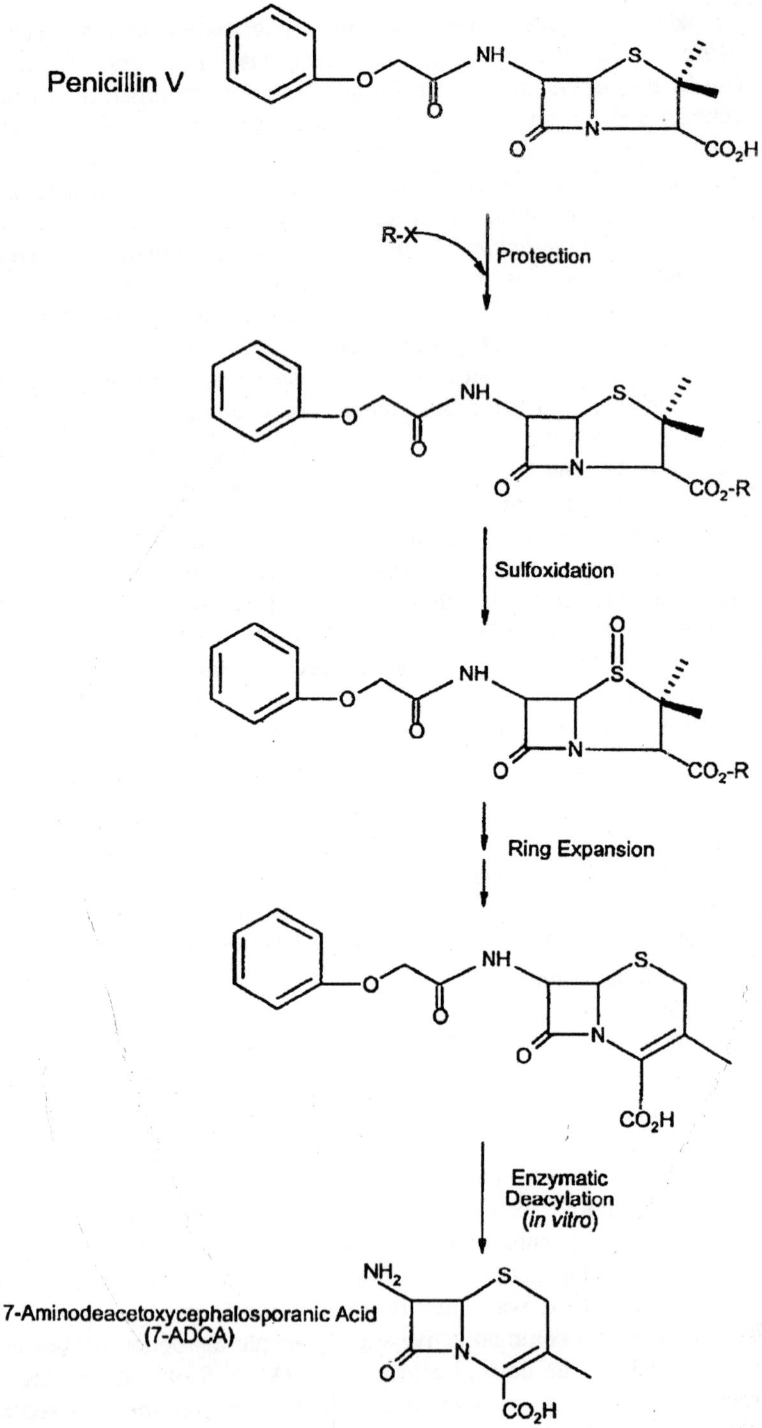

Penicillin V

R-X

Protection

Sulfoxidation

Ring Expansion

Enzymatic Deacylation (*in vitro*)

7-Aminodeacetoxycephalosporanic Acid (7-ADCA)

Fig. 19.2. The current chemical process for the production of 7-amino-deacetoxy-cephalosporanic acid.

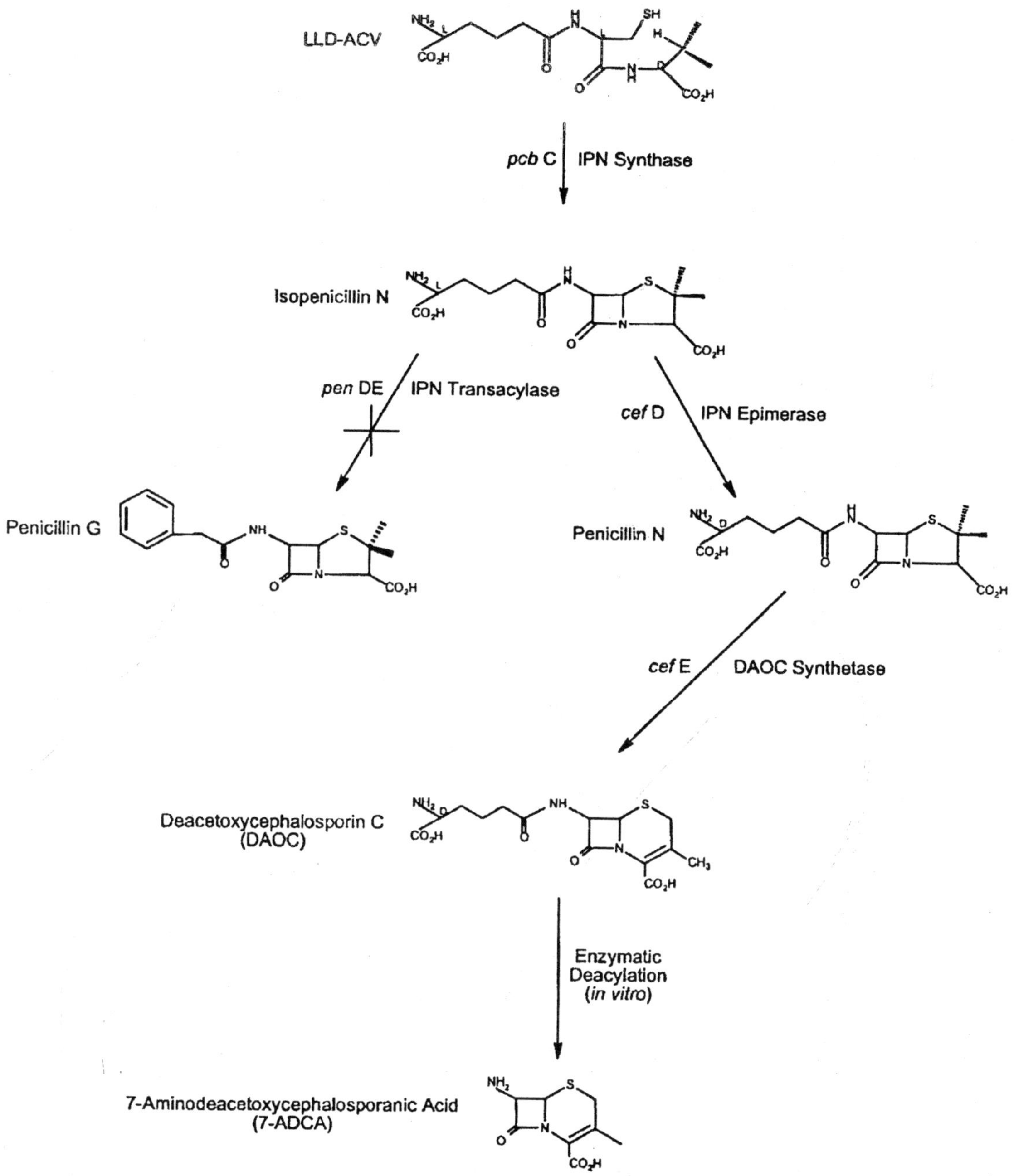

LLD-ACV

pcb C IPN Synthase

Isopenicillin N

pen DE IPN Transacylase

cef D IPN Epimerase

Penicillin G

Penicillin N

cef E DAOC Synthetase

Deacetoxycephalosporin C (DAOC)

Enzymatic Deacylation (*in vitro*)

7-Aminodeacetoxycephalosporanic Acid (7-ADCA)

Fig. 19.3. Metabolic engineering for deacetoxycephalosporin production in P. chrysogenum expressing the S. clavuligerus cefD and cefE genes.

previously reported, 4-fold higher than the parent *S. clavuligerus*, and about 75% of the activity of an industrial strain of *C. acremonium*. A similar tactic was used by Bovenberg et al to construct hybrid genes using the promoter and terminator regions of the *P. chrysogenum pen*DE gene and the *cef*E ORF from either *S. clavuligerus* or *Nocardia lactamdurans*. The *pen*DE promoter and terminator regions

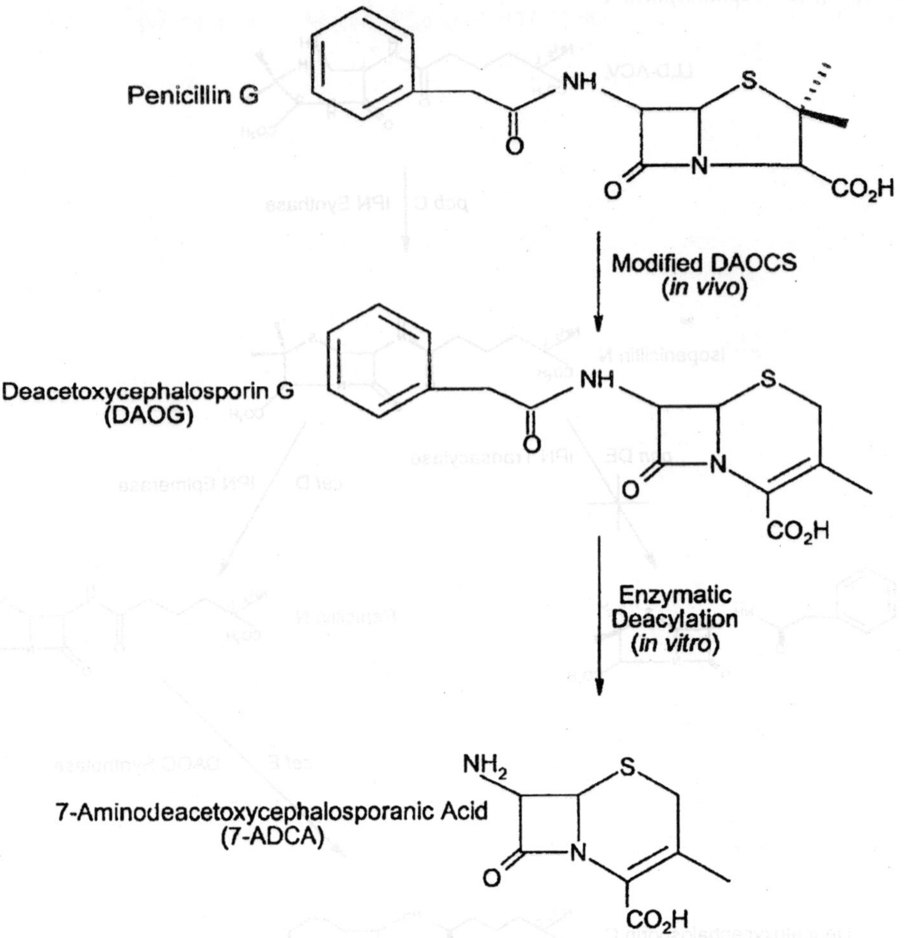

Fig. 19.4. Metabolic engineering for ring expansion of penicillin G in P. chrysogenum expressing a modified S. clavuligerus DAOCS.

ensure expression of DAOCS after formation of isopenicillin N. Sutherland et al. reasoned that because IPNS and DAOCS were members of the same family of oxidase enzymes, they might share sequence similarity in the binding pockets for their respective substrates. In an elegant set of experiments, they analyzed the binding site of the L-α-aminoadipyl side chain of ACV from the structurally characterized *A. nidulans* IPNS and identified homologous amino acids in *S. clavuligerus* DAOCS responsible for binding penicillin N. Using site-directed mutagenesis, the *S. clavuligerus cefE* gene was modified to accept penicillin G as its primary substrate. *P. chrysogenum*, transformed with the modified gene hybridized as described above, successfully produced DAOG.

Production of Adipyl-7-ADCA

Yet another process for producing 7-ADCA utilizing expression of CPC pathway genes in *P. chrysogenum* was described by Conder et al. and Crawford et al. The process involved the generation of adipyl-6-amino penicillanic acid (adipyl-6-APA) by feeding disodium adipate in place of potassium phenoxyacetate to fermentations of *P. chrysogenum*, *in situ* ring expansion to adipyl-7-ADCA, followed by *in vitro* deacylation to the final product. The authors successfully gambled on the expandability of adipyl-6-APA *in vivo*, considering that *in vitro* expansion of the substrate was marginally detectable in one report using purified *C. acremonium* DAOCS/DACS and not detectable in other reports. Hybrid genes containing the promoter region from glyceraldehyde-3-phosphate dehydrogenase (GAP),*pcb*C (IPNS) or β-tubulin from *P. chrysogenum* fused to the *cef*E ORF of *S. clavuligerus* were constructed. Transformants were screened for the production of adipyl-7-ADCA and, although all isolates expressed mRNA for the hybrid gene and produced adipyl-6-APA, the level of product varied from undetectable to relatively high levels. The authors could not correlate product formation to gene copy number, and they concluded that expression was influenced more by site of gene integration than by the promoter sequence fused to the *cef*E ORF adipyl-7-ADCA. Finally, traditional strain improvement techniques with the highest-producing transformants significantly improved adipyl-7ADCA production, and the authors predicted a commercially viable process. In related work, Crawford et al. described the production of 7-aminocephalosporanic acid (7-ACA), another important intermediate in semisynthetic cephalosporin manufacture, in adipate fed *P. chrysogenum* transformed with a hybrid gene containing the *C. acremonium cef*EF gene.

The application of traditional microbiology, mathematical modeling, biochemical engineering, analytical chemistry, mutagenesis, and screening significantly improved the production of CPC by fermentation of *C. acremonium* from the early 1950s through the 1970s. With the advent of recombinant DNA technology combined with new, readily available analytical techniques and sophisticated enzyme biochemistry in the early 1970s, an unparalleled understanding of the biosynthetic process for CPC production was realized. Reducing or eliminating rate limitations in the biosynthesis of CPC through the application of gene cloning resulted in yield increases in production strains where the traditional methods were no longer proving to be successful. Cloning and expression of several CPC biosynthetic genes in *P. chrysogenum* has led to the novel, economical, and environmentally desirable biosynthetic routes to important precursors for the production of semi-synthetic cephalosporins. Interestingly, the traditional methods of fermentation optimization and strain improvement are successfully improving production of the semisynthetic cephalosporin intermediates by the newly created cephalosporin-producing *P. chrysogenum* strains. Metabolic engineering for improved biosynthetic production of intermediate and end products for economically important antibiotics has been firmly established as indicated by the pioneering work described in this chapter. Similar advances are discussed in other chapters of this book, and we believe that these gene/enzyme methodologies will be commonly applied to the production of other existing as well as newly discovered antibiotics in the future.

The authors had the privilege of working with Sir Edward P. Abraham and note with sadness the passing of this historically important scientist. EPA, as we affectionately knew him, helped elucidate the structure of penicillin during World War II. In 1940, with E. Chain, he discovered the β-lactamase enzyme. In the 1950s and early 1960s, with G.G.F. Newton and others, he discovered the cephalosporin antibiotics and described their isolation from the fungus provided to Oxford by Guiseppe Brotzu, culminating in the elucidation of the structure for CPC. EPA provided Lilly scientists with purified isopenicillin N synthetase, thereby enabling, via reverse genetics, the first cloning and characterization of the *pcb*C gene and the expression of recombinant IPNS in *E. coli*. Working with us, he helped demonstrate the transformation of *P. chrysogenum* with hybrid *cef*D and *cef*E genes from *S. clavuligerus* and the production of cephalosporins by the recombinant *P. chrysogenum*. Thus, his scientific career spanned the beta-lactam antibiotic story from first discovery to modern metabolic engineering. Throughout our interactions with him, he exhibited a mentoring, humble manner that inspired us and belied the greatness of this man from Oxford, England.

20

COSMETICS AND THEIR RELATION TO DRUG

Under the Food, Drug, and Cosmetics Act, the Food and Drug Administration (FDC) of the United States has the authority to regulate foods, prescription (Rx) drugs, over-the-counter (OTC) drugs, and cosmetics. The FDA also administers a second statute, the Fair Packaging and Labeling Act. In order to administer this complex task, the FDA depends on the legalistic and statutory definitions of drug and cosmetics in the FDCA. Nevertheless, the public's interpretation of what constitutes a drug or a cosmetic may differ somewhat from that of regulatory agencies. Philosophically and historically, a cosmetic is a product that nelps improve external appearance and has the ability to hide, or at least distract from, unwanted stigmata or skin defects.

A product that changes the color of hair is a cosmetic, as is a product intended to increase the skin's tendency to tan by exposure to sun. This traditional view remains ingrained in the consumer's mind but may not be judicially valid. A change in hair color, for example, can be effected by the following: (1) a wig, which might be viewed as an article of clothing; (2) a variety of dyeing processes, which are properly identified as cosmetic changes; and (3) possibly by a variety of ingested or topically applied substances that gradually alter the hair follicle's ability to synthesize melanin, which should be classified as a drug effect. The common goal of these three approaches is to effect a change in appearance, the key objective of all cosmetics. The method by which this goal is achieved differentiates the three hair "coloring" processes and makes a product a drug or a cosmetic. This can create some confusion, as is demonstrated by a consideration of sunscreen products. Sunburn prevention by topical products was for years considered within the scope of cosmetics, even though ultraviolet-B (UV-B) light absorbers were incorporated into these "*cosmetics*."

The cosmetic industry responded rather calmly when the FDA's review of OTC drugs included suntan preparations and sunburn preventives. What for years had been a cosmetic suddenly became a drug by legislative or administrative fiat. The FDA's rationale is justifiably based on the concept that sunburn prevention is prevention of disease. Adding an ingredient that enhances the ability of melanocytes to produce melanin in the skin would be viewed as a cosmetic by the user. The FDA is likely to accept cosmetic (color change, appearance) claims for such a product, but a definition of a drug would become mandatory if the melanin is claimed to protect against sunburn. The implication that a parasol intended to prevent exposure to sun is a medical device has not been judicially examined. One must recognize that the differentiation between cosmetics and drugs is complex and is blurred by the interplay of consumer perception, commercial interest, and statutory interpretation by regulatory agencies, with the ultimate decision in the hands of the judiciary. For these reasons, differences between drugs and cosmetics are discussed in the next section on the basis of existing U.S. laws, the product's composition, and safety and efficacy. Laws and rules covering the distinction between cosmetics and drugs differ from country to country. For this reason, marked divergence from U.S. practices will be noted in this survey.

Comparison on the Basis of Law

Definitions

The sharpest distinction between a drug and a cosmetic is based on the statutory definitions in the Federal Food Drug and Cosmetic Act. Cosmetics are clearly defined as: (1) articles intended to be rubbed, poured, sprinkled, or sprayed on, introduced into, or otherwise applied to the human body or any part thereof for cleansing, beautifying, promoting attractiveness, or altering the appearance and (2) articles intended for use as a component of any such articles; except that such term shall not include soap.

On the other hand, drugs are defined as follows: The term drug means: (A) articles recognized in the official United States Pharmacopoeia, official Homeopathic Pharmacopoeia of the United States or official National Formulary or any supplement to any of them; (B) articles intended for the use in the diagnosis, cure, mitigation, treatment, or prevention of disease in man or other animal; (C) articles (other than food) intended to affect the structure or any function of the body of man or other animals; and (D) articles intended for use as a component of any articles specified in clause (A), (B), or (C); but does not include devices or their components, parts, or accessories.

Table 20.1. List of products (recognized as cosmetics)

Baby preparations	Creams, lotions, oil, powders, shampoos
Bath preparations	Bubble baths, capsules, oils, salts, soaps and detergents, tablets
Cleansing preparations	Creams, douches, liquids and pads, lotions, personal cleansing products
Dentifrices	Aerosols, breath fresheners, liquids, mouthwashes, pastes, powders
Fragrance products	Colognes and toilet waters, deodorants, fragrances, perfumes
Hair products	Depilatories, dressings, dyes and colors, grooming aids, lighteners, miscellaneous rinses, permanent waveproducts, shampoos, sprays, straighteners, tints, tonics, wave sets
Makeup preparations	Blushers, eyebrow pencils, eyeliners, eye makeup preparations, eye makeup removers, eye shadows, face powders, facial makeups, fixatives, foundation makeups, leg and body paints, lip glosses, lipsticks, mascaras, rouges
Miscellaneous products	Paste masks, powders (men's, women's, talcums)
Shaving preparations	Aftershaves, beard softeners, shaving creams (aerosol, brushless lather), preshaves
Skin care preparations	Body and hand preparations (moisturizers), eye creams, face and neck preparations, fresheners and astringents, suntan gels

These definitions may differ from the interpretation of the consumer or from generally accepted usage, but courts will adjudicate exclusively on the basis of these statutory definitions. It is clearly the intent of the product, not necessarily its performance, that is used judicially to classify a product as a drug or as a cosmetic. A skin-care product intended to beautify by the removal of wrinkles is both a cosmetic (alters the appearance) and a drug (affects a body structure). Historically and intuitively, the requirements for a drug are more stringent than those for a cosmetic, and the regulatory agency and the courts tend to apply the more stringent requirement to a product that may be perceived to be both a drug and a cosmetic. Some of the products are considered drugs or quasi-drugs in other countries.

Food and Drug Administration's Tasks

The FDA is authorized to enforce the FDCA and the FPLA. The FDA's tools include inspection and seizure, which may be applied equally to drugs or cosmetics. The FDCA prohibits the use (or presence) of poisonous or deleterious substances. Their presence makes a cosmetic "*adulterated*" or "*misbranded*." In this regard, no significant distinction is made between drugs and cosmetics. Similarly, good manufacturing practices (GMPs) are applicable to drugs and with minor changes to cosmetics. Products that are manufactured under conditions that are in violation of the GMPs may become subject to seizure. In recent years, the FDA has not initiated formal cases against violators of cosmetic regulations; instead, the FDA has relied on so-called Warning Letters to obtain compliance without recourse to complicated legal action.

In contrast to Rx drugs, OTC drugs and cosmetics are not subject to pre-clearance. Preclearance is specifically designed to prevent the introduction of dangerous or undesirable drug entities into the market. The restrictions on ingredients are most severe in the case of OTC drugs and preclude introduction of untested drugs or combinations. In fact, a "new chemical entity," which might be entirely suitable for introduction as an OTC drug, requires workup via the new drug application (NDA) process. The approval of Rx and OTC drugs by the FDA is, in principle, based on the performance of the drug entity. Efficacy against the disease, bioavailability, and lack of adverse side effects are of primary importance. Thus, judicious choice of drug excipients is required for all drug approvals. Nevertheless, in the absence of an FDA- approved list of cosmetic ingredients, the cosmetic manufacturer has the responsibility to provide products that are not injurious to the user under the expected conditions of use. Some ingredients are specifically restricted, and a regulation requiring safety substantiation exists. These will be discussed in the section entitled "Restrictions on the Use of Ingredients."

Color Additives

Color additives are of particular importance to the formulation of cosmetics. Dyes and pigments not only make products more attractive but also are vital to any product that is intended to alter the color of any part of the body. Color additives are regulated meticulously by the FDA, and only some general information on the current regulatory status of colorants in the United States can be provided.

Certified color additives are synthetic organic dyes that are described in an approved color additive petition. Each manufactured lot of a certified dye must be analyzed and certified by the FDA prior to usage.

Color lakes are pigments that generally consist of an insoluble metallic salt of a certified color additive deposited on an inert substrate. These lakes are subject to the color additive regulations of the FDA and must be certified by the agency prior to use.

Color additives that are not classified as certified color or color lakes are identified as *non-certified color additives*. Each of these substances is the subject of an approved color additive petition, but individual batches do not require certification by the FDA prior to use.

The fourth major class of color additives is *hair colorants*. These compounds or their mixtures may be used only to color scalp hair and may not be used in the eye area. Use of these colorants is "exempt," that is, the so-called coal-tar hair dyes may be sold with cautionary labeling, directions for preliminary (patch) testing, and restrictions against use in or near the eye.

Soap Exclusion

Soap is specifically excluded from cosmetics in the FDCA, and no cosmetic or drug regulations are applicable to soap. The FDCA fails to define the term *soap*, but the FDA has ruled that a product is a soap if the bulk of the non-volatile matter is the alkali salt of a fatty acid and if its detersive properties are due exclusively to the fatty acid salt. In addition, the product must be labeled as a soap. A product is identified as a shampoo when it consists, e.g., only of aqueous potassium oleate. It then must conform to cosmetic regulations.

The term *soap* thus has two meanings. The first is the FDA's definition, which is used for legal purposes. The second is the generic sense, whereby soaps may refer to cleansing products that may not meet the specifics of FDA's definition. Such products must, therefore, be labeled as cosmetics. The Federal Trade Commission (FTC) and the Consumer Products Safety Commission (CPSC) handle the regulatory control for soaps.

Comparison on the Basis of Composition

Drug Ingredients Versus Cosmetic Ingredients

On the basis of the Drug Efficacy Study Implementation (DESI) review, which began in 1962, the FDA ultimately concluded that of about 16,000 claims made for 3400 Rx drugs, only about 2300 drugs were effective for at least one indication. Today, Rx drugs must undergo the NDA process, which, for all practical purposes, is a critical preclearance procedure. As the work on the DESI review neared completion, the FDA initiated the so-called OTC review in 1972. The FDA classified some 250,000 drugs into about 55 therapeutic groups. The panels that reviewed each group had the responsibility to establish the safety and efficacy of each OTC drug and to restrict claims for these drugs to those the panel considered appropriate for a given drug or combination of drugs. It is apparent that the marketability of a drug—Rx or OTC—requires the presence and bioavailability of an identifiable drug entity that can be expected to exert some therapeutic benefit. No such legal requirement for the use of raw materials exists in cosmetics. As a rule, the presence of and claim for any component in a cosmetic that may have a therapeutic effect converts such a cosmetic into a drug.

The FDA has classified the following topically applied products as OTC drugs on the basis of safety and efficacy review of the drug(s) constituents:

1. Acne products
2. Antidandruff products
3. Antimicrobial products
4. Antiperspirant products
5. Astringent products
6. Oral care products
7. Skin-protectant products
8. Sunscreen products
9. External analgesic products

In other countries, some of these products are considered cosmetics.

Some of the actives used in the past in such products have been classified as Category I, i.e., safe and effective. Usage of these agents and the claims made for the finished product make these products OTC drugs, not cosmetics.

The activities of the OTC panels are not yet completed, although most of the tentative final reports have been published. However, no definitive rulings have been made or subjected to judicial review. It appears at this time that the ingredients reviewed by the OTC panels can be used in cosmetics as excipients and the like. To repeat, their use, together with drug or therapeutic claims, transforms the cosmetic into a drug, in which case the labeling and claim structure must conform to those established for OTC drugs. The designation "*cosmetic*" places almost no restriction on the use of components.

However, claims for therapeutic efficacy convert any cosmetic into a drug, as interpreted by the FDA. The regulations do not restrict the use of a drug substance for purposes unrelated to its drug status.

Cosmetics and their Relation to Drugs

Restrictions on the Use of Ingredients in Cosmetics

The review of active drugs by the OTC panels was limited to relatively few drug entities, but the cosmetic industry employs thousands of ingredients, including many of plant and animal origin. Many typical cosmetic ingredients are identical to the components used in Rx and OTC drugs, but only very few cosmetic ingredients are subject to restrictions by the FDA. These include mercury compounds, except those used as preservatives in products intended for use in or near the eye. Others are bithionol, vinyl chloride, halogenated salicylanilides, zirconium compounds in aerosol products, chloroform, chlorofluorcarbon propellants, and hexachlorophene. With regard to cosmetic ingredients, the FDA has placed the responsibility for substantiating their safety squarely on the producer. Such safety substantiation also includes finished products. Each ingredient used in a cosmetic product and each finished cosmetic product shall be adequately substantiated for safety prior to marketing. Any such ingredient or product whose safety is not adequately substantiated prior to marketing is misbranded unless it contains the following conspicuous statement on the principal display panel: Warning—The safety of this product has not been substantiated.

These regulatory activities and the need to demonstrate to the public that the cosmetic industry as a whole is prepared to accept responsibility prompted the Cosmetics, Toiletries and Fragrance Association (CTFA) in 1976 to establish the Cosmetic Ingredient Review (CIR) for the purpose of evaluation and review of the safety of the ingredients used in cosmetics. The CIR process established a system for prioritizing ingredients based on frequency of use, concentration used, area of use, frequency of application, use by sensitive subgroups, likelihood of biologic activity, and consumer complaints. This is a scientific review of worldwide data, and non-voting members from industry and consumer groups participate in the deliberations. In order to speed up the review process and to avoid duplication, the CIR expert panel may defer study of substances that are already under review by other safety programs. The most important of these are those by the Research Institute for Fragrance Materials (RIFM) and the Flavor and Extract Manufacturers Association (FEMA). The former establishes the safety of fragrance components; its funding and concept permit expenditures for safety testing of substances. The latter addresses issues related to the safety of individual flavor materials. The reviews by the CIR panel are available from the CTFA and have appeared over a period of years in the Journal of the American College of Toxicology.

Although the CIR process is sponsored by the CTFA, the latter will conduct safety studies for substances considered crucial to the survival of the cosmetic industry. The CTFA will also establish and pay for research required to confirm the stability, chemical purity, and safety of various cosmetic ingredients. These activities are part of the cosmetic industry's technically oriented self-regulation program. Similar programs exist in the pharmaceutical industry. RIFM has recommended discontinuance of the use of acetylethyl tetramethyltetralin, 6-methylcoumarin, musk ambrette, and musk ketone. Another self- imposed ingredient restriction concerns the use of potential nitrosating agents in products containing various (secondary) alkanol amines, in light of the hazard of nitrosamine formation. In the European Union, the use of tri- and di-ethanolamine is restricted.

One of the key self-regulatory procedures in the cosmetic industry is the voluntary reporting process of adverse reactions. The program is intended to provide data on the type and frequency of adverse reactions reported by consumers or by their medical advisors to the industry. It is an important means of detecting problems that are not treated in hospital emergency rooms (i.e., documented in the National Electronic Injury Surveillance System, NEISS) or do not reach poison control centers.

Practical Aspects

For practicing formulators, the border between cosmetics and drugs is not clear. Drug entities for which claims are made on the label differentiate drugs from cosmetics. However, the same or chemically similar excipients and formulation aids are widely used in cosmetics and drugs. Finally, one must recognize that cosmetics may include groups of substances not normally found in drugs. Substances considered drugs by U.S. law have been excluded from the table. This listing is not comprehensive and is presented for illustrative purposes only. The overlap on the basis of ingredient usage is apparent from an examination of column 3.

Labeling of Cosmetics

An important ingredient-related topic is cosmetic ingredient labeling. Advocates of consumers' rights have suggested that the public would benefit from full disclosure of the composition of cosmetic products. Pursuant to the regulations by the FDA and the FPLA, all cosmetics are now required to carry the following information on labels: (1) a statement of the identity of the product; (2) a statement of the net quantity of contents; (3) a statement of the name and place of business of the manufacturer, packer, or distributor; (4) a list of the ingredients included in the product in order of predominance; and (5) cautionary or warning language.

Except the aforementioned labeling for item 4, similar requirements exist for Rx and OTC products at the time of this writing. Labeling of all constituents in OTC drug products is still under consideration. The listing of ingredients in cosmetics must be in descending order of predominance, with some exceptions for components present as minor constituent and color additives. In order to achieve uniformity for identification, the CTFA has continuously created shorthand nomenclature for all cosmetic ingredients. The "naming" process is similar to that employed by USAN. Many names and chemical descriptions of cosmetic ingredients have been reviewed and accepted by the FDA (for the purpose of using these names on labels). As a result, cosmetics in the U.S. are now labeled in accordance with the nomenclature and the rules of the International Nomenclature of Cosmetic Ingredient Dictionary. This approach has been accepted in the E.U., where the same names (with minor modifications) are used. "Harmonization" of names is a continuing process to make these names linguistically acceptable throughout the world.

Comparison on the Basis of Safety and Performance

Safety

Users know that, as a rule, Rx drugs are more likely to cause adverse side effects than OTC drugs. This is an obvious result of the nature and of the distribution system for these products. Prescription drugs are administered under the supervision of a physician, who has the responsibility and moral obligation to monitor the patient's progress. However, OTC drugs may be used ad lib by the uninformed, who may not always be competent to diagnose the underlying disease or to recognize adverse side effects. In this respect, cosmetics resemble OTC drugs except that cosmetics are used repeatedly and over extended periods of time. Thus, the requirements for the safety of cosmetics should be, in fact, much more stringent then those for many drugs. The level of side effects or adverse effects that can be tolerated by manufacturers of cosmetics is virtually nil. Of particular concern is the sensitizing potential of components during prolonged and repeated use. Photosensitization is another phenomenon that has led to the removal of some cosmetic ingredients from the list of routinely employed substances.

Elegance

Elegance is not a primary concern in the case of Rx drugs but impacts marketing of OTC drugs and helps to ensure patient compliance. By contrast, any feature that detracts from the elegance (appearance, odor, texture, etc.) of a cosmetic interferes with its marketability and acceptance. As a matter of fact, cosmetic elegance is the essential attribute of a successful cosmetic product.

Performance

Performance is the one issue in which cosmetics and drugs are different. Drug efficacy is assessed on the basis of cure or prevention of disease. The FDA has established that cosmetic products that exert therapeutic effects are drugs. As a result, some traditional cosmetics were converted into drugs via the OTC panel process. Any performance claims for these OTC products are limited to the wording approved during the OTC review process.

Claims for (non-drug) cosmetics may be, for example, fashion-oriented (color), beauty-oriented (hiding of blemishes), or texture-oriented (emollient or lubricant). These, and related claims, are easily perceived and can be readily documented. More complex issues arise when cosmetic claims are made for age-related or reparative skin-care preparations. In the past, various regulatory agencies have been permissive with regard to cosmetic puffery claims. More recently, claims made for some cosmetics suggest to consumers that the product may exhibit a drug-like effect, as defined by statute. A Commissioner of Food and Drugs has labeled these claims "daring." Advertising copy that implies that a product nourishes the skin, is active, causes tingling, tightens the skin, discourages wrinkle formation, is prepared by a pharmaceutical company, or performs like a face-lift may be false and misleading if the product does not perform. On the other hand, the product is considered a drug if it performs as claimed. Aside from drug results, claims for skin or hair benefits require documentation for commercial purposes (advertising and promotion). Thus, claims for performance are likely to run afoul of FTC rules. In the E.U., however, claims for efficacy require substantiation by regulation. Guidelines for documenting cosmetic performance exist in Europe but not in the United States. On the other hand, the FDA has a powerful tool for stopping unsubstantiated claims. A claim for wrinkle "removal," even on a temporary basis, may make a cosmetic product into a drug. Thus, the cosmetic industry is as tightly controlled as the Rx industry. Whenever a new indication for an existing drug constituent is claimed or whenever a drug-like claim is made for any ingredient, a new drug application is required.

Shelf Life

Cosmetic preparations need not be labeled for out-dating. This does not imply that cosmetic products must (or do) exhibit indefinite stability. The physical and chemical stability of cosmetics is routinely studied by the same procedures as those used for Rx or OTC drugs. Since cosmetic products do not contain active drug entities, the chemical stability of any component may be critical to the performance of the product: The components of a fragrance product require monitoring; the performance of a hair-waving preparation may depend on alkalinity and the chemical integrity of the reducing agent.

Physical stability affects cosmetic elegance, for example, by the breaking of an emulsion. Moreover, physical stability may also affect efficacy, as is the case during settling of a pigment in a nail lacquer that might then no longer be readily redispersible. A similar type of instability may occur as a result of the settling of an antiperspirant compound in a suspension aerosol. In these cases, neither the cosmetic (nail lacquer) or the OTC drug (antiperspirant) performs as claimed and may be considered misbranded or mislabeled. As a rule, therefore, the demands of chemical and physical stability are similar for drugs and cosmetics. Under certain circumstances, the demands on physical stability may be especially critical as, for example, in hand and body lotions that have to perform under tropical conditions after having been exposed to the heat of the sun on the beach or after storage under arctic conditions in a ski hut.

The criteria for microbiologic cleanliness of cosmetic products are especially complex. Like a drug, a cosmetic is deemed adulterated if: (1) it bears or contains any poisonous or deleterious substance which may render it injurious to users on the conditions of use as are customary or usual; (2) it contains in whole or in part of any filthy, putrid, or decomposed substance; and (3) if it has been prepared, packed, or held under unsanitary conditions where it may have become contaminated with filth, or whereby it may have been rendered injurious to health.

Cosmetic companies adhere to FDA-mandated GMPs or to GMPs promulgated by the CTFA with regard to housekeeping, cleaning, and sanitizing of equipment, and purity of raw materials and process water. Water is a particularly important component of finished cosmetics. Its purity is closely monitored to avoid the inadvertent introduction of contaminating biota into products. The GMPs established by the FDA are available in 21 CFR, Part 211, and the CTFA has published similar recommendations in the form of Quality Assurance Guidelines for Cosmetic Manufacture.

The final check on purity is on the finished product. The high water content and the inclusion of nutrients for unwanted microbiota make cosmetics subject to microbiological contamination. Thus, topical OTC products and cosmetics require preservation and a final check before distribution. Preservative systems and GMPs usually ensure delivery of essentially uncontaminated cosmetics. The microbiologic requirements recommended by the CTFA include the following: (1) baby products: less than 500 microorganisms/g; (2) eye products: less than 500 microorganisms/g; (3) oral products: less than 1000 microorganisms/g; (4) all other products: less than 1000 microorganisms/g; and (5) pathogens should be absent.

The use of preservatives to achieve the desired low levels of contaminating microorganisms is required. Some liquid cosmetic products do not support the growth of microorganisms (e.g., alcohol-based after-shave), while others are excellent growth substrates (e.g., a protein-containing hair conditioner). Because consumers frequently introduce microorganisms during normal product use, some cosmetic manufacturers may require that their products be self-sterilizing. This is a difficult task and not always achievable. A final check for levels of microorganisms is, nevertheless, desirable.

Relation to Health-Care Providers

Like the drug industry, the cosmetic industry requires animal toxicology and human testing to establish the safety of its products. As a rule, most cosmetic products are quite innocuous upon ingestion, even though they may cause laxation or act as emetics. The industry makes a deliberative effort not to market products that might elicit toxic syndromes when ingested or applied topically. The former type of problem is usually handled by poison control centers and routinely (in 90% of all cases) involves ingestion by children. The number of fatalities was reported as nil between 1971 and 1978.

Dermatologists see many patients who have used cosmetic products properly but still report adverse reactions. The cosmetic industry is conscious of the need to provide products that do not elicit irritation or allergic responses during use. For this reason, the cosmetic industry depends on all types of patch and related testing by dermatologic laboratories to establish the safety of a given product in a predictive fashion. A whole battery of test protocols is available, and hundreds of subjects are tested routinely by dermatologists before product marketing.

Topical drugs and cosmetics have the potential of penetrating the skin. In the case of a topical drug (e.g., an antiinflammatory steroid), localized permeation may be a desirable feature. Penetration of cosmetics into and through the skin may elicit undesirable effects, especially since consumers may apply two or more products to the same site. Thus, in contrast to topically used Rx drugs, cosmetics should be retained on the skin with minimal penetration. Dermatologists also recommend cosmetics to patients as, for example, in cases of dry or chapped skin. Clearly, the cosmetic industry–physician–user relationship is not very different from that existing in the drug industry.

Cosmetic or Drug?

Formulators and marketers require an answer to the question of whether a given product is a cosmetic or a drug. Some of the answers are almost obvious. In the United States, a product is a drug if a drug claim is made for the preparation. The inclusion of a new chemical entity on which a therapeutic claim is based requires filing of a NDA; a product containing such a substance is automatically viewed as a drug. A typical example is a suntan product that adds an UV light- absorbing substance that was not reviewed by the OTC panel but was previously used as a sunscreen. Although the product in question was labeled as a drug, the FDA ruled that this clearly constituted use of an unapproved new drug substance. The addition of an OTC-reviewed sunscreen into a cosmetic makeup preparation— without claims for sun-protective action but with the indication that the product contains a sunscreen for the purpose of reducing UV light-induced skin aging— could be considered a drug use in the United States.

A soap to which an OTC Category I antimicrobial agent has been added is converted into a drug. This raises an interesting secondary issue. Soaps may be tinted with non-certified color additives. This inclusion of the antimicrobial requires not only drug labeling but also reformulation with approved colorants. As a rule, the status of the product is determined by the claims made for it and its intended purpose. The use of aluminum chloride, a Category I OTC antiperspirant, as an astringent probably does not confer drug status on the product. It was already noted that certain OTC Category I skin protectants, such as petrolatum, can be used freely in cosmetics as long as no drug claims are made for the product. Numerous other issues might arise, and each one might require specific adjudication. An example is the use of an approved sunscreen in a cosmetic product to preserve it against UV light deterioration. Since the intent of the sunscreen's use is clearly not drug related, the product will probably be considered a cosmetic. Cosmetics and drugs are distinctly different on the basis of U.S. law. In principle, cosmetics may not contain ingredients that treat or prevent disease or alter the structure or function of the human body. The objective of cosmetics is limited to the enhancement of appearance. The ingredients used in cosmetics to a large extent are the same as those employed in drugs, with the exception of components that are intended to cure, alleviate, or prevent disease. The demands on product stability and manufacturing practices are essentially the same for cosmetics and drugs. Finally, important differences are seen in judging the performance of cosmetics and of drugs. Consumers assess cosmetics based on the products' performance vis-à-vis the demand for better appearance. On the other hand, drugs are assessed on their ability to prevent or improve a disease state.

21

Clinical Supplies Manufacture

The Federal Food, Drug, and Cosmetic Act (the Act), Title 21, U.S. Code, section 301 et. seq., establishes that a drug shall be deemed to be adulterated if "...the methods used in, or the facilities or controls used for, its manufacture, processing, packing, or holding do not conform to or are not operated or administered in conformity with current good manufacturing practice to assure that such drug meets the requirements of this article as to safety and has the identity and strength, and meets the quality and purity characteristics, which it purports or is represented to possess." This requirement is generally referred to as "CGMP" (current good manufacturing practice), or simply "GMP."

The requirement as written in the law is obviously very broad. It does not define the specific steps manufacturers must take to comply, or the controls that must be in place to ensure compliance. A later section of the Act gives the Secretary of Health and Human Services authority to promulgate regulations for the efficient enforcement of the Act. The FDA, acting in accordance with this authority, has promulgated regulations found in Title 21 of the Code of Federal Regulations (CFR) that sets forth the definitions to be used in specifying GMP requirements for all drugs (21 CFR Part 210) and the procedures and controls necessary for manufacturing of finished pharmaceuticals (human and veterinary), found in 21 CFR Part 211. Part 211 of the regulations is what is generally meant by the term "CGMP" or "GMP" (the acronym GMP will be used in this text). While FDA gives consideration to prevailing practice in regulated industry before specific requirements are written into the regulations as being "current, good practices," FDA's final basis used to establish GMP requirements is whether the practice is "feasible and valuable" in assuring drug safety, quality, and purity. We also point out that the final GMP regulations are the product of notice and comment rule-making through publication, first as a proposal in the Federal Register. The affected public, including the industry, has an opportunity to comment on the proposed rule before it is finalized.

Because the regulations apply to all "*finished pharmaceuticals*," and because of the statutory requirement to comply with GMP, there is no question that the regulations apply in a binding manner to the manufacture of clinical supplies. Nevertheless, a debate has existed for many years, and even continues today, regarding exactly how and in what respects a company may differ in its approach to the application of GMP regulations to clinical supplies vs. full-scale commercial production.

Background Information

Clinical supplies, also known as clinical trial materials, are those investigational new drug products intended for administration in human or veterinary (animal) patients during clinical trials. In many respects, there is no difference between the equipment and technology employed to manufacture clinical supplies and that used for commercial production. In other respects, for example, production scale, robustness of the manufacturing process, labeling for clinical trial materials, expiration period (and hence the need for supporting stability data), final container, and even formulation and dosage form, there are important differences that should be taken into account when designing appropriate GMP controls for clinical supplies.

Placebos used in medical treatment to bring about a therapeutic effect without a pharmacologically active ingredient, or placebos used as study controls in clinical trials for new drugs are also subject to the requirements in the current good manufacturing practice regulations (GMP). Because they lack any active ingredient, placebos clearly cannot be tested for potency, but their inactive composition can be confirmed. This and other considerations unique to placebos also call for some degree of interpretation of GMP.

Clinical supply manufacturing operations are those areas involved in the manufacture of Phase I–IV clinical trial materials, and may include laboratory (or table-top) scale activities, operations performed in a pilot plant (with batch sizes generally larger than lab scale, but smaller than commercial scale), clinical supplies produced in facilities manufacturing commercially approved products, as well as clinical supplies produced at contract manufacturing sites.

The GMP regulations apply to investigational new drug products produced for clinical trials in humans or animals, whereas those activities earlier in the product development life cycle such as "*basic research* " discovery or preclinical experimentation are not subject to GMP requirements.

FDA Inspections of Clinical Supply Manufacturers

Under the Federal Food, Drug, and Cosmetic Act, the FDA has the authority to "...enter, at reasonable times, any. . . establishment in which food, drugs, devices or cosmetics are manufactured, processed, packed, or held...". This authority clearly includes sites that manufacture or conduct analysis of clinical supplies (for lot release, stability, or in connection with failure investigations). The term "*reasonable time*" has been interpreted by the courts to mean any time-regulated operations are taking place, regardless of date, day of the week, or time of day or night. Inspections are typically not preannounced, but may be in certain cases.

In practice, FDA only occasionally inspects clinical supply manufacturing sites. However, that should not result in a false sense that an FDA inspection will never take place. Manufacturing sites should always be prepared to undergo FDA inspections. Factors that may cause FDA to inspect clinical supply manufacturers include: Review in connection with a pre-approval inspection of the commercial manufacturing site; routine inspections of contract manufacturers who manufacture only clinical supplies; inspections resulting from observed product defects, especially when such defects are linked to adverse reactions in patients (such as contaminated parenterals); in reaction to recalls of clinical supplies; or other factors. The FDA inspections of manufacturing operations for clinical supplies used in Phase III trials are more likely than for operations producing Phase I or Phase II clinical trial material.

Each site should have ready access to a person or persons highly knowledgeable in FDA inspection procedure who can prepare personnel for the inspection and manage it from the company's perspective when it occurs. It is not the purpose of this article to explain in detail how to manage an FDA inspection, but the authors highly recommend that key personnel at each site receive relevant training in preparation for an FDA inspection, and prepare detailed policies and procedures concerning the handling of FDA inspections.

Understanding and Using FDA Documents

To properly interpret and apply GMP requirements to a specific context require some research and a good deal of judgment. This process can be greatly aided by reference to a variety of FDA documents in the public domain. Examples of useful documents include: Guidelines; the so-called Points to Consider documents issued by the Center for Biologics Evaluation and Research (CBER); Compliance Policy Guides; Inspection Technical Guides; Compliance Program Guidance Manuals; and others.

A key document for interpretation of GMP in a clinical supply setting is FDA's 1991 Guideline on the Preparation of Investigational New Drug Products (Human and Animal). This Guideline illustrates when drug development activities are subject to GMP requirements, the degree of compliance expected at certain stages of drug development, and FDA guidance for several important sections of the GMP regulations.

FDA's position on the applicability of GMP to clinical supplies was clearly articulated in the Preamble to the September 29, 1978 revision of the Drug GMPs that stated: "GMP regulations apply to the preparation of any drug product for administration to humans or animals, including those still in investigational stages. It is appropriate that the process by which a drug product is manufactured in the development phase be well documented and controlled in order to assure the reproducibility of the product for further testing and for ultimate commercial production."

Compliance Policy Guides are FDA internal documents that provide precedent for GMP (and other) enforcement decisions by FDA's field offices. They are found on the "Field Operations" or "ORA" (Office of Regulatory Affairs) pages on FDA's website under the heading "Compliance References."

Points to Consider documents are topical policy statements by CBER on subjects such as viral inactivation, transgenic animals, and other specialized technology subjects. Compliance Programs provide FDA investigators with procedural guidance for performing inspections in a wide variety of industries.

Industry publications and seminars can also provide useful information, but users should be wary of placing too much weight on "*podium policy*" statements by FDA officials or reading inspection citations issued to other companies. These sources may be misleading when the reader may not know all the facts surrounding any statements.

Selected GMP Systems as Applied to Clinical Supplies

Quality Organization

21 CFR 211.22 is the regulation that sets forth the responsibilities of the "Quality Control Unit" (QCU). There is no difference in the required roles and responsibilities of the QCU in the manufacture of clinical supplies vs. commercial products. The FDA considers the presence of an adequately staffed and trained QCU, empowered with authority to carry out its responsibility effectively, as a critical factor in GMP compliance.

Companies should be aware that "*Quality Control Unit*" is a generic term, and the company-specific terminology may differ from the term QCU. For example, in most companies, this unit is referred to as Quality Assurance (QA). Other common terms include Regulatory Compliance, QA/QC, or in some cases, the Regulatory Affairs group fulfills many, if not all, of the listed QCU functions. In very small companies or "virtual" firms, the QCU may be as small as one person, while in large companies the number of QCU employees may be quite large, and the quality organization may have several subdivisions. Thus, the name given to the QCU and its members is not as important as the authority to implement the required roles and responsibilities.

The regulation requires that the QCU be responsible for the following, at a minimum:

1. Dispositioning (approval or rejection) of components, containers, closures, in-process materials, packaging, labeling, and finished products.
2. Review of production records to assure that no errors have occurred.
3. If errors have occurred, they have been fully investigated.
4. Approval or rejection of standard operating procedures (SOPs) and specifications.

5. Approval or rejection of changes.
6. Oversight of contracted manufacturing operations (including testing).
7. Approval or rejection of all activities having a potential impact on the safety, purity, potency, quality, and efficacy of the products being manufactured.

The FDA expects (and many other regulatory authorities require) that the QCU will have full independence from other units. This is to provide the maximum degree of assurance that the QCU's decisions will be free of conflicts of interest and other impediments. Normally, the expectation is that the head of the QCU will report to a very senior level person of the company, and that there will not be a situation where the head of the QCU reports to manufacturing, marketing, or other similar functions.

The GMP requires that the QCU should have a qualified laboratory. This may be an in-house laboratory that is part of the QCU itself, or it may be an outside contractor or another company site laboratory. Here again, there is an expectation of independence of the laboratory from manufacturing or other units, in order to assure the maximum degree of objectivity in the data that are generated.

Master (and Batch) Production and Control Records

The specific requirements for master production and control records, and batch production and control records outlined in sections 21 CFR 211.186 and 21 CFR 211.188, respectively, also apply to clinical supplies. Despite these requirements, the level and amount of available documentation for early developmental batches will generally be much less when compared to commercial products, until the manufacturing process becomes more fully defined. Batch production and control records for clinical batches produced will have an increased amount of notes, changes, and other information handwritten on them during execution of clinical batches. The amount of this extraneous information usually coincides with the stage of development for the drug product (e.g., early phase production = more notes and changes), and may include the following:

1. Notes of any situations arising during production.
2. Problems that occurred.
3. Modifications made to the formulation, processing step sequence, processing parameters, or equipment set points.

This information that is annotated on executed master production and control records should be evaluated, reviewed and, if necessary, approved, and incorporated utilizing an established change control system. In many cases, master production and control records used in the production of clinical supplies start out as "*batch cards*," which are sometimes printed on a heavier stock paper that may be colored (e.g., blue or green), in order to differentiate them as related to R&D production operations, and not commercially manufactured products.

Buildings and Facilities

While buildings and facilities are required to be of suitable size and construction, as well as maintained in a good condition for both approved products and clinical supplies, the level of protection these areas are required to provide is dependent upon the activities taking place inside a respective area. For example, sterile fill operations necessitate, among other things, high-efficiency particulate air (HEPA)-filtered air, temperature and humidity controls, and Class 100 (Class A) environmental conditions. It would be inappropriate to perform aseptic filling operations for even Phase I clinical supplies in a non-environmentally controlled laboratory suite under a hood certified to meet Class 100 conditions. As it will be noted later in this article, there is little to no difference in matters of sterility assurance when comparing clinical trial materials to approved products. Similar discretion should also be exercised for operations such as dispensing, mixing, and packaging because FDA expect buildings and facilities used to manufacture clinical supplies are the same as those for commercial products.

Equipment

As with buildings and facilities, equipment must also be of suitable size and construction, as well as suitably located to facilitate its operation, maintenance, and cleaning (21 CFR 211.63). While there is clearly no difference in regulatory requirements for equipment used to manufacture clinical supplies, when compared to commercial manufacturing (e.g., equipment must be maintained and cleaned at appropriate intervals, measurement devices calibrated, qualified, and operating according to written and approved procedures), cleaning is especially important, in as much as many compounds encountered during drug development are of unknown toxicities that pose additional risks. Generally, fully established and validated cleaning procedures will not be in place during Phase I and II clinical supply manufacture. However, the actual cleaning regimen should be robust enough to minimize the potential for contamination or product carry-over. This may be accomplished via visual inspection, or possibly by verification through actual sampling and analytical testing. Finally, 21 CFR Part 211.105 requirements regarding identification of equipment used in the manufacture of clinical trial material can be satisfied with a single sign, or placard, denoting the material in question, the phase of production, and batch number.

Control of Incoming Materials

General requirements related to incoming materials, which include components, drug product containers, and closures, include establishing and following written procedures for the receipt, identification, storage, handling, sampling, testing, and approval (or rejection) of said items (21 CFR 211.80). Research and development organizations will typically have receiving functions and areas that are separate from those used to receive incoming materials for commercial manufacturing operations. The quantities of components, drug product containers and closures, and the containers holding them are generally smaller when compared to the volumes and sizes of incoming materials received by commercial operations.

It is important to note that FDA expects incoming materials used in the manufacture of clinical supplies to be released by the Quality Unit (21 CFR 211.22). Attempts to circumvent the established receiving operation in order to expedite use of these materials should be avoided. Equally important is the requirement to ensure proper storage and segregation of incoming materials, such that quarantined, released, and rejected items are easily identified, and there is some level of separation among them. Different lots or item numbers of similar materials should not be comingled during storage, in order to avoid inadvertent mix-ups with their use in manufacturing (21 CFR 211.80). Finally, incoming components (e.g., raw materials) used to manufacture clinical supplies must be tested for identity using a specific identity test (if available). Specifications should be established and confirmed for each lot of components, drug product containers, and closures received (21 CFR 211.84 and 21 CFR 211.94), and all other provisions of 21 CFR Part 211, Subpart E, Control of Components and Drug Product Containers and Closures not noted in this section also apply to clinical supply manufacturing operations.

Qualification and Validation Activities

Qualification activities are normally associated with buildings, facilities, utility systems (e.g., water, air handling, Clean-in-place/Steam-in-place (CIP/SIP), and compressed gases) major equipment (including laboratory instrumentation), whereas validation likely is in reference to those confirmatory tasks related to processes and analytical methods. In simplistic terms, validation (and qualification) can be defined as documented evidence that a process, activity, or piece of equipment can consistently meet its predetermined acceptance criteria and quality attributes. This section will be dedicated towards outlining the requirements for validation of manufacturing processes, as the requirements for buildings, facilities and equipment, and the validation of cleaning processes have been discussed in previous sections.

The FDA has indicated that during development, processes are expected be validated, and this should be completed to the "*extent possible.*" Challenges with earlier stages of development include fewer batches from which to establish physicochemical characteristics (including toxicity and potency), processing parameters, and commensurate equipment set points. There is also a greater reliance on in-process monitoring and testing, and final product testing for Phase I, II, and possibly early Phase III clinical supply manufacture. This more intensive monitoring and testing is needed to supplant full process validation, where multiple batches have not been produced under replicated conditions. Once, as FDA puts it, "a growing body of scientific data and documentation" reaches a point, complete validation of the manufacturing process will be required.

While blending times and tablet press parameters may not be fully established for early phase clinical supply manufacturing of solid oral dosages, those variables have a much lower potential to directly affect product safety than sterility, endotoxin contamination, or objectionable types and levels of particulates do for sterile, parenteral clinical supplies. Because clinical supplies can be incompletely characterized, and are usually given to patients already in weakened conditions, those processes and their related validation data necessary to guarantee patient and product safety (e.g., sterilization and aseptic fill) are expected to be in place as early as Phase I clinical supply manufacture.

Production and Process Controls

Written procedures are required to be established and followed for production and process controls as specified in 21 CFR Part 211.100. Because the specific requirements regarding handling of changes, deviations, and equipment identification are addressed in other sections of this article, and all other provisions of Subpart F are required in order to meet CGMP requirements for clinical supplies, this section will focus on the other aspects of Subpart F that provide unique challenges during clinical supply manufacture. Yield calculations are not only required according to 21 CFR Part 211.103, but they also provide some measure of process, phase, or step consistency when compared on a batch-by-batch basis. This information may prove useful when continuing process development, process optimization, or in the investigation of any process problems encountered during clinical supply production. Actual yields and percentages of theoretical yield also one of many important measures used to evaluate the validation of a manufacturing process.

Time limitations on production may not be fully known or established during early clinical supply development. However, those operations that are time-sensitive such as mixing or blending times, and drying times should be supported by data that are obtained through developmental studies. Arbitrarily assigning time limits without the benefit of any data, or the working knowledge of the operation in question, should be avoided, and can result in costly developmental errors and product delays.

Reprocessing can be defined as the repeating of a defined step or sequence of steps outlined in a master production and control record, in order to achieve a predetermined endpoint. Written procedures should be established and followed for any reprocessing steps or operations that are incorporated into a developed manufacturing process. The effectiveness of any reprocessing activity should be demonstrated through validation studies and should be fully supported by data.

Sterility Assurance

During inspections, FDA places a great deal of emphasis on the following systems they feel most directly will impact the safety and efficacy of sterile products manufactured, namely:

1. Sterilization processes for the drug itself, any components, container/closures, product-contact equipment, and surfaces
2. Depyrogenation processes
3. Water systems

4. Air handling systems
5. Environmental monitoring programs
6. Handling of incoming components
7. Packaging and labeling operations
8. Laboratory controls
9. Lyophilization (if applicable).

In general, the above-mentioned, including procedures, systems and, if applicable, validation should be in place for clinical supply manufacturing operations. This would include validation of processes such as sterilization, depyrogenation, and lyophilization; qualification of water and air handling systems; establishing and following procedures for: environmental monitoring programs, handling of incoming components, packaging, and labeling operations; and CGMP compliance for laboratories performing analyses of raw materials, in-process and final product samples, environmental monitoring activities, and testing in support of clinical supply manufacturing. Additionally, those processes or activities that are product-specific (e.g., sterilization, depyrogenation, the manufacturing process for the finished drug product itself, and analytical testing related to raw materials, in-process and final product testing) should be validated to what has been previously noted as the "*extent possible*." For example, in the case of sterilization processes such as terminal sterilization using moist heat, all of the following validation and process control requirements would be necessary in order to avoid exposing a patient to a risk of non-sterility:

1. Equipment that is qualified, maintained, and calibrated.
2. Empty chamber heat distribution studies.
3. Heat penetration studies that are product and load pattern-specific.
4. Challenges with biological indicators.
5. Process controls and monitoring typical for steam sterilization (e.g., time, temperature, and pressure).

Similar logic can be applied to sterilization by filtration or depyrogenation by means of dry heat. In these and other cases, there will be little to no difference in the level of compliance necessary when comparing clinical supply manufacturing to that for the manufacturing for commercially approved products.

Change Control

Change control is one of the GMP systems that is applied somewhat differently in clinical supply manufacture than it is in the manufacture of commercial products. Change control does not have a separate and distinct section in the GMP regulations; however, the management of change is referenced or mentioned in several GMP sections.

In commercial manufacturing, the purpose of change control is two-fold:

1. Keep validated systems functioning in a validated state.
2. Maintain the accuracy of approved submissions to regulatory agencies.

In the manufacture of clinical supplies, normally, manufacturing processes are not robust (and therefore not completely validated) until Phase III, sometimes not until the later stages of Phase III. Therefore, the goals of change control in clinical supply manufacture are somewhat different. Those goals should include:

1. Assurance that equipment (including computer systems and software), which has been qualified (installation, operational, and performance qualification), is maintained in a qualified state.
2. Support systems (such as water for injection, air handling systems, compressed gases, vacuum, clean-in-place systems, and others) are likewise maintained in a qualified state.

3. Any significant modification of the Chemistry, Manufacturing, and Controls section of the IND is noted, and, where applicable, the approved submission is supplemented to provide for the change.
4. Key changes in the development of formulation, dosage form, manufacturing process, cleaning procedures, and other key operations are identified for the purpose of documenting them as part of the development history.
5. When significant numbers of batches are manufactured using replicate processes (usually in late Phase III trials), changes are evaluated in order to determine if process development is complete, and validation should commence.

Laboratory Controls

The majority of 21 CFR 211.160 (laboratory controls) and subsections can be applied in the same manner for clinical supplies as for commercial products. An exception, in many cases, is the time by which analytical methods validation is required. For new chemical entities or significant formulation changes, new analytical methods may need to be developed. As with manufacturing processes, until such methods are robust it is difficult (or impossible) to validate them to the full extent that is expected for commercial products. The factors normally considered in analytical methods validation include:

1. Specificity
2. Sensitivity
3. Linearity
4. Repeatability
5. Robustness
6. Ruggedness
7. Limit of detection
8. Limit of quantitation.

Analytical method validation should track closely to the stages of development of the method itself. However, it is not realistic to expect complete and thorough validation of the method until its development cycle is complete. An exception to this would be a situation where an accepted compendial method is applied to clinical material (such as a dissolution test or release testing of a compendial component). In these cases, companies must be prepared to demonstrate that consistent acceptable results can be obtained when using the compendial method in the company's laboratory (also known as methods verification). The obvious difference is that a compendial method is not a proprietary method, having been developed fully in a collaborative process. Therefore, transfer of a compendial method to a clinical supply context does not differ from a similar transfer to a commercial product.

Methods for the investigation of out-of-specification (OOS) results should be similar to what is required for commercial manufacturing. However, it is recognized that in many cases, specifications may be less exact and methods may still be under development; therefore, it may be considerably more difficult to determine assignable causes for OOS findings related to clinical supplies.

When considering OOS investigation procedures for clinical supplies, manufacturers must keep certain basic principles in mind. Those basic principles include:

1. OOS results must not be arbitrarily dismissed simply because they are unexpected and present obstacles to release of materials.
2. Consideration must be given as to whether analyst error, equipment malfunction, inappropriate reagents, or some other detectable and assignable cause was the reason for an OOS result.
3. Consideration must be given as to whether a detectable process error or non-process related (employee) error was the reason for the OOS result.

4. There must be a documented rationale for resampling or retesting, including documentation of the reasonableness of the number of retests that are needed to overcome an OOS finding.
5. Averaging of results should be avoided when the purpose of the test is to reveal variability in a batch (such as blend uniformity or content uniformity testing) because averaging tends to hide variability.
6. If averaging is employed, OOS results must be included along with within-specification findings, unless they may be discarded by an approved statistical outlier test (either approved in the compendia or in the IND).

Training records for analysts should demonstrate that they have the necessary combination of education, training, and experience to perform the specific methods they are assigned to perform. Stability testing will be guided mainly by the conditions approved in the IND. However, the manner in which the stability program is managed should be similar to that required for commercial products. For example (not an all inclusive list):

1. Procedures to ensure that stability samples are correctly collected and are representative of the batch.
2. Procedures to ensure that chambers are qualified (temperature mapped) and monitored for environmental parameters.
3. Procedures to ensure that test intervals are consistently met.
4. Procedures for the development of stability-indicating analytical methods.
5. Complete, clear, and accessible records of all testing, including the preservation of raw data.

Deviations and Failure Investigations

As with commercial manufacturing, product or process deviations, or the failure of any clinical batch or any of its components to meet any of its specifications must be handled by approved procedures and thoroughly investigated (21 CFR 211.192). The investigation report should include, among other things:

1. Nature of the deviation or failure
2. Date
3. Affected batch or batches
4. Root cause determination
5. Impact analysis
6. Recommended corrective actions
7. Approval by the Quality Unit.

Apart from being product or process-related, deviations can also be procedural in nature, meaning that certain requirements of a specific SOP were not adhered to. Sometimes the terms "unplanned" and "planned" deviations are also used. Unplanned deviations include those events, activities, or actions that are non-intentional. An example of an unplanned deviation could include shutdown of processing equipment during the manufacture of a batch due to safety concerns. Planned deviation, on the other hand, is a term that is not favorably looked upon by FDA. A conscious decision not to follow written procedures, manufacturing instructions, or other records required under the predicate rule is, at the very least, a CGMP issue. The FDA expects that deviations will be fully and thoroughly documented, including any decisions made and by whom.

In the clinical supply setting, systems and procedures should be established and followed for handling deviations and performing investigations. For deviations, this would also include trending (either according to defined categories such as equipment, process, etc. by product line or other predefined criteria), timely resolution of the issues, and re-evaluation of process or equipment parameters and specifications, procedural requirements, or other items bearing on the quality or purity of the finished drug product. This re-evaluation is especially important during new product development, where less information may be known about the drug product being studied, the method of manufacture, process capabilities, or sensitivities of test methods. In these and other cases, improperly or incorrectly defined product or process attributes could contribute to an artificially high deviation rate, and more importantly, could suggest that additional product development work is needed.

Complaints and Adverse Reactions

Section 211.198 of the GMP regulations sets forth the requirements for reporting and investigating complaints. This section is intended to assure that when a manufacturer is notified of a product defect, a thorough investigation will be performed to determine the cause of the defect, and whether a recall of the product from the marketplace should be initiated. Of course, these activities are all aimed at protection of patients from harm caused by defective products.

When the product in question is intended only for use in clinical trials, the fundamental purpose of the regulation, protection of patients from defective products, must still be of primary concern. However, the quantity of product at risk, and its limited distribution will impact the process of complaint investigation. For example, the generally smaller amount of product involved may make it difficult to identify low-level occurrences of manufacturing defects. The limited and more tightly controlled system of distribution of clinical trial supplies, however, will likely facilitate and limit the recall process should that be deemed necessary.

Complaints of adverse reactions to clinical supplies are typically seen as reportable events that impact the safety or efficacy of the test article. Companies should give consideration to the possibility that an increase in the frequency or severity of adverse reactions may be linked to a manufacturing defect. For example, a product that has been formulated such that it is super- potent in its final form can be expected to produce adverse reactions of greater severity or frequency than if it was properly formulated. Labeling mix-ups can have devastating impact on patients, or, at minimum, may seriously affect the validity of a clinical trial. Therefore, the following elements should be included in the complaint assessment system:

1. Complaints of observable (physical) defects should be promptly and thoroughly investigated to determine the root cause of the defect and the probable scope of its occurrence.
2. Complaints of unusual or severe adverse reactions, or significant and unexpected increases in the number of adverse reactions (including marked lack of efficacy) should be evaluated to determine whether manufacturing errors may have caused or contributed to the observed effects.
3. When a product defect is identified, the evaluation should include a health hazard assessment by a qualified person, usually a physician. The FDA's recall policy regulations contain a suggested rubric for performing a health hazard assessment.
4. Product defect complaints and adverse reaction data and trends should be periodically compared to determine if there is any correlation between unexpected numbers, types or severity of adverse reactions, and the number and type of reported product defects.
5. As with commercial products, careful records of reported complaints, their investigation and resolution are critical to GMP compliance.

Technology Transfer Plans and Reports

Technology transfer plans and reports are used by a research and development organization in order to document their official "transfer" of a newly developed or recently upgraded product/process from the developmental area and facilities to an operations unit and site, usually located in separate buildings, or at an entirely separate and different manufacturing sites. While the format and content has not been formally prescribed by FDA, companies generally include the following information in these documents:

1. Definition of responsibilities for key departments; documentation review, approval, and storage requirements.
2. Summary of developmental activities completed.
3. Summary of scale-up activities; summary of formulation, synthesis, process, and analytical method changes; establishment of impurity specifications; establishment of critical process parameters; identification of validation plans and activities.
4. Definition of component, container/closure, and product attributes.
5. Analytical methods development and validation summary.
6. Descriptions, specifications, design parameters and requirements of facilities, and major equipment and utility systems.
7. Definition of the manufacturing process.
8. Stability and expiry dating information.
9. Change control.
10. Reprocessing.
11. Cleaning processes, including methods development and validation of the processes and methods.
12. Summary of Regulatory Affairs activities, including regulatory commitments, key data and information to be summarized in regulatory filings.

Data Integrity Considerations

The integrity of GMP data should be a vital part of any company's compliance scheme. The term "data integrity" generally means that the raw (source) data and associated data summaries and reports are truthful, accurate, legible, indelible, complete, and readily accessible. This applies whether the data are in hard copy (paper) form or electronic form. The GMP rules allow for the preservation of data through photocopying or other optical reproduction process (microfilming, optically scanning, etc.); however, original documents should be preserved whenever possible.

The fundamentals of good data recording practices should be observed in clinical supply manufacturing in exactly the same manner as required for commercial materials. Those fundamentals include the following:

1. Data, and the identification of those responsible for it, should be recorded contemporaneously, or as close to the time of execution of a step or an observation as is practical. Transfer of data from one form to another should be minimized, and should include one hundred percent verification for accuracy by a second person. This serves to enhance the accuracy of the data.
2. Hard copy documents should be recorded in indelible ink. Errors are inevitable, and when they occur, the original entry should be struck out with a single line, initialed and dated, the correct information entered, and a brief explanation of the error should be appended as directed by the document and associated procedures.
3. Data should always be recorded on forms designed for the specific purpose. Extraneous notations on loose slips of paper should be strictly prohibited in a GMP environment.
4. Log books, laboratory notebooks (when used), batch production and control records, qualification and validation protocols and reports, investigations of deviations and failures, and other GMP documentation must be carefully identified, controlled, and archived in a manner that will facilitate its prompt retrieval.

5. Electronic records (and electronic signatures, if used) must comply with the provisions of 21 CFR Part 11. It is beyond the scope of this article to explain "Part 11" compliance in total, however, the general principle is to construct and maintain electronic records with the same degree of accuracy and linkage to the originator as is achieved with hard copy documents. Each company choosing to use electronic data capture techniques and electronic signatures must thoroughly understand Part 11 and ensure compliance with this regulation.
6. Each company should have a policy that strictly prohibits the deliberate falsification, mutilation, obliteration, or destruction of raw data and associated GMP documentation. Companies must insist on strict adherence to such policies and should take aggressive disciplinary action when lapses are detected. Failure to do so may subject the company and its corporate officers to severe regulatory sanctions, including criminal prosecution under the Federal Food, Drug, and Cosmetic Act, or the general criminal laws of the United States. Even inadvertent (non-deliberate) acts that result in loss of data or records should be prevented, and, if they occur, they should be promptly and thoroughly investigated.
7. Establishing and following policies and procedures for good documentation practices, numerical rounding, significant figures, and directed audits to ensure the integrity of data contained in records or other documents prior to submission of applications to FDA).

22

Dental Products

A considerable number of products are now recommended for use in the oral cavity. Products for caries control are widely used and include fluorides in dentifrices and mouthwashes. Plaque control is achieved through the use of chemical agents such as chlorhexidine and quaternary ammonium compounds. Mechanical products for plaque control include dental floss, toothpastes, and mouthwashes. Products also exist to combat halitosis, act as topical anesthetics, desensitize sensitive teeth, act as tooth-bleaching agents, and assist in reducing xerostomia. More recently, products designed for the local delivery of antimicrobial agents to the oral cavity have also been made available. These, and other products, are reviewed in this article.

Caries Control Using Fluorides

Over 300 million people worldwide now consume optimally fluoridated water. The U.S. Public Health Service has established recommended levels for fluoride concentrations in water supplies in accordance with mean annual temperatures. The daily intake of fluoride not only comes from drinking water but also from food consumed or prepared with fluoridated water. Also, crops are frequently fertilized with phosphate fertilizers of high soluble-fluoride content, and food products including bone in animal feeds contain fluoride. Naturally fluoridated foods and water have been ingested for decades with no serious side effects. In addition, public fluoridation has been widespread in this country for over 30 years without serious adverse effects. The incidence of mottled enamel, one of the earliest and most sensitive signs of fluoride toxicity, has not increased significantly in the past 15 years of water fluoridation. The safety and efficacy of fluoride has definitely been established, with no scientific evidence against fluoridation.

Mechanism of Action

The mechanism by which fluoride prevents caries is not clearly understood. It is known that the fluoride ion (F^-) can replace the hydroxyl ion (OH^-) in hydroxyapatite, the major crystalline structure of enamel. The substituted crystal, called fluorapatite, is more resistant to acids, such as those produced by plaque bacteria, than the original hydroxyapatite. As the tooth develops and enamel is formed, ingested fluoride is incorporated into the enamel. Therefore, because enamel develops its outer layer first, more fluoride can be expected to be deposited on the outer layers as compared to the inner layers. It is this surface enamel layer containing fluoride that imports, in part, caries resistance to a tooth. Topical fluorides also become incorporated into enamel and provide protection against acid. A number of studies have now shown that topical fluorides may be most beneficial in early enamel caries and that there is an increased uptake of fluoride in early lesions, with some tooth remineralization occurring. This finding has caused some investigators to label fluoride as a remineralizing agent as well as a caries inhibitor. The incorporation of fluoride into enamel can be represented as a chemical reaction:

$$Ca_{10}(PO_4)_6(OH)_2 + F \rightarrow Ca_{10}(PO_4)_6F_2 + 2(OH)^-$$

Dental plaque also tends to concentrate fluoride. This could increase possible antienzymatic activity. Some caries protection from this may be expected. Additionally, studies have suggested that topical application of fluoride may also reduce smooth surface plaque, with a resulting beneficial effect on the periodontal tissues. In areas where there is no fluoridation of the community water supply, fluoride may be added to school water. This is not a substitute for community water fluoridation because fluoride intake from birth is important. In some areas where fluoride is absent from drinking water, the school water supply has been fluoridated as much as 4.5 times the level usually recommended for community water levels. These studies, conducted for 12 years in fluoride-deficient areas, revealed a 40% reduction in DMF surfaces. Essentially, no undesirable fluorosis resulted from this procedure. However, it should be noted that ingestion occurred only during part of each day and only on school days. This level (4.5 ppm) from birth (during major formation of permanent teeth) would cause undesirable fluorosis with continued intake.

Therapeutic Effects

Fluoridated water

The administration of fluoride in drinking water at concentrations of approximately 1 ppm significantly reduces dental caries. The anticaries benefits are similar to those due to natural fluoride in drinking water. Fluoridated drinking water produces the following: a 60% lower dental caries rate, a 75% decrease in the loss of 6-year molars, and a 90% reduction in the incidence of proximal caries of the four upper anterior teeth. Evidence suggests that greater inhibition of caries occurs when teeth receive fluoride throughout the calcification period. Therefore, maximum benefit may be expected from the continued use of fluoridated drinking water.

Dietary supplements/tablets

Maximum benefits to both deciduous and permanent teeth may result from daily fluoride supplements from infancy until approximately 13 years of age, at which time all permanent teeth except the third molars should have erupted. Because cariostatic benefits may tend to diminish gradually after fluorides are discontinued, periodic applications of topical fluorides may then be necessary. The use of dietary fluoride or topical applications of fluoride depends partly on the age of the child. Dietary supplements of fluoride are best for very young children, whereas topical fluoride applications are preferred for older children with permanent teeth. Younger children who are highly susceptible to caries may benefit from both measures. The natural level of fluoride in drinking water where the child lives should be known before dietary fluoride is prescribed. At present, it is suggested that fluoride supplements be limited to where drinking water contains 60% or less of the optimal level of fluorides recommended for community water in the geographic area.

As a precaution, no large quantities of sodium fluoride should be stored in the home. It is recommended that no more than 264 mg of sodium fluoride be dispensed at any one time, which is enough for at least a 4-month period. Each package dispensed should also bear the statement: Caution—store out of the reach of children. Although the optimal level of fluoride in drinking water is well documented, there is no established allowance for fluoride administered once a day. The standard allowance is 1 mg/day for a child over 3 years of age and one-half this amount for a child between the ages of 2 and 3. A more accurate method to use in calculating the daily fluoride needs of a child is to administer a dose based on the child's weight, for example, .025 mg/lb of body weight. However, for all children over 6 months of age, the dose should not exceed 1 mg/day of fluoride ion regardless of weight. In order to avoid the possibility of unesthetic dental fluorosis, the prescribed dietary allowance should be reduced in proportion to the fluoride levels in the drinking water. These allowances are for children over 6 years of age. The allowances should be reduced for children 6 years of age and under.

Table 22.1. Adjustment of prescribed fluoride relative to natural content of drinking water for children over 6 years of age

Water fluoride (ppm)	*Adjusted allowance sodium fluoride (mg/day)*	*Provides fluoride ion (mg/day)*
0.0	2.2	1.0
0.2	1.8	0.8
0.4	1.3	0.5
0.6	0.0	0.0

For children under 6 months of age, experts question the value of prescribing fluoride supplements. Dental caries have been prevented when fluoride tablets were administered in a school-based program. After two or more years of fluoride ingestion, protection against dental caries ranged from 20–40%. In an extended trial of fluoride tablets reported in the literature, there was a 36% reduction in dental caries after 8 years.

Table 22.2. Adjustment of prescribed fluoride ion relative to natural content of drinking water for children under 6 yr of age

	Content of water fluoride		
Patient's age	*0–0.3 ppm*	*0.3–0.6 ppm*	*>0.6 ppm*
0–6 mon	0.0	0.0	0.0
6 mon–3yr	0.25	0.0	0.0
3–6 yr	0.50	0.25	0.0

The use of fluoride tablets can provide both a preeruptive (endogenous) effect and a posteruptive (topical) effect. Therefore, tablets should be chewed or dissolved in the mouth and the teeth rinsed with the resultant solution before swallowing. One advantage of fluoride tablets compared to water fluoridation is that a specific dosage of fluoride is delivered. One disadvantage is that dietary supplements of fluoride taken once a day are rapidly cleared from the body.

Breast-feeding

Fluoride levels in human breast milk have been found to be less than 0.05 ppm. This concentration remains constant, regardless of drinking water and maternal plasma levels. Thus, breast-fed infants who receive no formula bottle feedings ingest considerably less fluoride than infants receiving formula mixed in 1 ppm fluoridated water. Fluoride supplementation for breast-fed infants should be considered. The administration of fluoride supplements to expectant mothers in an effort to benefit the teeth of the offspring has been evaluated in several studies. The evidence, however, is not sufficiently conclusive to warrant recommendation.

Vitamins

Vitamin preparations containing sodium fluoride are also available as drops, tablets, and chewable tablets. These forms of supplementation are useful in areas where the water supply contains less than 0.6 ppm, and they offer a way to provide fluoride to the child, if the parents are conscientious in dispensing the required amount daily and if the child does not object to taking oral medications. In recommending vitamins with fluoride, it is mandatory that one know the fluoride content of the child's water supply, as well as the fluoride content of the vitamin being recommended.

Topicals

Fluoride can be applied topically in various forms, offering the practitioner a number of options to choose for his or her patients. Topical agents are of lesser value in a caries reduction program when they are used in fluoridated communities. However, when used in non-fluoridated areas, they are more effective. In such areas, they often are the only form of fluoride therapy available. The dosage forms of topical fluoride currently available include varnishes, dentifrices, solutions, gels, mouthwashes, and prophylaxis pastes.

Table 22.3. Various topical fluoride preparations

Preparation	*Form*	*Formulation*
Acidulated phosphate fluoride	Topical solution	1.23% in 1% phosphoric acid
	Topical gel, foam	1.23% in 1% phosphoric acid
	Mouthrinse	0.02–0.04%
	Prophylaxis paste	1.2%
Amine fluoride	Dentifrice	1.6%
	Mouthrinse	2.5%
Sodium fluoride	Topical solution	2%
	Mouthrinse	2.5%
	Foam	0.2%
	Varnish	5% (every 3–6 months)
Sodium monofluorophosphate	Dentifrice	0.76–0.8%
Stannous fluoride	Topical solution	8%
	Mouthrinse	0.1%
	Prophylaxis paste	8%
	Dentifrice	0.4%
	Gel	0.4%

Dentifrices

The earliest fluoride dentifrices contained sodium fluoride. However, the fluoride was biologically unavailable because the calcium in the dentifrice abrasive bound the fluoride and thus inactivated it.

Although a number of dentifrices containing fluoride are on the market, not all provide available fluoride because the abrasive systems that some dentifrices contain inactivate the fluoride. Therefore, the product may contain as much fluoride as any other dentifrice but it is not available. Also, if the product has a short shelf life, it will be ineffective if poor marketing gets it to the consumer too late.

For these reasons, only dentifrices approved by the Council on Scientific Affairs of the American Dental Association (ADA) should be recommended. These products are listed in that association's publications and carry the ADA seal on their packaging.

Currently accepted dentifrices contain sodium monofluorophosphate, sodium fluoride, or, less frequently, stannous fluoride, all of which reduce caries by approximately 25% when used daily. In some clinical studies, stannous fluoride dentifrices stained teeth, particularly in pits and fissures. This stain is related to the tin in this compound, which adheres to plaque. The significance of this staining and its esthetic problems have resulted in a decreased usage in dentifrices. Stannous fluoride dentifrices are marketed in a plastic container because a reaction of stannous ions at an acid pH occurs when conventional soft metal tubes are used. The composition of some popular toothpastes is important for a proper understanding of this topic. With the exception of extra strength products, the various dentifrices are formulated to provide 1000 ppm of fluoride. Since children ingest most of the fluoride toothpaste when they brush their teeth, only a pea-sized amount should be placed on the brush.

Stannous fluoride

Dentifrices containing stannous fluoride as an active ingredient are no longer widely marketed; however, these formulations were the first to be evaluated for caries-reducing properties. Effectiveness in caries reduction varied from 23 to 34%. One stannous fluoride dentifrice containing a patented stabilized form of stannous fluoride is marketed with a claim of both caries and gingivitis reduction. However, this product is not ADA accepted. Currently, there are no ADA-approved, over- the-counter dentifrices containing stannous fluoride. However, there are a number of ADA accepted stannous fluoride prescription products approved for application by the dentist or by the patient.

Amine fluoride

Clinical data from several long-term studies in Europe have demonstrated the effectiveness of the use of a dentifrice containing organic amine fluorides. The amine fluorides also have strong plaque-reducing properties. However, although the amine fluorides may be more effective for caries reduction than other forms of fluoride, the FDA has not allowed these products to be extensively tested in this country.

Sodium fluoride

Sodium fluoride as an ingredient in dentifrices has been the subject of a number of clinical investigations. Recent studies of sodium fluoride dentifrices formulated to ensure ready availability of fluoride ions have shown anticaries benefits similar to those obtained in clinical caries trials with dentifrices containing stannous fluoride and sodium monofluorophosphate. Clinical caries trials conducted under well- controlled, daily supervised brushing conditions have reported reductions in dental caries of approximately 25–48%.

Sodium monofluorophosphate

A number of clinical studies have been conducted with dentifrices containing 0.76% monofluorophosphate (MFP). The data from these controlled clinical studies of sodium MFP dentifrices have indicated reductions in dental caries ranging from approximately 17–42%. Two studies indicating effectiveness were conducted in fluoridated communities. In clinical studies comparing this form of fluoride with sodium fluoride, the findings for caries reduction have been similar. Unlike dentifrices containing sodium fluoride, dentifrices containing MFP are compatible with a number of abrasive systems; this is one of the reasons why there are more ADA-accepted products in this category.

Solutions and Gels

In children, a reduction of 30–40% in dental caries is seen with the following: 2% sodium fluoride, 8% stannous fluoride, and acidulated phosphate-fluoride products. No one agent appears to be superior to any other when used as directed. Solutions of 8% stannous fluoride have been used to reduce caries. As with the other agents, the teeth are polished, dried, and isolated, and a 4-min application follows. The disadvantages of this solution are that it must be freshly prepared, some tooth discoloration (as discussed under dentifrices) has occurred, and it has an unpleasant taste that is difficult to mask.

Topical concentrated fluoride solutions are useful in children with high caries activity because they may have both a caries-arresting property and one of caries prevention. The frequency of application varies with the caries activity of the child. For children with an average incidence of caries, it can be applied annually between the ages of 3 and 13.

When gels are used, they are placed into a tray that is placed against the teeth so that the gel flows around all surfaces. Best results have been reported with custom-fitted trays. It has been estimated that about one-third of the total fluoride placed in a tray is actually available for uptake by teeth. The remainder is simply a filler for the tray, some of which is swallowed. The value of topical fluorides on adults has not been established. However, some studies have suggested that the acidulated phosphate fluoride types may offer some caries protection. Recent reports have suggested that polishing of teeth is not necessary prior to the topical application of fluorides. These studies have stated that deplaquing of teeth with a toothbrush is adequate and offers the advantage of not removing surface fluoride from tooth structure. This concept may be valid, and future investigations in this area should be encouraged.

Fluoride mouthwashes

Substantial research has been performed on the caries- inhibiting effect of fluoride mouthrinse products. The effectiveness of these topically applied fluorides varies with patient compliance. The daily use of fluoride rinses by young children should be carefully monitored, and it should be noted that the ADA does not recommend the use of fluoride mouthrinse for children under 6 years of age. Moreover, because these products, when brought into the home, present a potential danger, the ADA Council on Scientific Affairs has recommended that these rinses should not exceed 300 mg of sodium fluoride. Fluoride mouthrinse solutions for use in school or community programs, however, are available in larger volumes, based on the assumption that storing and dispensing of the products in public settings will be closely monitored. The potential dangers involved with unsupervised ingestion of these products should be made known to both parents and children.

Studies evaluating the effectiveness of mouthrinses containing sodium fluoride have shown the usefulness of these agents for children living in non-fluoridated areas. Most studies have been conducted using a mouthrinse containing approximately 0.05% sodium fluoride used daily or a 0.2% sodium fluoride used weekly. The Council on Scientific Affairs has accepted a number of fluoride mouthrinses. All products discussed below have ADA Council on Scientific Affairs acceptance. Some mouthrinses are marketed as a concentrate for dilution to recommended levels. If concentrates are used, special care should be exercised to keep them out of the reach of children. The products are not packaged in glass containers, because the pH becomes more alkaline in glass. Plastic is the container of choice. Examples of prescription and non-prescription products follow.

ACT

This product is an aqueous solution of 0.05% sodium fluoride. It also contains 8% glycerin, 7% alcohol, a detergent, a preservative, saccharin, coloring, and flavoring agents. It is intended to be used on a daily basis and is available without prescription.

Fluorigard

This product is available as a rinse containing an aqueous solution of a 0.05% sodium fluoride, 15% glycerin, 5% alcohol, a detergent, a preservative, saccharin, coloring, and flavoring agents. It is intended to be used on a daily basis and is available without a prescription.

Fluorinse

This product contains 0.2% sodium fluoride as the active ingredient. It also contains a detergent, a preservative, flavoring, and color agents. It is intended to be used on a daily basis and is available without a prescription.

Phos-Flur oral rinse supplement

This product is an aqueous solution containing 0.044% sodium fluoride, 0.055%, phosphoric acid, 1.35% sodium biphosphate, and flavoring and coloring agents. It is intended to be used once daily and is available by prescription.

Desensitizing Agents

A number of studies have reported that topical fluoride application may reduce dental hypersensitivity. These results have been found when concentrated dosage forms have been applied ranging from 8% stannous fluoride gels to 33.3% sodium fluoride paste. It has been shown that commercial dentifrices containing stannous fluoride may also decrease dental hypersensitivity. Also, a combination of stannous fluoride and potassium nitrate is marketed by one manufacturer to reduce sensitivity. Varnishes containing sodium fluoride have also been shown to reduce dental hypersensitivity.

Chemical Agents for Plaque Control

A number of chemical agents have been evaluated over the years in terms of their antimicrobial effects in the oral cavity and the importance of these effects on oral health. In 1986, the establishment by the ADA of guidelines for acceptance of these products has served to stimulate properly designed clinical studies for evaluating potential therapeutic agents.

Products that have earned the ADA's seal of acceptance are Peridex, Listerine, some generic copies of Listerine, and Colgate Total. In this section, data on various available agents are presented according to chemical agent category. When the term *substantivity* is used, it refers to the ability of an agent to be retained in the area cavity and to be released over an extended time period with a continued antimicrobial effect.

Chlorhexidine

Of the products included in this report, chlorhexidine appears to be the most effective agent. Long-term studies in over 700 subjects showed reductions in plaque averaging 55% and in gingivitis 45%.

The mechanism of action of chlorhexidine is related to a reduction in pellicle formation, alteration of bacterial absorption and/or attachment to teeth, and an alteration of the bacterial cell wall so that lysis occurs. Chemically, it is classified as chlorhexidine digluconate and the U.S. Adopted Name (USAN) designation is chlorhexidine gluconate. It has high substantivity. Adverse effects reported included staining of teeth, reversible desquamation in young children, alteration of taste, and an increase in supragingival calcified deposits. Long-term and microbiologic studies do not demonstrate the development of resistant strains. It is sold in the United States in a 0.12% concentration as a prescription mouthrinse (Peridex, PerioGard, and generically), which contain 11.6% alcohol with a pH of 5.5 and is approved by the ADA for control of plaque and gingivitis. Recommended usage is twice daily.

Fluorides

Fluorides are purported to have some antiplaque properties. The most widely used topical fluorides are stannous fluoride, acidulated phosphate fluoride, and sodium fluoride. Of the fluorides, short-term studies of stannous fluoride have been promising. However, long-term published studies showed lower plaque scores, but the differences were not significant. No effect on gingival health was noted with the exception of one study. With stannous fluoride, the mechanism of action appears to be related to an alteration of bacterial aggregation and metabolism.

In summarizing the properties of this agent, it can be stated that it has moderate substantivity, that the antibacterial activity may be related to the tin ion, and that a 0.4% concentration may be the most effective. Stannous fluoride is the most toxic of the products considered and has the shortest shelf life. Adverse effects have been taste and black stain lines on teeth. Usage of once or twice daily favors compliance. Stannous fluoride is most often available as an aqueous gel.

Stannous fluoride products are accepted by the ADA for their ability to deliver fluoride but have not been approved for their plaque-reducing properties. Examples of accepted products are Activux Basic Control, Gel-Kam, Gel-Tin, Perfect Choice, Pro-Dentx, Schein Home Care, and Super-Dent.

Oxygenating Agents

In evaluating the efficacy of oxygenating agents, one must evaluate the endpoints selected for efficacy and their measurement. Oxygenating agents have anti- inflammatory properties. Therefore, less bleeding on probing, a major sign of inflammation, would be expected following their use, but the bacteria producing the disease process would not necessarily have been reduced. Peroxides are found in dentifrices in combinations with sodium bicarbonate in concentrations of 1.5% or less. Also, they are found in bleaching agents discussed later in this chapter. As long-term studies of the effect of oxygenating agents are unavailable and short-term studies offer contradictory findings, questions of safety have been raised with regard to chronic use.

Phenolic Compounds

Listerine

Short-term studies of phenolic compounds have shown plaque and gingivitis reductions averaging 35%, and long-term studies have shown plaque reduction averaging 35% and gingivitis reduction averaging 30%. The only product in this category that has been adequately studied is Listerine. Listerine is a mixture of essential oils—thymol, menthol, a eucalyptol, and methylsalicylate. The mechanism of action appears to be related to alteration of the bacterial cell wall. This product is uncharged and has a low substantivity. Adverse effects reported have been a burning sensation and bitter taste. It is available in a 21.6–26.9% alcohol vehicle with a pH of 4.2. Recommended usage is twice daily, and the ADA accepts the product and some of its generic copies for the control of plaque and gingivitis.

Plax

Only short-term, clinical studies with small numbers of patients have been published. These pilot studies suggested some reduction in plaque when this product was used as a prebrushing rinse. Effects on gingivitis have not been reported. Additional long-term studies have questioned the efficacy of this product to reduce plaque and gingivitis. The active ingredient is stated to be sodium benzoate. However, the product also has about 30% of some of the ingredients (oils) found in Listerine. It contains 7.5% alcohol. Usage is as a prebrushing rinse. It is not ADA accepted.

Quaternary Ammonium Compounds

Quaternary ammonium compounds have been evaluated in a number of short-term studies relative to their effect on plaque and gingivitis. In these studies, an average plaque reduction of 35% has been reported, with mixed effects on gingival health. A 6-month study has been reported showing a 14% reduction in plaque and a 24% reduction in gingivitis. Cepacol, Scope, and Advanced Care Viadent are well-known representatives of this group, each with concentrations of approximately 0.05% cetylpyridium chloride. In addition, Scope contains 0.005% domiphen bromide. The mechanism of action is related to increased bacterial cell wall permeability, which favors lysis, decreased cell metabolism, and a decreased ability for bacteria to attach to tooth surfaces. These agents are categorized as being cationic, which favors their attraction to anionic surfaces of teeth and plaque. They are surface-active agents that alter surface tension and have some substantivity. Adverse effects have been some tooth staining and a burning sensation in the oral cavity. These agents are available in a 14–18% alcoholic vehicle with a pH range of 5.5–6.5. Recommended usage is twice daily, and they are not ADA accepted.

Sanguinarine

Short-term studies of sanguinarine have shown some plaque and gingivitis reduction. In the long-term studies of the product in a dentifrice form, no significant reduction in plaque or gingivitis occurred, with the exception of one study in which the product was used as a dentifrice and as a mouthrinse.

The proposed mechanism of action is by alteration of bacterial cell surfaces so that aggregation and attachment is reduced.

Sanguinarine (benzophenathradine) is derived from the bloodroot plant (*Sanguinaria canadensis*). The extract concentration in the product is 0.03%, which equals 0.10% sanguinarine. It also contains 0.2% zinc chloride. The product may be cationic, and the degree of substantivity is unclear. Adverse effects have been a burning sensation and a question of epithelial cell dysplasia. It is available as Viadent toothpaste and Viadent mouthrinse. The mouthrinse pH is 4.5, the dentifrice pH is 4.8, and the alcohol content of the rinse is 11.5%. It is not ADA accepted.

Triclosan

Triclosan (2,4,4'-Trichloro-2'-hydroxdiphenyl ether) is a new antiplaque/antigingivitis agent available in dentifrices. The addition of a copolymer, vinylmethyl-ether maleic acid (Gantrez), has been shown to improve the effectiveness of triclosan by enhancing its retention (substantivity) by hard and soft surfaces. This formula (Colgate Total) has been approved by the FDA for sale in the United States, and is ADA accepted. Claims allowed are for the reduction of plaque, gingivitis, calculus, and caries. Studies as early as 1973 showed that this chemical agent had a broad spectrum, antimicrobial effect against a wide range of gram-positive and gram-negative bacteria found in the mouth. The minimal concentration of triclosan for oral pathogens is 0.3 mg/ml. Triclosan' s antibacterial activity is not affected by anionic agents, such as lauryl sulfate, which are essential to dentifrice and mouthwash formulations—a fact that broadens its range of use. In doses lower than 0.5%, taste perception is minimally affected; however, at concentrations of greater than 0.5%, undesirable effects on taste occur.

Zinc citrate

This agent is found in some tartar control dentifrices and also has some plaque- and gingivitis-reducing properties as found in Mentadent and Advanced Care Viadent. ADA does not accept dentifrices with this ingredient for reducing plaque and gingivitis.

Mechanical Products for Plaque Control

Good control of plaque is accomplished by mechanical procedures, which include brushing, flossing, and professional prophylaxis. A professional cleaning is recommended at least twice a year to remove plaque and tartar (calculus), both supragingivally and subgingivally.

Brushing

A recent survey of brushing habits in the United States showed that only 60% of the public follow a strict brushing regimen. Clearly, motivation and education are needed in this area. For the average adult, a soft brush with rounded bristles is most efficient in removing plaque from supragingival tooth surfaces (with the exception of the surfaces between the teeth). Most bristles are made of nylon, and the bristle ends are rounded. Subgingival plaque can be removed only to a depth of a few millimeters. For patients with a highly developed gagging reflex, a child's toothbrush is recommended. In addition, these patients sometimes find that placing a small amount of salt on the tongue is helpful in checking the desire to gag.

Studies of toothbrushing methods indicate that thoroughness is more important than technique. In the United States, the most widely used technique is one in which the bristles are directed into the gingival crevice at a 45° angle, and a gentle, jab-jiggle action is used. The motion is elliptical, rather than a back-and-forth scrubbing. Power toothbrushes are of special value for people who have motor coordination problems or difficulty in properly removing plaque by manual brushing. For children, the novelty effect of the powered brush is sometimes of motivational value. Also, a number of studies have shown advantages of 10–15% better plaque removal than manual brushing.

Flossing

Surveys find that only 25% of the population questioned use dental floss regularly. Flossing is essential for removal of plaque from the surfaces between teeth and under the gumline, where the toothbrush does not reach. Because plaque has a propensity to build up in these areas, some dentists feel that flossing is actually more important than brushing. Patients who do not have the manual dexterity to use dental floss can use the various types of dental floss holders or powered interdental cleaners. Dental floss is available in waxed, lightly waxed, and unwaxed varieties. Most dentists feel that lightly waxed and unwaxed types are the most efficient in plaque removal. If the floss shreds or splits during use, this may be a sign of decay between the teeth or a defective filling margin. However, new flosses have been introduced that do not shred and are easier to use. The first of these new flosses was Glide Floss, followed by similar products from Colgate and Oral B.

Disclosing Agents

Disclosing agents are dyes similar to those in food colorings that, when introduced into the oral cavity, color the supragingival plaque and make it easily visible. Various dyes are available in both liquid and tablet form. They are used in the dental office and at home both to increase the patient's awareness of plaque and to demonstrate where self-care has been ineffective in removing plaque.

Toothpastes

The majority of toothpastes advertised as specially formulated to control plaque contain (in addition to fluoride) a foaming agent and a mild abrasive, both of which facilitate plaque removal. However, the only toothpaste accepted by the ADA as possessing an active ingredient with proven ability to prevent or control plaque formation and reduce gingivitis is Colgate Total, with Triclosan as the active ingredient. Toothpastes claiming to be effective against plaque are simply more effective than brushing without any toothpaste because the use of toothpaste motivates people to brush longer and more thoroughly. In fact, it is mainly the mechanical action of brushing that removes plaque.

Toothpastes are effective as vehicles to deliver fluoride and Triclosan to the tooth surface, and although fluoride may have some effect against plaque bacteria and their enzymes, its major effect is to make the tooth surface more resistant to destruction by plaque bacteria. With the exception of Colgate Total, other tooth-pastes are accepted by the ADA for their fluoride content and effectiveness against tooth decay but not for their plaque–and gingivitis-reducing properties.

Other Oral Hygiene Aids

A number of devices aid in the removal of plaque from surfaces between teeth, around bridgework, and in other areas that are difficult to reach. The limitation of many of these devices is that they are effective for control of supragingival plaque but, at best, can remove subgingival plaque only to a depth of few millimeters. Therefore, they are of minimal value against subgingival plaque located deeper within the gingival crevice, as is the case in periodontal disease.

Various oral irrigators on the market remove some loosely attached plaque and particles of debris present around teeth and dental appliances, including braces. Because they are not effective in removing all attached plaque, they are not substitutes for brushing and flossing; rather, they should be used as adjuncts to these procedures. In addition, oral irrigators are limited in their ability to reach subgingival plaque. However, the introduction of subgingival applicator tips allows solutions to be delivered 6–7 mm apically.

Some studies have suggested that irrigators may alter plaque composition by eluting bacterial endotoxins. Patients with severely inflamed gum tissues should be cautioned to use irrigators at low pressures to guard against tissue laceration (if the tissue is severly inflammed), which may aggravate the existing problem.

Tartar (Calculus)-Reducing Products

A number of products, both dentifrices and mouth- rinses, are available for reduction of supragingival calculus (tartar) in dental patients. Calculus reduction has been shown with dentifrices containing pyrophosphates, zinc salts, triclosan, and papain. The incidence of calculus formation ranges from 45 to 66%, with some variation between males and females and different age groups. Although supragingival calculus is not a major etiologic agent for gingivitis or periodontitis, its surface porosity provides an environment for plaque formation. In addition, it serves as a plaque-delivery system by holding plaque against gingival tissues. Although plaque formation has been well correlated with gingivitis and periodontitis, a similar correlation for calculus has not been reported. For this reason, the ADA does not offer an acceptance program for products that reduce calculus formation because this is considered to be a cosmetic issue, rather than an issue of disease. The mechanism of action of the calculus-reducing chemicals is related to the latter's ability to inhibit crystal growth and interrupt the transformation of calcium phosphate (found in foods and saliva) into dental calculus. This effect may occur as follows:

1. The agents complex on the tooth surface to block receptor sites for calcium phosphate that precipitates from saliva and chemically absorbs to initiate calculus formation.
2. This same receptor site blockage also occurs in the calculus matrix as it begins to form.
3. The pyrophosphate complexes combine with free calcium in saliva to inhibit the attachment at the tooth surface (probably a secondary mechanism).

Because these products offset mineralization, there has been concern over demineralization of teeth. All manufacturers have addressed this issue and have reported that this has not been a problem, probably because of the positive effect of fluoride on remineralization of dentin and enamel. Some patients cannot use tartar control toothpastes containing pyrophosphates because they develop tooth sensitivity and sloughing of tissue. These adverse effects have not been reported with nonpyrophosphate-containing tartar control products such as those made by Den-Mat Corporation.

Crest tartar control dentifrice

This dentifrice contains 3.4% tetrasodium pyrophosphate and 1.37% disodium dihydrogen pyrophosphate to reduce calculus. Also, 0.243% sodium fluoride is included for caries reduction and prevention. It was the first calculus-reducing dentifrice introduced into the United States. On the basis of various clinical studies, a reduction of 30–40% can be expected. It has also been shown to significantly reduce the tooth staining seen in some patients who use chlorhexidine.

Crest tartar control mouthrinse

This mouthrinse provides 1.6% ionic pyrophosphate from di sodium and tetrasodium pyrophosphate to act against calculus formation and 0.05% sodium fluoride as a caries-reducing agent. Data on the extent of calculus and caries reduction were not available when this article was written because the product was in test market.

Colgate tartar control dentifrice

This product contains 5% tetrasodium pyrophosphate and a polymeric fatty acid with the company-patented name of Gantrez as the calculus-reducing agents. Also, 0.243% sodium fluoride is included for caries reduction and prevention. On the basis of various clinical studies, a calculus reduction of 35–50% can be expected. It is equal to Crest in terms of calculus reduction, with some clinical studies even suggesting a superiority to Crest.

Colgate tartar control mouthrinse

This mouthrinse contains tetrasodium pyrophosphate and tetrapotassium pyrophosphate, which provide 1% ionic pyrophosphate. It also contains 0.02% fluoride. Calculus reduction has been reported to be 35–40% with twice-a-day rinsing, with no claim made for caries reduction.

Listerine tartar control mouthrinse

This mouthrinse contains 0.09% zinc chloride to reduce calculus and also contains the same ingredients as Listerine mouthrinse.

Rembrandt mouth-refreshing rinse

This product has been shown to reduce tartar due to a formulation of surface-active agents and citroxain, a form of papain.

Targon

This mouthrinse reduces staining due to a formulation of surface-active agents. With the introduction of these products, the practitioner is offered a variety of dosage forms and flavors. If one decides to recommend a calculus-reducing agent, the product selection should be based on the product the patient likes to use best and one that will not diminish his awareness of the importance of plaque control. For example, if he is not already using a mouthrinse, would its introduction de-emphasize the mechanical methods of brushing and flossing as a means of plaque and/or calculus reduction?

HALITOSIS

Local factors, systemic factors, or a combination of both can cause halitosis. It is estimated that 80% of all mouth odors are caused by local factors within the oral cavity, and these odors are most often associated with caries, gingivitis, and periodontitis. Oral malodors occur because of the action of various microorganisms on proteinaceous substances, such as, exfoliated oral epithelium, salivary proteins, food debris, and blood. Studies have shown that saliva from individuals who are free of dental disease produces malodor less rapidly than saliva from patients with dental disease. It has also been observed that after prolonged periods of decreased salivary flow and abstinence from food and liquid malodors tend to be most severe.

Various oral bacteria produce products that are degraded to a number of compounds, foremost of which are sulfides and mucoproteins. These compounds have been most often associated with oral malodor. Specifically, it appears that oral malodor usually results from the bacterial-mediated degradative processes of methyl mercaptan and hydrogen sulfide in oral air. Ammonia is also produced but does not appear to contribute significantly to halitosis. It has even been suggested that ammonia production may improve the odor of mouth air. Control of halitosis is directed at its etiology. If systemic factors are the problem, a medical consultation is indicated. If local factors are responsible, efforts should be directed toward their elimination. However, for many patients, systemic or local factors cannot be identified. Tongue scraping has been shown to reduce malodor in some patients. Mouthwashes and dentifrices can serve an esthetic function by reducing halitosis. They can accomplish this by masking malodors, acting as antimicrobial agents, or both. There are no ADA-accepted products to reduce halitosis at this time.

TOPICAL ANESTHETICS

Topical anesthetic agents are selected for their ability to diffuse into the oral mucosa. Because many anesthetics used effectively for nerve block or infiltration do not adequately cross the mucosa, they cannot be used for topical anesthesia. The concentration of anesthetic used for surface application is 2–5%. The rate of onset of topical anesthesia ranges from 2 to 5 min, is of relatively short duration, and has minimal effects deep to the area of application. One exception is a mucosal patch containing 10.4 mg of Lidocaine that gives anesthesia deep into the gingiva after a 5-min application period. Systemic absorption of topical anesthetics applied to the oral mucosa is rapid, and blood levels may approach those seen following injection. Several drugs used as topical anesthetics are not readily soluble in water but are soluble in organic solvents. They are, thus, prepared in alcohol, propylene glycol, polyethylene glycol, volatile oils, and other vehicles suitable for surface application. Their slower absorption rates make them safer for topical use on abraded or lacerated tissue. They produce anesthesia for short periods.

Topical anesthetics are useful to temporarily relieve the pain of ulcers, wounds, and other injured areas. The topical use of anesthetic agents before injection may produce superficial anesthesia. They are also of value in taking impressions or intraoral radiographs in patients with an excessive gag reflex.

Patients who are allergic to parenterally administered local anesthetics will also be allergic to topical application of these agents. In addition, as the agents may be absorbed into the systemic circulation, careless application of excessive amounts can result in signs of systemic toxicity. Symptoms of toxicity should be treated, as they would be for injectable agents. One can minimize the absorption of these agents by limiting the concentration of the drug, the area of application, and the total amount applied. In general, for topical anesthesia, one should use no more than one-fourth to one-half the maximum recommended dosage for injection of the agent. Some topical anesthetic preparations are marketed in spray containers. These containers make it difficult to control the amount of material expelled and to confirm the agent was applied to the desired site. If these agents are applied to the posterior part of the mouth, a patient may inhale enough of the aerosol spray to provoke a toxic reaction. Use of topical anesthetics on the posterior pharynx may alter the swallowing reflex.

Benzodent

This ester-type anesthetic is poorly absorbed. Because it contains benzocaine, which has a low water solubility, it is prepared in a base containing petrolatum and sodium carboxymethylcellulose. Eugenol is included for its antiseptic and anodyne properties. Hydroxyquinoline sulfate is a preservative. This ointment can be directly applied to abraded or ulcerated lesions with minimal systemic effects. It is sometimes used to temporarily relieve denture sores and painful lesions.

Hurricaine

This ester-type anesthetic also contains benzocaine and is prepared in a polyethylene glycol base with flavoring agents added. It is available as a liquid, gel, or spray. The propellant for the spray is A 70.

Butyn

This ester-type anesthetic contains butacaine, with benzyl alcohol as a preservative. It is available as an ointment. The maximum dose is 5 ml of a 4% solution or 200 mg.

Cetacaine

This ester-type anesthetic is a combination of tetracaine HCl (2%), butyl aminobenzoate (2%), and benzocaine (14%). Benzalkonium chloride and cetyl dimethylammonium bromide are included as surface-active agents to facilitate the passage of benzocaine into the mucosal tissues. Tetracaine is rapidly absorbed through biologic membranes and requires no facilitating agents. Because of its high toxicity and absorption, agents containing tetracaine should be used with caution and should not be placed under dentures. Spraying this agent is dangerous because the patient may inhale the aerosol. The maximum amount to be applied is 20 mg or 1 ml of a 2% solution. Cetacaine is available as a liquid, ointment, spray, or gel.

Xylocaine

This amide-type anesthetic contains a lidocaine base in a monoaqueous vehicle. It is available as a 2% viscous product containing lidocaine 2%, sodium carboxymethylcellulose, sodium saccharin, methylparaben, propylparaben, flavors, and purified water. It is also available as a liquid containing 4% methylparaben, sodium hydroxide, and flavoring agents. Another dosage form is a 5% ointment containing lidocaine 5%, polyethylene glycol, propylene glycol, and flavoring. The maximum dose is 300 ml of a 5% liquid form or 15 ml of the 2% viscous preparation.

Dentifrices and Sensitive Teeth

Sometimes a patient will complain of teeth that are hypersensitive to heat and cold. These teeth usually have exposed root surfaces, sometimes with a loss of cementum. Most teeth, when in an ideal position in the mouth, have only the enamel surface exposed to the oral cavity. On occasion, such teeth may even respond with pain to extreme heat or cold. However, in true dentinal hypersensitivity, the response to thermal and tactile changes is more pronounced, sometimes eliciting severe pain. Root surface exposure that allows contact with stimuli may occur because of gingival recession or following periodontal therapy.

Several theories have been advanced to explain the mechanism of dentinal hypersensitivity: innervation of the dentinal tubules, permitting transmission of impulses to the pulp, or the presence of lymph fluid in the dentinal tubules. In the latter case, exposure of dentin results in increased colloidal pressure on the tubules (thereby increasing pressure on the odontoblastic cells). Also proposed is a hydrodynamic mechanism involving the movements of tubular fluid in either direction, which elicits pain in the nerves of the pulp. Although no one theory has been proved, occlusion of the dentinal tubules by various methods brings relief. Various dentifrices are recommended for the treatment of sensitivity, with some success.

The greatest success occurs with dentifrices containing 5% potassium nitrate, and some fluoride-containing dentifrices. Recently, a dentifrice containing potassium nitrate and stannous fluoride has been introduced to treat this problem (Colgate). The primary mechanisms postulated for these dentifrices are that they occlude dentinal tubules, preventing stimuli from the oral cavity from irritating the dental nerve via these tubules. Also, those containing potassium may depolarize nerve fibers resulting in decreased impulse conduction and an associated decrease in pain. For maximum effect, a patient must use only one of these dentifrices for at least a month. If no benefit occurs after a month, a different dentifrice should be recommended or other methods employed. Topical varnishes containing sodium fluoride have also been shown to reduce dentinal hypersensitivity (e.g., Duraphat and Fluor-Protect) as well as reduce root surface caries.

Bleaching Agents

Tooth-bleaching agents can be classified as to whether they are used for external or internal bleaching and whether the procedure is performed in the office by a dentist or at home by a patient. For tooth bleaching, hydrogen peroxide (H_2O_2) is used alone at levels of 30% or at 10–22% levels in a stable gel of carbamide peroxide (urea peroxide) that breaks down to form hydrogen peroxide (3.35% H_xO_2 from 10% carbamide peroxide), urea, ammonia, and carbon dioxide. The FDA has not approved peroxide solutions for use as a home bleach, however.

Internal Bleaching

Internal bleaching produces reliable results when used to eliminate intrinsic stains in dentin caused by blood breakdown products or endodontics or for stains in receded pulp chambers. Internal bleaching is always an in-office procedure.

External Bleaching

External bleaching is indicated for teeth that are disclosed from aging, fluorosis, or staining due to the effects of tetracycline. External bleaching can be applied by the dentist or staff or can be applied by the patient in home-use bleaching. When dentist-administered and home-use bleaching are both used, it is called "*dual bleaching.*"

Dentist-applied external bleaching can be done with periodic repetitions of an office-bleaching agent using Superoxol or 30% H_2O_2. An etching gel containing phosphoric acid applied to selected dark areas increases the penetration of the bleach. Light is used to produce heat, which accelerates the bleaching process. External bleaching may need additional treatment every 1–2 years to touch up relapses. Severely stained teeth may require more frequent retreatment. Home bleaching, supervised by the dentist, is done by the patient at home using a custom-made carrier that holds the bleach against the patient's teeth. After the desired result is achieved, overnight use on a periodic basis (1–4x month) can maintain the lightening that has been achieved.

External bleaching is seldom permanent, lasting approximately 1–4 years, after which teeth gradually return to their original color. Usually the younger the patient, the longer the bleaching will last. The more difficult it is to bleach a tooth, the more likely it is to discolor again. Bluish–gray stains seem to reappear more quickly than yellow stains. Because reoccurrence of staining is unpredictable, promises about longevity should not be made. Internal bleaching usually lasts longer than external bleaching.

Whitening Formulas

Whitening of teeth can occur by two mechanisms. One method is mechanical, in which an abrasive is used to remove debris from the tooth. The other method involves either the use of peroxides, which react with water to form free oxygen radicals that help to whiten the teeth or a combination of mechanical and chemical actions. This latter mechanism is found with bleaching agents and is longer lasting than whitening procedures.

XEROSTOMIA

The widely held belief that saliva production significantly decreases with age is not well supported in the literature dealing with this subject. Aging does not appear to play a major role as a single contributing factor in causing xerostomia. However, senior citizens may receive medication that produces the side effect of xerostomia. The aged also develop medical problems that can diminish salivary production. For these reasons, most of the studies of xerostomia have focused on older patients. One study reported a direct correlation between the intake of anticholingergic drugs, sedatives, and hypnotics and xerostomia. Over 400 drugs have been identified as potential reducers of salivary flow by acting on the cholinergic (parasympathetic) system either directly or indirectly. Another study found that the use of drugs producing xerostomia increases with age and, as expected, is highest in institutionalized patients. There are over 30 classifications of prescription and non-prescription medications that can reduce salivary flow.

Other factors that can cause xerostomia are systemic disorders and radiation. These factors must be considered in the differential diagnosis of xerostomia.

Clinical Problems with Xerostomia

Clinical problems associated with reduced salivary flow include difficulty chewing foods, reduced denture retention, recurrent caries, root surface caries, and oral candidiasis (low grade). When any of these conditions are found in a patient, regardless of age, reduced salivary flow should be considered in a differential diagnosis of the problem.

Treatment

Treatment of patients with reduced salivary flow should include the following: (1) drug and dosage changes by the patient's physician in consultation with the patient's dentist; (2) use of artificial saliva in a spray form; (3) use of mouth moisturizers and lip balms; (4) use of sugarless hard candy; (5) frequent sipping of water; (6) use of decaffeinated products; (7) use of pilocarpine (Salagen) 3–5 $\times$ daily; and (8) inclusion of citrus and pineapple flavors in the diet.

Local Delivery of Antimicrobial Agents

In the past decade, significant research and product innovations have focused the attention of dental practitioners on the concept of the local application of antimicrobials to treat periodontal diseases. Three local delivery agents are now available in the United States, and two additional products are available in other parts of the world. Though the rationale of antimicrobial approaches to treatment is evident, their limitations have also been evident. With systemic therapy, it may be difficult to achieve bacteriostatic or bactericidal antibiotic concentrations in pockets without using doses that evoke systemic side effects. The development of bacterial resistance is also an issue. The rise of antibiotic resistant, disease-producing bacterial strains is currently a major public health concern. Prolonged, repetitive courses of antibiotics for recurring dental infections is discouraged, because such practice can more readily lead to the development of resistance. Preferably, the cause of the infection should be eliminated rather than merely "managed" with antibiotics. Once antibiotic therapy is initiated, however, the importance of compliance with dosage and duration of treatment must be stressed with the patient. With poor patient compliance, under-dosing may occur, which, in turn, can favor the emergence of resistant bacteria.

Controlled Medication Delivery

The limitations of systemic therapy have prompted extensive research for the development of alternative delivery systems. Local, controlled delivery systems are available to release pilocarpine to the eye for a week after single placement for treatment of glaucoma. The oral cavity offers another relatively accessible disease site for localized therapy. In localized therapy for periodontal disease, the concern is the difficulty in reaching deep pockets and sustaining bacteriostatic or bactericidal levels long enough to be effective but not causing the development of resistance.

Tetracycline-containing fibers (Actisite)

The first local delivery product available in the United States, one which has been extensively studied, is an ethylenevinyl acetate copolymer fiber, diameter 0.5 mm, containing tetracycline, 12.7 mg/9 in. When packed into a periodontal pocket, it is well tolerated by oral tissues, and for 10 days, it sustains tetracycline concentrations exceeding 1300 μg/ml, well beyond the 32–64 μg/ml required to inhibit the growth of pathogens isolated from periodontal pockets. In contrast, crevicular fluid concentrations of only 4–8 μg/ml are reported following systemic tetracycline administration, 250 mg, 4× daily for 10 days (total oral dose, 10g). Thus, controlled site-specific tetracycline delivery can achieve a bactericidal effect at approximately 1/1000th of the dose administered systemically.

Studies demonstrate that the tetracycline fibers, applied with or without scaling and root planing, reduce probing depth, bleeding on probing, and periodontal pathogens and provide gains in clinical attachment level. Such effects are significantly better than those attained with scaling and root planing alone or with placebo fibers. The fibers used in conjunction with scaling and root planing have also provided a statistically significant improvement in probing depth reduction and clinical attachment level gains of over 60% and in bleeding on probing reductions over scaling and root planing alone at 6 months after therapy. Actisite was the first local delivery system cleared by the FDA for the adjunctive treatment of recurrent periodontal disease. Although 6-month studies have demonstrated their value, longer-term studies are needed.

Chlorhexidine delivery system (PerioChip)

A newer development in controlled local delivery, one that utilizes the antiseptic chlorhexidine as the antimicrobial agent, has been introduced in a number of countries and was recently cleared by the FDA for use in the United States. This delivery system, Perio-Chip, was developed in Israel and has been tested in the United States as well as in Europe.

The PerioChip is a small chip (4.0 × 5.0 × 0.35 mm) composed of a biodegradable hydrolyzed gelatin matrix into which has been incorporated 2.5 mg chlorhexidine gluconate per chip. It is rounded on one end and inserts easily and in less than a minute into periodontal pockets that are 5 mm or greater in depth. The PerioChip releases chlorhexidine and maintains drug concentrations in the gingival crevicular fluid greater than 100 μg/ml for at least 7 days, concentrations well above the tolerance of most oral bacteria. Because the PerioChip biodegrades in 7–10 days, a second appointment for removal is not needed. Studies with the PerioChip were as long as 9 months. At 9 months, significant decreases were observed in probing depth from baseline favoring the active chip plus scaling and root planing compared with controls (scaling and root planing only): chlorhexidin chip plus scaling and root planing, -0.95 ± 0.05 mm; placebo chip plus scaling and root planing, -0.69 ± 0.05 mm ($p = 0.00056$); scaling and root planing alone -0.65 ± 0.05 mm ($p = 0.00001$). The proportion of pocket sites with a probing depth reduction of 2 mm or more was increased in the chlorhexidine chip group compared with scaling and root planing alone, a difference which was statistically significant on a per patient basis ($p < 0.0001$). Improvements favoring the chlorhexidine chip compared with controls were also observed for clinical attachment levels at 9 months, improvements that were significant when the data were pooled ($p < 0.05$). Bleeding on probing was reduced in the active chip group compared with both controls, differences which were significant in one of the two studies ($p < 0.05$) and when the data were pooled ($p = 0.012$).

The results of these studies suggest that the Perio Chip may be a valuable adjunct to scaling and root planing in the treatment of periodontal disease. This product is easily placed, requires no appointment for removal, and provides reductions in probing depths similar to subgingivally placed antibiotics now available in various countries across the world. In addition, a major advantage of this system is that its active agent is an antiseptic instead of an antibiotic.

Subgingival Delivery of Doxycycline (Atridox)

Atridox is a recently developed gel system that incorporates the antibiotic doxycycline (10%) in a syringeable gel system. An animal study in beagle dogs initially suggested some benefit to locally delivered doxycycline, and it is used in the veterinary population.

A recent 9-month, multicenter study was designed to study the effects of subgingivally placed doxycycline compared to subgingival placement of the vehicle and an herbal agent (Sanguinaria). No scaling or root planing was performed in any of the groups, and there was no untreated group. The patients were instructed in oral hygiene and randomly assigned to one of three groups: vehicle control, 5% sanguinarine in the vehicle control, and 10% doxycycline in the vehicle control.

Treatment with doxycycline was more effective than the other treatments at all time periods, with the exception of the 3-month clinical attachment level value. Also, when the authors evaluated the effect based on initial probing depth, the differential effect in the doxycycline group in comparison with the other two groups was greater as pretreatment probing depth increased. For the doxycycline group, the reduction in clinical attachment level at 9 months showed a gain of 0.4 mm compared to vehicle control, the reduction in probing depth was 0.6 mm greater than vehicle control, and the reduction of bleeding on probing was 0.2 units greater than vehicle control. Although the differences were small, they were statistically significant. The patient's oral hygiene scores (plaque index) averaged between 0.7 and 1.1 in all three groups throughout the study. Although resistance was not evaluated in this study, the local application of doxycycline has previously been reported to show transient increases in resistance in oral microbes and no overgrowth of foreign pathogens.

Data have recently been presented from two multicenter clinical trials. All treatment groups showed clinical improvements from baseline over the 9-month period. The results for all parameters measured were significantly better in the doxycycline group compared with vehicle control and oral hygiene only. Compared with scaling and root planing, the effects of doxycycline on clinical attachment level gain and probing depth reduction were equivalent. Clinical study results suggest a potential periodontal benefit from the subgingival application of doxycycline. However, the value of this agent as an adjunct to scaling and root planing is untested. This product is cleared by the FDA for use in animals and humans.

Host Modulation

In 1998, the first non-antimicrobial drug to treat periodontal disease, Periostat, was approved by the FDA. Nonetheless, in the antibiotic family, the dose of the drug used is too low to kill bacteria. Periostat acts through its effects on inhibition of metalloproteinases, such as, collagenase and gelatinase. The therapeutic objective is to modulate the inflammatory host response. Periostat, available as a 20 mg capsule of doxycycline hyclate, is prescribed for use by patients twice daily. The mechanism of action is by suppression of the activity of collagenase, particularly that produced by polymorphonuclear leukocytes. Although this drug is in the antibiotic family, it does not produce any antimicrobial effects because the dose of 20 mg twice daily is too low to affect bacteria. As a result, resistance to this medication cannot develop. Four double-blind, clinical, multicenter studies in over 650 patients have demonstrated that Periostat improves the effectiveness of professional periodontal care and slows the progression of the disease process.

23

VIRTUAL SCREENING

Identification of viable chemical leads is one of the key tasks of the early stage of drug discovery. Historically, the lead discovery phase was mainly supported by in vivo experiments that usually resulted in compounds with acceptable efficacy and suitable pharmacokinetic profile at least in animal models. On the other hand, however, lead optimization was slow and rarely successful that gave significant role to serendipity. Because in vivo based, purely intuitive approaches yielded hardly predictable results; drug discovery faced a paradigm shift in the early 1980s. Limitations of animal models and the lack of the molecular mechanism were found to be critical factors when analyzing attrition rates that initiated research groups to introduce in vitro tests at the frontline of discovery programs. Application of rational approaches was also facilitated by in vitro screening supplying reliable data-sets for the first time for computer aided drug discovery (CADD) methods. In vitro assays serve the basis of structure- activity relationship that drives medicinal chemistry during active-to-hit and hit-to-lead processes. Dramatic developments in molecular biology, detection methods, computer technology, and robotics made high-through-put in vitro screening (HTS) to be a characteristic tool of lead discovery. In the 1990s, the brut-force HTS was the ultimate technology of lead discovery. Today, however, it became clear that productivity of lead discovery could not be increased by screening more compounds against more targets even in more and more sophisticated assays. In addition to limitations in target validation, assay development, compound and data quality and despite ultra high throughput, the number of available, or ever synthesized compounds is still negligible relative to the drug-like chemistry space. Random screening should, therefore, be replaced by methodologies that combine the capacity of HTS approaches and the rational basis of CADD techniques. Virtual screening (VS) methods exemplify this idea, as high-throughput CADD tools are capable to investigate huge compound collections in reasonable time and cost.

Application of the HTS technology requires the selection of the target, the development of the assay, and the definition of the screening library in a suitable format. In vitro HTS campaigns are then typically performed in a highly automated environment and generates huge amount of data that should be stored, treated, and analyzed. In these contexts, VS techniques can be considered as "*in silico*" analogues of in vitro HTS technologies. After defining the target, VS also requires the development and optimization of the prediction technique (i.e., the in silico analogue of the assay) applied for affinity predictions. Databases that serve as screening library should be preprocessed to use in VS. The screening process itself is performed in the computer memory and should, therefore, be fully automated while generating data similar to HTS data-sets both in quantity and quality. In addition to similarities between the procedures, HTS and VS have a common conceptual framework as well.

Both methods have limited accuracy that is compensated by the number of compounds investigated. VS and HTS, are rather classification techniques that separate actives from inactives, than a method of choice when quantifying biological affinity. These methods could identify candidates rather than validated hits. Some of the promising candidates could never be validated, these are false positives. Both high-throughput technologies surely miss some active compounds that are called "*false negatives.*" Although every reasonable effort should be done to minimize false positive and negative rates, the common philosophy behind these techniques suggest that if we identify even a single interesting compound, then false positives and negatives can be tolerated.

Finally, candidates identified by HTS or VS should be experimentally validated before starting active-to-hit and hit-to-lead processes. The most characteristic difference between HTS and VS is that the former identifies the candidates experimentally, while the latter derives them computationally. The computational strategy applied in VS suggests that: (i) it could be more effective in time, resource, and cost; (ii) it could explore a significantly larger part of the drug-like chemistry space; and (iii) it could yield higher hit rate than random screening. Although these potential advantages suggest VS being more favorable than HTS, comparative studies demonstrated that these approaches are rather complementary than competitive. In one hand, VS techniques could be useful when designing target specific screening libraries. On the other hand, distinct structural classes identified by VS and HTS are clearly the observations that most straightforwardly support complementarities between VS and HTS. While the underlying disciplines of HTS are bioinformatics and biochemistry, VS is based on cheminformatics and computational chemistry.

In fact, there are computational approaches–most of them are CADD methods–already applied in drug discovery that were transformed to VS tools. Similar to CADD techniques VS methods can be divided into ligand-based and structure-based approaches. Ligand-based techniques operate exclusively in the small molecule space using chemical and biological information encoded in known active compounds to identify new candidates with similar properties. Structure-based methods require the three-dimensional structure (3-D) of the target protein that is used for docking small molecules into the binding site. Evaluation of binding modes and protein-ligand interactions finally allows ranking of docked compounds by their binding affinity. This entry summarizes the background of both approaches, gives case studies for supporting practical applications, and collects success stories to demonstrate capabilities.

Data Base Filtering

Physicochemical Filters

One of the early physicochemical filters is the famous rule-of-five (ROF) introduced by Lipinski et al. ROF is based on the distributions of easily accessible and interpretable physicochemical properties obtained from known drugs. Compounds fulfilling ROF do not violate more than one rule out of the followings: molecular weight (MW) < 500, calculated log P (clogP) < 5, number of hydrogen bond acceptors (HBA) < 10, and number of hydrogen bond donors (HBD) < 5. These ranges of properties define a chemistry space containing molecules without serious absorption, distribution, metabolism, and elimination (ADME) problems that are expected to be orally bioavailable. This chemistry space is usually referred as drug-like space and its content is called drug-like molecules. Consequently, drug-likeness of compound libraries (both virtual and physical) can be easily investigated by assessing their members by ROF. In addition to properties included to ROF, Oprea proposed further limitations in features when searching for drug-like molecules. His analysis suggested that the number of rotatable bonds (RB) should be lower than eight while the number of rings ideally smaller than four. Kelder et al. introduced polar surface area (PSA) as a relevant descriptor for predicting oral bioavailability. PSA was defined as the sum of the van der Waals surface of polar atoms including oxygen, nitrogen, and sulfur with attached hydrogens. PSA showed significant impact on membrane penetration including intestinal (PSA < $140A^2$) and blood–brain barrier permeabilities (PSA < $80A^2$). As PSA can be approximated from the 2-D structure, these approaches are now considered as filtering methods for VS of large compound libraries. Although purely statistical approaches are still dominating on this field, Gillet, Willett, and Bradshaw used a genetic algorithm (GA)-based weighting scheme for property and shape descriptors when discriminating between drugs and non-drugs.

The concept of lead-likeness has been established by Hann and Oprea, analyzing lead molecules and corresponding drugs. Comparative studies on leads and drugs revealed that leads are typically less complex molecules than drugs. Consequently, their physicochemical properties should differ significantly from that of the drugs. In fact, effective leads have lower MW and clogP, have a smaller number of rings (RNG), and RB. The original ROF was therefore modified to rule-of-three (ROT: MW < 300, clog P < 3,H-bond donors (HDO) < 3, rotatable bond (RTB) < 3) by Astex reflecting to the reduced complexity of leads. Based on these findings, Leach et al. established a filtering scheme of MW < 350, RTB < 6, number of heavy atoms < 22, HDO < 3, high-activity moleucle (HAC) < 8, clogP < 2.2 when selecting compounds for reduced complexity screening. Surveying medicinal chemistry literature Oprea and coworkers have drawn less strict conclusion, when formulating the criteria of lead-likeness MW < 460, –4 < LogP < 4.2, RTB < 10, RNG <4, HDO < 5, HAC < 9.

As similar to HTS, the basic objective of VS is to identify interesting starting points for medicinal chemistry programs. We believe that lead-likeness would be a useful concept for filtering compound libraries before more sophisticated approaches. Nevertheless, it should be emphasized that limits applied for both drug-like and lead-like compounds are based on statistical analyses of known examples. Although these simple filters demonstrated significant classification accuracy when discriminating drugs and non-drugs, leads and drugs–their fully empirical nature warns against unconditional applications.

Functional Group Filters

Functional group filters are mainly utilized to remove unstable, reactive, toxic, or otherwise unsuitable compounds from compound libraries. The rapid elimination of swill (REOS) method. introduced by Vertex was the first realization of this concept. REOS effectively combines physicochemical filters with a set of functional group filters. Databases are first subjected to property filtering similar to ROF that is followed by checking a set of rules based on the presence of functional groups expected to be problematic. It is important to note that REOS allows the user to customize each functional group filter as well as the set of rules applied.

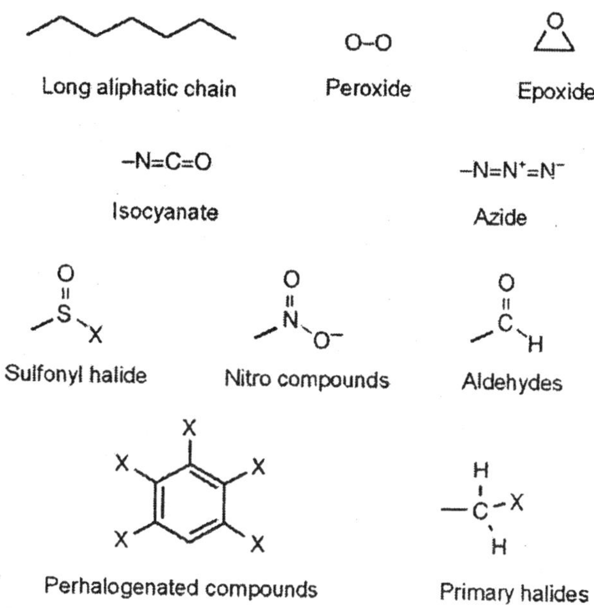

Fig. 23.1. Examples of functionalities filtered out by REOS.

Hann et al. used a similar, multilevel approach when pooling compounds for HTS. These authors applied three types of filters. Basic filters were used to remove molecules with non-drug-like features. Next functional group-based hard filters were utilized comprising filters for reactive functional groups, unsuitable leads (i.e., compounds which would not be initially followed up), and unsuitable natural products (i.e., derivatives of natural product compounds known to interfere with common assay procedures). Finally, soft filters represented by a GA trained to identify unsuitable compounds that the other filters would fail to find. This algorithm scores compounds for drug-likeness, relative to a training set classified by medicinal chemists. Andrews and coworkers used a set of 200 drug molecules to derive a set of "*intrinsic binding energies*" for the 10 functional groups. The inherent binding affinity of compounds was then estimated by summing the intrinsic binding energies and subtracting an entropic factor. Muegge, Heald, and Brittelli described a functional group filter to discriminate between drugs and non-drugs. The authors assigned a score to each molecule that is based on the presence of fragments typically found in drugs. Each non-overlapping drug-like fragment counts one point in this scheme. Molecules with a score between two and seven are classified as drugs, otherwise they are classified as non-drugs. As it was noted that CNS active compounds are relatively small and typically contain only a single pharmacophoric group, they defined a second filter. This filter ensured that compounds containing a single drug-like functional group could only be classified as drugs if they contain one of the distinguished groups.

Topological Filters

It is generally accepted that structural similarity to known drugs significantly increases the drug-like character of compounds. Therefore, molecular topology of known drugs in comparison to non-drugs served as suitable starting point for a number of approaches. One group of methods utilized neural networks for discriminating between drugs and non-drugs. Compounds in drug databases such as World Drug Index (WDI), Comprehensive Medicinal Chemistry (CMC), and MDL Drug Data Report (MDDR) and databases of chemical suppliers (typically Available Chemical Directory; ACD) were represented by structural descriptors. Sadowski and Kubinyi reported the application of Ghoose–Crippen atom types as input neurons, while the output neuron was set to one for drugs and zero for non-drugs when training the net by 5000 WDI and 5000 ACD compounds. The trained net was able to classify about 80% of test compounds.

Murcko and coworkers reported a similar approach based on drugs collected from CMC and non-drugs from ACD. Molecules were represented by 166 binary ISIS keys and the authors added further physicochemical descriptors, including MW, number of HBD and acceptors, number of RBs, aromatic density, clog P, and one additional descriptor reflecting the degree of branching. A Bayesian neural network (BNN) was trained using 3500 molecules from both the CMC and the ACD databases. The trained network was then tested on CMC and ACD compounds that were not included in the training set. A subset of the MDDR library was used for external validation. The classification accuracy of both CMC and ACD approached 90%, while external validation revealed 78% of the MDDR compounds being drug-like.

Frimurer et al. also reported a neural network based approach trained on a larger dataset. These authors partitioned the MDDR database into drug- like (compounds that have progressed to at least Phase I of clinical trials) and lead-like (compounds labeled as "*Biological Testing*") sets. Diversity selection from these sets resulted in 4400 MDDR drug-like compounds (3000 training and 1400 test compounds), and 90,000 ACD compounds (60,000 training and 30,000 test molecules) dissimilar to the drug-like set. The 60,000 lead-like MDDR compounds were used exclusively for external validation. All compounds were represented by 77 CONCORD atom types and three further descriptors including the number of atoms, number of heavy atoms, and total charge. Predictive power of the trained neural network was first assessed in the test set. Using a threshold of 0.15 as a criterion to discriminate between drugs and non-drugs, the neural network was able to classify 88% of the MDDR drug-like set and ACD databases correctly. External validation on lead-like compounds predicted 75% of these molecules as drug-like. Although neural network based methods are extremely fast and successfully identified the majority of known drugs, these models are hardly interpretable for medicinal chemists and, therefore could rather be used as high-throughput filters than driving chemistry to the drug-like space.

Wagener and Geerestein applied recursive partitioning to distinguish of drugs and non-drugs. Analyzing tolerated and non-tolerated functional groups in both WDI and ACD databases the authors were able to recognize almost 75% of drug-like molecules in MDDR and CMC databases.

Limited number of structural frameworks represented in known drugs can also be used for the identification of drug-like compounds. In their pioneering work, Bemis and Murcko analyzed shapes of existing drugs and identified drug-like molecular frameworks. A graph-theoretical approach was used to decompose molecules into fragments. Rings and linkers together form the framework, while acyclic side chains were removed. Based on this analysis, the authors concluded that almost the 50% of known drugs in the CMC could be described by only the most frequent 32 frameworks. The diversity of drug-like side chains was found to be similarly low, only 20 different side chains account for over 70% of all the side chains appeared in CMC.

It is interesting to note that this approach is also useful for designing target-based libraries when the topological framework analysis is applied to active compounds within a target family. One realization of this concept is the retrosynthetic combinatorial analysis procedure (RECAP) algorithm that was also utilized for the analysis of drug-like fragments. RECAP first identifies active or drug-like fragments using retrosynthetic analysis applying any of the 11-retrosynthetic reactions defined. In the next step, the resulting fragments are usually clustered and transformed into monomers that can be used for designing targeted libraries. As fragments were extracted from known actives, it is expected that compounds enumerated from the derived monomers will be also active and are synthetically accessible because of the retrosynthetic approach applied. A similar method, TOPology-Assigning System (TOPAS) has been reported by Schneider et al. These authors developed an evolutionary algorithm for fragment-based de novo design. This stochastic method utilizes a set of ~25,000 fragments that serves as building blocks obtained by a rule-based fragmentation procedure applied to 36,000 known drugs.

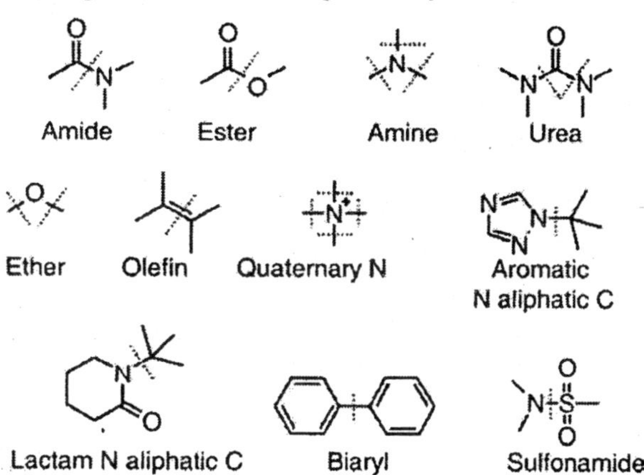

Fig. 23.2. Retrosynthetic reactions defined in RECAP.

LIGAND-BASED SCREENING

Similarity Searches

Similarity searching is one of the simplest methodologies of ligand-based VS, when screening databases against a query using chemical similarity principles. During a similarity search, the query molecule is compared to members of the database and a similarity measure is calculated quantifying the similarity between the query and each molecule in the screened database. For 2-D similarity searches, the query structure and members of the screened database are typically represented by molecular fingerprints that encode molecular structure and properties in binary format. Each bit of the fingerprint detects the presence or absence of molecular fragments or connectivity pattern, can encode descriptor value ranges or binary transformed descriptors. Fingerprints can be divided into two major groups: structural keys and hashed fingerprints. Structural keys associate a specific descriptor (structural fragment or property) with each bit, while hashed fingerprints assign overlapping bit segments to descriptors.

Generation of structural keys requires a predefined fragment library that collects the fragments searched in each molecule of the database. MACCS key (MDL Information Systems) is a typical example for a structural key. In contrast, there is no fragment library needed for hashed fingerprints. These fingerprints are derived algorithmically from all possible linear paths of the limited number of connected atoms. Paths define a pattern of atoms and bonds that are used to generate a set of bits during the hashing procedure that typically produces 4–5 bits per pattern. Although hashed fingerprints are not physically interpretable, they show highly characteristic bit patterns for molecules. Bit strings vary in length and complexity but Daylight and UNITY are the most popular hashed fingerprints used in similarity searches.

Analysis of molecular similarity is based on the quantitative determination of the overlap between fingerprints of the query structure and all database members. As descriptors of a given molecule can be considered as a vector of real or binary attributes, most of the similarity measures are derived as vectorial distances. Tanimoto and Cosine coefficients are the most popular measures of similarity In addition to binary descriptors, molecular holograms are also useful for similarity searches. Similar to fingerprint, hologram is a vector that contains numerical properties, e.g., number of occurrences for atoms or fragments.

3-D similarity searches utilize 3-D information including shape, steric, and electrostatic properties obtained for the query molecule and the database screened. High-throughput molecular alignment techniques of this kind superpose all database entries onto the query molecule. FlexS, one of the most popular approaches, keeps the query rigid and considers test molecules as flexible when offering several alternative superpositions–each scored and ranked by similarity. Genetic algorithm similarity program (GASP) is a superposition tool using GA that handles both the query and the test molecules as flexible. Wild and coworkers described an alignment tool utilizing GA-based fitting of molecular electrostatic potential fields. In MIMIC, Mestres, Rohrer, and Maggiora represented molecules as sets of Gaussian functions, modeling property fields. Alignment is optimized and scored assessing the overlap between corresponding fields. Rapid overlay of chemical structures (ROCS) performs a shape-based superposition using a Gaussian representation of the molecular volume and allows to combine 2-D and 3-D similarity.

Pharmacophore Searches

Pharmacophore mapping

Pharmacophore is an arrangement of steric and electrostatic features in the 3-D space that are crucial for the biological action. These kinds of feature- based pharmacophore models were found to be useful for ligand-based VS because they can effectively fish very different chemotypes from virtual libraries. Pharmacophore models usually consist of a number of pharmacophore points including a group of atoms, or features such as HBDs and HBAs, charged groups, hydrophobic centers, and corresponding geometric constraints. Pharmacophore features can be derived from both the structure of the target protein or from the collection of known ligands.

Structure-based pharmacophores are typically explored by analyzing binding site interactions formed between ligands and protein atoms within the active site of the target. In addition to direct structural information, site directed mutagenesis data are also useful when identifying most important residues responsible for ligand binding. LigandScout uses ligand-bound target structures to extract structure-based pharmacophore models. Hydrogen bonding features, as well as electrostatic and hydrophobic interactions, are utilized to derive the most important interactions within the active site. Starting from the protein structure, LUDI generates interaction sites that are preferable to occupy for ligand atoms. This methodology is the basis of the structure-based focusing (SBF) technique available in Cerius2. The identification of the interaction sites by LUDI is followed by the clustering of interaction vectors. The obtained clusters are the starting point for generating the pharmacophore hypothesis. POCKET realizes a similar approach to LUDI when identifying grids within the active site to characterize favorable ligand interactions. Considering the flexibility of the active site, Carlson et al. suggested a molecular dynamics approach when generating a diverse set of protein conformations to develop structure-based pharmacophore models. Reflecting to multiple potential binding modes, geometric constraints between pharmacophoric points are here defined as ranges rather than values. Pharmacophore constraints can include not only distance, angles, and dihedrals, but also excluded volumes; surface volumes and spatial restraints might also be used in the UNITY program. Molecular Operating Environment (MOE) also allows queries containing locations of features, chemical groups, or shape constraints.

In the absence of structural information on the target, pharmacophore could be developed using a set of actives that are expected to realize similar binding modes when interacting with the target. Ligand-based pharmacophore generation that is also called as pharmacophore mapping usually consists of three elementary steps. In the first step, the pharmacophore features, common in all of the actives, are identified. The second step involves the generation of putative bioactive conformations that might be explored by the actives. Finally, alignments of these conformations are prepared that ensure matches of pharmacophore features. Identification of possible bioactive conformations is clearly the greatest challenge in pharmacophore mapping. There are two basic strategies to achieve this goal. The first one generates only low energy conformations for all of the actives and then searches for common features. The other one, however, enumerates all possible conformations of each ligand and evaluates the orientation of pharmacophore features previously identified.

Although pharmacophore mapping can be completed manually in simple and straightforward cases, most of the applications require the automated generation of pharmacophore. There are several software suites available for this purpose. HipHop and HypoGen are both featured by the Catalyst package. In Catalyst, the random search algorithm used for the identification of low energy conformers is conducted with a pooling function that allows the in-depth coverage of the conformational space. Features are then identified by analyzing the surface accessibility of the actives followed by the definition of the pharmacophore using the absolute coordinates of all conformations. HipHop is useful to generate qualitative hypotheses, while HypoGen is the method of choice for more predictive quantitative models. The initial model is based on the features of the two most active molecules that serve as a starting point to generate all the possible pharmacophores. Models are then evaluated by analyzing the overlay between the pharmacophore hypotheses and the geometric arrangement of features in all conformations of the actives.

For quantitative models, Catalyst assigns weight descriptors to each feature that correspond to its importance in explaining the biological activity. Disco and Disco-Tech, both characterize actives by ligand and site points. Ligand points include HBDs and HBAs, and hydrophobic and charged features. Site points are generated on the basis of complementarity principles using the atomic coordinates of the corresponding ligand atom. Similarly to the Catalyst approach, a set of low energy conformers is first generated that are aligned as rigid objects. Alignment of the conformers represented by interfeature distances to a reference molecule having the fewest conformation is carried-out by a click detection algorithm. Disco produces a ranked list of hypotheses that contains all of the common features identified in actives. Alignment parameters calculated by Disco drive the users to select good quality pharmacophore maps. In GASP, the conformational analysis of actives takes place on the fly that is followed by the assignment of pharmacophore features including both the ligand points and site points. The molecule with the least number of features serves as reference.

The alignment procedure is carried out by a GA utilizing chromosomes that encode dihedrals of RBs in all actives and mapping of the reference's pharmacophore features to other actives. The fitness function generates conformations for each active that are then fitted to the reference using the mapping information. The best possible overlay is achieved by calculating the internal van der Waals energy of each molecule, the number, and similarity of the overlaid features in combination of the volume integral of the overlay.

Pharmacophore search

The pharmacophore model obtained by the mapping procedure allows 3-D database searching. Database searching can identify actives in different chemotypes relative to those utilized for pharmacophore generation. This procedure is often termed as scaffold hopping or lead hopping that is not limited to lead discovery programs but might contribute to back-up/follow-up strategies.

Pharmacophore searches are usually realized in two steps. Search algorithms first check the availability of pharmacophore features encoded in the query and next they evaluate the overlay of the spatial arrangement of features and the query. The fastest way of the second step is matching database entries as rigid objects. As flexible molecules can adopt a number of different low energy conformations, this set of conformers should be precomputed before screening. Another option for rigid searches is the on the fly generation of conformers that is followed by the subsequent structural alignment. Conformational flexibility is more explicitly considered in flexible 3-D searches that, however, require significantly higher resources. Pharmacophore queries that include constraint ranges could partially compensate conformational changes occurring upon ligand binding. There are a number of codes available for database searching. 3D-SEARCH divides the searches into two parts, a fast pre-screen using an inverted key system and a slower atom-by-atom geometric search using the Ullman algorithm. Features to handle angle/dihedral constraints and to take into account "excluded volume" are implemented as part of the geometric search. Catalyst utilizes both multiconformer databases and the on the fly conformer generation. ChemDBS-3D generates low energy conformers that are filtered by conformational rules. Root mean square (RMS) deviation from the pharmacophore constraint can be minimized by torsional minimization. The flexible 3-D search available in UNITY realizes this concept based on the Directed Tweak algorithm that could match the constraints of the query. A recent review by Langer and Wolber compares these technologies when used for pharmacophore searches.

Case Study: Ligand-Based VS against Kv1.5 Potassium Channel

Peukert et al. reported VS experiments using different ligand-based techniques against the voltage-dependent potassium channel Kv1.5. In their first attempt, the authors utilized similarity searching to identify new actives. A potent indane derivative first published by Eli Lilly was used as a query in a 2-D similarity search performed in UNITY. Compounds in the corporate collection were represented by 2-D UNITY fingerprint and the fingerprint of the query was compared to that of the library members. Compounds with Tanimoto coefficient larger than 0.8 were considered to be similar and was subjected to biological testing. This protocol led to the identification of a structurally novel hit with moderate potency (9.5 μM) and limited chemical stability. Suboptimal physicochemical properties and stability prompted the authors to replace the central naphthalene moiety that resulted in the discovery of a good

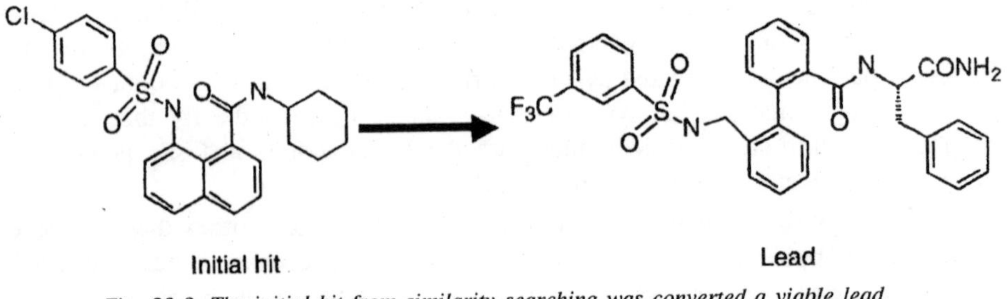

Cl O S O N O N F3C O S O N N O CONH2

Initial hit Lead

Fig. 23.3. The initial hit from similarity searching was converted a viable lead.

quality lead with improved potency (4.8 μM). Optimization of this lead was supported by solid phase parallel synthesis that enabled the authors to identify a set of highly potent and selective Kv1 .5 potassium channel blockers.

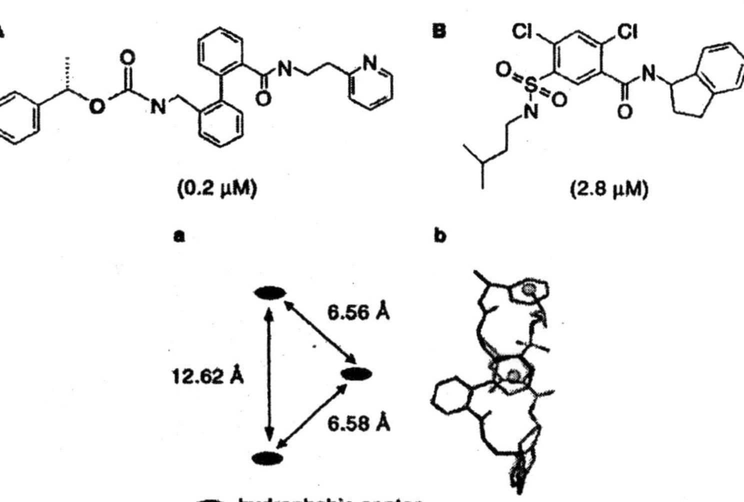

Fig. 23.4. Definition of the pharmacophore query for the Kv1.5 channel.

Structure-activity information gained for this compound series and also that obtained in a parallel lead optimization program allowed the development of a pharmacophore model for Kv1.5 potassium channel blockers. Seven potent molecules from each series were used to derive the model that consists of three hydrophobic centers in a triangular arrangement. The seven compounds were first subjected to an exhaustive conformational search utilizing the Monte Carlo (MC) Multiple Minimum algorithm as available in MacroModel. The resulting conformers were then clustered using distances between the potential pharmacophore features. A minimum energy conformation in each of the clusters was used as input to DISCO algorithm. DISCO models were visually inspected and one of them was used as a 3-D query in the subsequent UNITY 3-D flexible search.

The performance of this ligand-based VS tool was first evaluated against an in-house set of known Kv1.5 potassium channel blockers. This test revealed that the methodology was able to retrieve 58% of known actives. VS was performed on the Aventis compound collection and identified 4234 virtual hits that were first subjected to filtering. Compounds with reactive or non-tolerated features regarding the Kv1.5 potassium channel inhibitory activity, with non-drug-like character, as well as known blockers were removed during this process. The final set of 1975 compounds was submitted to hierarchical clustering that resulted in 27 clusters in total. Representatives of the available 18 clusters were tested against Kv1.5 potassium channel that identified one structurally novel compound with an IC_{50} of 5.6 μM. This hit was considered as a starting point for optimization that led to the identification of a series of compounds with remarkable activity (best IC_{50} was found to be 0.5 μM) and acceptable pharmacokinetics.

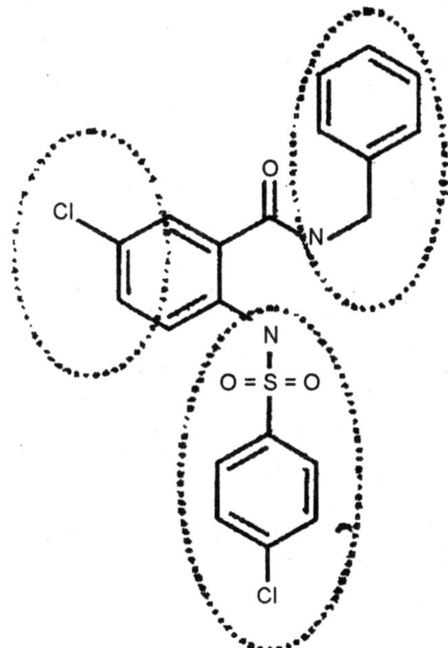

Fig. 23.5. The structurally novel lead identified by the pharmacophore search.

In the final round, the authors reported the development of a structure-based pharmacophore that was also used for VS. To achieve this goal, a homology model of the Kv1.5 potassium channel has been developed. The pore domain of the target protein was built using the crystal structure of the bacterial KcsA channel. A single subunit of the Kv1.5 channel was generated by the COMPOSER program as implemented to SYBYL software that was used to create the tetrameric structure arrangement of the target protein. The resulting model was then subjected to structural refinement using a two-step minimization protocol and it was validated by a number of protein analysis tools including PROCHECK, WHATCHECK, and MATCHMAKER. The binding site was identified by applying geometrical criteria on the validated model using the putative active site for spheres (PASS) algorithm. Visual inspection of PASS results led to the selection of a binding site that has been further characterized by the GRID force field. Pharmacophore features were derived by the calculation of molecular interaction fields using the hydrophobic, the amide nitrogen, and the carbonyl oxygen probes. Local minima of the fields were visually inspected and the selected minima of GRID energy maps in addition to the exclusion volume defined by protein atoms were used to define the pharmacophore query. This structure-based pharmacophore was utilized for a UNITY Flexsearch-based VS that resulted in 3102 hits in total. Drug-like filters, as well as partial match constraints (at least 3 out of the 12 features), were applied. Compounds with reactive or non-tolerated features regarding the Kv1 .5 potassium channel inhibitory activity were removed. After visual inspection of the hits by medicinal chemists, the authors identified 244 compounds that were subjected to in vitro screening. Biological evaluation of the hits revealed 19 actives in total including 5 compounds with an inhibition concentration (IC_{50}) under 10 μM, while the best compound having an IC_{50} of 9 μM. As all of the ligand-based efforts described in these papers were carried out on the same screening library (i.e. the Aventis compound repository), hit rates of different approaches could directly be compared.

Based on this comparison, one can conclude that pharmacophore search–both with ligand-and structure- based pharmacophores–outperformed 2-D similarity search. Although the two latter techniques gave similarly good result in hit rate, the authors found no overlap between their hit lists. Comparing the number of chemical series identified it is clear that screening by the structure-based pharmacophore hypothesis outperformed the ligand-based approaches. It should be noted, however, that the effectiveness of different VS protocols obviously depends on the target and the quantity and quality of structural and structure-activity relationship (SAR) information actually available. The multiple chemotypes identified by different strategies suggest the usefulness of parallel VS programs against the same target but with different approaches.

Structure-based VS

The functions of drug molecules and protein targets are regulated by the principles of molecular recognition. The rational drug development requires the understanding of molecular recognition in terms of structure and energetics. Structure-based VS tools study the binding between the ligand and protein structures with respect to structural and energetic considerations. In the earlier era of the structure-based drug discovery process, the low resolution of protein structures and poor computational power hindered the rapid improvement of the method. Today, these techniques have experienced a comeback because drastic changes occurred.

Genomics have resulted in a huge number of potential therapeutic targets that are available for investigation. However, learning the sequence of a genome is a long way from understanding its biological function. Predictions of protein function can be attempted from the knowledge of the structure alone or other additional information can be used to gain information about functional predictions. In many respects, it is still early days for seeing the fruits of this process in the products offered on the market by pharmaceutical companies. Therefore, there are still large investments in functional genomics, HTS methodologies, combinatorial chemistry, predictive ADME methods, and structural biology.

VS, and structure-based VS, has emerged as an inexpensive and straightforward method for identifying lead molecules. The investments in structural biology prompted the improvement of structure-based VS. Structure-based VS involves explicit molecular docking of each ligand into the active site of the target protein. Hereby, a predicted binding mode is produced, and then the quality of the fit of the molecule in the active site is scored. This scoring information is used to rank the compounds and only the top solutions can be investigated further. Without the need of completeness, we discuss the most state-of-the art structure-based VS that are generally used at pharmaceutical industries during the drug discovery process. Our attempt was also to give a picturesque overview on the structure-based VS process and show its effectiveness or its failures through a case study and some success stories during the CADD processes.

Preparation of Protein Structures

The first step in the structure-based VS process is to obtain the coordinates of a protein. Generally, structures solved by X-ray crystallography or nuclear magnetic resonance (NMR) are used, but protein structures, which have difficulties in the crystallization process e.g., membrane proteins such as G-protein coupled receptors (GPCR) can be modeled based on homology. Currently, 3-D structure information can be generated for up to ~56 % of all the known proteins. However, there is considerable controversy concerning the real value of homology models for structure-based VS. Recently published results on ligand-supported homology modeling might be able to provide reasonable quality homology models that are suitable for structure-based VS.

The definition of the active site is needed for docking into a target protein because scanning the entire surface of the protein would hardly be feasible with most of the currently used docking algorithms. On the other hand, ignoring biochemical information or structural data on the active site is unreasonable, although, in some cases information about binding sites is not available. These cases-binding sites can be identified by algorithms detecting geometric cavities, or algorithms based on physicochemical and geometrical characterization. The preparation of the active site depends on the docking tools being used. This step involves the addition of hydrogen atoms avoiding atomic clashes; assignment of appropriate protonation states of titratable residues and correct tautomers of histidine residues, and involvement of structural water molecules in the binding cavity. The conformational flexibility in the active site has to be evaluated. Commonly used docking methods, however, are able to consider the flexibility to a limited extent. Therefore, the selection of the target structure is a crucial point in the docking procedure, so target-binding sites should be as representative as possible, mimicking a real and general binding conformation.

Docking Algorithms

In spite of the fact that only a specified part of the target protein is considered during the docking procedures, the representation of atomic coordinates is not a practical choice. Thus geometric space descriptors alone or combined with physicochemical descriptors, sphere images and interaction points/surfaces are commonly used instead. Otherwise, a complete representation of ligands in atomic coordinates is definitely feasible. The central problem in ligand handling is the flexibility. Two generally used strategies can be applied: whole molecule and fragment-based methods. Earlier rigid docking, when the whole molecules are docked, was commonly used. An extension of rigid body docking is the incorporation of conformational flexibility. Historically, the DOCK algorithm addressed rigid body docking using a geometric matching algorithm to superimpose the ligand onto a negative image of the binding pocket. Important features that improved the algorithm's ability to find the lowest energy-binding mode, including force field-based scoring, on the fly optimization, an improved matching algorithm for rigid body docking, and an algorithm for flexible ligand docking, have been added over the years. This multiconformer docking can be an effective tool, however, for flexible molecules that have significantly higher number of conformers it may not be straightforward. Fragment-based methods provide an alternative solution for the docking problem; molecules are dissected into fragments that can be docked individually, either separately or incrementally. Now there is a driving force to treat protein flexible because ligands requiring larger conformational changes in the active site upon binding cannot be placed correctly by these methods. The degree of the applied flexibility varies in a wide range. Small adjustments of rigid structures, explicit side chain flexibility, or the use of protein ensembles are very popular methods, however, the full consideration of flexibility still remains as the domain of the molecular dynamical simulations.

Systematic methods

These kinds of algorithms make an attempt to explore all the degrees of freedom but face the problem of combinatorial explosion:

$$N_{\text{conformations}} = \prod_{i=1}^{N} \prod_{j=1}^{n_{increment}} \frac{360}{\theta_{i,j}}$$

$\theta_{i,j}$-the size of incremental rotational angle j for bond i

N-the number of rotatable bonds

Thus ligands are often incrementally built within the active site. The principle of the FlexX algorithm is that, physicochemical properties provide the most useful information for ligand placement. Once a set of favorable placement of the base fragment (the core part of the ligand from where the incremental construction starts) has been computed, the ligand building can be started. The incremental construction is formulated as a tree search problem. As the search tree grows exponentially, a complete search is definitely not feasible to calculate. Instead the binding energy values, approximated by the scores, which are represented by the interior nodes, can be used to guide the search. Conversely, DOCK 4.0 algorithm divides ligands into rigid (core fragment) and flexible parts (side chains); the core parts are docked prior to the flexible parts. The steric complementarity is the guideline during the ligand construction. Another method of systematic search is the use of databases of pregenerated conformations. Conformations are calculated once and the search problem is reduced to a rigid body docking procedure. This is the main concept of FLOG docking program.

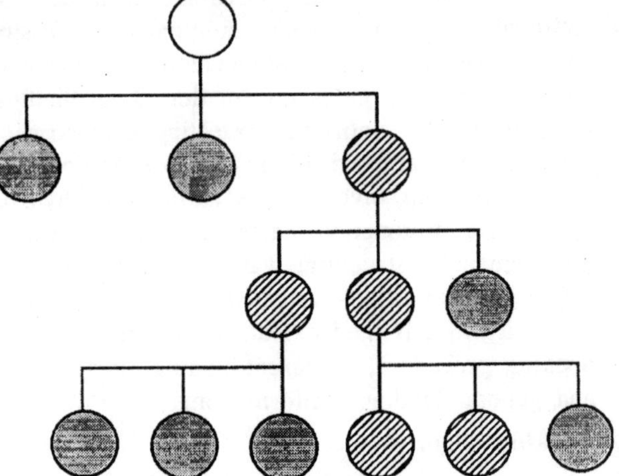

Fig. 23.6. The schematic representation of the search tree. Red nodes indicate energetically unfavorable conformations during the ligand building.

Random or stochastic methods (MC, GA, and tabu search)

The most widely used random approaches are the MC, genetic, and tabu search algorithms. MC algorithms generate initial random conformations of a ligand in the binding cavity then calculate scores for these initial configurations. The generation and scoring of configurations are repeated until the Metropolis criterion, which is used to determine whether the new configuration is retained. According to the Metropolis criterion, the new solution is accepted if the score of the new configuration (E_{new}) is better than the older one's (E_{old}). If the configuration is not a new minimum, it has to pass the Boltzmann-based probability function test, otherwise the solution is rejected.

$$P = \exp\left[\frac{-(E_{new} - E_{old})}{kT}\right]$$

P - probability for the acceptance of the new configuration

Internal coordinated mechanics (ICM) uses global MC minimization docking procedure, describes both the relative positions of two molecules and their conformations by a uniform set of internal variables and uses a pre-calculated grid of interaction energy values to speed up the computation. GAs form a class of computational problem solving methods adapting the main principles of biological competition and population dynamics. GAs are stochastic optimization methods; the problem is encoded generally in the language of genetics.

Initially, a random population is generated that composes a set of the potential solutions for a given problem. The members of the population are represented by chromosomes; the genes correspond to certain variables. When docking into protein structures, the variables for translation, rotation, and torsion angles are encoded in the chromosome. Then genetic operators (crossing over and mutation) are applied for the generation of new populations. The members of the new population are decoded and the estimation of the binding free energy is evaluated. The generation of new populations is terminated when a fixed number of population generation or a given score is reached. A prominent example for the GA using docking algorithms is the genetic optimization for ligand docking (GOLD) program. Its special characteristic is the direct encoding of H-bonding motifs. The latest version of AutoDock uses a Lamarckian GA, which is a combination of a traditional GA with local search method to perform energy minimization.

Besides MC and GA methods, further heuristic algorithms have been developed for the docking problem. Tabu search was found to perform well and provided a straightforward searching strategy of the PRO_LEADS program. This method operates on randomly generated positions and these positions are examined on the basis of the tabu list. This latter list contains pregenerated solutions and provides restriction on the search process. A random move of the ligand is "tabu" if it generates a solution that is not sufficiently different from the stored ones, unless its energy is more favorable, therefore, the revision of the search space is avoided.

Simulation methods (molecular dynamics and energy minimization)

Molecular dynamics simulation methods are currently the most popular approaches. This method is for the analysis of protein flexibility and dynamic properties of molecular systems. With respect to docking, these simulations could provide a realistic view of the docking process, however, these calculations are still out of reach. Therefore, dynamical simulations during the docking process are limited to the protein-ligand complexes. Molecular dynamical simulations are often unable to cross high-energy barriers as well, so an attempt is generally made to simulate different parts of a complex at different temperatures or molecular dynamical simulations can be started from different starting ligand positions. In contrast to molecular dynamical studies, energy minimization methods are rarely used as search techniques but often complement other methods such as MC methods. DOCK performs an energy minimization step after fragment addition, followed by a final minimization step before scoring.

Scoring Functions

The interaction between protein and ligand is a reversible equilibrium reaction. The quantity to characterize this reaction is the free energy of binding. Binding free energy values with reasonable accuracy can only be calculated requiring large computational resources. For scoring thousands of ligands, functions to estimate the binding free energy must be computed fast and without much computational power. Generally used scoring functions estimate the binding free energy for only one position/ conformation, and all of them share the assumption that the full energy term can be decomposed into a sum of terms.

However, the free energy of binding is a state function so, in a strict physical sense, additivity is not allowed. These scoring functions at low computational cost are suitable for the calculation of an estimation of the binding free energy. Three main classes can be separated: force field-based methods, empirical methods, and knowledge-based methods.

All fast scoring functions share several deficiencies. First of all most of them are fitted to or derived from some kind of experimental data. Consequently, the functions reflect the accuracy of these measurements. Molecular size can influence the scores as well, generally the larger the molecule the better the score is, however biological measurements do not support this observation. As scoring functions are derived from X-ray structures, only the favorable interactions are rewarded but unfavorable interactions are not penalized because information from the crystal structures cannot be obtained. Uncertainties in the protonation states and the involvement of water in ligand binding further complicate scoring. Some of the failures can be corrected using consensus-scoring schemes, when the disadvantages and advantages of the various scores might provide a combination, which is able to describe the main characteristics of the protein-ligand binding.

Force field-based scoring functions

The force field is a function expressing the energy of a system as a sum of e.g., diverse molecular mechanics terms. Non-bonded energy terms of molecular mechanics force fields were first used to score protein-ligand complexes. The binding energy between a ligand and a protein is most often estimated by the summation of the electrostatic and van der Waals energy terms. Standard force field scoring functions have major limitations because they were developed to model enthalpic gas phase contributions to structure and energetics, and do not involve solvation and entropic terms either. These scoring functions are restrained by the fact that in VS, significant steric clashes cannot be avoided because the energy terms have steep form at short interatomic distances, the Lennard– Jones potentials used for modeling van der Waals interactions can lead to very strong repulsion, therefore, these terms are often scaled down. Recently developed scoring functions contain entropy terms to increase the potential of specific molecular recognition, H-bonding are often designed in different ways. Below, two generally applied scoring functions are detailed in terms of use.

The GOLD score (G-score) is based on the work of Jones et al. and concentrates on H-bonding interactions. The H-bonding term contains desolvation of donors and acceptors. A pairwise dispersion term involves the contribution of hydrophobic interactions and a molecular mechanical equation is used to calculate the internal energy of the ligand. Therefore, this scoring function performs well when polar interactions are dominant and has difficulty with ligands that are primarily non-polar in nature.

Gold Score

Protein-ligand:

$$E_{vdW} + E_{\text{H-bond}} = \sum_{\text{protein}} \sum_{\text{ligand}} \left[\left(\frac{A_{ij}}{d_{ij}^8} - \frac{B_{ij}}{d_{ij}^4} \right) + \left(E_{da} + E_{ww} \right) - \left(E_{dw} + E_{aw} \right) \right]$$

Internal-ligand:

$$E_{vdW} + E_{\text{torsion}} = \sum_{\text{ligand}} \left(\frac{C_{ij}}{d_{ij}^{12}} - \frac{D_{ij}}{d_{ij}^6} \right) + \sum_{\text{ligand}} \frac{1}{2} V \left[1 + \frac{n}{|n|} \cos(|n|\omega) \right]$$

where A_{ij}, B_{ij}, C_{ij}, and D_{ij} are van der Waals parameters for atoms i and j, and d_{ij} is the interatomic distance. E_{da}, E_{ww}, E_{dw}, E_{aw} are the donor–acceptor individual energy values, V is the torsional barrier, $|n|$ is the periodicity, ω the torsion angle.

GOLD score is the original GOLD scoring function implemented in GOLD docking program package. An optional H-bonding energy term can be added.

Protein-ligand:

$$E_{vdW} + E_{\text{electrostatic}} = \sum_{\text{protein}} \sum_{\text{ligand}} \left[\left(\frac{A_{ij}}{d_{ij}^{a}} - \frac{B_{ij}}{d_{ij}^{b}} \right) + 332 \frac{q_i q_j}{\varepsilon(d_{ij}) d_{ij}} \right]$$

Internal-ligand:

$$E_{vdW} + E_{\text{electrostatic}} = \sum_{\text{ligand}} \left[\left(\frac{A_{ij}}{d_{ij}^{a}} - \frac{B_{ij}}{d_{ij}^{b}} \right) \right] + 332 \frac{q_i q_j}{\varepsilon(d_{ij}) d_{ij}} + E_{\text{H-bond(optional)}}$$

where q_i and q_j are atomic partial charges and $\varepsilon(d_{ij})$ is a dielectric function.

Dock score (D-score) considers both electrostatic and hydrophobic contributions to the binding energy but entropic terms. A distance dependent dielectric attenuates polar interactions.

Protein-ligand:

$$E_{vdW} + E_{\text{electrostatic}} = \sum_{\text{protein}} \sum_{\text{ligand}} \left[\left(\frac{A_{ij}}{d_{ij}^{12}} - \frac{B_{ij}}{d_{ij}^{6}} \right) + 332 \frac{q_i q_j}{\varepsilon(d_{ij}) d_{ij}} \right]$$

$\varepsilon(d'_{ij})$ - a distance-dependent dielectric function

The scoring function implemented in DOCK Version 4.0:

Protein-ligand:

$$E_{vdW} + E_{\text{electrostatic}} = \sum_{\text{protein}} \sum_{\text{ligand}} \left[\left(\frac{A_{ij}}{d_{ij}^{a}} - \frac{B_{ij}}{d_{ij}^{b}} \right) + 332 \frac{q_i q_j}{\varepsilon(d_{ij}) d_{ij}} \right]$$

Empirical scoring functions

Empirical type functions form the second group of the scoring functions. The binding energy is approximated by a weighted sum of explicit hydrogen bonding and hydrophobic contact terms. Many additional terms and different functional forms are used for the scoring. Some functions describe H-bonds with, e.g., distance terms while others penalize angular deviation from the idealized values. The binding free energy can be estimated as: $\Delta G_{\text{bind}} \cong \sum \Delta G f_i$, where f_i corresponds to a weighting factor and ΔG_i represents an interaction term. The weighting factors are obtained from regression analysis using experimentally determined binding energies and 3-D structural information. The appeal of empirical scoring functions is that their terms can be simple to evaluate but they are based on approximations similar to force field functions.

The disadvantage of this class of scoring functions is the dependence on the dataset used for the regression analysis and fitting. Empirical scores contain a rotor term, which estimates entropy penalties on binding from a weighted sum of the number of RBs in ligands. Currently used terms involve an incomplete description of solvation/desolvation energy upon ligand binding. In the next paragraph, three of the most commonly used scoring functions are discussed in terms of their use.

LUDI separates the H-bonding term into neutral and ionic H-bonds and calculates the hydrophobic contributions based on the molecular surface area.

$$\Delta G_{\text{bind}} = \Delta G_{\text{H-bond}} \sum_{\text{H-bond}} f(\Delta R, \Delta \alpha)$$
$$+ \Delta G_{\text{ionic}} \sum_{\text{ionic}} f(\Delta R, \Delta \alpha)$$

$$+\Delta G_{\text{hydrophobic}} \sum_{\text{hydrophobic}} \left|A_{\text{hydrophobic}}\right|$$

$$+\Delta G_{\text{rotor}} N_{\text{rotor}} + \Delta G_0$$

where $A_{\text{hydrophobic}}$ is the molecular surface area, ΔR is the deviation from the ideal H-bond length, $\Delta\alpha$ is the deviation from the ideal H-bond angle, ΔG_0 is a regression constant.

FlexX score is based on Bohm's work. This equation is basically the ΔG for an ideal H-bond, ionic, aromatic, etc., interaction, adjusted by a penalty function that depends on the deviation from the ideal geometric values of two interacting elements.

$$\Delta G_{\text{bind}} = \Delta G_{\text{H-bond}} \sum_{\text{H-bond}} f(\Delta R, \Delta\alpha)$$

$$+\Delta G_{\text{ionic}} \sum_{\text{ionic}} f(\Delta R, \Delta\alpha)$$

$$+\Delta G_{\text{aromatic}} \sum_{\text{aromatic}} f(\Delta R, \Delta\alpha)$$

$$+\Delta G_{\text{contact}} \sum_{\text{contact}} f(\Delta R)$$

$$+\Delta R_{\text{rotor}} N_{\text{rotor}} + \Delta G_0$$

ChemScore is based on a diverse training set of 82 receptor-ligand complexes. It uses four terms that estimate contributions to binding energy from lipophilic interactions, metal-ligand binding, hydrogen bonding, and loss of ligand flexibility. ChemScore is more accurate and robust than many other widely used functions.

$$\Delta G_{\text{bind}} = \Delta G_{\text{H-bond}} \sum_{\text{H-bond}} f(\Delta R, \Delta\alpha)$$

$$+\Delta G_{\text{metal}} \sum_{\text{metal}} f(\Delta R, \Delta\alpha)$$

$$+\Delta G_{\text{lipo}} \sum_{\text{lipo}} f(\Delta R)$$

$$+\Delta G_{\text{rotor}} \sum_{\text{rotor}} f(P_{nl}, P'_{nl}) + \Delta G_0$$

where P_{nl} and P'_{nl} are the fraction of non-lipophilic atoms on either side of the frozen bond.

Knowledge-based scoring functions

In knowledge-based functions, the "knowledge" that is implicitly encoded in the protein-ligand complexes is tried to be captured. These scores are based on the concept of the inverse formulation of the Boltzmann law:

$E_{ij} = -kT \ln(p_{ijk}) + kT \ln(Z)$

E_{ij} – potential of mean force

p_{ijk} – probability density

Z – partition function

This approach has been applied to assemble potentials from databases of protein structures to score protein models in the context of protein structure predictions. To establish a function for scoring, the *i*, *j*, and *k* variables are assigned to protein and ligand atom types and their interatomic distances. The occurrence frequency of their contacts is a measure of the energetic contribution to the binding.

DrugScore and potential of mean force (PMF) are popular implementation of this type of scoring functions:

DrugScore:

$$\Delta W = \gamma \sum_{\text{protein}} \sum_{\text{ligand}} \Delta W_{ij}(r) + (1-\gamma) \times \left[\sum_{\text{ligand}} \Delta W_i(\text{SAS}, \text{SAS}_0) + \sum_{\text{protein}} \Delta W_j(\text{SAS}, \text{SAS}_0) \right]$$

SAS — solvent accessible surface area

W_{ij} — distance-dependent pairwise potential

γ — adjustable weight factor

Parametrized pairwise potential PMF score:

$$\text{PMF} = \sum_{\text{protein}} \sum_{\text{ligand}} A_{ij}(d_{ij})$$

$$A_{ij}(d_{ij}) = -k_B T \ln \left[f^j_{\text{volume\_corr}}(r) \frac{\rho^{ij}_{\text{seg}}(r)}{\rho^{ij}_{\text{bulk}}} \right]$$

k_B - Boltzmann constant

$f^j_{\text{volume\_corr}}(r)$ - ligand volume correction factor

$\rho^{ij}_{\text{seg}}(r)$ - the number density of a ligand-protein atom pa of type *ij* at a certain atom pair distance *r*

ρ^{ij}_{bulk} - the number density of a ligand-protein atom pair of type *ij* in a reference sphere with a radius of 12Å

Post-processing

Filters such as the ones used for preparing the input screening databases can also be applied here. Although after docking, this step does not save time, e.g., compounds not suitable for further drug development can be filtered out. Currently used scoring functions are inadequate for the precise binding affinity predictions. Therefore, additional postprocessing strategies are often advised to apply for the minimization of the number of false positives in the ranked database and to propagate the true hits to the top of the list.

A popular strategy is the consensus scoring. In this approach, scoring functions first can be separately applied for selection of the best docked position and then for ranking the best positions. The top ranking molecules then can be rescored by other scoring functions, and can be ranked again. Scoring functions can be weighted, so a linear combination of the scores can also be applied. An appropriate scoring scheme for the particular protein target can be worked out. Several variety of consensus scoring approaches have been frequently applied to increase the performance of VS.

Besides the consensus scoring and 1-D filters (MW, log P etc.) can decrease the artificial enrichment, which occurs as larger molecules are usually scored better. Thereby normalized scores can be calculated with e.g., solvent accessible surface, MW etc., so as to compensate the large molecular surface.

From the visual inspection of the docking solutions to the involvement of solvation or entropic effects, scores are often corrected to improve the prediction of the binding free energy and as a direct consequence the enrichment of active compounds.

Case Study: VS for Checkpoint Kinase-1 Inhibitors using Knowledge-Based VS

Kinase inhibitors have recently become a major area of drug discovery and structure-based design. Novel inhibitors for kinase targets such as cyclin-dependent kinase, and epidermal growth factor receptor kinase have recently been discovered. As many 3-D structures are publicly available for kinases, they seem to be an ideal target for VS studies. Although only a few case studies have been published in the pharmaceutical industry, VS is often performed for kinase targets. As kinases share a conserved ATP binding site, the discovery of truly novel inhibitors can be limited. The existence of the conserved ATP binding sites does suggest that a general VS strategy can be employed in searching for kinase inhibitors.

Lyne et al. proved an evidence for the above assumption using knowledge-based strategy for checkpoint kinase-1 (ChK-1). Their strategy exploits the chemical and structural information available for kinase inhibitors. Compounds with a minimal kinase-binding motif were docked; only then the docked poses were rescored using a scheme customized for a kinase, the CDK-2. High scoring compound were further investigated visually and selected for biological testing. Thirty-six effective inhibitors out of the 103 best ranking compounds were found.

The screening library was first prepared for docking. The preprocession of this database involved a filtering step of molecules having MW greater than 600 Da, and having rotatable bonds more than 10. Large, non-drug-like, and flexible molecules were excluded. Flexible molecules are often docked improperly using the FlexX algorithm. Tautomeric and protonation states of the ligands were generated using Leather face. 3-D coordinates were computed using Corina. Compounds without an appropriate kinase-binding motif were filtered out by using Plurality (H-bond donors/acceptors).

The ChK-1 crystal structure was protonated at crystallization pH. Active site contained all the residues within 6.5Å of the bound inhibitor. Essential pharmacophore constraints for the Cys87 (backbone NH) and Glu85 (backbone CO) residues were given.

CDK-2 was chosen as a surrogate for ChK-1 because more activity data were available for the CDK-2 that time. An enrichment study using a screening database of 8000 inactive and 100 of active compounds was performed. Three hundred docked poses per molecule were saved. For rescoring, the Cscore module of SYBYL was used. Z-scores were calculated for all the possible scoring functions combinations:

$$Z = \sum_i \frac{x_i - \bar{x}}{\sigma}$$

where x is the raw score for a pose, $\bar{x}$ average raw score for all the poses, and σ is the standard deviation for all the raw scores. For CDK-2 PMF and FlexX, scoring functions were found to give the best enrichment factors (EF). Thus this scoring scheme was applied for ranking the docked solutions for ChK-1. Enrichment factor (EFs) assess the quality of the rankings:

$$\text{EF}(\%) = \left(\frac{N_{\text{active}(\%)} / N_{(\%)}}{N_{\text{active}} / N_{(\text{all})}} \right).$$

where EF(%) is given at the percentage of the ranked database, $N_{\text{active}(\%)}$ is the number of active compounds in a selected subset of the ranked database, $N_{(\%)}$ is the number of compounds in the subset, and N_{active} and Nall are the number of active molecules and the number of compounds in the screening database. EF were not scaled, i.e. absolute values depend on the ratio of active and inactive molecules and should be compared to the maximum (ideal) achievable EFs.

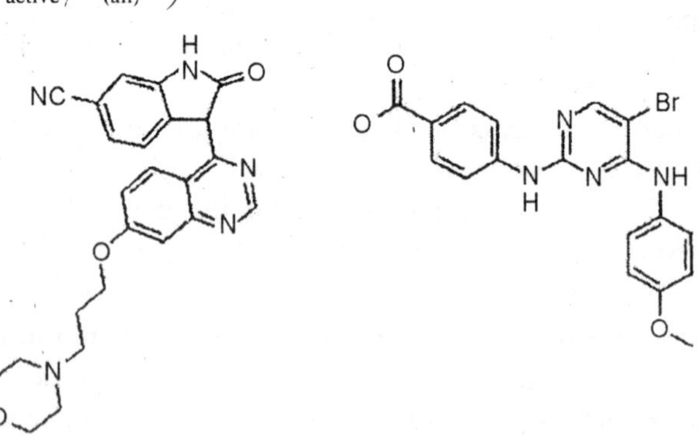

Fig. 23.7. Two examples of the hits found by virtual screening for ChK-1.

This study proves to be a successful case study in the field of protein kinase inhibition with ATP competitive compounds. The hit rate was

36%, and was achieved by screening 103 compounds. Hits corresponded to four chemical classes. These are the results for this particular study only and it is not premised that these could be observed in general with VS for protein kinases. However, this study gives a proof of the applicability of this strategy in other VS study performed for protein kinases.

Success Stories

Improvements in docking algorithms and the increasing number of scoring functions have resulted in a large number of successful VS studies. In this section, a collection of successful screening stories is described. Besides experimental high-throughput screening, VS has emerged as a knowledge-based alternative that can be applied in drug discovery. Recently published studies have revealed that the two approaches are rather complementary than competitive. Owing to the involvement of ever increasing numbers of compounds in today's drug design projects, there is a high demand for efficient computational screening tools. Progress has been made in the quality and speed of VS methods but there is still much room for further improvement. VS offers an approach with requirements opposite to those of experimental screening, which is mainly technology-driven ignoring the structural properties of the target. Nevertheless, VS depends on factors determining binding to the target. Structural information of target proteins and generation of reasonable binding modes of the ligands can serve for prediction of binding affinities. Either structure-based or ligand-based screening can be used to scan large virtual compound libraries.

The applicability of VS generally depends on the target selected for investigation. Recently published success stories demonstrate that these two approaches can be applied simultaneously or in a screening cascade to find quality hit or lead molecules. Large databases containing hundreds of thousands or millions of compounds can be focused or filtered, therefore, e.g., compounds with a special character are enriched resulting in a database with a reduced size. As the docking programs still need large computational power and the currently used scoring functions are not sophisticated enough to operate as a sole criterion for the final hit selection from a list of hundreds of thousands of molecules, there is a need to concentrate on information in a database containing, e.g., filtered compounds. These screening cascades are generally applied and hit rates of recently published success stories provide clear evidence for their effectiveness in drug discovery projects. Considering the current drug discovery landscape, establishing more effective target identification and validation strategies appears to be as important as making progress with VS and predictions of in vitro and in vivo characteristics. Any of these areas has significant potential for computational approaches and the opportunity to streamline the discovery process. As the amount of the experimental data grows, the computational models can be developed and tuned in an easier way. The most straightforward in lead discovery if virtual and experimental approaches are complementary applied.

24

IMAGING OF LUNG DEPOSITION

Inhalation aerosols have been successfully used to deliver drugs to the lung for local and systemic therapeutic effects. In vivo evaluation of pharmaceutical inhalation products is achieved by gamma scintigraphic imaging of the aerosol deposited in the lung. Imaging provides direct information on the amount and location of the drug deposited in the lung after inhalation. This local bioavailability, rather than the systemic bioavailability after absorption, is pertinent to drugs that act directly on the lung. For drugs that act systemically, the deposition site affects the rate and extent of absorption. As a result, lung deposition using gamma scintigraphy has been proposed for bioequivalence studies of aerosol products. The deposition data can further be linked to the clinical response and in vitro particle size distribution, adding a new dimension to the interrelationship between them. To measure lung deposition by imaging, the aerosol must be first labeled or tagged with a suitable radionuclide. Radiolabeling techniques have been developed for current inhalation products including nebulizers, propellant-driven metered dose inhalers (MDIs), and dry powder inhalers (DPIs).

Lung imaging is achieved using a gamma camera, which creates an image of the gamma rays emitted by the radionuclide in the lung. In the past, numerous lung deposition studies on radiolabeled aerosol products have been carried out using planar imaging by which only the anterior or posterior two-dimensional view of the lung is obtained. However, as the lung is a three-dimensional object, spatial distribution of the aerosol in the lung can be best obtained using tomographic (rather than planar) imaging such as single photon emission computed tomography (SPECT), a technique for producing cross- sectional images of the radionuclide distribution in the body. This is achieved by imaging the lung at different angles (e.g., 64 or 128 images at 180 or 360°, respectively) around the thorax using a rotating gamma camera, followed by computational image reconstruction.

RADIOLABELING PHARMACEUTICAL AEROSOLS

It is a prerequisite that the pharmaceutical aerosols be suitably radiolabeled before any lung scintigraphic imaging can commence. Ideally, the drug can be directly radiolabeled, that is, chemically by substitution of an atom in the drug molecule with a radioactive isotope. This can be achieved using positron emitters such as C-11, N-13, and O-15 atoms. Positrons are positively charged electrons, which, when combined with an electron, produce two gamma rays with equal energy (511 keV) emitted at 180° to each other. Theoretically, as C, N, and O atoms are present in all organic molecules, they can be used to label virtually any drug. In reality, the use of these atoms is limited by their short half-lives (20, 10, and 2 min for C-11, N-13, and O-15 atoms, respectively) relative to the time taken for manipulating the drug (including organic synthesis for radiolabeling and successive processing for product characteristics assurance such as particle size distribution of the aerosol particles). Furthermore, to produce these positron emitters, it is necessary to have a nearby cyclotron facility, which means that the process involves extra cost. So far, only three antiasthmatic compounds have been successfully radio- labeled by positron emitters: ipratropium bromide (Br-77), triamcinolone acetonide (C-11), and fluticasone proprionate (F-18). As Br-77 will dissociate from ipratropium in water, tracking ipratropium in the body still requires proper labeling of the molecule itself with a positron emitter. This is indicative of the difficulties of direct radiolabeling.

Because of the aforementioned limitation, gamma emitters have been employed to radiolabel the drug indirectly for gamma scintigraphy. In this case, the radiolabel associates with the drug by physical means instead of chemically incorporating into the drug molecule via covalent bonds. Hence, instead of being a direct chemical approach, it is indirect radiolabeling. Technetium-99m is the most commonly used pure gamma emitter for indirect radio labeling of pharmaceutical aerosols. The gamma ray of ^{99m}Tc has sufficient energy (140 keV) to penetrate body tissues without significant absorption or scattering, but when it reaches the detector of the gamma camera, it is absorbed and converted into light photons, thus optimal for gamma camera imaging. The half-life of ^{99m}Tc is 6 hr, which is long enough for handling and imaging, but not too long to increase the radiation dose to the subject unnecessarily. As a result, ^{99m}Tc is used for the majority of nuclear medicine imaging studies. Once inhaled into the lung, ^{99m}Tc can have a much shorter biological half-life, depending on the physical form. As diethylenetriamine pentaacetic acid or DTPA complex, it will be absorbed rapidly from the lung into systemic circulation, followed by glomerular filtration in the kidney to the bladder where it is excreted in the urine, and the whole process can take less than 2 hr, if the subject drinks plenty of water.

Regardless of the type of aerosol products to be radiolabeled, a fundamental requirement in radiolabeling aerosol products is that the radiolabel must associate with the drug in such a way that not only the radiolabel distribution matches the drug distribution, but also that the radiolabel distribution matches that of the unlabeled aerosol product.

Nebulizer Solutions

Nebulizer solutions are by far the simplest among the aerosol products, and radiolabeling is achieved by simply mixing the radionuclide with the drug solution. As the radionuclide and the drug are uniformly distributed in the solution and provided that no precipitation of the ingredients occurred, each nebulized aerosol droplet would contain both radioactivity and drug in proportion to the droplet size. Technetium-99m, complexing with DTPA or human serum albumin, is widely used as the radionuclide. Sodium pertechnetate is not suitable as the free anion, like iodide, has a high affinity for the thyroid. Lung deposition of nebulized salines and drug solutions including nedocromil sodium, salbutamol, fenoterol, ipratropium bromide, carbenicillin, pentamidine isethionate, flunisolide, liposomes containing beclomethasone dipropionate, interferon gamma, and cyclosporine have been studied using this radiolabeling technique of mixing the radionuclide with the drug solution.

Propellant-Driven MDIs

Historically, there are three major methods of radiolabeling suspension MDIs, developed by Few, Short, and Thomson, Newman et al., and Kohler, Fleischer, Matthys. The first two were initially developed for polymeric particles but were later modified for drugs.

Early in 1970, Few, Short, and Thomson radio- labeled polystyrene particles for a mucociliary clearance study. The radiolabeled aerosols were produced by a spinning-disk generator. The technique involves the key steps of extracting sodium pertechnetate ($Na^{99m}TcO_4$) into chloroform as tetraphenylarsonium (TPA) pertechnetate, followed by evaporation of the chloroform. A solution of polystyrene is added to the radioactive residue and dispersed. This technique has subsequently been adopted by other workers for radiolabeling pharmaceutical MDIs of sodium cromoglycate. It is important to note that in this technique, the complexing agent TPA chloride is classified as poisonous. Although the actual amount of the compound inhaled is in the nanogram range, safety to the researchers and the subjects inhaling the aerosols has to be carefully ensured.

Another way to radiolabel the pharmaceutical MDI is to use Teflon particles with a size distribution similar to that of the drug of interest. This was carried out in 1981 by Newman et al., who employed Teflon particles of mean size 2 ± 0.4 μm to mimic the MDI aerosols of bronchodilators. Hence, the Teflon particles were used as a surrogate for the drug. The Teflon particles were almost monodisperse and were produced by a spinning-disk aerosol generator. However, this approach is limited by the physicochemical characteristics of the Teflon particles being different from those of the drug particles. Furthermore, the aerosol particle size distribution of the Teflon may not match that of the drug. By coadministering a physical mixture of the radiolabeled Teflon particles with the drug salbutamol, the lung deposition and clinical response had been monitored simultaneously.

The first attempt to radiolabel drug particles (instead of polymers like polystyrene or Teflon particles) for pharmaceutical aerosols was carried out on fenoterol and salbutamol by Kohler, Fleischer, and Matthys. However, it was later found that their method would change the particle size distribution of the labeled aerosol, resulting in a coarser aerosol than the unlabeled product. After subsequent improvement by Summers et al., this method has become widely used for radiolabeling MDIs. It is preferred over other methods, as it does not involve extraction with TPA chloride and chloroform.

It is worth noting that each of the above-mentioned radiolabeling methods can be further modified for the study need. For example, the drug particles can be suspended in the organic phase containing the radiolabel and spray-dried, followed by reconstitution in the propellants, as has been carried out on salbutamol sulfate.

Although the radiolabeling methods have been widely used, the mechanism of association between the radiolabel and the drug particles has been studied only recently. The study by Farr on MDI systems indicated that in the chlorinated fluorocarbons (CFC) formulation, the radiolabel $^{99m}TcO_4^-$, being hydrophilic, would associate with hydrophilic domains including the surface of hydrophilic drug particles and the interior of surfactant reverse micelles. There is a need to extend the study to other systems, such as hydrophobic drugs and non-CFC propellants.

DPI

A method of wide application to radiolabeling dry powders is by adsorbing the radiolabel on the particles in a suitable liquid. The drug particles are wetted with a non-solvent containing the radiolabel, followed by evaporation of the solvent, leaving the radiolabel on the surface of the drug particles. This method has been applied to radiolabel terbutaline sulfate, budesonide, and formoterol. Factors influencing the radiolabeling of dry powder formulations include the physicochemical nature of the drug, choice of non-solvent for the drug, solubility of radiolabel in the non-solvent, moisture level, electrostatic charge, and the number of processing steps. Unfortunately, the details still remain largely as proprietary information and are not available in the literature. For example, exactly how the spherical agglomerates of budesonide powder are to be wetted with the ^{99m}Tc solution to ensure reproducible radiolabeling has not been reported.

Alternatively, a method resembling can be used, provided that the drug (e.g., terbutaline sulfate) to be radiolabeled does not dissolve in $CHCl_3$. After the filtrate (the $CHCl_3$ phase containing the ^{99m}Tc-TPA) is collected and added to the drug powder, the $CHCl_3$ is then evaporated (e.g., at 70°C), leaving the radiolabel with the powder. The powder is ready for filling into the DPI. Bronchodilators (salbutamol and terbultaline sulfate) and prophylactics (nedocromil sodium) for asthma along with lactose carriers have been successfully labeled by this technique for lung deposition studies.

An earlier method of radiolabeling dry powders (mainly sodium cromoglycate) involved spray-drying. The basic principle can be considered the same as the one for MDIs in that radiolabeled particles were produced by evaporation of radiolabel-containing atomized droplets. The method is straight-forward, but suffers the limitation that the spray-dried particles may not be physicochemically the same as those in the commercial products, because milling rather than spray-drying is normally used for micronization of the drug particles. Spray-drying, following ^{99m}Tc adsorption to the surface of the particles, has also been used to prepare radiolabeled cromoglycic acid and nedrocromil powders.

Technegas is another form of ^{99m}Tc, which can be used to radiolabel drug particles. Sodium pertechnetate is combined with carbon to form nanoparticles, which primarily has been used for lung ventilation studies. Recently researchers have adsorbed Technegas onto the surface of DPI particles to use in lung deposition studies. This technique offers the ability to achieve high levels of specific activity (MBq/mg) for the powder along with fast processing times (e.g., 10 min). However, there is still some concern over the long-term safety of administering carbon nanoparticles to the various sites of the lung.

The exact mechanism of association between the radiolabel and the drug particles is unknown and is generally regarded as a surface-coating phenomenon. However, the surface is proportional to the square of the particle size, whereas the volume (drug mass) is proportional to the cube of the particle size. It follows that to have a match between the radiolabel and drug mass in the aerosol, the radiolabeled particles must exist as agglomerates rather than as single particles.

Measuring the subjects' inhalation patterns during a scintigraphic study can be important, especially considering that many DPIs are dependent on inspiratory flow for aerosol generation. This can be measured using an inline spirometer or calibrated flowmeter connected to oscilloscope. The critical flow parameters that may affect the aerosol generation are peak flow rate, total volume of inhalation, initial acceleration, and time of inhalation. These parameters are becoming more commonly measured to help explain any variation or flow dependency. Depending on the study aims, controlling the patterns with restriction valves may be needed to obtain consistent flow profiles.

Quality Control of Aerosols

It is imperative that the radiolabeling process be sufficiently validated before the aerosols are administered to human subjects. This includes identifying the purity and form of the radiolabel if complex extractions are performed. As mentioned previously, it is important to ensure that the particle size distribution of the radiolabeled aerosol is similar to that of the unlabeled aerosol, which is most commonly accessed using an impaction method to determine the aerodynamic size. Depending on the process, it may also be necessary to perform the quality check on the day of study prior to inhalation of the aerosol. Dose uniformity is important for MDIs and reservoir DPIs; thus knowledge of the dosing needs to be established. Assessment of the physical characteristics such as particle morphology and crystallinity, which can affect dispersion of dry powders, is required to ensure that the radiolabeling process has not altered these parameters.

Microbial contamination of aerosol products is of major concern, as contaminated aerosols entering the human airways may lead to infection. This is especially important when aqueous solutions or compressed air are used in the labeling process. Autoclaving and using hospital grade disinfectants on equipment used in the radiolabeling process along with a suitable environment (good manufacturing practice or cleanroom facility) may help to minimize the risk of contamination. The use of inlet air filters on spray drying equipment is also recommended. External testing laboratories are able to test the aerosol product against the British Pharmacopoeia or other regulatory standards for microbial requirements on inhalation products. Yeast, mould, and total viable aerobic count must all be less then 10^2 cfu/g with no pathogens present.

Radiotracer Imaging of Lung Deposition

Nuclear medicine scintigraphic imaging provides a powerful tool for studying drug delivery and the use of the gamma camera for the non-invasive measurement of aerosol deposition and clearance is well established. The gamma camera allows the formation of an image of the radiotracer distribution in the patient or subject. The gamma camera detector consists of a collimator in front of a scintillating crystal, which is coupled to an array photomultiplier tubes and then the gamma camera electronics and computer. The collimator acts like a lens and only allows gamma rays within a specified angle to reach the scintillation crystal, which converts the energy of the gamma rays to light photons. The light photons are converted to electrical signals by the photomultiplier tubes. Electronic processing of the signals from the photomultiplier tube then provides position information of the detected gamma ray, which is used to build up an image of the radiotracer distribution in the subject in computer memory. The image formed by the gamma camera is a compression of the three-dimensional radiotracer distribution into a two-dimensional image and is usually referred to as planar imaging. Planar imaging is well established for lung deposition studies, being considered the "industry standard" and method of choice, and indeed has provided valuable insight into the performance of aerosols and aerosol delivery devices as well as interventions and pathologies that affect lung aerosol clearance through, for example, mucociliary clearance. However, compressing the three-dimensional radioaerosol distribution in the lungs into a two-dimensional image is a major drawback. This limits the ability to assess regional distribution of the aerosols in the lungs, and this may become particularly critical if the lung deposition data are to be used for bioequivalence comparisons.

Images of the three-dimensional tracer distribution in the lungs can be produced by SPECT. Single photon emission computed tomography involves taking typically 60–120 projection images at regular angular increments, while the gamma camera is rotating around the patient covering 360°. The projection images are then reconstructed into transverse slices that provide images of the three-dimensional aerosol distribution in the lungs. The stack of transverse slices reconstructed from the SPECT projections describes the volumetric distribution of the radiotracer in the lungs and can be reformatted into coronal, sagittal, or other oblique sections as required. Coronal slices as shown in Fig. 1 are most commonly employed, as they provide intuitive comparison with anterior and posterior planar imaging. Single photon emission computed tomography has been used to measure lung deposition in a number of studies, and SPECT has proved superior to planar imaging in discriminating between deposition in lung parenchyma, large and small airways and for assessing regional aerosol distribution.

Positron emission tomography (PET) is another tomographic technique using radiotracers, labeled with positron emitters. Positron emitters include ^{13}N, ^{15}O, ^{11}C, and ^{18}F, sometimes referred to the elements of life, and these radioisotopes are particularly suitable for incorporating into the drug molecule, thus allowing not only the deposition of the drug, but also its absorption and clearance from the lungs to be studied. However, as mentioned earlier, owing to the short half- life of positron emitters (^{13}N—10 min, ^{15}O—2 min, ^{11}C—20 min, and ^{18}F—110 min), ready access to a close by cyclotron and radiochemistry facility is required. This has restricted the wide spread use of the PET in aerosol studies. However, with the rapid growth of PET cyclotrons to meet the demand of the rapid expansion of clinical PET, access to this technology has improved considerably.

Quantification of Aerosol Deposition and Clearance

Assessment of aerosols and aerosol delivery devices requires accurate estimations of not only was the activity deposited in the lungs, but also in other regions such as oropharynx and stomach. For clearance measurements, such as mucociliary clearance, absolute estimates of activity are not required. Instead, the method should be able to confirm initial deposition of the aerosol to, primarily, the ciliated airways and provide good differentiation between central and peripheral regions to allow their respective clearances to be determined. Acquisition frame has to be sufficiently fast to allow clearance to be accurately followed, particularly during the fast initial clearance of aerosols from the lungs.

Estimation of in vivo activity for both planar and SPECT studies requires corrections for both attenuation and scatter. Attenuation occurs when gamma rays are absorbed by body tissue before reaching the gamma camera detector. This causes a reduction in detected activity, which depends on the amount of tissue between the source of the gamma photons and the detector. Gamma rays lose part of their energy and change direction owing to Compton interactions in the tissue, which is referred to as scatter. Scatter causes mispositioning of the detected counts and blurring in the image, as well as loss in quantitative accuracy as it causes a relative increase in detected photons in areas with increased amounts of tissue between the source of the photons and the detector.

Attenuation correction requires estimates of the amount of the tissue and its density between the gamma emitting source and the detector. Because of the heterogeneous nature of the thorax (lungs, bone, and soft-tissue) with quite different densities and attenuating properties, uniform attenuation cannot be assumed in the thorax. Thus for proper attenuation correction, attenuation has to be measured. Attenuation information can be obtained by a transmission scan with an external gamma-emitting source, or can be derived from anatomical imaging such as CT or MRI. To avoid uncertainty in the alignment between the emission and attenuation data, transmission data is ideally acquired simultaneously with the emission data, which also avoids extending the study time associated with a separate transmission data acquisition. A number of simultaneous emission/transmission techniques have been implemented for SPECT including scanning line source and fan beam collimators. For planar imaging, simultaneous emission/transmission scanning is not usually performed. Attenuation is assessed by measuring transmission using a sheet source of activity or introducing a known amount of activity into the lungs by intravenous injection of labeled particles that lodge in the capillaries of the lungs.

A number of different scatter correction techniques have also been developed, including methods based on multiple energy windows, as well as based on the transmission data and Monte Carlo modeling techniques. All of these can be applied to SPECT data, but planar imaging scatter correction is limited to the multiple energy window techniques. Attenuation correction is essential for quantitative aerosol deposition measurement, but scatter correction can sometimes be avoided by suitable phantom calibration of activity measurement. Planar activity quantification techniques have to make assumptions about the distribution of activity as a function of depth. Use of geometric mean of anterior and posterior images reduces but does not eliminate the dependence of activity estimation on the three-dimensional distribution entirely. For planar aerosol deposition studies, it is usually assumed that activity is distributed uniformly throughout the lungs and errors can be introduced when this assumption does not hold, for instance, for aerosols with pronounced central airway depositions. As SPECT provides images of the three-dimensional activity distribution, no such assumptions are required.

Planar vs. SPECT

While it is acknowledged that SPECT has the potential for better assessment of regional aerosol distribution, the main drawbacks attributed to SPECT are high radiation dose and long image acquisition times. This can potentially lead to significant clearance of the aerosols from the lungs during the SPECT study, confounding interpretation of total and regional lung deposition.

A survey of planar and SPECT imaging studies found that similar radiation doses were associated with planar than with SPECT studies. The radiation detriment to the subject from a given study is quantified by the effective dose, which not only depends on the amount of radioactivity in the lungs, but also depends on the total inhaled radioaerosol activity. The total inhaled amount of activity was approximately 50 MBq on each occasion, but the fraction delivered to the lungs differed substantially between the studies. The effective dose was 0.3 mSv on each occasion based on total administer activity of 50 MBq of ^{99m}Tc-DTPA for a total effective dose of 0.9 mSv for the three studies. It has been customary in planar studies to inhale radioaerosols until a set count rate of about 2000 cps is reached in the lungs. To achieve a count rate of about 2000 cps with the camera used for this SPECT study, approximately 40 MBq of activity would need to be deposited in the lungs. Based on the fractions delivered to the lungs, total inhaled activity would have to be 100, 190, and 565 MBq for the three studies respectively, resulting in effective doses of 0.6, 1.1, and 3.4 mSv, respectively for a total effective dose of 5 mSv from the three studies. Hence careful consideration to radiation dose must not only be given to SPECT studies but also to planar studies.

Activities >10 MBq deposited in the lungs provide adequate SPECT images of the lungs with a 2 min SPECT acquisition protocol described below. The use of less than 5 MBq still allowed the activity in the lungs to be accurately quantified. This allows the limiting of total inhaled activity to about 50–100 MBq for SPECT studies when an appreciable fraction (>10%) of the radioaerosol deposits in the lungs. The effective dose associated with that is 0.3–0.6mSv for ^{99m}Tc-DTPA and 0.6–1.3 mSv for ^{99m}Tc-pertechnetate. For comparison, most clinical nuclear medicine studies and diagnostic radiology procedures are associated with effective doses of several to 10s of mSv, and radiation dose from natural sources of background radiation is about 2–3 mSv in a year, depending on the geographical location. While the effective dose associated with SPECT studies is small, there is considerable scope for reducing inhaled activity below 10 MBq and as low as 1 MBq. Thus if a low dose planar study provides the required information, then use of a higher dose SPECT study would need to be questioned. Conversely, if a low dose planar study does not provide all the required information, but a moderate dose SPECT study does, a SPECT study is advised, as a suboptimal planar study exposes the subject to unnecessary radiation.

Traditionally, lung SPECT studies have been associated with long acquisition times of 15–30 min. Significant clearance of the radiolabel from the lungs may occur, during the SPECT study, through absorption or mucociliary clearance, particularly for radiotracers with fast clearance, such as ^{99m}Tc-pertechnetate, with lung half-clearance times of only about 10-15 min. Clearance potential not only leads to an underestimation of activity deposited in the lungs, but also reconstruction artifacts.

Current generation multidetector gamma camera systems allow complete SPECT studies to be collected in as little as 10 sec and have been used for quantifying tracer uptake and clearance for a range of applications. Application of fast, dynamic SPECT has also been demonstrated in the lungs, with SPECT frame rates of 1 min for aerosol deposition and clearance studies and as low as 30 sec for measuring the wash-out of ^{133}Xe from the lungs. Even at these fast SPECT frame rates, adequate SPECT images can be obtained while maintaining a low radiation dose to the subject. Thus these techniques have overcome the limitation of long SPECT study times and make them suitable for SPECT measurement of aerosol deposition and clearance. However, multidetector SPECT cameras are recommended to achieve these short study times. With the widespread clinical use of dual detector systems, this should not be a major issue.

Quantitative SPECT regimes are well established and rely on fewer assumptions about, e.g., three-dimensional activity distribution than planar activity quantitation approaches. While phantom studies can be used to assess accuracy of activity quantitation, these may not entirely reflect the accuracy achieved in human subjects. Mass balance calculations, where the initial activity loaded into the delivery device is compared to the activity in the subject estimated by the imaging technique plus the residual activities in the device and exhalation filter, can provide a good indication of the in vivo activity quantitation. With our quantitative fast SPECT technique, the recovered activity as a percentage of initial device activity was 102 ± 7% (n = 40) for a range of different protocols using both liquid and dry powder aerosols. Thus the accuracy of SPECT is at least as good as the "around 10%" quoted for planar studies. It has been suggested that the accuracy of planar activity estimation may be affected by differences in central distribution vs. peripheral distribution. No such distribution effect has been observed with our SPECT studies. In addition, careful attention has to be paid to attenuation and scatter correction with planar imaging to avoid large errors. It is unclear at this stage whether SPECT offers any significant advantage over planar imaging for total, as distinct from regional, activity quantitation as both techniques appear to provide quantitation with an acceptable accuracy.

Data Analysis

Image processing

No or limited processing of planar images is required before they can be analyzed with region of interested analysis. Formation of geometric mean images from anterior and posterior views reduces the dependence of the activity distribution with depth and improves quantitation. In addition attenuation correction factors have to be estimated according to the selected validated method for activity quantitation. In contrast, the acquired SPECT projections have to be reconstructed before volume of interests can be defined. Quantitative SPECT reconstruction with attenuation and scatter correction is required if aerosol deposition is to be quantitated. The main algorithms used for SPECT image reconstruction are filtered back projection and iterative reconstruction. The main advantage of filtered back projection is its computational efficiency and speed. This not only causes artifacts in the image, but can also bias the activity quantitation. Iterative reconstruction techniques avoid the streak artifacts and also can easily incorporate attenuation and scatter correction as part of the reconstruction. The main disadvantage of higher computational burden and long reconstruction times has been largely eliminated by the development of accelerated algorithms and the speed of current generation nuclear medicine computers. Further advantages of iterative reconstruction are improved noise properties and more control over noise, which is particularly important for the fast SPECT acquisition times proposed for aerosol studies. Thus iterative reconstruction is the clear method of choice for fast lung SPECT studies.

Drawing of the Lung Region

Assessment of regional lung aerosol deposition mandates reliable and reproducible definition of a region over the right lung for planar studies. As variations in aerosol deposition precludes using the aerosol image for lung region of interest (ROI) definition, either a ventilation image using ^{81m}Kr or ^{133}Xe or a transmission image is used to manually draw the right lung ROI which is then superimposed on the aerosol deposition image. The whole lung region can then be further subdivided into apex and basal regions, or for estimation of the penetration index (PI), into central, peripheral, and intermediate regions. However, there is no consensus on how the size and shape of the regions should be defined, and both rectangular and lung shape regions have been used in the past. Peripheral regions should contain more small airways, while in the central region, large, conducting airways should dominate to allow assessment of relative aerosol deposition in the small and large airways. In planar imaging, there is considerable overlapping of lung structures, and hence planar imaging only provides a crude and insensitive measure of peripheral vs. central airway deposition. However, the PI from planar images has proven to be a useful index for detecting marked differences in deposition patterns, particularly as the subjects act as their own controls.

Early regional analysis of SPECT data has been limited to applying planar image definition techniques to a central, thick coronal slice extracted from the SPECT data. However, this does not take full advantage of the information contained in the SPECT data. Automated definition of the right lung volume of interest from the simultaneously collected transmission data has been achieved using thresholding and morphological operators. Alternatively, coregistered anatomical imaging has been proposed to define the right lung volume outline. The lung volume of interest can then be divided into concentric shells, which can be related to airway generations. Central and peripheral lung regions are then defined by combining appropriate number of inner and outer shells, respectively. As has been demonstrated, this approach has proven to be more sensitive to detecting changes in regional aerosol deposition than planar imaging.

Future Directions of Lung Deposition Studies

Planar imaging will continue to provide useful information about aerosol deposition and clearance and will be sufficient for a range of applications. Fast SPECT has been shown to be feasible for aerosol studies and is likely to provide additional insight and information about aerosols and delivery devices. With the large expansion of clinical PET, PET applications to aerosols, particularly labeling of the active drug molecules and following their fate in vivo is likely to grow. Most PET scanners recently installed are combined PET/CT system, taking full advantage of the complementary information provided by the coregistered functional and anatomical information. A hybrid SPECT/CT system, with a low end CT, has been available from one manufacturer for a number of years. Recently, two more gamma camera manufacturers have announced SPECT/CT systems with high end, multi- slice CTs. The CT images from these scanners not only provide information for attenuation correction, but also show great potential for more precisely defining and characterizing regional lung deposition, provided an additional radiation dose from the CT can be obtained.

Radiolabeling of nebulizer solutions, propellant-driven metered-dose inhalers, and dry-powder inhalers is generally well documented. For some dry-powder inhalers the procedure may still be lacking sufficient details to ensure reproducible radiolabeling. Deposition of radiolabeled aerosols in the lung has been mainly measured by planar imaging. Tomographic imaging using SPECT can provide three-dimensional information about the spatial distribution of the aerosol in the lung. The recent development of the fast dynamic SPECT has made it the method of choice for aerosol imaging.

25

RADIOCHEMICAL METHODS OF ANALYSIS

In nuclear medicine, drugs containing radioactive metals, metal complexes, and metal conjugates are used for diagnosis and therapy of various diseases. Radioactive materials used as pharmaceuticals are not only small organic and inorganic molecules but are also macromolecules such as monoclonal antibodies and antibody fragments that are attached to radioactive metals. Nuclear medicine has become a $12 billion medical industry, and more than one-third of the hospitals in the United States currently use radioisotopes for such procedures. It is anticipated that diagnostic procedures in the United States are likely to exceed 20 million by the end of 2000. The successful use of radiochemicals needs a basic understanding of radiation, radioactivity, and the nature and characteristics of instruments to detect and quantitate radiation. This article addresses these applications related to radioactivity and radiochemical methods of measurement.

ATOMIC STRUCTURE, NUCLEAR STABILITY, AND RADIOACTIVITY

Atomic physics describes the structure of atoms in complex mathematical terms of quantum mechanics. However, the model of the atom as described by Niels Bohr in 1913 is very simple, pictorial, and more than adequate for a basic understanding of the phenomenon of radioactivity. Bohr's planetary model of the atom consists of a dense positively charged nucleus surrounded by negatively charged electrons (e) in orbits of well-defined energy states. The nucleus consists of positively charged protons and neutral particles called neutrons. The protons and neutrons are held together by very a strong nuclear force of attraction, effective at very close distances (approximately 10^{-13} cm). These strong forces for each nucleus are computed in terms of binding energy. The electroneutrality of the atom is maintained by the orbital electrons, which are equal in number to that of the protons. This number is called the atomic number, Z. The masses of the atoms (A) and other particles are described in terms of atomic mass units (amu). The amu is defined as 1/12th the mass of a carbon atom with atomic mass of 12.0000. Any configuration of protons and neutrons is called a nuclide. There are three nuclides of the element hydrogen with atomic number 1.

The notation is used to indicate the nuclide of an element. The three nuclides of hydrogen are called isotopes of hydrogen. Tritium with an N/Z ratio of two is unstable. When the N/Z ratio becomes higher, the nucleus become unstable and results in the disintegration of the nucleus so as to achieve a stable N/Z ratio and therefore a stable nucleus. This process is called radioactive decay. This radioactive process can be spontaneous in some naturally occurring nuclides; then these elements are said to be naturally radioactive. When such instability is brought about by bombarding stable nuclides with high-energy particles, it is called *artificial radioactivity*. Of nearly 3000 known nuclides of elements, which are either man-made or natural, 287 nuclides of 83 elements are stable; the rest are unstable to varying degrees. The unstable nuclides disintegrate to form stable nuclides with release of energy and nuclear particles. Binding energy and nuclear stability are found to be dependent on the ratio of number of neutrons to protons (*N/Z* or *n/p* ratio). To be stable, at least one proton is required. The most stable heavy nuclide is, with 83 protons and 126 neutrons ($N/Z = 1.5$). In general, when the *N/Z* ratio is greater than 1.6, the radioactive nuclide readjusts to a stable ratio of *N/Z* with the release of energy and particles of matter. The three nuclides of hydrogen are called isotopes. Other members of the nuclide family are isobars and isotones.

Radioactive Decay

Different radioactive species undergo disintegration at different rates. The rate of this decay or activity is characteristic of the individual nuclide and is proportional to the number of radioactive nuclides present at the beginning of this time interval. The proportionality constant is called the decay constant and is denoted by λ. The decay constant is a measure of the probability that a certain radioactive nucleus will disintegrate within a specified time interval. These disintegrations are characteristic of the nuclide and are unaffected by pressure, temperature, concentration, and other physical or chemical properties of the radionuclide. This rate constant is conveniently denoted in terms of $t_{1/2}$, or halflife. The halflife of a radionuclide is the time required for the sample activity to decrease to half its initial value. $t_{1/2}$ is related to rate constant (λ) as follows:

$$\lambda = 0.6932/t_{1/2}$$

In fact, less than 1% will be radioactive in seven halflives, and after 10 halflives, greater than 99.9% of the radioactive nuclide will have lost its activity. The halflife refers to that of a pure nuclide. In a sample containing mixtures of disintegrating radionuclides, the total activity is the sum of the separate activities. From a plot of relative activity against time, the individual halflives can be computed. However, in practice, this can be realized for mixtures containing 3 or <3 nuclides. Other commonly used terms in nuclear medicine and pharmacy are average (mean) halflife, biological halflife, and effective halflife. Average half-life is the mean lifetime of a nuclide, and it is equal to $1.44 \times t_{1/2}$. Biologic halflife, tb, is the time required for the body to eliminate half the administered dose by normal biological process of elimination. Effective halflife (t_{eff}) is a measure of how fast the body eliminates the radioactive material by the combination of biological elimination and radioactive decay:

$$1/t_{eff} = 1/t_b + 1/t_{1/2}$$

Unit of Activity

The fundamental SI unit of activity is the Becquerel (Bq). One Bq is equal to one disintegration per second (dps). Because this is a very small unit, it is more often expressed in kilobequerels or kBq. However, the older historical unit of activity C_i is normally used for radio- pharmaceuticals. The Curie was defined in terms of the number of disintegrations per second of 1 g of ^{226}Ra and is equal to 3.7×10^{10} dps. Other commonly used units are millicurie and microcurie (mC_i and μC_i). The unit of C_i represents absolute activity (*A*). However, relative activity *R* is proportional to the efficiency of the counting device. The device reports in counts per minute.

$R = qA$; q = efficiency quotient. Sometimes specific activity, in terms of radioactivity per unit mass of an element or radiolabeled compound or unit volume of solution is also specified. In these case, the mass or volume should be clearly specified.

Decay Processes

The radioactive decay process involves the emission of radiation, which is dependent on the mode of decay of the particular radionuclide. Radiation resulting from any decay process can be classified as alpha (α), beta (β), gamma rays (γ), and/or other emissions.

α-Particles

Alpha (α)-particles are doubly charged, highly energetic helium nucleus. α-Particles originate in the nuclei of heavier atoms. The emission involving α-Particles is the most efficient process for a radionuclide to attain stability because the nuclide loses both charge and mass. Because α-Particles are very heavy (7400 times of that of an electron) and doubly charged, they attract electrons from the surrounding medium when they pass through a medium. This results in the ionization of the medium. An α-Particle loses energy, slows down, and finally becomes a helium nucleus. In each ionization process, it loses 34 eV per event. For example, a loss of 3.4 MeV of energy causes 100,000 ionization events. These particles travel very short distances, called the range. Because they are extremely efficient in ionizing, they lose energy very rapidly. This range is approximate 4 cm in air and a few thousandths of a centimeter in biological tissues. Because of this tremendous amount of energy transfer, α-Particles can cause extensive damage to organs and tissues when they are exposed to this radiation. Generally, α-Particles arise during the natural decay of elements with a Z value greater than 83. A typical alpha decay process is represented below:

$$^{238}_{92}U \rightarrow {}^{234}_{90}Th + {}^{4}_{2}He + \text{Energy}$$

β-Particles

A β-Particle is a high-velocity nucleon ejected out of a decaying nucleus. β-Particles have the rest mass (0.000548amu) of an electron. If it is negatively charged, it is called a negatron and if positively charged, it is called apositron. In common usage, β-Particle emission refers to the negatron (β^-) and β^+-Emission is called positron emission. For example, the decay of $^{32}_{15}P$ to $^{32}_{15}S$ results in the emission of β^-, antineutrino, and release of energy. The difference in the masses of the two nuclides, 0.001836 amu (31.965675 for P – 31.9638390 for S), results in the release of energy equivalent to 1.70 MeV. Part of this energy is used up in the ejection of particles, and the remaining is used in the release of antineutrino. Because no other energy is emitted, ^{32}P is called a pure β-Emitter. Sometimes some portion of the energy difference may be retained in the nucleus, and consequently the nuclide resides in a nuclear excited state. The excited nucleus may lose the excess energy and return to the stable ground state in the form of electromagnetic radiation (gamma-rays). β-Particles are emitted with variable energy from zero to the maximum of the difference in energy between the parent and daughter nucleus. The variability in energy arises from the distribution of energy between the β-Particle and the antineutrino.

Negatively charged β-Particles are emitted when the radionuclide has more neutrons than required by the number of protons for stability. Sometimes more than one β-Particle may be emitted. For example, ^{131}I decays with the emission of six β-Particles and 14 γ-Rays of different energies:

$$^{131}_{53}I \rightarrow {}^{131}_{54}Xe + \beta^- + \beta^- + \gamma$$
$$+ \text{ antineutrino} + \text{Energy}$$

Nearly 100% of all these decay processes correspond to β-Particles of energy 0.61 MeV and γ-Radiations of energy 0.364 MeV. The decay to form stable nuclides may involve the formation of many unstable intermediate radionuclides. For example, the decay of $^{127}_{50}Sn$ to $^{127}_{53}I$, shown below, involves the formation of a number of intermediate nuclides:

$$^{127}_{50}Sn \rightarrow {}^{127}_{51}Sb \rightarrow {}^{127}_{52}Te \rightarrow {}^{127}_{53}I$$

In general, β^-- and β^+-Particles penetrate deep into the medium; however, they do not cause damage to tissues and organs. Radionuclides that decay by β-Particle emissions are used very extensively in nuclear medicine for diagnostic and therapeutic applications. Positron-emitting nuclides are used in nuclear medicine for diagnostic purposes. β^+-Emitting radionuclides are under active study for use in radiotherapy. An example of a decay process involving emissions of positrons follows:

$$^{15}_{8}O \rightarrow {}^{15}_{7}N + {}^{0}_{1}\beta^+$$

γ-Rays (γ)

During the disintegration of the nucleus, part of the energy is used in the creation of excited-state radionuclide. In the excited state, the nuclide is unstable. The release of energy while the excited nucleus returns to the ground state appears as electromagnetic radiation. These radiations are called γ-Rays. γ-Emission is common when the difference between the excited state and the lowest energy ground state nucleus is greater than 100 keV. Because γ-Emission iselectromagnetic radiation, there is no change in the neutron number or mass number or atomic number. Therefore, invariably, γ-Radiation is always preceded by a nuclear decay reaction involving emission of α, β^-, β^+ particles.

γ-Rays are high-energy electromagnetic radiation such as X-Rays with no electrical charge. γ-Rays are different from X-Rays in that they differ with respect to their origin. X-Rays originate from orbital electrons, whereas γ-Rays originate from the decay of a nuclide. The γ-Rays also ionize the medium by striking orbital electrons with high energy and by knocking the electrons out of the atom. These ejected electrons cause secondary ionization referred to as indirect ionization. The degree of penetration of γ-Rays is extremely high. There are at least seven different processes by which γ-Rays can interact with matter. However, the processes associated with γ-Ray interaction or production, which are pharmaceutically relevant, are electron capture, isomeric transition, and internal conversion. These are briefly discussed below.

Electron capture is a decay process in which an orbital electron loses energy and becomes absorbed into the nucleus. As a result, outer-shell electrons jump to fill the inner-shell vacancy resulting in an electron orbit reshuffling. This process result in the release of X-Rays, and these electrons are subsequently absorbed and result in the release of weakly bound orbital electrons. These are called Auger electrons. When the decay process involves in positron emission, it is almost always followed by electron capture. As a result of nuclear reaction, an excited radionuclide (with energy >100 keV) loses energy by de-excitation:

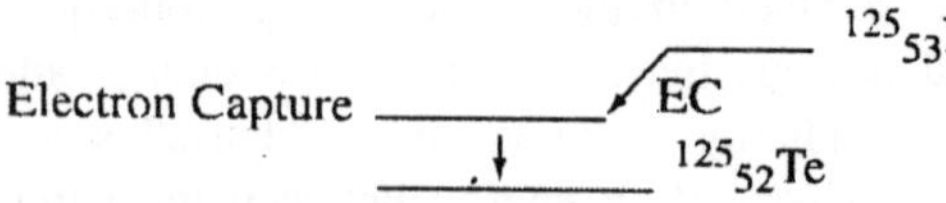

$^{125}_{53}I$

Electron Capture ↙ EC

↓ $^{125}_{52}Te$

More often, these occur in multiple steps with the release of γ-Ray photons of multiple energy. Thus, the resulting γ-Ray spectrum is unique to the decaying radionuclide; this uniqueness, therefore, is used to identify the unknown nuclide. γ-Rays with no mass and charge can penetrate into matter and bring about other chemical reactions in the system. γ-Rays are widely used in nuclear medicine.

An excited radionuclide may remain in several excited states before reaching ground state. However, transitions can occur within these excited states with the emission of γ-Rays. These transitions are called isomeric transitions. When these isomeric transitions are significantly long-lived, these are called metastable states. An example of the decay process is shown below. (↘-increase in Z, ↙-(left arrow) decrease in Z)

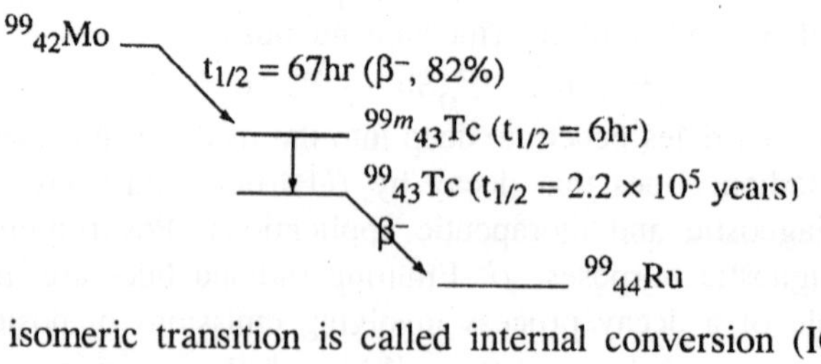

$^{99}_{42}Mo$

↘ $t_{1/2}$ = 67hr (β^-, 82%)

$^{99m}_{43}Tc$ ($t_{1/2}$ = 6hr)

↓

$^{99}_{43}Tc$ ($t_{1/2} = 2.2 \times 10^5$ years)

↘ β^-

$^{99}_{44}Ru$

A process alternative to isomeric transition is called internal conversion (IC). In some cases, the γ-energy is absorbed by a K-shell (inner) electron. This electron is ejected out with lower energy. This ejected electron is the internal conversion electron, and the process is called internal conversion. Some diagnostic and therapeutic radionuclides with corresponding half lives are given below.

Diagnostic raidonuclides. ($t^1/_2$ in units as indicated are given in parentheses.) $t^1/_2$ hours: ^{67}Cu (62.0); ^{67}Ga (78.3); ^{90}Y (64.1); ^{117}In (67.9); ^{99m}Tc (6); ^{201}Tl (72) {β-particles}-*t* min; ^{11}C (20.4); ^{13}N (10.1); ^{15}O (2.0); ^{18}F (1.9); ^{68}Ga (68.0); and ^{82}Rb (1.25) {β^+}.

Therapeutic radionuclides. $t^1/_2$ days: D; ^{32}P(14.3); ^{47}Sc (3.4); ^{67}Cu (2.6); ^{64}Cu (0.5); ^{90}Y (2.7); ^{105}Rh (1.5); ^{111}Ag (7.5); ^{117m}SN (13.6); ^{131}I (8.0); ^{149}Pm (2.2); ^{153}Sm (1.9); ^{166}Ho (1.1); ^{177}Lu (6.7); ^{186}Re (3.8); ^{188}Re (0.7).

Radiation Detection and Measurement

Interaction of Radiation with Matter, Ionization Chamber, and GM Counters

The detection and quantitation of nuclear radiation are based on its interaction with material contained in the detector. Ionization of the gas particles in the medium and scattering are the two most common types of interaction of radiation with matter. Radiation causes darkening of photographic emulsion, ionization of a gas or a mixture of gases, or fluorescent scintillation. In radiology, exposure and observation of the photographic film are most commonly used. When α-Particles with high kinetic energies impinge on gases enclosed in a chamber, they produce approximately 40,000 ($\pm$ 10,000) ion pairs per cm. The range of α-particles is short (approximately 6 cm in air and 2 μM in lead); β-Particles have longer and irregular paths and produce approximately 100–700 ion pairs per cm. A typical ionization chamber, consists of a sealed tube containing helium, neon, or gas–air mixtures placed in a space between two electrodes. The incoming particles create ion pairs; the ions are separated and collected at the electrodes of opposite charge. Electrons are collected at the anode. The number of such ions collected at each electrode is also a function of the applied voltage across the electrodes. If the response is measured in terms of pulse height (proportional to the number of electrons collected), a plot of this value against applied voltage will exhibit a characteristic response. The different regions are explained below. Region I is called the recombination region. In this region, ion pairs produced increase linearly as a function of applied voltage (< 100V) as recombination is proportionately decreased. This is not a useful region for measurement. In region II (100–400V), pulse height attains a plateau because all ions formed are collected. This region is used in ionization chambers to measure energies of γ-Rays and X-Rays. This region is also used for identification of α- and β-Particles because the height at which plateau occurs is characteristic of the nature of the particle. Dose meters and dose rate meters, which measure high-intensity radiation fields, operate in this region. In region III (400–800 V), the number of pulses produced is proportional to the intensity of radiation. The size of the pulses counted gives a measure of the primary ionization produced. In this region, the

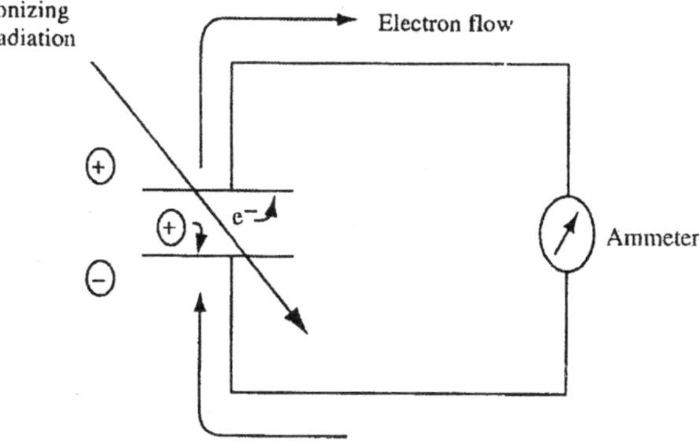

Fig. 25.1. Block diagram of a simple air ionization chamber.

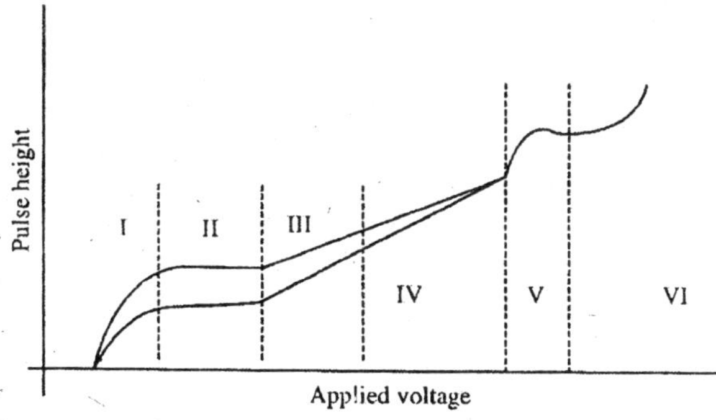

Fig. 25.2. Pulse higher versus applied voltage response.

primary electrons are accelerated with high gain in energy. This high energy causes additional secondary electrons to be generated as a result of interaction with gases in the ionization chamber. These secondary electrons cause further ionization. The net effect is pulse amplification; the size of the amplification is of the order of 100–10,000 times that of the size of the ions initially produced in the ionization chamber.

Region IV (applied voltage 800–1000V) is limited proportional region and is not important for purposes of detection. When the applied voltage is between 1000 and 1500 V, the size of the pulse is no longer proportional to the initiating event. However, each pulse corresponds to a single event. The counters that operate in this region are called Geiger–Mueller counters or GM counters. The GM counters are very sensitive. Because of the high gain involved, these are used primarily in regions where the radioactivity is of very low intensity, (e.g., radioactive contamination). The readings are given in milli-, micro-, or Roentgens/h or in counts per minute. In the GM counter, ionization produced spreads to the entire gas. Therefore, the counter may not respond to a succeeding second incoming pulse before a recovery time of approximately 100– 300 μs. This dead time for recovery is unusually high compared with the dead time for the proportional counter, which is approximately 1 μs. Secondly, because a fixed amount of gas is present in the chamber, the purity of the gas in the chamber decreases. Therefore, the GM counter has to be calibrated frequently, using standard ^{226}Ra or ^{137}Cs sources per Nuclear Regulatory Commission (NRC) requirements. Above an applied voltage of 1500 V, continuous discharge occurs, and this is not useful for any measurement.

Scintillation Detectors

When radiation interacts with certain substances called fluors or phosphors, it produces a flash of light called scintillation. The scintillation is then detected using a sensing element, amplified, sorted, and recorded by counting. The scintillation-detecting instruments include well counters, scanners, thyroid probes, and scintillation cameras called Auger cameras. In addition, all these instruments consist of a collimator (excluding well counters), photomultipliers, a high-voltage power supply, an amplifier, a gain control unit, a pulse height analyzer, and instruments or computers for appropriate display modes. The scintillation cameras also contain coordinate-positioning (x,y) circuits.

Solid-state detectors

These detectors are made of semiconducting materials. In these detectors, solid-state electrodes are made from Li doped with Si or Ge. The resolution is approximately 1–2 keV for 1 MeV γ-Rays and sometimes provides a greater than 10-fold improvement over NaI (Tl) scintillation detectors, described below. These are commercially available and more often used in research-grade instruments.

Liquid Scintillators

The sample radionuclide is dissolved in a liquid scintillator called the scintillation cocktail. It consists of two principal components. The first is a primary solvent such as toluene, xylene, or 1,2,4-Trimethylbenzene (pseudocumene). The second component is the fluor solute, 2,5-Diphenyloxazole (PPO) that emits UV light at ~380 nm. The cocktail may also contain one or more the following:

1. A secondary solvent such as dioxane to improve solubility of aqueous samples or surfactants such as sodium dodecylbenzenesulfonate as emulsifier.
2. A secondary scintillator to shift the wavelength of photons emitted (~380 nm) to the wavelength response of some photomultiplier tubes (PMT, ~420 nm).
3. One or more adjuvants for purposes of suspending or solubilizing biological tissues.

Photomultiplier (PM) tubes

The PM tube has a light-sensitive electrode called the photocathode. It emit electrons when photons strike it. The electrons are then accelerated from the photocathode to the anode of PM tube by the application of approximately 1000 V in steps of approximately 100 V by a series of electrodes called the dynodes. In the PM tube, secondary electrons are produced, resulting in pulses of 10^5 to 10^8 electrons. Typically a photo- tube with 10 dynodes delivers approximately 410 electrons. This gain or amplification is dependent on the dynode voltages.

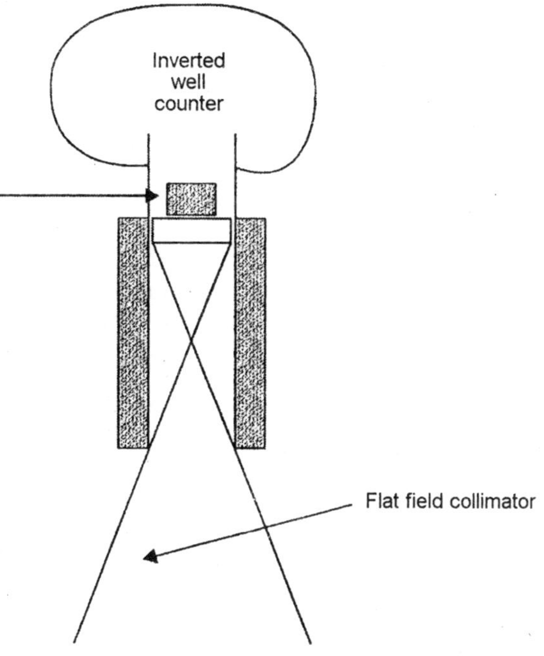

Fig. 25.3. A typical well counter used in nuclear medicine.

Preamplifier

Even though such a large number of secondary electrons are generated, these are not adequate to generate enough current. The voltage pulse is amplifed by a factor of 4–5 by the preamplifier without loss of power. The preamplifier also provides the driving force necessary to prevent loss in the several feet of connecting cables.

Linear amplifier

The pulses received from preamplifier have wide variation in energies of the particles. The gain in the amplifier is of the order of 8000 such that a 1 mV signal is amplified to approximately 8 V while still maintaining the proportionality of the energy delivered by the particle (more often γ-Ray) to the detectors. The amplified pulse is then delivered to pulse height analyzer.

Pulse height analyzers (PHA)

The pulses that emerge from the amplifier usually have different amplitudes owing to differences in energies. These analyzers are essentially energy sorters. Single-channel PHAs count pulses of a given amplitude, whereas multichannel analyzers (MCAs) scan whole energy range and record the pulses in each channel. For example, by using an MCA, γ-Ray spectrum can be recorded and, thus, these instruments that use MCAs are called γ-Ray spectrometers. MCAs may have as many as 4000 channels.

X- Y-positioning circuits

These are unique to scintillation cameras, known as Auger cameras, used in nuclear medicine studies. Approximately 19–91 PMTs are mounted on a Na(Tl) crystal used in the camera. These crystals are typically- thick. The number of PMTs, which are optically coupled to the back of the crystal, is determined by the size and shape of the crystal. A maximum amount of light will be received by the PMT nearest to the point of interaction compared with the other PMTs, which are positioned differently. The amount of light received in these PMTs is proportional to the solid angle subtended by the PMT. Therefore, X–Y-positioning of the camera has to be controlled and known so that X–Y-coordinate of the γ-Ray interaction can be assessed accurately. These data are stored in a computer and then processed or recorded on Polaroid or X-Ray films.

Efficiency of detection in scintillation detectors

In gas-filled as well as scintillation detectors, the observed count rate is typically less than the actual decay rate of the radionuclide. The efficiency of detection may differ from particle to particle under identical conditions using the same type of detector. The factors that affect the efficiency of detection are operating voltage, resolving time, geometry of the instrument used in relation to the position of the sample with respect to the detector, scaler, energy resolution, absorption by cells, and sometimes constituents of the sample itself. For example, the scintillation cocktail sometimes reduces counts considerably. This effect is known as quenching. For accurate measurements of radioactivity, appropriate correction for quenching is required.

Frequent calibration of the instruments with the use of appropriate standards is required to make suitable allowances for decreases in the efficiency of the instruments. Such calibration standards are available from the National Institute of Standards and Technology (NIST). Other sources traceable to NIST standards through active program of participation in comparison measurements also provide such standards. The United States Pharmacopeia (USP) also provides nuclear decay data for new calibration standard. USP 24 lists $t^1/_2$, energy of photons, and number of photons per disintegrations, for the following radionuclide standards: ^{137}Cs, ^{137m}Ba, ^{22}Na, ^{60}Co, ^{57}Co, ^{54}Mn, ^{109}Cd, ^{109}Ag, and ^{129}I.

Tomographic Imagers

Tomography is a process in which three-dimensional images are constructed using a large number of two- dimensional slices of images from an object. Computed tomography uses rigorous mathematical algorithms to reconstruct these images. When radionuclide emissions are used, it is called emission tomography. Two common techniques are now used to obtain images using emission tomography, namely, single photon emission computed tomography (SPECT) and positron emission tomography (PET). In SPECT, γ-Emitting nuclides are used, whereas in PET, positron-emitting nuclides are used. In the SPECT system, an object is photographed using many Auger cameras at a number of small angles (between 3 and 10°) around the object. The total span may be between 0 and 180° or between 0 and 360°. Because the rotating cameras provide two-dimensional digital images, these are stored as 64 × 64 matrix (for 180° span) or as 128 × 128 matrix (for 360° span) digital information. The Auger cameras use NaI (Tl) crystals in the detector heads. In PET, positron-emitting radionuclides are used. Each positron emitted from these radionuclides travels through tissues, deposits energy, and finally is annihilated by interaction with an electron. The annihilation results in the formation of two photons traveling in opposite directions (180° apart) with energy of 0.511 MeV. Two Auger cameras are placed 180° apart but at the same distance from the object. Each camera detects a photon at the same time. By appropriately moving cameras in pairs, the data are collected over many angles and stored in 64 × 64 or 128 × 128 matrix. Thus, this electronic collimation brought about by simultaneous detection increases sensitivity and reduces the need for use of collimators as in SPECT. Additional advantages of PET include easy availability of radionuclides with short halflives of isotopes of elements commonly found in organic molecules (such as F, N, C, and O).

Analysis of Radiochemicals

Radiochemical methods of analysis are considerably more sensitive than other chemical methods. Most spectral methods can quantitate at the parts-per-million (ppm) level, whereas atomic absorption and some HPLC methods with UV, fluorescence, and electrochemical methods can quantitate at the parts-perbillion (ppb) levels. By controlling the specific activity levels, it is possible to attain quantitation levels lower than ppb levels of elements by radiochemical analyses. Radiochemical analysis, inmost cases, can be done without separation of the analyte. Radionuclides are identified based on the characteristic decay and the energy of the particles as described in detection procedures presented above. Radiochemical methods of analysis include tracer methods, activation analysis, and radioimmunoassay techniques.

Tracers and Tracer Methods of Analysis

Radiochemical tracers or radiotracers are compounds labeled with radioisotopes. For tracer methods, the compound to be measured or a suitable reagent is radiolabeled. A measurement of the redistribution of tracer within such a sample–reagent reaction system provides the required quantitative analytical information. Major advantages of tracer methods are high sensitivity, simplicity, and speed. Radiotracers are more commonly used for following mechanisms of biological and/or chemical processes or if there is need to eliminate complicated separation procedures, especially in biological processes.

Isotopic dilution analysis

In isotope dilution analysis, a known amount of radio- labeled compound with known specific activity is spiked to a known amount of an unknown mixture containing the same compound made up of stable isotopes. Then, the components of the radiotracer-diluted samples are mixed thoroughly to form a homogeneous mixture. This istopically diluted mixture, with known levels of dilution, is then suitably treated to isolate a small amount of the desired constituent. The radioactive isotope content of the isolated portion is determined by measuring its specific activity. From the specific activities of the tracer before and after dilution, the concentration of the component in the mixture can then be calculated. The major advantage is that these isolation procedures need not be quantitative; however, it is necessary that the compound isolated should be pure enough for an activity determination. Isotope dilution analyses are used for determination of inorganic trace elements and for the determination of organic compounds in biological systems. If separations are required and the radioisotope concentration is not adequate to bring about separation, dilutions can be accomplished by using a non-radioactive compound (or carrier) with similar chemical behavior. For example, if radio strontium is to be precipitated and it is in low amounts such that it cannot be quantitatively precipitated, it can be coprecipitated along with a calcium salt by the addition of calcium before precipitation. An alternative procedure to isotope dilution, reverse or inverse isotope dilution, can be used to determine the quantity of radioactive compound by dilution with an inactive compound. This procedure is applicable when a system contains an unknown amount of isotopically labeled substance of known specific activity.

Radioisotope exchage

For understanding mechanisms and kinetics of organic or biological reactions, non-radioactive atoms in molecules or ions are allowed to exchange with appropriate radiolabeled compound. After chemical exchange between a labeled compound and the test sample (the chemical form of the element being different in the two solutions, e.g., iodine in CH_3I vs $^{131}I^-$ in labeled sodium iodide), the specific activity of the element becomes the same in the sample and reagent. A measured decrease in the activity of the reagent or increase in the activity of the sample can then be related to the amount of element present in the sample. Isotopic exchange methods of analysis are very sensitive, rapid, and specific. Isotopic exchange plays a very important role in pharmacokinetic studies. For example, a drug molecule may be labeled with tritium to follow the drug distribution. Exchange of tritium with an unlabeled compound or with a water molecule in the vicinity may lead to erroneous interpretation of the drug distribution if suitable precautions are not taken to avoid potential isotopic exchange reactions.

Radiotracers as radiopharmaceuticals: Methods for radiopharmaceutical analysis

When radiolabeled compounds (radiotracers) are used for diagnostic and therapeutic purposes, it is called a radiopharmaceutical. A radiopharmaceutical should be easily produced, inexpensive, readily available, have relatively short halflife, and preferably should be a γ-Emitter with an energy between 30 and 300 keV. Such a γ-Emitting nuclide should invariably decay by electron capture or isomeric transition. When positron-emitting nuclides are used, they must have specific localization in the desired organ or tissue and should not result in undue radiation exposure. Radiotracers, used as pharmaceuticals, are produced in one of two ways: either as a product of nuclear fission reactions or as a product of nuclear reactions induced by high-energy accelerator particles or neutrons. Particle accelerators are instruments that cause nuclear reactions by bombarding target nuclides with highly accelerated and energized particles such as protons, deutrons, and electrons. For production of radiopharmaceuticals, on-site accelerators called cyclotrons are used. For production of positron-emitting radionculides linear accelerators are used. Readily transportable instruments, which serve as sources for short-lived radionuclides, are called *generators*. Typically, in a generator, a long-lived parent nuclide is allowed to decay to a short-lived daughter radionuclide. Using differences in chemical properties, the daughter nuclide is separated from the parent.

A radiopharmaceutical is a radioactive chemical used as a pharmaceutical. Therefore, as pharmaceuticals, they should have proper ionic strength, pH, isotonicity, and osmolarity. In addition to chemical purity, radionuclide purity and radiochemical purity also have to be demonstrated. The radionuclide purity refers to the ratio of the amount of radioactivity corresponding to that of desired radionuclide to the total amount of radioactivity owing to other isotopes and other isotopic impurities. Radionuclide purity is determined by measuring halflives and other characteristics of radiation of the radionuclide. Radiochemical purity refers to the fraction of total radioactivity in the desired form. Radiochemical impurities are general chemical impurities formed by the chemical as a result of decomposition of the chemical entity, whereas all the resulting impurities may still be radioactive. Potential decomposition pathways are the same as for any other pharmaceutical. Examples include acid and base hydrolysis products, oxidized and reduced species, additional radiolysis products, and photochemical and thermal decomposition products of the chemical. For example in many ^{99m}Tc-labeled complexes, free unreacted $^{99m}TcO_4^-$ and hydrolyzed ^{99m}Tc are radiochemical impurities. A number of analytical methods can be used to detect and determine radiochemical impurities. For example, when separating the impurities from radiochemical compound of interest using HPLC, if a radiochemical detector is used, all the radioactive impurities that are separated can be quantitated, and radiochemical purity can be ascertained. These include but are not limited to distillation, precipitation, paper, thin layer, gel chromatography, HPLC, ion exchange, solvent extraction, and other separation and purification techniques. The techniques and principles of these techniques are the same as for any other pharmaceutical.

Activation analysis

Activation analysis is a process in which a target trace element in a sample matrix is irradiated with particles in a nuclear reactor. As a result, an activated radionuclide is formed. The characteristic particles or γ-Rays emitted are used for qualitative identification and, more often, for quantitative measurement. The most common activation analysis is neutron activation analysis (NAA). In this technique, a sample containing the element is irradiated with neutrons in a reactor. After irradiation, γ-Emissions ensue from the decaying radionuclide. These are quantitated by using appropriate semiconductor radiation detectors. Detecting γ-Rays of a specific energy identifies the radionuclide. These particular energy values correspond to unique energies characteristic of the decaying radionuclides. For example, when ^{24}Na decays to ^{24}Mg, the γ-Rays released have unique energies of 1.268 and 2.754 MeV. A plot of γ-Ray counts versus energy yields a γ-Ray spectrum; the area under the curve is proportional to the radioactivity of the sample. The rate at which γ-Rays are emitted is proportional to the concentration of the radionuclide. When a large number of elements in a single sample matrix are analyzed using appropriate instruments for quantitation, without separation of the elements, it is called instrumental neutron activation analysis. When there is spectral interference in the sample matrix and if chemical separation is carried out to isolate the element, it is called radiochemical neutron activation analysis. When other charged particles are generated for analysis by activation, it is called charged particle activation analysis (CPAA). CPAA is applied to the determination of elemental concentration in surface layers. All methods of activation analysis are very accurate and sensitive, and a precision of approximately 2% RSD is easily attainable. Detection limits in parts per per billion or lower, depending on the element and sample matrix, are easily attainable. As many as 60 different elements that can form radionuclide can be analyzed using NAA.

Radioimmunoassay

Radioimmunoassay (RIA) is a technique based on the formation of antigen–antibody complex. This technique essentially involves the application of isotope dilution analysis. An antigen is typically a protein of molecular weight greater than 10,000 that stimulates the production of antibody in an animal body. The antigen subsequently binds with the antibody. Antigen is usually measured in the patient's sample, and the antigen becomes the analyte. To an antibody, a mixture of labeled and unlabeled antigen is added in excess such that the quantity of antibody needed to bind is allowed to be insufficient. As a result, both types of antigen compete with the limited amount of antibody in the sample. The reaction in an RIA mixture can be described as follows.

$$\begin{matrix} Ag* & & & \\ & +Ab & \underset{k_2}{\overset{k_1}{\rightleftarrows}} & Ag*-Ab+Ag \\ Ag & & & Ag-Ag+Ag \end{matrix}$$

k_1 and k_2 are rate constants; equilibrium constant K = k_1/k_2.

To a constant amount of labeled antigen and antibody, increasing amounts of unlabeled antibody are added. The initial amount added is still in excess of the antibody needed for binding. As a result of competing reactions of the labeled and unlabeled antigen, the greater the concentration of the unlabeled antigen added, the less is the amount of bound labeled complex (Ag^*–Ab complex) and hence greater is the free (unbound) antigen. After incubation to equilibrium at a specified temperature and time, unique to the system, separation of the free labeled Ag^*, the fraction of the bound labeled antigen is determined by measuring the activity of the radioactive nuclide. By plotting the percent of bound labeled antigen versus the concentration of antigen added, the concentration of the unknown antigen can be determined. Several radionuclides such as ^{14}C, ^{3}H, ^{131}I , ^{32}P, ^{75}Se, ^{59}Fe, ^{99}Mo, and ^{57}Co have been used for RIA. However, ^{125}I is the most commonly used radionuclide for RIA. The earliest method of separation included electrophoresis and chromatography. However, today RIA kits are marketed by commercial manufacturers with detailed description of the principles of the method, methods of use, sensitivity, precision, and limitations of use for specific uses. The RIA methods are very rapid, sensitive, specific, and inexpensive, especially for large biological samples in complex sample matrices.

The RIA technique is applied in assays of hormones, steroids, peptides, aminoglycosides such as to bramycin and gentamycin, insulin, many immunoglobulins, different types of viral heptitis, plasma catecholamines, angiotension-converting enzymes, many vitamins including vitamine $B_{12,}$ human growth hormones, many folate derivatives, and others. Many commercially available RIA kits, unique to each kit, contain series of standards with known concentrations of unlabeled antigen, a vial of suitable labeled antigen, a vial of antibody solution, and appropriate precipitants or other analytical aides.

Radiation Safety

When radiation energy is absorbed by tissues, depending on the dose received, rupture of chemical bonds occurs that causes damage to cells and tissues. Such damage may not be clinically apparent even for years if the absorbed dose is small. Radiation damage is measured in terms of absorbed dose. Dose is defined as the energy imparted to a material per unit mass. The SI unit of dose is called Gray, or Gy (joules/Kg). The traditional unit is rad. One Gy = 100 rads. However, the effectiveness of all radiations is not the same. The effectiveness is dependent on the nature of the particle, the thickness of the tissue or organ, and the characteristics of the material or organ to which such a dose is administered. Thus, to account for such differences in effectiveness, another term, called dose equivalent, is used. The SI unit of dose equivalent is Sievert, which is numerically equivalent to Gy multiplied by the appropriate weighting factor corresponding to biological tissue or organ. For example, the weighting factor (W_R) for many tissues is 0.3, whereas it is 0.03 for bone surfaces. The radiation weighting factor is also dependent on the energy of the particles. For example, for neutrons with less than 10 keV, W_R, = 5, whereas it is equal to 20 for neutrons greater than 100 keV.

For purposes of administered dose of a radiopharmaceutical, the package insert contains a table that lists dosage for the "average" patient as a function of administered activity. This information may be used for calculation of radiation dose. If needed, a medical physicist will calculate administered dose based on Medical Internal Radiation Dose (MIRD) committee recommendations.

External exposure to ionizing radiation as a result of occupation is measured using dosimeters. Three different types of dose monitors are commercially available. They are pocket dosimeters, film badges, and thermoluminescent detectors (TLDs). Pocket dosimeters are GM counting-based digital dosimeters, which provide immediate reading. Film badges are the least expensive and most popular. Using appropriate filters in the film holder, accurate readings to exposure to different particles can be measured. The major disadvantage with film badges is the waiting period required for developing and processing films. In TLDs, the radiation received is stored in holders containing crystals of LiFor manganese-activated calcium fluoride. Subsequently, during measurement, the crystals are heated to required temperatures such that they emit light. When measured, the emitted light provides a measure of absorbed dose.

Regulatory Requirements

The regulations of various advisory groups and government organizations have to be met in handling, use, and disposal of radioactive material and radio- pharmaceuticals. These include the FDA, NRC, Department of Transportation (DOT), Environmental Protection Agency (EPA), and Occupational Safety and Health Administration (OSHA). Of these, the FDA regulates safety, stability, efficacy, and toxicity of the radiopharmaceuticals; NRC regulates all reactor-produced by-products regarding use, handling, disposal, and radiation safety and protection of workers and the public using the facilities. Title 10 of the Code of Federal Regulations, 10 CFR 20, contains the regulations for radiation protection, whereas 10 CFR 35 addresses medical uses of radioactive materials. Title 49, 49 CFR, addresses packaging and transportation of radioactive materials. In addition, all USP requirements have to be met for a radiopharmaceutical.

The International Committee on Radiation Protection (ICRP) and the National Committee on Radiation Protection (NCRP) provide radiation dose recommendations for adoption to other regulatory agencies. The NRC requires that licensees follow the ALARA philosophy regarding radiation exposure. ALARA is an acronym for as low as reasonably achievable. Under the ALARA concept, when radiation exposure of a worker exceeds 1 0% of the allowed occupational limit, an investigation is required. If it exceeds 30%, investigation and corrective action are necessary per NRC requirements. As with any other pharmaceutical, radiotracers used as pharmaceuticals are subject to all regulatory requirements. The radiopharmaceutical manufacturer must, at a minimum, satisfy the requirements of the NRC and the FDA.

INDEX